2G4/$79.50

D0930555

PAUL and JUHL'S

Essentials of ROENTGEN Interpretation

JOHN H. JUHL, M.D.

Professor of Radiology
University of New Mexico School of Medicine, and
Chief of Radiology
Veterans Administration Medical Center
Albuquerque, New Mexico

formerly
Professor and Chairman
Department of Radiology
The University of Wisconsin Medical School
Madison, Wisconsin

PAUL and JUHL'S
Essentials of
ROENTGEN
Interpretation

FOURTH EDITION

HARPER & ROW, PUBLISHERS

PHILADELPHIA

Cambridge
New York
Hagerstown
San Francisco

1817

London
Mexico City
São Paulo
Sydney

The author and publisher have exerted every effort to ensure that drug selection and dosage set forth in this text are in accord with current recommendations and practice at the time of publication. However, in view of ongoing research, changes in government regulations, and the constant flow of information relating to drug therapy and drug reactions, the reader is urged to check the package insert for each drug for any change in indications and dosage and for added warnings and precautions. This is particularly important when the recommended agent is a new and/or infrequently employed drug.

10   9   8   7   6   5   4

Fourth Edition. Copyright © 1981 by Harper & Row, Publishers, Inc. All rights reserved. No part of this book may be used or reproduced in any manner whatsoever without written permission except in the case of brief quotations embodied in critical articles and reviews. Printed in the United States of America. For information address Medical Department, Harper & Row, Publishers, Inc., East Washington Square, Philadelphia, Pennsylvania 19105.

Library of Congress Cataloging in Publication Data

Paul, Lester W
    Paul and Juhl's essentials of roentgen interpretation.

    Bibliography.
    Includes index.
    1. Diagnosis, Radioscopic.   I. Juhl, John H.
II. Title.   III. Title: Essentials of roentgen interpretation.
RC78.P3   1981   616.07′572   80-20938
ISBN 0-06-142143-X

In Memory of
Helen B. Juhl
and
Lester W. Paul

CONTENTS

SECTION III
THE ABDOMEN AND GASTROINTESTINAL TRACT

SECTION IV
THE URINARY AND FEMALE GENITAL TRACTS

SECTION V
THE CHEST

SECTION VI
THE FACE, MOUTH, AND JAWS

PREFACE

The rapid changes in diagnostic radiology, which include the wide use and acceptance of CT scanning of the central nervous system, mandate another revision of this volume. This is a formidable task, undertaken with some trepidation since I am working alone this time. I discuss CT scanning briefly, outline its indications in central nervous system conditions, and include a few illustrative examples of CT brain scans. Because the advance of ultrasonic scanning has changed the pattern of imaging in several areas, I make mention throughout the text of the use of this modality in conjunction with the discussion of the appropriate organ or disease. Otherwise, I do not include ultrasound, since it is beyond the scope of this volume. As in previous editions, I have revised the bibliography, deleting some of the older references and adding newer ones.

All of the chapters have been revised, some of them rather extensively. Additions to the text include the following: stenosis of the spinal canal, absence and hypoplasia of a vertebral pedicle, idiopathic juvenile osteoporosis, chronic symmetric osteomyelitis, diffuse cystic angiomatosis, Gaucher's disease, malignant fibrous histiocytoma, effects of frostbite on bone, scoliosis, diffuse idiopathic skeletal hyperostosis (DISH), subcutaneous fat necrosis, lissencephaly, pituitary microadenomas, multifocal leukoencephalopathy, the tethered conus, small left colon syndrome, inspissated milk syndrome, intestinal pseudo-obstruction, giant sigmoid gas cyst, omphalocele, transjugular cholangiography, infusion tomography of the gallbladder, choledochal cyst, choledochocele, cholangiolytic hepatitis, pyogenic cholangitis, diffuse esophageal spasm, cricopharyngeal achalasia and chalasia, double contrast examination of the stomach, "double channel" pylorus, abetalipoproteinemia, potassium depletion states, myxoglobulosis; renal amyloidosis, scleroderma, myeloma and sarcoidosis; the kidney in hemophilia, agnogenic myeloid metaplasia and S-hemoglobinopathy; cyclophosphamide cystitis, cystitis glandularis, malakoplakia, placenta membranacea, spontaneous ovarian amputation, bead-chain cystourethrography, congenital lobar emphysema, pulmonary isomerism, Legionnaire's disease, pulmonary infection in the compromised host, epiglottitis, acute laryngotracheobronchitis, bronchial mucocele, bronchocentric granulomatosis; paraquat lung, pulmonary blastoma, immunoblastic lymphadenopathy, Behcet's syndrome and the lung, lymphomatoid granulomatosis, necrotizing sarcoidal granulomatosis, hypoplastic left heart syndrome, diffuse pulmonary hemangiomatosis, pulmonary varices, cardiac pacemakers, classification of cardiomyopathies, computed tomography of the orbit and eye, inverting papilloma of maxillary sinus, odontogenic keratocyst, adenomatoid odontogenic tumor, static bone cavity (Stafne), and osteoblastoma of the jaw.

Many of the illustrations are new and others are made from new negatives and prints in order to improve their quality. I am very grateful to a number of colleagues who have aided in the collection of new illustrations. They include Drs. Mary Ellen Peters, Andrew B. Crummy, Joseph F. Sackett, Charles M. Strother, Sue A. Hausserman, Roger A. Kimmel, Jon I. Abrahams, Michael Katz, Daniel Arndt, and Sultan Bhimani.

I also wish to express my thanks to the colleagues who reviewed sections of the manuscript. Dr. Crummy reviewed the chapter on the cardiovascular system, Drs. Sackett and Strother the chapters on intracranial diseases and the spinal cord, and Dr. Albert J. Alter the chapter on the urinary tract.

Gretchen Van Alstyne, Barbara Juhl, and Ellen Moore compiled an extensive list of references which were reviewed for this revision. Most of the photographic work has been supervised by Walter C. Fumuso. Cheryl Bradley has helped with the assembly of illustrations and has done some of the typing. Miss Lorena Carmichael, who typed all of the first three editions, has also assisted with the typing. The bulk of the manuscript has been typed by Margaret Koehler, without whose superb skills this revision would have been much more difficult. My appreciation and thanks are extended to all of these invaluable people.

Finally, I wish to thank the publisher's staff, who have been very patient and helpful through some very trying times.

John H. Juhl, M.D.

FROM PREFACE TO
FIRST EDITION

In preparing this volume, it has been our aim to organize and to set
down as concisely as possible what we consider to be the basic facts
of roentgen interpretation. Designed to bridge the gap between the
elementary text and the multiple-volume reference work, it will, we
believe, serve equally well as a review source for the practicing physician and surgeon, for those taking postgraduate training in one of
the specialties, and as a textbook for the undergraduate medical student.

We have discussed briefly the roentgen anatomy of the various
divisions of the body. The descriptions of disease processes are con-
cise, with discussions of clinical and pathologic features limited to
the information necessary to clarify the roentgen observations. The
emphasis necessarily is restricted to roentgen diagnosis. All the common and most of the unusual conditions and diseases with positive
roentgen findings are included. Roentgen differential diagnosis has
been emphasized in the more common diseases. Methods of roentgen examination are described, particularly those dealing with the
more complicated diagnostic procedures such as bronchography and
myelography. The care of the patient before and after such investigations is important, and the referring physician should have some
idea of what the examination entails and the way in which it is conducted. Technical methods are likely to vary somewhat from one institution to another; those described here are used by us at University Hospitals and give a general concept of the procedures and what
they entail. We have avoided discussions of controversial matters, indicating only either the existence of controversy or the present lack
of knowledge about some subjects.

Because of the variable patterns and the changing character of
disease processes, often from day to day, it is possible only to illustrate the signs most frequently encountered. The illustrations have
been chosen to present as many facets as possible, but the reader
should be aware that only infrequently can a single roentgenogram
portray all of the possible variants.

References have been selected carefully to direct the reader to
a wide range of literature; books and articles have been chosen that

contain more extensive bibliographies than it would be advisable to include in a book of relatively restricted size such as this.

We have been fortunate in having a group of associates who have been willing to give freely of their time to aid us in many ways. Dr. Edgar S. Gordon has reviewed two chapters (on the osseous system and the abdomen and gastrointestinal tract) and offered valuable criticisms. Dr. D. Murray Angevine has done the same in the chapter dealing with diseases of the joints. Dr. Theodore C. Erickson kindly read two chapters covering diseases of the brain and spinal cord; Dr. Helen Dickie reviewed the chapters dealing with diseases of the lungs; and Dr. Richard H. Wasserburger, the cardiovascular system. To these and many others who gave us advice and encouragement go our most heartfelt thanks.

Dr. Margaret Winston prepared several drawings. Dr. Arthur Chandler, Jr., prepared those for the chapters dealing with diseases of the cardiovascular system and the lungs. Other members of our staff who aided us in many ways during the preparation of the manuscript and the selection of illustrative material include Drs. Charles Benkendorf, Robert F. Douglas, Joyce Kline, Lee A. Krystosek, M. Pinson Neal, Jr., and John F. Siegrist. The photographic work has been under the supervision of Mr. Homer Montague who has personally prepared most of the illustrations. To him goes the credit for the faithful reproduction of the roentgenograms. The typing has been done by Miss Lorena Carmichael with assistance from Mrs. Charlotte Helgeson. Their careful workmanship has made our tasks easier.

Finally we wish to thank the publisher, Mr. Paul B. Hoeber, for his many courtesies and the excellent co-operation we have received at all times. In particular, Mrs. Eunice Stevens of the publisher's staff deserves our gratitude. Her enthusiasm and her skillful guidance have been invaluable aids.

Lester W. Paul, M.D.
John H. Juhl, M.D.

PAUL and JUHL'S

Essentials of
ROENTGEN
Interpretation

INTRODUCTION

DISCOVERY OF ROENTGEN RAYS

The discovery of roentgen rays (x-rays) by Wilhelm Conrad Roentgen, Professor of Physics at the University of Würzburg, Germany, on November 8, 1895, marked the beginning of a new era in medical science. For the first time it became possible to "see through" the intact skin and superficial tissues and to visualize the bones and deeper structures of the body. Improvements in the crude equipment of the early days followed and, with the tremendous interest generated throughout the world by the news of the discovery, it was only a short time before methods became available for the study of the body cavities and the visceral structures. The fascinating story of Professor Roentgen's discovery and of the many other scientific advances that preceded it and made it possible is beyond the scope of this book; they have been the subject of numerous articles and books, and every student is urged to read the complete story. Following shortly after Roentgen's contribution came the discovery of the radioactivity of uranium by Becquerel and the isolation of the element radium by the Curies. Thus was completed the birth of a new science. Radiology, the name applied to this science, is one of the youngest of the medical specialties and yet in the 85 years since its origin it has completely revolutionized the diagnosis and treatment of many diseases, established entirely new concepts of living anatomy and physiology, and has become a tool of research in many phases of scientific endeavor, often in fields remote from the practice of medicine.

The rays that Professor Roentgen discovered he called x-rays—"x" representing the unknown. It was only a short time, however, before investigations by Roentgen himself determined some of the fundamental properties of the rays and, combined with the investigations of many others through the years, they no longer belong in the category of the unknown. Because of this and to honor their discoverer it has become common usage to refer to them as roentgen rays rather than x-rays and this term will be used throughout this book.

DEFINITION

Roentgen rays are a form of electromagnetic energy of very short wave length (0.5 to 0.06 Å or less). An angstrom unit (Å) is a measure of length, one angstrom being 10^{-8} cm (one hundred-millionth cm). The place of roentgen rays in the electromagnetic spectrum is shown in the accompanying diagram (Fig.I-1). Because of their short wave lengths they have the ability to penetrate matter and it is this characteristic that makes them of use in the study of body tissues. In order to understand some of the fundamental properties of roentgen rays it is advisable to review briefly the ways in which they are formed.

PRODUCTION OF ROENTGEN RAYS

Roentgen rays are formed by the sudden stopping of high-speed electrons. This is accomplished by passing a high-voltage electric current across the terminals situated within a highly evacuated glass bulb (Fig.I-2). One of the terminals is called the cathode and it consists essentially of a tungsten wire filament that can be heated to incandescence by a separate current, and of a focusing collar around the filament to direct the electron beam toward the other terminal, called the anode. The anode consists of a heavy rod or bar of copper on the face of which is set a small button usually made of tungsten. The face of the anode is called the target. The basic principle of operation of a modern roentgen-ray tube depends upon the fact that metals when heated to incandescence give off free electrons. When the filament in the tube is heated in this manner a cloud of electrons forms about it. When a high-voltage current is applied to the terminals of the tube so that a negative charge is applied to the heated filament and a positive charge to the anode, the electrons will be repelled from the cathode and forced toward the anode. The electrons travel at very high speed and the stream continues as long as the current is applied. These high-speed electrons are known as cathode rays. The focusing collar around the filament focuses the stream of electrons so that they strike the button of tungsten set in the face of the target. This face is set on a slant of approximately 20 degrees from the long axis of the anode stem. The area where the electron beam impinges on the target is called the focal spot and it is here that the roentgen rays are emitted. The size of the focal spot varies in different tubes but usually measures from 0.3 to several millimeters in diameter. The velocity of the electrons in the beam depends upon the

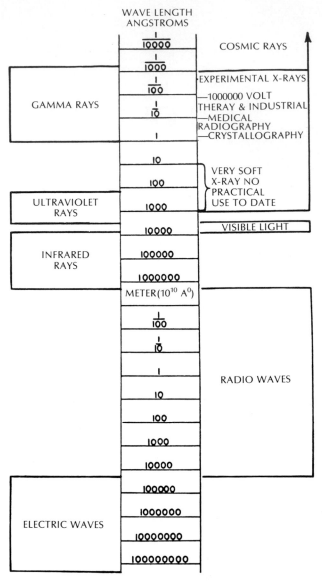

Fig. I-1. Diagrammatic representation of the electromagnetic spectrum illustrating the relative position of roentgen rays (x-rays) in relation to the other forms of electromagnetic energy. (*Courtesy General Electric X-ray Corporation, Milwaukee, Wisconsin.*)

voltage applied to the terminals. The number of electrons available at the filament depends upon the heat of the filament. The cathode-ray output of the filament therefore can be regulated easily by controlling the heat of the filament. When high-speed electrons are stopped by the tungsten target the major portion of their energy is transformed into heat and only a small part, less than 1%, into roentgen rays. One of the reasons why tungsten is used in the target is because of its relatively high melting point. Copper is used for the stem of the anode because of its heat-transmitting properties (Fig. I-3). Various methods are used to dissipate the heat including circulating water, radiator fins attached to the outside of the anode stem, and immersion and cooling of the tube with oil. Most diagnostic roentgen-ray tubes now are of the oil-immersed and oil-cooled type. In order to increase the operating capacity of the tube and keep the focal spot size at a minimum, rotating anode tubes are commonly used (Fig. I-4). The anode consists of a disc that is rotated during the exposure. The beam of electrons is focused within a small area along the rim of the disc. Since the disc is rotating during the time that it is being struck by the electron beam, successive areas of metal along the rim of the disc are brought into the beam and its effect therefore is distributed around the edge of a circle instead of at a single point. The voltages used in diagnostic roentgenology vary from about 25,000 to 150,000 volts (25 to 150 kV). In therapeutic radiology, voltages as low as 85,000 are used in the treatment of superficial lesions, but for the therapy of lesions involving the deeper structures of the body much higher voltages are employed, and these vary from 200,000 to those in the multimillion-volt range.

The majority of the cathode rays striking the target are slowed down gradually and their energies are transformed into heat. Only a relatively small percentage of the total electrons in the beam are stopped suddenly; it is these that have their energies transformed into roentgen rays. Because some of the radiation is produced below the surface of the target, it may be absorbed by the tungsten before it can be radiated into space. Actually, about half of the radiation produced at any given time is absorbed in this manner. The remainder is emitted from the face of the target through an arc of 180°. Because roentgen rays cannot be focused, only a small portion of this beam can be utilized; this portion is confined to a rather narrow windowlike opening in the metal cover housing the roentgen-ray tube. The beam often is further reduced in size by the use of metal diaphragms or cones.

CHARACTERISTICS

Roentgen rays travel in straight lines at the speed of light. When a beam of rays passes through matter its intensity is reduced by absorption. This is true even for a gas such as air although the amount of absorption is small. The denser the matter, the greater the amount of absorption. Roentgen rays also cause ionization of the substances through which they pass and it is this property, the ionization of gas, that is utilized to measure the intensity of a given beam. In addition to being able to penetrate matter and to be absorbed by it, there are several other characteristics of this form of radiation that make it useful in the study of the body structures.

PHOTOGRAPHIC EFFECT

A photographic film is affected by roentgen rays the same as it is by visible light. The sensitized silver emulsion turns black when it has been exposed to the radiation and the film is subsequently processed by development and fixation. When a film protected from light is placed beneath an object, for example a hand, and a beam of roentgen rays of suitable intensity and wave length is passed through it, an image will be produced in the emulsion and brought out by the developing process that will be an accurate representation of the variable densities of the tissues through which the beam has passed. Thus the bones, because they absorb more of the radiation than do the soft tissues covering them, will appear as light areas surrounded by the darker soft tissues. The density of the bones is not uniform and cortex, being more compact than the cancellous bone in the medullary cavity, appears lighter on the film. It is this selective absorption by the body tissues that results in an image of the part on the film. This is, in effect, a two-dimensional representation of the structures within a three-dimensional object. All variations in density overlying a single point will appear as a single composite shadow.

FLUORESCENCE

Another important property of roentgen rays is their ability to cause fluorescence of certain crystalline substances, such as barium platinocyanide, zinc sulfide, and calcium tungstate, or, in other words, the energy is transformed into visible light. This property is used in fluoroscopy. A fluoroscopic screen consists of a piece of cardboard coated with a thin layer of one of the fluorescent materials such as calcium tung-

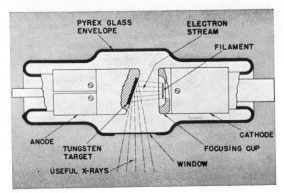

Fig. I-2. Diagram of a fixed-focus type of diagnostic roentgen-ray tube. (*Courtesy General Electric X-ray Corporation, Milwaukee, Wisconsin.*)

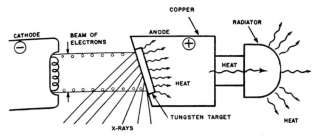

Fig. I-3. Diagram illustrating the basic operating principles of a roentgen-ray tube. (*Courtesy General Electric X-ray Corporation, Milwaukee, Wisconsin.*)

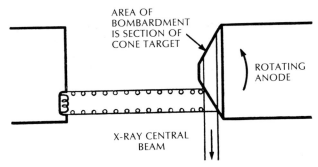

Fig. I-4. Diagram to illustrate the operation of a rotating target tube. The electron beam from the cathode is focused on a small area of the rotating anode so that the area of bombardment is a circular band on the slanted face of the target. By this means heat is distributed over a fairly wide area, allowing the focal spot to be kept small. (*Courtesy General Electric X-ray Corporation, Milwaukee, Wisconsin.*)

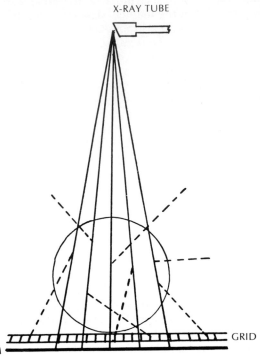

Fig. I-5. Diagram illustrating the principles of a grid used to absorb secondary radiation arising in the structure being examined. The vertical lead strips (**solid black lines**) are separated by wood spacers. The lead strips are placed so that only radiation arising at the target of the tube (primary radiation) or traveling in the same direction as the primary beam can pass through the grid to affect the film emulsion. The scattered radiation (**broken lines**) will be absorbed by the lead strips. Lead is very effective in absorbing radiation while wood absorbs very little. Properly constructed grids are very effective in removing unwanted radiation. When a beam of roentgen rays is passed through matter the effect is much the same as when ordinary light passes through fog. The scattering of the radiation causes a blurred image and loss of detail.

state in finely divided form. When a part of the body is placed between a tube emitting roentgen rays and such a screen, an image of the part is formed by visible light on the surface of the screen. In contrast to the shadows produced on a film, the denser structures appear the darkest since they absorb more of the rays and prevent them from striking the screen. In radiography, fluorescent screens are used to intensify the effect of the roentgen-ray beam. This is done by enclosing the photographic film in a hinged holder known as a cassette. The part of the cassette that will face the roentgen-ray tube is made of a substance, such as aluminum or bakelite, which absorbs very little radiation. A fluorescent screen is mounted on the inner surface of each of the leaves of the cassette and the film is placed between them. When the cassette is closed the screens are brought into close contact with the film. The film used in roentgenography differs from ordinary photographic film in that the celluloid base is coated with sensitized emulsion on both sides. When the loaded cassette is exposed to roentgen rays, not only is there a direct effect of the rays upon the film but the image also is registered by means of the visible light from each of the screens. By using intensifying screens the blackening effect of the radiation is increased on the order of 20 times that obtained without screens.

SCATTERING

When roentgen rays pass through matter, not only is some of the radiation absorbed but the character and quality (wave length) of the emergent beam are altered. Some of the rays are deflected and have their directions altered; also, new radiation is produced within the substance. The total effect is known as scattering. Scattered rays may be projected in any direction. Scattered radiation strikes the fluoroscopic screen or the photographic film from many directions other than that of the primary beam. The result is a more or less uniform blackening of the film emulsion with a consequent loss of sharpness and detail of the images. Scattered radiation serves no useful purpose in diagnostic roentgenology and every effort is made to eliminate it or reduce its intensity. This is accomplished by the use of a device known as the Potter-Bucky grid. This consists of a thin grid made of alternating strips of lead and wood set on edge. These are arranged so that they lie in the radii of a circle, the center of which will be the focal spot of the tube. When the grid is placed between the part being examined and the film, only that radiation traveling in a straight direction from the focal spot of the tube can pass through the spaces between the lead strips (Fig. I-5). Radiation arising in the body tissues or elsewhere and traveling in any direction but in a line between the focal spot and the film will be absorbed by the metal strips. When the grid is stationary the metal strips cause lines on the film. To eliminate these the grid is kept in motion during the exposure; this blurs the shadows of the lines and they become invisible. Fog also can be reduced by limiting the beam of radiation to as small an area as possible. This is done by means of lead diaphragms placed close to the window of the tube or by means of metal cylinders or cones that limit the size of the beam. For some uses, such as with portable equipment at the bedside, a very thin "wafer" grid is available. The lead strips are so fine that the lines on the film are not objectionable. Stationary thin grids of this type are not as efficient in eliminating scatter as the movable grids but they do clean up fog sufficiently to make their use worthwhile.

BIOLOGIC EFFECTS

The effect of radiation upon living cells has received intensive study. That roentgen rays affect living cells makes them useful in the treatment of malignant tumors and other conditions, a subject entirely beyond the scope of this book. It is emphasized that roentgen rays can be lethal to normal tissues, that dangers arise not only from the absorption of relatively large amounts of radiation over a short period of time but also from cumulative effects of very small amounts received over a period of months or years. In diagnostic roentgenology certain exposure limits have been devised that should not be exceeded. Roentgen rays, being a form of ionizing radiation, can add measurably to the total amount of radiation to which the population, as a whole, may be exposed. The fears expressed by geneticists and others concerning the long-range effects of exposure to small amounts of radiation from atomic sources need to be kept in mind but should not unduly influence the use of roentgen rays when properly indicated for the diagnosis and treatment of disease. Anyone who uses roentgen-ray equipment should be familiar not only with its operating characteristics, particularly the intensity of radiation emitted under given conditions, but should be fully aware of the hazards of overexposure and the ways to prevent it.

EQUIPMENT

Modern roentgen-ray generators and the accessories required in diagnostic roentgenology often are complicated devices but the basic principles of construction and operation are not difficult to understand. Only these simplified features will be discussed in this section (Fig. I-6).

ELECTRICAL CIRCUITS

The essentials of a roentgen-ray generating circuit consist of the following.

1. A source of alternating current. Usually this is 220-volt, 60-cycle current, although portable units are designed to operate at the bedside on standard 110- to 120-volt circuits. Alternating current is necessary in order that it may be stepped up by means of a transformer to the high voltages needed to produce roentgen rays.

2. A method for regulating the voltage. This is usually accomplished by a device called an autotransformer by means of which the voltage supplied to the high-tension transformer can be altered without changing the amperage to any great extent.

3. A step-up transformer to increase the voltage of the secondary circuit into the 25- to 130-kV range.

4. A means of rectifying the high-voltage current. A roentgen-ray tube acts most efficiently when direct current is used to energize it. The tube itself can act as its own rectifier as it does in many portable units. As long as the anode does not become heated to incandescence, the flow of current between the terminals will be, to a large extent, unidirectional since the only source of electrons to allow current flow is at the cathode end. For greater efficiency, however, it is desirable to have the high-tension alternating current rectified to direct current before it is supplied to the tube. This is done by special rectifying vacuum tubes often called valve tubes because they allow passage of electrical current in only one direction.

5. A means for controlling the quantity of the current flowing through the tube. As indicated in an earlier paragraph this is accomplished by controlling the heat of the tube filament. The filament circuit is a separate one and usually is operated at a low voltage of 10 to 12 volts.

6. Means for protecting against electrical shock and stray radiation. Because of the high voltages employed in the production of roentgen rays, special shockproof cables are used to convey the high-tension current from the transformer to the roentgen-ray tube and the tube is immersed in oil. The tube is made rayproof by a metal casing that encloses it and allows rays to escape only through a window placed beneath the target.

FLUOROSCOPES

Fluoroscopy consists in viewing the image produced when roentgen rays strike a fluorescent screen. In order to prevent damage to the skin of the patient and

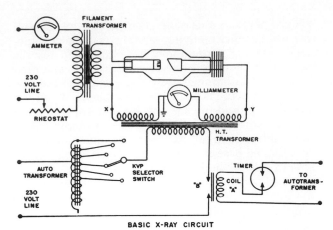

Fig. I-6. Diagram of a basic roentgen-ray generating circuit. In this diagram alternating current is supplied to the terminals of the roentgen-ray tube, which acts as its own rectifier (see text). This type of circuit is used in most portable units that operate from ordinary 110- to 120-volt circuits. Most other roentgen-ray generators use rectifying tubes between the secondary of the high-tension transformer and the roentgen-ray tube to change the alternating current to direct current. The autotransformer is used to control the voltage supplied to the high-tension transformer and this, in turn, will determine the voltage in the secondary circuit of the transformer. The filament transformer controls the current that heats the filament of the roentgen-ray tube and this determines the quantity of electrons available for bombardment of the target. (*Courtesy General Electric X-ray Corporation, Milwaukee, Wisconsin.*)

because roentgen-ray tubes cannot be operated at high current and voltage values for more than a few seconds at a time, fluoroscopy is carried out with a low current value, usually on the order of 3 to 4 mA.* The intensity of the screen illumination is so low that the retina must be dark-adapted before adequate visualization is obtained. Normally this requires a period of about 20 minutes in the dark and this waiting period is essential if satisfactory visualization of the fluoroscopic image is to be obtained. Most fluoroscopes are incorporated into tables that can be tilted from the horizontal to the erect position, often through an arc of 180 degrees. The roentgen-ray tube is placed beneath the radiotransparent table top, the latter being made of bakelite or similar material that has a low degree of absorption of roentgen rays. The fluoroscopic screen is mounted in a frame above the table, the screen and tube being attached to one an-

* One milliampere (mA) equals 1/1000 ampere.

other so that they can be moved in unison from one end of the table to the other. The screen is covered with a panel made of leaded glass to protect the operator from the direct beam of rays. Movable lead shutters are available that can be used to limit the beam to a small area. Usually incorporated in the screen mounting is a device that will allow a film cassette to be brought into place between the patient and the screen so that the image may be recorded on film whenever desired. Roentgenograms made under fluoroscopic control are often referred to as "spot films."

Photofluorography. It is possible to photograph the image produced on a fluoroscopic screen since it is registered in visible light. This procedure is known as photofluorography. The camera and the fluoroscopic screen are enclosed in a lightproof hood so that only the illumination from the screen can enter the aperture of the camera. Photofluorography has been used in the past as a method for mass screening of chests for detection of pulmonary tuberculosis. This use has largely been abandoned. Photofluorography of the thicker and denser parts of the body, particularly of the abdominal viscera, has not been very successful until recently because of the long exposure times required. Cameras now are available that are sufficiently "fast" for use of this method in radiography of the stomach and intestinal tract as well as of other abdominal viscera. Photofluorography is now used extensively in barium studies of the gastrointestinal tract.

Image Intensification. The faint illumination of the fluoroscopic screen requires a period of dark adaptation on the part of the examiner and, once adapted to the dark, vision is by means of the retinal rods rather than the cones. Rod vision enables the retina to detect the low intensities of light but detail is poor; this is a function of the retinal cones. To enable fluoroscopy to be performed in a lighted room without adaptation to the dark requires a considerable amplification of the fluoroscopic intensity. A device known as an image intensifier is capable of increasing the intensity of the fluoroscopic illumination from 200 to 1000 or more times. This is accomplished by means of electronic amplification using a special electron vacuum tube. In most current models the scanning area of the tube is limited to a field of from 5 to 9 inches in diameter. The larger tube is of a satisfactory size for fluoroscopy and cinephotography. The unit also is rather bulky and the reduced image at the eyepiece of the tube needs to be magnified by lenses and mirrors before it can be viewed with comfort.

The degree of amplification of the illumination is such, however, that fluoroscopy can be carried out in a lighted room without any adaptation. In fact, in order to obtain the benefit from cone vision, adaptation is to be avoided. Pulsation of vessels in the thorax and of the cardiac chambers can be seen to better advantage. The image can be recorded directly on movie film by attaching a standard movie camera to the eyepiece of the image amplifier tube, and "slow-motion" movies can be made. It is also possible to televise the image substituting a television camera for the movie camera. The image then can be viewed on a monitor by a number of persons at one time, either in the same room as the fluoroscope or, by means of a closed circuit, transmitted to television receivers in distant class or conference rooms.

At the present time the image intensifier finds its greatest usefulness in certain phases of gastrointestinal roentgenology, in cardiac catheterization, in angiographic examinations, and in research investigations on certain physiologic actions where motion plays a part (the act of swallowing, the study of gastric peristalsis, and similar phenomena). Image intensification has exerted a profound influence on the practice of diagnostic roentgenology.

FURTHER OBSERVATIONS
MAGNIFICATION AND DISTORTION

It is important for the student beginning the study of the use of roentgen rays in diagnosis to realize that certain laws dealing with light with which he is familiar also hold true for this type of radiation. There is always some magnification of the object being examined, depending upon its distance away from the film. The farther it is away from the film and the closer to the tube the greater the magnification of its image on the film. Only when a relatively thin part such as a finger is placed in close contact with the film is there absence of appreciable magnification. Because roentgen rays obey the inverse square law (the intensity varies inversely with the square of the distance from the source) the tube–film distance must be kept within certain limits, otherwise the length of exposure must be prolonged unduly. Thus doubling the distance of the tube from the film requires a fourfold increase in roentgen-ray intensity to achieve the same degree of film blackening. For most parts of the body this distance varies from 30 to 40 inches and the part to be examined must be kept as close to the film as possible. Chest radiography is carried out routinely at a distance of 6 feet because not much radiation is required to penetrate the air-filled lungs and by using the longer distance a more accurate representation of cardiac size is obtained. The image of an object often is distorted because not all parts of it are at the same distance from the film.

Because roentgen rays are not produced at a point source, the farther an object is from the film the more unsharp will its borders become. In a previous paragraph it has been pointed out that the focal spot where roentgen rays are emitted in the tube must be of a measurable size, usually on the order of 1 to 2 mm, because of the intense heat generated at the point where the cathode rays strike the target. Other factors being equal, the tube with the smallest focal spot will produce film images with the greatest detail; also the capacity of such a tube (the amount of current that can be passed through it and therefore the quantity of roentgen rays that can be produced before damage is caused to the tube) will be curtailed correspondingly (Fig. I-7).

TERMINOLOGY

The terms "roentgenogram," "radiograph," "x-ray film," and "x-ray negative" are synonymous but the first is preferred. These terms refer to the finished film that has been exposed to roentgen rays and then records in black and white or in varying shades of gray the structures through which the roentgen-ray beam has passed. The commonly used term "x-ray plate" has no place in modern terminology since it refers to the early days of roentgenology when glass photographic plates rather than flexible cellulose films were used as the recording media.

STANDARD POSITIONS

For most examinations it is essential that at least two views be obtained, preferably at right angles to each other. The observation of any object is facilitated by observing it from more than one vantage point. The two-dimensional character of the roentgen-ray image makes it possible for a dense structure to overlie a less dense part and thus completely obscure it. The size and shape of an object and the relationship of one object to another cannot be appreciated from a single projection. Standard positions usually consist of frontal and lateral views. If for the frontal projection the anatomic structure of greatest interest lies closest to the posterior surface of the body, the part is placed so that its posterior surface is closest to the film holder. This is done to improve detail of the object being examined. Since the beam of roentgen rays will pass through the body traveling in an an-

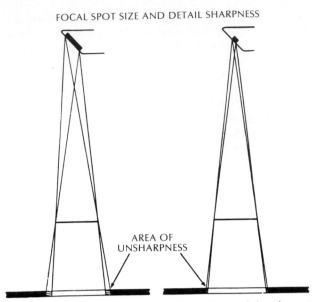

FOCAL SPOT SIZE AND DETAIL SHARPNESS

AREA OF UNSHARPNESS

Fig. I-7 Diagram illustrating the effect of focal spot size on detail sharpness. This is known as the penumbra effect. For a given focal spot size, detail also will be influenced by the distance of the object being examined from the film. (*Courtesy General Electric X-ray Corporation, Milwaukee, Wisconsin.*)

teroposterior direction, such an exposure is described as an anteroposterior view (AP view), the designation indicating the direction taken by the roentgen ray beam in relation to the body surfaces. Lateral views are designated as right or left lateral, depending upon which side is nearer to the film. Oblique positions (usually 45 degrees of obliquity) also are in frequent use and these are described according to the relation of the body surface to the film. Thus in a right anterior oblique view of the chest the patient would be facing toward the film holder with the tube behind him and with the right anterior surface of the body against the film holder.

At times it is impossible to obtain satisfactory projections except in one plane and some anatomic parts are difficult to examine in more than one direction. For the study of complicated anatomic structures, such as the base of the skull or other portions of the cranial vault, it often is advisable to make stereoscopic roentgenograms. Stereoscopy is a method whereby a three-dimensional image may be visualized from a two-dimensional film. The method consists of making two exposures of a part, the two films being in the same relative position to the part at the times of exposure but the tube is shifted a distance approximately equal to the interpupillary distance of the eyes. These films are viewed in a steroscope, which consists of two viewing boxes and a set of mirrors so arranged that one eye sees one film while the other eye sees only the second film. Since the films were exposed from slightly different angles, the eyes view the film images from different points of view and the brain registers the composite image as one with depth, or in other words as a three-dimensional object. The principle of roentgen-ray stereoscopy does not differ in any way from that with which most individuals are familiar when dealing with photography.

RADIATION HAZARDS IN DIAGNOSTIC ROENTGENOLOGY

The use of roentgen rays for diagnostic purposes has increased at a rapid rate since their discovery by W. C. Roentgen in 1895. Radiologists have long been aware of the hazards of ionizing radiation, and protective measures have been developed and used for years. The National Council on Radiation Protection has made recommendations regarding methods of protection and maximum permissible radiation dosage.* The dose has been gradually decreased through the years to the current permissible weekly level of whole body radiation of 100 mR per week, 400 mR per month, 1250 mR per 13-week period, and 5000 mR per year for workers for whom radiation is an occupational hazard.

Radiation exposure is measured in roentgens. The roentgen is the amount of radiation that produces a specific amount of ionization in 1 cm^3 of air at standard conditions. The rad is the unit of absorbed energy or dose. One rad is equal to 100 ergs per gram of tissue, and, in the discussion of roentgen-ray dosage, 1 rad is equal to 1 R of exposure. The rem is the unit of absorbed dose, which takes into account the relative biologic effect of varying types of ionizing radiation; for roentgen rays, 1 rem can be considered equivalent to 1 R.

The effects of radiation usually considered are somatic and genetic because of the difference in doses necessary to produce injury and also because of the importance of genetic effects of radiation on an entire population. The somatic effects may be local or general. Local injuries can be avoided by the proper use of radiographic and fluoroscopic equipment. Very few

* National Council on Radiation Protection, Reports No. 17, 33 & 34. NCRP Publications. P.O. Box 4867, Washington, D.C. 20008

general effects have been documented in humans as a result of diagnostic x-rays, but there is some evidence that the incidence of leukemia is doubled in children of mothers who during pregnancy have had roentgen pelvimetry and have thus been exposed to small doses of general body radiation. There is some evidence suggesting that the incidence of leukemia in radiologists is higher than in other physicians who are not exposed to as much radiation. Among the survivors of the Hiroshima and Nagasaki atomic bomb explosions, the incidence of leukemia was increased roughly in inverse proportion to the square root of their distance from the hypocenter of the explosion. The great majority of those developing leukemia had complaints referable to radiation exposure; the dose rates were high, far beyond those used in diagnostic roentgenology. There is evidence to suggest an increase in carcinoma of the thyroid in patients who have received therapeutic irradiation of the thymus in infancy.[6] Animal experimentation has shown that whole body irradiation can shorten life, but the doses used have been relatively large. There is no conclusive evidence to show any shortening of the life span even in radiologists who are exposed to much more radiation than would be received by a patient as the result of diagnostic use of roentgen rays.

The genetic hazards must be considered on the basis of the entire population rather than on the basis of individual exposures. The genetic effect of radiation is based on the production of mutations, the majority of which are undesirable. The number of mutations produced is directly proportional to the gonadal dose, regardless of intensity or time lapse between exposures. This means that 100 R delivered in one sitting has the same genetic effect as the same dose given in small amounts over a long period of time.[2] Some recent evidence shows, however, that there may be some gonadal cellular recovery following small doses of radiation. The committee on genetic effects of atomic radiation of the National Academy of Sciences[10] has estimated that a total dose of 30 to 80 R to the gonads of the entire population would be required to double the existing mutation rate in humans. The committee has used a doubling dose of 50 R as a basis for their calculations of long-range genetic effects. It has further suggested that, up to the age of 30, the general public receive no more than 10 R over and beyond the background of radiation from natural causes. It considered this dose to be reasonable, although not entirely harmless. These figures may require revision in later years. In the meantime it is necessary to use all possible measures to keep the gonadal dosage from diagnostic use of roentgen rays to the lowest possible limit.

Radiation dosage in various roentgen diagnostic procedures has been measured by numerous investigators and has been the subject of a number of reports. Actual dosages recorded vary considerably in these reports. For example, the dose to the female gonads in pelvimetry ranges from 150 mR (1 mR equals 0.001 R) to 7500 mR, and the dose to the fetus during pelvimetry ranges from 2000 mR to 9000 mR or more. In contrast to this, the gonadal dose in a routine posteroanterior examination of the chest ranges from no detectable radiation to 0.36 mR, while the skin dose to the posterior chest wall ranges from 8 to 190 mR.[7] In the Department of Radiology of University Hospitals, where a high kilovoltage technique is used, the average skin dose to the chest is 27 mR. Doses in fluoroscopy are considerably higher and range from 5 to 10 R or more per minute of exposure.

When the hazard of radiation injury is recognized, it is possible to take precautions to decrease the amount of radiation to the patient, particularly to the gonads, since the gonadal effect is of the greatest long-range importance to the entire population. In most planned and definitely indicated radiologic examinations, the benefit to the patient outweighs the potential hazards, so that no procedure should be condemned when there are indications for it. On the other hand, unnecessary procedures should be avoided. For example, routine roentgen pelvimetry cannot be justified, but in a given individual the value of pelvimetry may far outweigh its potential hazard. The physician who uses radiographic or fluoroscopic equipment should know the output of the equipment and should know how to use it.

A number of specific measures can be taken to decrease the amount of radiation:

1. Filtration. A minimum of 2 mm of aluminum filtration should be used on all fluoroscopes and radiographic units. This results in significant reduction in radiation to the skin in the center of the beam.

2. Cones. Cones or collimating devices of various sizes can be used to limit the exposure to the area undergoing examination.

3. Voltage. The highest voltage consistent with good technique is recommended because it reduces the total radiation exposure.

4. Distance. Radiation dose is inversely proportional to the square of the distance from the source (target of x-ray tube). It is therefore important that the maximum distance consistent with good technique be used in radiography and that the tube be at least 18 inches from the nearest part of the patient in fluoroscopy.

5. Protective devices. Various commercial devices are available to protect those parts of the body not in the area of interest. Lead–rubber aprons or sheets can be used to cover most of the body during dental roentgenography or in examination of the extremities. Special leaded strips can be made to cover the female pelvis and male gonads when the hips or adjacent femurs are being examined.

6. Films and screens. High-speed intensifying screens and fast films should be used to reduce dosage. Rare earth screens that significantly reduce radiation required for various procedures are now available.

7. Image amplifiers. These devices are now in general use, and the apparatus now available reduces the dosage significantly in fluoroscopic procedures.

8. Fluoroscopy. Because of the high dosage to the patient, fluoroscopy should be held to a minimum. The lowest amperage consistent with adequate visualization and the smallest fluoroscopic field compatible with visualization should be used. In addition, a built-in timer with an automatic shut-off device should be employed.

All physicians should be aware of the potential danger of ionizing radiation, although necessary radiographic procedures can often be carried out with little or no gonadal exposure if proper precautions are taken. The protection of the gonads is particularly important in the population below the age of 30. The pregnant woman must also be protected, and procedures that irradiate the fetus in utero should be held to a minimum. Non-emergency roentgenography should not be done on women when there is a possibility of pregnancy.

REFERENCES AND SELECTED READINGS

1. CHAMBERLAIN WE: Fluoroscopes and fluoroscopy (Carman lecture). Radiology 38:383, 1942

2. CROW JF: Genetic considerations in establishing radiation doses. Radiology 69:18, 1957

3. FILES GW: Medical Radiographic Technique, 2nd ed. Springfield, IL, Thomas, 1951

4. GLASSER O: Dr. W. C. Röntgen. Springfield, IL, Thomas, 1945

5. GLASSER O, QUIMBY EH, TAYLOR LS, WEATHERWAX JL: Physical Foundations of Radiology, 3rd ed. New York, Hoeber, 1961.

6. HODGES PC: Health hazards in the diagnostic use of x-ray. JAMA 166: 577, 1958

7. LAUGHLIN JS, MEURK ML, PULLMAN I, SHERMAN RS: Bone, skin and gonadal doses in routine diagnostic procedures. Am J Roentgenol 78: 578, 1953

8. LEWIS EB: Leukemia and ionizing radiation. Science 125: 578, 1953

9. MORGAN RH: Protection from roentgen rays. Am J Med Sci 226: 578, 1953

10. NATIONAL RESEARCH COUNCIL: The Biological Effects of Atomic Radiation. Washington DC, National Academy of Sciences, 1956

SECTION I

THE OSSEOUS SYSTEM

1

DISTURBANCES IN SKELETAL GROWTH AND MATURATION

Roentgen examination is the key to the diagnosis of many skeletal abnormalities, and it is essential that skeletal radiographs be studied carefully in order that the maximum amount of information may be obtained from the examination. Each bone included must be examined on an anatomic basis, including the cortex, the medullary canal (cancellous bone or spongiosa), the periosteum, and the articular planes. The size, shape, position, and alignment in relation to other parts of the skeleton are determined. In children the epiphysis and epiphyseal line or physis must be examined. If ossification centers are small or are not yet present, alignments are very difficult to assess and it may be necessary to obtain films showing the opposite extremity in similar projections. The soft tissues adjacent to the bones are examined, particularly when there is history of injury or the possibility of infection in which obliteration of normal soft-tissue lines or distention of a joint capsule by fluid may be of particular importance. When disease is present it is important to determine whether single or multiple bones or joints are involved as well as the distribution of the lesions when they are multiple. The presence and type of bone destruction and bone production, the appearance of the edges or borders of the bone disease, and the presence or absence of cortical expansion and of periosteal reaction must also be noted. The findings are then correlated with the clinical history and the age and sex of the patient to arrive at a logical diagnosis that may be firm in some instances; in other cases a differential diagnosis must be made since the exact diagnosis cannot be determined and, in other instances, differentiation of a benign from a malignant condition may be the only information possible to obtain.

OSSIFICATION OF THE SKELETON

At birth the shafts of the long tubular bones are ossified but the ends, with a few exceptions, consist of masses of cartilage, the *epiphyses*. Cartilage is relatively radiolucent as compared to bone and has the same general density as the soft tissues. Thus at birth the ends of the bones are separated by radiolucent spaces representing the cartilaginous epiphyses. At variable times after birth, one or more ossification centers appear in the epiphyses (*epiphyseal ossification centers* or EOC). The exceptions occur in the distal femoral and proximal tibial epiphyses where ossification centers appear during the last 1 or 2 months of intrauterine life. The short tubular bones are similar to the long except in having an epiphysis at only one end. The carpal bones are cartilaginous at birth. In the tarsus, normally, ossification centers are present at birth for the calcaneus, navicular, and talus. The other tarsal bones are cartilaginous. For the vertebrae three ossification centers are present, one for the body and two for the arch. Shortly after birth the two halves of the lamina fuse, beginning first in the lumbar area and ascending to the cervical. Union of the arches to the bodies begins in the third year of life and is completed about the seventh year. Here fusion begins in the cervical area and is completed in the lumbar. The cranial bones have ossified but remain separated by fibrous tissue sutures. The individual pelvic bones are present but separated by cartilaginous plates or epiphyseal masses.*

The few epiphyseal ossification centers present at birth, particularly that for the distal femur, are useful indicators of skeletal maturity and since these often can be recognized in roentgenograms of the mother's abdomen during the last month of gestation they also serve as valuable indicators of fetal maturity.

The process of bone formation in cartilage is known as endochondral ossification. The bones grow in length by this means. Some bones are formed in membrane; the bones of the cranial vault are principal examples of this process. In the mandible and clavicle, ossification occurs both in cartilage and in membrane. The tubular bones grow in their transverse diameters by bone formation by the osteogenic cells of the inner layer of the periosteum. This is a form of bone formation in membrane. Since the cortices of the bones are formed in this way and the cortex makes up the bulk of a tubular bone, it can be appreciated that much of the mass of the skeleton is formed in membrane.

THE BONES IN INFANCY AND CHILDHOOD

After an epiphyseal ossification center appears at or near the center of the epiphysis it gradually enlarges

* Only the briefest résumé of this important subject will be given here in order to define some of the terms that are used in describing the bones during the developmental period. For a more complete discussion the references listed at the end of the chapter should be consulted.

and takes on the shape that is distinctive for the end of that particular bone. In some areas there is more than one ossification center and they may appear at different times (*e.g.,* the distal humerus). The ossified epiphysis remains separated from the shaft by a cartilaginous disc or plate known variously as the epiphyseal plate, growth plate, or physis. The epiphyseal plate gradually becomes thinner as growth proceeds until it finally ossifies, the epiphysis fuses to the shaft and growth in length is complete (Fig. 1-1).

The times of appearance of the various epiphyseal ossification centers are good indicators of the skeletal age of the individual during infancy and early childhood. Similarly, the times of fusion of the epiphyses can be used as indicators of skeletal age during late adolescence.

The end of the shaft of a tubular bone is bounded by a thin radiopaque line or zone, the *zone of provisional calcification*. This is the area where mineral salts are deposited temporarily around the degenerating cartilage cells. Subsequently blood vessels grow into the lacunae left by the degenerated cartilage cells bringing with them the osteoblasts. These are specialized connective tissue cells, one of whose main functions is the production of osteoid. Osteoid is the organic matrix in which mineral salts are deposited to make bone. Osteoid also is relatively radiolucent and any large amount of it will cause the bones to appear more translucent than is normal. As osteoid is formed the zone of provisional calcification, which has acted as a framework for bone formation, disappears on the shaft side and is replaced by trabecular bone. It is replaced on the epiphyseal side so that, normally, it never disappears until the epiphysis fuses to the shaft. It is seen in roentgenograms as a narrow radiopaque line or zone marking the end of the shaft. The area at the end of the diaphysis where active bone formation is taking place is known as the metaphysis and includes the zone of provisional calcification. There is a zone between the metaphysis and epiphysis, termed the *physis*, containing reserve cartilage, proliferating cartilage cells, and vacuolating cartilage cells. The latter are adjacent to the calcified cartilage or zone of provisional calcification. It is rather frequent during childhood to see one or more thin opaque lines crossing the shaft near its ends. These are commonly known as "growth lines" and, while there may be other causes for them, it is probable that in most cases they indicate a temporary cessation of orderly

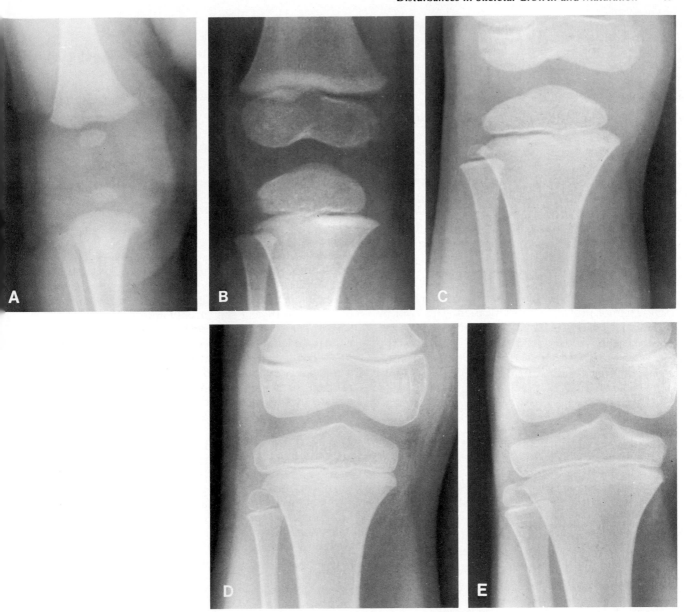

Fig. 1-1. A. One-year-old child. Normal ossifications at the knee are largely cartilaginous, but there are small ossification centers for the femur and tibia. The remainder of the space between bone ends is cartilaginous. **B.** Child 2 years of age. The ossification centers have grown considerably. The zone of provisional calcification produces the wide transverse lines at the metaphyses. **C.** Child 5 years of age. The epiphyses have developed to a point where the ends of the bones resemble those of an adult. A cartilaginous plate remains between the epiphysis and metaphysis, the physis or epiphyseal line or plate. **D.** In this 8-year-old child the epiphyseal line remains distinct and the femoral condyles are approaching the adult shape. **E.** In this 10-year-old child there has been further ossification in the physis (epiphyseal line). Longitudinal growth continues until the physis disappears and the epiphysis fuses to the metaphysis.

ossification brought about by one or more episodes of systemic illness.

In summary, the following are definitions of some of the terms used in describing the bones during infancy and childhood (Fig. 1-2):

1. Epiphysis. The cartilaginous end of a bone.
2. Physis. The cartilaginous zone between the epiphysis and the calcified cartilage. It also is known as the growth plate or the epiphyseal plate. When it has become thin as a result of growth it sometimes is called the epiphyseal line.
3. Metaphysis. The end of the shaft of a tubular bone where active bone formation takes place.
4. Diaphysis. The shaft of a tubular bone.
5. Epiphyseal ossification center (EOC). The ossified portion of an epiphysis.
6. Zone of provisional calcification. The layer or zone of deposition of mineral salts at the end of the shaft that serves as a framework for the deposition of osteoid. It is seen in roentgenograms as a thin white line or narrow zone.
7. Osteoid. The organic matrix formed by the osteoblasts and which, when mineralized, becomes bone.
8. Endochondral ossification. The process whereby bone is formed from cartilage.
9. Intramembranous ossification. The process whereby bone is formed from membrane without a cartilaginous stage; periosteal and endosteal growth are included.
10. Apophysis. An accessory ossification center that develops late; it forms a protrusion from the end or near the end of the shaft of a long bone. Apophyses usually serve as attachments for muscles or ligaments and do not contribute much to the length of a long bone.

SKELETAL MATURATION

Radiographic determination of skeletal maturation (bone age) is a very useful clinical tool, but there is controversy regarding the various methods of assessment. The most well-known and widely accepted method is that of Greulich and Pyle,[4] described in their book *Radiographic Atlas of Skeletal Development of the Hand and Wrist.* The accuracy of this

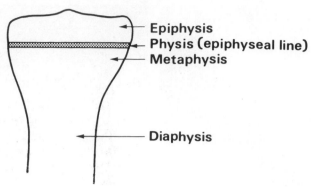

Fig. 1-2. The anatomic divisions of the end of a typical growing bone are shown in this diagram.

method is such that its use as the sole method of assessment is sufficient in most instances. Its accuracy can be exhanced by proper training. As a rule the use of the metacarpal and phalangeal centers is more accurate than that of the carpal centers. Exclusion of carpal centers has no effect on replicability and usually does not decrease the accuracy of the method. If further evaluation of skeletal maturation is necessary and indicated, Kuhns and Finnstrom's [8] method, described in their published article *Standards of Ossification in the Newborn,* will be found useful in premature infants and in the newborn. Standards described by Garn, Rohmann, and Silverman[3] are useful in infants and young children. Figure 1-3 shows the centers of maximum predictive value and ranks them in the order of the greatest correlation value. Tanner and associates[13] also have reported a method of assessing skeletal maturity along with prediction of adult height. Their method is too time-consuming for regular clinical use but may be employed as an alternate one in difficult situations, particularly for predicting height. Standard radiographic atlases have been compiled by Pyle and Hoerr[11] for the knee and by Hoerr, Pyle, and Francis[5] for the foot and ankle. Appearance and fusion time of various centers in the hand, wrist, and other bones are listed in Tables 1-1 and 1-2.

DISTURBANCES IN SKELETAL GROWTH AND MATURATION (Table 1-3)

The relationship of the endocrine glands to the growth and maturation of the skeleton is a very important one. Roentgen examination of the growing skeleton may give valuable information concerning

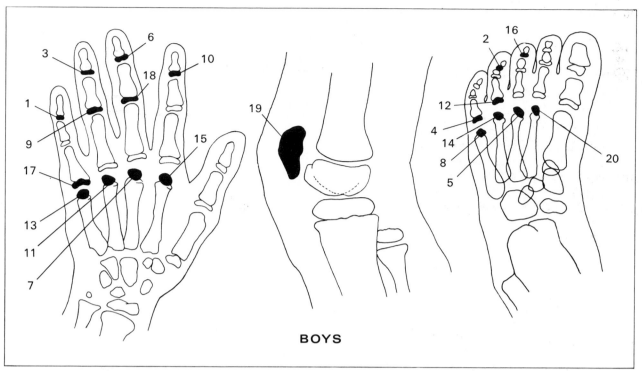

BOYS

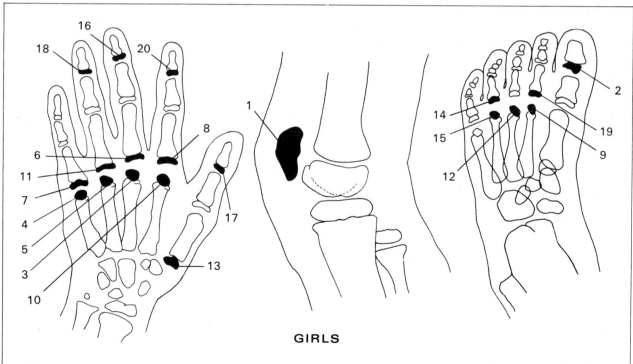

GIRLS

Fig. 1-3. The 20 centers of maximum value in predicting skeletal maturation in the hand, foot, and knee are shown in these diagrams. The numbers indicate the order of the greatest correlation value. (Garn, S. M.: In Medical Radiography and Photography. Radiography Markets. Rochester, Eastman Kodak Company, 1967. With permission of Stanley M. Garn, Ph.D.)

Table 1-1. Ossification Time Table (Females)

CENTERS PRESENT	HAND AND WRIST	FUSION (IN YR)	OTHER BONES	FUSION (IN YR)
At birth	Capitate (birth to 3 mo)		Distal femur	17
	Hamate (birth to 3 mo)		Proximal tibia	16 to 17
			Proximal humerus (occasionally)	17½ to 20
			Calcaneus	
			Talus	
			Cuboid	
End of 1 yr	Prox. phalanges II, III, IV	15	Coracoid, scapula	14 to 16
	Metacarpal II, III	15	Capitellum	14 to 15
	Distal radius (9 to 12 mo)	17	Proximal femur (1 to 6 mo)	16 to 17
			Distal tibia (1 to 7 mo)	16 to 17
			Distal fibula (1 to 7 mo)	15½ to 17
			Cuneiform III (3 mo)	
End of 2 yr	Triquetrum (18 to 24 mo)		Metatarsals	17 to 20
	Prox. phalanges I, V	15	Prox. phalanges toes (1 to 2½ yr)	18
	Mid. phalanges II, III, IV	14½	Mid. phalanges toes	
	Dist. phalanges I, III, IV, V	13½	(½ to 2½ yr)	18
	Metacarpals I, IV, V	15		
End of 3 yr	Dist. phalanx II	13½	Proximal fibula (2 to 4 yr)	17½ to 20
	Mid. phalanx V	15	Cuneiform I, II (½ to 2½ yr)	
	Lunate (30 to 36 mo)		Tarsal navicular (1 to 3 yr)	
			Dist. phalanges toes (1½ to 4 yr)	18
			Greater trochanter (1½ to 3 yr)	16
End of 4 yr	Greater multangular (36 to 42 mo)		Med. epicondyle humerus	
	Lesser multangular (42 to 50 mo)		(2 to 5 yr)	20
	Navicular (42 to 50 mo)		Patella (2 to 3½ yr)	
End of 6 yr	Distal ulna	16½	Proximal radius (3 to 5½ yr)	14 to 15
End of 8 yr	Pisiform (variable and unreliable)		Trochrea humerus (7 to 9 yr)	14
			Second calcaneal (5 to 12 yr)	12 to 22
End of 10 yr			Less. trochanter (9 to 14 yr)	16
			Tibial tuberosity (10 to 13 yr)	19
			Olecranon (8 to 11 yr)	14 to 15
End of 13 yr			Lat. epicondyle humerus (11 to 14 yr)	20
End of 15 yr			Inner border scapula	20
			Secondary centers pelvis	21+
End of 17 yr			Medial end clavicle	25

NOTE: Figures in parentheses indicate range of normal variation in time of appearance.

the presence or absence of disturbances of these glands, particularly the thyroid, pituitary, and gonads. Delay in the times of appearance of epiphyseal centers, in their growth and their fusion, may result from deficient secretion by one or more of these glands. Hypersecretion may accelerate these processes. Table 1-3, prepared by Graham, indicates a number

of glandular disturbances and their effect on skeletal maturation.

The more important endocrine conditions that may alter the rate of skeletal growth are considered briefly in the paragraphs to follow and the ways in which roentgen examination can be useful are described.

(*Text continues on p. 23.*)

Table 1-2. Ossification Time Table (Males)

CENTERS PRESENT	HAND AND WRIST	FUSION (IN YR)	OTHER BONES	FUSION (IN YR)
At birth	Capitate (birth to 3 mo) Hamate (birth to 3 mo)		Distal femur Proximal tibia Proximal humerus (occasionally) Calcaneus Talus Cuboid	18 to 19 18 to 19 21
End of 1 yr	Distal radius (12 to 15 mo)	18	Coracoid, scapula Capitellum, humerus Proximal femur (2 to 8 mo) Distal tibia (1 to 7 mo) Distal fibula (1 to 7 mo) Cuneiform III (6 mo)	14 to 16 14 to 15 18 17½ to 19 17½ to 19
End of 2 yr	Prox. phalanges II, III, IV, V Mid. phalanges III, IV Dist. phalanx I Dist. phalanges III, IV Metacarpals II, III, IV	17 16 to 17 15 15½ 17	Prox. phalanges toes (1 to 2½ yr)	17 to 18
End of 3 yr	Triquetrum (24 to 32 mo) Mid. phalanx II Prox. phalanx I Metacarpel I Metacarpal V Lunate (24 to 36 mo)	16 17 15½ 17	Metatarsals Mid phalanges, toes (1 to 4 yr) Cuneiform I, II (1 to 3½ yr)	18 to 20 18
End of 4 yr	Mid. phalanx V Dist. phalanges II, V Greater multangular (40 to 48 mo)	16 15¼	Great. trochanter (2½ to 4 yr) Prox. fibula (2½ to 5 yr) Tarsal navicular (1½ to 5½ yr)	16 19
End of 6 yr	Lesser multangular (60 to 66 mo) Navicular (60 to 66 mo) Distal ulna (60 to 66 mo)	17½	Medial epicondyle (5 to 7 yr) Patella (2½ to 6 yr) Dist. phalanges, toes (3½ to 6½ yr) Prox. radius (3 to 5½ yr)	20 18 15
End of 8 yr	Pisiform (variable and unreliable)		Trochlea, humerus (7 to 9 yr)	14
End of 10 yr			Less. trochanter (9 to 13 yr) Olecranon (8 to 11 yr) Secondary calcaneus (5 to 12 yr)	16 14 to 15 12 to 22
End of 13 yr			Tibial tuberosity (10 to 13 yr) Lat. epicondyle, humerus (11 to 14 yr)	19 20
End of 15 yr			Secondary centers, pelvis Inner border scapula	21+ 18 to 20
End of 17 yr			Medial end clavicle	25

NOTE: Figures in parentheses indicate range of normal variation in time of appearance.

Table 1-3. Abnormalities of Skeletal Maturation*

CONDITION	BONE AGE	STATURE	COMMENTS
CENTRAL and GENERAL			
Hyperpituitarism (giantism)	N or (↓), may fuse late	↑ ↑	eosinophilic adenoma, acromegalic if late
Hypopituitarism (pan-, pituitary dwarfism)	↓ ↓ may never fuse	↓ ↓	? "normal" early
Primordial dwarfism (genetic, constitutional)	N or (↓)	↓	
CNS disorders			(2° to neoplasm or other disease)
Pinealoma	↑	↑, adult ?N	Especially males
Fibrous dysplasia	↑	↑, adult ?N	especially females
Craniopharyngioma	↓	↓	
Hypothalamic dysfunction	↑ or ↓	↑ or ↓	many associations, i.e., obesity
Exogenous obesity	N or (↑)	N or (↑), adult N	
Malnutrition and/or Chronic disease	(↓)	(↓), adult may be N	
Chrondro-osseous dysplasias and Syndromes	↓ occasionally	↓ ↓ occasionally	rarely advanced, many die early
GONADS			(may be 2° to gonadotropin ↑ ↓)
Hypergonadism (hyperplasia, neoplasm)	↑ ↑, fuse early	↑ ↑, adult ↓	
Hypogonadism			
Eunuchoidism	N or (↓), fuse late	↑, long extremities	intrinsic, castration, 2° to disease
Pituitary	N	↓	not panhypopituitarism
Gonadal "dysplasias"			
Turner's syndrome	N or (↓), fuse late	↓	XO types, hypomineralization
Kleinfelter's syndrome	N or (↓), fuse late	↑, long extremities	XXY types
Abnormal sexual differentiation	(N)	(N)	pseudohermaphrodite types
Sexual developmental variations			
Delayed adolescence	(↓), then N	↓, adult N	
Premature pubarche	(↑), then N	↑, adult N	
Premature thelarche	N or ?(↑)	N	
Constitutional precocity	(↑), then N	↑, adult N	
ADRENALS			(may be 2° to ACTH ↑ ↓)
Cortical insufficiency (Addison's disease)	(↓)	(↓)	like a chronic disease
Cortical hyperactivity (Cushing's disease)	↓ occasionally	↓	cortisol ↑, hypomineralization
Adrenogenital syndrome (hyperplasia, neoplasm	↑ ↑ ↑, fuse early	↑ ↑, adult ↓	usually masculinizing, rarely feminizing
THYROID			(may be 2° to thyrotropin ↑ ↓)
Hypothyroidism			
Congenital (Cretinism)	↓ ↓ ↓ ↓	↓ ↓ ↓, infantile	epiphyseal dysgenesis hypermineralization
Acquired	↓	↓	
Hyperthyroidism	(↑)	(↑), adult N	? hypomineralization
PARATHYROIDS			
Hyperparathyroidism (1° or 2°)	(N)	(N)	hypomineralization
Hypoparathyroidism	(N)	(N)	hypermineralization
(Pseudohypoparathyroidism)	(N)	↓	associated with XO types

* Modified from Graham CB: Radiol Clin North Am 10:198, 1972.

Legend: N = normal   ↑ = advanced   ↓ = retarded
               (N) = probably normal   (↑) = possibly advanced   (↓) = possibly retarded

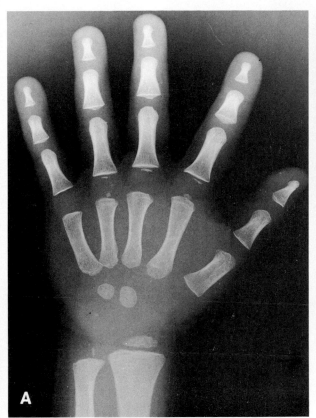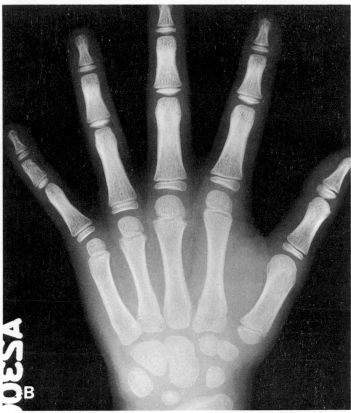

Fig. 1-4. Cretinism. **A.** Hand of an 8-year-old cretin shows delay in ossification. Compare with **B,** the hand of a normal 8-year-old child.

HYPOFUNCTION OF THE THYROID GLAND

Cretinism

Deficiency of thyroid secretion on a congenital basis and present at birth is known as cretinism. The roentgenologic characteristics are as follows:

1. The time of appearance of ossification centers is greatly delayed and growth of them, once they appear, is slow. No other disorder causes as severe a delay in ossification as cretinism (Fig. 1-4).

2. The centers that do ossify often are malformed and irregular in shape.

3. Certain epiphyses, notably those for the proximal ends of the femurs, show a tendency to ossify from numerous small irregular centers rather than from a single one as they normally should. The epiphysis does not grow properly and the femoral head develops a flattened shape (Fig. 1-5). It may resemble rather closely the flattened and fragmented epiphysis of osteo-

chondrosis (Legg–Perthes' disease) or that seen in patients with Morquio's disease, and in those with dysplasia epiphysialis multiplex. These conditions are discussed in Chapter 2. Roentgen examination also is useful in the follow-up study of cretins who are under treatment and the progress of skeletal development is a good index of the efficacy of therapy.

4. Dental defects, delay in the development and eruption of the teeth, tend to parallel the delay in ossification of the skeleton. The teeth that do erupt are structurally abnormal and subject to caries.

5. Stunting of growth may not be very obvious during infancy but, as the child becomes older, the thyroid deficiency if not treated will result in dwarfism.

6. Other findings noted in cretinism include: (*a*) increased thickness of the bones of the cranial

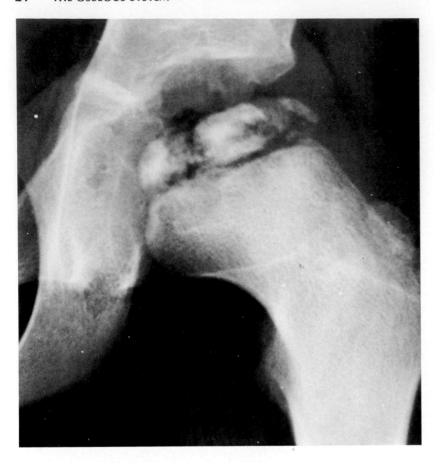

Fig. 1-5. Cretinoid epiphysis. The epiphysis for the femoral head is ossifying from multiple centers. The femoral neck is broad.

vault, narrow diploic space, and a brachycephalic shape; (b) shortening of the skull base; (c) the fontanelles may remain open for an abnormally long time and wormian bones along the sutures may be present; (d) in severe involvement, some degree of flattening of the vertebral bodies ("bullet-shaped") may be noted and a thoracolumbar gibbus with forward slipping of one vertebra on another may occur, and disc spaces are wide; (e) slipping of a capital femoral epiphysis (Fig. 1-6); (f) underpneumatization of the sinuses and mastoids; and (g) prognathous jaw.

In childhood hypothyroidism the abnormality observed in the skeleton is related to skeletal maturation. Osteosclerosis of the base of the skull and thickening of the lamina dura appear to be limited to patients with a bone age between 1 and 3 years. Wormian bones may be present early in skeletal development but usually disappear when the bone age reaches 5 years. Dense metaphyseal lines may be present very early in life, but they tend to disappear at a bone age of approximately 6 months. Epiphyseal disturbances, particularly in the femoral head, persist beyond the bone age of 8 years. It is interesting that some retardation of skeletal growth has been reported in a high percentage of patients with Perthe's disease, but there is evidently no correlation between the severity of the process and the degree of skeletal retardation.

In many adult cretins little or no residual skeletal deformity persists even though insufficient or no treatment was given.

Juvenile Hypothyroidism

When the thyroid deficiency occurs after birth as an acquired disease, the process usually is less severe than it is in cretinism. The term "juvenile hypothyroidism" is used to designate this form of the disease. The roentgen signs will usually be limited to some degree of delay in ossification. In determining the significance of alterations in skeletal age it must be re-

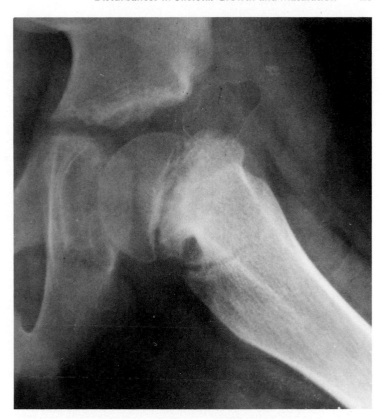

Fig. 1-6. Slipped capital femoral epiphysis in a patient with juvenile hypothyroidism. Note the irregularity of the metaphysis.

membered that there is a considerable range of normal variation, and that there is a difference according to sex, females maturing more rapidly than males. It is good practice to allow a variation of 3 months, plus or minus, during the first year of life, and up to 1 year at the end of puberty before considering the skeletal age to be abnormal. This will prevent the unnecessary treatment of children with potent preparations for supposed hormonal deficiency when none exists.

In chronic cases the metaphyses may appear irregular, somewhat suggestive of rickets. Slipping of the capital femoral epiphyses has been observed (Fig. 1-6). In more severe cases, the roentgen findings may be similar to those of cretinism.

HYPERFUNCTION OF THE THYROID GLAND

Hyperthyroidism occurring during childhood will cause some acceleration of skeletal development but it seldom is a striking alteration and frequently the skeletal age will remain within or close to the normal range. In chronic cases, particularly in older children, there often is generalized demineralization of the skeleton.

Meema and Schatz[10] observed cortical striations related to decrease in density of the cortex in the fingers in 50% of patients with moderate to severe thyrotoxicosis. The striation, however, is nonspecific, since it is also found in children with acromegaly, those with involutional osteoporosis, and sometimes in those who are normal. As a rule the amount of bone mass loss is directly proportional to the duration of untreated hyperthyroidism.

Thyroid acropachy is a rare manifestation of hyperthyroidism which produces periosteal reaction; it is discussed in Chapter 10, The Superficial Soft Tissues.

HYPOFUNCTION OF THE PITUITARY GLAND

Decreased function of the pituitary gland during childhood leads to generalized disturbance in bone growth and maturation since the pituitary is concerned with bone growth both directly and indirectly through the thyroid gland and the gonads. The epiphyseal centers are slow in appearing and delayed in uniting; at times union may never take place (Fig. 1-7). Since epiphyseal closure is closely related to go-

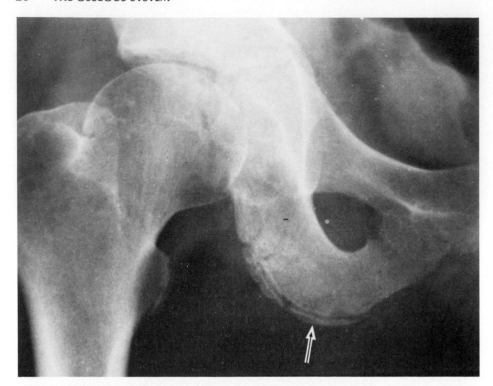

Fig. 1-7. Hypopituitarism. The epiphyseal plate for the ischial tuberosity **(arrow)** has not fused in this 30-year-old female pituitary dwarf.

Fig. 1-8. Acromegaly. The cranial bones are thickened, and the nasal sinuses enlarged. The sella turcica is moderately enlarged by an eosinophilic adenoma of the pituitary gland **(arrow).**

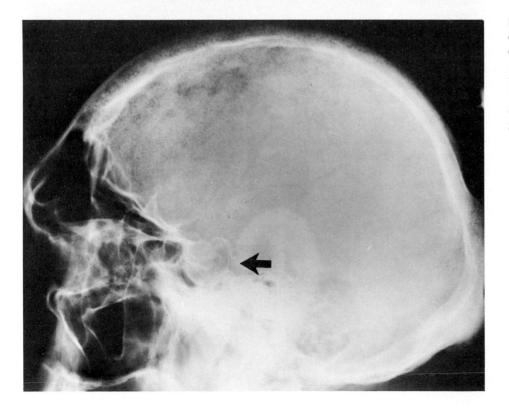

nadal function this is generally considered to be an indication of secondary hypogonadism. The bones do not grow normally in length or breadth so that the patients are small in stature, usually well proportioned and with normal mentality, but sexually immature. This condition is known as the Lorain type of pituitary dwarfism.

In many patients there is delay in eruption of the teeth, which tend to become impacted because their size is not affected. Since the arrest of skeletal growth occurs during childhood when the cranial vault is relatively large compared to the facial structures, this disproportion may persist into adulthood. Patients with the clinical signs of hypopituitarism and normal or increased height have been reported. Slipping of the capital femoral epiphysis has occurred in some patients with the disease.

The incidence of slipped femoral capital epiphysis is increased in patients with hypopituitarism who are treated with growth hormone.

Decrease in sellar size has been noted in some patients but there still is uncertainty about the significance of the "small" sella particularly when only measurements of the height and anteroposterior diameter are made on a lateral view of the skull. If the width also is measured, then volume determinations can be made and the results may be more meaningful. It should be noted that small sellas have also been found in association with some other types of dwarfism.

HYPERFUNCTION OF THE PITUITARY GLAND

Increased secretion by the eosinophilic cells of the anterior lobe of the pituitary gland, either as a result of an adenomatous tumor or from simple hyperplasia, leads to acceleration of bone growth. If this condition develops before growth has ceased it will result in gigantism. If it begins after adulthood has been reached it causes acromegaly.

Acromegaly

Increase in length of the bones does not occur in acromegaly, at least to any significant degree, if the disease develops after endochondral bone growth has ceased. Certain well-defined skeletal changes do appear, however, which are characteristic of the disease.

Skull. The cranial bones become thickened and of increased density. The diploë may be obliterated and the cranial bones have the density and appearance of cortical bone. Hyperostotic thickening may develop on the inner table causing the internal surface of the vault to appear shaggy. The nasal accessory sinuses become enlarged and the mastoids overpneumatized. The prognathous jaw, one of the obvious clinical features of acromegaly, can be demonstrated. There may be enlargement of the external occipital protuberance. The sella turcica may or may not be enlarged. In most patients some enlargement is noted and this is caused by pressure erosion from the eosinophilic adenoma that is present. The increase in sellar size seldom is as pronounced as that caused by chromophobe adenoma of the pituitary. The characteristic changes of acromegaly in the cranial bones are shown in Figure 1-8.

Long Bones. While not increased in length the long bones often become enlarged at their ends. This is demonstrated to best advantage in the hands and feet. The heads of the metacarpals and metatarsals become enlarged with irregular bony thickenings along their margins. Diaphyseal width usually remains normal. In some younger patients, however, the shafts of the short tubular bones are narrowed from accentuated growth in length and abnormal resorption along the shafts. The terminal tufts of the distal phalanges enlarge, forming thick bony tufts with pointed lateral margins. These curve proximally and may actually impinge against the phalangeal shafts. Hypertrophy of the soft tissues leading to the typical square, spade-shaped hand can be visualized. Measurement of the heel-pad thickness has been used as an indicator of the increase in soft tissues.[7] This distance is measured from the inferior surface of the os calcis to the nearest skin surface. In the normal this should not exceed 21 mm. However, more recent observations indicate that, in many obese individuals, heel-pad thicknesses over 21 mm will be found and the same is true of some other persons not overweight. It cannot, therefore, be considered as a completely specific sign. In some patients there is widening of the joint spaces owing to hypertrophy of the articular cartilages. This is best demonstrated in the metacarpophalangeal joints. Degenerative changes in the joints manifested by marginal spurring and sclerosis of articular margins may be seen even in relatively young patients. The general texture of the bones becomes coarsened (Fig. 1-9).

Spine. Calcific spurs may form along the margins of vertebral bodies particularly in the thoracic region and this may be very extensive. The vertebral bodies may actually increase in their anteroposterior diame-

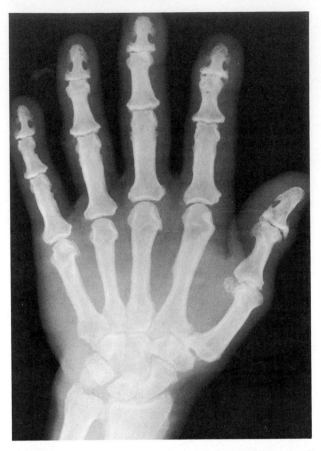

Fig. 1-9. Acromegaly. The terminal tufts of the distal phalanges are enlarged. There are spurlike bony projections adjacent to the joint surfaces near the ends of many of the phalanges.

ters. "Scalloping" or increased concavity of the posterior aspect of the vertebral bodies occurs in a number of patients. It is most prominent in the lumbar spine. There frequently is an increase in the thoracic kyphosis causing an increase in the anteroposterior diameter of the chest. There is a compensatory accentuation of the lumbar lordosis. The intervertebral discs may be of increased height owing to overgrowth of cartilage.

Gigantism

The roentgen features of gigantism are essentially those of an excessively large skeleton because skeletal growth is accelerated and this happens before the epiphyses close. Additionally there usually are the signs of acromegaly and, if the disease continues to

be active after adult life is reached, the acromegalic aspects increase. The sella may or may not enlarge.

HYPOGONADISM

Deficiency of gonadal secretions occurring before skeletal growth has ceased results in delay of epiphyseal closure, therefore the long bones become elongated and slender. The most familiar clinical condition in which this is seen is that which follows surgical removal of the gonads, or atrophy of them from disease, and is known as eunuchoidism. Delayed fusion of the epiphyses is seen in hypopituitarism and is believed to be caused by secondary hypogonadism in these instances. In contrast to the appearances in eunuchs, the bones in hypopituitarism are small and short, leading to dwarfism.

ACCELERATED MATURATION OF THE SKELETON

Acceleration of skeletal maturation usually is associated with general precocious development and early puberty. Among the conditions in which this is found are the following:

Albright's Syndrome. This syndrome consists of widespread osseous lesions of fibrous dysplasia and pigmented areas (café-au-lait spots) in the skin. In females there may be precocious sexual development, rapid skeletal growth, and early fusion of the epiphyses. As a result the patients usually show some degree of dwarfism. These latter changes do not occur in males. Fibrous dysplasia is discussed more fully in Chapter 2.

Granulosa Cell Tumor of the Ovary. This tumor causes precocious puberty and the skeletal system responds by early closure of the epiphyses.

Pineal Tumor. Tumors of the pineal gland may cause precocious puberty in males. Skeletal maturation is accelerated.

Hyperfunction of the Adrenal Cortex in Childhood. This may affect both sexes. In females it causes virilism; in males, sex characteristics are intensified and puberty develops early. The epiphyses fuse prematurely and the patients tend to be dwarfed.

Several rare syndromes have also been recorded in which there is accelerated skeletal maturation. Most of these patients have multiple defects such as facial abnormalities, motor inadequacy, and mental deficiency.

DELAYED MATURATION OF THE SKELETON

In addition to the abnormalities of the gonads and of the pituitary and thyroid glands, delay in skeletal maturation has been reported in persons with congenital heart disease in whom it appears to be related to low oxygen tension since the most severe delays are found in patients with the more severe cyanotic heart diseases. Dietary deficiencies and a number of chronic illnesses, including renal disease and celiac disease, have long been known to result in delay in skeletal maturation. Ionizing radiation may also cause a delay in skeletal growth. Doses as low as 2500 rads have been known to produce diminution in bone growth when administered to children under the age of 6 years.

REFERENCES AND SELECTED READINGS

1. Doyle FH: Radiologic assessment of endocrine effects on bone. Radiol Clin North Am 5: 289, 1967
2. Follis RH Jr, Park EA: Some observations on bone growth, with particular respect to zones and transverse lines of increased density in the metaphysis. Am J Roentgenol 68: 709, 1952
3. Garn SM, Rohmann CG, Silverman FN: Radiographic standards for postnatal ossification and tooth calcification. Med Radiogr Photogr 43: 45, 1967
4. Greulich WW, Pyle SI: Radiographic Atlas of Skeletal Development of the Hand and Wrist, 2nd ed. Stanford, Stanford University Press, 1959
5. Hoerr NL, Pyle SI, Francis CC: Radiographic Atlas of Skeletal Development of the Foot and Ankle. Springfield, IL, CC Thomas, 1962
6. Jackson DM: Heel-pad thickness in obese persons. Radiology 90: 129, 1968
7. Kho KM, Wright AD, Doyle FH: Heel-pad thickness in acromegaly. Br J Radiol 43: 119, 1970
8. Kuhns LR, Finnstrom O: New standards of ossification of the newborn. Radiology 119: 655, 1976
9. LeMay M: The radiologic diagnosis of pituitary disease. Radiol Clin North Am 5: 303, 1967
10. Meema HE, Schatz DL: Simple radiologic demonstration of cortical bone loss in thyrotoxicosis. Radiology 97: 9, 1970
11. Pyle SI, Hoerr NL: A Radiologic Standard of References for the Growing Knee. Springfield, IL, CC Thomas, 1969
12. Roche AF, French NY: Differences in skeletal maturity levels in the knee and hand. Am J Roentgenol 109: 307, 1970
13. Tanner JM, Whitehouse RH, Marshall WA et al: Assessment of Skeletal Maturity and Prediction of Adult Height (TW2) Method. London, 1975
14. Weitersen FK, Balow RM: The radiologic aspects of thyroid disease. Radiol Clin North Am 5: 255, 1967

2

THE OSSEOUS DYSPLASIAS

The osseous dysplasias consist of a group of disorders characterized by an abnormality in the growth of cartilage or bone or of both.[1] The most recent classification of constitutional diseases of bone is shown in Table 2-1. The classification developed by Rubin[26] has received some acceptance. It was based upon the division of growing bone into four zones: epiphysis, physis or growth plate, metaphysis, and diaphysis. It was considered that the basic disturbance in most of the dysplasias occurred in one of these zones. Each group of dysplasias (epiphyseal, physeal, etc.), was further subdivided into hypoplastic and hyperplastic types. McKusick[17] has emphasized the hereditary nature of many of these diseases. More recently Aegerter and Kirkpatrick[1] have presented a classification based largely on the morbid physiology of the cells involved.

It should be noted that in many of these diseases considerable change in the roentgen appearances may occur from infancy to adulthood. Also, many have congenita and tarda types so that a description of the abnormal findings at one age period may not be correct for another.

Many of the osseous dysplasias are briefly described in this chapter, but much clinical and genetic data have not been included because of space restrictions. The interested reader is referred to *Bone Dysplasias* by Spranger, Langer, and Wiedemann,[30] to *Roentgen Diagnosis of Diseases of the bone* (2nd ed.) by Edeiken and Hodes,[4] and to *Orthopedic Diseases* (4th ed.) by Aegerter and Kirkpatrick.[1]

In the discussions to follow a classification is not attempted but, in general, the listing as given by Aegerter and Kirkpatrick[1] is used with some additions and changes.

Radiographic examination of the skeleton is essential for accurate diagnosis of the osseous dysplasias and a precise diagnosis forms a solid basis for genetic counseling.

Table 2-1

**Special Report:
International Nomenclature of Constitutional Diseases of Bone**

INTRODUCTION

The description and separation of new disorders necessitated the creation of an International Nomenmclature of Constitutional Diseases of Bone which was first developed in Paris in 1969. Because of the rapid progress in the delineation and classification of these disorders, the international nonemclature was revised in May 1977. This new list includes the clearly identified forms of a single disease or defect. "Other forms" means that other forms of the disorder exist which, as yet, have not been defined well enough to include.

This revision endeavors to modify the previously proposed terms as little as possible, and its primary goal has been to introduce the names of a certain number of new conditions which have been defined since the original conference. it is necessary to emphasize that the essential purpose of this nomenclature is to unify the terminology used in this field in different parts of the world. It is not intended to be a classification of skeletal disorders, and the subdivisions proposed are devised only to clarify the presentation of the various disorders.

Among the changes which have been made, attention is directed to the elimination of the term "dwarfism" which seemed somewhat offensive to the patients or their families. Thus the term "diastrophic dwarfism" has been replaced by "diastrophic dysplasia." Moreover, the constitutional disorders of growth have been eliminated from the current list because it seems that they truly do not correspond to constitutional skeletal disorders; it has been proposed that another committee develop a nomenclature of syndromes in which these conditions ought to be included. Among constitutional disorders of growth, only those in which skeletal involvement is predominant as a manifestation have been retained and these are listed among the dysostoses. Metabolic disorders which involve complex sugars have been designated, insofar as is possible, by the responsible enzymatic defect. By virtue of the pathogenetic uncertainties which surrounded mucolipidosis II and III, these terms are retained in the nomenclature for the time being.

This nomenclature has been elaborated by a group of experts who met in Paris in May 1977 at the request of P. Maroteaux. The meeting was held under the aegis of the European Society for Pediatric Radiology and the National Foundation–March of Dimes. Participants included J. Dorst, C. Faure, A Giedion, J. Hall, H. J. Kaufmann, K. Kozlowski, L. Langer, L. Lenzi, P. Maroteaux, A. Murphy, A. K. Poznanski, D. Rimoin, J. Sauvegrain, F. Silverman, J. Spranger, R. Stanescu, and V. Stanescu.

OSTEOCHONDRODYSPLASIAS
Abnormalities of cartilage and/or bone growth and development.

Defects of growth of tubular bones and/or spine
A. Identifiable at birth
  1. Achondrogenesis type I, parenti-Fraccaro
  2. Achondrogenesis type II, Langer-Saldino
  3. Thanatophoric dysplasia
  4. Thanatophoric dysplasia with clover-leaf skull
  5. Short rib-polydactyly syndrome type I, Saldino-Noonan (perhaps several forms)
  6. Short rib-polydactyly syndrome type II, Majewski
  7. Chondrodysplasia punctata
    a. Rhizomelic form
    b. Dominant form
    c. Other forms, excluding symptomatic stippling in other disorders (e.g., Zellweger syndrome, Warfarin embryopathy)
  8. Campomelic dysplasia
  9. Other dysplasias with congenital bowing of long bones (several forms)
  10. Achondroplasia
  11. Diastrophic dysplasia
  12. Metatropic dysplasia (several forms)
  13. Chondroectodermal dysplasia, Ellis Van Creveld
  14. Asphyxiating thoracic dysplasia, Jeune
  15. Spondyloepiphyseal dysplasia congenita
    a. Type Spranger-Wiedemann
    b. Other forms (see B, 11-12)
  16. Kniest dysplasia
  17. Mesomelic dysplasia
    a. Type Nievergelt
    b. Type Langer (probable homozygous dyschondrosteosis)
    c. Type Robinow
    d. Type Rheinhardt
    e. Other forms
  18. Acromesomelic dysplasia
  19. Cleidocranial dysplasia
  20. Larsen syndrome
  21. Otopalatodigital syndrome
B. Identifiable in later life
  1. Hypochondroplasia
  2. Dyschondrosteosis
  3. Metaphyseal chondrodysplasia type Jansen
  4. Metaphyseal chondrodysplasia type Schmid
  5. Metaphyseal chondrodysplasia type McKusick
  6. Metaphyseal chondrodysplasia with exocrine pancreatic insufficiency and cyclic neutropenia
  7. Spondylometaphyseal dysplasia
    a. Type Kozlowski
    b. Other forms
  8. Multiple epiphyseal dysplasia
    a. Type Fairbanks
    b. Other forms
  9. Arthroophtalmopathy, Stickler
  10. Pseudoachondroplasia
    a. Dominant
    b. Recessive
  11. Spondyloepiphyseal dysplasia tarda
  12. Spondyloepiphyseal dysplasia, other forms (see A, 15-16)
  13. Dyggve-Melchior-Clausen dysplasia
  14. Spondyloepimetaphyseal dysplasia (several forms)
  15. Myotonic chondrodysplasia, Catel-Schwartz-Jampel
  16. Parastremmatic dysplasia
  17. Trichorhinophalangeal dysplasia
  18. Acrodysplasia with retinitis pigmentosa and nephropathy Saldino-Mainzer

Disorganized development of catilage and fibrous components of skeleton
1. Dysplasia epiphyseal hemimelica
2. Multiple cartilagenous exostoses
3. Acrodysplasia with exostoses, Giedion-Langer
4. Enchondromatosis, Ollier
5. Enchondromatosis with hemangioma, Maffucci
6. Metachondromatosis
7. Fibrous dysplasia, Jaffe-Lichtenstein
8. Fibrous dysplasia with skin pigmentation and precocious puberty, McCune-Albright
9. Cherubism (familial fibrous dysplasia of the jaws)
10. Neurofibromatosis

Abnormalities of density of corticol diaphyseal structure and/or metaphyseal modeling
1. Osteogenesis imperfecta congenita (several forms)
2. Osteogenesis imperfecta tarda (several forms)
3. Juvenile idiopathic osteoporosis
4. Osteoporosis with pseudoglioma
5. Osteopetrosis with precocious manifestations
6. Osteopetrosis with delayed manifestations (several forms)
7. Pycnodysostosis
8. Osteopoikilosis
9. Osteopathia striata
10. Melorheostosis
11. Diaphyseal dysplasia. Camurati-Engelmann
12. Craniodiaphyseal dysplasia
13. Endosteal hyperostosis
    a. Autosomal dominant, Worth
    b. Autosomal recessive, Van Buchem
14. Tubular stenosis, Kenny-Caffey
15. Pachydermoperiostosis
16. Osteodysplasty, Meinick-Needles
17. Frontometaphyseal dysplasia
18. Craniometaphyseal dysplasia (several forms)
19. Metaphyseal dysplasia, Pyle
20. Sclerosteosis
21. Dysosteosclerosis
22. Osteoectasia with hyperphosphatasia

DYSOSTOSES
Malformation of individual bones singly or in combination.

Dysostoses with cranial and facial involvement
1. Craniosynostosis (several forms)
2. Craniofacial dysostosis, Crouzon
3. Acrocephalosyndactyly, Apert (and others)
4. Acrocephalopolysyndactyly, Carpenter (and others)
5. Mandibulofacial dysostosis
   a. Type Teacher-Collins, Franceschetti
   b. Other forms
6. Oculomandibulofacial syndrome, Hallermann-Streiff-Francois
7. Nevoid basal cell carcinoma syndrome

Dysostoses with predominant axial involvement
1. Vertebral segmentation defects, including Klippel-Feil
2. Cervicooculoacoustic syndrome, Wildervanck
3. Sprengel anomaly
4. Spondylocostal dysostosis
   a. Dominant form
   b. Recessive forms

5. Oculovertebral syndrome, Weyers
6. Osteoonychodysostosis
7. Cerebrocostomandibular syndrome

Dysostoses with predominant involvement of extremities
1. Acheiria
2. Apodia
3. Ectrodactyly syndrome
4. Aglossia-adactyly syndrome
5. Congenital bowing of long bones (several forms) (see also osteochondrodysplasias)
6. Familial radioulnar synostosis
7. Brachydactyly (several forms)
8. Symphalangism
9. Polydactyly (several forms)
10. Symphalangism
11. Polysyndactyly (several forms)
12. Camptodactyly
13. Poland syndrome
14. Rubinstein-Taybi syndrome
15. Pancytopenia-dysmelia syndrome, Fanconi
16. Thrombocytopenia-radial-asplasia syndrome
17. Orodigitofacial syndrome
    a. Type Papillon-Leage
    b. Type Mohr
18. Cardiomelic syndrome, Holt-Oram (and others)
19. Femoral facial syndrome
20. Multiple synostoses (includes some forms of symphalangism)
21. Scapuloiliac dysostosis, Kosennow-Sinios
22. Hand-foot-genital syndrome
23. Focal dermal hypoplasia, Goltz

IDIOPATHIC OSTEOLYSES
1. Phalangeal (several forms)
2. Tarsocarpal
   a. Including Francois form (and others)
   b. With neophropathy
3. Multicentric
   a. Hajdu-Cheney form
   b. Winchester form
   c. Other forms

CHROMOSOMAL ABERRATIONS
Specific entities not listed.

PRIMARY METABOLIC ABNORMALITIES
Calcium and/or phosphorus
1. Hypophosphatemic rickets
2. Pseudodeficiency rickets, Prader, Royer
3. Late rickets, McCance
4. Idiopathic hypercalcuria
5. Hypophosphatasia (several forms)
6. Pseudohypoparathyroidism (normo- and hypo-calcemic forms, including acrodysostosis)

Complex carbohydrates
1. Mucopolysaccharidosis, type I (alpha-L-iduronidase deficiency)
   a. Hurler form
   b. Scheie form
   c. Other forms
2. Mucopolysaccharidosis, type II, Hunter (sulfoiduronate sulfatase deficiency)

3. Mucopolyaccharidosis, type III San Filippo
   a. Type A (heparin sulfamidase deficiency)
   b. Type B (N-acetyl-alpha-glucosaminidase deficiency)
4. Mucopolysaccharidosis, type IV, Morquio (N-acetylgalactosamine-6-sulfate-sulfatase deficiency)
5. Mucopolysaccharidosis, type VI, Maroteaux-Lamy (aryl sulfatase B deficiency)
6. Mucopolysaccharidosis, type VII (beta-glucuronidase deficiency)
7. Aspartylglucosaminuria (aspartyl-glucosaminidase deficiency)
8. Mannosidosis (alpha-mannosidase deficiency)
9. Fucosidosis (alpha-fucosidase deficiency)
10. GM1-gangliosidosis (beta-galactosidase deficiency)
11. Multiple sulfatase deficiency, Austin, Thieffry
12. Neuraminidase deficiency (formerly mucolipidosis I)
13. Mucolipidosis II
14. Mucolipidosis III

Lipids
1. Niemann-Pick disease
2. Gaucher disease

Nucleic acids
1. Adenosine-deaminase deficiency and others

Amino acids
1. Homocystinuria and others

Metals
1. Menkes kinky hair syndrome and others

This, the most recent classification of Constitutional Diseases of Bone was developed by a Committee formed by the European Society for Pediatric Radiology and the National Foundation—March of Dimes. (Am J Roentgenol 131:352–354, 1978)

STIPPLED EPIPHYSES

Other names applied to this dysplasia include *punctate epiphyseal dysplasia, dysplasia epiphysealis punctata, chondrodystrophia calcificans congenita, Conradi's disease,* and *chondroangiopathia calcarea seu punctata.* Some authorities consider stippled epiphyses to be the *congenita* form of multiple epiphyseal dysplasia and others have commented on the possible relationship of this disorder and multiple epiphyseal dysplasia, spondyloepiphyseal dysplasia, and epiphyseal hyperplasia. Infants frequently are stillborn or die within the first year of life of associated anomalies or of intercurrent disease. The disease is genetically transmitted as autosomal recessive.

The characteristic roentgen finding is the presence of numerous small, round, opacities in the unossified epiphyseal cartilages (Fig. 2-1). In some patients, the spots appear to extend into the adjacent

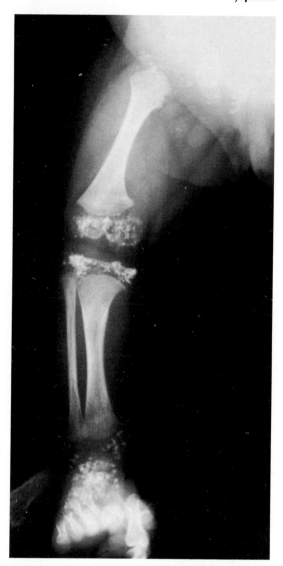

Fig. 2-1 Stippled epiphyses. Numerous tiny, dense foci were noted throughout the cartilages of the skeleton. They were most numerous in the right lower extremity. The bones are shorter than normal. (Paul LW: Am J Roentgenol 71: 941, 1954. Copyright 1954 American Roentgen Ray Society. Reproduced by permission)

soft tissues. They also have been found in other cartilages such as the nasal septum, larynx, and trachea. Stippling of the vertebral cartilages is common in the more severe cases. The extremities may be dwarfed and flexion deformities also may be present. The femur and humerus are most likely to be shortened.

In many patients there have been congenital cataracts, saddle nose, hyperkeratotic dermatoses, and failure of proper mental and physical development. If the infant survives it is said that in some cases the foci may ossify and then merge to form a fairly normal epiphyseal center.

In one of our patients, followed for 9 years,[22] dwarfing was severe in the right lower extremity and stippling was extensive throughout the cartilages of the body. The spots gradually disappeared. Normal-appearing ossification centers formed which seemed to have no relationship to the abnormal foci. Eventually the epiphyses developed an essentially normal shape. An exception was the proximal femoral epiphysis in the dwarfed right lower extremity. This center was late in appearing and when it did appear it remained small and malformed. Also a left convex thoracic scoliosis developed owing to failure of growth of the right sides of the midthoracic vetebrae. In addition, the fingers and toes may be short and stubby. The carpal and tarsal bones may be normal or show some irregularity in shape.

Chondrocalcification similar to that seen in this disorder also has been noted in the rare *cerebro-hepato-renal syndrome,* except that the calcified foci are most marked in the patellae and may be limited to these bones. Other findings in this syndrome as listed by Poznanski and associates[24] include (*1*) marked flaccidity, (*2*) abnormal facies, (*3*) cataracts, (*4*) flexion contractures of the extremities, (*5*) small cortical renal cysts, (*6*) fibrosis of the liver with increased deposits of hemosiderin, and (*7*) abnormality of the cerebrum including lissencephaly and sudanophilic leukodystrophy.

MULTIPLE EPIPHYSEAL DYSPLASIA

The characteristic finding in this dyspasia is the presence of multiple ossification centers for the affected epiphyses giving them a fragmented appearance. The epiphyses may be enlarged and the ends of the long bones may be somewhat flared. The involvement may be limited to a single epiphysis, a pair of epiphyses, or all epiphyses throughout the body. Symmetric involvement of the capital femoral epiphyses is common. Knock-knee or bow-leg deformity may be present and flexion deformities at the knee joint may be seen. The tibias usually are curved. A coronal cleft in the patellas (*i.e.,* "double-layered patella") has been described[9] as a fairly consistent and characteristic finding in the tarda form.

The vertebrae may be flattened in the thoracic spine with irregular end-plates. The skull is normal. Dwarfing of the extremities, resembling achondroplasia, is present in many and becomes more obvious as the child grows (the pseudoachondroplastic type). The long bones appear to be short and thick. The thickness is an illusion rather than real because of the shortening. An upward sloping, from within out, of the distal articular surface of the tibia is present in about one-half of the patients. The carpal and tarsal bones are often irregular and the digits stubby. In many patients, however, the hands are normal.

The patients usually are brought to the attention of a physician after they begin to walk because of their peculiar waddling gait. Eventually the multiple centers merge and then unite to the shaft. Irregularity of the articular plates frequently persists (Fig. 2-2) and leads to the early development of degenerative joint disease, particularly in the hip joints. At this stage it usually is impossible to determine what the primary disorder was since the other epiphyseal dysplasias may also result in early degenerative joint disease. In mild cases (the *tarda* form of Rubin) the disorder may not be recognized until the arthritic changes bring the patient to the physician. The disease is considered to be transmitted as an autosomal dominant with complete penetrance but variable expression.

In differential diagnosis, the lack of characteristic changes in the skull and pelvis serves to exclude achondroplasia. The normal vertebrae is significant in excluding Morquio's disease. When the heads of the femurs alone are involved, bilateral Perthes' disease and the epiphyseal dysgenesis of cretinism must be considered.

EPIPHYSEAL HYPERPLASIA

This disorder also has been called *dysplasia epiphysealis hemimelica* (Fairbank) and *tarsoepiphyseal aclasis.* It is essentially an eccentric overgrowth of an epiphysis of a long bone or a small bone of the foot forming an irregular bony mass along one side of the affected epiphysis. Only a single epiphysis is involved; in the great majority of patients it is the talus, followed by the distal femur and distal tibia, that is involved. Other areas less frequently affected include the upper tibia, upper fibula, lesser trochanter of the femur, and the tarsal navicular and first cuneiform. The bony mass may be attached to the adjacent epiphysis or exist separately. It is usually first noticed during childhood and is asymptomatic until the mass interferes with joint function. Pathologically, the le-

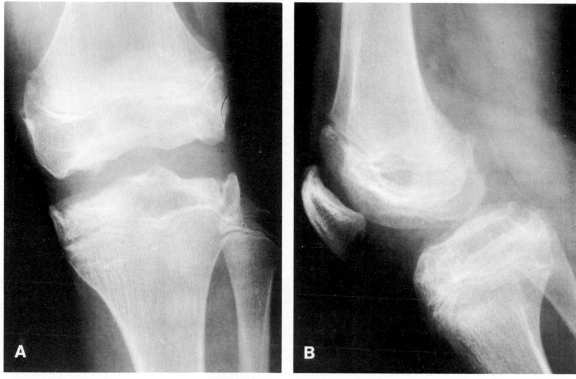

Fig. 2-2. Multiple epiphyseal dysplasia in an adolescent. The articular surfaces are irregular as visualized in frontal **(A)** and lateral **(B)** projections. The joint abnormality often leads to the early development of degenerative joint disease.

sion is said to be identical with an exostosis or osteochondroma. However, most authorities agree that these latter lesions do not arise from epiphyses.

SPONDYLOEPIPHYSEAL DYSPLASIA

The term *spondyloepiphyseal dysplasia congenita* has been used synonymously with Morquio's disease. However, Morquio's disease is now considered to belong to the group of mucopolysaccharidoses. In spondyloepiphyseal dysplasia (SED), growth of extremities and vertebrae is affected and it has been suggested that it is a transitional form between achondroplasia and Morquio's disease. Dwarfism is one of the major features of the childhood form of the disease while precocious degenerative joint disease is the chief finding in adults. The childhood form has also been called *pseudoachondroplastic spondyloepiphyseal dysplasia;* the latent type, *spondyloepiphyseal dysplasia tarda.*

As with many of the other dysplasias, the roentgen signs vary with the age of the patient. In the congenital form, as described in the literature,[29] there is at birth and during early infancy a general delay in ossification. Ossification centers for the distal femurs, proximal tibias, and the calcanei and tali usually are absent and the pubic bones show similar delay. Flattening of the vertebral bodies (*i.e.,* platyspondyly) is present and the posterior parts of the bodies are more decreased in height than anteriorly. The acetabular angles are small. There may be flaring of the anterior ends of the ribs and the thorax is broad and bell-shaped. Lateral bowing of the femurs is frequent. The long tubular bones are shortened with various epiphyseal and metaphyseal abnormalities. In later infancy and early childhood, delay in ossification of the pubis and the femoral heads and necks persists. The vertebral bodies remain flattened and have an ovoid shape in lateral views. Anterior hypoplasia of one or more vertebral segments often is pronounced at the thoracolumbar junction. In the pelvis there is a lack of the normal iliac flare and the ilia appear small in their cephalocaudal dimensions. There is little or no acetabular slant.

In later childhood thre is accentuation of the dorsal kyphosis and lumbar lordosis and scoliosis may develop. There is lack of normal ossification of the odontoid process and platyspondyly persists. Ossification of the pubis lags behind the normal, the acetabular roofs are more horizontal than normal and the Y cartilage is wide. Ossification of the femoral heads is still retarded and when they do appear there may be multiple ossification centers.

In the adult there is persisting platyspondyly, hypoplasia of the odontoid, and dysplasia of the proximal femurs with a varus deformity. The hands and feet remain relatively normal. The degree of dwarfism varies from patient to patient and results from both vertebral and long-bone changes.

The most difficult diagnostic problem is that of Morquio's disease. Differentiation is based upon its mode of inheritance, *i.e.*, as a dominant trait, its manifestation at birth, the different roentgen changes, the lack of corneal clouding, and the absence of keratosulfaturia.

In the latent or *tarda form of SED,* the disease often is not recognized until adulthood when precocious degenerative joint disease causes the patient to see a physician. At this stage it may be impossible to recognize the cause of the joint disease as the other epiphyseal dysplasias may lead to similar degenerative changes.

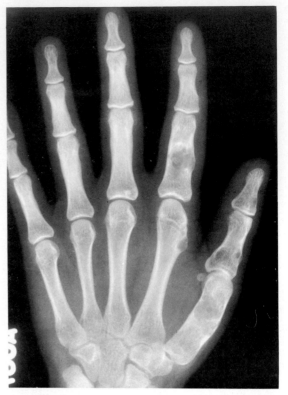

Fig. 2-3. Enchondromatosis involving the hand. The lesions have caused expansion of the shafts. Only the first and second digits are involved.

ENCHONDROMATOSIS (OLLIER'S DISEASE)

The basic lesion in this dysplasia is the enchondroma, described as a hamartomatous proliferation of masses of cartilage within the bone.[1] Thus these lesions are radiolucent although spotty areas of calcification within them are common. In some cases the lesions are limited to one extremity or to the extremities on one side of the body. The name, Ollier's disease, has been applied to this form. Even when widely disseminated, the involvement may be more severe on one side of the body than on the other. The masses of cartilage and calcified cartilage are found in the ends of the shafts and cause an irregular, club-shaped enlargement of the shafts' ends. The femur and tibia are most often or most severely involved. Stunting of growth of the affected member is common and, at times, a unilateral shortening of one leg has brought the patient to the physician. The epiphyses are not involved. The spine and skull usually are normal. The iliac crest and the vertebral border of the scapula have been affected in some of the patients with more severe involvement.

In the long bones the lesions may appear as elongated, radiolucent streaks extending in the direction of the long axis of bones and involving the metaphysis and adjacent diaphysis. In the hands and feet the lesions tend to be globular and cause considerable expansion of the bone (Fig. 2-3). At other times the lesion will involve the entire shaft of one of these short tubular bones.

With growth, the lesions appear to migrate into the shaft. Eventually they may ossify but residual deformity persists.

Malignant transformation of an enchondroma into a chondrosarcoma can occur, particularly in the lesions in the long tubular bones, and this is one of the common causes of chondrosarcoma in later life.

Maffucci's syndrome consists of a combination of enchondromatosis and multiple cavernous hemangiomas that may be widely distributed throughout the body. The presence of calcified thrombi (phleboliths) may allow roentgen recognition of the vascular lesions. The disease is rare.

There is risk of sarcomatous transformation of angiomatous lesions as well as of chondrosarcoma.

HEREDITARY MULTIPLE EXOSTOSES (OSTEOCHONDROMATOSIS; HEREDITARY DEFORMING CHONDRODYSPLASIA)

This dysplasia is characterized by the presence of numerous osteochondromas at the ends of the shafts of the tubular bones and in other bones preformed in cartilage. The disorder is inherited as an autosomal dominant trait with complete penetrance in males and reduced penetrance in females, so it usually passes from the father to his children. Males are affected over females about three to one. The lesions are not present at birth but usually are first discovered during childhood and, as a rule, are asymptomatic unless they cause pressure upon other structures. They are most common at the sites of greatest growth, *i.e.,* at the knee, shoulder, and wrist. Their number may vary from a few to hundreds, but they are usually bilaterally symmetric. Small lesions in the hands and feet are noted in some patients and the metacarpals and metatarsals may be shortened; in others, the hands and feet are normal. Lesions occur in the pelvic bones, the ribs, scapula, vertebrae, and, very rarely, in the base of the skull.

The characteristic lesion is a broad-based, bony outgrowth with the apex pointing away from the nearest joint (Fig. 2-4). It consists of a cortical shell surrounding a core of cancellous bone. The cortex of the lesion merges smoothly with the normal cortex of the bone, and the growth is covered by a layer of cartilage that acts as an epiphyseal plate. This is not visible in roentgenograms. Occasionally the lesion is more pedunculated, with a narrow base and a bulbous outer extremity containing lucent areas of cartilage and stippled areas of calcification similar to the solitary osteochondroma. The osteochondromas originate in the metaphyseal region of the long tubular bones and cause the end of the shaft to be thickened and club-shaped.

In about one-third of the patients there is a characteristic deformity of the forearm due to shortening and bowing of the ulna which does not extend far enough distally to take part in formation of the wrist joint. Another characteristic deformity occurs in the necks of the femurs. The neck is grossly thickened, particularly on the undersurface, caused by irregular, bony overgrowth, sometimes likened to candle gutterings (Fig. 2-5). The fibula may be shortened and stunting of growth of other bones is seen in the more severe cases.

Growth of the osteochondromas continues throughout childhood and usually ceases when the nearest epiphysis fuses. Malignant degeneration can occur and is said to have an incidence of about 5%. When an osteochondroma, after a stationary asymptomatic period, begins to enlarge and becomes painful, sarcomatous degeneration should be suspected.

DIASTROPHIC DWARFISM

This dysplasia was first reported by Lamy and Maroteaux in 1960. It is inherited as an autosomal recessive trait. Characteristics include delay in appearance of the epiphyseal centers, subluxation of various joints (especially the hips), scoliosis, and clubfeet.

The long bones are short and thick with widened metaphyses, simulating achondroplasia. In the hands, the bones are short and rectangular, especially the thumb and it may project at a right angle to the other digits ("hitch-hiker's thumb"). The metacarpal of the thumb also may have an ovoid shape. The bones of the feet show changes similar to those in the hands. In addition there is bilateral clubfoot deformity.

The epiphyseal centers are late in appearing and, when they do appear, are apt to be flat and abnormal in shape. In most patients, laxity of ligaments and tendons cause subluxation of the joints. Bilateral dislocation of the hips is common. The subluxations are not present at birth but develop after the child begins to walk. Scoliosis and kyphosis also appear at about the same time. Other bones, including the vertebrae, the skull, and the pelvis, are normal. The tarsal bones may be distorted because of the equinovarus deformity but otherwise are normal.

The differentiation from achondroplasia, in the average patient, is not difficult if all findings are taken into consideration. The normal appearance of the skull, vertebrae, and pelvis is significant.

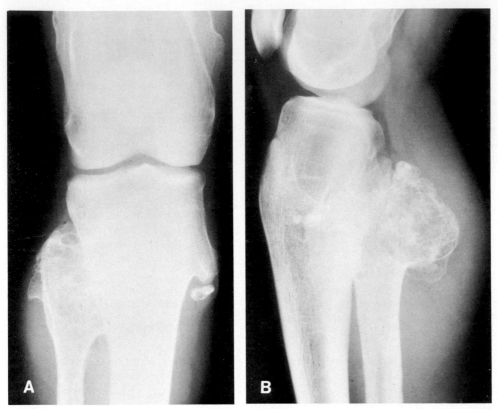

Fig. 2-4. Hereditary multiple exostoses. The lower femur and the upper tibia and fibula are involved. In addition to the exostoses there is a lack of modeling of the ends of these long bones.

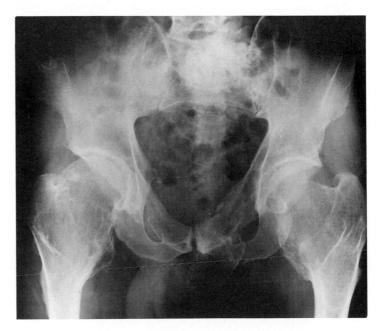

Fig. 2-5. Hereditary multiple exostoses in an adult illustrating the characteristic appearance of the upper ends of the femurs in this disease. The broad neck with irregular bony overgrowths along the inferior surface is typical. There is also a large osteochondroma overlying the upper sacrum and another arising from the left pubis.

THANATOPHORIC DWARFISM

This rare dysplasia was first recognized as a distinct entity in 1967. Previously it probably was mistaken for a severe type of achondroplasia because of its many similar features including dwarfing of the long tubular bones with a relatively long trunk, a prominent forehead with a short skull base and depression of the nasal root, small square iliac wings with horizontal acetabular roofs, a narrow thorax with short ribs, and a decrease from above downward of the interpedicular distances in the lumbar spine. Distinguishing features that have been pointed out[10] include extreme flattening of the vertebral bodies which appear waferlike and with thick intervertebral spaces, very short limb bones with bowing, especially in the lower extremities, and with no reported cases of involvement of other members of the family with the same disorder.

The infants have been stillborn or have died shortly after birth possibly from respiratory failure owing to the short ribs and narrow thorax. However, the cause of death has not been clearly established in most of the patients.

ACHONDROPLASIA

Achondroplasia is an hereditary, congenital disturbance caused by inadequate endochrondral bone formation leading to dwarfism. It is transmitted as an autosomal dominant trait. Bone formation in membrane is not affected. It is the most common form of dwarfism. Achondroplasia has been recognized since antiquity. Many of the affected became court jesters and today many obtain employment in circuses and sideshows as clowns.

Characteristically, the short limb bones contrast with the nearly normal length of the trunk. The facies also is characteristic with a prominent skull vault, saddle nose, and prognathous jaw. Writers frequently comment on the fact that achondroplasts all look as if they belonged to the same family. The following are the most typical changes in the skeleton.[1, 14, 26]

Skull. The skull is brachycephalic in shape with a short base and a relatively large vault with frontal bulging. This is owing to the fact that the base is preformed in cartilage while the vault is of membranous

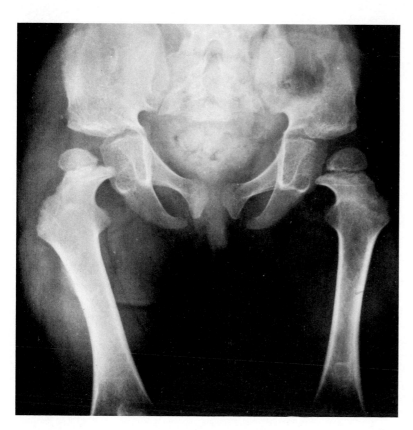

Fig. 2-6. Achondroplasia. Note the short, square-shaped ilia, the short sacrosciatic notches and pubic bones, and the large, shallow acetabula. The sacrum articulates low on the ilia. There is subluxation of the proximal femoral epiphyses and the femurs are short and relatively broad.

origin and thus not affected in growth. Communicating hydrocephalus is said to be common but is seldom severe enough to cause mental retardation. The mandible, also, shows relatively normal growth and thus appears prognathous.

Vertebrae. The length of the spinal column may be normal or nearly so but vertebral development is not normal. In infancy the bodies may be quite thin and the intervertebral disc spaces as thick as or thicker than the bodies. The pedicles are short and thick and the posterior surfaces of the bodies are concave. In the lumbar area the interpedicular distances narrow progressively from above downward instead of increasing normally. The net effect is a stenotic spinal canal which, in adult life, may lead to severe neurologic symptoms, especially if herniated disc or degenerative joint disease develops. The lumbar lordosis is increased and the lumbosacral angle becomes more acute than is normal. The sacrum tends to be tilted upwards. One or several vertebrae at the thoracolumbar junction (T12 to L3) may be wedge-shaped and crowded backward.

Pelvis. Characteristic changes occur in the pelvis. The ilia are short and square. The sacrosciatic notch is small. The ischial and pubic bones also are short and broad. The acetabular angles are decreased in infancy. The sacrum articulates low on the ilia (Fig. 2-6).

Long Tubular Bones. The shortening of these bones is responsible for the dwarfism. The humerus and femur tend to be relatively more affected than the distal bones of the extremities. The diameter is usually normal but the bones appear thick because they are short. The ends of the shafts are flared. The zone of provisional calcification may be smooth or irregular. At times there is a sizable V-shaped notch in the metaphyses and the epiphyseal centers may be partially buried in the metaphyses—ball-and-socket epiphyses (see Fig. 2-9). The fibula often is longer than the tibia causing an inversion of the foot. Bowing of the long bones is common. The distal ends of the femoral shafts tend to be tilted upwards, laterally (Figs. 2-7 and 2-8). Langer and associates[14] have described a rectangular-shaped translucent area in the upper end of the femur caused by an unusual thinning of the bone in its anteroposterior diameter.

Short Tubular Bones. These bones show changes similar to those in the long bones. They are short and

appear thick and the fingers tend to be of similar lengths, *i.e.,* the so-called trident hand (Fig. 2-9). Ball-and-socket epiphyses are common.

Other Bones. The carpal and tarsal bones are normal. The scapula is short and the sternum may be thick and short. The ribs are short causing a decrease in the anteroposterior diameter of the thorax.

In the differential diagnosis of achondroplasia, in

Fig. 2-7. Achondroplasia. Lower extremities of an infant showing short and thick bones. The metaphyses are irregular with an upward-outward slant of the distal femoral metaphyses. The thickening is more apparent than real, since the extremities are very short.

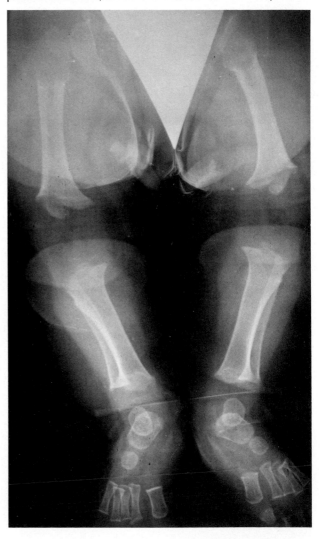

In addition, thanatophoric dwarfism probably should be included as it is considered by some authors to be a separate disease and not a severe form of achondroplasia. The roentgen changes in these dysplasias, including differential features, have been considered elsewhere in this chapter.

Fig. 2-9. Achondroplasia in a child. The bones of the hand are short and broad, and there are ball-and-socket epiphyses at the distal ends of the metacarpals. Note the flaring of metaphyses, particularly involving the radius and ulna.

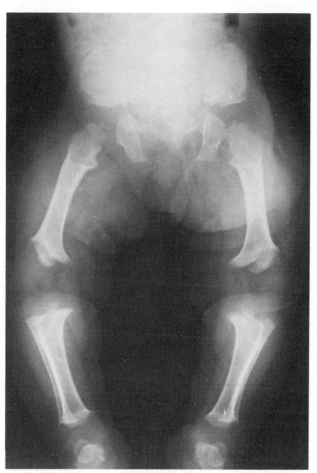

Fig. 2-8. Achondroplasia in an infant. The distal ends of the femoral shafts are tilted upward and laterally with laterally placed epiphyses. The bones are short.

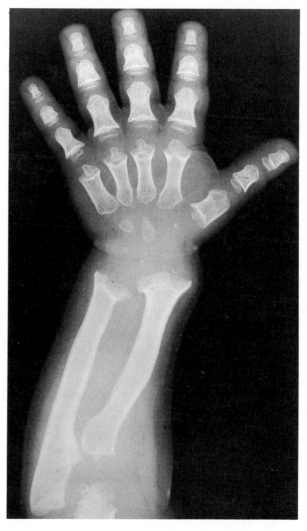

addition to the pseudoachondroplastic forms of multiple epiphyseal dysplasia and spondyloepiphyseal dysplasia as described by Rubin,[26] the following entities have been listed by Silverman.[27]

1. Metaphyseal dysostosis
2. Cartilage-hair hypoplasia
3. Hypochondroplasia
4. Ellis-van Creveld syndrome (chondroectodermal dysplasia)
5. Asphyxiating thoracic dystrophy
6. Diastrophic dwarfism
7. Dysplasia epiphysealis punctata (stippled epiphyses)
8. Metatropic dwarfism

HYPOCHONDROPLASIA

According to most authors, incomplete or mild forms of achondroplasia do not occur. These cases, although uncommon, have been termed *hypochondroplasia* to distinguish them from achondroplasia. The skull in these patients may be normal or nearly so, but the interpedicular distance may decrease slightly from L1 to L5. The pelvis is small and lordosis may be present. Shortening of the tubular bones is less than in achondroplasia. These bones are proportionately shortened in contrast to disproportionate shortening in achondroplasia.

METAPHYSEAL CHONDRODYSPLASIA (CARTILAGE-HAIR, METAPHYSEAL DYSOSTOSIS, CARTILAGE-HAIR DYSPLASIA)

This dysplasia was found by McKusick[17] among the Old Order Amish of Eastern Pennsylvania and Canada. Dwarfism is noted at birth owing to shortening of the tubular bones of the extremities and it is said that adults seldom exceed 4 feet in height. The epiphyses are normal and the skull is normal, an important point in differentiating this dysplasia from achondroplasia. The hair is fine, sparse, short, and brittle and is said to be characteristic of this dysplasia. Other findings include flexion deformities at the elbows, hyperextensibility of the wrists and fingers, an excessively long fibula and pes planus. The fingers are greatly shortened. The intelligence is not affected. Genetically the disorder is autosomal recessive. At maturity the roentgen findings at the ends of the bones resemble metaphyseal dysostosis.

METAPHYSEAL DYSOSTOSIS

In 1934, Jansen reported a case of dwarfism which resembled achondroplasia except that the skull and epiphyses were normal. The disorder was characterized roentgenologically by a rachitic rosary, coxa vara, genu valgum, and anterior bowing of the femurs. The growth plates of the tubular bones were thickened and irregular owing to extensions of cartilage into the metaphyses.

In 1949, Schmid reported patients having similar but much less severe changes. Most writers, including Schmid, have considered the two types to be variants of the same dysplasia. The Schmid type is relatively common; 21 cases were reported from our department in 1964.[18] The spine and skull are not affected so that the dwarfism is of the rhizomelic type as seen in achondroplasia. The skeletal changes are not present at birth but appear between 3 and 5 years of age. Dwarfism is relatively mild compared to the Jansen type. Bowing of the legs is marked and patients have a waddling gait. Mild to moderate inhibition of growth of all cylindrical bones is present; there is bilateral coxa vara and a tendency for epiphyseal slipping. The hereditary nature of the disease now is well established. It is transmitted as an autosomal dominant trait. Irregularity of the zones of provisional calcification resembles rickets and is caused by extensions of cartilage into the metaphyses (Fig. 2-10). There has been discussion in the past as to whether these cases actually are atypical examples of

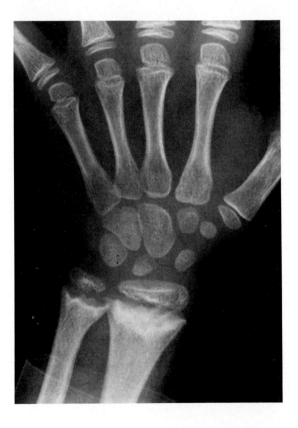

Fig. 2-10. Metaphyseal dysostosis. The metaphyses of the radius and ulna are concave and irregular. Similar changes were present in the metaphyses of the other long tubular bones. The bones of the hand are not affected.

vitamin-D refractory rickets. In contrast to rickets, the epiphyseal ossification centers usually are normal and the diaphyses, except for bowing, are roentgenologically normal.

METATROPIC DWARFISM

This is one of the recently defined entities that cause dwarfism and which may have been confused, in the past, with achondroplasia.[16] Roentgen changes are apparent at birth with shortening of the long tubular bones and hyperplastic, greatly flared metaphyses (chondrodysplasia). There is overconstriction of the midshafts so that the bones have a dumbbell shape. Epiphyseal ossification centers are delayed in appearance and when they do appear are deformed. The ribs tend to be short with a narrow chest. Kyphoscoliosis is present and there is some degree of platyspondyly, *i.e.,* flattening of the vertebrae. In the pelvis the iliac wings are short, the sacroiliac notches are short and deep, and the acetabula are horizontal. As the child grows older there is lengthening of the long bones, more than is seen in achondroplasia. However, the platyspondyly and the kyphoscoliotic curvature worsen and the child changes clinically from what appears to be achondroplasia to an appearance resembling spondyloepiphyseal dysplasia. In this connection it is to be noted that the base of the skull is not foreshortened and the interpedicular distances in the lumbar spine usually remain normal, findings which aid in differentiating this dysplasia from achondroplasia during infancy.

THE MUCOPOLYSACCHARIDOSES

The mucopolysaccharidoses consist of a group of metabolic diseases. In addition to the skeletal, other tissue systems are involved. Each is characterized by the excretion in the urine of abnormal amounts of one or more mucopolysaccharides and in an abnormality in the elaboration and storage of these substances.[1] The following types have been defined according to the mucopolysaccharide involved, their mode of genetic transmission, and their clinical and roentgen features.[17, 28]

The Mucopolysaccharidoses (McKusick[17] classification, 1972)

Type I-H. Hurler syndrome
Type I-S. Scheie syndrome
Type I H/S. Hurler/Scheie compound

Type II A. Hunter syndrome, severe
Type II B. Hunter syndrome, mild
Type III A. Sanfilippo syndrome A
Type III B. Sanfilippo syndrome B
Type IV. Morquio syndrome
Type V. Vacant
Type VI A. Maroteaux–Lamy syndrome, classic form
Type VI B. Maroteaux–Lamy syndrome, mild form
Type VII B. Glucuronidase deficiency

From a roentgen point of view, Morquio's disease and Hurler's disease (gargoylism) are the most important. The others differ one from another chiefly in their nonroentgen manifestations.

MORQUIO'S DISEASE

This dysplasia also has been called *Morquio–Brailsford disease* and *chondro-osteodystrophy.* The disease is rare and is characterized by dwarfism, kyphosis, and severe disability. The dwarfism is caused primarily by shortness of the spine although some degree of shortening of the long tubular bones is common. Both sexes are affected equally and it is hereditary and familial, the genetic transmission being autosomal recessive. Consanguinity has been noted in some histories.

Vertebrae. The most characteristic change is universal platyspondyly, a flattening of the vertebral bodies. The disc margins are irregular and roughened and an anterior, central, tonguelike projection is seen in the thoracolumbar region (Fig. 2-11). Also undergrowth and posterior displacement of one vertebra on another is usually present at the thoracolumbar junction. This results in a sharp angular kyphosis, one of the significant clinical observations. The intervertebral discs may be thick early in life, but later are reduced in height.

Long Tubular Bones. Epiphyseal ossification centers may be multiple and often are irregular. They are late in appearing but mature normally. The degree of dwarfing of the long bones is variable; in some patients they are of normal lengths. The zones of provisional calcification are irregular and the metaphyses are broad. The proximal femur is often the most severely affected. Delay in appearance of the capital epiphysis, fragmentation, flaring, and irregularity of the metaphysis and subluxation at the hip are common (Fig. 2-12). The acetabulum has a coarse outline and it may be enlarged and deepened.

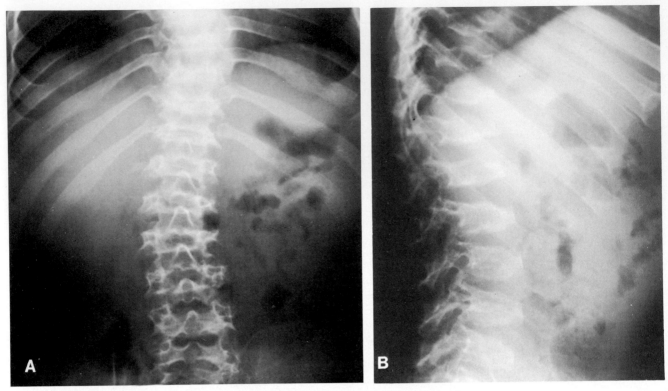

Fig. 2-11. Morquio's disease. Anteroposterior **(A)** and lateral **(B)** view of the lower thoracic and lumbar spine. The flattening of the vertebrae and the irregularity of disc surfaces are evident. The anterior central beaking can be seen in the lower thoracic bodies in the lateral view. The lower ribs are narrowed at their vertebral ends.

Fig. 2-12. Morquio's disease. Characteristic changes in the pelvis and proximal femurs include the "wine-glass" contour of the pelvis, the large, irregular acetabula, the small, poorly formed femoral epiphyses, and the broad femoral necks. The ilia are flared, and the femurs are partially subluxed.

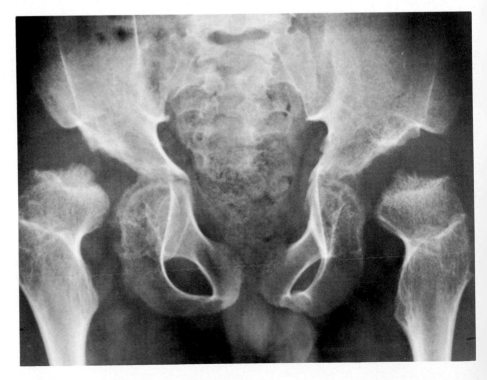

Short Tubular Bones. These bones often are short with irregular epiphyseal ossification centers. The second, third, fourth, and fifth metacarpals often taper at their ends. The metatarsals are affected similarly (Fig. 2-13).

Flat Bones. The ilia flare laterally and the acetabular cavities are enlarged and have rough margins. Rubin[26] describes the ribs as "canoe paddles," the vertebral end being narrow while the remainder is broad.

Other Findings. The skull and facial bones are normal, another significant finding in the differentiation from achondroplasia. A hypoplastic or absent odontoid process is seen in many patients. The carpal and tarsal bones are late in appearing and, later, may have irregular or angular shapes.

The head appears large in relation to the size of the trunk. The lower extremities are more undeveloped than the trunk and the trunk more so than the head and the upper extremities. The joints appear widened and some of the large joints are hypermobile owing to laxity of muscles and tendons. However, flexion deformities also occur in the elbows, hips, and knees caused by the epiphyseal distortions. The hands are held in ulnar deviation. The first symptoms usually are noted at the time that the child begins to sit, stand, or walk. The disorder is due to an abnormality in the elaboration and storage of the mucopolysaccharide (MPS), keratansulfate.

Recently there have been several reports of a form of this disease, usually of lesser severity, in patients who do not excrete keratansulfate.

HURLER'S DISEASE (GARGOYLISM)

This disorder is usually first noted after the first year of life. Clinical characteristics include a large, bulging head, flared nostrils, flat nasal bridge, hypertelorism, and corneal opacities leading to blindness. One of the significant clinical findings is hepatosplenomegaly, often of considerable degree. The lips are thick and the tongue large. The teeth are poorly formed. The stature is dwarfed. The facial appearance has been likened to that of a gargoyle, hence the designation, *gargoylism.* The genetic transmission is autosomal recessive. The disorder results in excessive urinary excretion of dermatan sulfate and heparan sulfate.

Recently, patients have been reported in whom roentgen and clinical findings of Hurler's disease have been present but no abnormal mucopolysaccharide excretion could be domonstrated.[32]

Skull. The skull often is scaphocephalic owing to premature closure of the sagittal and metopic sutures. The anteroposterior diameter of the sella is lengthened with an anterior depression, described as shoe-shaped or J-shaped (Fig. 2-14). The sinuses and mastoids are poorly pneumatized. The mandible is short and thick and the articular surfaces of the condyles are often concave, one of the characteristic findings. Hyperostotic thickening of the frontal and occipital areas may develop but the base does not become sclerotic.

Ribs. The ribs, especially the lower, are broad and flat.

Long Tubular Bones. The upper extremities are more involved than the lower; the latter may be normal. The humerus is short and the shaft widened and a constriction with a coxa vara-like deformity of the humeral neck may be seen (Fig. 2-15). The radius

Fig. 2-13. Morquio's disease. Hand and wrist of the same patient illustrated in Figure 2-11. There is moderate tapering of the proximal ends of the second, third, fourth, and fifth metacarpals.

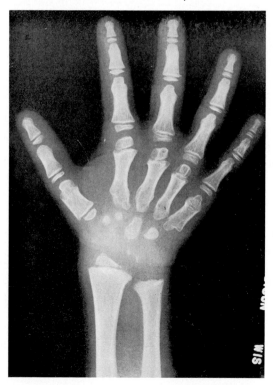

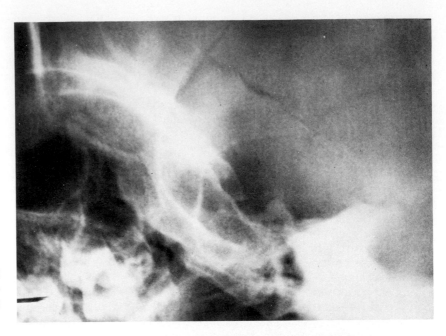

Fig. 2-14. Hurler's disease. Lateral view of the skull showing the anterior depression of the tuberculum (J-shaped sella).

Fig. 2-15. Hurler's disease. The humerus shows a constriction of the neck, a varus deformity, and expansion of the mid and distal portions of the shaft.

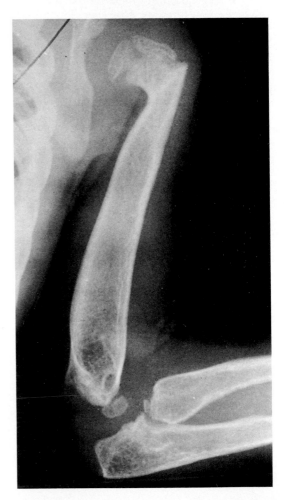

and ulna show similar changes and the distal metaphyseal surfaces tend to be tilted toward one another (Fig. 2-16). The femoral neck is constricted and there is a coxa valga deformity at the hips. The epiphyseal ossification centers are often flattened and irregular.

Short Tubular Bones. The appearance of the hands usually is characteristic. The bones have a coarse texture with wide shafts and the metacarpals in particular have conical or pointed proximal ends (Fig. 2-17). Similar changes may be seen in the feet or they may be relatively normal.

Vertebrae. There is an angular kyphosis or gibbus at the thoracolumbar junction with one or several of the bodies hypoplastic and with an anteroinferior beak (Fig. 2-18). Posterior displacement of one vertebra on the one above or below is often present at the level of T12 to L1. The intervertebral disc spaces are intact.

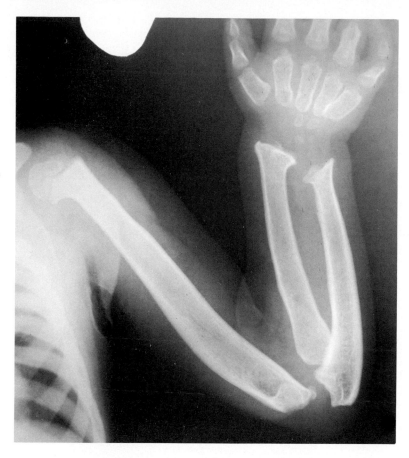

Fig. 2-16. Hurler's disease. Left upper extremity. In addition to the expanded shafts, the distal metaphyses of the radius and ulna are tilted toward one another. The metacarpals are characteristic, and there is delayed ossification of epiphyses at the elbow and wrist as well as of the centers for the carpal bones.

Flat Bones. The pelvis may resemble achondroplasia during early infancy, but in those that survive its appearance comes to resemble that of Morquio's disease (Fig. 2-19).

Other Bones. The carpal and tarsal bones may be late in appearing and then may show irregular or angular contours. The clavicle may be thickened. The teeth are poorly developed.

OTHER MUCOPOLYSACCHARIDOSES

The other mucopolysaccharidoses mentioned above appear to be variants of Hurler's disease. They differ from one another chiefly in their clinical manifestations and the mucopolysaccharide involved, rather than in specific roentgen characteristics. In the *Hunter* syndrome the skeletal changes and mental

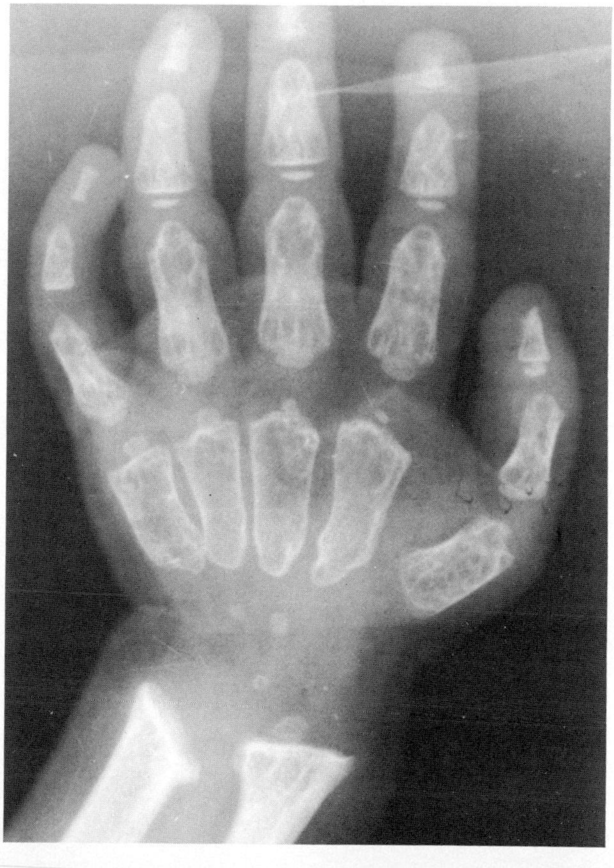

Fig. 2-17. Hurler's disease. The hand and wrist show characteristic changes as described in the text.

retardation are less severe than in Hurler's disease. There is no corneal clouding and the genetic transmission is X-linked recessive instead of autosomal recessive as in Hurler's.[28] In the *SanFilippo* syndrome the skeletal changes are mild and there is no corneal clouding. However, mental retardation is severe. The genetic transmission is autosomal recessive. In the *Maroteaux–Lamy* syndrome, skeletal changes are severe and there is corneal clouding. However, the mentality is not affected. In the *Scheie* syndrome, bone changes are mild with normal mentality, clouded corneas, and congenital heart disease (aortic regurgitation). The genetic transmission is the same in all of these syndromes, autosomal recessive, except for Hunter's syndrome in which it is X-linked recessive. In Morquio's disease the mucopolysaccharide involved is keratan sulfate. In the others it is heparan sulfate, alone or in combination.[17]

THE MUCOLIPIDOSES

Spranger and Wiedmann[31] classified this group of autosomal recessive conditions as follows.

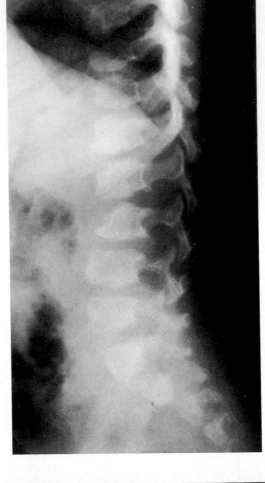

Fig. 2-18. Hurler's disease. The lumbar spine shows the anteroinferior beaking of L3 and mild angular kyphosis and malalignment of L2 on L3. The vertebrae are moderately flattened.

Fig. 2-19. Hurler's disease. The contour of the pelvis resembles Morquio's disease, but the femoral epiphyses are better developed. The acetabula are shallow. There is moderate constriction of the femoral necks.

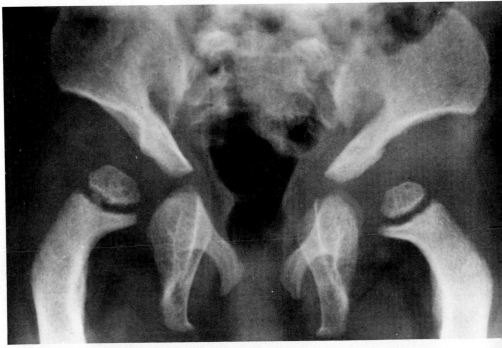

Mucolipidosis I. (formerly Lipomucopolysaccharidosis). This resembles a mild form of Hurler's syndrome with moderate progressive mental retardation, calvarial thickening, biconvex vertebrae, hypoplasia of acetabular roofs, and mild expansion and prominent trabeculation of the ribs and short tubular bones. It is transmitted as an autosomal recessive trait.

Mucolipidosis II. This also simulates Hurler's disease but has much more severe clinical and radiographic features than does type I. There is severe psychomotor retardation, pelvic dysplasia with hip dislocation, diaphyseal expansion of the tubular bones (often with thin cortices and bowing, shortening and undermodelling, and epiphyseal dysplasia), and short anteroposterior diameter of vertebral bodies with biconcavity of end plates and concavity of anterior aspects. The tubular bones of the hands and feet are short with marked retardation of ossification and diaphyseal expansion.

Mucolipidosis III (Pseudo-Hurler Polydystrophy). The clinical evolution of this condition is much slower than that of the Hurler syndrome. It is characterized by short stature, coarse facies, restricted joint motion, corneal opacities, minimal to moderate mental retardation, and, sometimes, aortic valve disease. Roentgen features consist of severe pelvic dysplasia, hypoplastic ilium with shallow acetabulum, and coxa valga. The vertebral anomalies consist of irregular upper and lower plates, hypoplasia of the dorsal portion of the thoracic vertebral bodies, and anterior hypoplasia of the lumbar bodies. The disc spaces are irregularly narrowed.

OSTEOGENESIS IMPERFECTA (OSTEITIS FRAGILITANS; FRAGILITAS OSSIUM CONGENITA; OSTEOPSATHYROSIS IDIOPATHICA; BRITTLE BONES)

Osteogenesis imperfecta is a rare hereditary disorder characterized by an unusual fragility of the bones leading to multiple fractures often from a trivial

Fig. 2-20. Osteogenesis imperfecta, infantile type. This newborn baby has multiple fractures.

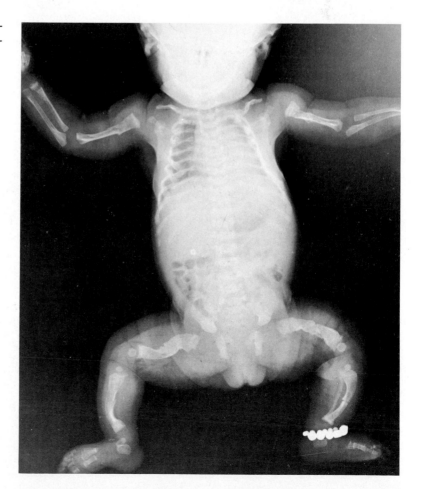

cause. The underlying difficulty is that the collagen fibers are abnormal, probably as a result of incomplete maturation. In the bones, there is a disorder of osteoblastic activity. These abnormalities result in fragile bones, thin skin and sclera, poor teeth, and hypermobility of the joints. There are two forms of the disease: (1) osteogenesis imperfecta congenita and (2) osteogenesis imperfecta tarda. In the former the disorder develops *in utero* and is noted at birth, the infant being born with multiple fractures. Mortality is high, resulting from intracranial hemorrhage at birth or from recurrent respiratory infections in the first 2 years of life. In the tarda type the disease is first noted during childhood because of the unusual tendency for fractures. The joints are lax, dislocations are frequent, deafness caused by otosclerosis becomes apparent, and the teeth are discolored, fragile, and break easily. Blue sclera also becomes more apparent, evidently owing to the intraocular pigment which shows through the thin sclera.

Skull. In the congenital type the cranial bones are largely membranous at birth. If the infant survies, ossification progresses slowly leaving wide sutures and multiple wormian bones (*mosaic skull*). Still later the sutures become of normal width. In older children a bulge in the temporal region is said to be characteristic.

Long Bones. In the congenital form the infant usually is born with multiple fractures of the long bones (Fig. 2-20). The shafts are wide and appear short owing to the multiple fractures and the width of the bones. However, the cortices are thin. In the tarda type the width of the bones is reduced and they appear thin and gracile. The ends appear wide and the zones of provisional calcification may be denser than normal. The trabeculae are diminished in size and number; the cortices are thin. There often is extensive deformity owing to fractures and previous fractures which have healed (Fig. 2-21). The epiphyses are normal.

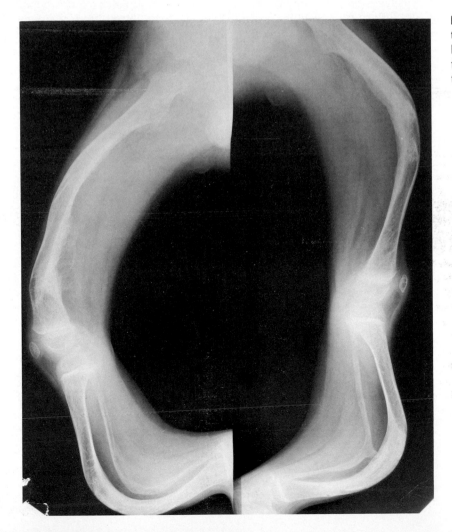

Fig. 2-21. Osteogenesis imperfecta tarda. The misshapen bones have been caused by multiple healed fractures and abnormal softness of the bone.

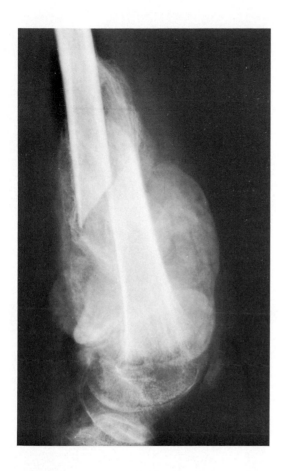

Of considerable interest is the tendency for fractures to heal with excessive callus formation (Fig. 2-22). This may be so extensive that a malignant tumor may be suspected.

Osteogenesis imperfecta tarda is largely an autosomal dominant disorder but a small autosomal recessive group also probably exists in the congenital form.

OSTEOPETROSIS (ALBERS-SCHÖNBERG DISEASE; OSTEOSCLEROSIS FRAGILIS; MARBLE BONES)

Osteopetrosis is a rare dysplasia characterized by an unusual density or radiopacity of the bones. Although dense to roentgen rays, the bones are brittle and fracture readily. The disease may be discovered at birth or shortly thereafter, or not until adulthood. As with most of the other dysplasias the earlier the disease is found the more severe it is likely to be. In the infant, all of the bones may be affected, having a uniformly dense, structureless appearance with complete obliteration of normal trabecular architecture. The medullary canal is obliterated by dense sclerosis and merges with the cortex. The density of the bones is thought to be the result of failure of normal removal of old bone while new bone continues to be formed. Growth is often stunted; myelophthisic anemia may become severe and lead to death. Jaundice, hepatosplenomegaly, and cranial nerve palsies are common. Death often occurs within the first year of life. In the infantile (congenita) form the disease has been found in utero and the baby may be stillborn. This form is transmitted as an autosomal recessive trait, while the adult form may be either autosomal dominant (majority) or recessive.

In the adult form the disease may first come to attention of a physician because of a fracture of a long bone. Characteristically, these fractures are of transverse type. Or there may be a history of repeated fractures during childhood. Another presenting symptom may be an unexplained anemia. These patients often suffer from carious teeth and dental or jaw infections.

Short Bones. Fractures involving these bones are less frequent than in the long bones. Otherwise they show similar changes.

Vertebrae. Growth of the vertebrae is normal but they are osteoporotic with thin cortical margins. Compression fractures are frequent and multiple bodies may show biconcave disc surfaces, *i.e.*, fish vertebrae. The intervertebral disc spaces may be widened. Scoliosis is frequent.

Flat Bones. The pelvis may show changes in shape secondary to the osteoporosis and protrusio acetabuli is common. Fractures of the ribs also are common. Here, as elsewhere, the fractures heal readily, often with exuberant callus.

Other Findings. The teeth are often small, deformed, and the pulp chambers and root canals obliterated. Dislocations of the larger joints may occur secondary to the laxity of the ligaments and hypertonicity of the muscles.

Skull. The base shows the most marked sclerosis but all of the cranial bones may be involved. The sinuses and mastoids may show complete lack of pneumatization. The cranial foramina are encroached upon leading to various cranial nerve palsies such as blindness and deafness. The teeth are late in erupting and develop caries early. Dental infection may lead to osteomyelitis of the jaw. The lamina dura, the cortical margin of the tooth socket, may be unusually thick and dense and the disease may be suspected from dental roentgenograms.

Vertebrae. These bones are uniformly involved by the sclerosis and there may be impingement on the spinal nerves. In the adult or latent type of sclerosis may be limited to the upper and lower surfaces ("sandwich vertebrae"; "rugger jersey spine").

Other Bones. In the long and short tubular bones the sclerosis is usually uniform in the infantile form. Occasionally there may be alternating bands of sclerotic and normal bone at the ends of the shafts. The trabecular pattern is completely obliterated. The length of the bones is usually normal but is occasionally shortened. Characteristically the ends of the bones are club-shaped owing to failure of normal modeling (Fig. 2-23). The epiphyseal ossification centers are dense but they mature normally. In the adult the increased density often is limited to bands of sclerosis at the ends, sometimes alternating with bands of normal density. The bones of the hands and feet are involved the same as the long tubular bones. The sternal ends of the clavicles may be widened.

PYKNODYSOSTOSIS

This disease is often confused with osteopetrosis because of the generalized dense, sclerotic appearance of the bones.

In the *skull* there is a failure of closure of the cranial sutures and fontanelles and numerous wormian bones are present (Fig. 2-24). The skull has a dolichocephalic shape due to bossing. The mandibular rami are hypoplastic with loss of the normal mandibular angle which is characteristic. Sclerosis and thickening of the cranial and facial bones may be severe. The sinuses may fail to develop, particularly the frontals, and the mastoids often are not pneumatized. The *hands* arc short and stubby with partial agenesis or aplasia of the terminal phalanges (Fig. 2-25). The *vertebrae* are sclerotic and there is a lack of fusion of

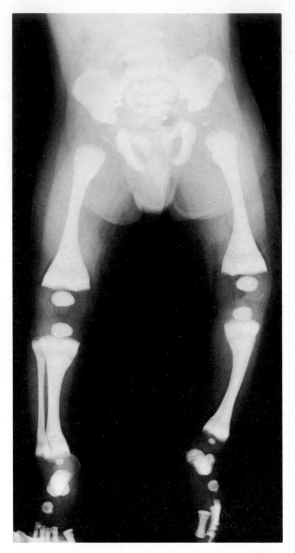

Fig. 2-23. Osteopetrosis in an infant. The bones throughout the skeleton are chalky white. No trabecular architecture was visible on the films. Translucent bands can be visualized crossing the ends of the shafts, representing periods of more normal ossification as the bones grew in length. The metaphyses are large and club-shaped, owing to a failure of modeling as the bones increased in length.

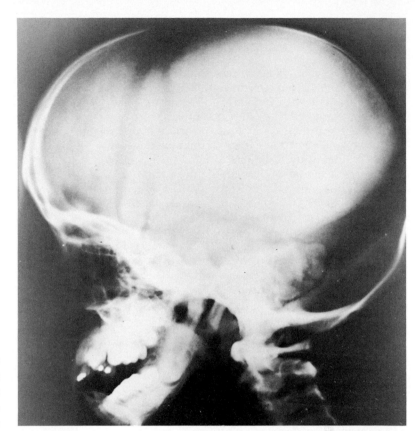

Fig. 2-24. Pyknodysostosis. Lateral view of the skull demonstrates the sclerotic cranial bones, large unossified areas especially along the lambdoid sutures, and the loss of the mandibular angle.

Fig. 2-25. Pyknodysostosis. The bones of the hand and wrist are uniformly increased in density. There is tapering of the distal phalanges with loss of terminal tufts.

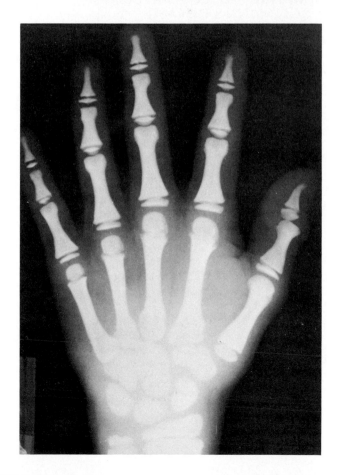

the neural arches in some. Fractures are extremely common and in the long bones they are of the transverse type. The stature is reduced and deformity from old fractures may lead to further shortening of the long tubular bones. Dental caries occur frequently.

METAPHYSEAL DYSPLASIA (PYLE'S DISEASE; CRANIOMETAPHYSEAL DYSPLASIA)

In this dysplasia the basic disturbance appears to be a failure of modeling of the cylindrical bones. The changes are often most noticeable at the lower ends of the femurs and upper ends of tibias and humeri leading to a club-shaped enlargement often referred to as having an "Erlenmeyer flask" appearance. The cortices at the ends of the bones are thin and thus the bone is most subject to fracture.

In the hand there is distal flaring of the metacarpals and proximal flaring of the phalanges. Marked thickening of the ribs, clavicles, and ischial and pubic bones is present and there may be minimal vertebral flattening. Skull findings include a distinct supraorbital bulge and sometimes there is mild hyperostosis of the cranial vault. Minimal prognathism and a rounded, obtuse mandibular angle may also be present.

The disease is transmitted as an autosomal recessive trait and consanguinity has been noted in the histories of many of these individuals. Some authors[7] separate craniometaphyseal dysplasia from Pyle's disease. Clinically, there is hypertelorism and broadening of the root of the nose in craniometaphyseal dysplasia. The bone sclerosis at the root of the nose leads to nasal obstruction. Temporal bone changes often lead to deafness and sometimes to focal paralysis. Frontal, paranasal, and occipital sclerosis or hyperostosis is present and diaphyseal sclerosis is a common feature. There is no thickening of ribs, clavicles, and ischial and pubic bones. Metaphyseal flaring is less than in metaphyseal dysplasia.

DIAPHYSEAL DYSPLASIA (ENGELMANN'S DISEASE; PROGRESSIVE DIAPHYSEAL SCLEROSIS)

The major manifestations of this dysplasia consist of symmetric cortical thickening in the mid-diaphyses, particularly of the femur and the tibia. The lesion tends to progress and eventually involve most of the diaphysis. The epiphyses and metaphyses are spared. The disorder may begin in early childhood with a difficulty in walking and a shuffling or waddling gait being the first sign. The cortical thickening begins subperiosteally but, with failure of resorption within, the medullary canal may be encroached upon leading to anemia and hepatosplenomegaly. The disease also progresses to involve other bones as the child grows older and, in some, may involve the short bones of the hands and feet as well as the bones of the trunk, skull, and face. The base of the skull may become thick and dense with its subsequent impingement on the cranial nerves. The vault is seldom involved except for frontal and occipital bossing. The muscles tend to be flabby and weak. Dental caries is often present. In a small percentage of patients the skin has been noted to be thick and dry and the hair scanty. The mentality is not affected.

In 1949, Ribbing described the occurrence of a dis-

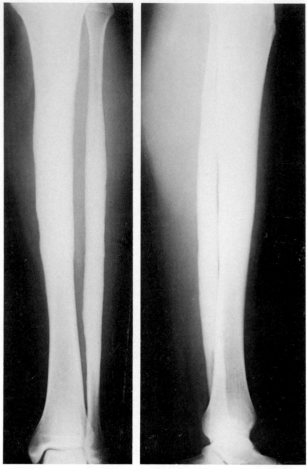

Fig. 2-26. Hereditary multiple diaphyseal sclerosis. The patient has rather similar lesions in both femurs and one radius. The patient's son also has changes characteristic of Engelmann's disease.

order in siblings consisting of a dense diaphyseal sclerosis not unlike that seen in Engelmann's disease. He believed it to be a separate entity, however, because of the late onset of symptoms and the familial nature, which had not been recorded in Engelmann's disease before that time. Two similar cases occurring in brothers have been reported from our department (Fig. 2-26).[23] Subsequently we examined the father of these two patients and found mild involvement in some of the long tubular bones. Also we later examined the son (age 5) of one of the original patients and found an appearance typical of Engelmann's disease. We believe, therefore, that the two disorders, Engelmann's disease and Ribbing's disease are

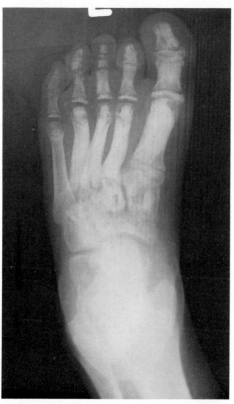

Fig. 2-27. Melorheostosis. Dense sclerosis of the first to fourth metatarsals and phalanges of the great toe of the left foot is evident. Similar changes were present along the inner side of the long bones of the left leg and the left side of the pelvis.

closely related, the latter probably being the adult or latent type of the former. The condition is transmitted as an autosomal dominant trait with a wide variability of expression.

MELORHEOSTOSIS

This disorder presents as an irregular thickening of the cortex along one side of a bone or the bones of one extremity. The thickening may be external, internal, or both (Fig. 2-27). The appearance has been likened to molten wax flowing down the side of a candle. If an extremity is involved the pelvis (or shoulder girdle) on the affected side is likely to show similar thickening. The onset may be in infancy or not until late adolescence, *i.e.,* at age 20. The presenting symptom is pain which may be severe. The disease does not appear to be hereditary. If it begins early in life the epiphyses may fuse prematurely causing shortening of the involved extremity. The lesions usually cease progressing when skeletal growth is complete. Regression has not been noted. The disease is rare, less than 50 cases having been reported in the literature.

OSTEOPOIKILOSIS (OSTEOPATHIA CONDENSANS DISSEMINATA)

This is an asymptomatic disorder characterized by the appearance of numerous small, round or oval densities in the ends of the long bones (Fig. 2-28), the small bones of the hands and feet, and in the acetabulum. The lesions are composed of dense, compact bone. They are discovered by chance on roentgen examination for some other condition. The disorder is transmitted as an autosomal dominant trait and has been discovered in newborns as well as in the fetus in utero. The lesions may increase or decrease in size and number during the period of active bone growth and have been noted to disappear altogether. In the acetabulum, when numerous and oval in shape, the lesions tend to radiate toward the hip joint. Solitary sclerotic foci of the same nature are common throughout the appendicular skeleton and pelvis and are known as *compact islands* or bone islands. While usually small, an occasional compact island measuring more than a centimeter in diameter is seen. When observed over a period of several years or longer, compact islands have been noted to increase or decrease in size. Such a lesion may be mistaken for a sclerotic focus of metastatic carcinoma.

OSTEOPATHIA STRIATA (VOORHOEVE'S LINES)

This process is similar in many ways to osteopoikilosis but, instead of rounded foci, consists of striae of dense bone extending toward the nearest joint. In children the striae begin at the epiphyseal line and extend for a short distance into the diaphysis. In the acetabulum the striae have a "sunburst" appearance, fanning outward toward the iliac crest. Any or all of the long bones and the pelvis may be involved. The lesions are asymptomatic and are discovered by chance.

FIBROUS DYSPLASIA

This disease usually begins during childhood and is characterized, pathologically, by replacement of normal bone undergoing physiologic lysis by an abnormal proliferation of fibrous tissue.[1] The disease may involve a single bone (monostotic), the bones of one extremity, or be widely distributed throughout the skeleton (polyostotic). There is some predilection for the long bones of the extremities but any bone may be involved.

In the monostatic form, the femur, tibia, and ribs are the most common sites. The lesions are usually diaphyseal but may extend into the metaphysis. Most of them are discovered as the result of a pathologic fracture.

The polyostotic form is much less common than the monostatic and is usually associated with café-au-lait spots. Most patients have a fracture through a site of the disease at some time. In about one-third of females with the polyostotic form, sexual precocity occurs (Albright's syndrome); it is very rare in males. Other endocrine abnormalities are present in some of the patients. Acceleration of skeletal growth and maturation is fairly common, and thyroid enlargement, toxic and nontoxic, is found in about one-fourth of the patients. Acromegaly and parathyroid hyperplasia are rare associated conditions.

Roentgen Observations. The individual lesions vary from one to another. In some the appearance is that of a well-defined lucent area or "cyst." The cavity is filled with fibrous tissue rather than fluid so that it does not represent a true cyst (Fig. 2-29). The affected bone may have a "milky" or "ground-glass" appearance with absence of normal trabeculation (Fig. 2-30). The margins often are ill-defined but, in the "cystic" variety, a thin sclerotic rim may bound the lesion (Fig. 2-31). The cortex may be eroded from within and the bone locally expanded (Fig. 2-32). This predisposes to fracture. The fracture heals with ample periosteal callus. Cases of fibrous dysplasia have been reported showing a sequestrum within an apparent "cavity" in a long bone.[25] In severe and long-standing disease the bones may be bowed or misshapen, some of which may be the result of previous fracture. Thus the upper end of the femur characteristically shows a "shepherd's crook" deformity and coxa vara with lateral and anterior bowing of the shaft. Bending also occurs because of the fibrous tissue replacement of normal bone.

In the skull the lesion appears as a somewhat multilocular cystlike area involving the diploic space and

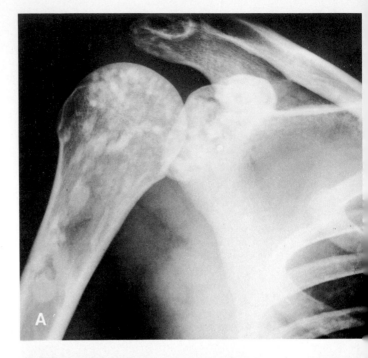
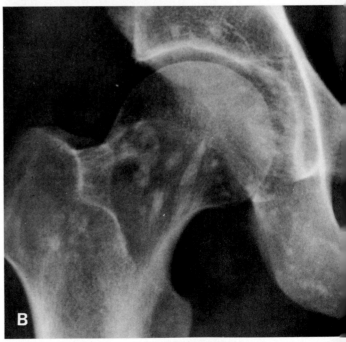

Fig. 2-28. Osteopoikilosis. **A.** The islands of dense bone in this patient were widely distributed throughout the skeleton in the bones adjacent to the joints. **B.** The bony islands in this patient are not quite as dense as in those in patient **A,** but were widely distributed.

Fig. 2-29. Fibrous dysplasia, monostotic form. The lesion in the neck of the femur appears cystic, but abnormal bone is noted continuing well into the upper diaphysis where the signs of abnormality fade gradually until normal-appearing bone is evident.

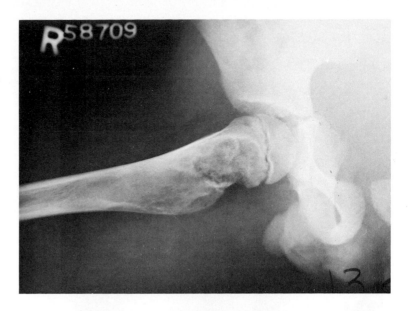

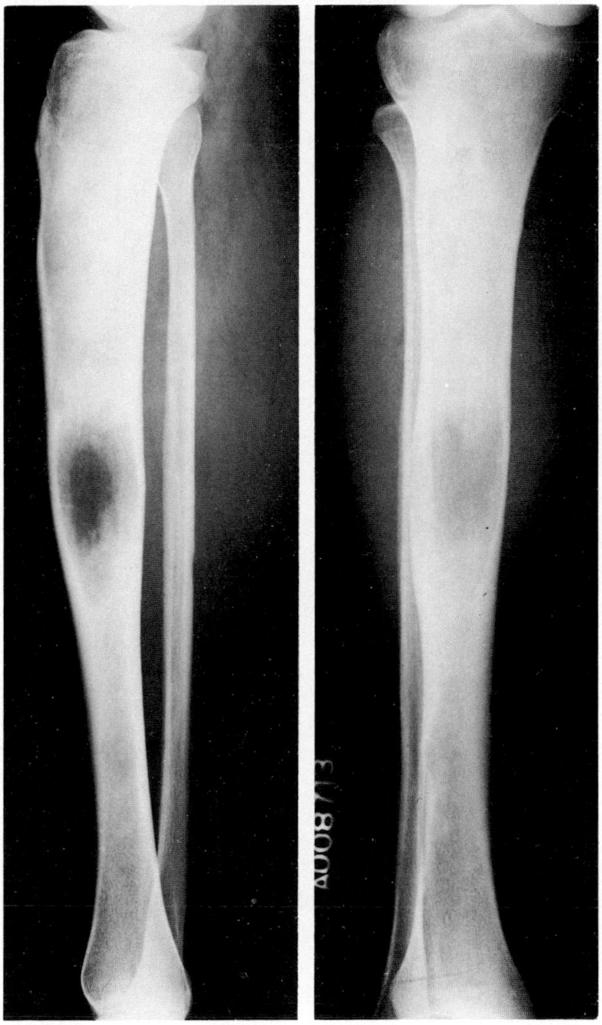

Fig. 2-30. Fibrous dysplasia. There is loss of normal trabeculation with uniform density above and below the central cavity which contains fibrous tissue, not fluid. The extreme upper and lower ends of the tibia appear normal.

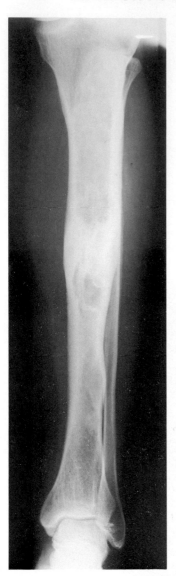

Fig. 2-31. Fibrous dysplasia. There is a mixture of cystlike rarefaction and sclerosis in the shaft of the tibia as well as expansion of much of the upper half of this involved bone.

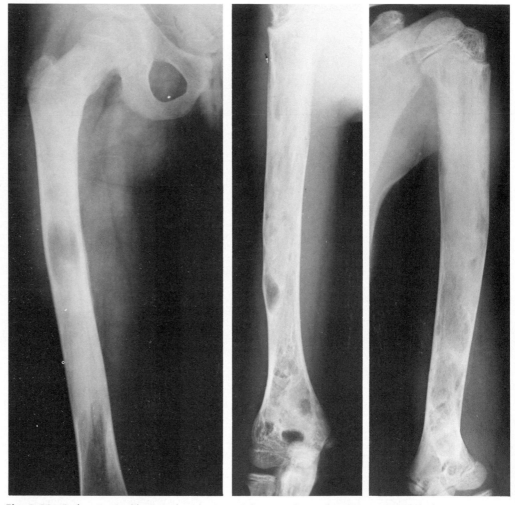

Fig. 2-32. Polyostotic fibrous dysplasia. Widespread involvement of the skeleton was present in this patient who had lesions in most of the long bones. This demonstrates the variation in the pattern of disease in this condition.

Fig. 2-33. Fibrous dysplasia of the skull. The lesion in the posterior parietal area consists of areas of irregular rarefaction and some sclerosis. In tangential view the lesion involved the diploë with expansion of the inner and outer tables of the skull.

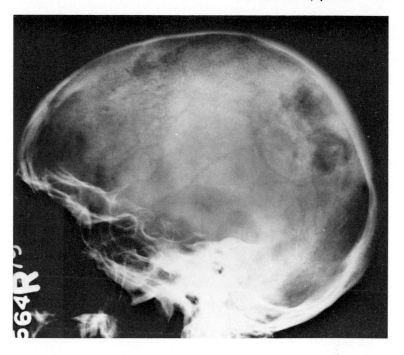

expanding the tables (Fig. 2-33). The margins are somewhat sclerotic and the boundary of the lesion not sharply defined. When fibrous dysplasia involves the base of the skull and the facial bones, the appearance is different. It causes a marked sclerosis and thickening. The sinuses may be obliterated. In the base the similarity to meningioma may cause difficulty in diagnosis and, at times, arteriography or CT scan may be necessary. Involvement of the facial bones is similar to that in the base of the skull with thickening and sclerosis (Fig. 2-34). This appearance is known as *leoniasis ossea* and, while there are other causes for it, fibrous dysplasia is probably the most frequent lesion responsible.

In the differentiation from meningioma, the lack of dilated vascular grooves leading to the area of the bone lesion has been considered a significant finding. However, a few patients with fibrous dysplasia have been reported in whom enlarged, tortuous grooves were found so that the occurrence of dilated vessels cannot be considered entirely specific for meningioma when sclerotic or "mixed" lesions are present. Of greater importance is the lack of involvement of the inner table in fibrous dysplasia and its occurrence in meningioma.

When skeletal involvement is extensive there may be severe crippling and deformity. Solitary lesions or disease of lesser magnitude may cease to progress

Fig. 2-34. Fibrous dysplasia of the zygoma and maxilla on the left. The marked thickening of the bone has encroached upon the maxillary sinus and the floor of the left orbit.

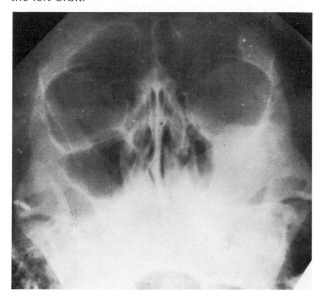

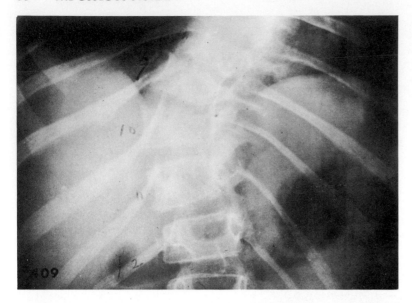

Fig. 2-35. Neurofibromatosis. There is sharp scoliosis in the lower thoracic spine. Vertebrae are malformed, and the lower ribs are thin, particularly on the left side.

when skeletal growth is complete and may cause little or no permanent disability or deformity. Sarcomatous degeneration has been reported as a complication of fibrous dysplasia but appears to be very uncommon.

HEREDITARY FIBROUS DYSPLASIA OF THE JAWS (CHERUBISM)

This condition was first described by Jones in 1933 in four of five siblings. The lesion appears as multilocular, radiolucent, cystic areas expanding the jaw. This causes rounding of the facial featues, hence the term "cherubism." The lesions involve the mandible bilaterally with or without posterior maxillary disease. The entire mandible, except the condyles, may be involved. Maxillary involvement is less frequent and less severe than mandibular disease and probably does not occur without lesions in the lower jaw. While the exact cause is unknown, it has been suggested that the disease represents an hereditary form of fibrous dysplasia.

NEUROFIBROMATOSIS (VON RECKLINGHAUSEN'S DISEASE)

This disease entity was first described by von Recklinghausen in 1882. It is a disease of the supporting tissues of the nervous system. While skin tumors are the most prominent feature, the disorder may involve other systems including the endocrine, gastrointestinal, and skeletal. The present discussion is concerned chiefly with the latter. In addition to skin nodules, brownish pigmented areas (café-au-lait spots) occur frequently. The extent of the disease may vary considerably but there is a tendency for it to slow or stop when skeletal growth is completed. It is said that about 10% of the lesions may become malignant (neurofibrosarcoma). There is an increased frequency of meningiomas in patients suffering from von Recklinghausen's disease.

Skeletal Lesions. Kyphoscoliosis is common in the spine. The scoliosis is usually a sharp, angular one and its cause often is obscure since associated neurofibromas are not found (Fig. 2-35). The vertebrae often are wedge-shaped at the height of curvature. The ribs often are thin and have been likened to a "twisted ribbon." In the long bones, pressure from an adjacent tumor may cause a small local excavation in the cortex, the so-called "pit" or "cave" defect. A neurofibroma may arise within bone causing a sharply outlined area of radiolucency. Another peculiar manifestation of the disease is localized enlargement of a part such as a finger or one extremity (focal giantism). The bone, except for its greater size, appears normal. In the skull, absence of part of the orbital wall may cause unilateral exophthalmos, often pulsating in type. There may be absence of the clinoid processes of the sella on the affected side. As with some of the other bone changes (*e.g.*, scoliosis) an associated tumor need not be present and the loss of bone is not caused by pressure erosion. Localized thinning along the lambdoid suture has been reported. A neurofibroma may affect a cranial nerve, particularly the acoustic, causing enlargement of the corresponding foramen.

Lateral intrathoracic meningocele is found with some frequency in neurofibromatosis. It presents as a rounded mass projecting into the thoracic cavity along the spine and is usually associated with considerable deformity of the contiguous vertebrae including kyphosis, scoliosis, and erosions of vertebral bodies, arches, and ribs. Scalloping of the posterior surfaces of one or more vertebral bodies is common in association with other spinal deformities. It has been shown that scalloping can occur in neurofibromatosis without any associated tumor or other mass to account for it.

A neurofibroma of a spinal nerve root often is of dumbbell shape having intraspinal and extraspinal extensions. This type of tumor is prone to erode the contiguous vertebral pedicles and, in the thoracic area, a paraspinal mass may be seen. A neurofibroma of an intercostal nerve causes a mass density along the thoracic wall and often there is pressure erosion of adjacent ribs and localized widening of the rib interspace (see Fig. 7-42). It should be noted that a solitary neurofibroma may occur in many different areas of the body without the other stigmata of von Recklinghausen's disease. (See section on Neurofibroma, Chapter 7.)

Periosteum is often abnormal and appears to be easily stripped in some patients, leading to subperiosteal hematoma which later calcifies.

Pseudarthrosis. During the newborn period (occasionally noted at birth) a pathologic fracture may occur through one of the weight-bearing bones, usually the distal one-third of the tibia. The fracture fails to heal, the ends of the fragments become pointed or smoothly rounded, and pseudarthrosis results. In about one-half of these patients stigmas of neurofibromatosis, such as café-au-lait spots, may be present. When observed early the lesion appears as a gradual local lysis of bone with failure to replace the desossified bone by normal bone.[1] In some the fracture heals temporarily but refractures when weight bearing is attempted. Some authorities have contended that intraosseous neurilemmoma is responsible for the lesion but most investigators believe that it represents an ununited fracture, perhaps related to the abnormal periosteum sometimes present in neurofibromatosis (Fig. 2-36).

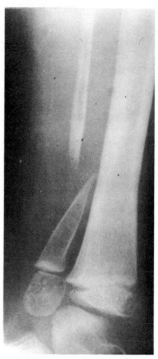

Fig. 2-36. Pseudarthrosis of the fibula in a patient with neurofibromatosis.

MISCELLANEOUS DYSPLASIAS
DYSCHONDROSTEOSIS

This entity was first reported by Leri and Weill in 1928. Its major abnormality is at the wrist where a lesion similar to or the same as Madelung's deformity occurs (see "Madelung's Deformity," Ch. 3). Some believe that Madelung's deformity and dyschondrosteosis are one and the same. Others point out that, while the lesion at the wrist corresponds to Madelung's deformity, there also are other findings in most patients.[8] Among these is shortening of the forearms and legs (middle-segment dwarfism). Genu varum is also found and occasionally an exostosis occurs on the tibia. Dyschondrosteosis is transmitted as an autosomal dominant trait.

MARFAN'S SYNDROME (ARACHNODACTYLY)

Marfan's syndrome is a disease of connective tissue caused by an individual's inability to manufacture normal collagen or one of the constituents of colla-gen.[1] It involves the heart and aorta and one of its common manifestations is aneurysm formation, usually of the ascending aorta and of dissecting type. The affected individuals are tall and slender, usually over 6 feet in height. The muscles are poorly devel-oped with poor tone. Thus the joints may be hyper-mobile, there may be dislocation of the hips, genu re-curvatum, dislocation of the patella, and pes planus. Ectopia lentis is common.

The bones are of normal density but long and gra-cile. Their thickness is normal but the increased length gives an illusion of thinness. In the hands, elongation of the bones leads to a characteristic ap-pearance (*arachnodactyly*) described as "spider-like" (Fig. 2-37). Scoliosis is frequent. The skull often has a dolichocephalic shape owing to increased length of the base. There is a decrease in subcutane-ous fat so that the individuals appear emaciated. There often is pectus excavatum. The hereditary na-ture of the disease has been established in many pa-tients. The syndrome is transmitted as an autosomal dominant trait.

HOMOCYSTINURIA

Homocystinuria[17] is an inborn error of metabolism that simulates Marfan's syndrome. However, it is transmitted as an autosomal recessive trait. The medium-sized arteries are involved. Osteoporosis is present; arachnodactyly is found only occasionally.

CLEIDOCRANIAL DYSOSTOSIS

In most patients with cleidocranial dysostosis the skull and clavicles are involved but other structures may be affected as well. The skull usually has a brachycephalic shape. The sutures remain open and numerous wormian bones are present. Permanent patency of fontanelles is usually seen. Often the ante-rior fontanelle particularly is large and extends forward between the frontal bones with the metopic suture failing to close (Fig. 2-38). The foramen mag-num is large and shows a forward and downward slant. The mandible is prognathous but the maxilla is hypoplastic as are other facial bones. The malar, lac-rimal, and nasal bones may be deficient. The palate tends to be narrow with a high arch. The sinuses often are small.

Another major abnormality is deficiency of or ab-sence of the clavicles (Fig. 2-39). Because the clavi-cle ossifies from three centers, any part may be ab-sent so that there are many variations in the

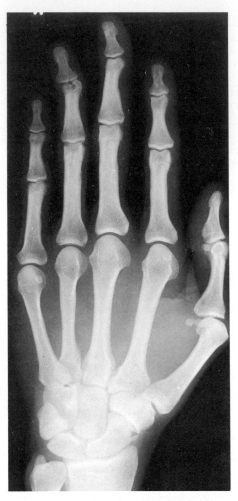

Fig. 2-37. Arachnodactyly (Marfan's syndrome). Note the long, slender bones, particularly the proximal phalanges. The deformity of the fourth finger is sec-ondary to old trauma.

appearance of these bones. Clinically the deficiency of the clavicles allows the individual to approximate the shoulders anteriorly, a significant feature of the disease.

The radius may be short. There may be extra epiphyses for the metacarpals and phalanges. Occa-sionally the second metacarpal is unusually long with a steplike shortening of the third, fourth, and fifth metacarpals.

In the pelvis the bones are often underdeveloped and the symphysis pubis may be unusually wide. The sacrum and coccyx may be malformed or the coccyx may be absent. Coxa vara is noted at the hips.

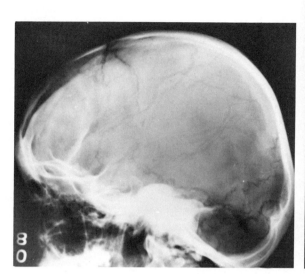
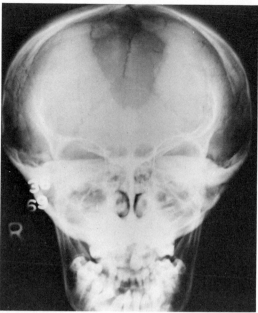

Fig. 2-38. Cleidocranial dysostosis. The anterior fontanel is open and greatly enlarged. The basal angle of the skull is flat. There are numerous wormian bones adjacent to the lambdoidal suture, and some of the teeth are malposed.

Fig. 2-39. Cleidocranial dysostosis. This is the same patient as shown in Figure 2-38. Note the defects in the clavicles and the midline spina bifida occulta involving the upper three thoracic vertebrae.

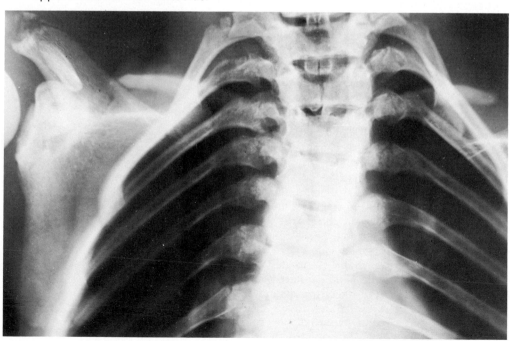

Changes in the feet are often similar to those noted in the hands. Scoliosis, lordosis, or kyphosis may be seen in the spine and failure of fusion of the arches has been observed.

The teeth usually are abnormal. There may be retention of deciduous teeth, delay in eruption of permanent teeth, faulty implantation, and dental caries. Dentigerous cysts have been reported in some patients.

Cleidocranial dysostosis is transmitted as an autosomal dominant trait.

CONGENITAL PSEUDARTHROSIS OF THE CLAVICLE

This entity is rare and does not appear to be related to cleidocranial dysostosis even though it consists of a clavicular defect. The defect is usually slightly lateral to the midpoint of the clavicle so that the sternal fragment is larger than the acromial. The adjacent ends are usually enlarged and covered by thin cortical bone. There is a false joint between the ends. Clinically there is a painless lump on the clavicle that may become more conspicuous as the child develops, and there is unusual mobility of the shoulders. The right side is almost invariably involved when the lesion is unilateral, but occasionally the involvement is bilateral. Most of the reported cases have not been familial, although a few families in which numerous members have this condition have been described. The defect does not represent an ununited intrauterine fracture.

CHONDROECTODERMAL DYSPLASIA (ELLIS–VAN CREVELD DISEASE)

This rare disorder has probably been misdiagnosed in the past as achondroplasia. It was first defined as a distinct entity by McKusick[17] who found cases among the Old Order Amish people of Pennsylvania. He considered the disease to be transmitted as an autosomal recessive trait. Cardiac anomalies (atrial septal and ventricular septal defects being the most frequent) have been found in about 60% of these patients. The ectodermal component of the syndrome is manifested by small, friable nails, defective dentition, and, in a few cases, alopecia.

The changes in the skeleton are usually characteristic. Fusion of the hamate and capitate bones in the wrist is often present. Polydactyly and syndactyly are almost universal. These changes involve the ulnar side of the hand so that a partially or completely formed sixth metacarpal is fused to the fifth. Its distal

end, however, is free so that there is a sixth digit (Figs. 2-40 and 2-41). Cone epiphyses are common during childhood (see section on "Peripheral Dysostosis"). Shortening of the long tubular bones characteristically becomes more severe distalward. Thus the tibia and fibula are much shorter than the femur and the distal phalanges more dwarfed than are the proximal. The distal end of the radius and proximal end of the ulna are somewhat enlarged. Also, the radial head may be flared and frequently dislocated at the elbow. The proximal end of the tibia also is widened and the epiphysis offset medially. A small exostosis on the upper inner cortex of the tibia is frequently present. The intercondylar notch of the femur is shallow and the tibial spine is small.

The teeth are delayed in appearance and then are small, defective, and irregularly spaced. In the pelvis the iliac crest tends to be flared but the pelvis of many of these patients is normal. The same is true of the vertebrae, ribs, and skull.

Fig. 2-40. Ellis-van Creveld disease in a woman. There is progressive shortening of the bones going distally from the wrist with polydactyly, syndactyly, and carpal fusions. (Courtesy Dr. M. Pinson Neal, Jr., Richmond, Virginia)

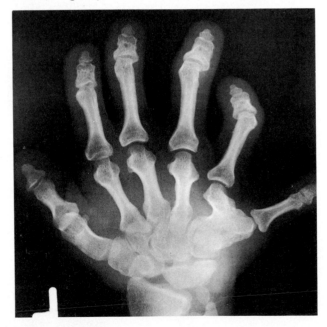

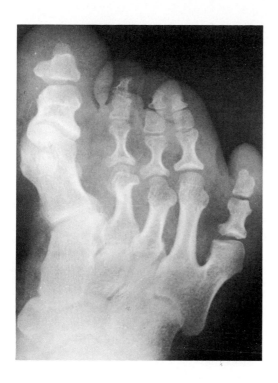

Fig. 2-41. Foot of the patient with Ellis-van Creveld disease illustrated in Figure 2-40. (Courtesy Dr. M. Pinson Neal, Jr., Richmond, Virginia)

found in association with various abnormalities, the Ellis–van Creveld disease being only one of such syndromes.

TRICHO–RHINO–PHALANGEAL DYSPLASIA

This condition is characterized by slow-growing, brittle hair; early loss of hair; bulbous or pear-shaped nose; and long philtrum.[7] Short phalanges with cone-shaped epiphyses are similar to those in individuals having peripheral dysostosis. There is growth retardation leading to short stature. The mandible may be hypoplastic, scoliosis or lordosis may be present, and the scapulae are often winged.

MESOMELIC DWARFISM (NIEVERGELT SYNDROME)

This syndrome is characterized by dwarfism caused by marked shortening of the lower extremities, particularly the tibia which is often grossly deformed, with exostoses resulting in a triangular shape. Multiple tarsal synostoses with atypical clubfoot deformity may also be present. The ankle may resemble a ball-and-socket joint because of a rounded superior aspect of the talus. Upper-extremity involvement is less severe and consists of radioulnar synostosis with subluxation of the radial head at the elbow.

ENDOSTEAL HYPEROSTOSIS (VAN BUCHEM DISEASE)

This condition, transmitted as an autosomal recessive trait, is characterized by symmetrical sclerosis of the skull, mandible, and clavicles. In the diaphyses of the bones of the extremities, endosteal thickening tends to widen the cortex but does not increase the diameter of the bone. The medial aspects of the clavicles tend to be increased in diameter, however.

ASPHYXIATING THORACIC DYSTROPHY

This dysplasia was first reported by Jeune in 1955 in two infant siblings who died of respiratory distress associated with a small, and relatively immobile, thorax. The major roentgen abnormalities[12, 23] consist of very short ribs and a variable degree of shortening of the long tubular bones with metaphyseal notching.

PERIPHERAL DYSOSTOSIS

This uncommon entity, described by Brailsford in 1948 and also by Singleton, Daeschner, and Teng in 1960, has been considered by some to be only a mild form of the Ellis–van Creveld disorder. The characteristic roentgen changes are limited to the short tubular bones of the hands and feet which are short and broad and with cone-shaped or ball-and-socket epiphyses. The term *cone epiphysis* refers to an epiphyseal center that is partially or completely buried in the metaphysis, and usually has the shape of a cone. A *ball-and-socket epiphysis* is similar except that the center is more rounded than cone-shaped. The terms, however, are often used interchangeably. Supernumerary epiphyses and pseudoepiphyses are often present. Cone-shaped epiphyses also have been found in a number of other conditions including (*1*) cleidocranial dysostosis, (*2*) Ellis–van Creveld disease, (*3*) tricho-rhino-phalangeal syndrome, (*4*) osteopetrosis, (*5*) epiphyseal hyperplasia, (*6*) Apert's syndrome, (*7*) pseudohypoparathyroidism, (*8*) achondroplasia, (*9*) multiple hereditary exostoses, and (*10*) no recognizable cause.[20]

The tendency among investigators working in this field is to consider peripheral dysostosis as a symptom rather than a specific entity and one that may be

The ribs project horizontally and may be so short as to barely reach the anterior axillary line. The shortened ribs reduce the volume of the thorax and are responsible for the respiratory distress. The cardiac silhouette often appears large but this is probably an illusion because of the smallness of the thorax. In the pelvis the ilium is shortened in its inferosuperior diameter, the acetabular roof is broad and there may be a deep V-shaped notch in it. The disease frequently is fatal with the infant dying from respiratory complications. Associated renal disease has been reported and, in some patients with less severe skeletal changes, renal failure may be the cause of death.

It should be noted that short ribs with a narrow thorax occur in some other dysplasias including achondroplasia and thanatophoric dwarfism and that other changes common to achondroplasia may be seen in asphyxiating thoracic dystrophy and thanatophoric dwarfism. Some investigators still believe that these latter two entities may represent only the severe form of achondroplasia in which the infants often die early in life usually owing to respiratory embarrassment.

As case reports of this disease accumulate, it is evident that a number of these infants may survive, some for many years, so that it is no longer considered as uniformly lethal in the neonatal period as formerly believed.

REFERENCES AND SELECTED READINGS

1. AEGERTER E, KIRKPATRICK JA JR: Orthopedic Diseases, 4th ed. Philadelphia, WB Saunders, 1975
2. CAMPBELL CJ, PAPADEMETRIOU T, BONFIGLIO M: Melorheostosis. A report of the clinical roentgenographic and pathological findings in 14 cases. J Bone Joint Surg [A] 50: 1281, 1968
3. COMINGS DE, PAPAZIAN C, SCHOENE HR: Conradi's disease. Chondrodystrophia calcificans congenita, stippled epiphyses. J Pediatr 72: 63, 1968
4. EDEIKEN J, HODES PJ: Roentgen Diagnosis of Diseases of Bone, 2nd ed. Baltimore, Williams & Wilkins, 1973
5. ELMORE SM: Pycnodysostosis. A review. J Bone Joint Surg [A] 49: 153, 1967
6. FELMAN AH, KIRKPATRICK JA: Madelung's deformity. Observations in 17 patients. Radiology 93: 1037, 1969
7. GORLIN FJ, COHEN MM JR, WOLFSON J: Tricho-Rhino-Phalangeal Syndrome. Am J Dis Child 118: 595, 1969
8. HENRY A, THORBURN MJ: Madelung's deformity. A clinical and cytogenic study. J Bone Joint Surg [B] 49: 66, 1967
9. JUBERG RC, HOLT JF: Inheritance of multiple epiphyseal dysplasia tarda. Am J Hum Genet 20: 549, 1968
10. KEATS TE, RIDDERVOLT HO, MICHAELIS LL: Thanatophoric dwarfism. Am J Roentgenol 108: 473, 1970
11. KETTLEKAMP DB, CAMPBELL CJ, BONFIGLIO M: Dysplasia epiphysialis hemimelica. A report of 15 cases and a review of the literature. J Bone Joint Surg [A] 48: 476, 1966
12. KOHLER E, BABBITT DP: Dystrophic thoraces and infantile asphyxia. Radiology 94: 55, 1970
13. LANGER LO JR: Dyschondrosteosis, a hereditable bone dysplasia with characteristic roentgenographic features. Am J Roentgenol 95: 178, 1965
14. LANGER LO JR, BAUMANN FA, GORLIN RJ: Achondroplasia. Am J Roentgenol 100: 12, 1967
15. LANGER LO JR, CAREY LS: The roentgenographic features of the K. S. mucopolysaccharidosis of Morquio (Morquio-Brailsford disease). Am J Roentgenol 97: 1, 1966
16. LAROSE JH, GAY BB JR: Metatropic dwarfism. Am J Roentgenol 106: 156, 1969
17. MCKUSICK V: Heritable Disorders of Connective Tissue, 4th ed. St. Louis, Mosby, 1972
18. MILLER SM, PAUL LW: Roentgen observations in familial metaphyseal dysostosis. Radiology 83: 665, 1964
19. NEUHAUSER EBD, et al: Diastematomyelia: transfixation of the cord or cauda equina with congenital anomalies of the spine. Radiology 54: 659, 1950
20. NEWCOMBE DS, KEATS TE: Roentgenographic manifestations of hereditary peripheral dysostosis. Am J Roentgenol 106: 178, 1969
21. PAUL LW: Hereditary multiple diaphyseal sclerosis (Ribbing). Radiology 60: 412, 1953
22. PAUL LW: Punctate epiphyseal dysplasia (chondrodystrophia calcificans congenita): report of a case with nine year period of observation. Am J Roentgenol 71: 941, 1954
23. PIRNAR T, NEUHAUSER EBD: Asphyxiating thoracic dystrophy of the newborn. Am J Roentgenol 98: 358, 1966
24. POZNANSKI AK, NASANCHUK JS, BAUBLIC J et al: The cerebro-hepato-renal syndrome (CHRS). Am J Roentgenol 109: 313, 1970
25. PRATT AD, FELSON B, WIOT JF et al: Sequestrum formation in fibrous dysplasia. Am J Roentgenol 106: 162, 1969
26. RUBIN P: Dynamic Classification of Bone Dysplasias. Chicago, Year Book Medical, 1964

27. SILVERMAN FN: A differential diagnosis of achondroplasia. Radiol Clin North Am 6: 223, 1968

28. SILVERMAN FN: Pediatric radiology. In McLaren JW (ed): Modern Trends in Diagnostic Radiology, 4th ed. New York, Appleton-Century-Crofts, 1970

29. SPRANGER JW, LANGER LO JR: Spondyloepiphyseal dysplasia congenita. Radiology 94: 313, 1970

30. SPRANGER JW, LANGER LO JR, WIEDEMANN HR: Bone Dysplasias. An Atlas of Constitutional Disorders of Skeletal Development. Philadelphia, WB Saunders, 1974

31. SPRANGER JW, WIEDEMANN HR: The genetic mucolipidoses; diagnosis and differential diagnosis. Human Genet 9: 113, 1970

32. STEINBACH HL, et al: The Hurler syndrome without abnormal mucopolysacchariduria. Radiology 90: 472, 1968

33. TASKER WG, MASTRI AR, GOLD AP: Chondrodystrophia calcificans congenita (dysplasia epiphysalis punctata). Am J Dis Child 119: 122, 1970

3

MISCELLANEOUS SKELETAL ANOMALIES AND SYNDROMES

ACCESSORY BONES AND OSSIFICATION CENTERS

Certain accessory bones and centers of ossification that fail to unite are found rather frequently in the skeleton. An accessory bone represents either a supernumerary ossicle not ordinarily found in the skeleton or a bony process or secondary center for the tip of a process that has failed to fuse and remains as a separate bony structure. An accessory bone may be mistaken for a pathologic condition, particularly a fracture, and a knowledge of its distribution and frequency is of some importance.

Differentiation of Anomalous Bones from Fractures

A fracture line is ragged along the margin and it is invariably irregular. Anomalous fissures are characterized by smooth margins, rounding of the edges, and a line of cortex along the entire surface. A chip fracture will have an irregular surface at the line of fracture and there is a defect in the adjacent bone corresponding to the avulsed chip. Fresh fractures are always accompanied by swelling of the contiguous soft tissues. Accessory centers and anomalous bones are commonly bilateral. Examination of the corresponding part of the opposite extremity is helpful in doubtful cases.

THE FOOT AND ANKLE

The foot is a common site for the appearance of accessory bones (Fig. 3-1) and the following are the most frequent:

Os Trigonum. This accessory ossicle occurs in about 10% of individuals. It is a separate center for the posterior process of the astragalus to which the astragalofibular ligament is attached. Its shape varies from a small triangular fragment to one more rounded or oval. The division from the astragalus may be incomplete. A fracture of a long posterior process of the astragalus may resemble an os trigonum. Differentia-

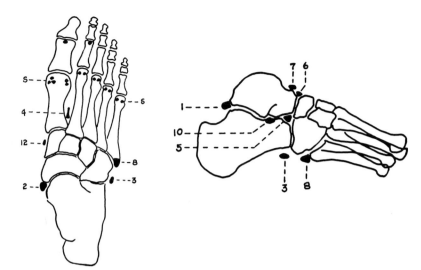

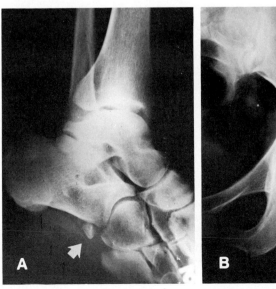

Fig. 3-1. Common accessory ossicles in the foot. **(1)** Os trigonum; **(2)** os tibiale externum; **(3)** os peroneum; **(4)** os intermetatarseum; **(5)** calcaneus secondarius; **(6)** supranavicular; **(7)** secondary astragalus; **(8)** os vesalianum; **(10)** os sustentaculi; **(S)** sesamoid bones (the **small black dots** over the metatarsal heads and proximal phalanges of first and second toes represent the most frequent sites of the sesamoid bones, but they may occur in other locations). Number **9** is not included for purposes of clarity.

tion depends upon the factors listed in the preceding paragraph.

Os Tibiale Externum. This ossicle represents the unfused tuberosity on the medial proximal side of the tarsal scaphoid (navicular). It is sometimes called the divided scaphoid or an accessory scaphoid. It is a common variation and is usually bilateral.

Os Peroneum (Peroneal Sesamoid). The os peroneum is a small ossicle found in or adjacent to the ten-don of the peroneus longus just lateral to and below the os calcis and cuboid (Fig. 3-2). It is found in about 8% of individuals. Occasionally there may be two or even three separate ossicles representing a bipartite or tripartite sesamoid.

Os Intermetatarseum. This is a small bone having the form of a tiny rudimentary metatarsal found between the proximal ends of the first and second metatarsals; its frequency is about 10%.

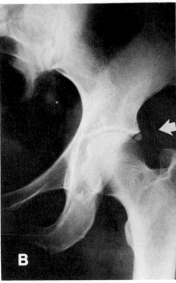

Fig. 3-2. A. Os peroneum. **B.** Os acetabuli.

Calcaneus Secondarius. The secondary os calcis is a small, irregular bony mass found at the upper anterior end of the os calcis where it articulates with the astragalus and navicular. It is seen to best advantage in oblique roentgenograms of the foot; its frequency is about 2%.

Supranavicular (Pirie's Bone). This is a small, triangular bone occurring at the proximal superior edge of the navicular and articulating with the astragalus and navicular. It is relatively common and can easily be mistaken for a fracture.

Secondary Astragalus. The secondary astragalus is a small rounded bone found just above the head of the astragalus; it is seen only in lateral views of the foot. It should not be confused with the supranavicular, which lies between the astragalus and scaphoid.

Os Vesalianum. This is a rare accessory bone found just proximal to the head of the fifth metatarsal. It should not be mistaken for the lateral epiphysis of the metatarsal head, which is a normal finding (see below).

Epiphysis for the Head of Metatarsal V. This bony center is not an anomaly but is a constant epiphysis that appears in individuals at about the age of 13 years and unites shortly thereafter. It is a flat bony center found along the lateral side of the proximal end of metatarsal V. It often is irregular in shape but its long axis parallels the long axis of the metatarsal. A fracture in this location is also common but the line of fracture invariably extends across the long axis of the shaft, the fracture surfaces are irregular, the soft tissues overlying the area are swollen, and the proximal fragment often is displaced or rotated.

Os Sustentaculi. This is a rare, small, wedge-shaped bone that comprises the upper posterior end of the sustentaculum tali.

Cuboideum Secondarium. This is another rare bone. It represents the cuboid divided into two portions.

Paracuneiform. Only a few instances of the presence of this bone have been reported. It is a small rounded ossicle lying along the medial aspect of the internal cuneiform and is seen to best advantage in anteroposterior roentgenograms of the foot.

Os Subtibiale. The os subtibiale is a separate ossification center for the tip of the medial malleolus.

Os Subfibulare. Corresponding to the subtibiale, this is a separate center for the tip of the lateral malleolus. It varies from a tiny rounded ossicle to a fairly large triangular fragment. It is best seen in anteroposterior views of the ankle joint. Some of these apparent accessory ossicles around the ankle joint may be old chip fracture fragments that have smoothed off and have united with fibrous rather than bony union. Others may be foci of ossification that have formed as a result of soft-tissue injury. It often is impossible to determine the nature of such an ossification in the ankle area from a single roentgen examination. Because of the frequency of injury to the ankle one must always consider the possibility of an apparent ossicle of this type being secondary to injury rather than an anomalous ossification center.

THE KNEE

Bipartite Patella. The patella may be divided into two or even more segments. The smaller segment or segments are usually located along the upper outer quadrant of the patella. The recognition of this anomaly is important as it may be mistaken for fracture. In approximately 80% of the cases the anomaly is bilateral.

Fabella. The fabella is a small sesamoid bone very frequently found in the tendon of the lateral head of the gastrocnemius muscle at the level of the knee joint. It may become enlarged and roughened in the presence of degenerative disease of the knee joint.

THE HIP

Os Acetabuli. The os acetabuli is a round or oval ossicle lying along the upper rim of the acetabulum (see Fig. 3-2). This is not the anatomic os acetabuli that forms in the Y-shaped triradiate acetabular cartilage, but is either an ununited epiphyseal center or a sesamoid bone. There is normally an epiphyseal center or centers for the upper rim of the acetabulum that appear at about the age of 13 and that undergo fusion with the acetabulum within a very short time. Failure of this epiphysis to unite results in some cases of this so-called roentgenologic os acetabuli. In other instances a small sesamoid may be found in this area, usually situated more laterally than the epiphysis but called by the same name.

THE SHOULDER

Os Acromiale. The os acromiale is the unfused tip of the acromion process. It represents a normal secondary ossification center that fails to undergo fusion. The incidence of this anomaly has been reported as from 1% to 6% but we have seen it infrequently.

THE ELBOW

Patella Cubiti. The patella cubiti is a small bony center that forms at the tip of the olecranon process of the ulna. Some authorities contend that there are no proved accessory centers at the elbow and that this is actually an example of osteochondritis dissecans (see Ch. 8).

THE WRIST AND HAND

The variations in the wrist are numerous; Pfitzner listed 33 possible carpal elements. They are less common clinically than those in the foot. The most important ones are listed here (Fig. 3-3).

Os Centrale. This is a small ossicle situated on the radial side of the os magnum (capitate). In the embryo this is a frequent cartilaginous center and it may persist into adult life as a separate ossicle. Frequently the cartilaginous os centrale does not ossify but remains as a separate cartilage fragment visible only as a distinct notch or space on the outer side of the os magnum.

Divided Scaphoid (Navicular). The carpal scaphoid may be found in two parts with a transverse fissure through the center. It may be difficult to determine whether this is an anomaly or an old ununited fracture since fractures of this bone are notorious for their failure to unite with bony union. Eburnation of edges, roughness, and cystlike areas along the line of the fissure favor the diagnosis of an ununited fracture. When the fissure is the result of an anomaly the bone otherwise is normal.

Radiale Externum. The radiale externum is an infrequent small ossicle lying just distal to the styloid process of the radius.

Os Triangulare. This is a small bone found at the tip of the ulnar styloid. It can be differentiated from frac-

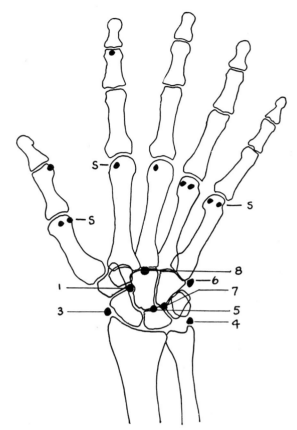

Fig. 3-3. Diagram illustrating the most frequent accessory ossicles in the hand and wrist. **(1)** Os centrale; **(3)** os radiale externum; **(4)** os triangulare; **(5)** epilunatum; **(6)** os vesalianum manus; **(7)** epipyramis; **(8)** os styloideum; **(S)** the most frequent sites for sesamoid bones in the hand. Number **2** is not included for purposes of clarity.

ture of the styloid process by the fact that the styloid is of normal length without the addition of this fragment.

Epilunatum. The epilunatum is a separate center for the dorsal tip of the semilunar (lunate).

Os Vesalianum Manus. This is a small bone in the wrist that corresponds to a similar one in the foot and is found at the proximal end of the fifth metacarpal. It is a rare anomaly.

Epipyramis. The epipyramis is a small ossicle that occurs between the os magnum, unciform, and cuneiform. This is another of the uncommon variants in the wrist.

Os Styloideum. The unfused styloid process of the third metacarpal is known as the os styloideum. It projects from the dorsal side of the base of the third metacarpal and is usually visualized best in true lateral projections of the wrist. It is a rather frequent anomaly.

CARPAL AND TARSAL FUSIONS

Fusions have been found in nearly every possible combination in the carpal and metacarpal regions and in the corresponding portion of the foot. In many instances they are associated with other anomalies but they may occur as isolated findings. Some of these are hereditary and familial. In the foot, certain types of tarsal fusion are important clinically because of the symptoms produced. Examples include talocalcaneal or calcaneonavicular fusions. The term "calcaneonavicular bar" is sometimes applied to the latter. Special oblique projections may be required for adequate demonstration of these fusions.

CONGENITAL VARIATIONS IN THE SKULL AND FACIAL BONES

WORMIAN BONES

Wormian bones are small separate ossicles found between the sutures of the skull; they are most frequent near the junction of the coronal and lambdoid sutures (Fig. 3-4). They are of no clinical importance as a rule but are often associated with other anomalies of the skeleton. A particularly large ossicle is occasionally seen forming the superior portion of the occipital bone; this is known as the Inca bone.

SKULL DEFECTS WITH MENINGOCELE

A meningocele of the skull represents herniation of a meningeal sac through a defect in the skull and is of fairly frequent occurrence. The sac may contain only the meninges and cerebrospinal fluid or it may contain a variable amount of brain tissue. The size of the defect in the skull varies greatly and occasionally it may be very large. Meningoceles occur in the midline of the skull and the most frequent situation is in the occipital region. In some cases the defect communicates with the foramen magnum and in others there is absence of one or more of the upper cervical arches (occipitocervical meningocele). Less frequently, cra-

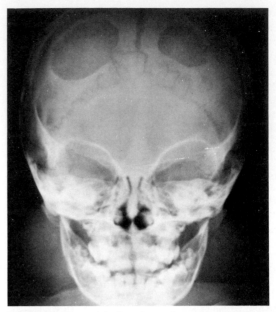

Fig. 3-4. Congenital enlarged parietal foramina. Note wormian bones along lamboidal sutures.

Fig. 3-5. Lacuna skull (Lückenschadel). The translucent areas represent thin bone separated by ridges in the inner table. The condition can be distinguished from the "beaten silver" appearance caused by increased intracranial pressure by the normal size of the skull and the presence of normal vault sutures.

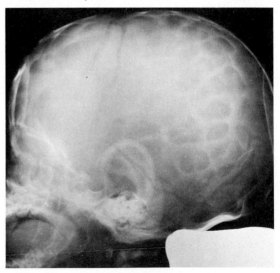

nial meningocele occurs in the anterior aspect of the skull in the region of the glabella and, rarely, in the base of the skull.

CONGENITAL PARIETAL FORAMINA

The parietal foramina are two tiny channels in the posterior parts of the parietal bones close to the midline, possibly for the passage of the parietal arteries. However, in most there are no associated arteries or veins. They probably represent an ossification anomaly without relation to vessels or to skeletal disease. Very rarely, similar defects may be found in the frontal or in the occipital bone. Rarely, these may be greatly enlarged up to several centimeters in diameter (see Fig. 3-4). They may communicate across the midline, forming a dumbbell-shaped defect. There is a distinct hereditary tendency for the occurrence of enlarged parietal foramina. They are of no clinical importance but may be mistaken for trephine holes or for destruction caused by disease.

LACUNA SKULL (LÜCKENSCHÄDEL)

In association with a spinal meningocele and occasionally seen as an isolated defect without meningocele, the cranial bones may show excessively prominent lakelike depressions of the inner table that give the skull a relief-map appearance (Fig. 3-5). The skull is thinned in the depths of the depressions, which are surrounded by smooth ridges. There may be complete bony defects in some areas. In addition to the spina bifida and meningocele there often are other skeletal deformities, particularly in the spine and ribs. The cause of the skull changes is unknown; theories that have been suggested include increased intracranial pressure during intrauterine life, and a congenital ossification defect of the cranial bones. In some patients the entire skull is involved. More frequently the changes are confined to the posterior aspect of the vault or at least are the most prominent in this region. If the lacuna skull is an isolated defect and not associated with other lesions that might cause early death, there is a gradual disappearance of the abnormality and the skull, after a period of several years, tends to assume a normal appearance.

PREMATURE FUSION OF THE SUTURES (CRANIOSYNOSTOSIS)

The sutures of the skull usually remain open until middle life or later and may never completely fuse. When they fuse prematurely before growth is complete the skull becomes deformed; if fusion is exten-

sive and occurs early enough in life, increased intracranial pressure may result as the brain continues to grow. Growth of the skull is largely a reflection of growth of the brain and most of this (80%) occurs during the first 3 years of life. The brain is reported to double its weight during the first 7 months of life and to triple it in 30 months. Premature fusion of the sutures developing during the first year of life, therefore, is more significant than a similar occurrence during later childhood. While one or more of the sutures may be fused at the time of birth, it is more frequent to find them open with the fusion occurring some time later. A suture that is going to close prematurely often will show some thickening or heaping up of bone along its edges when the suture is viewed end on. The normal sutures in the newborn are poorly defined with the edges of the bones fading gradually into the suture area. When the margins of the bones are sharply defined and the suture lines easily visualized during very early infancy, the possibility of imminent fusion is considerable. Once a suture has fused, growth proceeds in whatever direction possible unless all sutures fuse simultaneously; then severe signs of increased intracranial pressure are to be expected (Fig. 3-6). These signs include prominence of convolutional markings on the inner table of the skull ("beaten-silver" appearance), separation of any suture or sutures that may remain open, and erosion of the sella—a late sign (rare). It is important to recognize the more severe forms of craniosynostosis during early infancy, preferably during the first year of life, because surgical measures are available that will prevent undue deformity of the skull from developing.

In addition to primary premature closure of the sutures, craniosynostosis occurs as a secondary phenomenon in a variety of diseases and dysplasias.[10] Other fusion anomalies such as carpal and tarsal coalition, radioulnar synostosis, syndactyly, or vertebral fusion may occur in association with cranial fusions in the absence of other anomalies.

Craniosynostosis may be classified[38] into the following: 1) fusion of all sutures, 2) fusion of multiple sutures, and 3) fusion of one suture. The resultant cranial deformity is dependent upon the suture or sutures involved and which fuses first.

Fusion of All Vault Sutures (Microcephaly of Varying Degrees)

When all the vault sutures close early and at about the same time there results an abnormally small head (microcephaly) with roentgen signs of increased intracranial pressure (deep impressions on the inner table of the skull and erosion of the sella). This type of craniosynostosis is not very frequent and defective development of the brain is a more common cause of a microcephalic skull. As has been noted, unless growth of the brain proceeds in a normal manner, enlargement of the skull will not occur. In these patients with defective brain growth the skull is abnormally small but the sutures remain visible. The bones of the vault, instead of showing increased convolutional impressions and being unusually thin, may actually be thicker than normal. Even under these circumstances the sutures may fuse early, but signs of increased pressure do not develop since there is a failure of the brain to grow.

Fusion of One or More Transverse Sutures

Fusions of one or more transverse sutures are characterized by an unusually high vertex and an increased vertical diameter of the skull because growth in an anteroposterior direction is stopped or delayed by closure of the suture(s). The resultant deformity is termed **turricephaly (oxycephaly).** The premature fusion may be limited to the coronal suture, to the coronal and the lambdoid, or it may affect all the vault sutures. When all the sutures are found to be fused and the skull still has a turricephalic shape it

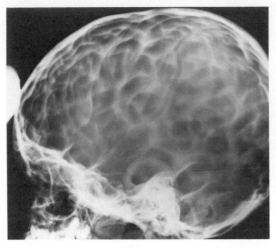

Fig. 3-6. Craniosynostosis. Premature closure of all the vault sutures has caused the deepening of the convolutional impressions on the inner table, indicating that there is chronic increase in intracranial pressure. This is caused by growth of the brain within the unyielding skull. Note complete absence of suture lines that normally should be present in childhood.

Fig. 3-7. Scaphocephaly. In this defect the head is long and narrow, and growth occurs mainly in an anteroposterior direction. This is caused by premature fusion of the major part of the sagittal suture. The lateral vault sutures remain open.

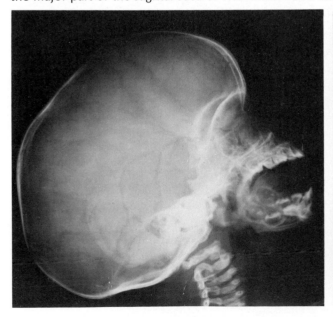

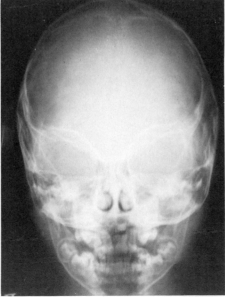

usually indicates that the fusion began in the lamb-doid and that the other sutures fused at a later date. Increased convolutional impressions are often seen in the frontal area in this condition and they may be widespread in the more severe cases (the impressions probably do not actually correspond to the convolutions of the brain, but the term "convolutional impression" has come into wide use). With more extensive fusion there may be the clinical signs of increased intracranial pressure including exophthalmos, mental retardation, convulsions, headaches, and failing vision. Several cases have been reported in which an abnormal-appearing sella turcica was found in association with an oxycephalic skull leading to the erroneous impression of a pituitary tumor.[18]

Fusion of the Sagittal Suture

Early closure of the sagittal suture allows growth predominantly in an anteroposterior direction. This type of skull is called *dolichocephalic* (scaphocephalic). When viewed from the front the scaphocephalic skull is triangular in shape with its base broadened and its vertex more or less pointed (Fig. 3-7). When viewed from the side the appearance sometimes resembles a canoe with upward bulging anteriorly and posteriorly and a central depression.

Unilateral Fusion of One or More Transverse Sutures

Early unilateral closure of one or more of the transverse sutures results in an asymmetrical skull, one side being smaller than the other. This condition is known as *plagiocephaly*. Few skulls are completely symmetrical and minor degrees of visible asymmetry are moderately frequent. As with other forms of craniostenosis, the significance of these lesser changes is doubtful because lack of growth in one direction can be compensated for in another. It is only when the fusion is present at birth or develops during the first year or two of life that the distortion in shape of the skull may become sufficient to be of clinical importance. When there is unilateral closure of one coronal suture the orbit develops an elliptical shape with an upward slanting of the outer roof (Fig. 3-8). This is a characteristic finding even when the evidence of sutural closure is not too obvious. There is also elevation of the ipsilateral sphenoid wings and the calvarium becomes flattened on the side of closure. The nasal septum may be directed obliquely upward toward the involved side. Early treatment is aimed at preventing exophthalmos, loss of vision, and to correct cosmetic deformities.

Fusion of the Metopic Suture

Some investigators believe that the malformation termed *trigonocephaly* is caused by intrauterine closure of the metopic (interfrontal suture). This results in a congenital malformation of the skull in which there is a small, pointed forehead. This, together with an increase of the biparietal diameter, gives the skull a triangular or egg-shaped configuration. While the majority of patients with trigonocephaly are otherwise normal, in some there is an associated malformation of parts of the forebrain. In these there may be other anomalies such as a deformed nose, an undivided nasal cavity, absence of the premaxilla, and microcephaly. Hypotelorism, with the orbital cavities close together, is another common associated finding. Trigonocephaly usually is more obvious on clinical inspection than on roentgen examination.

Miscellaneous Fusions

Cruzon's Disease (Craniofacial Dysostosis). This is a form of craniosynostosis inherited as an autosomal dominant trait. The sutural closure most often affects the coronal leading to a brachycephalic skull. However, other sutures may fuse first so that the skull shape is variable. In some it shows the features of a trigonoscaphocephaly. There is hypoplasia of the facial bones. Hypertelorism, exophthalmos, and a divergent squint are present. The nose is beaked (parrot nose). Mental deficiency has been described in some patients.

Apert's Syndrome (Acrocephalosyndactyly). Apert's syndrome consists of abnormalities of the skull, hands, and feet. Clinically there is an unusually high-peaked forehead; wide-spaced, bulging eyes; and a flat face with a short nose. The skull is brachycephalic in shape with a short anteroposterior diameter, a wide transverse diameter, and a high-peaked skull with maximum height between the anterior and posterior fontanels due to premature fusion of the transverse vault sutures. The palate is narrow with a high vault. The other prominent feature of the dysplasia is syndactyly, which is usually complicated (Fig. 3-9). The synostoses may occur between the metacarpals, metatarsals, or phalanges of various digits. The visual appearance has been termed "mitten hands" or "stocking feet" because of the extensive soft-tissue fusions. Also, there may be fusion of two or more segments of the same digit or multiple digits. The thumb is short, often with fused phalanges, and deviated radially. Phalanges of the fingers are also short and often fused. The capitate and hamate may also be fused.

Cloverleaf Skull (Kleeblattschädel) Syndrome. In this rare syndrome there is premature fusion (before birth) of multiple skull sutures including the coronal, lambdoid, squamous, and sagittal. The result is a bizarre, trilobed or cloverleaf-shaped skull.[1] Additionally there are severe exophthalmos, hypertelorism, and shallow orbits. The nose is beaked with a depressed bridge and the ears are low in position. There is hypoplasia of the maxillae with a relative prognathism of the mandible. Abnormalities of the teeth are frequent and there is macroglossia. Of interest are changes in the appendicular skeleton that resemble achondroplasia and aid in differentiation from Cruzon's disease. Ankylosis of some of the large joints and bowing of the tibias have been described. Webbing of the toes, an equinovarus deformity, and spadelike thumbs have been noted in some. The cause is unknown. Most of the patients have died early in life.

Cephalic Index. The cephalic index is a useful indicator of skull shape. It is obtained by dividing the maximum width of the skull by its length and multiplying by 100. The normal index varies between 65 and 75. If the cephalic index is above 75 the skull is relatively short for its width and this is called brachycephaly. If the index is below 65 the opposite condition is present and the skull is long for its width; this is known as dolichocephaly. In connection with premature fusion of the sutures, the oxycephalic or turricephalic type of skull is usually a form of brachycephaly since the anteroposterior diameter is short compared to the width. In scaphocephaly, however, the length of the skull is increased for the breadth and thus the skull is of dolichocephalic shape. In addition to being caused by premature closure of the sutures, brachycephalic and dolichocephalic skulls may result from other factors, including racial and hereditary influences. Mentally and physically re-

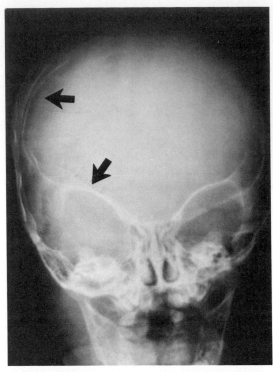

Fig. 3-8. Plagiocephaly. Note elliptical shape of the right orbit **(lower arrow)** and piling up of bone along the right coronal suture **(upper arrow).**

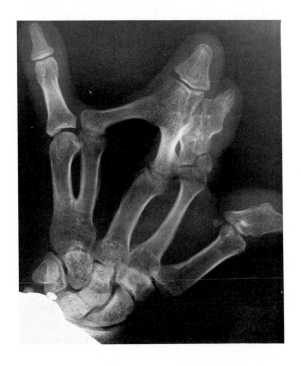

Fig. 3-9. Apert's syndrome. The hand shows extensive fusion anomalies. Similar changes were present in the feet, and the skull showed the typical changes of the syndrome.

tarded infants who do not or cannot sit up at the normal time and thus are kept on their backs for months often develop brachycephalic skulls because of molding of the soft cranial bones.

OCULAR HYPERTELORISM AND HYPOTELORISM

In *ocular hypertelorism (Greig's syndrome)* the orbital cavities are more widely spaced than they are normally. The condition is encountered with a variety of associated anomalies including mental retardation, syndactyly, renal hypoplasia, webbing of the neck, congenital heart anomalies, high-arched palate, cleft lip and palate, hypoplasia of the maxilla, macroglossia, microdontia, and Sprengels' deformity.[23] Hypertelorism also is seen in association with various types of craniosynostosis and craniofacial dysostosis. The cause is unknown but it has been suggested that there is overdevelopment of the lesser wings of the sphenoid and a relative underdevelopment of the greater wings. Most cases of hypertelorism can be recognized on frontal roentgenograms of the skull. In borderline cases the measurements devised by Hansman can be used.[19]

Hypotelorism indicates that the orbital cavities are closer together than they are normally.

MANDIBULOFACIAL DYSOSTOSIS (TREACHER-COLLINS SYNDROME)

In this entity there is hypoplasia of the facial bones. The malar bones may be underdeveloped or completely absent (Fig. 3-10). The zygomatic arches are often incomplete. A receding hypoplastic mandible has been present in most of the patients whose case history has been reported and is a distinguishing feature. The palpebral fissures are oblique. Defects of the auricles, stenosis or absence of the external auditory canals, and middle ear defects are part of the syndrome in some patients.

Goldenhar's Syndrome. This entity also is known as *oculoauriculovertebral dysplasia.*[8] There is unilateral hypoplasia or absence of the zygomatic arch, hypoplasia or aplasia of the maxillary sinus on the same side, and a low position of the orbit. There is minimal to marked unilateral hypoplasia of the mandible and hypoplasia of the temporal bone with decreased development of the mastoid. Atresia of the external auditory canal and absence of the ossicles with hypoplasia of the middle ear may also occur. The unilateral

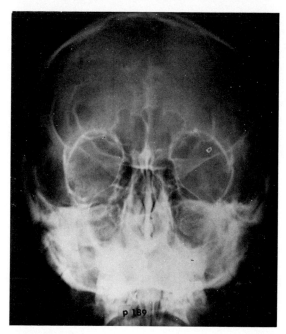

Fig. 3-10. Treacher–Collins syndrome. Note complete absence of both zygomatic arches.

nature of the defects allows differentiation from the Treacher–Collins syndrome. Multiple anomalies of the vertebrae are present including hemivertebrae, fused vertebrae, scoliosis, spina bifida, decreased interpedicular distance, and decreased disc spaces. There are often multiple rib fusions, usually on one side. The odontoid process may be elongated. In the hand, absence or hypoplasia of the first metacarpal and hypoplasia of the distal phalanges may be noted.

PORENCEPHALY

Porencephaly represents a defect in the cerebral structures, which appears as a cystlike cavity either communicating with the ventricles or separated from them by only a thin layer of tissue. It is found most commonly near the central fissure but may occur elsewhere in the brain. Porencephaly may be either congenital or acquired; the latter usually is the result of trauma occurring at or shortly after birth. In many cases, when the patient has reached late adolescent or early adult life, plain roentgenograms of the skull reveal a unilateral decrease in size of the skull, depressions on the inner table with local thinning of the diploë, and an overdevelopment of the sinuses, particularly of the ethmoid cells on the side of the cyst.

Such changes in the cranial bones always suggest the possibility of an underlying porencephaly, but similar findings are observed in unilateral cerebral atrophy without actual cyst formation. During encephalography or ventriculography, after gas has been introduced into the subarachnoid space and the ventricular system, the cyst may fill; this type of procedure offers the maximum diagnostic information.

ANENCEPHALY

In anencephaly there is an almost complete absence of the skull and brain and the anomaly is incompatible with life. The cranial bones that are present form an ill-defined mass. The chief importance roentgenologically lies in the detection of this condition in utero and the diagnosis can be made without difficulty on roentgen examination of the mother when ossification of the fetal skeleton has developed sufficiently for the bones to be visualized. This usually occurs during the fifth or sixth month of gestation.

PLATYBASIA

In platybasia the base of the skull is unusually flat. *The normal basal angle* is formed by drawing lines from the nasofrontal suture and the anterior lip of the foramen magnum to the tuberculum sellae. This angle has an upper limit of normal of about 140 degrees. Basal angles above 140 degrees indicate some degree of platybasia. Flattening of the base of the skull in itself is of no importance but it frequently is caused by an invagination of the occiput into the base (basilar invagination). In turn, basilar invagination may be a developmental anomaly or it may be caused by abnormal softening of the bones as a result of disease. McGregor's line is drawn from the posterior margin of the hard palate to the lowermost point of the occiput. When the tip of the odontoid extends more than 6.5 mm (approximately) above the line, a diagnosis of basilar impression or invagination can be made. Among the conditions that predispose to basilar invagination are Paget's disease (Fig. 3-11) and osteomalacia. Congenital assimilation of the atlas has been thought to be associated with basilar impression, but this is not usually the case since there may be no basilar invagination in patients with fusion of the atlas to the occiput (Figure 3-12). However, when either *basilar invagination* or *cervico-occipital fusion* is present, the foramen magnum may be decreased in size and deformed in shape and thus cause pressure upon the cord or medulla, with the development of clinical signs and symptoms.

SINUS PERICRANII

Occasionally a large vein extends through the skull, forming a localized soft-tissue swelling in the scalp. Characteristically the swelling becomes larger when the patient lowers his head or when the intracranial pressure is elevated from any cause such as sneezing or coughing. It decreases in size or disappears when the head is held upright. This condition is known as sinus pericranii. The opening in the skull through which the venous channel extends may be large enough to be visible in skull roentgenograms and then is seen as a smooth, rounded defect. The diagnosis is readily apparent when the clinical signs are elicited.

DERMOID TUMORS

A dermoid tumor of the scalp may have an intracranial extension through a small defect in the cranial bone or the major portion of the tumor may be in the cranial cavity with a small stalk projecting through the skull. Dermoids are found in or very close to the midline. The character of the skull defect is not diagnostic in skull roentgenograms and it may appear similar to the defect of sinus pericranii or that of a small craniocele or meningocele. At times there will be only a small dermal sinus lined by squamous epithelium, but at any point from the skin to the meninges and sometimes into the cerebellum or fourth ventricle the sinus may expand as a result of the formation of an epidermoid or dermoid cyst.[31] The occiput in the region of the inion is the most frequently involved area in the skull. Radiographic findings consist of a midline occipital bony defect ranging from 2 to 3 mm to 1 cm or more in size, often associated with a soft-tissue mass in the scalp. The margins are distinct and slightly sclerotic. The tumor is presumably the result of incomplete or faulty separation of cutaneous ectoderm from neuroectoderm in early development. It must be differentiated from encephalocele, which it may resemble very closely, and from an emissary vein. A useful distinguishing feature is its oblique course through the occipital bone. At times, an intradural epidermoidoma is found in the same area; absence of the bony channel and lack of soft-tissue mass usually make this differentiation.

PARIETAL THINNING

An area of thinning of the bone is seen infrequently in the superior portion of one or both parietal bones. When viewed tangentially the inner table is seen to

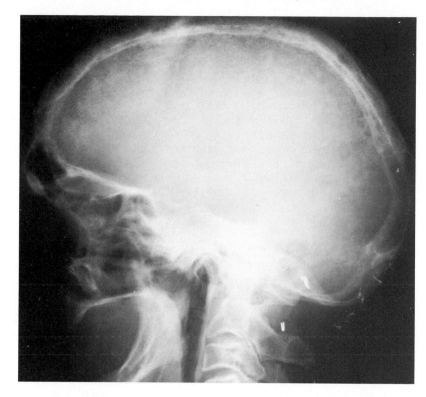

Fig. 3-11. Platybasia caused by Paget's disease of the skull. The basal angle is nearly 180 degrees (normal is 140 degrees). The deformity in this patient is caused by the softness of the cranial bones allowing the skull to be molded along the upper part of the cervical spine. A suboccipital craniectomy has been performed for decompression.

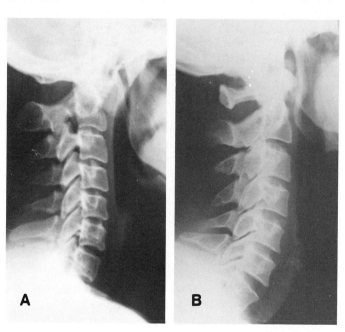

Fig. 3-12. Congenital cervico-occipital fusion. **A.** The first cervical vertebra is fused to the occiput, only a part of its arch being visible. **B.** Lateral view of the normal cervical spine (compare with **A**).

be normal but the diploë is absent in the area of thinning and the internal and external tables are fused. The defect extends in an anteroposterior direction and may be in the form of a distinct groove, which is easily palpated. It is usually bilateral but may be unilateral. It is usually found in the elderly (often associated with osteoporosis). Rarely it occurs in young adults. Tangential film will show the local thinning of the parietal bone with preservation of the inner table. Lateral views show a poorly defined elongated area of decreased density in the superior aspect of the parietal area which is not marginated. The condition is of no clinical importance and is not a cause of symptoms.

BATHROCEPHALY

In bathrocephaly, overgrowth of the apex of the occipital bone superiorly when viewed from the side, is seen to project posterior to the parietal bones. Its only importance lies in the fact that it may be mistaken for a depressed fracture.

ANOMALOUS PARIETAL SUTURES

Rarely the parietal bone may be divided symmetrically or asymmetrically by 1) an anomalous vertical suture between the sagittal and squamosal sutures, 2) an anomalous horizontal suture between the coronal and lambdoidal sutures, or 3) an oblique suture isolating a triangular portion of parietal bone to form what appears to be a large wormian bone.[32] Also there may be one or more small wormian bones along the course of the anomalous suture. Also the suture may be incomplete. Normally the parietal bone ossifies from a single center, therefore the sutures described here evidently indicate development of two centers that persist into adult life. Suture lines can be differentiated from skull fractures by the serration and sclerosis usually associated with cranial sutures; however, differentiation may be difficult in neonates, requiring a follow-up study for confirmation.

CONGENITAL VARIATIONS IN THE SPINE

Many developmental anomalies are found in the spinal column. Because of the important part that the spine plays in weight-bearing, some of these lead to clinical symptoms while others are only incidental findings and of importance only because they may be confused with changes resulting from trauma or disease.

DEVELOPMENT OF THE SPINE

Because of its importance in roentgen interpretation, a summary of the development of the spine as described by Ehrenhaft is given here. The column of cells derived from the entoderm around which the vertebrae develop is called the notochord. During the early weeks of embryonic life this forms a long rounded column extending from the hypophyseal pouch to the lower end of the primitive spine. It is the central structure around which the vertebrae are formed. Without going into the more precise details concerning vertebral development it is sufficient to recall that the mesenchyme surrounding the notochord undergoes segmentation with the formation of zones of densely packed cells, called scleromes, separated by less dense zones. The scleromes develop processes that form the anlagen for the vertebral bodies, the neural arches, and the transverse processes or ribs. Eventually the notochord is completely surrounded by the processes arising from the scleromes and the primitive vertebrae are formed. With further development the notochord becomes more and more squeezed into the regions that will become the intervertebral discs. The anlage for the vertebral body is divided initially into two lateral halves by an extension of the perichordal sheath. Centers of chondrification begin on either side of the sheath. The cartilage centers fuse, but for a time there is left a remnant of the sheath in the center of the cartilaginous body, known as the mucoid streak. This is continuous with the remnants of notochord that come to lie within the disc regions. These masses of notochordal cells, with the addition of mucoid material, fibrous tissue, and hyalin cartilage cells, form the nucleus pulposus of the fully developed disc. Notochordal cells can be identified in the nucleus until the age of adolescence or even later. During early life and until about the age of 25 to 30 years the nucleus forms a semifluid, noncompressible substance that is of great importance in absorbing shocks and in distributing the stresses to which the spine is subjected. During the period of its development the intervertebral disc is supplied by blood vessels derived from the periosteal vessesls as well as by some extending into the disc from the vertebral bodies. The latter vessels penetrate the cartilage plate surrounding the nucleus pulposus. Along with other degenerative changes that begin in the disc shortly after birth, these vessels regress and eventually disappear. Where the vessels penetrated the cartilage plates of the disc, defects in chondrification result and these may persist throughout life. They form weakened areas through which protrusion of disc material into the vertebral body can occur. These herniations are known as Schmorl nodes (Fig. 3-13). The discs become avascular during the third decade of life and the nucleus pulposus gradually is replaced by fibrous tissue.

While the remnants of notochord enclosed within cartilage will disappear as the disc becomes avascular, there are areas where small masses of fetal notochord may persist throughout life. These are found most frequently in the region of the clivus at the base of the skull and in the sacrococcygeal area. It is in these locations that tumor known as chordoma is prone to develop. Remnants of notochord sometimes persist where the mucoid streak entered the disc. These are visible roentgenologically as smooth, cup-shaped or concave defects centrally situated on the disc surface of one or more of the vertebral bodies. Usually the defects are multiple and they are seen most frequently in the lower part of the thoracic and upper part of the lumbar spine. Such defects represent weakened areas with thinning or, at times, a complete deficiency of the cartilage plates of the disc. They are in effect a congenital or developmental type of Schmorl node. In some instances larger masses of notochordal tissue remain, causing larger defects on the disc surface of the vertebral bodies. As has been noted, gaps in chondrification of the disc may form where the cartilage was perforated by vessels arising from the vertebral body. These weak areas predispose to traumatic protrusion of disc material. So long as the herniated material is composed only of cartilage the defect may be difficult or impossible to visualize in roentgenograms. Usually, with the passage of time, reactive sclerosis forms around the herniated cartilage nodule and it then becomes visible. Traumatic Schmorl nodes usually occur near the center of the disc surface of the body but may be situated eccentrically. The defect is concave and the wall of sclerosis usually is distinct. Thinning of the intervertebral disc space may or may not accompany herniation of disc material. Thinning of the disc in these patients is caused not so much by the actual loss of disc material as it is by the associated degenerative changes that may either precede or follow the herniation. With degeneration the disc loses turgor and elasticity and its total volume is reduced.

Ossification of the vertebral body begins at 3½ to 4 months of fetal life from two separate centers. These do not correspond to the two centers of chondrification mentioned above but rather are situated dorsally and ventrally to one another. Shortly after their appearance they fuse to form a single center for each vertebral body. The neural arch ossifies from two centers, one for each lateral half. At birth the vertebra

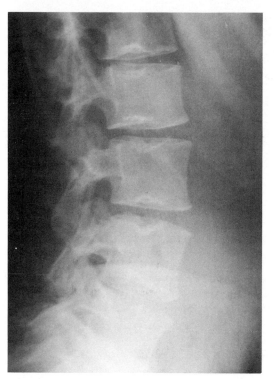

Fig. 3-13. Schmorl nodes. There are shallow, concave defects in the upper and lower disc surfaces of several lumbar vertebrae.

consists of three separate ossification areas, one for the body and two for the arch, and these are separated by zones of cartilage. Shortly after birth the two halves of the laminae unite, beginning first in the lumbar area and ascending to the cervical. Union of the arches to the bodies begins during the third year of life and is completed by about the seventh year. In this instance, fusion begins in the cervical region and is completed in the lumbar. At the time of puberty, secondary ossification centers appear for the tips of each of the vertebral processes and a ringlike epiphyseal plate for the upper and lower edges of the bodies also begins to ossify (Fig. 3-14).

FUSION OF VERTEBRAE

Fusion or partial fusion of two or more vertebral bodies is a frequent occurrence. Usually such fusion can be differentiated from that resulting from disease by the fact that the sum in height of the combined fused bodies is equal to the normal height of two vertebrae less the intervertebral disc space; the bony structure is normal except for the fusion; in cases of partial fusion it is the anterior aspect that fuses while

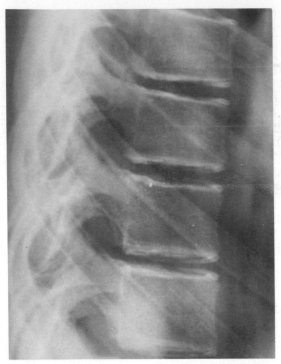

Fig. 3-14. Normal "ring" epiphysis of the vertebrae. Lateral view of midthoracic spine of an adolescent.

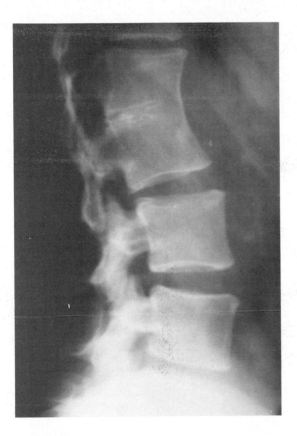

a rudiment of the disc remains in the posterior portion. This condition sometimes is called *Block vertebra* (Fig. 3-15). Clinical symptoms ordinarily are not associated with vertebral fusion except as listed under the two following headings.

Occipitocervical Fusion

This consists of a fusion or partial fusion of the atlas and the occiput. Associated with this there usually is deformity of the foramen magnum, which is often decreased in size and irregular in shape, and frequently a platybasia deformity of the skull. This has been discussed in the section "Platybasia" (see Fig. 3-12). In most normal individuals the upper edge of the odontoid process of the second cervical vertebra lies below a line drawn between the posterior margin of the hard palate and the posterior rim of the foramen magnum (Chamberlain's line) in a lateral roentgenogram of the skull and cervical spine. At times, in the normal individual, the odontoid projects slightly above this level, perhaps as much as 5 to 7 mm; when there is fusion of the first cervical vertebra and the occiput, the odontoid also is situated close to the occiput and will invariably extend above this line. McGregor's line also can be used. This is drawn from the upper surface of the posterior edge of the hard palate to the most inferior part of the floor of the posterior fossa, *i.e.,* the occipital curve. Normally, the tip of the odontoid does not project more than 4.0 mm above this line. There are several other lines that have been proposed to indicate abnormal elevation of the odontoid in its relation to the skull, but the two mentioned are the most commonly used. In some cases there is almost complete assimilation of the first cervical into the occiput with complete bony fusion of these structures. Because of the narrowing that results in the upper cervical spinal canal and at the level of the foramen magnum, pressure on the cord and medulla may result and these patients often develop symptoms simulating multiple sclerosis, lateral sclerosis, syringomyelia, and other neurologic disorders. Other bony anomalies lower in the cervical spine may cause cord compression leading to neurologic disorders. Tomography is useful in detection of arch anomalies of this type, since bone protruding into the spinal canal is readily observed.

Fig. 3-15. Congenital fusion of two lumbar vertebrae ("block vertebrae"). A remnant of the intervertebral disc is present posteriorly.

Klippel–Feil Syndrome

This syndrome is essentially an extensive fusion of the cervical spinal segments. There is numerical variation in the cervical vertebrae with more or less complete fusion into one bony mass or with multiple irregular ossified segments present. The upper dorsal vertebrae may be affected in the same way and there often are spina bifida defects as well as other skeletal anomalies (see Fig. 3-31). Males and females are affected equally. The classic physical signs include apparent absence or shortening of the neck with a lowering of the hairline on the back of the neck and limitation of motion of the head. Other signs and symptoms that may be present include torticollis, mirror movements, facial asymmetry, dorsal scoliosis, difficulty in breathing or swallowing, and hearing deficiencies. Klippel–Feil syndrome is sometimes associated with congenital elevation of the scapula (see Fig. 3-31).

NARROWING OR STENOSIS OF THE SPINAL CANAL

Congenital narrowing of the spinal canal may be caused by local overgrowth or hypertrophy or thickening of the laminae and pedicles, or, in some instances, the narrowing or stenosis may involve several segments such as in the narrow lumbar spinal canal syndrome in which there is developmental narrowing of the anteroposterior and interpedicular diameters of the lower two or three lumbar vertebrae. In the latter instances the laminae tend to be oriented vertically with a small interlaminar space. This latter syndrome does not appear to be familial. An anteroposterior diameter of 16 mm or less on the standard lateral lumbar spine film which reflects an actual diameter of less than 13 mm is used by Robertson and associates[28] in the diagnosis of this syndrome. Similar narrowing may occur in the cervical canal and less commonly in the thoracic canal.[4]

HEMIVERTEBRA

Failure or improper development of a lateral half of a vertebral body results in a hemivertebra. Embryologically the fault probably lies in an absence of one of the lateral centers of chondrification. A hemivertebra has a triangular shape when viewed in the anteroposterior roentgenogram and it causes an acute lateral angulation of the spine. A hemivertebra in the thoracic region has only one rib, that on the side of the ossified center. Associated with a hemivertebra there may be numerical variations in the ribs, fusion of two or more ribs, and rudimentary development of some of the others. Except for the scoliotic deformity that it causes, a hemivertebra is of no clinical importance (Fig. 3-16).

MIDLINE CLEFTS

Rarely the two lateral centers of chondrification for a vertebral body fail to fuse and a cleft persists in the midsagittal plane, dividing the body into two lateral halves. More frequently the cleft is only partial, resulting in a rather characteristic shape that is described as "butterfly vertebra" (Fig. 3-17). Another anomaly consists in a partial or complete cleft in the coronal plane, separating the vertebral body into anterior and posterior portions. Either the anterior or posterior half of a vertebral body may fail to develop and the result is a ventral or a dorsal hemivertebra. A dorsal hemivertebra is more common and because of its wedge shape and absence of normal ossification anteriorly a sharp gibbus deformity in the spine results.

Anterior midline cleft of the C1 arch may simulate a vertical odontoid fracture. This is extremely rare

Fig. 3-16. Congenital hemivertebrae in the thoracic spine of an infant. Three hemivertebral segments are visualized.

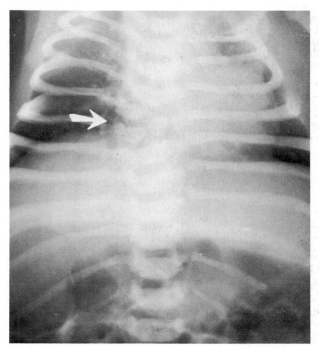

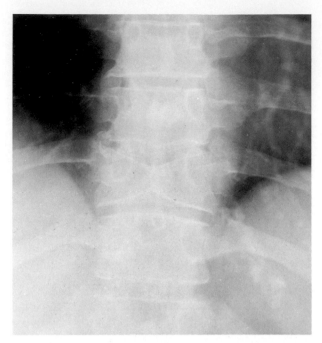

Fig. 3-17. Partial sagittal cleft of the tenth thoracic vertebra ("butterfly vertebra").

and is presumably associated with the presence of two centers for the anterior arch rather than the usual single center. Failure of fusion of the two centers results in the cleft.

The presence of a vertical cleft or ossification defect in the midline of a vertebral arch is common in the lumbosacral region or at other transitional areas in the spine. This condition is known as *spina bifida manifesta* when there are associated soft-tissue defects or when there is a meningocele; *spina bifida occulta* when no visible soft part malformation exists. Spina bifida occulta is frequent in the cervical spine where it involves the axis (C1) in 3% of all spines. Rarely there may be absence of all of the posterior arch of C1 except for a small ossification in the region of the posterior tubercle. Only slightly less common is spina bifida occulta of the first thoracic vertebra. Rarely an anterior cleft of the atlas associated with a posterior defect results in a bipartite first cervical vertebra. Spina bifida occulta is also very frequent in the lumbosacral region, affecting either the arch of the fifth lumbar or the first sacral segment. It is doubtful if any symptoms are caused by the defect in most cases. If there is an associated anomalous development of the articular processes or a partial fusion of adjacent vertebral bodies, such as sacralization of

the fifth lumbar or lumbarization of the first sacral segment, it is possible that localized weakness of the spine may result and become manifest after severe exertion. Some orthopedists place more emphasis on this condition than others and its importance as a cause of low-back disability is not entirely settled.

NEURAL ARCH DEFECTS

Cleft formation between the superior and inferior articular processes of a vertebra is frequent, the incidence being reported as from 6% to 7%. The clefts usually are bilateral and they predispose to the forward displacement of one vertebra upon the other. When clefts exist without displacement the condition is known as *spondylolysis*. If displacement is present it is termed *spondylolisthesis* (Fig. 3-18). This condition is observed most frequently at the lumbosacral joint where the clefts occur in the arch of the fifth lumbar; occasionally the fourth lumbar is affected. Rarely, spondylolysis occurs in the cervical spine, usually associated with spina bifida of the same level. Spondylolisthesis may also be present when the defect is bilateral. C6 is the most common cervical site. The amount of displacement varies widely in different cases. Meyerding's classification of the degree of spondylolisthesis is a useful one (Fig. 3-19). In a lateral roentgenogram the superior surface of the sacrum is divided into four equal parts. A forward displacement of the fifth lumbar up to one-fourth the thickness of the sacrum is called a first-degree spondylolisthesis, half the thickness a second-degree spondylolisthesis, and so on. Complete displacement of the fifth lumbar on the sacrum with the body of the fifth actually lying in front of the upper sacrum can happen. This is termed a fourth-degree spondylolisthesis. Because the clefts are present between the superior and inferior articular masses, the arch is not attached to the vertebral body by bony support and it is described as a "floating arch." When clefts are present the vertebral body often is decreased in size, particularly in its anteroposterior diameter. The arch may be generally small and poorly developed. Midline spina bifida is sometimes present. Most investigators are now of the opinion that lateral arch defects of this nature are acquired rather than being of developmental origin and have considered birth trauma with a failure of bony union at the sites of the arch fractures as a possible etiologic factor. Also, a chronic stress or fatigue fracture has been implicated in some cases while, in others, acute injury is the likely cause. Those who have described these defects as being of developmental origin consider them to result from

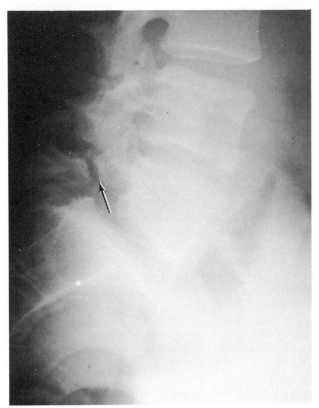

Fig. 3-18. Spondylolisthesis. Lateral view of the lumbosacral area showing a forward displacement of the fifth lumbar vertebra on the sacrum. Note the clefts in the arch between the upper and lower articular processes **(arrow).** The anteroposterior diameter of L5 is smaller than that of the other vertebrae.

Fig. 3-20. Transitional vertebra. The fifth lumbar is partially sacralized. Its left transverse process is broad and articulates with the sacrum. The right transverse process remains free.

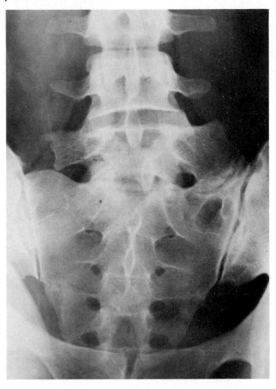

Fig. 3-19. Diagrams illustrating Meyerding's classification of spondylolisthesis. The superior surface of the sacrum is divided into four zones. The diagrams, from left to right, illustrate first-, second-, third-, and fourth-degree spondylolisthesis.

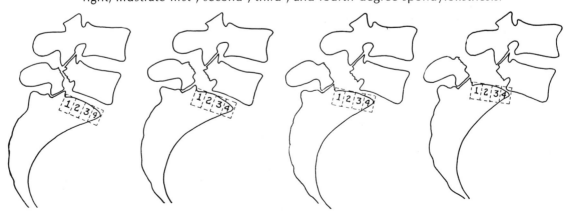

the presence of two ossification centers for each side of the arch with subsequent failure of fusion. However, the accumulated evidence indicates an acquired origin in most cases.

UNFUSED CENTER FOR ARTICULAR PROCESS

A small, triangular bony mass may be found at the tip of one or more of the inferior articular processes of the vertebrae. This represents an ununited ossification center and it can be confused with a fracture. Isolated fracture of this process is very unusual without an associated fracture of the body or neural arch. A similar center occasionally is seen for the superior articular process but is much less frequent.

TRANSITIONAL VERTEBRA

At the junctions of the various major divisions of the spine a vertebra may take on part of the characteristics of both divisions. This is most frequent at the dorsolumbar and the lumbosacral areas. The first lumbar, and rarely the second, may have rudimentary ribs articulating with the transverse processes. The fifth lumbar may be partially sacralized, often with one transverse process fused with the sacrum, the other being free and with only a rudimentary disc between them (Fig. 3-20). The first sacral segment may become partially lumbarized in the same manner. When the transition is complete there will be six lumbar vertebrae or thirteen dorsal and four lumbar or various combinations. As a rule an addition of a segment to one division of the spine will be corrected at another level.

The seventh cervical vertebra may have ribs attached to its transverse processes. The ribs may be only short, nubbinlike structures or they may be long enough to articulate with the sternum. Frequently the rib is fused with the first dorsal rib or it forms a pseudarthrosis with it. Even when the rib is short a fibrous band may extend from its tip to the first rib or to the sternum and be a source of pressure upon the brachial plexus or the subclavian artery. There may be only one rib or the condition may be bilateral.

DIASTEMATOMYELIA

This is a rare anomaly of the vertebrae and the spinal cord, usually consisting of a vertical division of the cord or the cauda equina, the two portions being separated by an osseous or fibrocartilaginous septum. This septum is attached anteriorly to one or more of the vertebral bodies. Frequently there is anomalous ossification of the vertebrae; the interpedicular spaces are widened at the site of the defect. Diastematomyelia is found most frequently in the lumbar part of the spine, less commonly in the thoracic region. The lesion is clincally significant and the patient will show evidence sooner or later of impaired innervation to the lower extremities. Dimpling of the skin, local pigmentation, or excessive hair may be present over the area at birth. Occasionally there is an associated meningocele. Roentgenograms of the spine show widening of the neural canal over several segments and often a fusion or partial fusion of vertebral bodies. Other abnormalities commonly associated include kyphosis, scoliosis, spina bifida, hemivertebrae, abnormal fusion of laminae and narrowing of intervertebral spaces. If the septum dividing the cord is ossified it may be visualized in anteroposterior views as a vertical thin bony plate lying in the midline of the neural canal. When an iodized oil such as Pantopaque is injected into the spinal subarachnoid space the defect caused by the septum is readily demonstrated (Fig. 3-21). This procedure of myelography is discussed more fully in Chapter 12.

SACRAL AGENESIS; THE CAUDAL DYSPLASIA SYNDROME

Absence of part or all of the sacrum is an uncommon but not rare anomaly. There is a high incidence of neurogenic bladder in these infants with the complications of vesicoureteral reflux, hydronephrosis, and infection. Occasionally, patients with agenesis of the sacrum or of the lumbar vertebrae or both show a more severe neurologic deficit below the level of the vertebral anomaly which may be complete. The changes associated with sacral agenesis have been termed the *caudal dysplasia syndrome.* [13] In addition to neurogenic bladder, in the more severe cases there may be abduction and flexion deformities of the lower extremities with popliteal webbing so that the legs cannot be straightened. The appearance of the lower extremities has been described as "froglike" or as having a "stuck-on" appearance. Most patients have an equinovarus deformity of the feet and, less frequently, dislocation of the hips. Anomalies in other systems that may be present include renal agenesis, congenital heart disease, imperforate anus, cleft lip or palate, and microcephaly. The upper extremities usually are normal. The increased frequency of this syndrome in infants of diabetic mothers has been commented upon in the literature.

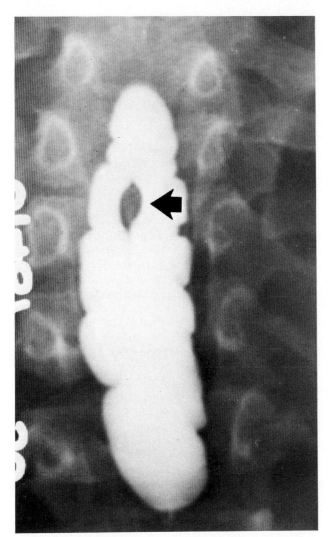

semble the deformity produced by a fracture. Recognition of the increased height together with the normal texture and appearance of the bone will aid in preventing error. Secondary ossification centers appear at the tips of all the vertebral processes; occasionally one or more of these fail to unite and will persist into adult life as a separate bony fragment. Anterior herniation of the nucleus pulposus may cause a separation of a triangular, smooth, bone fragment which apparently represents the ring apophysis. It then fails to unite. This results in a triangular bony mass along the anterior border with a corresponding defect in the adjacent vertebral body and is known as *limbus vertebra* (Fig. 3-22). A discogram[15] may be used to confirm the presence of the anterior disc herniation in these patients. The vertebral bodies may be unusually wide for their heights, the

Fig. 3-22. Limbus vertebra. There is an unfused ossification center along the upper anterior border of the fourth lumbar vertebra. This should not be mistaken for fracture. It is found most frequently in the lumbar area.

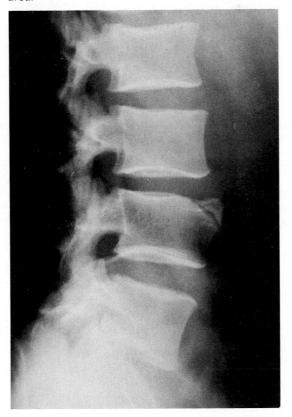

Fig. 3-21. Diastematomyelia. Oil myelogram illustrating the central defect in the oil column caused by the bony spur **(arrow).** Note the widened interpediculate distances of most of the vertebrae at and below the level of the spur. Fusion anomalies are also present.

MISCELLANEOUS ANOMALIES

Many other variations in development may be found in the spine. The vertebral bodies may be abnormally tall or one or more may show an increased height with the adjacent ones normal. Occasionally a vertebra may be of unusual height in its posterior aspect while the anterior part is normal. This causes it to appear wedge-shaped in the lateral view and to recondition being termed "platyspondyly." This is often associated with other anomalies, particularly of the spinal cord (see section on Diastematomyelia) and in the mucopolysaccharidoses (see Ch. 2).

Absence or hypoplasia of a pedicle is occasionally observed in the cervical spine. Absence of a lumbar pedicle with compensatory hypertrophy of the opposite pedicle has been reported but is exceedingly rare. The hypertrophy of the opposite pedicle differentiates this anomaly from acquired pedicular lesions. Furthermore, there are other associated congenital anomalies such as persistent synchondrosis between the two halves of the arch, short vertical cleft in the opposite pedicle or an adjacent one, and, usually, hypoplasia of ipsilateral arch elements. The intervertebral foramen is widened, and there is posterior displacement of the maldeveloped lateral mass. Absence or hypoplasia of a pedicle must be differentiated from erosions caused by neurofibromatosis, metastatic tumors, vertebral artery aneurysm, and from arch fractures.

Moderate to severe local flattening or thinning of a pedicle at the twelfth thoracic or first lumbar level, either unilaterally or bilaterally, is a common anatomic variant.[4] The inner margin may be straight, convex, or occasionally, concave, while the outer margin may be flat or concave. A slight increase in the interpedicular distance at the involved level is common, despite the absence of mass within the spinal canal.

Several anomalies may involve the lamina chiefly in the thoracic and lumbar spine including absence of an inferior articular process, hypoplasia of an inferior articular process, absence of the lamina, and a notch in the inferior lamina which is usually present bilaterally.

CONGENITAL VARIATIONS OF EXTREMITIES, THORAX, AND PELVIS

In addition to the ununited ossification centers and supernumerary bones referred to previously, a large number of malformations may involve parts of the skeleton. Many of these are obvious on clinical examination and roentgen study is useful only to make a record of the anatomic changes. Among these are such easily recognized defects as absence of a part and the presence of supernumerary digits. A few of these defects deserve mention because they may be confused with acquired disease and others cause significant deformities and interference with functions.

DIASTASIS OF PUBIC BONES

This condition is ordinarily found associated with exstrophy of the bladder, epispadius, and other lower urinary tract anomalies. It may also be associated with cleidocranial dysostosis. However, it has also been reported in a family with no other anomalies.[30]

CONGENITAL SYNOSTOSIS

A congenital synostosis consists of a fusion of two or more bones. It is a frequent anomaly in the thorax where there may be a partial fusion of several of the ribs. This may affect any part of the rib but is more frequent in the lateral portions and at the vertebral ends. In the latter location the fused ribs may cause a dense shadow along the mediastinum which may, on casual inspection of thoracic roentgenograms, be interpreted as a mass in the mediastinum or the lung.

The proximal ends of the tibia and fibula occasionally are fused. Another uncommon site of fusion is at the proximal ends of the radius and ulna; this results in an inability to supinate the forearm. In some cases there is an associated dislocation of the head of the radius (Fig. 3-23).

Fusion of the vertebral bodies has been discussed in the previous section dealing with the spine.

The *calcaneonavicular bar* is a bony bridge, complete or incomplete, between the os calcis and the navicular and it may lead to the clinical condition referred to as "peroneal spastic flatfoot" or "rigid flatfoot." The latter term is perferred since the rigidity of the tarsus is the result of bony fixation and not of spasm. The bony fusion may occur at any point between the two bones but is most frequent along the anteromedial aspect. The bony bridge may be incomplete with a fibrous or cartilaginous type of union present. Other tarsal bones may be fused to one another and the general class of these fusion anomalies is known as *tarsal coalition* (Fig. 3-24). Because of the unusual rigidity of the fused joints, clinical complaints of pain may ensue, particularly when unusual stresses are placed upon the foot.

CONGENITAL DISLOCATION OF THE HIP

The hip is the most frequent site of congenital dislocation. It is six to ten times as common in females as in males, the left hip is involved more often than the right in the ratio of 3:2, and it is much more frequent in whites than in Blacks. It is unusual for dislocation to be present at birth; rather displacement occurs gradually during the first year of life. Because it has

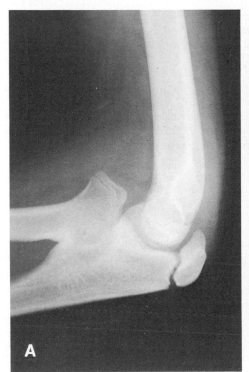
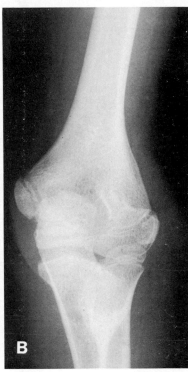

Fig. 3-23. Congenital radioulnar synostosis with congenital dislocation of the head of the radius. There is bony fusion between the dislocated radius and the ulna.

Fig. 3-24. Calcaneonavicular bar **(arrow).**

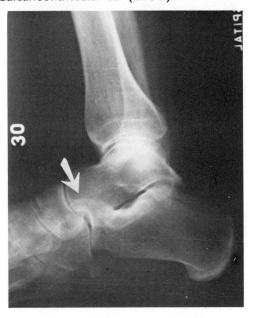

been believed that faulty development of the hip joint and its associated structures was responsible for the dislocation, the term "hip joint dysplasia" has come into common use to denote the conditions that may be present before actual dislocation has developed. However, it is no longer believed by most writers on the subject that the fault lies in lack of proper development or hypoplasia of the bony structures of the hip, particularly the acetabulum. Rather, most investigators consider the fault to be in the supporting soft tissues of the hip joint with the primary abnormality being relaxation of the joint capsule. Shortening or tightening of the muscles which activate motion across the joint is considered by some to be the result rather than the cause of the dislocation. Others, however, consider this to be one of the primary causes along with increased relaxation of the fibrocartilaginous structures, so that when stress is applied dislocation will result. The diagnosis of the predislocation stage during the newborn period is often difficult both clinically and roentgenologically. Caffey and his associates[6] seriously doubt the existence of a dysplastic or predislocation phase, at least in a form that can be recognized by clinical or roentgen examinations.

According to Doberti and Manhood[9] the head of

the femur, even though still cartilaginous, will produce a shallow concavity or fossa on the superior wall of the acetabulum through muscular traction and pressure. The floor of the fossa is bounded by a sclerotic margin which aids in identifying it in the neonatal period. Identification of this shallow fossa aids in determining the position of the cartilaginous femoral head. If it lies within the inner one-third of the acetabular roof, the head is considered to be in normal position. If situated more laterally, the head is considered to be in abnormal position and the hip dysplastic.

Roentgen examination of the hips for a suspected hip joint dislocation should include an anteroposterior roentgenogram of the pelvis obtained with the patient's legs straight or slightly flexed at the knee and with the toes pointing forward, and a so-called "frog" view. In this position the thighs are flexed, externally rotated and maximally abducted with the feet brought together in the midline. Careful positioning is necessary to make certain that the hips are symmetrically placed in relation to the film cassette and the roentgen-ray tube so that one side can be compared with the other.

Roentgen Observations

Increased Acetabular Angle. The acetabular angle is in effect a measure of the slope of the upper half of the acetabular wall. The method of determining it is shown in Figure 3-25. For some time it has been considered that the normal acetabular angle for a newborn infant should be approximately 25 degrees with

an upper limit of 30 degrees. The acetabular angle as shown in Figure 3-25 is determined by drawing a line along the iliac portion of the acetabular roof to its point of intersection with a line drawn through the centers of both acetabula. An angle above 30 degrees was considered as significant for the presence of hip joint dysplasia that would in turn predispose to hip joint dislocation. Observations of Coleman and of Caffey and his associates,[6] based upon the measurement of a large number of infants, indicate that the

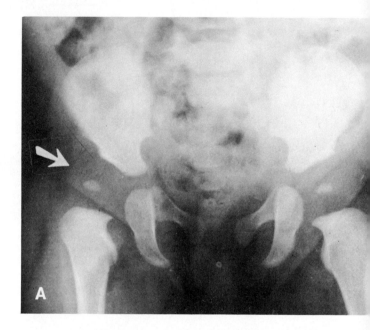

Fig. 3-25. Congenital dislocation of the right hip in an infant. **A.** Roentgenogram of the pelvis. **B.** Tracing illustrating the method for determining the acetabular angle. The line **A** drawn along the upper margin of the acetabulum represents the bony roof of the fossa, although, in an infant, the acetabulum is composed largely of cartilage. While the acetabular angle is larger on the right than on the left, this difference is not entirely diagnostic. The other findings indicate that subluxation is present, since the capital epiphysis is displaced laterally and very slightly superiorly. The line **H** is drawn through the centers of the triradiate cartilages of the acetabular fossae. The vertical lines **P** are drawn through the outer limits of the bony margin of the acetabular roof on either side perpendicular to the **H** line. Note that the right femoral epiphysis is located in a more lateral position than the left in this patient. The curved broken line **S,** or Shenton's line, is disrupted on the right and normal on the left.

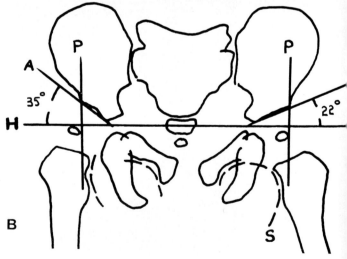

normal angles vary widely and that the upper limit of normal should be close to 40 degrees. These observations indicate that considerable caution should be exercised in the diagnosis of hip joint dysplasia based only upon the finding of an acetabular angle that measures more than 30 degrees. When only one hip is affected, the acetabular angle is more useful than when both are involved and a definite discrepancy in the angles on the two sides is an important finding. It should be noted in this regard that Caffey's figures indicate that the acetabular angle for the left hip is usually slightly larger than the right. The normal angle decreases considerably between birth and the age of 6 months and to a lesser degree between the ages of 6 months and 1 year.

The iliac angle also can be measured and, when added to the acetabular angle, gives the iliac index. The method for obtaining the iliac angle and index is given in Figures 3-36 and 3-37 near the end of this chapter.

Lateral Displacement of the Femur. An important finding in many cases is a lateral displacement of the femur in its relationship to the acetabulum. Because the ossification center for the head of the femur is not present at birth and does not appear normally until the age of 3 to 6 months, the neck of the femur must be used for this determination in the newborn. The distance of the upper inner margin of the femoral neck to a fixed point in the acetabulum, such as the inferior edge of the ischial portion, can be measured and, if one hip is normal and the other is displaced, there will be a measurable difference. Perkin's line, as shown in Figure 3-25, is useful when either one or both hips are involved. This consists of a vertical line drawn from the upper outer edge of the iliac portion of the acetabulum to intersect at a right angle the transverse line drawn through the centers of both acetabula. Coleman found that normally the beak of the femoral neck fell medial to this line in practically every case while in the majority of abnormal hips (60%) the femoral neck was situated lateral to this line.

Disruption of Shenton's Line. Shenton's line is a smooth, curved imaginary line formed by the inner margin of the femoral neck and the inner surface of the obturator foramen as shown in Figure 3-25. A lateral displacement of the femur may disrupt the smooth curve but usually it requires some degree of upward displacement before a significant break in the curve is seen.

Delayed Ossification of Femoral Epiphysis. The ossification center for the head of the femur appears normally between the ages of 3 to 6 months. In the presence of hip joint subluxation or dislocation the center may be delayed in appearance and when it does appear its growth lags behind the normal (Fig. 3-26). In the older infant a disparity in the size of the centers for the femoral heads should be viewed with suspicion as a possible indicator of subluxation on the side of the smaller center. Other signs must be present, however, before this finding can be considered of significance and as a solitary observation it need not be abnormal.

Later Stages. In older children and in adults, gross displacement usually is present and the diagnosis is made without difficulty (Fig. 3-27). In untreated subjects the head and neck of the femur do not develop properly, remaining small and hypoplastic. The acetabular fossa is very shallow, never having accommodated the femoral head. The head often impinges against the outer pelvic wall above and behind the shallow acetabulum and here a shallow pseudo-acetabular cavity may form.

Hip Joint Dysplasia in the Adult. is still somewhat debatable whether there is such an entity as hip joint dysplasia, that is, underdevelopment or hypoplasia of the acetabulum and partial subluxation of the femoral head. Some support for this opinion is given by the work of Doberti and Manhood referred to earlier.[9] Also, there are some hip joints in adults in which the acetabulum is small or shallow and the fit of the femoral head is poor. The early development of degenerative joint disease in these hips is common.

Other Congenital Dislocations

Congenital dislocations affecting joints other than the hip are infrequent. In the elbow joint dislocation of the radial head is seen occasionally. In these cases the radial head is displaced forward on the humerus. In some cases there is an associated congenital fusion of the dislocated radius with the proximal part of the ulna, the latter bone maintaining a normal relationship with the humerus (see Fig. 3-23). This lesion may be unilateral but more often is bilateral. With the passage of time it will be noted that the head of the radius fails to develop properly and the proximal end of the bone is smaller than the normal.

(Text continues on p. 93.)

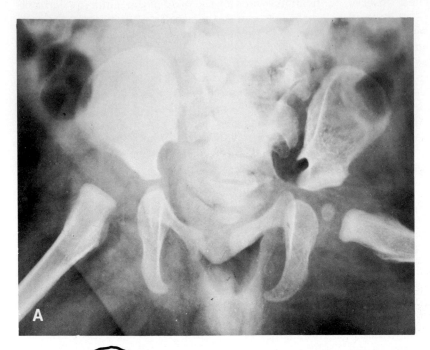

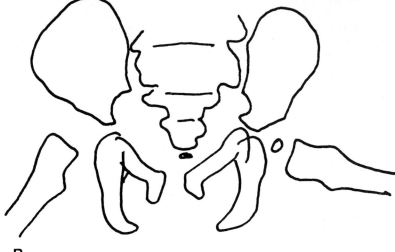

Fig. 3-26. Congenital hip joint dislocation illustrating the frog position with the thighs abducted and externally rotated. Note the absence of an ossified center for the right capital epiphysis and the poorly developed acetabular roof on this side, and an increased acetabular angle. The position of the femoral neck indicates the subluxation even though the femoral head is not visible. The patient also has extensive spina bifida in the lower lumbar and sacral spine. **A.** Roentgenogram of the pelvis. **B.** Tracing of the roentgenogram.

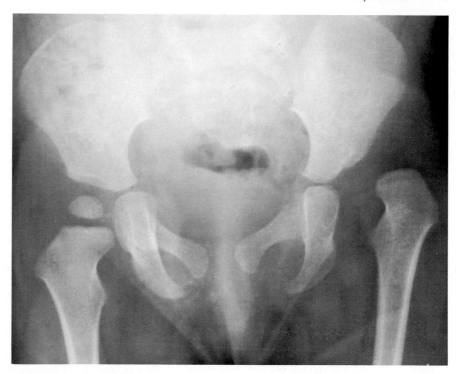

Fig. 3-27. Congenital dislocation of the left hip in an older child. The capital epiphysis has not developed an ossification center. The left acetabulum is hypoplastic with marked increase in the acetabular angle.

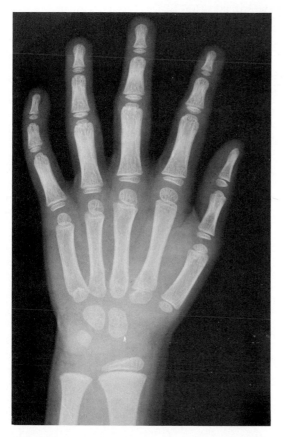

Fig. 3-28. Pseudoepiphyses and supernumerary epiphyses. The former are represented by incomplete clefts in the distal ends of the proximal phalanges and proximal end of the fifth metacarpal. The latter are present at the proximal end of the second metacarpal and the distal end of the first metacarpal.

MISCELLANEOUS ANOMALIES

Forked Ribs. The sternal end of a rib may be bifid or forked. The third and fourth ribs are most frequently involved.

Fenestrated First Rib. Fenestration of the first rib consists of a smooth, rounded opening in the anterior end of the rib. The significance of this deformity lies in the fact that it may be mistaken for a cavity in the lung in roentgenograms of the chest.

Supracondylar Process of the Humerus. This is a small bony spur found occasionally along the anteromedial border of the distal third of the humerus. It is directed distally and may form a foramen as in some of the lower animals.

Rhomboid Fossa of the Clavicle. Occasionally a well-marked concave depression is seen on the undersurface of the sternal end of the clavicle. This is a fossa for the attachment of the rhomboid ligament.

Pseudoepiphyses for the Metacarpals and Metatarsals. These are partial cartilaginous clefts appearing in the proximal ends of one or more of the lateral four or the distal end of the first metacarpal or metatarsal where normally no epiphyses are found. Less frequently the cleft is complete; these are termed *supernumerary epiphyses* (Fig. 3-28). It has been suggested that pseudoepiphyses and supernumerary epiphyses, especially when occurring in more than one bone, indicate the likely presence of other congenital stigmas or of disease acquired early in life. Some evidence has been presented to indicate that malnutrition during infancy or early childhood is important in the causation of these defects.

Kirner's Deformity (Clinodactyly). This deformity is an anterior and radial curvature of the shaft of the terminal phalanx of the fifth finger associated with a widening of the epiphyseal plate and partial dorsal displacement of the shaft on the epiphysis.[37] The epiphyseal margin adjacent to the growth plate is irregular. The entire distal phalanx may be shortened. The deformity may occur as an isolated defect, usually bilateral, or as a part of a more generalized growth disorder or dysplasia. It is more common in females than in males (66% of cases reported in the literature occurred in females).

Physiologic Bowlegs of Infancy. During early infancy a mild degree of bowleg deformity is physiological. In addition to an actual bowing of the bones, the bowed appearance is accentuated by the distribution of fat. It has been suggested that this bowing is the result of the normal internal tibial torsion that occurs during intrauterine life. Occasionally this bowing is accentuated to the point where it may be considered abnormal (Fig. 3-29) and the result of disease, particularly rickets or Blount's tibia vara (see Ch. 2). Differentiation from rickets can be made with assurance in most cases because the metaphyses are well ossified and none of the other findings seen in active rickets are present. It may not be possible to exclude the possibility of a healed rickets but, since this type of bowing usually comes to the attention of the physician during the first months or year of life, there seldom will have been time for rickets to have been present and to have undergone complete healing. Differentiation from Blount's tibia vara may be more difficult. In tibia vara the deformity is an angular one centered at the junction of the proximal metaphysis and epiphysis of the tibia; there is a broad beaklike projection of the inner side of the metaphysis within which are small islands of cartilage, and the tibial epiphysis tends to be triangular with the apex pointing medially. In physiologic bowing, both the tibia and femur are affected, the femur often showing more deformity than the tibia. Both the upper metaphysis of the tibia and the lower metaphysis of the femur show medial beaks but they are pointed rather than blunt. This type of bowleg deformity tends to correct itself and usually the legs have become perfectly straight by the time the child has reached the age of 4 to 5 years.

MADELUNG'S DEFORMITY

Madelung's deformity is a chondrodysplasia of the distal radial epiphysis. Some investigators believe that this deformity is a part of the dysplasia known as dyschondrosteosis (Ch. 2); others believe that it can occur as a separate deformity without other osseous stigmata; or it may be a minimal form of dyschondreostosis. It causes a curvature of the shaft of the radius, giving a bayonet-shaped deformity of the hand at the wrist somewhat as though there were an anterior dislocation of the hand. The reverse type also is seen but is very rare. The lesion usually is bilateral and the deformity is first noticed at about the beginning of adolescence. The characteristic roentgen findings include:

1. The radius is shortened in comparison to the length of the ulna.

2. There is lateral and dorsal curvature of the radius.

3. There is early fusion of the radial epiphysis on the internal side. This results in a tilting of the radial articular surface so that it faces internally and anteriorly more than normal. The epiphysis develops a triangular shape.

4. Because the radius fails to grow properly in length there develops a subluxation of the radioulnar articulation and the lower end of the ulna projects posterior to the radius.

5. The deformity of the radial articular surface leads to a derangement in alignment of the carpal bones. The carpus assumes the form of a pyramid with the apex pointing toward the radius and ulna and the base being formed by the carpometacarpal articulations (Fig. 3-30).

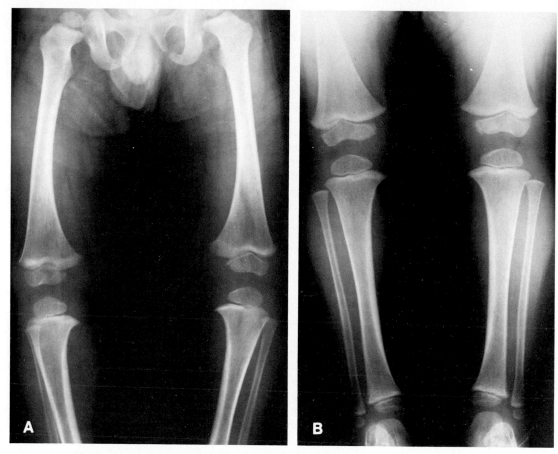

Fig. 3-29. Physiologic bowlegs. **A.** Initial views demonstrate moderate bowleg deformity. **B.** Approximately 1 year later the bowing has largely disappeared. Note that the bowing involves both femur and tibia.

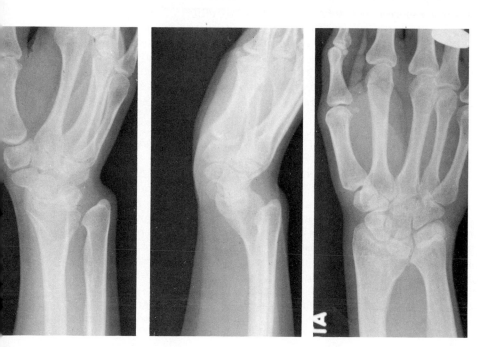

Fig. 3-30. Madelung's deformity.

SPRENGEL'S DEFORMITY

Sprengel's deformity also is known as congenital high scapula or congenital elevation of the scapula. The scapula is small, high in position, and rotated so that the inferior edge points toward the spine. The deformity may be unilateral or bilateral. A fusion of the cervical and upper thoracic vertebrae, the Klippel-Feil syndrome, is present in practically all cases (Fig. 3-31). This fusion anomaly may exist, however, without elevation of the scapula. In some cases there is a bony connection between the elevated scapula and one of the vertebrae, usually the fifth or sixth cervical. This bony connection is known as the *omovertebral bone* and it may join the scapula and the vertebrae by either bony or fibrous union (Fig. 3-32).

OSTEOCHONDROSIS DEFORMANS TIBIAE (TIBIA VARA; BLOUNT'S DISEASE)

Blount's disease is an infrequent cause of bowlegs during infancy and childhood. Its cause is uncertain but it often is classified with the osseous dysplasias. The possibility of ischemic necrosis as a causative factor has been considered by some investigators. Clinically there is a progressive nonrachitic outward bowing of the legs. The medial aspect of the upper tibial metaphysis is evidently the site of partial growth arrest resulting in medial flangelike broadening of the metaphysis in addition to shortening. This causes a rather sharp posteromedial slope of the medial tibial plateau. The amount of varus deformity depends on the angle of this slope.

The deformity actually is an angular one rather than a curved bowing, and is centered at the junction of the proximal tibial epiphysis and metaphysis (Fig. 3-33). For differential considerations see discussion of "Physiologic bowlegs of Infancy."

ONYCHO-OSTEO-ARTHRODYSPLASIA (NAIL–PATELLA SYNDROME, HEREDITARY ARTHRODYSPLASIA AND DYSTROPHY OF THE NAILS, J. W. TURNER SYNDROME)

This rare condition, transmitted as an autosomal dominant trait, is a complex disorder characterized by abnormalities of the fingernails, absence or hypoplasia of the patella, defects in the head of the radius, discoloration of the iris, and bony processes along the posterior surfaces of the iliac bones (iliac horns) (Fig. 3-34). Not all features of the syndrome need to be present in the individual case. The disorder affecting the nails varies from unusual thinning and small size to a complete absence of one or more of the nails. The thumb is involved most frequently and severely. The patellae are absent or small and hypoplastic. The femoral condyles, particularly the medial, may be unusually prominent and there may be a genu valga deformity. In the elbow, the head of the radius is poorly formed; in some subjects the radius is abnormally long so that the head projects behind the joint when the forearm is flexed. Less frequently, other bones show deformity in size and shape. The iliac horns are not a constant feature, but, in some of these patients, they appear to be the only abnormality. Fong was the first to report a case of this nature.[12] The lesions consist in bilateral, pointed, bony projections or exostoses extending posteriorly from the iliac bone. Increased hyperextension mobility of interphalangeal joints, flexion deformity of the hips, and genu recurvatum may be observed clinically.

PROGERIA

Progeria, also known as the *Hutchinson–Gilford syndrome*, is, essentially, premature senility developing in a child.[25] The infants appear normal at birth but the typical features become evident within the first few years of life. The appearance has been likened to that of "a wizened old man." There is loss of subcutaneous fat, alopecia, and atrophy of the muscles and the skin. The facies show a receding chin, beaked nose, and exophthalmos. There is premature arteriosclerosis in the coronary arteries and other vessels which leads to death during late childhood or early adolescence. The patients are dwarfed. Roentgen findings include hypoplastic facial bones, open cranial sutures and fontanelles, and dwarfism. The long bones are apt to be short, thin, and osteoporotic, and there is coxa valga which may be marked. A significant feature is acro-osteolysis of the terminal digits of the fingers and toes.

CHROMOSOMAL ABNORMALITIES

The normal human cell contains 22 pairs of somatic chromosomes, called autosomes, numbered from one through 22, and two sex chromosomes, XX in the female and XY in the male, for a total of 46. The somatic chromosomes are usually placed into seven groups: group A, numbers one through three; group B, 4 and 5; group C, 6 through 12; group D, 13 through 15; group E, 16 through 18; group F, 19 and 20; and group G, 21 and 22. The addition of a chromosome to one of the autosomal groups leads to one of the trisomy syndromes, the most common loca-

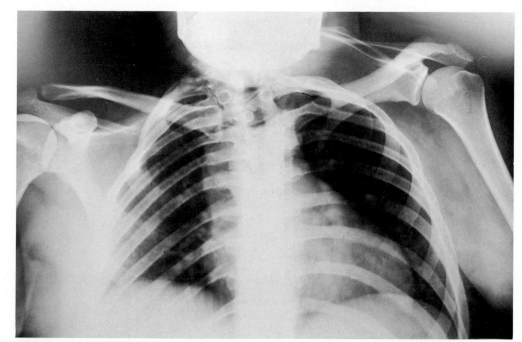

Fig. 3-31. Sprengel's deformity. The left shoulder is affected. There is an associated abnormality of ossification of the cervical and upper thoracic vertebrae with irregular segments fused together (Klippel–Feil deformity). These deformities frequently coexist.

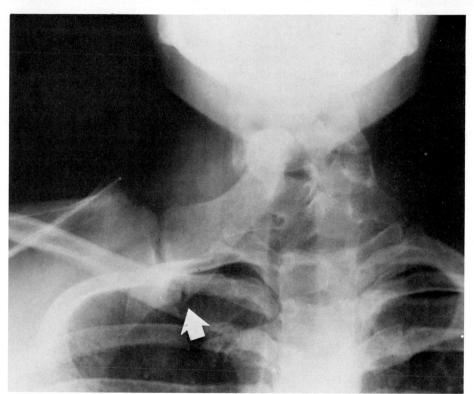

Fig. 3-32. The omovertebral bone in association with Sprengel's deformity and Klippel–Feil deformity. The bone forms an articulation with the scapula **(arrow)** and the arch of one of the cervical vertebrae.

tions being the 13–15, the 16–18, and 21–22 groups. Of the entities caused by abnormality of the sex chromosomes, Turner's syndrome is most likely to have significant roentgen findings.

TRISOMY 21 SYNDROME; MONGOLISM; DOWN'S SYNDROME

Mongolism is the result of an autosomal trisomy of chromosome 21. A number of skeletal stigmas have been described in mongolism, some of which are fairly specific and aid in recognition of the disease when clinical findings are equivocal, that is, during the early months of life. Among the skeletal anomalies that have been described are the following:

1. In the pelvis, during infancy the acetabular angles are flattened, the iliac bones large and flared and the ischia elongated and tapering (Fig. 3-35). The iliac index is decreased. The iliac index is said to be more significant than the acetabular angle in the diagnosis of mongolism. This index consists of the sum of the acetabular and iliac angles on both sides, divided by two. The method for determining the index is shown in Figures 3-36 and 3-37. In the newborn the normal iliac index has a mean value of 81 degrees with a range of 68 to 97 degrees. In mongolism the index has a mean value of 62 degrees with a range from 49 to 87 degrees. According to Astley[2] if the index is under 60 degrees, mongolism is very probable; if it is over 78 degrees, the child probably is normal. These changes are

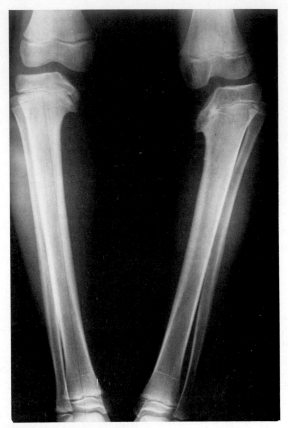

Fig. 3-33. Blount's disease. There is bilateral involvement with an angular deformity at the physis. The tibial shafts are straight and the femurs uninvolved.

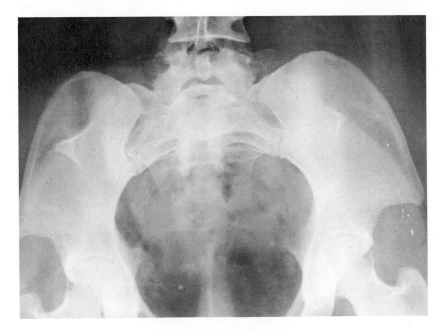

Fig. 3-34. Iliac horns in a patient with hereditary arthrodysplasia. Note the pointed projections along the posterior surfaces of the ilia.

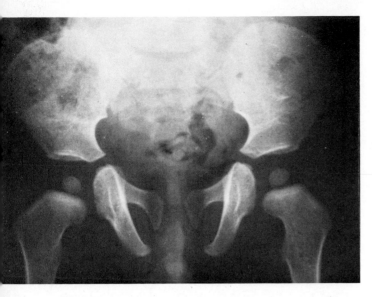

Fig. 3-35. Down's syndrome (trisomy 21). There is flaring of the ilia; elongated tapered ischia; and flattening of the acetabular angles.

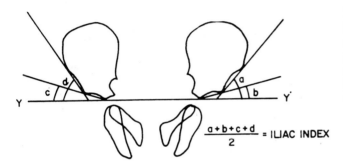

Fig. 3-36. Method for determining the acetabular and iliac angles and the iliac index. This index is the sum of the acetabular angles (**b** and **c**) and the iliac angles (**a** and **d**), divided by 2. The diagram illustrates the proper placement of the lines necessary for determining the various angles. (Tong ECK: Radiology 91: 376, 1968)

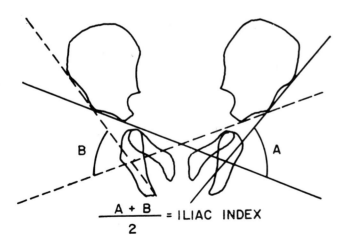

Fig. 3-37. Tong's method for determining the iliac index (**A** and **B** divided by 2). The measurement of the larger angles gives less chance for error than the method shown in Figure 3-36. (Tong, ECK: Radiology 91: 376, 1968)

most significant during the first 6 to 12 months of life.

2. Shortening of the middle phalanx of the fifth finger.

3. The manubrium sterni may ossify from two or three centers instead of one as is normal. This can be identified in a lateral view of the chest.

4. The lumbar vertebrae may be small in the anteroposterior diameter and increased in height.

5. Dental defects with anomalies of the teeth and delay in eruption have been noted frequently.

6. Coxa vara may be present.

7. Skull changes include: (*a*) the sphenoid is rotated up and back in relation to the clivus, (*b*) the bones of the calvarium are thin, (*c*) the palate has a high short arch, (*d*) the nasal sinuses are hypoplastic, (*e*) the interorbital distance is decreased (hypotelorism), and (*f*) closure of the cranial sutures may be delayed.

8. Subluxation of the atlas is common. The normal atlanto-odontoid interval in children has an upper limit of 5.0 mm.

9. Visceral anomalies include congenital heart disease, usually atrioventricular canal, an increased frequency of an aberrant right subclavian artery, and duodenal obstruction (duodenal atresia or annular pancreas).

TRISOMY 18 SYNDROME

Recent advances in cytogenetics have brought about recognition of several new syndromes of which the trisomy 18 syndrome is one of the most frequent. The abnormalities result from an extra chromosome for number 18. The clinical and roentgen findings include:[22] (*1*) Low-set, malformed ears and recession of the chin (mandibular and maxillary hypoplasia). (*2*) Ulnar deviation of the fingers with flexion deformities. When the fingers are forcibly extended the second and third fingers form a V-shaped notch. (*3*) Retarded bone age. (*4*) Short, hypoplastic first metacarpals. (*5*) Pseudoepiphyses for the metacarpals. (*6*) Equinovarus and "rocker-bottom" feet with hammer-toe deformities, short first toe, and hypoplastic distal phalanges. (*7*) Thin ribs and short, undersegmented sternum and an increase in the anteroposterior diameter of the chest. (*8*) Narrow transverse diameter of the pelvis due to anterior rotation of the ilia (antimongoloid pelvis). (*9*) Hypoplasia or absence of the medial third of the clavicle. (*10*) Hypoplastic dislocated femoral heads and with increased acetabular angles. (*11*) Thin cranial bones

with a prominent elongated posterior fossa and a shallow, J-shaped sella.

In addition, congenital cardiovascular disease is frequently present, usually a patent interventricular septum (VSD) or patent ductus arteriosis. Eventration of the diaphragm and malformation of the kidneys are relatively common. The latter defects include double ureters, multicystic kidneys, horseshoe kidneys, and hydronephrosis.

TRISOMY 13–15 SYNDROME

The genetic fault in this syndrome is an extra chromosome for the 13–15 group. It is less common than trisomy 18. The infants are usually small and do not thrive. Death often occurs during the first year of life. The ears are malformed and low set and there is micrognathia. Some of the skeletal stigmas resemble those found in the trisomy 18 syndrome but the major anomalies include craniofacial clefts, polydactyly, and syndactyly together with various anomalies of the viscera. Congenital heart disease is common, usually a ventricular septal defect with or without a patent ductus arteriosis and dextroposition. The skeletal anomalies include:[21] (*1*) Cleft palate. (*2*) Poorly ossified cranial bones with microcephaly. (*3*) Hypotelorism with small orbits, microphthalmia, and a sloping forehead. (*4*) Polydactyly and syndactyly with narrow distal phalanges. (*5*) Malformed ribs with asymmetry of the thorax. (*6*) Increased interpediculate distance in the cervical spine. (*7*) The fifth finger overlapping the fourth. (*8*) "Rocker-bottom" feet.

The visceral anomalies, in addition to heart disease, include: (*1*) Diaphragmatic hernia. (*2*) Genitourinary tract anomalies as seen in trisomy 18. (*3*) Umbilical or inguinal hernias. (*4*) malrotation of the colon. (*5*) Undescended testes. (*6*) Mental and motor retardation.

TURNER'S SYNDROME

Of the group of syndromes in which there is abnormal gonadal development, the one that may show significant roentgen findings is Turner's syndrome, or gonadal aplasia.[36] In this syndrome there is relative shortening of the fourth metacarpal in relation to the third and fifth. The *metacarpal sign* is determined by drawing a straight line tangential to the distal ends of the heads of the fourth and fifth metacarpals.[5] If this line passes through the head of the third metacarpal, the sign is said to be positive. Normally, the line will pass distal to the head of the third metacarpal. However, a positive sign occurs in some normals and in other growth disturbances so that it is not absolutely specific. The time of appearance of epiphyseal ossification centers is normal but fusion is delayed. Skeletal density is diminshed particularly in the wrist and foot. The proximal row of carpal bones assumes an angular configuration somewhat similar to Madelung's deformity with the apex pointing proximally. Various other abnormalities of the bones of the hands also have been described. At the knee, the medial femoral condyle is enlarged and the opposing tibial plateau is flattened or depressed. The medial part of the proximal tibial epiphysis may overhang the metaphysis and in some cases an appearance rather similar to Blount's disease has been noted. In the spine there may be scoliosis and the posterior arch of C1 may be hypoplastic. An appearance similar to Scheuermanns' disease also has been described. An increased carrying angle at the elbow, cubitus valgus, one of the significant clinical signs, also can be demonstrated radiographically (see Fig. 5-32).

OTHER SYNDROMES

A considerable number of syndromes have been described in the literature, often with eponymic titles, that include skeletal roentgenographic changes. Most of these are decidedly uncommon and limitations of space make it impossible to include them in this chapter. Most are of interest chiefly to pediatric radiologists and descriptions can be found in the more recent radiologic and pediatric literature or in books devoted to the subject.

REFERENCES AND SELECTED READINGS

1. ANGLE CR, McINTIRE MS, MOORE RC: Cloverleaf skull: Kleeblattschädel-deformity syndrome. Am J Dis Child 114: 198, 1967

2. ASTLEY R: Trisomy 17–18. Br J Radiol 39: 86, 1966

3. AUSTIN JHM, PREGER L, SIRIS E et al: Short hard palate in newborn. Roentgen sign of mongolism. Radiology 92: 775, 1969

4. BENZIAN SR, MAINZER F, GODDING CA: Pediculate Thinning: a normal variant at the thoracolumbar junction. Br J Radiol 44: 936, 1971

5. BLOOM RA: The metacarpal sign. Br J Radiol 43: 133, 1970

6. CAFFEY J, AMES R, SILVERMAN WA et al: Contradiction of the congenital dysplasia-predislocation hypothesis of congenital dislocation of the hip through a study of the normal variations in acetabular angles at successive periods in infancy. Pediatrics 17: 632, 1956

7. CONWAY JJ, COWELL HR: Tarsal coalition: clinical significance and roentgenographic demonstration. Radiology 92: 799, 1969

8. DARLING DB, FEINGOLD M, BERKMAN M: Roentgenological aspects of Goldenhar's syndrome: oculoauriculovertebral dysplasia. Radiology 91: 254, 1968

9. DOBERTI A, MANHOOD J: A new radiologic sign for the early diagnosis of congenital hip displasia. Ann Radiol 11: 276, 1968

10. DUGGAN CA, KEENER EB, GAY BB JR: Secondary craniostenosis. Am J Roentgenol 109: 277, 1970

11. FELMAN AH, KIRKPATRICK JA: Madelung's deformity. Observations in 17 patients. Radiology 93: 1037, 1969

12. FONG EE: Iliac horns (symmetrical bilateral central posterior iliac processes); case report. Radiology 47: 517, 1946

13. GELLIS SS, FEINGOLD M, TUNNESSEN WW JR et al: Caudal dysplasia syndrome (picture of the month). Am J Dis Child 116: 407, 1968

14. GERALD BE, SILVERMAN FN: Normal and abnormal interorbital distances with special reference to mongolism. Am J Roentgenol 95: 154, 1965

15. GHELMAN B, FREIBERGER RH: The limbus vertebra: an anterior disc herniation demonstrated by discography. Am J Roentgenol 127: 854, 1976

16. GORDON IRS: Microcephaly and craniostenosis. Clin Radiol 21: 19, 1970

17. GORLIN RJ, COHEN MM JR, WOLFSON J: Tricho-rhino-phalangeal syndrome. Am J Dis Child 118: 595, 1969

18. GRUNDY L, GAREE JA, JIMENEZ JP: Oxycephaly in the adult simulating pituitary tumor. Am J Roentgenol 108: 762, 1970

19. HANSMAN CF: Growth of interorbital distance and skull thickness as observed in roentgenographic measurements. Radiology 86: 87, 1966

20. JAMES AE JR: Tarsal coalitions and peroneal spastic flat foot. Australos Radiol 14: 80, 1970

21. JAMES AE JR, BELCORT CL, ATKINS L et al: Trisomy 13–15. Radiology 92: 44, 1969

22. JAMES AE JR, BELCORT CL, ATKINS L et al: Trisomy-18 syndrome. Radiology 92: 37, 1969

23. KEATS TE: Ocular hypertelorism (Greig's syndrome) associated with Sprengel's deformity. Am J Roentgenol 110: 119, 1970

24. KOONTZ WW JR, PROUT GR JR: Agenesis of the sacrum and neurogenic bladder. JAMA 203: 481, 1968

25. MARGOLIN FK, STEINBACH HL: Progeria. Hutchinson-Gilford syndrome. Am J Roentgenol 103: 173, 1968

26. MORRISON SG, PERRY LW, SCOTT LP III: Congenital brevicollis (Klippel-Feil syndrome). Am J Dis Child 115: 614, 1968

27. RECHNAGEL K: Dysplasia epiphysialis hemimelica. Acta Orthop Scand 29: 237, 1960

28. ROBERSON GH, LLEWELLYN HJ, TAVERAS JM: The narrow lumbar spinal canal syndrome. Radiology 107: 89, 1973

29. SALTER RB: Etiology, pathogenesis and possible prevention of congenital dislocation of the hip. Can Med Assoc J 98: 933, 1968

30. SCHEY WL, LEVIN B: Familial pubic bone maldevelopment. Radiology 101: 147, 1971

31. SHACKELFORD GD, SHACKELFORD PG, SCHWETSCHENAU PR et al: Congenital occipital dermal sinus. Radiology 111: 161, 1974

32. SHAPIRO R: Anomalous parietal sutures and a bipartite parietal bone. Am J Roentgenol 115: 569, 1972

33. SHOPFNER CE, COIN CG: Genu varus and valgus in children. Radiology 92: 723, 1969

34. SHOUL MI, RITVO M: Clinical and roentgenological manifestations of the Klippel-Feil syndrome (congenital fusion of the cervical vertebrae, brevicollis): report of eight additional cases and review of the literature. Am J Roentgenol 68: 369, 1952

35. SILVERMAN FN: Pediatric radiology. In McLaren JW (ed): Modern Trends in Diagnostic Radiology, 4th ed. New York, Appleton-Century-Crofts, 1970

36. SINGLETON EB, ROSENBERG HS, YANG SJ: The radiographic manifestations of the chromosomal abnormalities. Radiol Clin North Am 2: 281, 1964

37. STAHELI LT, CLAWSON DK, CAPPS JH: Bilateral curving of the terminal phalanges of the little finger. J Bone Joint Surg [A] 48: 1171, 1966

38. TOD PA, YELLAND JDN: Craniostenosis. Clin Radiol 22: 472, 1971

39. TONG ECK: The iliac index angle. Radiology 91: 376, 1968

40. WITTENBORG MH: Malposition and dislocation of the hip in infancy and childhood. Radiol Clin North Am 2: 235, 1964

4

METABOLIC, ENDOCRINE, AND RELATED BONE DISEASES

Bone is living tissue with old bone being removed constantly and replaced with new bone. Normally this exchange is in balance and the mineral content of the bones remains relatively constant. Under some conditions and as a result of certain diseases this balance may be disturbed. Generalized reduction in bone mass must be caused by decreased production of osteoid, decreased mineralization of osteoid, or an excessive rate of destruction or deossification of bone. The term *dystrophy,* a disturbance of nutrition either of mineral salts or organic components, should not be confused with the term *dysplasia,* which means a disturbance of bone growth. Certain metabolic and endocrine disorders result in bone dystrophy.

Osteopenia is a generic term used to indicate a decrease in skeletal density which may be local or general. Although the term *osteoporosis* has been and will probably continue to be used by clinicians and radiologists in this generic sense, it should probably be reserved to designate senile or postmenopausal atrophy of bone in which there is a quantitative decrease of bone. However, similar decrease may be caused by disuse, dietary deficiency, or endocrine imbalance, or, rarely, it may be a manifestation of a congenital anomaly.

Loss of mineral salts causes bone to become more radiolucent than normal. Increased radiopacity of bone can result from increased formation with new bone being laid down faster than old bone is removed. The same result will occur if there is interference with normal deossification, provided that bone formation continues at a normal rate. Various metabolic and endocrine diseases can cause one or more of these processes. The most common cause is osteoporosis associated with senility or the postmenopausal state. Similar quantitative reduction in bone density and in bone tissue may occur as a result of several abnormalities previously mentioned. The term osteopenia is being used to refer to them in preference to the term osteoporosis, largely because of our inability to distinguish between the various causes of bone rarefaction or radiolucency and because of the specific pathogenetic implications attached to the term osteoporosis. Therefore, osteopenia appears to be an acceptable and nonspecific descriptive term to designate general or regional skeletal rarefaction. Osteoporosis is used in this text to refer to the loss of bone matrix including the mineral and organic components in the conditions mentioned because it is still in common use. Radiographically, the bones are more radiolucent than normal. It is difficult to recognize lesser degrees in roentgenograms unless the process is localized and there is adjacent normal bone for comparison.

When osteoporosis is diffuse and generalized a considerable loss of bone is required before recognition is assured. Overexposed roentgenograms may give a false impression of osteoporosis. Because of these difficulties a number of methods have been devised to measure the mineral content of bone *in vivo* more accurately than can be done by observation of roentgenograms. This problem has been of recent concern because astronauts may spend considerable time in space in relative inactivity.[4, 22]

OSTEOPOROSIS

DISUSE OSTEOPOROSIS

To maintain osteoblastic activity at a normal level requires that the bones be subjected to a normal amount of stress and this demands muscular activity. Within a few weeks following fracture of a bone, localized osteopenia of the affected part begins to be discernible. This is more pronounced distal to the site of the injury. During childhood and adolescence, osteopenia following bone fracture is most pronounced in the metaphyses, apparently because of the increased blood supply at the sites where active bone growth is taking place. Even in adults it is likely to be most intense along the sites of the previous epiphyseal plates (Fig. 4-1). The cortical margin of the bone involved by the osteoporosis becomes thinned but never disappears completely, an important point in distinguishing disuse osteoporosis from destruction of bone caused by disease. The loss in bone matrix is largely the result of inactivity although hyperemia undoubtedly plays a part. Radiolucency tends to be uniform with loss of all trabeculae so that, when osteopenia is severe or long-standing, the bones develop a "ground-glass" appearance. This, combined with the thinned cortices, forms a characteristic pattern for osteoporosis. The same type of osteoporosis may develop following acute infections of the bone or of the soft tissues, or after immobilization.

Chronic disuse osteoporosis may develop gradually when due to a partial limitation of activity or it may be the continuation of an acute process. The bones involved show uniform radiolucency with a poorly

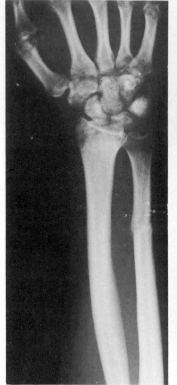
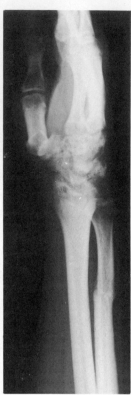

Fig. 4-1. Acute disuse osteoporosis. These views of the wrist obtained 6 weeks following fractures of the distal radius and more proximal ulna show severe loss of bone density particularly in the distal ulna but also in the distal radius, the carpals, and ends of the metacarpals.

defined trabecular structure and thinning of the cortex. The osteopenia may be limited to one extremity or to part of an extremity if the disuse has been limited to such an area, or it may be generalized throughout the skeleton if the body has been inactive. When the vertebrae are affected, the cancellous structure is lost, but the cortical margins remain distinct, the so-called "picture-frame" vertebrae. In disuse, the bone resorption exceeds formation resulting in a net loss of bone mass that is either local or general.

REFLEX SYMPATHETIC DYSTROPHY SYNDROME (SUDECK'S ATROPHY)[10]

This is a severe form of local osteopenia which usually follows trauma with or without fracture. It may also follow infection, peripheral neuropathy, central nervous system abnormality, or cervical osteoarthritis. In about 25% of the patients no predisposing disorder is recognized. The cause is not clearly understood, but abnormal neural reflexes leading to muscle atrophy, and sometimes to marked hypervascularity, are evidently the result of the stimulus of the inciting factor. Clinical manifestations consist of pain that is often severe resulting in far more disability than would be expected to follow the relatively minor injury. There are trophic changes in the skin which is smooth and glistening. The pain is often aggravated by immobilization, and the dystrophy tends to progress. Radiographic findings consist of diffuse and periarticular soft-tissue swelling with osteopenia that is also diffuse (Fig. 4-2). Cortical bone resorption is endosteal and intracortical in most patients and subperiosteal in about 50%. Articular erosions are also common. Magnification radiography shows endosteal scalloping and intracortical resorption that is identified by striation within the cortex. Linear resorption in the outer cortex may simulate periosteal new bone formation, a pseudoperiostitis. During the acute stage, the mottled appearance of the bones and the severe loss of bone density is striking. As the process becomes more chronic, the mottled appearance is lost and the bones assume a ground-glass, uniform loss of density. Sudek's atrophy develops at or distal to the area of injury, not proximal to it. After recovery the bones affected often show persisting coarse structure that may last for several years.

REGIONAL OSTEOPOROSIS

There are two general patterns of transient regional osteoporosis.[2] Transient osteoporosis of the hip is usually observed in young and middle-aged males but may involve females as well. Clinically there is gradual onset of hip pain with no antecedent history of injury. There may be some joint effusion, and, on biopsy, a mild, chronic synovitis may be observed. Recovery usually occurs spontaneously in 6 months or less. Radiographic findings consist of evidence of severe loss of bone density in the femoral head and to a lesser extent in the femoral neck and acetabulum. There is no narrowing of joint space.

Transient, painful osteoporosis of the lower extremities is a migratory type in which the knee, ankle, and foot are involved more commonly than the hip. Females are affected more often than males. There is gradual onset of regional pain and swelling accompanied by a rapid development of osteopenia, localized to the painful area. Pain often lasts as long as 9 months, and there may be subsequent involvement of other areas in the same or in the opposite extremity. Roentgenographic study reveals a decrease in bone density with no evidence of local destruction. The trabecular pattern is coarse and irregular and tends to change slowly with gradual return to normal over a period of several years. There are no alterations in calcium, phosphorus, or phosphatase. The cause is unknown.

Fig. 4-2. Sudeck's atrophy (reflex sympathetic dystrophy). There is severe loss of bone density which followed a fracture of the tip of the lateral malleolus which is ununited. Involvement is noted in the distal ends of the tibia and fibula, the tarsal bones, and the proximal end of the fourth and fifth metatarsals which are included. The cortical margins are thin but intact; the patchy and mottled character of the bone loss is characteristic. Note that the involvement of the tibia and fibula is confined to the bone ends.

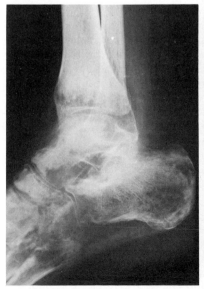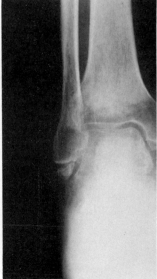

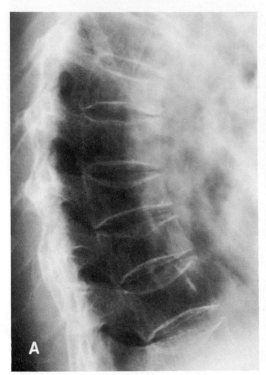
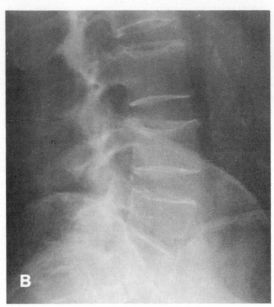

Fig. 4-3. Postmenopausal osteoporosis. **A.** There are multiple compression fractures resulting from the loss of structural strength of these vertebral bodies. The cortical margins are thin but stand out clearly as white lines marking the vertebral borders. **B.** In the lumbar spine, in addition to the compression which is minimal, there is some concavity of the superior vertebral bodies.

POSTMENOPAUSAL OSTEOPOROSIS

Following the menopause, some individuals develop a chronic osteopenia that may be sufficiently severe to cause fracture. The vertebral column and the pelvic bones are particularly susceptible to this form. Because of the pronounced loss of bone density, compression fractures of one or more vertebrae may result. The bodies in the mid and lower thoracic areas are most frequently affected. Fracture can occur after a very minor injury or during the course of normal activity. In severe forms of the disease, many of the vertebral bodies develop concave superior and inferior disc surfaces, giving what has been called a "fish" contour as seen in lateral roentgenograms (Fig. 4-3). Such deformity is caused by expansion of the intervertebral discs at the expense of the weakened vertebral bodies. An almost constant finding in association with the vertebral changes is the occurrence of calcific plaques in the abdominal aorta. The long bones show changes that may be more difficult to assess radiographically. The loss of cortical and cancellous bone may cause an apparent or real prominence of trabeculae and visible thinning of the cortex. If the sum of the two cortices of the midshaft of metacarpal, metatarsal, or long bones is less than one-half the diameter of the bone, osteopenia is present. Because the process is slow there is no periosteal irregularity, only mild endosteal scalloping and no cortical striation or tunneling.

SENILE OSTEOPOROSIS

The bones lose density with advancing age—part of the aging process. They become more brittle, fracture readily, and heal more slowly. Since many elderly persons are likely to be less active and dietary habits may be poor, a combination of factors can lead to severe osteoporosis with compression fractures of the vertebrae similar to those occurring in persons having the postmenopausal form of osteoporosis. It is obvious that in many persons showing chronic osteoporosis there may be more than one factor responsible and the dividing line between postmenopausal osteoporosis and the senile type of the disease often is not distinct. The roentgen findings are similar in both types and therefore are nonspecific as far as designating the cause of the osteopenia.

JUVENILE IDIOPATHIC OSTEOPOROSIS

This condition is manifested by an acute onset of osteoporosis that varies in severity. The age of onset varies from 5 to 17 years. The condition is self-limited in that it stabilizes, but bone density does not return to normal. When it is severe, there may be deformity secondary to bowing of the fragile bone and relatively short stature caused by vertebral compression fractures. The major change is usually in the metaphyseal area.

CUSHING'S SYNDROME

Osteopenia is one of the skeletal manifestations of Cushing's syndrome whether owing to administration of corticosteroids or to the spontaneous form of the disease. The latter may be caused by adrenocortical hyperplasia, or less frequently by adrenal cortical adenoma or carcinoma.[18] As a result of the demineralization the vertebrae are prone to collapse with multiple compression fractures leading to biconcave contours of the vertebral bodies (Fig. 4-4). There is marginal condensation especially along the upper surfaces of the compressed vertebrae, more than is commonly seen following vertebral compressions due to other causes. It has been suggested that this change is a manifestation of attempted repair with excess callus formation.[18] Rib fractures also are present, particularly in the anterior segments, and exuberant callus often forms around these. As is true with other fractures occurring in this syndrome, the fractures frequently are painless. Fractures of the pubic and ischial rami may occur, also frequently showing heavy callus.

Ischemic necrosis of the head of the femur and in the ends of other bones is another complication of the disease. The exact cause is not known. Because of the loss of bone the skeletal density is decreased. In the skull this may take the form of a granular rarefaction. Skull roentgenograms also may show an enlarged sella in patients with the uncommon cases of the syndrome that are secondary to a pituitary tumor. The lamina dura, the cortical margin of the tooth socket, may disappear. In children there may be delay in skeletal maturation.

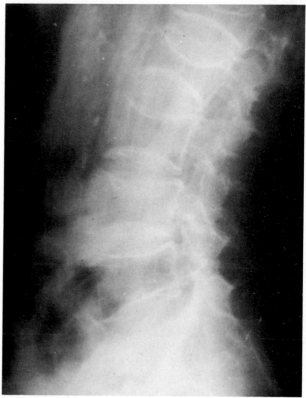

Fig. 4-4. Cushing's syndrome. There is compression of all of the lumbar vertebrae. Expansion of the intervertebral discs into the softened vertebral bodies causes a characteristic biconcavity of their upper and lower surfaces.

Nonskeletal roentgen manifestations include excess subcutaneous and intraabdominal fat and mediastinal widening from excess fat deposits. Extrapleural fat pads and epipericardial fat accumulations also may be seen in chest roentgenograms. Visualization of the enlarged adrenals often may be obtained by suitable techniques (see Ch. 20). In those cases secondary to a carcinoma of the adrenal glands, calcified deposits have been found in approximately 25% of the subjects.

MALNUTRITION AND RELATED CAUSES

Since protein deficiency or abnormal protein metabolism can cause osteoporosis, it may develop whenever there is severe malnutrition. Thus, osteoporosis and osteomalacia may both be present after periods of starvation. Osteoporosis may develop in persons with nephrosis as a result of loss of proetin. When diabetes is poorly controlled over a long period of time the bones become osteoporotic since these individuals use abnormal amounts of protein to make up for the inability to use glucose. Hyperthyroidism is another cause that is related to protein deficiency, probably owing to catabolic destruction of amino acids.

SCURVY

Infantile scurvy is a form of osteoporosis caused by a deficiency of vitamin C. This vitamin is necessary for normal osteoblastic activity; the organic matrix of bone cannot be laid down without it. Because of the lowered activity of the osteoblasts, the serum alkaline phosphatase usually is low or occasionally normal. The tendency for hemorrhage in this disease is said to be due to a lack of formation of intercellular cement substance in the capillaries. Scurvy is not a disease of the immediate postnatal period but is most frequent in children between the ages of 6 months and 2 years.

Roentgen Observations

1. There is a diffuse demineralization of the entire skeleton. The trabecular structure is lost and the cortices of the bone are thinned.

2. Zones of increased density develop at the metaphyses of the long bones and around the margins of the epiphyseal centers. As the cancellous bone of the center becomes more translucent than normal, the dense outer rim gives the appearance of a ring and this is a very significant finding in scurvy. This zone of density, known as the white line of scurvy, represents an abnormally wide zone of provisional calcification and it is caused by a failure of normal proliferation of cartilage cells so that the change from cartilage to bone becomes arrested.

3. On the shaft side of the metaphysis a zone of lessened density develops, forming a transverse band of rarefaction across the shaft. This is the area where active bone formation should be taking place but does not and the balance between bone formation and resorption is disturbed in favor of the latter. This is a weakened part of the bone and it is here that fracture may occur. The epiphysis and the zone of provisional calcification may be displaced because of such fracture. This zone of rarefaction is known as the *scurvy zone* (see Fig. 4-6). The scurvy zone often disappears as the epiphysis, together with the zone of provisional calcification, becomes impacted into the shaft. Lateral extension of the zone of

provisional calcification into the soft tissues for a short distance, forming spurlike projections, is a common finding (Fig. 4-5).

4. The "corner sign of scurvy" sometimes is an early and fairly characteristic change. It is a small area of rarefaction involving the cortex and spongiosa just proximal to the metaphysis on one or both sides of the shaft and it represents the early development of the scurvy zone (Fig. 4-6).

5. Healing of scurvy is shown first by the calcification of areas of subperiosteal hemorrhage. During the active stage of the disease, extensive hemorrhages may develop beneath the periosteum and elevate it. During infancy and childhood the periosteum is loosely attached to the cortex of the bone and it is elevated easily by

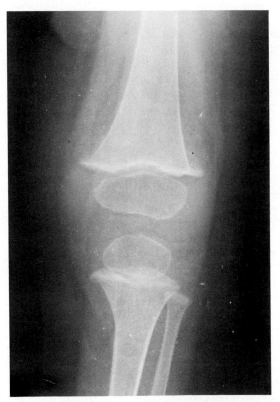

Fig. 4-5. Infantile scurvy. The white line of scurvy is particularly distinct in the metaphysis of the femur. Note the spurlike projection of the zone of provisional calcification laterally. The translucent scurvy zone is not visible because of the impaction of the shaft into the zone of provisional calcification.

hemorrhage beneath it. However, it is firmly attached at the end of the shaft and hemorrhage is limited at this point and it is here that the first deposition of calcium salts often occurs. Under adequate treatment, calcium is deposited throughout the area of hemorrhage, forming a dense shadow surrounding the shaft (Fig. 4-7). The scurvy zones recalcify. There is a gradual remineralization of the skeleton and the cortices regain normal thickness. As growth proceeds the thickened zone of provisional calcification appears to migrate in the shaft where it remains as a thin, dense, white line for a long period of time. In like manner a ring of density may

be visible within the epiphyseal center as normal bone forms around the edge of the old center ("ghost epiphysis" or "bone-within-a-bone"). The calcified subperiosteal hemorrhages gradually are absorbed. If epiphyseal dislocation did occur, the deformity will be corrected by growth and remodeling over a period of time.

OSTEOGENESIS IMPERFECTA

Osteogenesis imperfecta is a congenital form of osteopenia in which there is a defect or deficiency of osteoblasts. It is discussed in Chapter 2.

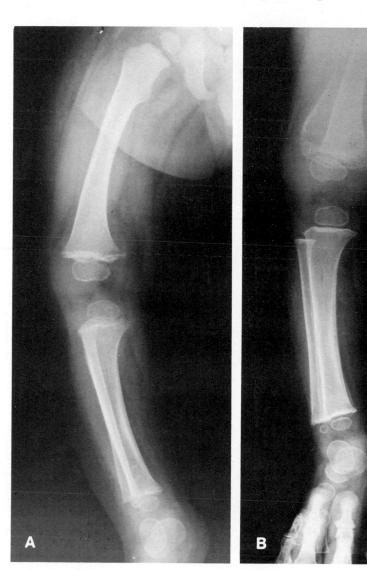

Fig. 4-6. Infantile scurvy. **A.** Lower extremity showing characteristic changes. Note the ringlike epiphyses. **B.** The same patient 2 weeks after treatment was begun. There is lateral displacement of the femoral epiphysis and healing is indicated by calcification in a large subperiosteal hematoma surrounding the femur.

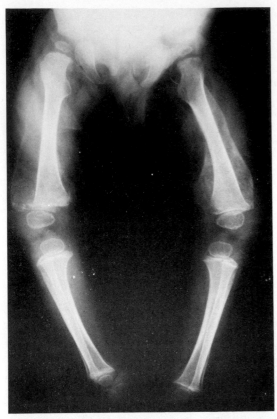

Fig. 4-7. Infantile scurvy. This roentgenogram was obtained shortly after the beginning of the patient's treatment. There has been epiphyseal fracture with lateral displacement of the right lower femoral epiphysis; large calcifying subperiosteal hematomas are noted, and ring contours of the epiphyses are distinct.

OSTEOMALACIA

Osteomalacia and rickets may be classified as to etiologic background as follows:[17]

    I. Deficiency
      A. Vitamin D
      B. Of calcium
      C. Of phosphorus
      D. Chelators in the diet
   II. Absorptive
      A. Gastric abnormalities
      B. Biliary diseases
      C. Enteric absorptive defects
  III. Renal tubular
      A. Proximal tubular lesions
      B. Proximal and distal tubular lesions
      C. Renal tubular acidosis (distal)
        1. Primary
        2. Secondary
  IV. Renal osteodystrophy
   V. Unusual forms
      A. With fibrous dysplasia
      B. With neurofibromatosis
      C. Associated with neoplasms
      D. Anticonvulsant medication
      E. Hypophosphatasia

Unless adequate amounts of calcium and phosphorus are available, proper calcification of osteoid cannot occur and the process of bone formation is arrested. Because removal of dead or devitalized bone continues, the balance is disturbed in favor of demineralization. When this happens during adult life the condition known as osteomalacia results. During childhood the effect on bone already formed is the same as in the adult. In addition, new bone being formed as a part of the process of growth is greatly altered and changes that are not seen in the adult become obvious. This form of osteomalacia is known as rickets. The two diseases, therefore, are essentially the same and the roentgen findings differ only because of the presence or absence of areas of actively growing bone (epiphyses and metaphyses).

The causes of osteomalacia are varied and include an inadequate intake or a failure of absorption of calcium, phosphorus, or vitamin D, singly or in combination. The importance of the first two in the proper mineralization of bone is obvious. The major effect of vitamin D is to increase absorption of calcium and phosphorus from the intestinal tract. It also may have a direct effect on bone. In addition to disturbances in the intake and absorption of calcium and phosphorus, certain renal diseases in which there is tubular insufficiency without glomerular involvement may cause osteomalacia.

INFANTILE RICKETS

Infantile rickets is osteomalacia occurring during infancy, usually because of a lack of vitamin D in the diet or of ultraviolet radiation (ultraviolet converts the sterols in the skin into vitamin D). This form of rickets is less prevalent than it used to be. It is found mainly in infants between the ages of 4 and 18 months. It is very uncommon during the first few months of life. The significant roentgen observations include the following:

There is a generalized demineralization of the skeleton, the bones having a coarse texture. In contrast to infantile scurvy, which is a form of osteoporosis, demineralization of the bone trabeculae occurs unevenly and those that remain stand out more prominently than is normal. Because of the poor mineralization of the bones, bowing of the weight-bearing bones will develop if the infant has begun to stand or walk. Even in the very young infant, fractures of the greenstick variety may occur. However, these are more likely to develop in the older child. If the rickets is very severe, transverse fissurelike clefts may form in the shafts of the long bones similar in all respects to the pseudofractures of osteomalacia in the adult (see section entitled "Osteomalacia" in this chapter).

The white line marking the ends of the shafts, the zone of provisional calcification, disappears and the metaphyses develop a very irregular appearance, becoming coarse and frayed. This is characteristic of rickets (Figs. 4-8 and 4-9). With failure of proper calcification of the newly formed osteoid in the metaphysis, the distance between the ossified portion of the epiphysis and the end of the shaft is increased. Modeling of the end of the bone, the normal reshaping that occurs as growth in length and width proceeds, is also interfered with and the ends of the shafts become broadened. Typically, a certain amount of cupping or concavity of the metaphysis

also develops although this finding is less constant than the others that have been described.

In severe rickets, thin stripelike shadows frequently develop along the outer cortical margins of the long bones. These resemble the periosteal calcifications of inflammatory type but actually represent zones of poorly calcified osteoid laid down by the periosteum, which would normally result in transverse growth of the bones.

Demineralization of the cranial bones occurs and, in the young infant, the suture margins become indistinct. The bones are soft and the skull is molded readily by pressure. The tendency for a piling up of poorly calcified bone leads to the formation of bosses or prominences, particularly in the frontal bone, and these become noticeable especially when healing has begun.

Also in severe disease, transverse fissurelike clefts may develop in the shafts of the long bones (Fig. 4-10), the axillary borders of the scapulae, the pubic rami, and other areas. These are called pseudofractures or Looser zones and are similar to those seen in osteomalacia of adults. The margins of the ossified epiphyseal centers become indistinct and in severe cases the centers may be difficult to visualize or even apparently disappear because of the pronounced decalcification (see Fig. 4-9).

Fig. 4-8. Infantile rickets. **A.** Note the poorly calcified, frayed metaphyses, particularly in the femur with fraying, cupping, and broadening. The coarse texture of bone is noted in the epiphyses as well as in the lower femoral shaft. **B.** Changes similar to those in **A** are noted in this wrist of another patient.

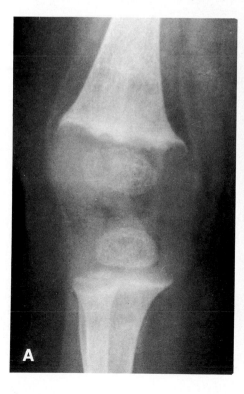 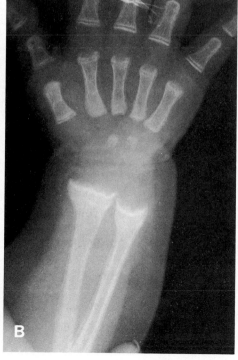

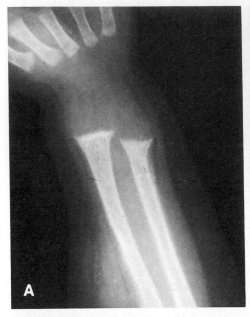

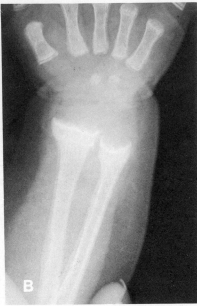

Fig. 4-9. Infantile rickets. **A.** This initial film shows evidence of broadening and some fraying of the metaphyses of the radius and ulna. **B.** Same infant as in **A** after 2 weeks of treatment. The metaphyses have partially recalcified and the osteoid, which was previously invisible, is now observed as transverse zones of calcification across the ends of the metaphyses. A minimal amount of subperiosteal calcification is also observed, and there are now two carpal ossification centers that were not identified 2 weeks earlier. The cupping persists but eventually disappears.

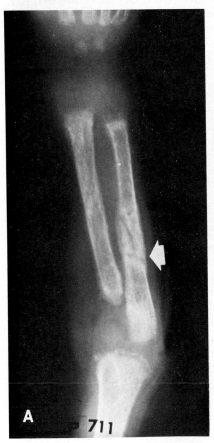

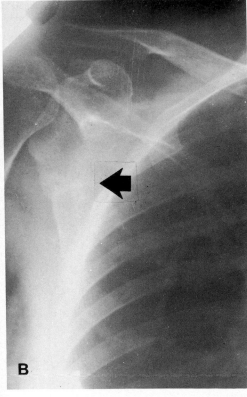

Fig. 4-10. A. Pseudofractures in a patient with active rickets. In addition to a transverse fissure line **(arrow)** there is an oblique one. The characteristic changes of florid rickets are present including coarse trabeculation and ragged, frayed metaphyses. **B.** An adult with osteomalacia. The **arrow** indicates pseudofracture of the axillary border of the scapula.

The changes noted in the metaphyses of the long tubular bones also develop in the sternal ends of the ribs and lead to the clinical sign of "beading." This is not specific for rickets as beading of the ribs, or the so-called rachitic rosary, is also seen in some other diseases.

The healing of rickets is shown by recalcification of the zone of provisional calcification. At first this is seen as a broad band of uniform density extending across the end of the shaft. Subsequently this is transformed into trabecular bone. Remineralization of the skeleton is a slow process and may take several months or even longer. The epiphyseal centers gradually regain normal density and sharpness of outline. The subperiosteal, poorly calcified osteoid is transformed into bone and the periosteal stripes disappear. If the bones have become bowed or otherwise deformed during the active stage of disease, the deformities are likely to persist. Thus when rickets has completely healed only the deformities from bowing or fracture will remain as evidence of the previous disease (Fig. 4-11).

OSTEOMALACIA IN ADULTS

The disease, osteomalacia, is the same as infantile rickets, but occurring after bone growth has ceased. In the United States, osteomalacia probably is caused most often by faulty absorption of the fat-soluble vitamin D and other substances from the intestinal tract because of the steatorrhea that occurs in the malabsorption syndromes, of which idiopathic sprue is the most common. Osteomalacia secondary to dysfunction of the proximal renal tubules (renal osteomalacia) is seen less frequently and dietary deficiency, the common cause of infantile rickets, also is infrequent in the United States. The basic roentgen abnormality is a generalized undermineralization of the skeleton. The texture of the bones is coarse, the same as is noted in rickets. This is caused by an irregular absorption of the bone trabeculae; the total trabecular structure of the bone is decreased but the primary trabeculae that remain stand out more prominently than is normal. In contrast to osteoporosis, the cortical borders of the bones may not be very distinct. Osteoporosis is characterized by a uniform undermineralization, when long standing, so that a ground-glass appearance results. This, combined with the sharply outlined cortices, aids in distinguishing osteoporosis from osteomalacia. Magnification or microradioscopy,[19] used in the study of hand bones in osteomalacia, demonstrates intracortical striations caused by local resorption or lack of mineralization. Because this change is not observed in osteoporosis, the procedure aids in the differentiation of these conditions. However, in severe osteomalacia

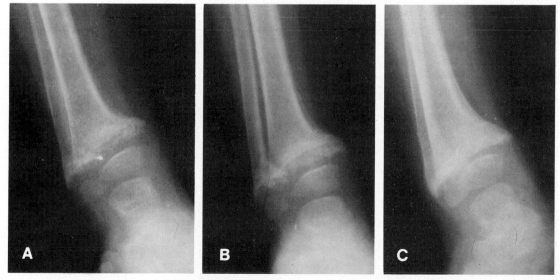

Fig. 4-11. Infantile rickets showing the result of therapy. **A.** Appearance at the beginning of treatment. **B.** The same patient 18 days later. The metaphyses are beginning to recalcify. **C.** Four weeks later. Healing is well advanced. There is bowing because the infant had started to walk before therapy was instituted.

there often is an associated osteoporosis so that the type of osteopenia may be difficult to evaluate. Because bone growth has ceased, the metaphyseal and epiphyseal changes that form a large part of the findings in infantile rickets are not observed. Pseudofractures are frequent and are highly characteristic of osteomalacia, although they may be found in a few other conditions. These are fissurelike defects or clefts extending transversely part way or completely through a bone. They represent fracture fissures filled with uncalcified osteoid and fibrous tissue. They are common along the axillary borders of the scapulae, the inner margins of the femoral necks, the ribs, the pubic and ischial rami, and the bones of the forearms. These fissures also are sometimes called Looser's zones.

The condition described by Milkman[20] and known as *Milkman's syndrome* is now considered to represent a mild form of osteomalacia in which the pseudofractures are particularly numerous. Some investigators now consider this syndrome to represent the form of osteomalacia caused by a dysfunction of the proximal renal tubules, either a persistence of vitamin D-refractory rickets from childhood or the result of some toxic agent such as plasma-cell myeloma, metal poisoning (including copper, *i.e.*, Wilson's disease), and glycogen storage disease, among others (see following section of this chapter).[1]

Because osteomalacia causes softening of the bones, they may bend or give way as a result of weight-bearing. In the pelvis there may be an inward bending of the pelvic sidewalls with deepening of the acetabular cavities (protrusio acetabuli) (Fig. 4-12). In the skull, softening of the bones may lead to a downward molding of the skull over the first and second cervical vertebrae. The basal angle of the skull is flattened and the condition is known as platybasia.

HYPOPHOSPHATEMIC VITAMIN D-REFRACTORY RICKETS

This condition has also been called rachitis tarda or late rickets because it is found in older children (beyond the age of 2½ years). It was formerly considered to be due to a high-tissue threshold for the effects of vitamin D since massive doses of the vitamin are necessary to effect a cure. It is now known that there are a number of proximal renal tubular abnor-

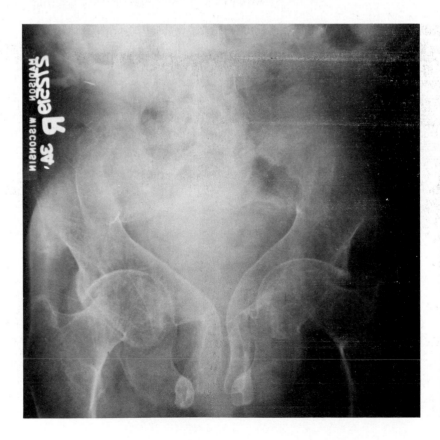

Fig. 4-12. Osteomalacia secondary to sprue. The bone loss is so severe that the osseous structures are difficult to outline. There is pronounced inward bowing of the lower pelvis, a characteristic in severe osteomalacia.

malities which cause hypophosphatemic rickets.[12] Four types have been reported. They are: 1) Classic vitamin D-resistant (hypophosphatemic) rickets or phosphate diabetes that is transmitted as a sex-linked dominant trait. Most children having this type of rickets fall below the third percentile in height by the age of 2 years; enlarged wrists and ankles, rachitic rosary, frontal bossing, and sometimes craniosynostosis are observed. 2) Vitamin D-resistant rickets with glycosuria in which there is an abnormal resorptive mechanism for glucose and inorganic phosphate, 3) Proximal tubular (Fanconi's syndrome) in which there is defective resorption of phosphate, glucose, and several amino acids. The rachitic lesions are severe, but this type appears to be less refractory to vitamin D thereapy than do the others, 4) A rare type of hypophosphatemic syndrome that does not become manifest until late adolescence or early adult life. It may be an acquired lesion, probably of toxic origin.

There are several syndromes in which proximal and distal renal tubules are involved. The proximal and distal Fanconi's syndrome is transmitted as an autosomal recessive trait and is probably unrelated genetically to the proximal Fanconi's sydrome. In children with this syndrome, rickets is usually severe with multiple fractures occurring in the first few months of life. There are several other lesions in which proximal and distal tubular abnormalities are found but these are very rare. The distal renal tubules are involved in renal tubular acidosis. In one form, bicarbonate is excreted in excess amounts with a reduced excretion of ammonia. In another, the acidosis results from loss of bicarbonate because of reduction in tubular resorption, and there is also increased excretion of sodium and potassium along with a decrease in water reabsorption resulting in severe dehydration. Over 70% of patients with chronic renal tubular acidosis have nephrocalcinosis.

Roentgen Findings. The roentgen findings are those of rickets but as the patients are older, bowing of the weight-bearing bones is greater, and shortening of the long bones leads to some degree of dwarfing (Figs. 4-13 and 4-14). There is anterior bowing of the femurs as well as lateral bowing. Coxa vara is common. The cupping and fraying of the metaphyses, loss of zones of provisional calcification, and coarse texture of the demineralized bones are the same as those of rickets. When the changes are mild, they are best demonstrated at the knees where widening of the epiphyseal line tends to be greatest on the medial sides of the distal femoral and proximal tibial me-

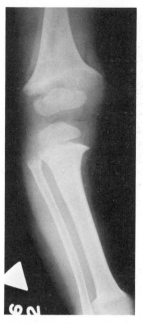

Fig. 4-13. Vitamin D-refractory rickets. The changes are the same as those seen in infantile rickets with additional findings of bowing and decrease in longitudinal growth of the bones.

taphyses. Pseudofractures or Looser's zones occur with more severe disease. Occasionally, the bones appear sclerotic instead of radiolucent. The disease may be mistaken for achondroplasia because of the dwarfing of the long bones. However, the characteristic changes of rickets and the lack of the typical skull and pelvic changes of achondroplasia should allow differentiation. The numerous other conditions causing rickets and osteomalacia usually produce symptoms and signs that aid in the diagnosis of the underlying cause of the bone changes.

HYPOPHOSPHATASIA

Hypophosphatasia is an inborn error of metabolism characterized by a low level of serum alkaline phosphatase and the presence of phosphoethanolamine in the urine and serum.

It is probably inherited as an autosomal recessive trait. The lack of adequate amounts of alkaline phosphatase causes failure of proper mineralization of osteoid and the result in the skeleton is an appearance similar to that of rickets or osteomalacia. The disease may be present at birth and has been discovered in utero in roentgenograms of the mother's abdomen.

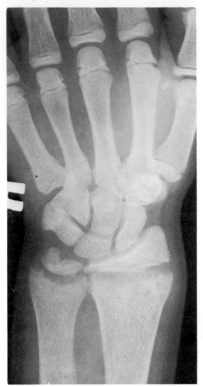

Fig. 4-14. Vitamin D-refractory rickets. Hand and wrist showing changes similar to those in the patient shown in Figure 4-13.

The earlier the disease is detected the more severe it is likely to be and infants born with it seldom survive more than a year or two. In these patients there is severe undermineralization of the metaphyses, the ends of which have a coarse, frayed appearance. The long bones in the newborn tend to be short and thin and to have a coarse texture. The bones of the cranial vault are largely unossified, and there is bulging of the anterior fontanelle. Fractures of the long bones may occur. In older children, the changes are similar but less severe and resemble infantile rickets (Fig. 4-15). If the patient survives and the cranial bones ossify, craniosynostosis often develops. Dwarfism also becomes a feature and a genu valgum deformity is common. Anterior and lateral femoral bowing, early loss of teeth, pseudofracture, and fractures caused by minimal trauma are common. Many of these patients improve spontaneously. In its mildest form, hypophosphatasia manifests itself chiefly by an increased tendency to fracture of the bones and a low serum alkaline phosphatase. The disease is very rare in adults.

The essential histologic feature is the presence of abnormal amounts of osteoid.

HYPERPHOSPHATASIA

According to Rubin,[23] other names applied to this condition are, *juvenile Paget's disease, hyperostosis corticalis deformans juvenilis, chronic idiopathic hyperphosphatasia congenita.* The serum alkaline phosphatase has been elevated in all reported cases. Clinical findings include lateral bowing of the femurs and muscular weakness. The mentality is normal. The disease probably has no relationship to Paget's disease.

Roentgen Findings. The characteristic finding is an extensive thickening of the diaphyseal cortex of all of the bones. The cortex is thickened both externally and internally and may, if the condition is severe, obliterate the medullary canal. Both the long and

Fig. 4-15. Hypophosphatasia in a child. There is deficient ossification of the metaphyses of the ulna and radius. The roughened, frayed appearance is particularly marked in the ulna. The changes are somewhat similar to those of rickets and were present in other long bones of this patient who had relatively minimal involvement. Note the pseudoepiphysis for the second metacarpal.

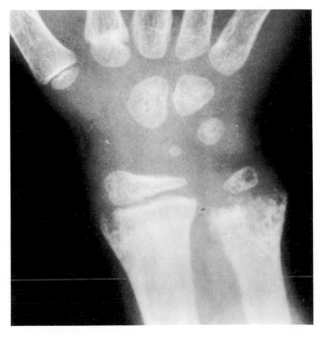

short tubular bones are affected. Bowing of the long bones is common. The bones of the cranial vault are thickened with patches of sclerosis. The pelvic bones may be of increased density. The carpal and tarsal bones are normal and the vertebrae show only minimal sclerosis.

VAN BUCHEM'S DISEASE

Rubin[23] classified this rare dysplasia as *chronic hyperphosphatasemia tarda*. It also is known as *hyperostosis corticalis generalisata*. However Van Buchem does not believe that the seven cases reported by him are related to chronic idiopathic hyperphosphatasia but instead represent a distinct dysplasia.[23] The onset appears to be later than in the *congenita* form, the ages of the patients ranging from 23 to 52 years. The disease was asymptomatic in the cases described by Van Buchem and associates. The major roentgen finding was a symmetrical, diaphyseal, cortical thickening of all of the long tubular bones, chiefly on the internal surface. The short tubular bones were involved in the same way. The femurs were not bowed. The epiphyses were spared. The cranial bones showed marked thickening of both vault and base. The maxillary sinuses and the mastoids were densely sclerotic. The mandible and clavicle were affected. There was diffuse sclerosis of the pelvic bones and the ribs were thickened when there was severe involvement elsewhere. Most of the patients did not show vertebral changes. As with the congenita form, the serum alkaline phosphatase was elevated in all of these patients, with calcium and phosphorus levels being normal.

HYPERPARATHYROIDISM

Hyperparathyroidism is an uncommon, although not rare, disease which results from either an adenoma of one or several of the parathyroid glands or a diffuse hyperplasia of these glands. Primary hyperparathyroidism usually is caused by an adenoma; secondary hyperparathyroidism, as in renal osteodystrophy, results from hyperplasia of the glands.[9] Primary disease occurs mainly during middle age although it has been found in the very young and the old. It is about twice as common in females as in males. The increased parathyroid activity leads to excessive secretion of parathyroid hormone which in turn causes (*1*) demineralization of the skeleton, (2) the occurrence of focal areas of bone destruction ("brown tumors"), and (3) decrease in the serum phospho-

rus level and increase in the serum calcium level, factors that eventually cause dystrophic and, later, metastatic calcification of the soft tissues, renal stones, nephrocalcinosis, and impairment of renal function.

It is believed that parathyroid hormone acts to increase the number of osteoclasts with resulting deossification of the skeleton. It also may diminish the reabsorption of phosphate from the glomerular filtrate by the proximal tubules, causing hyperphosphaturia and hypophosphatemia.[1] These are complex biochemical processes, however, and complete information about them is not available.

When the kidney threshold for calcium is exceeded this substance is excreted in the urine in increased amounts. Eventually renal stones may be formed and calcification of the kidney tubules may develop (nephrocalcinosis). When kidney function has been impaired in this way there is retention of phosphates and further calcium loss. Then the serum phosphorus level may rise to normal or higher and the calcium level falls.

The high serum calcium level may lead to calcification of other tissues which can be visualized roentgenographically, such as the blood vessels and articular cartilages. When the serum phosphorus level rises and the calcium falls as a result of renal impairment, the resulting high ionization product may cause further metastatic soft-tissue calcification.

Only about 5% of renal stones are caused by hyperparathyroidism but this disease should be a consideration when renal stones are found since it may be the cause of the presenting symptoms in some cases. Nephrocalcinosis can be caused by a number of different diseases including medullary sponge kidney, chronic pyelonephritis, sarcoid disease, vitamin D poisoning, or any other cause of hypercalcemia. Calcification of the articular cartilages occurs more frequently as a result of senescence or the pseudogout syndrome than it does from hyperparathyroidism, but, again, it may be a roentgen clue to the proper diagnosis which might not otherwise be suspected. Calcification in the walls of arteries may be seen even in the very young patient with hyperparathyroidism. The blood chemical findings include a normal or lowered phosphorus level, an elevated calcium level, and an elevated alkaline phosphatase level.

In patients with minimal skeletal disease, most of the bony structures may appear quite normal or, at the most, show a slight decalcification. An occasional cystlike lesion may be present and renal stones or nephrocalcinosis may be demonstrated. These findings are not specific enough to allow a diagnosis to be made but they may arouse the suspicion of the disease.

In patients with well-defined skeletal disease, some or all of the following findings will be present.

Generalized Skeletal Demineralization. The trabecular structure of the bones becomes hazy and indistinct, occasionally coarse and prominent. The cortical margins also become hazy and not well defined. In the skull, the bones develop a fine, granular appearance and the tables become indistinct (Fig. 4-16). This type of granular decalcification of the skull is a highly significant finding in this disease. The lamina dura, the cortical margin surrounding the tooth socket, disappears. Normally this is seen as a sharp, thin, white line surrounding the peridental membrane that attaches the tooth to the bone (Fig. 4-17). Loss of the lamina dura is not pathognomonic for hyperparathyroidism as some degree of it may be seen in osteomalacia and in other diseases. Dental roentgenograms are useful when the question of hyperparathyroidism arises.

Subperiosteal Resorption. This is a type of decalcification that is seen to best advantage in the phalanges but may be present elsewhere and seems to be a specific sign of the disease.[22] It consists of a fine, irregular loss of density along the outer margins of the cortices, especially of the middle phalanges (Fig. 4-18; see also Fig 4-23). The roughened surface has been described as lacelike. Fine-detail magnification radiography can detect subperiosteal resorption that is not visible on conventional films. Quantitative bone mineral analysis is even more accurate in detecting loss of mineral in this disease. In advanced disease there may be sufficient resorption to cause a general narrowing in width of the shaft, leaving the ends relatively intact (Fig. 4-19). In the distal phalanges, resorption of the terminal tufts may be an associated finding. Other areas where subperiosteal resorption may be found include the distal end of the clavicle (Figs. 4-20 and 4-21), the symphysis pubis, and the sacroiliac joints. In these areas there may be considerable loss of bone substance leading to a rough, frayed appearance. Erosions also may be seen at the calcaneal tendon insertions, the ischial tuberosities, and other bony prominences. The lamina dura absorption probably represents the same process.

Destructive Lesions. Localized destructive cystlike lesions of various sizes are frequent in this disease

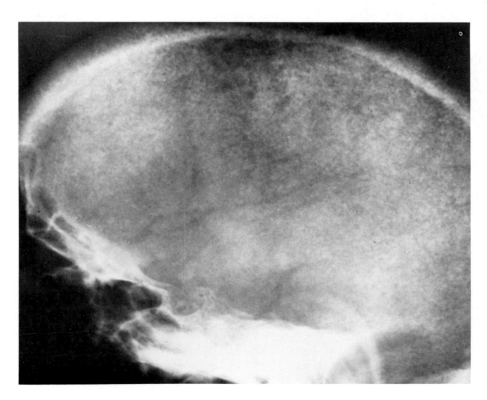

Fig. 4-16. Hyperparathyroidism. Note the granular appearance of the cranial bones with a decrease in overall density.

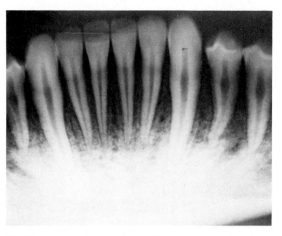

Fig. 4-17. Hyperparathyroidism. The anterior teeth of the lower jaw demonstrate nearly complete absence of the lamina dura, which is the cortex of the tooth socket. There is also loss of bone density in the alveolar ridge with the coarse trabecular pattern noted near the apices of the dental roots.

(Fig. 4-22). They are often referred to as "brown tumors." They are not true cysts but contain fibrous tissue, giant cells, osteoclasts, and decomposing blood.[1] The larger ones may be misinterpreted as giant cell tumors. This tumor is solitary and involves the end of a bone. Brown tumors may occur anywhere in the bone and often are multiple. The jaws, pelvis, and femurs are favorite sites but the lesion may be found in any part of the skeleton.

Pathologic Fracture. Fracture may result from the general weakening of the bone structure or because of localized destruction caused by a cystic lesion.

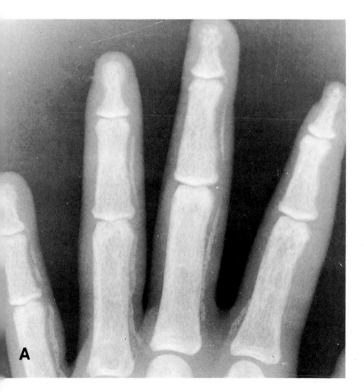

Fig. 4-18. Secondary hyperparathyroidism (renal osteodystrophy) in a 21-year-old woman with chronic renal insufficiency. **A.** There is subperiosteal resorption noted particularly along the lateral aspects of the shafts of the middle phalanges of the second and third digits. Bone texture is coarse with prominent trabeculae. Calcification in digital arteries is prominent, and there is vascular insufficiency leading to loss of soft tissues at the tips of the index and fourth fingers. **B.** The lumbar vertebral bodies show osteosclerosis that is most intense along the upper and lower borders.

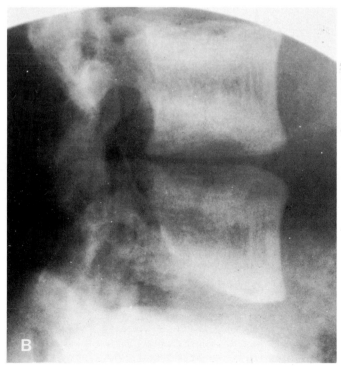

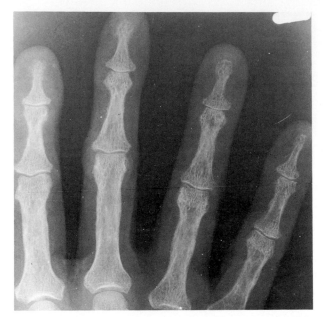

Fig. 4-19. Hyperparathyroidism. There is considerable thinning of the middle phalanges, particularly of the index and middle fingers. There is also a frayed appearance of the terminal tufts and general decrease in bone density.

Tissue Calcification. Calcium deposition in various structures, but particularly in the kidneys, is common. Calcium may be deposited in the joint cartilages; however, senescence and the pseudogout syndrome are more common causes of articular cartilage calcification. Premature calcification in the walls of the arteries is seen occasionally. Calcium deposition may occur in other tissues such as the pancreas and in the soft tissues around the joints. Calcification of the auricular cartilages has been noted.

Esophageal and Tracheal Displacement. In some patients the parathyroid tumor is large enough to cause recognizable deformity in outline of the trachea or esophagus or both. This may be found in the lower part of the neck or in the upper mediastinum. Barium study of the esophagus is a useful procedure in the evaluation of patients suspected of having a parathyroid adenoma since it will, at times, pinpoint the lesion, thus facilitating its surgical removal.

Osteosclerosis. In some of these patients, increased density or osteosclerosis may be found. This is seen most often in the subchondral and metaphyseal areas and is more frequent in the secondary form of the

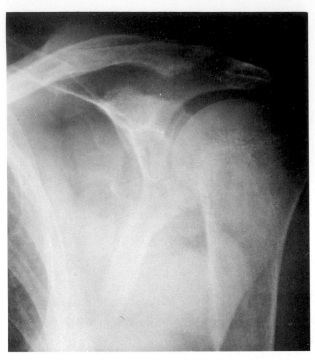

Fig. 4-20. Primary hyperparathyroidism in a patient with parathyroid adenoma. Note the erosion of the distal end of the clavicle causing apparent widening of the acromioclavicular joint space.

Fig. 4-21. Hyperparathyroidism. There has been loss of bone in the distal end of the clavicle. The **arrows** indicate the distal clavicle on the left and the medial acromion on the right.

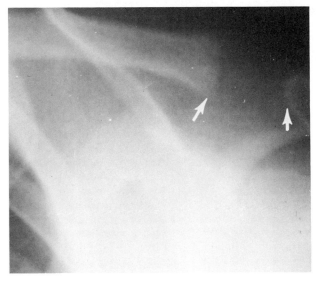

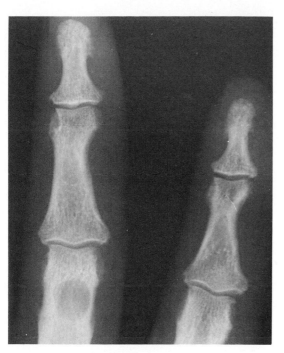

Fig. 4-22. Hyperparathyroidism. The cystlike rarefaction in the distal shaft of the proximal phalanx represents a brown tumor. Note also the concavity of the lateral shafts of the middle phalanges.

RENAL OSTEODYSTROPHY

This disease has been called renal rickets in the past but most investigators believe that the term "renal osteodystrophy" is preferable since much of the skeletal disease which develops is caused by increased parathyroid activity (secondary hyperparathyroidism). The exact pathogenesis is not clear. Recent investigations indicate that the intestinally active metabolite of vitamin D is generated in kidney tissue. As a result of certain renal diseases a decrease in this substance would inhibit the removal of calcium from the intestine causing hypocalcemia. This would, in turn, stimulate the parathyroids and lead to the clinical state of hyperparathyroidism. The low serum calcium level causes failure of normal mineralization of newly formed bone and thus the changes of both rickets and hyperparathyroidism develop. The metabolic effects are very complex, and the major manifestations may differ from one patient to another, depending upon a number of factors (Table 4-1).[12]

The skeletal disease usually does not become manifest before the patient is 2 years old. The kidney diseases responsible usually are congenital, such as polycystic disease, hypogenesis, or congenital obstructions of the ureters, bladder outlet, or urethra. Chronic pyelonephritis is frequently superimposed as a result of urinary tract stasis.[1]

Roentgen Findings. The roentgen findings are essentially a combination of those seen in rickets and hyperparathyroidism (Figs. 4-23 and 4-24). The latter include: (*1*) subperiosteal resorption (see Fig. 4-18), (*2*) generalized undermineralization, (*3*) brown tumors, (*4*) loss of lamina dura around the teeth. The rachitic changes are similar to those of infantile rickets (Figs. 4-25 and 4-26) except that epiphyseal subluxations may occur and a genu valgum deformity is common at the knee instead of a varus deformity.

If the disease begins early in life and the patient survives for a number of years, significant dwarfism occurs. Calcification in the walls of the arteries may be seen, even in the very young. Nephrocalcinosis may develop but renal stones are uncommon. If the disease develops later in life, dwarfism does not occur and the bone changes are mainly those of hyperparathyroidism. Osteosclerosis develops in some patients, chiefly at the ends of the bones and the superior and inferior margins of the vertebrae. It is more frequent than in the primary form of the disease. The reason why osteosclerosis develops is not clear. A substance elaborated by the thyroid, calcitonin, is

disease (renal osteodystrophy). In the spine the upper and lower margins of the vertebral bodies are affected ("rugger-jersey" appearance or "sandwich vertebra").

The differential diagnosis of hyperparathyroidism includes consideration of all the other diseases that cause generalized skeletal demineralization. While the final diagnosis usually rests upon the results of chemical examination of the blood and urine, together with the use of angiography and radioactive isotopes to localize and identify the tumor in some cases, two roentgen signs, when present, are considered to be highly reliable. The one, subperiosteal resorption of the cortices of the phalanges, and other areas such as the distal end of the clavicle, appears to be specific for the disease[22]; the other, loss of the lamina dura around the roots of the teeth, does occur in a few other conditions but is more distinct in hyperparathyroidism. Renal osteodystrophy (renal rickets) may cause changes identical with those seen in primary disease of the parathyroid glands. This is because of the secondary hyperplasia of the parathyroids and the skeletal changes of hyperparathyroidism become a significant feature of the disease.

Table 4-1 Bone and Soft-Tissue Changes in Chronic Glomerular Renal Disease*

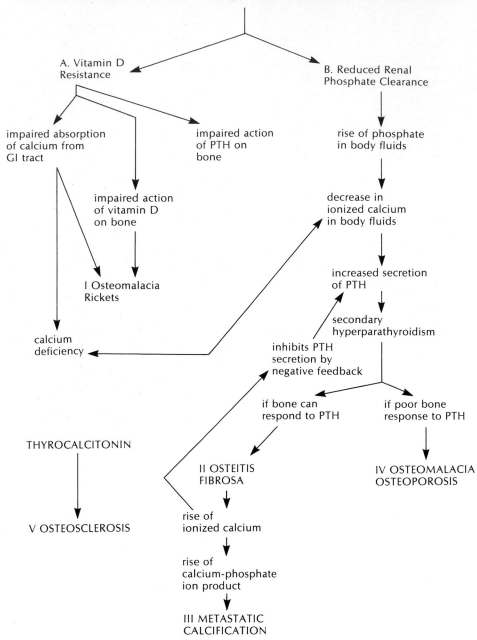

* Classification of bone and soft tissue changes in chronic glomerular renal disease. GI = gastrointestinal; PTH = parathyroid hormone; MET = metastatic. (Greenfield GB: Am J Roentgenol 116: 750, 1972)

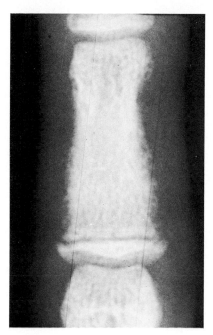

Fig. 4-23. Renal osteodystrophy. Note the loss of cortex of the middle phalangeal shaft in this child. The trabeculae appear to project into the surrounding soft tissues.

known to lower the serum calcium level and it may do so by preventing the normal removal of calcium from bone.

RENAL OSTEODYSTROPHY FOLLOWING RENAL TRANSPLANTATION

In addition to the signs of secondary hyperparathyroidism, a number of other skeletal changes have been demonstrated in patients who have had renal transplants.[13] Ischemic necrosis of the femoral head occurs in nearly one-half of those with skeletal changes. Subperiosteal resorption is also common, and pathologic fractures and brown tumors are also observed. In patients demonstrating osteosclerosis prior to transplantation, there may be an increase in the region of the superior and inferior vertebral end–plates, producing a rugger-jersey spine. Areas of osterosclerosis are also observed elsewhere in the skeleton, sometimes producing a somewhat irregular mixture of osteopenia and osteosclerosis. Large masses of periarticular metastatic calcification are also observed. Occasionally, extensive linear periostitis may involve the long bones. In addition to the hips, avascular necrosis may be observed involving

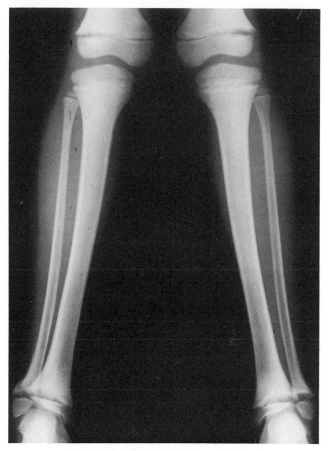

Fig. 4-24. Renal osteodystrophy. The metaphyses show changes resembling those of rickets. Note the tibia valga (knock knees).

the joint surfaces of other bones. This may be the result of steroid therapy, but some believe that it is a manifestation of secondary hyperparathyroidism.

HYPOPARATHYROIDISM

Hypoparathyroidism usually results from injury or accidental removal of the glands during thyroidectomy. Spontaneous idiopathic hypoparathyroidism occurs but is uncommon. The clinical symptoms are those that result from the hypocalcemia (parathyroid tetany). The serum calcium is low and the phosphorus elevated. Roentgen changes are relatively few and in some cases the skeletal system is normal. In others the bones have shown increase in density with widening of the cortices of the long bones. Infre-

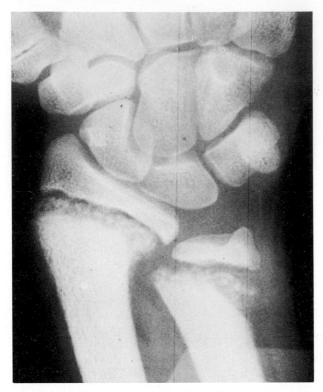

Fig. 4-25. Renal osteodystrophy. There are severe changes in the metaphysis of the radius and ulna with some medial epiphyseal subluxation.

quently the bones of the calvarium are thickened. In some patients, stippled areas of calcification occur within the brain. These tend to be symmetrically situated in the basal ganglia. This finding is not specific for hypoparathyroidism but is always suggestive of it.

PSEUDOHYPOPARATHYROIDISM (PH) AND PSEUDO-PSEUDOHYPOPARATHYROIDISM (PPH)

Pseudohypoparathyroidism (PH) is a congenital hereditary disorder characterized by a failure of normal response to parathyroid hormone.[25] There is hypocalcemia and hyperphosphatemia as in hypoparathyroidism and little or no response to the administration of parathyroid hormone. Most patients are obese and of short stature with a round facies, corneal or lenticular opacities, brachydactyly, and mental retardation.

Usually all of the tubular bones of the hands and feet are short, but some, especially the fourth and fifth metacarpals, are shorter than the others. Also they tend to be broad owing to lack of normal constriction of the midshafts. The terminal and middle phalanges tend to be relatively shorter than the proximal. Cone epiphyses are common and the epiphyseal plates are thin or, at times, partially fused at the apex of the cone when they first appear. Accelerated fusion is common in the hands and feet.

Calcified or ossified deposits may be found in the skin or subcutaneous tissues. Stippled calcification is often found in the basal ganglia or elsewhere in the brain, as in hypoparathyroidism. In some, the cranial bones are thickened and the skull has a brachycephalic shape. The interpedicular distances in the lumbar spine may decrease from above downward instead of showing the normal increase. The general skeletal density is decreased, apparently owing to osteoporosis, and the trabecular structure may be coarse. However, increased density has been reported in some patients and, apparently because of the hypocalcemia, the changes of secondary hyperparathyroidism may develop. In some infants the hands and feet have been normal but become abnormal as the child grows older.

Dentition often is abnormal including defective dentine, excessive caries, delayed eruption, and wide root canals. Other findings have been observed in some patients including coxa vara or valga, bowing of the long bones, and an occasional exostosis including one on the inner proximal tibia similar to that seen in the Ellis–van Creveld syndrome and in Turner's syndrome.

The hereditary nature of PH has been established. It is possible for some members of the family to show roentgen findings characteristic of the disease but with blood-chemistry studies showing normal values and no evidence of tetany. This entity has been called pseudo-pseudohypoparathyroidism (PPH) and is considered to be the partial expression of a disease of which PH is the complete syndrome.[25] Families showing only the characteristics of PPH have been reported and in some members the bone changes have been very minimal, such as a shortening of one or more of the metacarpals. There also is a lower incidence of intracranial calcification in PPH than in PH.

Among the entities to be considered in differential diagnosis are: (*1*) peripheral dysostosis, (*2*) chondroectodermal dysplasia, (*3*) multiple hereditary exostosis, and (*4*) Turner's syndrome.[25] These have, as

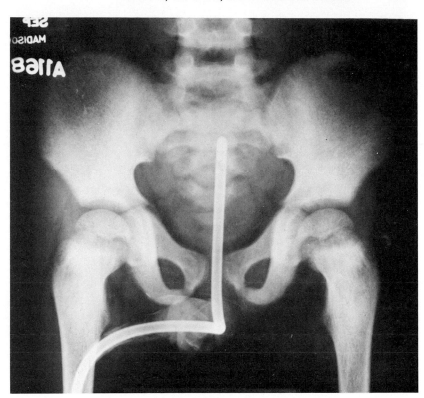

Fig. 4-26. Pelvis of the patient shown in Figure 4-24. The renal damage was caused by severe obstruction of the bladder neck.

a rule, other roentgen, clinical, and genetic findings that aid in differentiation. Short metacarpals and metatarsals also occur as isolated defects.

CALCIUM OXALOSIS

This is a rare inherited metabolic disease[6] in which calcium oxalate crystals cause extensive renal damage leading to renal failure. The crystals are found in soft tissues other than the kidney including the skin and subcutaneous tissues and the eye. The skeletal changes resemble those of secondary hyperparathyroidism. There are destructive areas of subperiosteal resorption and sclerotic bands producing the rugger-jersey changes in the spine. The same pattern is noted in the sternum. Striking findings are noted in the hands and knees; these consist of irregular, transverse, sclerotic metaphyseal bands in the distal femur and proximal tibia and fibula as well as in the distal radius and ulna. There is a drumstick configuration of the metacarpals, evidently a combination of narrowing of the diaphysis plus widening of the metaphysis. Renal calculi are common in patients with this disease, and diffuse, extensive renal calcification is also observed.

REFERENCES AND SELECTED READINGS

1. AEGETER E, KIRKPATRICK JA JR: Orthopedic Diseases, pp 235–242, 4th ed. Philadelphia, Saunders, 1975
2. ARNSTEIN AR: Regional osteoporosis. Orthopedic Clin North Am 3: 585, 1972
3. BROMER RS: Rickets. Am J Roentgenol 30: 582, 1933
4. CAMERON JR, MAZESS RB, SORENSON JA: Precision and accuracy of bone mineral determination by direct photon absorptiometry. Invest Radiol 3: 141, 1968
5. CAMP JD: Osseous changes in hyperparathyroidism. A roentgenologic study. JAMA 99: 1913, 1932
6. CARSEN GM, RADKOWSKI MA: Calcium oxalosis. Radiology 113: 165, 1974
7. DARLING DB, LORIDAN L, SENIOR B: The roentgenographic manifestations of Cushing's syndrome in infancy. Radiology 96: 503, 1970
8. EDEIKEN J, HODES PJ: Roentgen Diagnosis of Diseases of Bone, 2nd ed. Baltimore, Williams & Wilkins, 1973

9. GENANT HK, HECK LL, LANZL LH et al: Primary hyperparathyroidism. Radiology 109: 513, 1973

10. GENANT HK, KOZIN F, BEKERMAN C et al: The reflex sympathetic dystrophy syndrome: a comprehensive analysis using fine detail radiography, photon absorptiometry and bone and joint scintigraphy. Radiology 117: 21, 1975

11. GLEASON DG, POTCHEN EJ: The diagnosis of hyperparathyroidism. Radiol Clin North Am 5: 277, 1967

12. GREENFIELD GB: Roentgen appearance of bone and soft tissue changes in chronic renal disease. Am J Roentgenol 116: 749, 1972

13. GRIFFITHS HJ, ENNIS JT, BAILEY G: Skeletal changes following renal transplantation. Radiology 113: 621, 1974

14. HAFF RC, BLACK WC, BALLINGER WF II: Primary hyperparathyroidism: changing clinical, surgical and pathologic aspects. Ann Surg 171: 85, 1970

15. JACKSON DM: Heel-pad thickness in obese persons. Radiology 90: 129, 1968

16. JONES G: Radiological appearances of disuse osteoporosis. Clin Radiol 20: 345, 1969

17. MANKIN HJ: Rickets, osteomalacia, and renal osteodystrophy. J Bone Joint Surg [A] 56: 352, 1974

18. MCALISTER WH, KOEHLER PR: Diseases of the adrenal. Radiol Clin North Am 5: 205, 1967

19. MEEMA HE, MEEMA S: Improved roentgenologic diagnosis of osteomalacia by microradioscopy of hand bones. Am J Roentgenol 125: 925, 1975

20. MILKMAN LA: Pseudofractures (hunger osteopathy, late rickets, osteomalacia). Am J Roentgenol 24: 29, 1930

21. MURRAY RO: Radiological bone changes in Cushing's syndrome and steroid therapy. Br J Radiol 33: 1, 1960

22. PUGH DG: Subperisteal resorption of bone. A roentgenologic manifestation of primary hyperparathyroidism and renal osteodystrophy. Am J Roentgenol 66: 577, 1951

23. RUBIN P: Dynamic Classification of Bone Dysplasias. Chicago, Year Book Medical, 1964

24. STEINBACH HL: The roentgen appearance of osteoporosis. Radiol Clin North Am 2: 191, 1964

25. STEINBACH HL, YOUNG DA: The roentgen appearance of pseudohypoparathyroidism (PH) and pseudo-pseudohypoparathyroidism (PPH). Am J Roentgenol 97: 49, 1966

26. WHEDON GD, CAMERON JE (eds): Proceedings of the Conference on Progress in Methods of Bone Mineral Measurements. Washington DC, US Government Printing Office, 1970

5

TRAUMATIC LESIONS OF BONES AND JOINTS

While the presence of a fracture often is obvious on clinical examination, roentgenograms are essential to delineate the nature of the injury clearly, and only from roentgen examination can an accurate idea be obtained of the anatomic structures involved and the severity of the injury to them. In a great many instances, roentgen examination is necessary to determine whether a fracture exists or not because the clinical findings are not reliable. Conversely, there may at times be clinical evidence to suggest fracture, but roentgenograms fail to reveal it initially. As a general rule, when the slightest doubt exists concerning the presence or absence of a fracture of dislocation, roentgen examination should be performed. After reduction of a fracture, roentgenograms are needed to determine the accuracy of reduction, to furnish a record of the status of the fracture, and, later, to follow the progress of healing. The frequency of follow-up examinations to determine the degree of healing will vary widely, depending upon such factors as the type of fracture, the bone involved, the method of treatment employed, and the age of the patient, among others, so that no set rules can be given. A fracture being treated by means of skeletal traction may require daily examinations, at least until reduction has been accomplished. A fracture that has been reduced satisfactorily and the part placed in a cast should be examined immediately after the application of the cast and at intervals of several weeks thereafter until healing is sufficiently solid for use of the part. Oblique or spiral fractures need closer observation than transverse or impacted fractures because of the tendency for slipping of the fragments within the cast.

METHODS OF EXAMINATION

ROENTGENOGRAMS

It is usual in examining the bones for fracture to obtain at least two views made at right angles to one another. These are necessary in order to obtain a true perspective of the spatial relationships of the fragments (Fig. 5-1). At times the fracture line may be visible in only one of several projections and the examiner is not justified in saying that a fracture does not exist solely on observation of a single roentgeno-

127

gram of a part. Even with multiple exposures and technically good roentgenograms, a fine hairline fracture may escape detection until a reexamination some days later will show it clearly. The decalcification that occurs along the edges of the fracture fragments may make the fracture line more readily visible after a short period of time. Such fractures are seen occasionally in the carpal navicular and in the ribs. The term **occult fracture** has been used to denote this lesion, implying a fracture that may give clinical signs of its presence but which cannot be demonstrated roentgenologically until reparative changes have occurred.

Where two right-angle views are impossible to obtain, usually because of the condition of the injured patient, a third-dimensional image can be obtained by the use of stereoscopic roentgenograms. It is often impossible to secure completely satisfactory films of a severely injured patient at the time of the initial examination and only a general survey can be made to indicate the presence and extent of gross fractures. More detailed examination may be delayed until such complications as shock or internal injuries have received attention. In head injuries the damage to the brain often is of much greater importance than any associated fracture of the cranial bones; the desire to find out the extent of the patient's bone injuries should not influence the judgment of the physician in his care of the patient.

Terminology. When describing displacement of fracture fragments it is usual to refer to the displacement of the distal fragment in relation to the proximal, the latter being considered as the stationary part. Thus, one speaks of a posterior displacement of the distal fragment of the tibia on the proximal fragment rather than an anterior displacement of the proximal on the distal. The same method is used in describing dislocations, the distal extremity being considered to be the dislocated one. For example, all dislocations of the elbow joint are displacements of the bones of the forearm on the humerus. In describing angular deformity it also is usual to consider the distal fragment as being angled on the proximal. Unless otherwise modified, the term "medial angulation" refers to an inward angulation of the distal fragment on the proximal. For greater accuracy it is better to describe angulations in terms of convexity and concavity. In the example referred to above, where the lower fragment was turned inward on the proximal, the proper description would be a medical concave angulation of "x" degrees, or, if preferred, a lateral convex angulation of "x" degrees. Using the terms, "concave" and

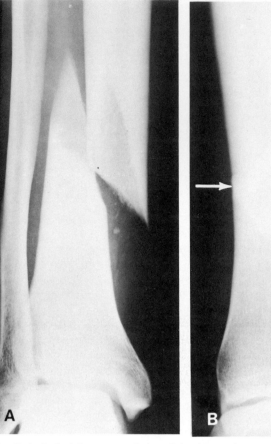

Fig. 5-1. Spiral fracture of the tibia. Note the amount of displacement in the anteroposterior view **(A)** and the lack of it in the lateral view **(B).** The zone of increased density on the lateral view indicates overriding **(arrow).**

"convex" will indicate clearly the nature of the deformity.

FLUOROSCOPY

At one time fluoroscopy was widely used to aid in the reduction of fractures because it enabled the orthopedic surgeon to manipulate the fragments under direct fluoroscopic vision. The danger of overexposure to radiation to the person doing the reduction is real. Many physicians in the past have developed severe reactions from repeated or prolonged exposure of the hands during the fluoroscopic manipulation of fractures. The danger of overexposure of the skin of the patient during a protracted reduction also must be kept in mind and is a definite hazard. Because of these harmful possibilities, fluoroscopy for this purpose is rarely employed. If it is used, certain precautions are essential: (*1*) The person operating the fluoroscope must be fully aware of the amount of radiation being delivered by the roentgen ray tube and equally aware of methods of protection. (2) A timing device should be incorporated in the roentgen-ray circuit to shut off the current automatically after a predetermined amount of time has elapsed. (3) All manipulation should be done with the fluoroscope turned off and it should be turned on for quick visual inspection only when the surgeon's hands have been removed from the field of exposure. (4) If repeated attempts at reduction become necessary, fluoroscopy should not be used. (5) An image intensifier should always be used.

TYPES OF FRACTURES

There are several ways in which fractures of the bones of the extremities can be classified. They can be divided into two major groups—open and closed fractures. An open fracture is usually spoken of as a compound fracture and this term is used to denote a perforation of the skin over the fracture. The importance of a compound fracture, of course, lies in the possibility of infection because of contamination at the time of injury, and this possibility must be taken into account when progress roentgenograms of a compound fracture are being evaluated. A closed fracture not infrequently is changed into an open one because of the need for surgical reduction, the placement of metal plates, bone grafts, or other fixation devices. While very infrequent with good surgical technique, there is always the possibility of such a fracture becoming infected.

Fractures also can be classified according to the mechanics of the stress that produces them and thus one finds such terms as torsion fractures, bending fractures, and shearing fractures used in descriptive terminology. While one can frequently suspect the nature of the force that caused the fracture from the roentgen appearances, this is not always the case and in general these terms are not commonly used in roentgenologic descriptions.

The following grouping of fractures is useful for descriptive purposes and the terms are those used in roentgen and clinical evaluation. Some fractures will not fit into a specific group because they show mixed features. For example, a compression fracture may also show evidence of comminution; the line of demarcation between an impacted fracture and a com-

pression fracture is not sharp; a Colles' fracture at the wrist is usually comminuted as well as impacted. These limitations must be kept in mind when one attempts to classify any specific fracture.

COMPLETE, NONCOMMINUTED FRACTURES

This term is used to designate a fracture that has caused a complete dissolution in continuity of the bone with separation of it into two fragments. The fracture is visualized in roentgenograms as a dark line or zone between the fragments and there may or may not be displacement.

Oblique, Spiral, and Transverse Fractures

According to the direction of the fracture line, the oblique, spiral, and transverse fractures can be recognized. Spiral and oblique fractures are common in the shafts of the long tubular bones (see Fig. 5-1). Transverse fractures are less frequent but can occur if the force producing the fracture is of the bending rather than the torsion type. A particular type of transverse fracture often occurs through abnormal bone, *i.e.*, a pathologic fracture. The line of fracture often extends directly through the bone at a right angle to the long axis and the ends of the fragments are smooth or at the most show only a moderate irregularity. Transverse fractures through normal bone are invariably ragged along the line of fracture.

Multiple Fractures

When two or more complete fractures involve the shaft of a single bone, they are spoken of as multiple fractures. Multiple fractures differ from comminuted fractures in that each fracture is a complete one leaving a fragment of intact shaft between them. In a comminuted fracture, one or more small fragments have been separated along the line of major fracture but these pieces, as a rule, do not represent a complete thickness of the bone.

Avulsion Fractures

An avulsion fracture consists of the separation of a fragment of bone that has been pulled away from the shaft. Usually avulsion fractures involve a tuberosity or bony process. Common examples are avulsion of the internal epicondyle of the humerus and avulsion fracture of the greater tuberosity of the humerus (Fig. 5-2). In other cases there may be avulsion of a fragment of cortex as a result of muscle or ligament

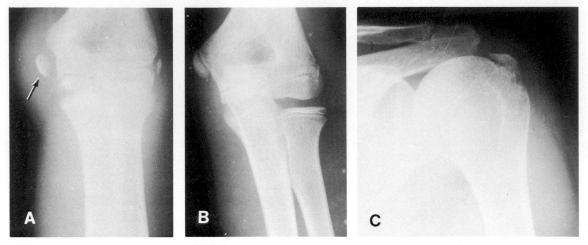

Fig. 5-2. Avulsion fractures. **A.** Avulsion fracture of the epiphysis for the medial epicondyle of the humerus **(arrow). B.** Normal elbow for comparison. **C.** Avulsion fracture of the greater tuberosity of the humerus.

pull occurring as part of a sprain. These are referred to as cortical avulsions or flake fractures and are frequent in the ankle area in association with severe sprains.

Chip Fractures

A chip fracture resembles an avulsion fracture and is a type of avulsion but the term usually is limited to denote the separation of a small fragment or chip of bone from the corner of a phalanx or other long bone. These fractures also are sometimes called corner fractures. They are very common in the fingers and the fragments often are very tiny. Chip fracture fragments do not always undergo bony union, but fibrous union generally takes place and unless the fragment was displaced considerably or was rather large there is usually little impairment of function.

COMMINUTED FRACTURES

A comminuted fracture is one in which, in addition to the major line of fracture that extends through the bone, one or more fragments have been separated along the edges of one or both major fragments. Occasionally the bone may be extensively shattered. More often the comminution is less severe and the fracture may follow a fairly distinct pattern. Thus one finds T, V, and Y fractures, the designation indicating the general appearance of the fracture lines. T fractures are frequent in the lower end of the femur with a transverse fracture extending through the bone just above the level of the condyles and a vertical

component forming the stem of the T extending into the joint and separating the condyles (Fig. 5-3). A Y fracture is rather similar; it is found occasionally in the lower end of the humerus. V fractures occasionally occur in the midshafts of the long bones.

A crush fracture is a special type of comminuted fracture seen in a distal phalanx and usually results from the finger being crushed in a door or between heavy objects. The terminal tuft often is broken into many small fragments that are spread apart slightly but generally not severely displaced. Crush fractures also may involve the os calcis as the result of a fall from a height, the patient landing on the heels. Usually there is considerable impaction also present and this type of fracture often is a mixture of comminution and impaction.

INCOMPLETE FRACTURES

In an incomplete fracture not all the bone structure gives way. Some of the trabeculae are disrupted completely but others only buckle or bend or remain intact. There may be an angular deformity but there can be little or no displacement.

Greenstick Fracture

The greenstick fracture is one of the common forms of incomplete fracture (Fig. 5-4). Only a part of the framework structure gives way, allowing a buckling or sharp angulation of the bone. The effect is similar to that obtained by trying to break a green twig. The simplest form may show only a slight buckling of the

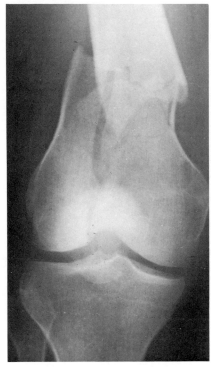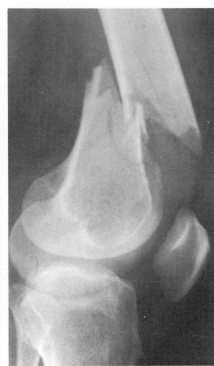

Fig. 5-3. Comminuted T-fracture of the lower end of the femur. In addition to the irregular transverse fracture through the shaft, there is a vertical fracture extending to the articular surface of the femur.

cortex and clinical symptoms may be negligible. Greenstick fractures are found almost exclusively during infancy and childhood. In older persons the bones are more brittle and this type of fracture does not occur. Greenstick fractures heal promptly.

Impacted Fracture

An impacted fracture usually is incomplete although there occasionally may be a complete disruption at the line of fracture with secondary impaction having occurred. In an impacted fracture the fragments are driven into one another either along the entire line of fracture or only along one side. A radiolucent fracture line is not seen in this type of fracture since the impaction completely obscures it. Instead, the line of impaction is denser than normal because of the condensed bony trabeculae within it. In addition, an impacted fracture can be recognized by the disruption of normal bone trabeculae and architecture at the site of impaction, by the sharp angulation of the cortical margin at least on one side of the fracture, and by the general disturbance of normal anatomic relationships. One of the frequent sites for impacted fracture is the neck of the femur. A type of impacted fracture frequent in the vertebrae and that also may involve some of the irregular bones, such as the os

calcis, is called a compression fracture. This is essentially the same as an impacted fracture but the latter term is usually limited to designate fractures occurring in the long bones, while the term "compression fracture" is applied to injuries involving the vertebrae or the bones of the carpus and tarsus.

Infractions

An infraction is a form of impacted fracture and the term is used to designate an injury of limited extent. Thus an impacted fracture of a metatarsal head in which there is a barely recognizable deformity might be designated as an infraction rather than a fracture. The term also is used to describe a minor localized break in the cortex of a bone that causes only slight local deformity. Local injury to a bone by a blunt object that causes only a small indentation or fragmentation of cortex can properly be called an infraction.

Buckling Fracture

This term is used to designate certain fractures that occur almost entirely in demineralized bone, chiefly secondary to severe osteoporosis. The bone breaks only part way through and there results a sharp angular deformity without lateral displacement. The effect can be likened to that obtained by sharply bending a thin rubber tube. Buckling fractures are caused by a bending type of strain. Porotic bone, being softer than normal bone, may give way in this manner. A normal bone suffering the same type of strain might not fracture at all or if it did the fracture would most likely be complete.

Penetrating Fracture

This term is used to indicate the type of bone injury that results from penetration by a sharp object such as a bullet or perforation by a sharp piece of metal. The injury is localized to a relatively small portion of the bone without a complete dissolution in continuity. The fracture therefore is properly included in the group of incomplete fractures, but frequently there is comminution with separation of small fragments at the site of injury. Some of these fractures are difficult to classify because they encompass various groups.

EPIPHYSEAL FRACTURES

During childhood a fracture may extend part way or completely through the epiphyseal plate at the end of a long bone and lead to displacement of the epiphysis on the shaft. This type of injury is frequent in the lower end of the tibia and in the distal end of the radius (Fig. 5-5). If the line of fracture is limited to the cartilage it will not be directly visible and its detection rests upon the evidence of epiphyseal displacement or upon variation in width of the epiphyseal line. In the absence of displacement, detection of a pure epiphyseal plate fracture is difficult; comparison with the opposite extremity is helpful in doubtful cases. In most cases the fracture does not remain confined to the cartilaginous plate but angles sharply into the bone so that a corner fragment of the shaft remains attached to the epiphysis and is carried along with it if the epiphysis becomes displaced. If there is no displacement, the oblique fracture line in the shaft can be recognized and indicates the nature of the injury.

Since the epiphysis is responsible for bone growth, injuries involving the epiphyseal growth plate may result in an alteration in length of the involved bone. In children, dislocations and ligamentous tears are uncommon. Injuries that cause these conditions in adults produce epiphyseal separation in the younger age group. The extent of the injury is important in assessing the likelihood of growth alterations. Prognosis depends on the degree of vascular damage, with growth disturbance paralleling the degree of arterial disruption.[10] The Salter-Harris classification is used commonly in describing these injuries of the epiphy-

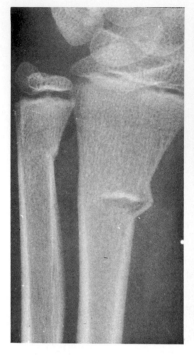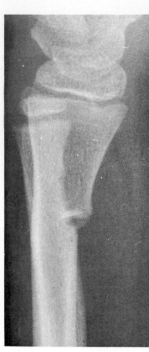

Fig. 5-4. Greenstick fractures of the radius and ulna in a child. There is some anterolateral buckling of bone, but the fracture line does not extend across the width of the shafts despite the slight angulation of the distal fragments.

seal plate (Fig. 5-6). Radiographic findings are distinct for each type and prognosis usually varies with the type. The[11] classification is as follows:

Type I: Pure epiphyseal separation. The line of cleavage is confined to the zone of hypertrophic cells within the epiphyseal plate. Since the fracture line is in cartilage, it is not visible radiographically; displacement of the epiphyseal ossification center is the only positive radiographic sign other than the presence of secondary soft-tissue swelling. The prognosis is generally favorable with no alterations in growth in most instances.

Type II: A fragment from the metaphysis accompanies the displaced epiphysis separating off a segment of bone on the metaphyseal side. This is by far the most common injury, compromising approximately 75% of cases. The most common sites are the distal radius which accounts for up to one half of all epiphyseal injuries. The distal tibia, distal fibula, distal femur, and ulna are involved in decreasing order of frequency. The prognosis in this injury is also generally favorable.

Type III: The fracture runs vertically through the epiphysis and through the growth plate. A portion of

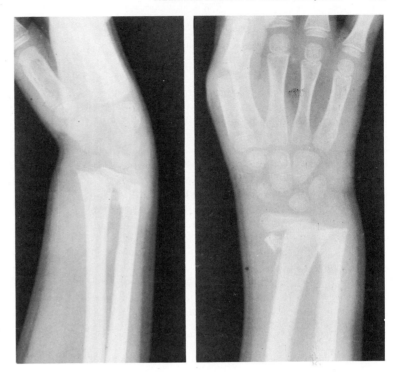

Fig. 5-5. Epiphyseal fracture–dislocation involving the distal end of the radius. The distal epiphysis, together with a fragment of the metaphysis, has been displaced posteriorly and laterally. This is a rather severe Salter-Harris type II injury. Note early callus in this 1-week-old fracture.

the epiphysis is detached and displaced. Usually the displacement is minimal without an associated fracture of the metaphysis. The most frequent site is the distal tibia. The prognosis is good if the fragment is replaced properly so that the joint surface does not become irregular.

Type IV: This is a vertically oriented fracture extending through the epiphysis and growth plate and into the metaphysis. The fracture fragment then consists of a portion of metaphysis, the growth plate, and epiphysis. The most common sites are the lateral condyle of the humerus in patients under age 10 and the distal tibia in those over age 10. Growth arrest and joint deformities are the distinct hazard in this type of injury although the incidence is reduced by proper reduction and fixation (usually surgical).

Type V: This rare injury is a result of crushing-type force, usually directed to the distal femoral or distal tibial epiphyseal centers. There may be no immediate radiographic alteration visible on the bone. Nearly 100% of those suffering this injury have some shortening and/or angulation as a result. Premature closure of an epiphyseal line and a slowing of the growth rate are the factors that result in deformity. Patients with a long interval between injury and cessation of growth must be followed for a minimum of 2 years before the possibility of these complications can be excluded.

Fig. 5-6. Diagram showing the end of the normal developing bone and the site of injury in the Salter–Harris classification of epiphyseal fractures.

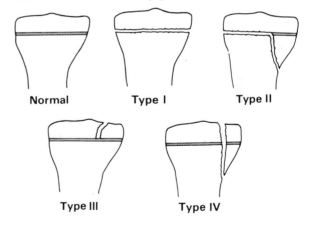

Normal   Type I   Type II

Type III   Type IV

PATHOLOGIC FRACTURES

A pathologic fracture is one occurring through diseased bone. It may occur in practically any of the forms described in the preceding sections. There are two types, however, which always suggest that a fracture has occurred through diseased bone: (*1*) A buckling fracture such as described previously. This usually happens when fracture involves osteoporotic bone. This type of fracture is rather frequent in osteogenesis imperfecta, which is a form of osteoporosis. If the angular deformity is not corrected, the bones become bowed (see Fig. 2-21). (2) A transverse fracture extending at right angles to the longitudinal axis of the bone with the ends of the fragments smooth or only slightly irregular (Fig. 5-7). In the presence of any fracture, the structure of the bone should be observed carefully for evidence of disease that may have predisposed to the injury. Occasionally a bone cyst, enchondroma, or other benign lesion is discovered because of the fracture. In adults a pathologic fracture may bring to light a focus of metastatic carcinoma or other significant local lesion of bone.

PSEUDOFRACTURES

These are transverse fissurelike defects that extend part way or completely through the bone. They are seen frequently in osteomalacia and are sometimes referred to as the "zones of Looser" or *Umbauzonen*. They are infractions of bone in which osteoid is formed in the defect but with failure of calcium deposition so that a fissure defect persists in the roentgenogram. Multiple pseudofractures of this type were described by Milkman in 1930 and the condition sometimes is designated as Milkman's syndrome. Most investigators now believe that this represents osteomalacia in which the pseudofractures happen to be a particularly prominent part of the disease (see Chapter 4, section on "Osteomalacia").

A similar type of transverse fracture is seen in Paget's disease, fibrous dysplasia, and osteogenesis imperfecta. Some authorities contend that these differ from the pseudofractures of osteomalacia in that they are true fractures that have healed by fibrous or cartilaginous union. Roentgenologically they are similar to the pseudofractures of osteomalacia but the basic change of the underlying bone disease (*e.g.,* Paget's disease) will be different and will lead to the correct diagnosis (Fig. 5-8). A pseudofracture may become complete following an injury and lead to dis-

Fig. 5-7. Pathologic fractures. **A.** Note irregular fracture line through the small cyst of the tibia. **B.** Comminuted fracture through a phalangeal enchondroma.

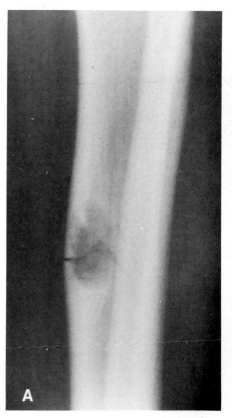
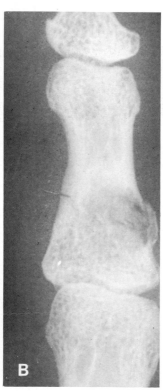
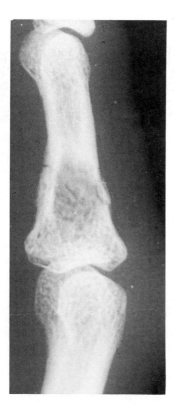

placement of fragments and the clinical signs and symptoms of fracture. Pseudofractures are probably very similar to the chronic fatigue fractures that occur in the metatarsals and other bones (see next section) and they probably develop in bone that is incapable of withstanding the stresses placed upon it. In normal bone, fissures will heal promptly. In abnormal bone, such as in osteomalacia, healing is delayed and the fissure persists as a roentgenologically visible defect.

CHRONIC STRESS OR FATIGUE FRACTURE

This is a type of fracture most frequently found in the metatarsals, particularly the second. It develops as a result of chronic foot strain. Following a brief period of pain and swelling, roentgenograms show changes which are usually characteristic. As a rule, the first sign is subperiosteal callus which tends to be faint, hazy, and fusiform. (Fig. 5-9). Within a few weeks this callus shadow becomes dense and generally at this time a faint line of fracture can be seen extending transversely through the bone. When the stress injury is near the end of a long bone or in a tarsal bone, the first sign may be sclerosis. Tomography is sometimes useful in demonstrating a fracture line when the diagnosis is in doubt. The lesion is considered to be a simple fracture that occurs in a bone unable to withstand the strains placed upon it but which is otherwise normal. The lesion also can develop as a result of abnormal stresses that have been applied for some time by muscle or ligament pull as part of an activity not ordinarily indulged in by the individual. It received the name *"march foot"* when it was first encountered in recruit soldiers after long marches. The line of fracture does not become visible for a week or two, or until decalcification along the fracture line makes it more prominent. Even then the fracture line may be very faint. The same type of fracture occasionally is found in other bones, particularly the inner upper margin of the tibia. Here the area of fracture may first appear as an incomplete transverse line of increased density with a small amount of periosteal calcification overlying it. This is a manifestation of early repair. In the os calcis the same finding, that of a linear zone of sclerosis, may be the first clue to the diagnosis. These fractures also have been described as occurring in the superior aspect of the femoral neck, the anterior portion of the first rib (Fig. 5-10), the upper end of the fibula, and the superior and inferior pubic rami. We have seen two examples of fatigue fracture involving the inner cortex of the tibia, several inches above the ankle

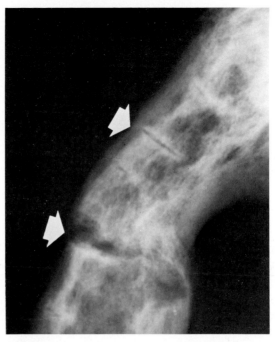

Fig. 5-8. Pseudofractures in Paget's disease. A portion of the femoral shaft showing severe Paget's disease with several incomplete transverse fissures **(arrows).**

joint, which developed in distance runners. When one finds a transverse line or band of increased density extending part way or completely through the end of either a long bone or one of the small bones, stress fracture should be considered the likely diagnosis.

Another stress-related injury appears to involve the pubis adjacent to the symphysis in athletes, the so-called osteitis pubis. There is gradual onset of local pain and tenderness at the symphysis. Radiographic findings are variable. In some instances a loss of subcortical bone at the inferior aspect of the symphysis, usually on one side is demonstrated; in others, the inferior aspect of the symphysis is also noted to be widened, but there is a sclerotic bone reaction.[6]

UNION OF FRACTURES

Most of the work on union of fractures has been done on experimental animals and, since changes are observed among various species, it follows that the process as it occurs in the human is not necessarily identical to that in animals. The process was described by Aegerter and Kirkpatrick on the basis of a

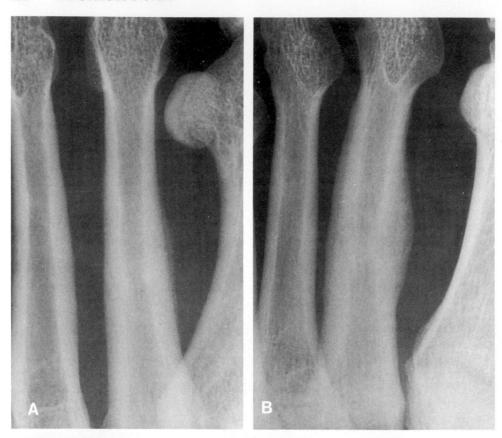

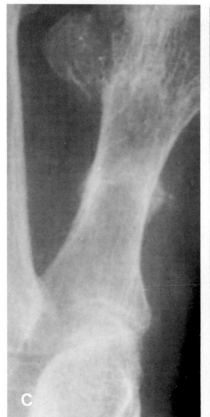

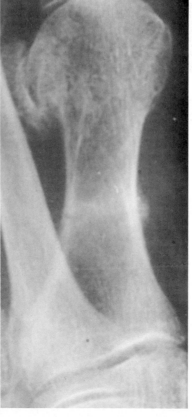

Fig. 5-9. Stress fractures. **A.** Note minimal subperiosteal calcification along the medial aspect of the shaft of the second metatarsal. **B.** One month later, fracture shown in **A** has considerable cortical new bone at the site of injury. **C.** Note subperiosteal callus and incomplete fracture line of the midshaft of the first metatarsal. (*Continued opposite page*)

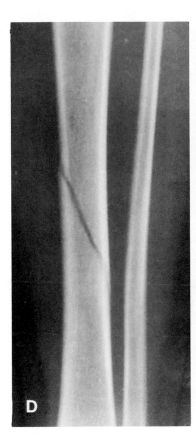
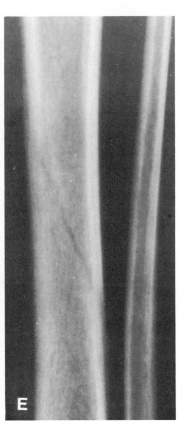

Fig. 5-9. (*Continued*) **D.** Oblique stress fracture of the midtibia. **E.** Six weeks later, fracture shown in **D** shows evidence of healing.

study of a series of fractured bones ranging in sequence from 6 hours to 116 days. This study was supplemented by surgical specimens and by a series of fractures in dogs. When a fracture occurs, the soft tissues are lacerated, the periosteum is usually torn, and vascular channels in the adjacent soft tissues are opened. These injuries result in hematoma as arterial blood flows into the tissues at the site of the trauma. Since the blood supply to the cells adjacent to the fracture is interrupted, these cells die and the edges of the fracture then consist of dead bone back as far as the junction of collateral vascular channels. A network of fibrin is precipitated in the clot and collagenoblasts penetrate the hematoma from the adjacent mesenchymal tissues. A network of endothelial buds is formed, and the hematoma is organized into a mass of granulation. The resulting hyperemia aids in the lysis of the dead bone, leaving an excess of mineral salts in the intercellular fluids.

Viable osteoblasts are beginning to produce osteoid during this time, and the new fibroblasts mature into osteoblasts and chondroblasts. Blood supply is diminished as collagen is laid down. Osteoid is laid down wherever there are fragments of old bone and it also forms on islands of newly formed cartilage. The osteoid soon becomes mineralized so that small masses of cartilage surrounded by fiber bone and osteochondroid can be found in the area. It is likely that fibroblasts first mature into chondroblasts, producing chondroid and with time the fibroblasts become osteoblasts that lay down intercellular substance which becomes osteoid. At times a large cartilage island persists, usually at the periphery of the area of healing. The chondroblasts mature, line up in columns as in the endochondral plate, and a line of provisional calcification is formed. The persistence of a cartilage island is not necessary or very common, however, in the healing of fractures.

There is also production of new bone between the periosteum and the old cortex and a solid mass of bone also replaces the marrow tissue. This new bone extends outward to merge with the outer callus bracing the shaft of a cylindrical bone from within and without. All of this new bone is termed *callus*.

At first the bone comprising the callus is largely fiber bone which must be replaced with adult bone

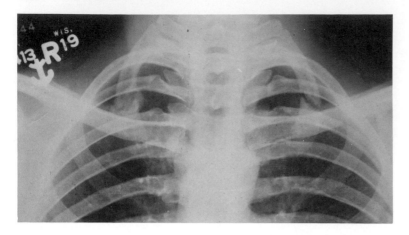

Fig. 5-10. Chronic stress fracture of the first ribs. Callus on the right obliterates the fracture line. No definite callus is observed on the left.

before it can withstand functional stresses. Strong adult bone moves into the area where strength is needed and the weaker fiber bone disappears. Lines of stress determine the shifting of bone so that the angulations of malposition may be straightened even when side-to-side rather than end-to-end approximation is attained as a result of fracture reduction. There is also a decrease in the bulk of the callus as the stronger adult bone replaces the weaker fiber bone. When periosteum is not devitalized, callus is formed more quickly than in fractures in which there is widespread periosteal destruction.

Cartilage appears to be formed in areas where there is no cortical bone and therefore no direct osteoid formation. Consequently, when fragments are separated, a ring of cartilage extends around the bone defining the fracture line. This forms the nidus from which extracortical callus forms. Movement of fracture edges tends to disturb the ring of cartilage and probably inhibits callus formation. Also, it is likely that motion produces multiple foci of osteochondroid formation leading to an increase in size of the callus which is often observed when there is motion at the fracture site.

ROENTGEN EVIDENCE OF BONE UNION

There is a great variation in the rate of healing of fractures and the rapid development of callus, as noted in fractures produced in the experimental animal, does not always occur in the human. The site of the fracture, the amount of displacement, and the age of the patient are a few of the factors that influence healing. In general, fractures heal at a much more rapid rate in infants and children than they do in adults (Fig. 5-11). There are several aspects of fracture healing noted in the description given in

preceding paragraphs that are of interest roentgenologically. The only change in the bones that can be recognized early is the decalcification of bone along the fracture edges. Usually this can be visualized within a week or two in most fractures and, because of it, the fracture line may become more prominent than it was immediately after the injury. A hairline fracture that may have been very difficult to visualize initially will usually become more obvious within a week or two. Uncalcified osteoid is not visible roentgenologically. If healing progresses normally, this uncalcified callus may be sufficiently solid to prevent motion between the fragments even though roentgenograms fail to show any signs of reformation of bone across the fracture. Failure to visualize calcified

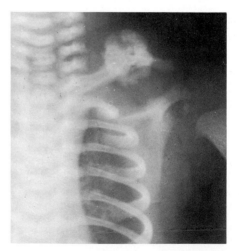

Fig. 5-11. Left clavicle was fractured at the time of birth. This roentgenogram, taken when the infant was 2 weeks old, shows a large amount of callus.

callus, therefore, does not necessarily indicate that the fragments are not held together. However, uncalcified osteoid callus is relatively soft and in weight-bearing bones will not allow use of the part; in the nonweightbearing bones, it may result in bending if support is discontinued. One must wait, therefore, until roentgenograms show calcified callus and, in the weight-bearing bones, this must become fairly dense and solid before the part can be used (Fig. 5-12).

Satisfactory progress of hearing of a fracture is shown in roentgenograms by the changes described in the following paragraphs.

Decalcification of Fragment Ends

Removal of bone along the injured surfaces of the fragments follows the injury within a matter of days. Definite evidence of such removal is sometimes not apparent in roentgenograms, particularly if the fragments are separated or displaced to any appreciable degree. The roentgen demonstration of decalcification of the ends of the fragments, however, is a favorable early sign that healing may take place in a normal manner, but its occurrence is no guarantee that bone union will develop.

Periosteal Callus

The most reliable roentgen evidence of beginning bone union is the visualization of calcified periosteal callus. This is seen at first as a faint hazy area of calcium density developing in the tissues adjacent to and directly overlying the borders of the fracture line. When this is sufficient to be visualized as a continuous zone of calcification extending from one fragment to another, it is reliable evidence that solid bone union will occur (see Fig. 5-12). With the passage of time, the periosteal callus shadow becomes increased in density and its outer margin more distinct. Eventually the callus becomes as dense as the normal cortex and in time it blends with the cortical margin and no longer remains as a distinct zone of density. The amount of visible periosteal callus varies greatly in different fractures. It is more extensive when there is displacement of fragments than when there has been accurate replacement and a close apposition of fragments. It is more prominent beneath large muscle masses and, in bones that are covered with little or no muscle, periosteal callus will be slight. This is noted in fractures of the phalanges, which often unite with little evidence of periosteal callus. It also is observed in fractures of the tibial shaft where heavy calcified

periosteal callus may form along the posterior and outer side of the fracture but with very little over the anterior surface. Fractures occurring through the intracapsular portion of the femoral neck will show no periosteal callus because there is no periosteum covering the bone at this site. Fractures of the skull also do not show periosteal callus because the periosteum does not have osteogenic properties in the bones of the cranial vault.

The amount and character of periosteal callus are satisfactory indicators as to when the part may be removed from traction or casts. Again the site and nature of the fracture must be taken into account. A fracture in an upper extremity that is nonweight-bearing will usually be held firmly enough for some degree of use when roentgenograms show a rather hazy periosteal callus shadow. In the lower extremity, however, such faint calcified callus is not enough and it is usually advisable to withhold any use of the part until the outer margin of the callus shadow has become sharp and continuous across the entire site of fracture. An impacted fracture may not require support as long as one that was not impacted.

While a large amount of periosteal callus may have formed around a fracture in which the fragments were not completely replaced in anatomic relationship, with the passage of time much of this will be absorbed peripherally and, particularly in children, there is a tendency for remodeling of the bone. The callus surrounding shaft fractures in children will disappear completely and, with growth and remodeling, even rather extensive deformity may be completely corrected.

Endosteal Callus

While periosteal callus is forming and calcifying, endosteal callus formation also is taking place. The roentgen visualization of endosteal callus is much less distinct because the early calcified callus is obscured by the bone surrounding it. Thus the fracture line may remain relatively clear even when periosteal callus can be visualized. However, in normal healing the line of fracture eventually becomes hazy and less distinct as calcified callus forms between the ends of the fragments and along the inner surface of the cortex. Eventually the fracture line disappears completely and the dense homogeneous shadow of endosteal callus is gradually replaced by trabecular bone so that a marrow cavity is reformed. In most fractures it is not necessary to wait for roentgen demonstration of recalcification of the fracture line before the part can be used. Occasionally a very accurate re-

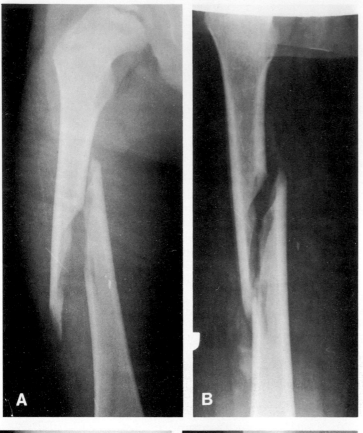

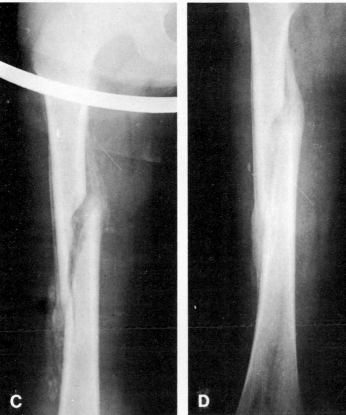

Fig. 5-12. Healing fracture. **A.** Roentgeno-grams taken immediately after the injury. **B.** In 2 weeks there is some hazy callus. **C.** At 4 weeks there is considerable callus. **D.** Three months after the injury there is a solid bridge of callus between fragments along the external surfaces, representing perios-teal callus. The fracture line itself is disap-pearing, indicating endosteal callus as well. (Courtesy of Dr. Ralph C. Frank, Eau Claire, Wisconsin)

placement of fragments has been accomplished so that even in the immediate postreduction roentgenograms the fracture line can barely be distinguished. In these cases one will find very little periosteal callus developing. Because the fracture line is indistinct from the very beginning, it may be difficult to tell when sufficient endosteal callus has formed to prevent motion. Usually sufficient decalcification will occur along the line of fracture to make it more clearly visible within a few weeks after the injury and the gradual fading of this line and its eventual disappearance are the roentgen indicators of satisfactory healing.

Reformation of Trabecular Bone

This is a late manifestation of bony union and represents the end stage of fracture repair. It indicates that the replacement of calcified callus by true bone has been accomplished. In certain areas, such as in the neck of the femur where there is no periosteal callus formation and where endosteal callus may be difficult to identify, the most certain evidence of bone union is the reformation of trabeculae that can be traced from one fragment to another without loss of continuity. Even in these examples, however, there is, as a rule, solid enough union before this observation can be made to allow use of the extremity.

Effects of Strain

The demonstration of a lack of motion between fragments in roentgenograms that were made while pressure was being applied in several directions is of considerable value in determining whether there is solid union. This is a useful procedure when routine roentgenograms and the results of clinical examination leave some doubt as to the presence of union. It is important that care be used in applying the pressure so that fresh callus will not be damaged or that precarious and early union not be disrupted.

Further Observations

Fractures occurring through diseased bone often heal surprisingly well. Fracture through a simple bone cyst in a child usually heals promptly and in the course of healing frequently initiates healing of the bone cyst. Even in osteoporotic bone, such as is found in osteogenesis imperfecta, healing may be prompt and often occurs with excessive periosteal callus. Even a fracture occurring through a focus of osteolytic metastatic carcinoma may heal partially

with callus in the face of a destructive malignant lesion. In these cases, of course, union is precarious and as the lesion increases refracture may occur.

Roentgen evidence of healing in fractures of compression type is difficult to evaluate. Because there is no true line of fracture visible initially and because these fractures usually occur in bones where little periosteal callus forms, it is very difficult to establish the progress of healing. This will be considered further in the discussion dealing with vertebral fracture. The healing of fractures of the cranial bones also will be considered in the section dealing with such fractures.

DELAYED AND NONUNION OF FRACTURES

GENERAL ASPECTS

When the rate of progress of healing of a fracture is slower than is normal for the particular type of fracture under consideration, but with healing eventually occurring, it is termed *slow* or *delayed union*. Some of the causes that are operative in production of nonunion of fractures also may be responsible for delay in union but with eventual healing taking place. Fractures unite more slowly in the aged than in younger adults and always heal more slowly in adults than they do in infants and children. The rapidity of callus formation and bone union in fracture occurring during birth is striking. For example, a birth fracture of a clavicle may develop a fusiform area of dense periosteal callus easily visualized in roentgenograms within 5 to 7 days after the injury (see Fig 5-11). The term *nonunion* refers to absence of bony union. Some fractures that fail to undergo bony union may unite with fibrous union and in certain areas this may be sufficient for practical purposes. In bone subjected to much use, and particularly in the weight-bearing bones, fibrous union is not adequate (Fig. 5-13). From roentgenograms it is impossible to determine whether solid fibrous union is present or not because the fibrous tissue joining the ends of the bones is relatively nonopaque.

Fractures in certain areas are noted for the frequency with which delayed or nonunion occurs. These include fractures at the junction of the middle and lower thirds of the tibia, the carpal navicular, the central third of the shaft of the humerus, and fractures in the lower third of the ulna.

The causes of nonunion include (*1*) infection, (*2*)

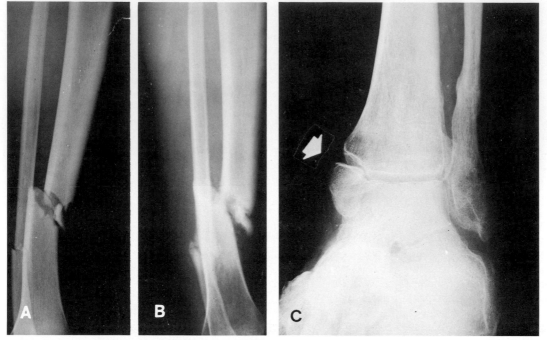

Fig. 5-13. Ununited fractures. **A.** Comminuted tibial fracture and transverse fibular fracture 3 weeks after injury. No callus is observed. **B.** Eight months later there is partial union of the fibula but no definite callus is noted bridging the tibial fracture. There is some eburnation of bone adjacent to the tibial fracture site. **C.** Old ununited fracture of the medial malleolus **(arrow).**

distraction of fragments,* (3) injury to the blood supply of one or both fragments, (4) improper fixation, (5) interposition of soft tissues between the fragment ends. Other causes include local bone disease at the site of fracture and, possibly, certain generalized conditions, such as osteomalacia, syringomyelia, and tabes among others.

ROENTGEN OBSERVATIONS

Roentgen evidence of nonunion depends upon the demonstration of one or more of the following changes:

Smoothness of Fragment Ends

A fracture that is not going to unite often shows, as the first evidence, the development of smoothness of the ends of the fragments that formerly were ragged

---

* Distraction refers to a separation or pulling apart of the fragments, leaving a gap between them. It is usually caused by excessive traction.

and irregular. This is first noticed along the margins, the sharp corners disappearing and being replaced by rounded borders. Eventually the end of each fragment heals over with cortical bone (see Fig. 5-13c).

Absence of Calcified Periosteal Callus

While visible periosteal callus is not necessary for satisfactory healing of a fracture, provided the ends are in close and accurate apposition or when the fracture occurs in an area where the periosteum is absent, such as in the intracapsular portion of the femoral neck, in most fractures some periosteal callus does become visible and its presence is a good indicator that union is commencing. Failure to demonstrate a periosteal callus shadow that is continuous across the external surfaces at the line of fracture should be viewed with suspicion. Not infrequently, periosteal spurs form along the margins of both fragments but these do not bridge across the line of fracture; rather, an irregular translucent line remains between them, which appears to be an extension of the fracture line.

Such periosteal callus is of no value in furnishing support because it does not offer a solid bridge (see Fig. 5-13).

Eburnation of Fragments

The fragment ends may undergo increasing sclerosis and eburnation when bony union fails to take place. The amount of eburnation varies from case to case but often the occurrence of sclerotic density in the fragment ends is the first evidence that bony union will fail to occur. The longer the duration of non-union, the more eburnated the fragments become. The fracture surfaces also develop a sclerotic appearance relatively early when the fracture has not been properly immobilized.

Motion between the Fragments

When roentgenograms are obtained with and without the application of pressure, or with pressure applied to one fragment in several directions, if there is lack of bony union, motion can be demonstrated. This is an excellent way to demonstrate absence of union in patients in whom the clinical examination gives indefinite results. As mentioned in a previous section "Effects of Strain," care should be exercised when pressure is made in an attempt to elicit motion so that early callus not be disrupted or that the bone not be refractured.

Pseudarthrosis

Occasionally a false joint is formed between fragments in the presence of nonunion. Usually this occurs as a result of incomplete fixation or with use of the part allowed before union has taken place.

OTHER COMPLICATIONS

DISUSE OSTEOPOROSIS AND SUDECK'S ATROPHY

Simple immobilization of a bone will result in a loss of osseous tissue; this is known as disuse osteoporosis (see Fig. 5-13). When there is, additionally, hyperemia, the osteoporosis is intensified at and distal to the level of hyperemia. Occasionally, following a fracture and sometimes after relatively minor trauma without fracture, there develops a more severe and painful form of osteoporosis known as Sudeck's atrophy (reflex sympathetic dystrophy). These conditions also are discussed in Chapter 4 (see Fig. 4-2). The roent-

gen differentiation between a simple disuse osteoporosis and Sudeck's atrophy depends to a large extent upon the severity of the demineralization. Simple disuse osteoporosis seldom causes more than a minimal to moderate degree of increased transparency of the bones that have been immobilized. Often this is more pronounced in the regions of the metaphyses in children, or in adults at the site of the previous epiphyseal plates. This is probably because of increased vascularity of the bone in this region. The bone loss develops gradually and usually can be noticed within several weeks after immobilization. There is a loss in density of the bones which may be uniform or mottled and that will, if immobilization is continued, develop, after a period of time, a ground-glass type of density.

INFECTION

A compound fracture may become infected. Following surgical procedures for the reduction of fractures, infection may develop. The appearances are essentially those of osteomyelitis with the occurrence of periostitis, irregular destruction of bone at the site of infection, and the formation of sequestra. The clinical evidences of infection usually are obvious and roentgenograms serve to establish the extent of involvement and the progress of the disease.

LATE JOINT CHANGES

When a line of fracture has entered the articular surface of a bone, injury to the articular cartilage results and not infrequently this is followed in time by the development of degenerative changes. This is particularly true in the weight-bearing joints and is seen most frequently in the knee and in the ankle. This condition sometimes is termed "traumatic arthritis" but it represents, essentially, degenerative joint disease that has been initiated by an acute trauma. The reader is referred to Chapter 9, "Diseases of the Joints," for a further consideration of this disease.

FRACTURES OF THE SKULL

The majority of fractures involving the bones of the cranial vault can be identified provided a sufficient number of technically good roentgenograms are obtained. A linear fracture of hairline type may stand out clearly only when the injured area was close to the film at the time the exposure was made. Such a fine fracture line in a part of the skull at a distance from the film may be completely invisible or nearly so because of the loss of detail that will occur. At times, with even the best of technique, linear fractures of the cranial vault will escape detection because of the thinness of the fracture line and its failure to be situated in a position where the roentgen beam passes directly through it.

Because many patients with head injuries are in serious condition, clinicians rightfully have stressed that roentgen examination should wait until other necessary emergency care of the patient has been given. The damage of the brain often is more important than the injury to the cranial bones. With some exceptions, and these often are obvious, fractures of the skull may not require immediate surgical treatment. Eventually, however, the individual who has had a severe head injury should have a complete roentgenologic study of the skull. If a fracture exists an effort should be made to determine if there is any depression of bone and the amount of such depression. This is best accomplished by means of tangential views so that the area of fracture is viewed on edge.

TYPES OF SKULL FRACTURE

Linear Fracture

A linear fracture is visualized as a sharp, dark translucent line, often irregular or jagged, and occasionally of branching character (Fig. 5-14). Linear frac-

tures often extend into the base of the skull and their inferior terminations become invisible. A linear fracture must be distinguished from suture lines and vascular grooves. A blood-vessel groove usually has a smooth curving course and is not as sharp or distinct as a fracture line. An old fracture of 6 months' duration or longer may resemble a vessel groove very closely and at times it is difficult or impossible to be certain about the nature of such a line. Suture lines generally have serrated edges. Occasionally the sagittal suture will appear as a straight dark line when viewed end-on in anteroposterior roentgenograms. The sutures between the temporal, parietal and occipital bones may also resemble fracture lines. The bilateral and symmetrical nature of the lines and their positions should enable the examiner to recognize them.

Ordinarily linear fracture without depression and without clinical signs of disturbed sensorium or neurological findings is of little significance. However, particularly in infants and small children, there may be soft tissue (usually meninges) interposed between fracture edges. This may lead to formation of a leptomeningeal cyst, meningocele or to a cicatrix between the skull and brain or meninges. Therefore, some believe that in children under age eight, a follow-up skull film twelve weeks after fracture is needed to avoid missing such complications which may result in an increase in width of the fracture ("growing fracture") and possible brain damage.

Fig. 5-14. Linear fracture of the skull. **A.** In this patient with a linear fracture of the parietal bone a faint fracture line extends posteriorly into the occipital bone **(arrow). B.** In this patient with the same type of fracture the fracture line extends into the posterior temporal bone from the parietal area **(arrows).**

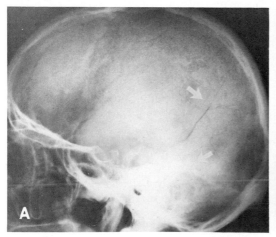 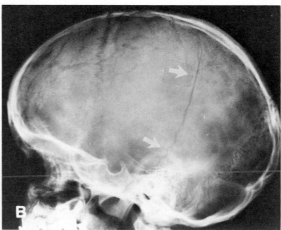

Depressed Fracture

After more severe trauma, particularly if the force has been localized to a small area of the skull, one or more fragments of bone may be separated and depressed into the cranial cavity. Such fractures often are stellate with multiple fracture lines radiating outward from a central point and with one or more comminuted pieces present. When viewed *en face* the line of fracture may appear denser than the normal bone because of overlap of fragments, the roentgen rays having to penetrate a double thickness of bone. Tangential views are essential to determine the amount of depression (Figs. 5-15 and 5-16).

Fracture Diastasis

Not infrequently a linear fracture follows a suture along at least a part of its course (Fig. 5-17). At times the entire fracture follows a suture. Usually there is some spreading of the suture where it is involved by the fracture so that it stands out more clearly than the normal, thus allowing the diagnosis to be made. Occasionally in transverse sutures, such as the coronal or lambdoid, one suture may, normally, appear wider than its mate. This may be caused by a slight tilting of the head from a true anteroposterior plane. The possibility of this normal variant should be kept in mind when fracture diastasis of a suture is a consideration. Even when a fracture does not involve a suture there may be some separation of fracture surfaces from a few millimeters up to a centimeter or even more. This type of fracture is seen most frequently during infancy and childhood and is called a *diastatic fracture.*

Basal Skull Fracture

Fracture limited to the base of the skull may be very difficult to visualize by roentgen examination. While this part of the skull can be shown in suitable projections, the clarity of detail may be poor and the anatomic structures comprising the base add to the difficulty in recognizing fracture lines. Many basal fractures will extend into the vault for at least a short distance and a part of the fracture will be visible. Tomography or body-section roentgenography often is useful in identifying a basal skull fracture when rou-

Fig. 5-15. Depressed comminuted skull fracture. **A.** Lateral view shows an irregular fracture line with an overlap causing increased density **(arrow). B.** The posteroanterior view indicates the extent of depression with inward displacement of the large bone fragment **(arrow).**

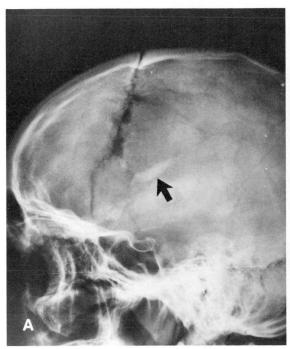
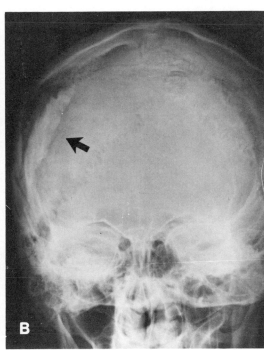

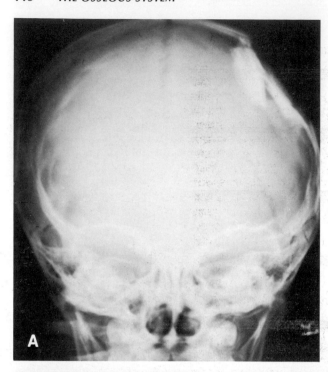

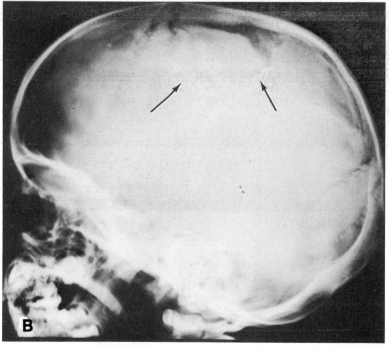

Fig. 5-16. Depressed skull fracture. The amount of depression of fragments is clearly shown on the frontal projection **(A). Arrows** outline the large fragment in the lateral projection **(B).**

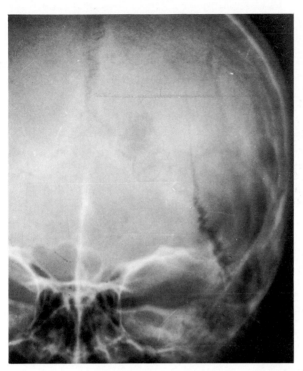

Fig. 5-17. Fracture diastasis of the skull. The fracture line follows the lambdoidal suture and then extends upward into the parietal bone on the left.

tine views fail to show it. Failure to demonstrate a basal skull fracture does not exclude the possibility of its presence and the clinical signs of such an injury may be more reliable than roentgen examination. A basal skull fracture may extend into the sphenoid sinus. If lateral roentgenograms are obtained with the patient sitting upright, an air–fluid level may be seen in the sinus. If the patient is unable to sit, a lateral view of the skull with a horizontal roentgen-ray beam and the film cassette placed alongside the head will demonstrate an air–fluid level if one is present. Clinical signs of injury also must be present, as infection also may cause an air–fluid level in the sinus.

Fracture through the planum sphenoidale may occasionally be simulated by an anatomic variant consisting of failure of fusion of the planum to the chiasmatic sulcus posterior to it. In failure of fusion, an oblique, smooth, radiolucent line extending from above downward and anteriorly is evident in the roentgenogram. In contrast, a fracture line is irregular and sharp, may be in any direction, and may be comminuted. Tomograms may be needed to make the differentiation.

HEALING OF SKULL FRACTURES

The time required for the disappearance of a skull fracture is extremely variable. A fracture in a young child usually heals promptly. The fracture line fades gradually and may disappear completely within several months. Fine hairline fractures heal more rapidly than those with a greater separation of surfaces. In older individuals, fracture lines tend to remain visible for longer periods of time and in some cases never completely disappear. Usually after several months the sharp edge of bone along the fracture line becomes indistinct. Gradually some recalcification develops with portions of the fracture becoming obliterated. A residual defect may remain more or less permanently as a hazy dark line that is easily mistaken for a vascular groove.

Complications

Cerebrocranial Cicatrix. If the dura is torn beneath an area of fracture it may become adherent to the bone along the margins of the fracture and allow the cerebral cortex to come into contact with the bone. An accumulation of cerebrospinal fluid may form in this space and develop into a leptomeningeal cyst. In other instances there are only the adhesions of the cortex and dura to the bone. Either condition predisposes to a gradual erosion of the bone overlying the cyst or cicatrix, apparently caused by the pulsating pressure of the blood vessels along the surface of the cortex. As indicated earlier this condition is seen most frequently in infants or young children. It occurs most commonly in the parietal area and following a diastatic type of fracture. The fracture may heal satisfactorily at first but within a few months erosion of bone along the line of fracture becomes apparent (Fig. 5-18). The bone often is destroyed sufficiently for a soft-tissue mass to bulge through the defect and to be obvious to inspection and palpation.

Pneumocephalus. If a fracture has extended through the frontal, ethmoid, or sphenoid sinuses, or the mastoids, air may enter the cranial cavity. If the dura and arachnoid have been torn, the air may find its way into the subarachnoid space and eventually reach the ventricles. This condition is known as post-traumatic pneumocephalus (Fig. 5-19). It is an uncommon but serious complication and can be recognized easily in roentgenograms because of the transparency of the air in contrast to the density of the surrounding brain tissue and cerebrospinal fluid.

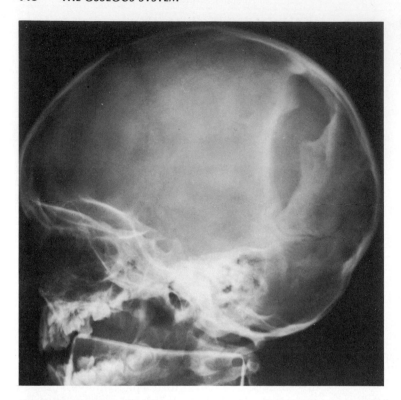

Fig. 5-18. Growing fracture caused by meningeal adhesions to the inner table. In this child a swelling was noted over the region of a previous fracture several months following the initial injury.

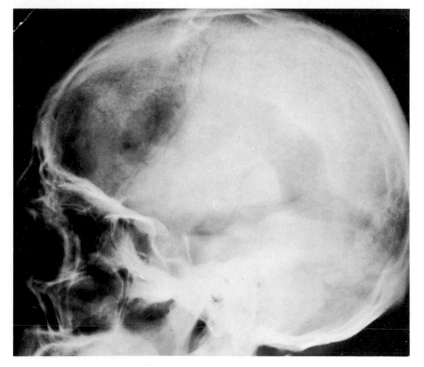

Fig. 5-19. Posttraumatic pneumocephalus. This patient had a fracture in the frontal sinus area. The presence of air indicates that the dura was torn and that air has entered the ventricular system.

After a compound-depressed fracture a brain abscess may form at or close to the site of brain injury. If gas-forming organisms are present the abscess may become visible as a gas- and fluid-filled cavity, the gas again offering the contrast needed to demonstrate it.

Subdural and Epidural Hematoma. These conditions are considered in Chapter 11, to which the reader is referred. A special type of hematoma formation not necessarily associated with fracture is known as *cephalhematoma*. This is found in newborn infants as a result of birth trauma. Usually caused by the application of forceps, injury to the external fibrous tissue covering of the skull is followed by formation of a hematoma beneath it. This forms a localized mass that subsequently undergoes calcification. It is visible then in roentgenograms as an area of increased density. When viewed tangentially the typical cephalhematoma is visualized as a homogeneous shadow of calcium density showing a sharply demarcated convex outer border, the margins of which merge smoothly with normal bone (Fig. 5-20). The bone beneath the area of calcification usually is normal. With the passage of time, a cephalhematoma tends to undergo gradual decrease in size and may disappear completely if small or, at the most, leave only an area of slightly thickened bone.

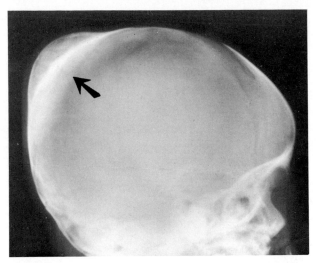

Fig. 5-20. Calcified cephalhematoma **(arrow)** following birth trauma. The dense calcified mass shown here gradually decreases in size and eventually disappears.

INJURIES INVOLVING THE VERTEBRAE

Any of the vertebrae may be fractured but most commonly vertebral fractures occur in the cervical part of the spine and in the mid and lower thoracic regions. The first and occasionally the second lumbar vertebrae also are frequently involved, but fractures of the lower lumbar bodies are less common unless the bone has been weakened by disease, particularly osteoporosis.

FRACTURES

Compression Fracture

The compression fracture is the most frequent type of injury involving a vertebral body. It is caused by an acute forward flexion of the spine and the damage usually is limited to the upper portion of the vertebral body and particularly to the upper anterior margin. The extent of compression varies, of course, depending upon the severity of the injury, from a very slight infraction of the upper anterior margin to rather extensive and general compression affecting the entire vertebral body (Fig. 5-21). A minor degree of com-

pression is difficult to recognize unless technically good roentgenograms are obtained and such a fracture usually can be observed only in a lateral view. It is seen then as a slight depression of the upper anterior disc surface coupled with a slight forward bulge of a small portion of the vertebral body along the superior anterior margin. There often is condensation of the bone extending inward from the marginal buckling, indicating the compression nature of the injury. The superior disc surface of the affected vertebral body usually is somewhat concave. With a more severe injury the concavity of the disc surface of the vertebra becomes more marked, and the loss in height and anterior wedging of the vertebral body are more severe. With the more extensive compression there usually is some loss in height of the vertebral body posteriorly as well as anteriorly, although the injury is generally more marked in the anterior aspect because of the lack of bony support at this point. Rather infrequently the injury is limited to the inferior surface of the vertebral body and, even less frequently, both surfaces are involved by compressions. Because of the damage to the disc surface there is a tendency for expansion of the intervertebral disc at the expense of the softened vertebra that accounts for the usual deformity. The lesser degrees of compression fracture usually show no significant alteration in the spinal curvatures but with a greater degree of compression there may be a definite gibbus deformity. With the more severe injury there often is

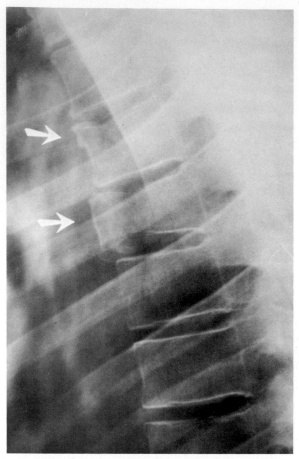

Fig. 5-21. Fractures of the thoracic spine. Anterior compression, some comminution, and anterior displacement of small fragment **(upper arrow)** and of the anterior one-third of a vertebral body **(lower arrow).**

some bulging of the posterior surface of the vertebral body into the spinal canal and this may be sufficient to produce signs and symptoms of cord compression. In the thoracic region in anteroposterior views, one occasionally sees a slight fusiform soft-tissue density adjacent to the fractured vertebral body, which represents a paraspinal hematoma. This seldom is very pronounced and it usually disappears within a short time after the injury.

Comminuted Fractures

With more severe injury, one or more vertebral bodies may be extensively crushed and fragmented and there may be associated fractures of the arch or processes (Fig. 5-22). In addition there may be varying degrees of subluxation or dislocation. The term "sub-

luxation" is used to designate displacement that is incomplete, while "dislocation" is used to indicate a complete displacement of one bone on the other. Subluxations are more frequent in the spine than are dislocations (Fig. 5-23).

Limbus Fracture

Small triangular fragments of the anterosuperior or anteroinferior aspect of vertebral bodies may result from either an avulsion by the anterior spinal ligament in an extension-type injury or by a bursting effect in a flexion-type injury. This is sometimes called a limbus or tear-drop fracture.

CERVICAL SPINE INJURIES

Fractures of the first cervical vertebra are usually caused by a force in an axial direction. A bursting or Jefferson fracture is produced by such a force. The fracture in the arch may be unilateral or bilateral and is usually posterior. There is often associated compression of the lateral masses with or without displacement of one or both on the axis. There may also be fractures of the transverse process. Rarely, horizontal fractures of the anterior arch have been reported; these usually have been associated with fractures of the odontoid process.

Fractures of the axis (C2) are produced by a hyperextension force such as that commonly experienced when the head or face hits the windshield or steering wheel in a motor vehicle accident. This is also the type of fracture that may be caused by hanging and is therefore sometimes termed "hangman's" fracture. In this injury there are bilateral fractures of the neural arch anterior to the inferior facets. The fracture lines are usually oblique and extend downward and anteriorly. Fractures tend to be relatively symmetrical, and there is often associated dislocation of C2 on C3. The anterior longitudinal ligament often ruptures and produces an avulsion fracture of the anteroinferior margin of C2 or the anterosuperior margin of C3. An additional roentgenographic finding is that of the presence of retropharyngeal soft-tissue swelling which is almost always present. Occasionally there is an associated fracture of the posterior aspect of the arch of C1 without displacement of C1 on C2.

A particularly important injury in the upper cervical spine is that of a fracture–dislocation involving the odontoid process, since an injury in this area may cause compression of the upper cervical cord and/or the medulla.

In the remainder of the cervical spine, flexion in-

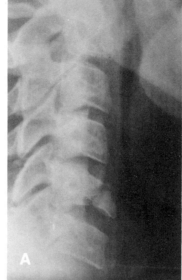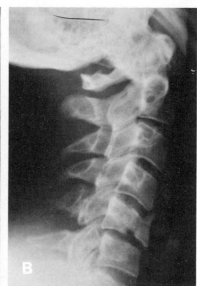

Fig. 5-22. Cervical vertebral fracture. **A.** Initial roentgenogram demonstrates fragmentation of the anterior aspect of the fifth cervical body as well as some compression. A little posterior displacement of the superior aspect of this body is also noted. **B.** Roentgenogram secured 6½ months later shows that the posterior relationships have improved. The anterior fragment is in better position and partial union is demonstrated by fading of the fracture line.

juries produce anterior compressions that are usually readily visualized on lateral roentgenograms. A horizontal zone of radiolucency can sometimes be observed on extension of the cervical spine in patients who have had an injury in which the disc is torn away from the vertebral end-plate. It resembles the vacuum phenomenon. Compression fractures of the lateral masses (articular pillars) are also reasonably common but are often missed. They are difficult to detect on ordinary anteroposterior and lateral films.[1, 16] Therefore, it is necessary to obtain anteroposterior and oblique films with caudad angulation or tomograms to detect them. Although compression fractures may be bilateral, a unilateral compression is the more common. It may be difficult, if not impossible, to determine the age of such pillar compression. In order to be certain that the changes are secondary to recent injury, a clear fracture line or sharp angulation with offset of cortical margins must be visible on the roentgenogram, preferably with a follow-up film demonstrating healing.

Torsion injuries may produce a rotatory type of subluxation in which one lateral mass or pillar may be displaced forward on the one below it and locked in a position of rotatory dislocation. This is usually associated with fracture of the posterior elements in one or more sites.

In patients with injuries of the cervical spine, it is important to be certain that all of the cervical vertebrae are included on the film. If possible, the upper portion of the first thoracic vertebra should be visible to determine its relationship to C7. Furthermore,

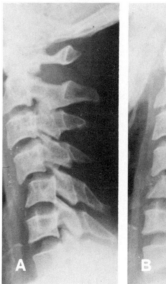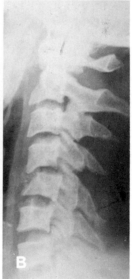

Fig. 5-23. Subluxation of the fourth on the fifth cervical vertebra. **A.** Film exposed immediately after the injury. Note the anterior offset of C4 on C5 resulting in reversal of the curve and angulation. **B.** Roentgenogram secured 2 months later shows the subluxation incompletely reduced, but there is now a little callus anteriorly, indicating the development of a calcific bridge between the vertebral bodies. Reduction was incomplete despite skeletal traction.

great care is needed in handling patients with suspected spinal injuries so as not to cause more extensive cord injury than may already be present. Therefore, it is wise to secure the lateral film for examination before additional views are obtained. Once it is determined that there is no subluxation or dislocation, anteroposterior, oblique, and caudal angulation views may be obtained. Often it is necessary to use tomography or computerized tomography to outline the fracture or fractures. Computerized tomography is particularly useful in the demonstration of bony fragments impinging on the spinal canal and, therefore, possibly on the cervical cord. This method of examination is also used for the other parts of the spine.

Whiplash Injury

Because of the increased frequency of automobile accidents the whiplash injury of the cervical spine has become of considerable importance. This type of injury follows a sudden deceleration of the body, as when an automobile in which the occupant is riding is stopped suddenly by collision. A similar type of injury may result when a stationary automobile is struck by a moving vehicle from behind, the head being snapped back and then pulled forward rapidly by muscular contraction. There is a considerable difference of opinion as to the importance of this so-called whiplash injury as a cause for clinical complaints and disability. When a definite compression fracture or subluxation between the lower cervical vertebrae can be identified in roentgenograms, the evidence of injury is obvious. When no fracture exists but the supporting ligaments have been injured, the diagnosis becomes more difficult and it may be impossible to state from roentgenographic evidence alone if such injury exists or not. Frequently, following a whiplash type of injury, roentgenograms will show a sharp reversal of the normal cervical lordotic curve at the fourth, fifth, or sixth cervical disc level, and, at times, a slight forward subluxation of the vertebra above on the one below the level of gibbus. If lateral views are obtained with the head in flexion and in extension, the reversed curve may not completely disappear during the maneuver, being increased with flexion and not entirely eliminated with extension of the head. These are suggestive signs of soft-tissue injury but they are not specific since a similar type of deformity is seen in association with other lesions that cause cervical muscle spasm. A similar deformity may occur with localized degenerative disease affecting one or more of the mid or lower cervical discs. Minor degrees of reversal of the cervical lordotic curve can be seen in normal individuals. A careful evaluation of the roentgenographic appearances with a consideration of the age of the patient, the duration of the injury, and the character of the clinical findings and complaints is necessary in cases of this nature.

In our experience, minor degrees of reversal of the cervical curve as well as minimal offsets of one cervical vertebra on another may be produced by voluntary muscle contraction and therefore presumably can be produced by muscle spasm secondary to pain without any actual ligamentous injury of the cervical spine.[7] This adds to the difficulty in assessing the significance of minor variations in the cervical spine. Care should be taken not to overemphasize these variations.

The cervical prevertebral fat stripe[17] represents areolar tissue in the retropharyngeal and retro-esophageal spaces anterior to the vertebral bodies. This radiolucent stripe parallels the cervical spine adjacent to the anterior spinal ligament. It normally extends down as far as the level of C6 where it slants anteriorly and is continuous with the areolar tissue behind the scalenus muscles. Above this level, it is usually seen in adults but may not be seen in children. Its displacement may indicate hemorrhage and edema as a result of cervical trauma with or without fracture, alerting the radiologist to look carefully for evidence of fracture. It is also helpful in determining whether or not the fracture is recent. It may also be displaced by masses originating within the vertebra.

THORACOLUMBAR SPINE FRACTURES

Upper thoracic spine fractures are usually associated with violent muscular action such as in convulsion. In the absence of such injury, compression of one of the upper four thoracic vertebrae should raise the possibility of an underlying pathologic condition such as tumor or metabolic disease. On the other hand, lower and middle thoracic spine fractures are caused by flexion injury. Posterior elements are usually not disrupted, but associated rib injuries with laceration of costal arteries may result in hematomas that are visible on films of the thoracic spine.

Most of the fractures of the thoracic vertebrae tend to be anterior compressions which are usually readily observed in lateral projections and may be observed on the frontal view. As indicated previously, upper lumbar compressions are not uncommon but lower lumbar compressions are unusual except in seat-belt injury.

Rapid deceleration injury resulting in acute flexion of the lower lumbar spine with a low fulcrum at the level of the seat belt may result in disruption of the posterior spinous ligament and may disrupt the facets and discs as well. This is often associated with horizontal fractures of posterior elements including the pedicles, transverse processes, laminae, and spinous processes. A horizontal fracture may also extend into the posterior aspect of the vertebral body. This may be accompanied by dislocation and by some compression of the anterior aspect of one or more lumbar vertebrae.

Occasionally, in a severe motor vehicle accident, a horizontal fracture of the ilium results when a lap-type seat belt is worn. Ordinarily, however, the width of the pelvis and that of the seat belt tend to distribute the force so that the pelvis is not fractured.

Fractures of the spinous processes may occur anywhere in the spine but are most common at the C7 level. Such a fracture is usually readily apparent on a properly exposed lateral film, but it also may be suspected when a double oval shadow of the spinous process is noted in the frontal projection. Fractures of transverse processes may occur in association with severe injury anywhere in the spine, but in the lumbar area they may be an isolated injury due to local trauma, either the result of muscle pull or of direct local injury. Radiolucent lines simulating fracture of transverse processes may be produced by the psoas shadow or, sometimes, by variations in the shadow of intraabdominal gas.

SACROCOCCYGEAL INJURIES

Sacral fractures are usually accompanied by fractures elsewhere in the pelvic ring. They are often subtle and may be observed only when slight alterations in the smoothly rounded contour of the superior aspect of one or more sacral foramina is disrupted. Coccygeal fractures are often difficult to diagnose because of overlying gas or fecal material in bowel. Furthermore, there is marked variation in the coccyx which may angle 90 degrees directly anteriorly from its junction with the sacrum.

Kümmell's Disease

This is a rare and somewhat equivocal lesion. It consists of a gradual compression of a vertebral body developing some time after an injury, there being no evidence of fracture immediately after the trauma. It has been considered to be caused by an ischemic necrosis resulting from interference with the blood supply to the vertebra. Some of these lesions probably are actually unrecognized fractures in which no deformity is apparent immediately after the injury but with collapse occurring as a result of continued weight-bearing without support, and it seems likely that most cases of so-called Kümmell's disease belong in this category.

FRACTURES AND DISLOCATIONS IN SPECIAL AREAS

Most fractures and dislocations are recognized easily in roentgenograms and cause little difficulty in diagnosis. For a detailed analysis of the various types of fractures and dislocations, the mechanical principles involved, the complications, the methods of treatment, and the processes of repair, the reader should consult one of the texts dealing specifically with these problems. Only those features of importance from the standpoint of roentgen examination and diagnosis will be considered in this section.

THE HAND AND THE WRIST
Colles' Fracture

This is the most common fracture in the wrist area and consists of a fracture through the distal 1 inch of the radius. The distal fragment is usually angled backward on the shaft with impaction along the dorsal aspect and with the impaction more severe on the outer side so that the hand tends to be in some degree of radial deviation. There frequently is an associated avulsion fracture of the styloid process of the ulna (Fig. 5-24). There often is comminution along the line of fracture and the distal radial fragment may be considerably fragmented. The injury is due, as a rule, to a fall on the outstretched hand. The resulting deformity is usually obvious on clinical examination and has been described as a silver fork or spoon deformity. In reduction of Colles' fracture it is important to reestablish as nearly as possible the normal anatomic relationships. The normal angle formed by the distal radial articular surface with the transverse and longitudinal axes of the bone is shown in Figure 5-25. Normally the articular surface is tilted anteriorly from the transverse axis of the bone approximately 10 to 15 degrees and it faces toward the ulnar side of the joint approximately 15 to 25 degrees in relation to the longitudinal axis. It is not always possible to reduce a Colles' fracture completely; even when reduction has been complete there is considerable difficulty in some cases in holding the frag-

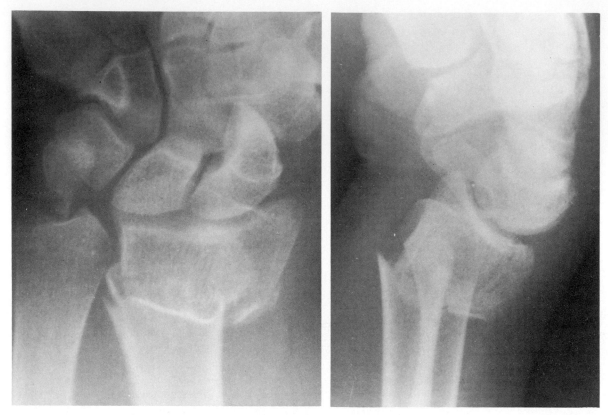

Fig. 5-24. Colles' fracture with some comminution and posterolateral impaction and posterior angulation of the radial joint surface. The ulnar styloid has been fractured off and is faintly visualized lateral to its normal position.

ments. Maintenance of reduction is favored if the hand is held in palmar flexion and ulnar deviation. A reverse type of Colles' fracture occasionally is encountered but it is rather infrequent; it consists in an anterior displacement and angulation of the distal fragment on the shaft.

Figure 5-26 shows a greenstick fracture of the distal radius and ulna with slight impaction which is anterior and thus the angulation is opposite to that seen in the usual type of Colles' fracture.

Fractures of the Navicular

Another common fracture in the wrist area is that involving the navicular (scaphoid). This is the most common fracture involving the carpal bones. The fracture usually is trasverse in type and occurs through the central part or waist of the bone (Fig. 5-27). Displacement of one fragment on the other may or may not be present. Frequently displacement

is slight or absent altogether so that the visualization of the line of fracture may be difficult. Roentgenograms must be of good quality and multiple views are required. The best projection to demonstrate a fracture through the waist of the navicular is made with the hand and wrist in an oblique position and with the hand placed in as much ulnar deviation as possible. This brings the navicular into profile. Union occurs by endosteal callus only. Nonunion of navicular fractures is common, or at least there is an absence of bony union. Fibrous union, however, may hold the fragments fairly well. After fracture of the navicular the proximal fragment may become avascular because the blood supply of the bone is derived chiefly through the distal portion. Ischemic necrosis of the proximal fragment becomes apparent as disuse osteoporosis develops in the bones around it. These bones become more transparent as there is a general loss of mineral components from them while the proximal fragment, having no blood supply, remains

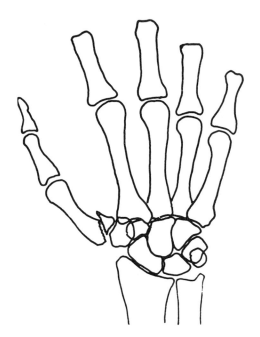

Fig. 5-25. Diagram of an anteroposterior roentgenogram of the wrist showing the usual angle formed by the radial articular surface with the long axis of the bone.

of normal density. Thus its shadow is denser than that of the viable bone. Subsequently the avascular fragment may undergo compression and fragmentation.

Other Carpal Fractures

The lunate fracture is a distant second to the navicular fracture in frequency. Triquetral and pisiform fractures are rare. The carpal tunnel view is valuable in observing pisiform and hamate fractures. In the distal row of carpals, capitate and hamate fractures are unusual and multangular fractures are exceedingly rare. Multiple carpal bone fractures occasionally occur in persons involved in moving vehicle accidents.

Dislocations

Dislocations at the wrist joint usually involve the lunate. This bone may be dislocated forward from the radius and from the rest of the carpal bones and the nature of the injury is usually recognized without difficulty in true lateral views of the wrist (Fig. 5-28). Less frequently a retrolunar (perilunate) dislocation

of the carpus is seen. In this injury the lunate maintains a normal relationship to the radius but the hand and all the rest of the carpal bones are dislocated backward on the lunate. The nature of this injury is recognized to best advantage only in lateral views of the wrist. There frequently is an associated fracture of the carpal navicular.

Isolated dislocation of the carpal navicular is very rare. If it is not corrected, significant disability may result. It is usually rotational. On the anteroposterior roentgenogram, loss of height of the navicular and widening of the space between it and the lunate, as well as a cortical ring shadow within the navicular outline, will be noted. In the lateral view, the long axis of the navicular will be seen in a horizontal position rather than the normal one which more nearly parallels the long axis of the radius.

Occasionally, one or more of the metacarpals dislocate on the carpus. The ulna may dislocate in either a dorsal or volar direction, but this is also uncommon. Other carpal dislocations, either single or multiple, are extremely unusual.

Radioulnar subluxation is another rare injury at

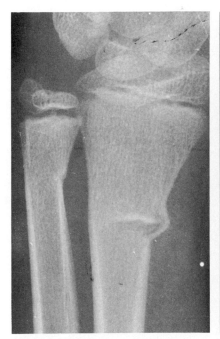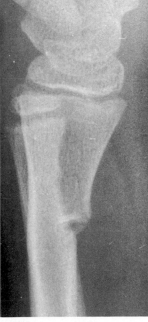

Fig. 5-26. Greenstick or incomplete fractures of the distal radius and ulna. Note that the slight impaction is anterior so that the angulation of the distal fragment is opposite to that observed in the Colles' fracture.

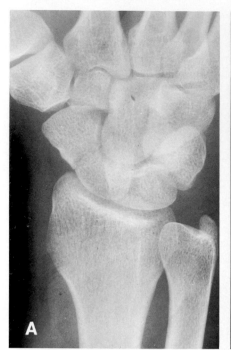
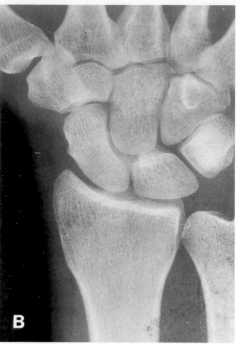

Fig. 5-27. Fracture of the carpal navicular. Note that the fracture line is observed on the oblique film **(A),** but not on the antero-posterior film **(B).**

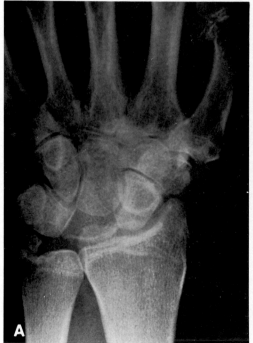
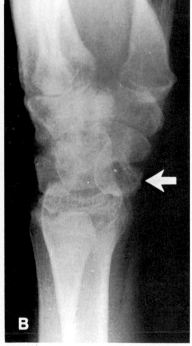

Fig. 5-28. Anterior dislocation of the carpal lunate. In the anteroposterior view **(A),** disruption of the normal joint space between the proximal and distal rows of carpals is noted. In the lateral view 2 **(B)** the lunate is seen to be displaced anteriorly **(arrow).**

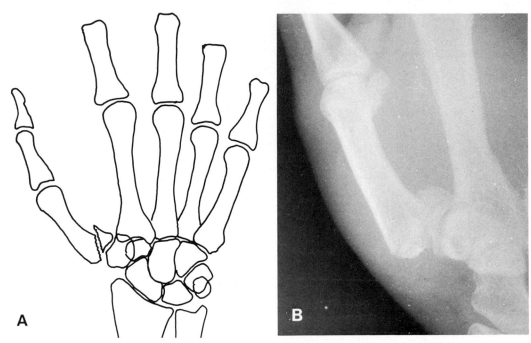

Fig. 5-29. A. Diagram illustrating the characteristic deformity in Bennett's fracture of the first metacarpal. **B.** Roentgenogram showing some impaction as well as lateral displacement of the shaft fragment in a Bennett's fracture.

the wrist. It is a rotatory subluxation in which the distal radius is rotated into a hyperpronated position on the ulna where it locks, apparently because the ulnar surface is irregular. On the roentgenogram, on the pronation view there is an apparent shift of the ulnar styloid laterally in contrast to its normal medial position in pronation.

Bennett's Fracture

Of the various fractures involving the metacarpals, one of the important ones is a Bennett's fracture. This consists of a triangular fracture through the proximal end of the first metacarpal with the line of fracture usually entering the articular surface. The triangular fragment consisting of the base of the bone remains in relationship to the multangular bone but the shaft is dislocated outward (Fig. 5-29). Fractures of other metacarpal bones are usually of oblique or spiral type and because of the slanting nature of the fracture line there often is overriding and foreshortening. Occasionally, fracture of the adjacent greater multangular bone is associated with a Bennett's fracture.

Anomalous Bones

In the interpretation of fractures involving the bones of the hand and wrist, attention must be paid to the possibility of mistaking an accessory ossification center or ununited epiphysis for a fracture fragment. The various accessory ossification centers that occur in this region are described in Chapter 3 to which the reader is referred for further information.

THE FOREARM AND ELBOW

Midshaft Fractures

When both bones of the forearm are fractured in their midportions a sufficient number of roentgenograms must be obtained so that the width of the interosseous space can be determined. Overriding of fragments is common at either one or both fracture sites and in the presence of overriding or, if there is much angular deformity, the fragments of the radius and ulna may come close together. If union occurs with a narrowed interosseous space there will be some limitation of pronation and supination. Occasionally, cross union occurs with a bridge of callus forming between the radius and ulna, and when this happens pronation and supination will not be possible.

Head of the Radius

Fracture of the head or neck of the radius is a common lesion and frequently the fracture is of the impacted type (Fig. 5-30). Roentgen evidence may consist only of a slight tilting of the plane of the articular

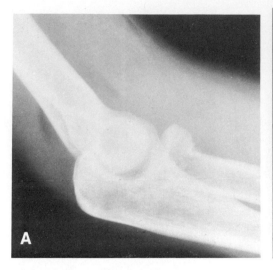

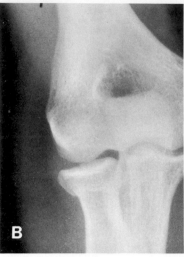

Fig. 5-30. Impacted fracture of the radial head. **A.** In the lateral view, note the lucency anterior and posterior to the lower humeral shaft, a positive fat-pad sign. **B.** The fracture is somewhat impacted resulting in a dense fracture line across the proximal radial shaft.

surface of the head in its relation to the longitudinal axis of the bone plus a slight buckling or sharp angular deformity of the cortical margin of the neck, usually along the outer aspect. With more severe injury the head may be comminuted and there often is a vertical fissurelike cleft extending through the articular surface, separating a small fragment from the outer margin. This may be displaced a variable degree or the line of fracture may be difficult to detect unless the roentgenograms are of good quality. Injury to the ends of the bones forming the elbow joint is accompanied by joint effusion. Normally there is a small accumulation of fat adjacent to the anterior surface of the lower end of the humerus. If the joint capsule is distended by fluid this fat pad will be displaced forward and upward (Fig. 5-31). Recognition of the abnormal position of the fat pad should cause the observer to search carefully for bone injury if it is not readily apparent.[4, 8] (Occasionally the fat pad cannot be seen in the normal person and in emaciated individuals it is not present.) There is a similar fat pad along the posterior surface of the humerus, but in the normal individual it lies largely within the olecranon fossa and is not visible in lateral views of the elbow. If the joint capsule is distended by fluid the pad is elevated and displaced posteriorly and then can be visualized. Displaced fat pads are a sign of joint distension and thus, in addition to trauma, should occur in any disease or condition in which there is synovitis (*e.g.*, rheumatoid arthritis).

In the absence of joint disease, no abnormal fat pads are ordinarily seen. Therefore, a positive fat pad sign almost always indicates trauma, and, in our experience, fracture of the radial head or proximal ulna

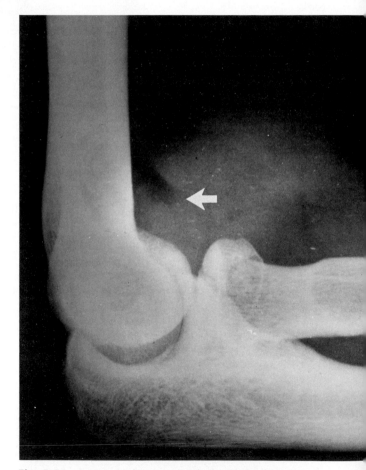

Fig. 5-31. Arrow indicates displacement of the anterior fat pad, indicating joint effusion secondary to the impacted fracture of the radial head.

is present in the vast majority of these patients. We obtain oblique views when no fracture is visible on anteroposterior and lateral projections in patients with a positive fat pad sign, and suggest a 2- to 3-week follow-up film when no fracture can be observed.

Dislocations of the Elbow Joint

Dislocation of the head of the radius occurs occasionally, chiefly in infants and children. In the adult, dislocation of the upper end of the radius sometimes occurs along with a fracture in the proximal portion of the ulna. This is known as a Monteggia fracture. The roentgen significance of this lesion lies in the fact that the radial dislocation may be overlooked.

Complete dislocations at the elbow joint almost invariably consist in a posterior dislocation of the radius and ulna on the humerus. Frequently small avulsion fractures are present in association with the dislocation or larger fragments may be broken off, particularly of the coronoid process of the ulna. Elbow joint dislocations are often followed by the occurrence of areas of calcification in and around the elbow joint—a posttraumatic myositis ossificans—and this may lead to considerable impairment of function even though anatomic relationships of the bones have been restored.

Fractures of the Elbow Area in Children

Because of the numerous ossification centers present in the elbow area during childhood, difficulty in interpretation of fractures is not infrequent. A knowledge of the appearance of the various ossification centers during the developmental period is essential in order to avoid errors. It is always helpful in doubtful cases to obtain roentgenograms of the opposite normal elbow joint and with these available it is usually possible to determine if fracture exists or not (see Fig. 5-2). In the very young infant, when most of the epiphyses at the elbow are still cartilaginous, injuries confined to them may be very difficult to detect until reparative changes develop in the form of periarticular calcification. In these patients, displacement of the fat pads, as noted above, offers a very valuable diagnostic clue at the initial examination.

One of the common fractures of childhood in the elbow region is a supracondylar fracture involving the humerus. This usually is the result of a fall on the outstretched hand with the elbow partially flexed

and, typically, there is a backward angulation or displacement of the condylar fragments on the humeral shaft. The condyles may be comminuted and the fracture may be of T type with a vertical component extending into the joint separating the condyles. In reduction of fractures involving the lower end of the humerus, an attempt is made to establish a normal carrying angle (Fig. 5-32). This is the angle formed by the longitudinal axis of the forearm in its relationship to the humerus. In the normal male this is approximately 170 degrees and in the normal female it is approximately 160 degrees (the forearm deviating laterally on the arm from 20 to 30 degrees).

The fractures are often of the greenstick or buckling variety associated with some impaction. In addition to restoration of the carrying angle, it is important that the normal anterior angulation of the capitellum be restored. More than 50% of this ossification center should lie anterior to a line drawn parallel to the anterior aspect of the anterior humeral cortex in the lateral view. Following reduction, it is wise to obtain a lateral view of the opposite (normal) elbow for comparison.

THE SHOULDER AREA

Dislocations

Dislocations at the shoulder are mainly of two types—anterior and posterior. In the anterior type, the humerus is displaced forward beneath the coracoid process and anterior to the glenoid of the scapula. It is also known as a subcoracoid dislocation (Fig. 5-33). Detection is not difficult in roentgenograms because of the gross distortion of anatomic relationships. This is the most frequent site and type of dislocation of any joint in the body. Repeated or "chronic" anterior dislocation of the shoulder is quite common. This condition can be diagnosed, or at least suspected, when the Hill–Sachs sign is present. This sign consists of an indentation or groove on the posterolateral aspect of the humeral head, probably produced by local fracture or repeated fractures of the head as it is compressed against the anteroinferior lip of the glenoid. This dislocation is best outlined on an anteroposterior view of the shoulder with the humerus in internal rotation. Associated with it there may also be a fracture of the inferior glenoid lip.

Posterior dislocation is much less frequent than the anterior type and more difficult to detect in standard roentgenograms. It comprises about 2% to 4% of shoulder dislocations. It is missed or misdiagnosed frequently. About one-half of these injuries result

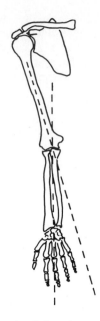

Fig. 5-32. Diagram illustrating the method for determining the carrying angle of the elbow joint and the normal angle.

from convulsive episodes while the remainder are produced by a direct blow to the anterior aspect of the humeral head or by a force transmitted along a flexed adducted and internally rotated humerus. The articular surface then lies posterior to the glenoid facing posteriorly, locked in internal rotation. An associated compression fracture resulting in flattening of the anterior surface of the humeral head may result; this may extend to form a deep groove or notch in the anterior aspect of the head if the dislocation continues to be unrecognized. The major problem lies in recognizing the possibility of a posterior dislocation on the anteroposterior roentgenogram. A positive rim sign is strongly suggestive of the diagnosis. This consists of an apparent widening of the space between the anterior glenoid rim and the medial aspect of the humeral head. Normally this space measures 6 mm or less; in posterior dislocation it is widened to as much as 13 or 14 mm. A positive rim sign is evident in most acute dislocations, but, because of the gradual indentation of the groove on the anterior aspect of the humerus, the space may narrow to a point where the rim sign is not positive in the more chronic dislocation. Occasionally a positive rim sign may be produced by lateral displacement of the humeral head due to causes other than dislocation, such as an accumulation of fluid within the joint or laxity of ligaments observed

in flaccid paralysis. Other helpful signs consist of: 1) absence of a half-moon overlap of the humeral head and glenoid; 2) position of the humeral head higher and, in some instances lower, than normal in relation to the glenoid fossa; 3) humeral head held in internal rotation; 4) flattening of the medial aspect of the humeral head representing a compression fracture of the anterior surface; and 5) in a few of the patients, linear fractures of the humeral head which are deemed to be the cause of disability. Once posterior dislocation is suspected, axillary or transthoracic roentgenograms usually confirm the diagnosis.

A 60% anterior oblique view of the shoulder can also be used to evaluate patients with suspected dislocation. In this projection, the scapula appears as a "Y." The acromion process is the posterior limb, the coracoid process the anterior limb, and the scapular body is the vertical limb. The glenoid is represented as a circular density at the junction of the limbs; the normal humeral head overlies it. In posterior dislocations the head is below the acromion; in anterior dislocations it is in a subcoracoid position. The anterior oblique view can be obtained very easily with the patient in the upright position but can also be secured with the patient supine, with the normal shoulder in a 60-degree posterior oblique position. If the patient can sit or stand, fluoroscopic positioning with spot filming is a convenient method of examination.

Approximately 20% of patients with dislocations of the shoulder also have an associated fracture. This may consist of an avulsion fracture of the greater tuberosity, a fracture of the neck of the humerus, or an injury to the anterior lip of the glenoid. These injuries should be watched for in any patient having a dislocation and roentgenograms always should be obtained after reduction of the dislocation because fractures frequently are more easily seen after normal relationships have been established.

Acromioclavicular Joint Injuries

The term "acromioclavicular separation" is used to describe the change in relationship between the clavicle and the acromion process. Actually a rupture or tear of the large coracoclaviclar ligament is more important than the soft-tissue injury adjacent to the acromioclavicular joint. The extent of a coracoclavicular separation has direct bearing upon the degree of acromioclavicular separation.

Subluxations or complete dislocations of the acromioclavicular joint are frequent injuries, particularly in athletes, and are caused by a fall on the shoulder. The dislocation may be incomplete and the lesion

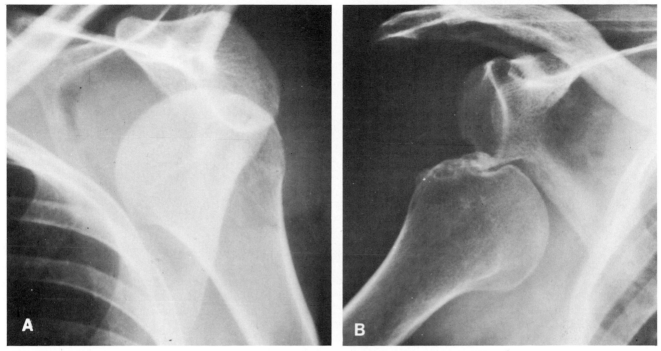

Fig. 5-33. A. Subcoracoid (anterior) dislocation of the humerus. The head lies anterior to the glenoid and beneath the coracoid process of the scapula. **B.** Chronic anterior dislocation of the shoulder. Note the indentation on the humeral head (Hill-Sachs) caused by a local infraction of the humerus at this point.

then is termed a subluxation (Fig. 5-34). This injury may not be evident on routine films and often requires comparison upright anteroposterior views obtained with 15- to 20-pound weights in each of the patient's hands. The joint is widened, but there is little or no upward displacement of the clavicle on the acromion process. When dislocation is complete the clavicle is displaced upward on the acromion and the ligaments attaching the clavicle to the coracoid process are ruptured. In evaluating the presence or absence of subluxation, the relationship of the under-surface of the clavicle to that of the acromion is important. The relative thickness of the acromion and clavicle varies in different individuals and the superior borders of these bones cannot be relied upon to indicate normal or abnormal relationships. The inferior surfaces, however, usually lie in the same plane. The width of the acromioclavicular joint space narrows gradually during life and becomes rather thin in the elderly individual because of degenerative changes in the cartilage. As with many other injuries, comparison with the opposite shoulder may be very

helpful in determining whether or not minor deformity exists.

Retrosternal Dislocation of Clavicle

Retrosternal dislocation of the clavicle is uncommon,[9] but prompt diagnosis is important because the posteriorly displaced clavicle may produce a considerable amount of morbidity including cough, dyspnea and dysphagia, voice change, and vascular compromise. On the other hand, the anterior dislocation does not compromise the mediastinal structures and is readily diagnosed clinically. Special horizontal-beam technique is required to make the diagnosis. The central beam is parallel to the table top, centered on the sternoclavicular joint, and directed along the axis of the clavicle. The arm near the x-ray tube is abducted over the head and a grid cassette is placed against the far shoulder, perpendicular to the beam. The normal clavicle is aligned with the manubrium while the dislocated one is projected posterior to it.

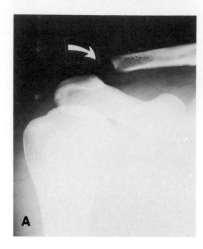

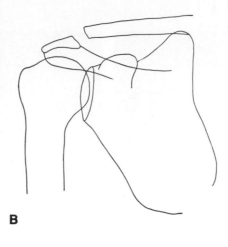

Fig. 5-34. Acromioclavicular separation. **A.** The joint is abnormally wide **(arrow)**. The clavicle is displaced upward in relation to the acromion process. **B.** Line drawing of this injury.

Fractures of the Scapula

Fractures of the scapula are not very frequent and are not too difficult to recognize in roentgenograms of the shoulder. There often are multiple fracture lines extending through the bone but healing usually occurs promptly. Unless a fracture extends directly into the glenoid there usually is little residual limitation of motion at the shoulder joint.

Fractures of the base of the coracoid process are often difficult to detect and may accompany acromioclavicular injuries, particularly in adolescents. The 60-degree anterior oblique view is useful in detection of this injury, but, in some instances, tomography is necessary to outline the fracture. Stress fracture at the base of the coracoid has been described in trapshooters.

Fractures of the Humerus

Fractures of the upper end of the humerus are usually divided into those involving the anatomic neck and those through the surgical neck of the bone. It often is difficult to classify fractures in this area according to this method because many times the fracture involves both the anatomic and the surgical necks. Fractures of the shaft of the humerus are of all varieties and this is one of the areas where delayed union or nonunion is rather common.

Fractures of the Clavicle

Most fractures involving the clavicle occur at the junction of the middle and distal thirds with a downward and forward displacement of the distal fragment on the proximal. Frequently there is separation of one or more comminuted fragments that may come to lie at a right angle to the long axis of the bone. Fracture involving the inner end of the clavicle is very uncommon as is dislocation at the sternoclavicular joint. Fractures occur in the outer end of the clavicle although they are less common than in the shaft proper. The fractures involving the distal end of the bone are often associated with subluxation of the acromioclavicular joint.

STERNUM AND RIBS

Fractures of the Sternum

Demonstration of fracture of the sternum requires technically good roentgenograms, particularly a true lateral projection. Many of these injuries result from automobile accidents, the driver being thrown against the steering wheel column. The fracture may be incomplete with only a slight angular deformity, or it may be complete with separation of the fragments and overriding of them. Tomography is often useful for clear delineation of the fracture.

Fractures of the Ribs

Complete fractures of the ribs with some degree of displacement of fragments usually can be identified without difficulty in roentgenograms obtained to show rib detail. Incomplete or greenstick fractures, occurring during childhood, and buckling fractures without displacement are more difficult to recognize. Hairline fractures also occur in the ribs and are very difficult to visualize at times. In some of these patients, reexamination after several weeks will show the presence of cloudy periosteal callus and evidence of a fracture line when none could be clearly identified in roentgenograms secured immediately after the injury. Visualization of hairline fractures is facilitated when the exact site of the suspected injury is known at the time the roentgenograms are made so that proper exposures can be obtained.

As a result of repeated and severe coughing spells, one or more fatigue type of fractures may occur in the lower ribs. These usually develop in the axillary arcs of the seventh, eighth, or ninth ribs and may or may not be a cause of pain. They have been discovered in roentgenograms of the chest in patients who have had no complaints referable to the fracture. As with fatigue fractures elsewhere, the line of fracture may be very indistinct at first and only become obvious after several weeks or after periosteal callus begins to form. These are termed "cough fractures."

Fracture in the anterior arc of the first rib also has been observed as a type of chronic fatigue fracture. As an example this fracture has been found in recruits after long marches carrying heavy packs and is believed to be due to abnormal stresses and strains on the rib with the development of a fatigue fracture very similar to those more commonly found in the metatarsal bones. These have been described earlier in this chapter (see Fig. 5-9).

FRACTURES OF THE PELVIS

Many types of fractures occur in the pelvic bones, depending upon the nature of the injury and its severity. The bones most commonly involved are the pubic rami on one or both sides; usually in association with pubic fracture there is a fracture of the sacrum on the same or contralateral side. The deformity of the sacral fracture often is minimal and may be overlooked unless roentgenograms are carefully inspected. Often a slight irregularity of one or more neural foramina may be the only sign of sacral fracture. Most other pelvic fractures can be identified without difficulty in roentgenograms of good quality. Since the pelvis is essentially a bony ring, fracture in one area should alert the observer to the possibility of another fracture of the ring or to subluxation or dislocation of the pubic symphysis or sacroiliac joint(s). In children a greenstick type of fracture is observed and its recognition may be difficult because of the rather minimal deformity that results. The examiner must pay careful attention to the trabecular architecture of the bone and to slight variations in contour of the various portions.

There are a number of avulsion injuries in the region of the pelvis and hips which usually occur as a result of muscle pull, particularly in young adults. In sprinters the anterosuperior iliac spine avulsions result from the pull of the sartorius or tensor fascia femoris muscles. Anteroinferior iliac spine avulsions may be due to rectus femoris pulls. The same is true of superior acetabular rim avulsions. The abdominal muscles may avulse fragments of the iliac crest. Hamstrings may cause an ischial tuberosity avulsion, while pull of the adductor muscles may produce injury in the region of the symphysis pubis and along the lateral aspect of the inferior ischial ramus. Greater trochanteric avulsions result from gluteal muscle pull, while lesser trochanteric avulsions may result from psoas major muscle pull.

Dislocation of the coccyx on the sacrum is a moderately common injury and can be identified usually without much difficulty in lateral roentgenograms. In some individuals the sacrum is unusually flat and forms a rather sharp angle with the lumbar spine instead of a smooth lordotic curve. In these persons, usually females, the coccyx points directly forward to form a right angle or, occasionally, even an acute angle with the sacrum. This is developmental and should not be confused with traumatic displacement.

FRACTURES OF THE UPPER END OF THE FEMUR

The various types of fracture affecting the upper end of the femur are shown in Figure 5-35. Those fractures occurring in the subcapital or transcervical area are intracapsular. There is an absence of periosteum in this region so that periosteal callus does not form and union occurs only by endosteal callus formation. Because of this and the poor blood supply in this part of the bone, union often is slow and occasionally nonunion results. Before the advent of modern methods of treatment with fixation devices, nonunion of femoral neck fractures was frequent. It is much less so at the present time. Fractures of the femoral neck may be either of abduction or adduction type. The difference is important because abduction fractures frequently are impacted along the superior aspect (see Fig. 5-35). Healing generally occurs without difficulty. Adduction fractures, on the other hand, are almost invariably associated with displacement of fragments. The femur often is held in external rotation so that the fracture surfaces are not in apposition (Fig. 5-36). Fractures through the intertrochanteric area usually heal with bony callus and without delay. Varying degrees of comminution are

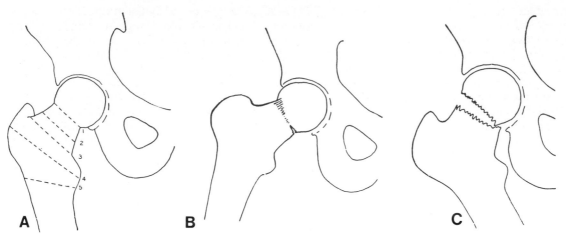

Fig. 5-35. Diagrammatic representations of fractures of the upper femur. **A.** The usual sites of fracture: **(1)** subcapital; **(2)** transcervical; **(3)** basocervical; **(4)** intertrochanteric; **(5)** subtrochanteric. **B.** Abduction fracture illustrates the usual impaction superiorly and distraction inferiorly. **C.** Adduction fracture. There is little tendency for impaction in this type of injury.

likely to be present and frequently the lesser trochanter is avulsed as a separate fragment (Fig. 5-37). From the point of view of roentgen diagnosis, femoral neck fractures can be recognized without difficulty, except the minor degrees of abduction-impaction fractures. In such a fracture there may be an absence of a distinct fracture line and the diagnosis depends upon demonstrating an angular deformity between the superior surface of the femoral head and the contiguous neck, some condensation where the bone has been impacted, and a valgus deformity with

an increased angle between the neck and head (Fig. 5-36A).

Dislocations of the hip are relatively infrequent lesions and the dislocation is usually a posterior one. It is easily recognized in roentgenograms. As with dislocations affecting other joints, it is important to search for evidence of avulson fractures and it is essential that roentgenograms be obtained after reduction in order to determine the adequacy of reduction and better to demonstrate small avulsion fractures if such be present.

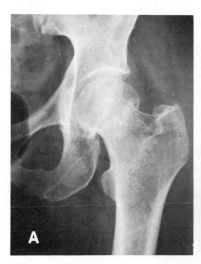
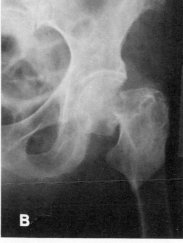

Fig. 5-36. A. Abduction fracture (subcapital) with impaction. **B.** Adduction fracture (transcervical). The shaft is in varus position and is externally rotated. The fracture surfaces are not in apposition.

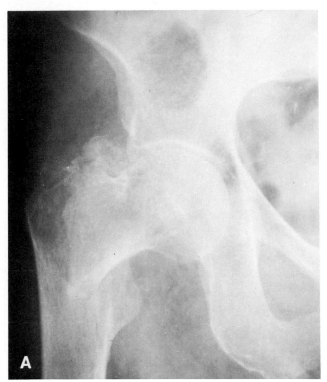
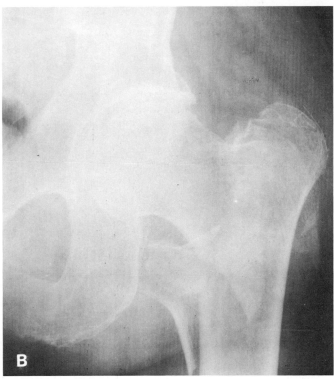

Fig. 5-37. Intertrochanteric fractures. **A.** The shaft is externally rotated with moderate abduction of the neck forming nearly a right-angle varus. **B.** There has been more comminution in this fracture. There is a large comminuted fracture of the greater trochanter, and the lesser trochanter is avulsed and fragmented.

FRACTURES INVOLVING THE KNEE

Condylar Fractures of the Femur

Supracondylar fracture of the femur is a frequent lesion and often there is a vertical fracture associated with the transverse one so that the condyles become separated. It is important to recognize this intra-articular component of the injury. The roentgen diagnosis of these fractures is not difficult (see Fig. 5-3).

Upper End of the Tibia

Most fractures involving the tibia are demonstrated without difficulty in roentgenograms. Again it is important that any fracture lines extending into the articular surface should be observed and the condition of the articular surface be noted. Fractures of the tibial plateau often result in depression of one of the condyles, leaving an irregular articular surface that predisposes to subsequent development of degenerative joint disease. The avulsion fractures of the inter-

condylar eminence of the tibia occur more commonly in children than in adults. Open reduction is not usually necessary in children unless the fragment is completely lifted out and separated from the adjacent bone. In adults, this fracture is often associated with injury of the cruciate ligament. Results of treatment may be improved by repair of the damaged ligaments in this group.

Lipohemarthrosis. In this condition, there is blood and fat in the joint space caused by intracapsular fracture which allows the blood and fat to extrude into the space.[2] The radiolucent fat floats on the blood and fluid in the joint and is observed as an area of lucency on a horizontal-beam film. It is found more often in injuries of the knee than elsewhere, but it has also been recognized in the shoulder. Therefore, when a fat–fluid level is noted on a horizontal-beam film of a joint, this usually indicates that there is a fracture into the joint. However, it is possible that a fat–fluid level can be manifest in association with se-

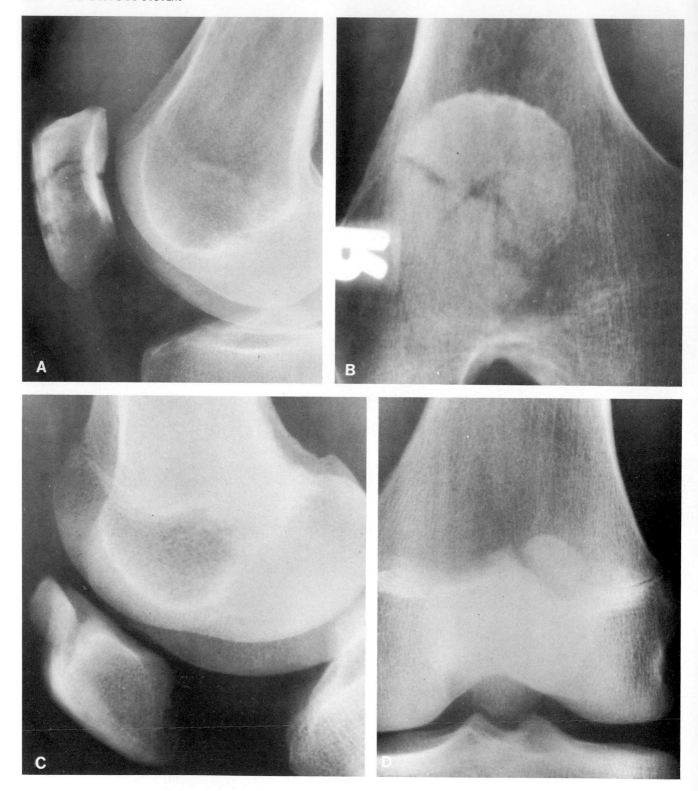

Fig. 5-38. (*Caption on opposite page.*)

vere injury, such as dislocation, without fracture. However, in these dislocations, small intra-articular fractures may be present although not visible radiographically.

Patella

Most fractures of the patella are transverse and separation of fragments may be severe because of the pull of the quadriceps muscle on the upper fragment (Fig. 5-38). Infrequently the line of fracture is vertical and may be visualized with difficulty unless oblique or tangential views of the bone are obtained. In dealing with injuries to the patella, care must be used not to confuse a bipartite or multipartite patella for a corner fracture. This anomaly consists of one or several unfused ossification centers that remain along the upper outer quadrant of the bone. The rounded corners of an anomalous center and the generally smooth cortical borders are in contrast to the irregular edges of a fracture fragment. The condition is bilateral in about 80% of cases.

Dislocation of the patella is rare. In nearly one-fourth of these patients, small longitudinal fractures along the medial aspect of the patella are present in addition to the dislocation.[5, 13] Presumably the fractures are caused by the trauma produced when the patella, which dislocates laterally, impinges upon the lateral aspect of the lateral femoral condyle. In many instances, fractures of the lateral femoral condyle may also be produced. Usually an axial or tangential view of the patella is necessary for the diagnosis of dislocation, but internal and external rotation of about 45 degrees is often necessary to outline the longitudinal fractures of the medial aspect of the condyle. These fractures may result in intra-articular loose fragments since they arise from the articular surface of the condyle and the patella. Therefore, this type of injury may be a frequent cause of loose bodies in the knee. Patellar dislocation usually results from trauma, but there are certain situations that tend to increase the risk. Dysplasia of the lateral femoral condyle resulting in a relatively flat anterosuperior surface in contrast to its usual lateral elevation is important. If this is present bilaterally, there may be bi-

lateral patellar dislocations. When the valgus angle is increased, the possibility of dislocation or subluxation is increased, and bilateral genu valgus may result in bilateral subluxation. Patellar size and shape may also be important, a small patella being more readily dislocated than one of normal size. Also, when there is a decrease in the transverse diameter and an increase in the anteroposterior diameter of the patella, the possibility of subluxation or dislocation is said to be increased. Once either has occurred, recurrences are common, often without injury or with trivial injury; therefore surgical repair in patients with recurrent dislocation may be necessary.

FRACTURES AND DISLOCATIONS OF THE ANKLE AND FOOT
The Ankle

Injuries involving the bones comprising the ankle joint are very frequent and the roentgen diagnosis is made without difficulty in most cases. No attempt will be made here to classify these fractures and dislocations, but it may be stated that a wide variety of injuries can occur. The simplest fracture is one involving only the lateral malleolus with or without a slight spreading of the mortise of the ankle joint (the tibiofibular articulation). More severe injuries lead to fractures of the medial malleolus and the posterior articular process of the tibia. Fractures of the posterior tibial process tend to be more readily seen on lateral roentgenograms obtained with slight external rotation (5 to 10 degrees) than on a true lateral film. These fractures may or may not be associated with dislocation. When dislocation exists, the foot is usually displaced posteriorly on the leg and the malleolar fragments tend to be carried backward with the foot (Fig. 5-39). As is true in fractures involving other joints, it is important to determine whether or not fracture lines enter the articular surface; if they do, whether or not the articular surface has been disrupted to any significant degree. In children, epiphyseal fracture may be difficult to recognize if there has been little or no displacement. As noted under the discussion of epiphyseal fractures, when a line of fracture extends through cartilage and does not affect bone it cannot be visualized readily unless it has caused some displacement of fragments. Usually the fracture does not remain in cartilage throughout its extent, but a corner fragment of bone, either of the shaft or of the epiphysis, remains attached to the cartilaginous plate and is displaced along with it. If the fracture is entirely through cartilage, a slight widening of the epiphyseal plate may be

Fig. 5-38. A and **B.** Undisplaced fracture of the patella. Note large soft-tissue density representing a large effusion in the suprapatellar portion of the joint space. **C** and **D.** Lateral and frontal views of a patient with bipartite patella showing the smooth, corticated surfaces in contrast to the fracture.

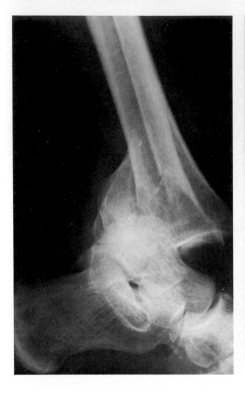

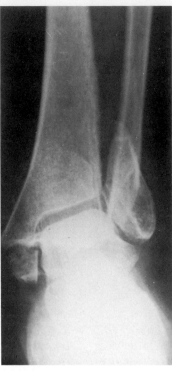

Fig. 5-39. Fracture-dislocation of the ankle. The distal malleolar fragments are shown to be displaced posteriorly with the foot. This represents a trimalleolar fracture with dislocation.

apparent. This can be recognized more easily if a film of the opposite normal foot is available for comparison.

In severe ankle injuries without evidence of fracture or dislocation, stress films should be considered since ligamentous tear or avulsion may not be apparent, and the resultant instability of the ankle joint may lead to later disability.

The Tarsus

Fractures of the Os Calcis. For the demonstration of fractures involving the os calcis, an axial view is required in addition to lateral and oblique projections of the bone. The more severe injuries to the bone can be visualized without difficulty because of the crushing and comminution, since most of these occur as a result of a fall from a height with the patient landing on the feet. Slight degrees of compression fracture may be difficult to recognize unless one is completely familiar with the normal appearance of this bone and in some cases it is advisable to compare the injured side with the opposite normal foot. A measurement of value in the examination of fractures of the os calcis consists in determining the tuber-joint angle (Boehler's angle) (Fig. 5-40). This is an angle formed by drawing two lines, one from the anterior superior margin of the bone and the other from the posterior superior margin to the highest point of the articular surface. These lines meet at an angle of 140 to 160 degrees in the normal individual. The complement to this angle is therefore 20 to 40 degrees. When there is impaction the tuber-joint angle of 20 to 40 degrees is reduced and may become zero or actually reversed (Fig. 5-41). In many fractures involving this bone there is injury to the subastragalar joint

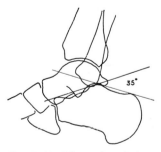

Fig. 5-40. The tuber-joint angle of the calcaneus. Diagram illustrates the method for determining this angle (Boehler's angle).

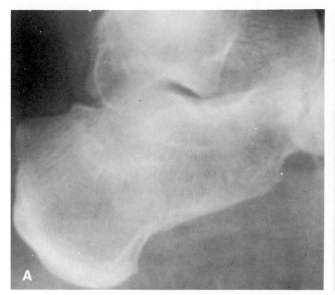 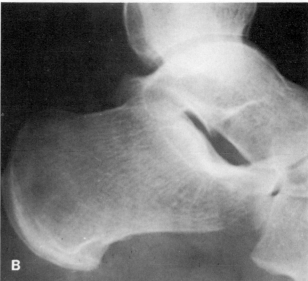

Fig. 5-41. A. Compression fracture of the os calcis showing loss of Boehler's angle. **B.** Normal os calcis showing preservation of the angle.

surfaces and the later development of a traumatic type of degenerative joint disease.

Fractures of the Astragalus. Any part of the astragalus may be involved by fracture and with the more severe injuries there often is accompanying dislocation. A fracture of a long posterior process must be distinguished from an accessory ossicle that occurs in this location, known as the os trigonum. An accessory ossicle usually has rounded margins, is bounded by cortex around the entire periphery, and is separated from the major part of the bone by a space of uniform width. A fracture of a process, on the other hand, will show irregularity of the margin where the process was separated from the bone, with an absence of cortex at this site; the soft tissues will be swollen around the area of fracture; and the fragment may be definitely displaced away from the bone.

Fractures through the neck of the astragalus are usually of vertical type occurring along the anterior part of its tibial articular surface. Fractures of this type often are followed by an ischemic necrosis of one or both fragments and the development of this complication should be watched for in serial roentgenograms (see Chapter 8).

Flake Fractures. In association with severe sprains of the ankle area, avulsion of one or more small flakes of cortical bone often occur where a ligament or ten-don was attached and partially or completely separated as a result of the injury. The demonstration of such small cortical flake fractures merely indicates the severity of the soft-tissue injury.

Fractures of the Metatarsals

The Fifth Metatarsal. Fractures involving the proximal end of this bone are frequent, usually following an inversion injury to the foot. Characteristically the fracture line extends transversely across the proximal end of the bone with separation of a triangular fragment (Fig. 5-42). This fracture must not be confused with a normal epiphysis that occurs at the proximal end of this metatarsal, appearing during adolescence and uniting within a few years. The epiphysis for this bone occurs on the outer side and the long axis of the epiphyseal center lies in the direction of the long axis of the bone. A familiarity with the appearance of this normal epiphysis will aid in preventing error in diagnosis (Fig. 5-43).

Fatigue Fractures of the Metatarsals. Chronic insufficiency or fatigue fractures of the metatarsals have been discussed under the heading "Chronic Stress or Fatigue Fracture."

Dislocations. There are a number of dislocations that may be observed in the foot.[20] These are usually

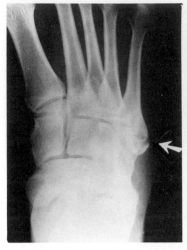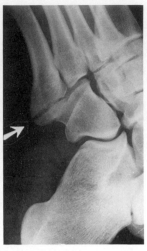

Fig. 5-42. Fracture of the fifth metatarsal. **Arrows** indicate the typical transverse fracture of the base of the fifth metatarsal without much displacement. This is a common result of inversion injury.

not difficult to diagnose roentgenographically, but they may be associated with avulsion or other types of fracture. Therefore, it is necessary to obtain multiple views, particularly after reduction when the fracture is often more readily visible. Dislocations in the foot and ankle include the following:

1. Subtalar dislocation. The ankle joint remains intact and the hindfoot is dislocated.
2. Total talar dislocation. This almost always results in ischemic necrosis since most of the talar surface is articular and the talus has no muscular attachments.
3. Dislocation of the forefoot on the talus and calcaneus.
4. Dislocation at the tarsometatarsal joints—complete or partial.
5. Dislocation at the metatarsophalangeal joints—complete or partial.
6. Dislocation of the interphalangeal joints. This often involves only one joint and is a minor injury compared with the others which usually imply a major injury.

THE BATTERED CHILD SYNDROME

In roentgenograms of the skeletons of infants one occasionally finds bizarre changes that appear to be the result of trauma.[15] These changes may be discovered while examining the infant for some totally unrelated condition and a history of injury may be unobtainable from the parents. In some cases this may be a deliberate misrepresentation; in others the low mentality of the parents may account for it. In still others the traumatic episode may not have been noticed by other members of the family. The possibility of deliberate mistreatment of the infant by a psychotic or an alcoholic parent must be borne in mind. The condition is known as the "battered child syndrome."

The infant skeleton responds to trauma more easily and with greater rapidity than the older child or the adult. The lesions vary considerably in their roentgen appearances. There may be separation of one or more small fragments from the corner of a metaphysis. Characteristically the metaphyseal margin of one or more bones may show an irregular or serrated appearance probably representing the effects of previous metaphyseal infractions. Skull fractures may be found in some of these patients and subdural hematoma may be one of the complications. Subluxation of one or more of the epiphyses, extensive subperiosteal calcification, or even a frank shaft fracture showing evidence of callus may all be present in the individual case. Typically, the lesions are likely to be found in multiple bones although there is no particular symmetry to the distribution and they vary a great deal in severity from one area to another. Among the conditions that must be considered in differential diagnosis are infantile scurvy, infantile cortical hyperostosis, osteomyelitis, and bone neoplasms. The proper diagnosis, in the absence of a history of injury, depends upon the irregular distribution of the lesions in the skeleton, the normal density and texture of the bones otherwise, the lack of clinical signs of infection or of other serious disease, the evidence of fragmentation, especially along the metaphyseal borders, and the presence of epiphyseal separations (Fig. 5-44). Also, there is often evidence of trauma of varying duration—some recent, some old and well healed. Lung contusions and lacerations have also been found associated with rib fractures.

In some cases the final diagnosis will depend upon the observation of prompt spontaneous regression and eventual healing.

CONGENITAL INDIFFERENCE TO PAIN

This is a rare disorder characterized by a congenital insensitivity to pain. The skeletal lesions are a reflection of this and consist in gross fractures or healing fractures, various forms of osteochondrosis or isch-

Fig. 5-43. In this patient the secondary ossification center is noted paralleling the lateral aspect of the proximal end of the fifth metatarsal. The irregular line between it and the shaft is roughly parallel to the shaft while the small, undisplaced fracture is at right angles to the shaft, the usual situation **(arrows).**

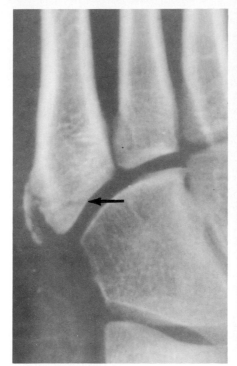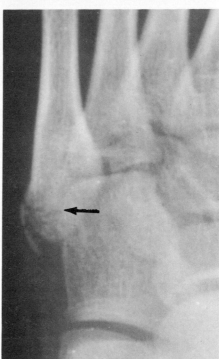

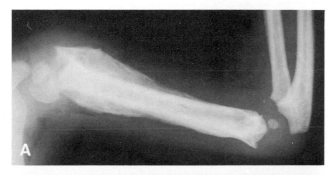

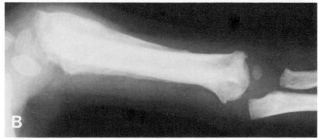

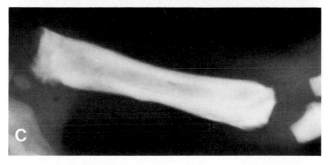

Fig. 5-44. Battered child syndrome. **A** and **B.** Note the extensive callus surrounding the proximal humeral shaft. The general thickening of this bone and the epiphyseal displacement indicate epiphyseal fracture. **C.** The more chronic changes of trauma in a battered child.

emic necrosis apparently owing to repeated minor traumas, and/or osteomyelitis in its various phases. In some cases the roentgen evidence of trauma is similar to that noted in the preceding paragraph, with metaphyseal infractions or "corner" fractures and reactive periosteal calcification. The inflammatory lesions are usually those of an infection of low virulence, with abscess formation. Necrosis of the distal phalanges has been reported, evidently the result of persistent cutaneous infections of the fingers. Other lesions that have been described include hydrarthrosis and subluxations.

REFERENCES AND SELECTED READINGS

1. ABEL MS: Clinical and roentgenological aspects of "occult" fractures of smaller elements of cervical vertebrae. Am J Surg 97: 530, 1959

2. ARGER PH, OBERKIRCHER PE, MILLER WT: Lipohemarthrosis. Am J Roentgenol 121: 97, 1974

3. BLICKENSTAFF LD, MORRIS JM: Fatigue fractures of the femoral neck. J Bone Joint Surg [A] 48: 1031, 1966

4. BOHRERS SP: The fat-pad sign following elbow trauma. Its usefulness and reliability in suspecting "invisible" fractures. Clin Radiol 21: 90, 1970

5. BRATTSTROM H: Shape of the intercondylar groove normally and in recurrent dislocation of patella. Acta Orthop Scan [Suppl] 68: 1964

6. HANSON PG, ANGEVINE M, JUHL JH: Osteitis pubis in sports activities. Physician in Sports Medicine 6: 111, 1978

7. JUHL JH, MILLER SM, ROBERTS GW: Roentgenographic variations in the normal cervical spine. Radiology 78: 591, 1962

8. KOHN AM: Soft tissue alterations in elbow trauma. Am J Roentgenol 82: 867, 1959

9. LEE FA, GWINN JL: Retrosternal dislocation of the clavicle. Radiology 110: 631, 1974

10. ROGERS LF: The radiography of epiphyseal injuries. Radiology 96: 289, 1970

11. SALTER RB, HARRIS WR: Injuries involving the epiphyseal plate. J Bone Joint Surg [A] 45: 587, 1963

12. SANDELL LJ: Congenital indifference to pain. J Fac Radiol 9: 50, 1958

13. SCHELLER S, MARTENSON L: Traumatic dislocation of the patella. Acta Radiol [Suppl] (Stockh) 336: 1974

14. SIEGELMAN SS, HEIMANN WG, MANIN MC: Congenital indifference to pain. Am J Roentgenol 97: 242, 1966

15. SILVERMAN FN: Unrecognized trauma in infants, the battered child syndrome and the syndrome of Ambroise Tardieu. Radiology 104: 337, 1972

16. VINES FS: The significance of "occult" fractures of the cervical spine. Am J Roentgenol 107: 493, 1969

17. WHALEN JP, WOODRUFF CL: The cervical prevertebral fat stripe. Am J Roentgenol 109: 445, 1970

18. WILSON ES JR, KATZ FN: Stress fracture. An analysis of 250 consecutive cases. Radiology 92: 481, 1969

19. WINFIELD AC, DENNIS JM: Stress fractures of the calcaneus. Radiology 72: 415, 1959

20. ZATZKIN HR: Trauma to foot. Semin Roentgenol 5: 419, 1970

6

INFECTIONS AND INFLAMMATIONS OF BONE

OSTEOMYELITIS

Osteomyelitis caused by pyogenic organisms may affect any bone at any age period. In the young it is usually the result of a hematogenous infection while in adults it is more often secondary to compound fractures, penetrating wounds, or surgical procedures such as the open reduction of fractures. While a variety of organisms can cause the disease, the most frequent is *Staphylococcus aureus*. Since the advent of antibiotics and chemotherapy, osteomyelitis has become a much less serious disease than it formerly was. The incidence of osteomyelitis also has decreased considerably. One of the reasons for this probably is the early treatment with antibiotics of lesions that may cause hematogenous osteomyelitis such as boils, carbuncles, and other localized infections. Frequently the lesion is brought under control at an early stage and roentgen findings may be minimal. However, cases of osteomyelitis, particularly in infants or children, are again being seen, although much less frequently than before, apparently owing to the development of resistant strains of organisms. In most cases the infection is aborted before much damage to bone has developed. Occasionally a small abscess cavity will remain, sometimes containing a sequestrum, indicating the amount of bone that was damaged by the initial assault of the infecting organisms. In any individual case the lesions may be single or multiple. In the child, in whom hematogenous infection is the rule, multiple foci of disease are relatively frequent. Hematogenous foci show a great tendency to develop in or near the metaphysis. The infection often is limited by the epiphyseal plate, but not necessarily so; it may extend through the plate or around the epiphysis into the adjacent joint and cause a pyogenic arthritis (Fig. 6-1).

The types of osteomyelitis are: (*1*) acute osteomyelitis, (*2*) chronic osteomyelitis, (*3*) bone abscess (acute, chronic, and Brodie's abscess), and (*4*) Garre's sclerosing osteitis.

ACUTE OSTEOMYELITIS

Normally there is a latent period of a week to 10 days between the time of onset of clinical symptoms of acute osteomyelitis and the development of definite

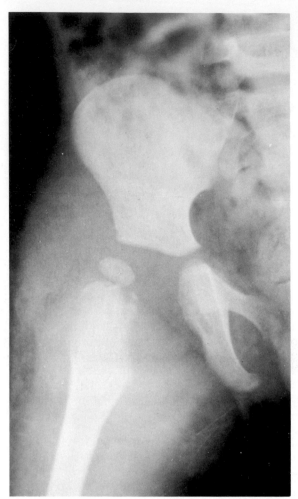

Fig. 6-1. Acute osteomyelitis of the proximal metaphysis of the femur with secondary involvement of the hip joint. There is little irregular loss of bone along the inner margin of the metaphysis indicating osteomyelitis. The femur is displaced laterally by the large joint effusion. There is rather marked soft-tissue swelling in the upper thigh.

roentgen changes in the bone. Because it is essential that adequate therapy be instituted as early as possible, one should not wait for the development of roentgen signs of bone disease in the presence of an acute virulent infection before instituting treatment.

The first roentgen evidence of the disease is a swelling of the soft tissues. Characteristically this is deep and adjacent to the bone and may be localized or extensive (Figs. 6-2, 6-3, and 6-4B). The early swelling is recognized because of displacement or obliteration of the normal fat planes adjacent to and between the deep muscle bundles.[2] At first the superficial fatty layer is unaffected but its outline soon disappears as the inflammatory reaction spreads. With skin infections, in contrast, the early swelling is superficial and usually a massive deep edema does not develop. The first evidence of disease in the bone usually is an area of indefinite rarefaction in the metaphysis. This is difficult to visualize unless the roentgenograms are of excellent quality. The rarefaction of the bone has a fine granular or slightly mottled appearance. The area of involvement is poorly defined. Associated with this or occasionally preceding it, there will be noted a slight amount of periosteal calcification laid down along the outer side of the cortex and paralleling it (Figs. 6-5, 6-6, and 6-7); swelling of the soft tissues around the involved area can be visualized. The limits of the bone lesion remain poorly defined throughout much of the acute stage and during the early course of the disease the extent of involvement appears much less than it actually is.

Within a short time, bone destruction becomes more prominent and this causes a ragged, moth-eaten appearance with foci of destruction intermingled with areas of apparently normal bone (Fig. 6-8). The periosteal calcification becomes more pronounced and the shaft at the site of the disease may be surrounded by a shell of calcification, known as the involucrum. Unless treated, the disease gradually progresses into the chronic stage. There is a considerable variation in the time required for development of the findings just noted. Among the factors involved are the virulence of the organism, the number of organisms present, the resistance of the host, the presence of an area or areas of increased local susceptibility such as local injury, and treatment of the host with antibiotics or other drugs.

In the neonate and the young infant, it is especially important to detect the subtle soft-tissue swelling early because there are transphyseal vessels present connecting the metaphyseal vascular system (derived from the nutrient artery of the diaphysis) to the epiphyseal vascular system. The vascular anastamosis is accomplished through "cartilage canals" making spread to the epiphysis and from there to the joint more likely than in the older child or adult in whom the transphyseal system has closed. Once the transphyseal system has closed, there is no connection between the metaphyseal system and the epiphyseal system of vessels. From the radiographic standpoint, it is often helpful to compare the suspected limb with the normal one, using soft-tissue tech-

Fig. 6-2. Acute osteomyelitis of the femur in an infant. **A.** Roentgenogram secured 7 days after the onset of fever and swelling of the thigh. Slight cortical destruction on the inner aspect of the upper femur and massive swelling of soft tissue of the thigh are evident. Also noted is lateral displacement of the femur, indicating effusion of the hip joint. **B.** Roentgenogram obtained 3 months later shows extensive periosteal calcification surrounding much of the shaft. Remnants of the old shaft are visualized within it. Several rounded or oval cavities, representing residuals of bone abscess, are seen in the proximal femur.

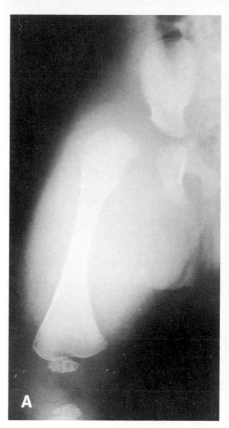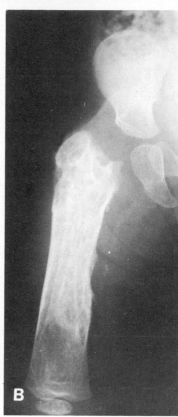

Fig. 6-3. Acute osteomyelitis of the acetabulum in an infant. **A.** Initial roentgenogram. Swelling of soft tissues and effusion of the hip joint were observed only by comparing this film with one of the opposite hip. **B.** Roentgenogram obtained 2½ weeks later reveals an area of poorly defined destruction in the roof of the acetabulum. **C.** Roentgenogram obtained 8 weeks after the onset shows increased density around the area of destruction, indicating sclerosis and healing. This was a staphylococcal infection.

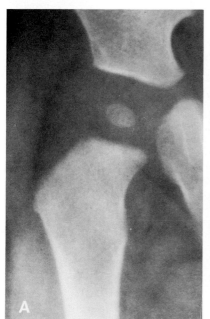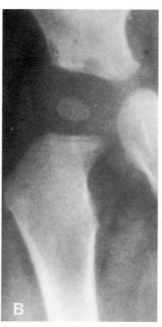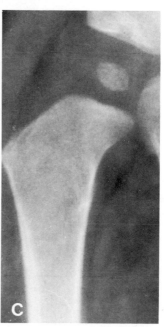

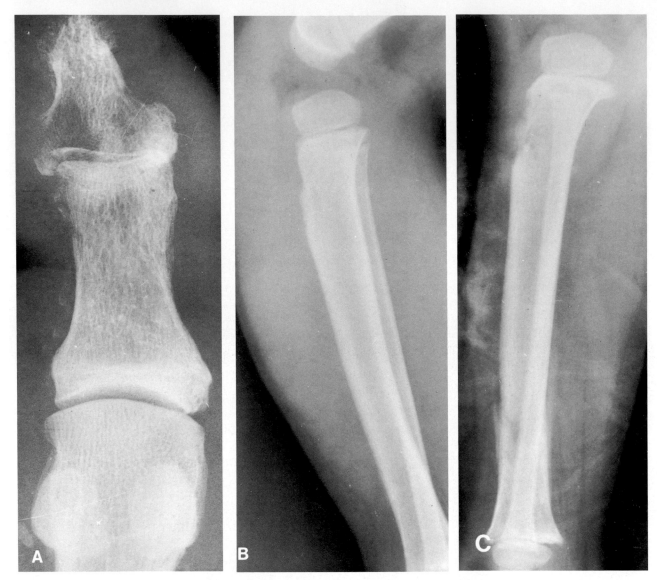

Fig. 6-4. A. Chronic osteomyelitis in a diabetic. Note destruction of the distal phalanx proximally with early changes in the lateral aspect of the distal end of the proximal phalanx. There is a little gas in the adjacent soft tissues, and calcification in arteries can be observed medial to the first digit. **B.** Acute osteomyelitis of the tibia. Initial film shows massive swelling of the soft tissues anterior to the upper three-fourths of the tibia extending up anterior to the knee. **C.** Nine days later there is noted some bone destruction of the proximal shaft and to a lesser extent of the lower shaft where there is also noted some periosteal calcification. A dressing is present producing some mottled densities anterior to the tibia.

niques to aid in detection of early subtle soft-tissue changes of osteomyelitis. It is estimated that, in neonatal osteomyelitis, involvement of the epiphyseal plate occurs as spread from the metaphysis in about 50% of the patients.

A number of special situations should be mentioned briefly in this discussion of acute osteomyelitis. *Staphylococcus aureus* is the most common causitive organism of the condition and involvement of the odontoid process by this organism has been reported to result in complete destruction of this process. After recovery the appearance may resemble

that of congenital absence of the odontoid process. However, there is usually limitation of motion and there may be ankylosis of the atlanto-axial joint. Complete destruction of the odontoid process has also been reported to be caused by tuberculosis and has resulted from trauma.

Acute osteomyelitis is common in heroin addicts. In these patients it may be local when secondary to an adjacent soft-tissue abscess, but more often it is hematogenous and there may be multiple sites of osseous involvement among which the vertebrae are the most common. Disc destruction as well as bone

Fig. 6-5. Acute osteomyelitis of the midfemoral shaft. **A.** Roentgenogram obtained 10 days following onset of pain and swelling. This anteroposterior view of the femur shows more subperiosteal calcification on the lateral than on the medial aspect with some cortical destruction laterally. **B.** Lateral view showing that the destruction extends and involves the anterior femoral cortex.

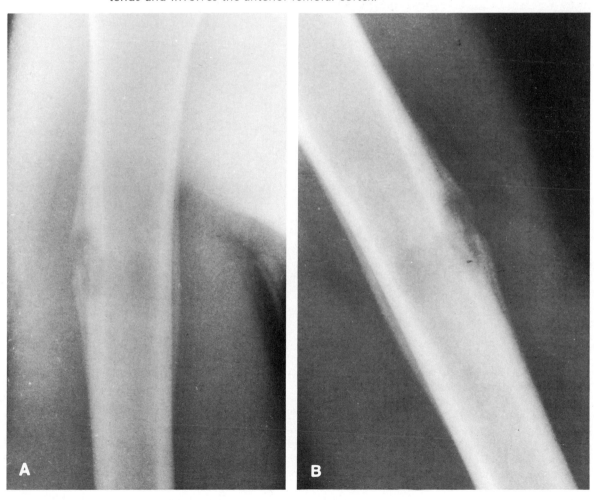

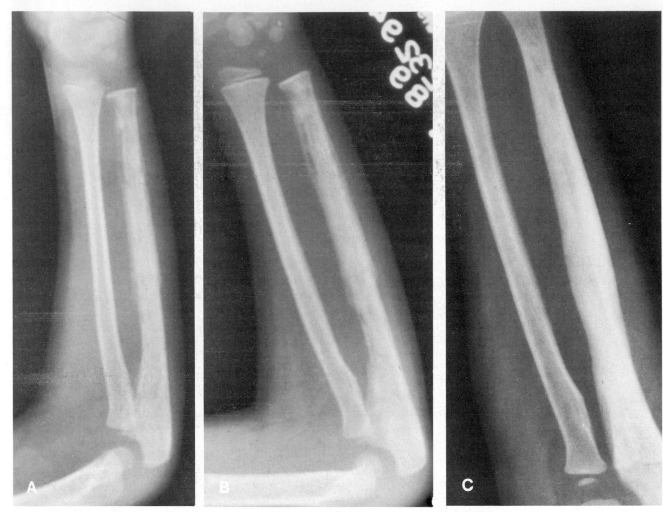

Fig. 6-6. Acute osteomyelitis of the ulna. **A.** Roentgenogram obtained 10 days after the onset of symptoms shows extensive permeative type of destruction of most of the ulna with a little subperiosteal calcification noted best distally. **B.** Roentgenogram obtained 1 week later shows that there has been an increase in the amount of subperiosteal calcification, but most of the areas of bone destruction persist. **C.** Roentgenogram obtained 6 months later shows some residual cortical thickening but no definite residual destruction.

destruction occurs and there is sometimes extension to form an epidural abscess.

Sickle cell disease is frequently complicated by acute osteomyelitis the causitive organism of which is *Salmonella* in approximately 80% of patients. Radiographic study reveals involvement of multiple and often symmetrical diaphyseal sites. The lesions are extensive and often involve the entire shaft. There are areas of longitudinal destruction, large sequestra including much of the shaft, and excessive sub-

periosteal new-bone formation (involucrum). Pathologic fractures are common. Differentiation from infarction without infection may be difficult in these patients with severe manifestations of sickle cell disease.

Acute osteomyelitis has also been reported following puncture of the os calcis to obtain blood in neonates. Staphylococcal septicemia associated with pulmonary and other visceral involvement may also be complicated by acute osteomyelitis. The latter may be

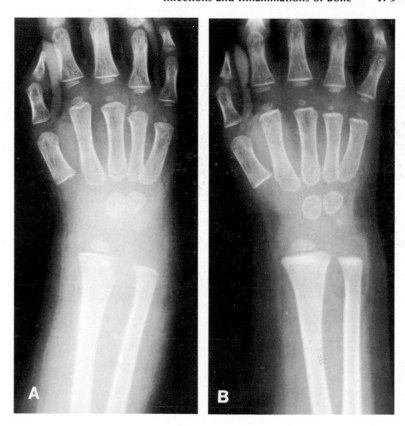

Fig. 6-7. Acute osteomyelitis of the distal radius in a child. **A.** Two weeks after onset of symptoms, poorly defined destruction of the medial aspect of the radial metaphysis and diffuse swelling of soft tissue are evident. **B.** Two months later, no distinct residual is noted. A superficial abscess had been drained and antibiotic therapy had been given.

overlooked in these acutely ill patients, but it must be treated, often by surgical drainage, to effect a cure. Radiographic findings are similar to those of acute osteomyelitis in other situations.

Another condition in which osteomyelitis occurs is *chronic granulomatous disease* of childhood[19, 21] which is characterized by infection, suppuration, and granuloma formation. There is a defect in the polymorphonuclear leukocytes in that they are able to ingest bacteria but cannot kill them. All other immune responses appear normal, including a normal amount of immunoglobulins in the plasma. When the neutrophils die, live bacteria and their toxic products are released. Bone infection is very common. It is similar to acute osteomyelitis initially but then tends to become markedly chronic with very little sequestration and very little sclerotic bone reaction. The destructive lesions tend to expand bone but usually do not break through the cortex. A secondary sign is a zone of rarefaction proximal to the growth plate similar to that sometimes observed in children with leukemia. The most common sites of involvement are the small bones of the hands and feet.

Fig. 6-8. Acute osteomyelitis involving the metaphysis and proximal shaft of the femur in a child. The patchy permeative type of destruction is often observed.

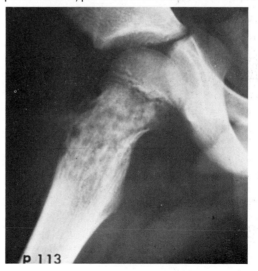

CHRONIC OSTEOMYELITIS

Chronic osteomyelitis is a continuation of the acute stage, there being no sharp line of demarcation between the two. *See* Fig. 6-4A. The patchy bone destruction becomes more pronounced but the limits of the lesion still remain poorly defined. If no treatment

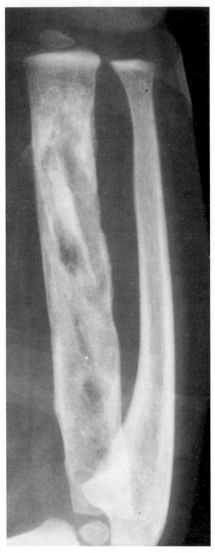

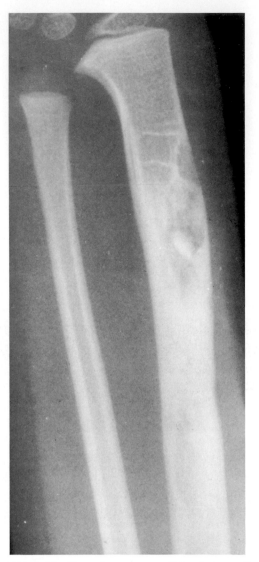

Fig. 6-10. Chronic osteomyelitis of the radius. There is an irregular cavity distally within which lies a dense sequestrum. Note the dense subperiosteal calcification, some of which has been incorporated into the cortex opposite the sequestrum.

Fig. 6-9. Chronic osteomyelitis. The entire radius has been involved. There are irregular cavities representing chronic abscesses and a large, dense sequestrum is noted within a long cavity in the distal end of the shaft. The general thickening of the bone is the result of chronic periostitis. The original cortex has been completely replaced.

is given the infection may extend to involve the entire shaft, the involucrum forming the main support.

Pieces of cortex die and become sequestra. These are evident in the roentgenogram as the areas of dense bone surrounded by zones of rarefaction. Because the sequestrum usually has lost its blood supply early in the course of the disease from vascular thrombosis and infarction it remains as dense as normal bone, standing out clearly from the demineralized bone around it (Fig. 6-9). Sequestra usually lie within abscess cavities (Fig. 6-10).

The end result of a chronic osteomyelitis after the infection has subsided is a thickened bone with a sclerotic-appearing cortex and a wavy outer margin (Fig. 6-11). The cortex may become so dense and thickened that the medullary cavity may not be apparent. Areas of defect where sequestra have been absorbed or removed surgically add to the general deformity of outline. If the infection becomes reactivated, and this is common, it is shown by the recurrence of deep soft-tissue swelling, by areas of hazy periosteal calcification, and by the development of relatively sharply outlined cavities within the bone representing abscess formation. It often is impossible to determine with any certainty by roentgen examination whether active infection is or is not present in an old osteomyelitis because of the irregular density and the marked sclerosis that may hide even large abscess cavities. It is in these cases that tomography is useful to visualize the interior of the bone to better advantage.

CHRONIC SYMMETRIC OSTEOMYELITIS

This is a rare disease which occurs in childhood. It is a very indolent process, tending to involve the metaphyses, usually in the femur and tibia at the knee.

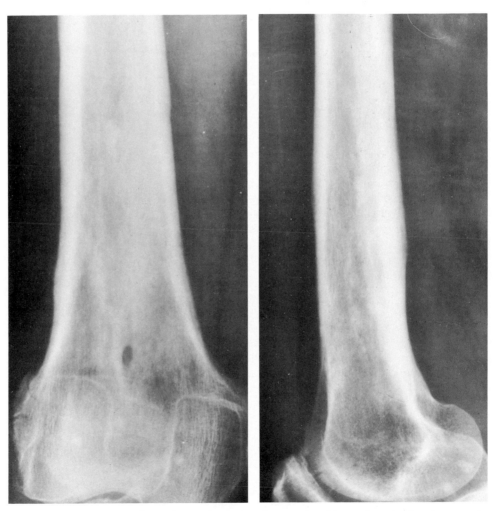

Fig. 6-11. Chronic osteomyelitis. The major feature in this patient is the dense sclerotic reaction in the posterior femoral shaft. The femoral cortex is slightly irregular and thickened, and there is some dense bone encroaching on the medullary canal.

The lesions are osteolytic. They tend to be rounded or oval and are surrounded by a thin sclerotic rim. Cortical breakthrough with resultant periosteal reaction occurs but is not common. In addition to the sites about the knee, the distial tibial metaphyses and distal ends of the clavicles tend to be involved. Generalized symptoms are minimal, but there may be short, febrile episodes. The sedimentation rate is moderately elevated, and there is often an increase in leukocytes. Histologic features are those of chronic inflammation, but organisms often are not isolated. Some authors believe that this condition is of viral origin. The course is very indolent and healing may not be complete for a number of years. There are usually no significant residua, however.

ACUTE BONE ABSCESS

The initial roentgen signs of an acute bone abscess are very similar to those of an acute osteomyelitis. Instead of the lesion extending to involve large areas of bone, it remains localized. The area of destruction becomes walled off by a zone of sclerosis and the lesion gradually becomes a chronic bone abscess. Acute bone abscess is a more frequent lesion than diffuse osteomyelitis because of the effect of penicillin and the other antibiotics in bringing the infection under control early in its course. The amount of bone destroyed will depend in large measure upon the time interval between the initial involvement by the infecting organisms and the onset of adequate therapy.

CHRONIC BONE ABSCESS

Chronic abscess may develop because the infecting organisms are of low virulence or it may be the continuation of acute abscess that has subsided into a chronic stage. It is characterized by a sharply outlined area of rarefaction of variable size, though often small, surrounded by an irregular zone of dense sclerosis (Figs. 6-12 and 6-13). Frequently one or more sequestra will be seen lying within the cavity and a dense shell of periosteal calcification often is present surrounding the region of the abscess.

BRODIE'S ABSCESS

The term "Brodie's abscess" has been used to indicate a form of chronic bone abscess of low virulence that has not gone through an acute stage. While such chronic bone abscesses do occur, it is probable that many of the lesions so diagnosed in the past were ac-

tually examples of osteoid osteoma (see Ch. 7). The symptoms may be similar, with intermittent episodes of pain and little constitutional reaction. From the standpoint of treatment and prognosis it makes little difference since both lesions can be cured by local excision.

GARRÉ'S SCLEROSING OSTEITIS

As originally described by Garré, this condition was a peculiar type of osteomyelitis which, after an acute and virulent onset, subsided without drainage or the formation of sequestra, leaving only a thickened,

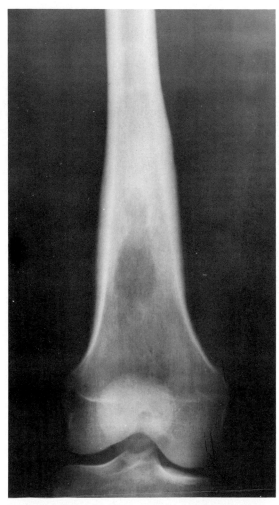

Fig. 6-12. Chronic bone abscess. The abscess cavity is seen as a well-demarcated area of rarefaction surrounded by sclerotic bone. The cortical thickening indicates previous periostitis.

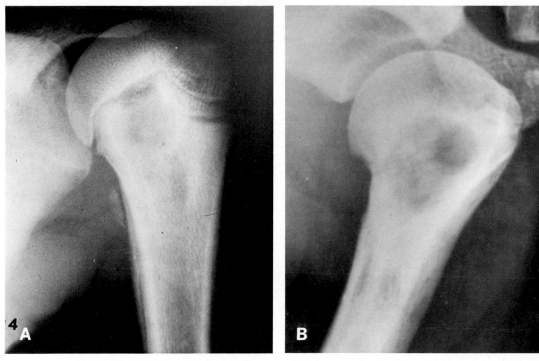

Fig. 6-13. A. Subacute bone abscess of the metaphysis. The cavity is surrounded by considerable sclerosis, and there is periosteal calcification extending for some distance down the humeral shaft. **B.** Chronic bone abscess in a similar location in an adult.

sclerotic bone. The term "Garré's sclerosing osteitis" is now used rarely to indicate chronic infection of bone of low virulence developing insidiously and leading only to a sclerotic reaction without any bone destruction or sequestration. Such a type of infection of bone is relatively rare and many lesions so diagnosed initially often turn out to be something else. If the possibility of other entities can be excluded the disease may be termed *chronic sclerosing osteitis.*

OSTEOMYELITIS IN SPECIAL AREAS

Flat Bones (Skull, Pelvis)

Osteomyelitis of the flat bones is characterized by a patchy type of destruction without sharp demarcation. In the skull, periosteal reaction is absent but a certain amount of sclerosis may be present. In the pelvis, periostitis occurs but the periosteal calcification is not as prominent as it is in the long bones. Sequestra form as in other bones and they show the same roentgen appearance.

Vertebrae

In pyogenic osteomyelitis of the vertebrae the roentgen changes may be slow in developing and the process may be chronic. The earliest roentgen change usually consists of a roughening or erosion of one surface of a vertebral body, most often along an intervertebral disc surface (Fig. 6-14A). The sharp cortical outline becomes lost and the edge of the bone has a frayed appearance. Narrowing of an intervertebral disc space is another relatively early finding and sometimes is the first manifestation of the disease. There appears to be a tendency for vertebral osteomyelitis to develop close to the intervertebral disc and, in some cases, the infection may be primary in the disc. In any event, spread to the contiguous vertebra is usual. If the disease progresses one or several bodies may develop a moth-eaten type of destruction with intermixed sclerosis (Fig. 6-14B and C). Periosteal reaction occurs fairly early in the disease and is seen as periosteal spurs along the disc edges of the vertebra or along the margins of the body. This reactive change, together with the sclerosis within the

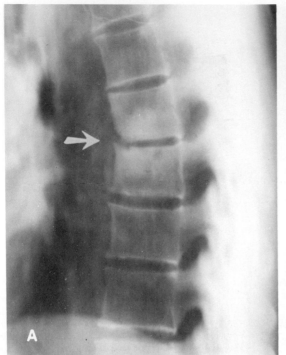

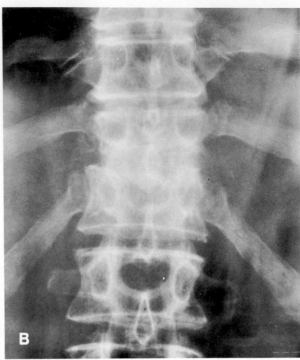

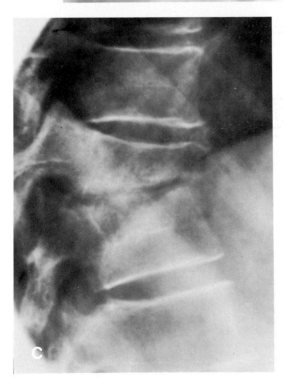

Fig. 6-14. A. Vertebral osteomyelitis. Tomogram shows the erosion of the anteroinferior edge of one body **(arrow)** with considerable sclerosis. There is very minimal disc narrowing. **B.** and **C.** A more destructive form of vertebral osteomyelitis. Irregular narrowing of the disc and extensive destruction of the inferior aspect of the vertebral body above it are noted best in the lateral view. There is a faintly visualized paraspinal mass noted on the anteroposterior view.

vertebral body, is of help in differentiating chronic pyogenic osteomyelitis from tuberculosis. The latter infection is characterized by its destructive nature, with little in the way of sclerotic reaction or periosteal calcification.

Nonspecific Spondylitis

The etiologic basis of this disease is not definitely known but many investigators believe that it is a very low-grade inflammatory process that involves an intervertebral disc and the contiguous surfaces of the adjacent vertebrae. Cultures usually have been sterile and organisms have not been seen on direct smear although scattered inflammatory cells have been found. Also, clinical signs of infection may be absent. The disease occurs both in children and adults and often no precipitating cause is evident. In some patients there has been a history of preceding mild trauma or infection 3 or 4 weeks before the onset of back pain. Roentgen findings resemble those described for osteomyelitis in the vertebrae, with thinning of an intervertebral disc space followed some weeks later by erosion of the disc surfaces of the adjacent vertebral bodies. In turn this is followed by a dense sclerotic reaction that may involve much of the vertebral body. The disease is self-limited and, after 3 or 4 months, healing usually has taken place with remineralization of the eroded vertebra. Some thinning of the disc may persist although with mild involvement it may return to normal thickness. It seems likely that this disease is similar to the one that develops after lumbar disc surgery or lumbar spinal puncture.

A similar disease is seen infrequently in children; this has been called *juvenile spondylarthritis* or *discitis*. Some investigators believe that it is a distinct entity and, while simulating the roentgen changes noted in the foregoing, it is not caused by an infection. Alexander[1] considers trauma to be the cause with disruption of the vertebral epiphyseal cartilaginous plate leading to disc thinning and vertebral erosion. Others maintain that it represents infection, however.

DIFFERENTIAL DIAGNOSIS

Benign Bone Tumors. These lesions, when they arise in the medullary canal, are very likely to cause expansion of the bone with thinning of the cortex. There is no periostitis or sequestration. A great many benign tumors are asymptomatic until fracture occurs through them. A significant exception is the osteoid osteoma as has been noted. Giant cell tumor also is a symptomatic lesion with the occurrence of pain and dysfunction early in the course of the disease. The roentgen appearance of this tumor, however, is not at all suggestive of osteomyelitis. The clinical signs of infection are absent in benign tumors.

Malignant Bone Tumors. Primary malignant bone tumors destroy bone as they grow. There are no sequestra. Periosteal calcification, if present, is much more irregular with a tendency for spicule formation at right angles to the cortex. Triangular shadows of periosteal calcification at the margins of the lesion, the so-called Codman triangles, are very suggestive of a malignant tumor but can be seen in some infections. Ewing's tumor may simulate infection closely and some of these lesions are extremely difficult to distinguish from infection based solely on the roentgen findings. The clinical history and symptoms should always be taken into consideration in evaluating roentgen changes and this is particularly true in Ewing's tumor. Even then the signs of infection may be mimicked by a neoplastic lesion and the nature of the process must depend upon biopsy. When the slightest doubt exists concerning the possibility of the presence of a malignant tumor, biopsy is indicated.

Other Infections. Tuberculosis, a number of fungus diseases, syphilis, and perhaps some viruses can produce bone lesions that may be difficult or impossible to differentiate from pyogenic osteomyelitis. However, there are usually some distinguishing features; these will be discussed in the following paragraphs.

TUBERCULOSIS

Tuberculosis of the shafts of the long bones is infrequent. However, in tuberculous disease of the joints the initial foci may be in the ends of the bones. This is particularly true of tuberculous joints in children in whom the initial lesion may be an abscess in the epiphysis or the metaphysis close to the joint. The bone infection is of hematogenous origin and pulmonary involvement is usually demonstrated. The clinical onset of the disease is insidious and the roentgen signs are those of a chronic nonvirulent infection. Tuberculosis may occur as a localized bone abscess or as a more diffuse osteomyelitis; the former is more frequent.

Roentgen Observations

Tuberculous Osteomyelitis. This lesion is usually a low-grade, chronic infection of bone which may be difficult to distinguish from pyogenic osteomyelitis on roentgen examination. The lesion is largely a destructive one and periosteal calcification is minimal or sometimes completely absent (Fig. 6-15). The amount of sclerosis surrounding areas of destruction also is slight, but in some instances may be moderate. Chronic draining sinuses are sometimes present. Soft-tissue swelling may be a prominent feature. There is a rather wide variety of manifestations. In some of these patients there may be medullary and cortical destruction, expansion of bone, and varying amounts of periosteal reaction. In others, there may be diffuse, uniform, honeycomb-like areas of destruction in which there may be pathologic fracture. Severe bone atrophy is often associated with the bone lesions. Muscle atrophy may also be severe in pa-

tients with chronic disease. At times the disease may progress very rapidly in contrast to its usual slow development. Disseminated tuberculous bone disease is not uncommon in heroin addicts, the incidence being much higher in addicts with pulmonary tuberculosis than it is in the general population with pulmonary tuberculosis. Ribs and spine are the most frequent sites of involvement in addicts. When draining sinuses are present secondary infection may be added and then the appearance is similar to that in pyogenic osteomyelitis. During infancy or childhood, tuberculous dactylitis is occasionally seen; this represents an infection involving one or more of the phalanges[10] (Fig. 6-16A). The diseased bone has an expanded appearance with irregular destruction of the bone architecture and absence of periosteal calcification. The lesion differs from syphilitic dactylitis, which is also encountered during infancy, in that the affected bone has an expanded appearance while in syphilis the bone is thickened as a result of periosteal

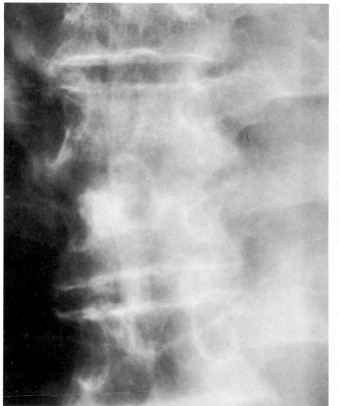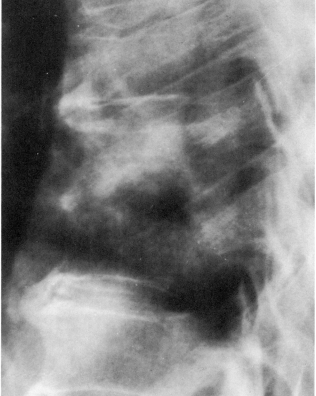

Fig. 6-15. Tuberculosis of the spine. There is destruction of the adjacent posterior aspects of two vertebral bodies with some loss of the disc space anteriorly. No appreciable sclerotic reaction is observed.

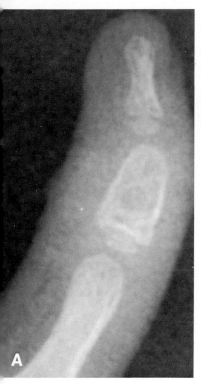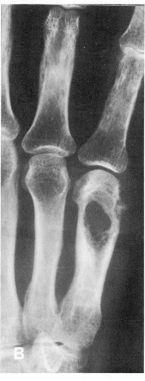

Fig. 6-16. A. Tuberculous dactylitis in a child. The middle phalanx is involved. The shaft is expanded, and there is irregular destruction of central cancellous bone. There is no evident periosteal involvement and there is considerable amount of soft-tissue swelling. **B.** Tuberculous abscess in the distal end of the fifth metacarpal. The cavity is clearly defined. There is some expansion as well as some sclerotic reaction proximal to the abscess.

calcification, which forms a dense shell around the shaft.

In children, there may also be involvement of long tubular bones in which there also may be bone expansion, a pseudocystic appearance, and sclerosis. As in adults there is ordinarily no formation of sequestra. At times the lesions may run a very indolent course and may be asymptomatic or nearly so.

Bone tuberculosis may occur in children as a complication of intradermal vaccination with BCG.[15] The time interval between vaccination and appearance of detectable bone lesions is rather short, ranging from 2 weeks to 2 months. The lesions are usually single and occur near the knee in the metaphysis of the femur or tibia. There is an eccentrically located area of destruction, often with cortical erosion and asso-

ciated soft-tissue inflammation and swelling. Periosteal reaction is slight if present. There is very little tendency to diaphyseal spread, but about a third of patients develop involvement of the adjacent epiphysis. When lesions are located in bones with a relatively thin cortex, such as the sternum, ribs, and tarsal bones, there tends to be marked destruction of the spongiosa and extensive spread of the disease. In these instances a multicystic appearance may develop as the disease becomes chronic or begins to resolve.

Tuberculous Bone Abscess. This is a chronic bone abscess, usually appearing as a sharply outlined cavity within the bone. The most common location is near the end of the shaft and, in children, sometimes involving the epiphysis. In contrast to a pyogenic bone abscess the tuberculous lesion has very little sclerosis around the cavity and there is usually an absence of periostitis (Fig. 6-17). Chronic draining sinuses are often present. Extension of the infection to involve the adjacent joint is a frequent complication and one that leads to the development of a tuberculous arthritis. This disease is considered more fully in Chapter 9. Subsequently the joint changes tend to obscure the lesion in the bone and to become the predominant clinical feature.

Atypical mycobacteria may also produce osteomyelitis. Most of the reported cases have been in children. Manifestations vary from an indolent chronic local bone lesion to a widespread dissemination with a fulminant course. The organism may be difficult to isolate. The osseous lesions usually respond satisfactorily to antituberculous therapy.

FUNGAL AND OTHER INFECTIONS

Fungal infections of bone are infrequent, the most common being blastomycosis, actinomycosis, and coccidioidomycosis. A lesion caused by one of these fungi can hardly be differentiated from other infections of bone. The lesion is likely to be a low-grade chronic infection with formation of a chronic bone abscess and draining sinus. The appearance of the abscess resembles tuberculosis in that it often is found in cancellous bone, is destructive in nature, and has little or no periostitis surrounding it. There also is little tendency for sclerosis to mark the boundary of the abscess in many cases (Fig. 6-18). Carter has listed some of the findings that are suggestive of mycotic disease: (1) Those lesions arising at points of bony prominence such as the edges of the patella, the

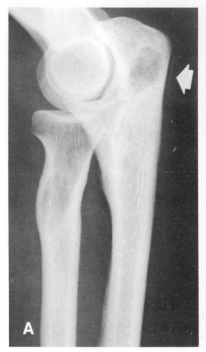
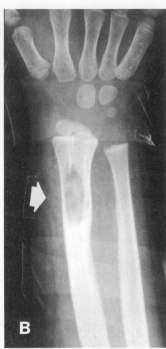

Fig. 6-17. Tuberculous abscess. **A. Arrow** indicates a cavity in the olecranon process of the ulna with very little reaction around it. **B. Arrow** indicates the abscess. There is a little more sclerotic reaction largely proximal to the cavity, than in **A.** There was also a draining sinus in this child.

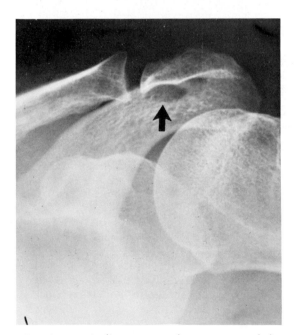

Fig. 6-18. Arrow indicates an abscess caused by North American blastomycosis in the acromion process. There is no sclerotic reaction in adjacent cancellous bone, and there is no periosteal reaction.

acromion or coracoid process of the scapula, the olecranon process, the styloid processes of the radius and ulna, the condyles of the humeri or the extremities of the clavicles, the malleoli, and the tuberosities of the tibiae. (2) Marginal solitary lesions of the ribs. (3) Localized destructive lesions of the outer table of the skull. (4) Destructive lesions of the vertebrae attacking indiscriminately the body, processes, or neural arch.

Coccidioidomycosis is endemic in certain areas of the country, notably the San Joaquin valley of California and in the arid zones of the Southwest. Blastomycosis is seen chiefly in the North Central states and actinomycosis has a rather similar distribution. Actinomycosis is noted for the way it extends across muscle and fascial planes, causing the development of deep and extensive sinus tracts. Bone involvement most frequently occurs secondary to soft-tissue invasion with a mixed destructive and proliferative reaction.

BLASTOMYCOSIS

Bones are involved in 25% to 50% of the disseminated form of the disease. The long bones, ribs, short tubular bones, and vertebrae are the most common sites. Facial bones are occasionally involved, but the skull is rarely affected. In about one-third of the patients, bone lesions are multiple. Epiphyseal involvement is common with rapid erosion into the adjacent joint and formation of fistulous tracts. In the spine, usually there is early disc involvement with frequent invasion of contiguous ribs and formation of a paraspinal abscess. In this invasive form, bone destruction is rapid, and there is very little reaction in the way of sclerosis or subperiosteal calcification. Occasionally the bone lesion is very indolent, expanding slowly and developing a sclerotic margin. The diagnosis depends upon the recovery of the organism.

COCCIDIOIDOMYCOSIS

Hematogenous dissemination is uncommon in this disease, but when it occurs the incidence of bone involvement is approximately 20%. Multiple bone lesions are the rule with the spine the most frequent site.[4, 5] The disc is usually spared or is involved late in the course of the process. Epiphyseal involvement of long bones is common, but there is very little tendency to extend into the adjacent joint. The major roentgen finding is destruction of bone and, in a chronic process, a sclerotic margin may develop late (Fig. 6-19). Subperiosteal calcification is uncommon. Paraspinal masses are common in vertebral disease and are often associated with involvement of ribs, pedicles, and transverse processes. Again, recovery of the organism is necessary to confirm the diagnosis.

CRYPTOCOCCOSIS

In cryptococcosis, osseous involvement is not common and usually occurs in patients with compromised defense mechanisms. The most frequent sites of involvement are the pelvis, ribs, and skull. The lesion tends to be lytic with reasonably discrete margins and little or no periosteal reaction.

PSEUDOMONAS OSTEOMYELITIS

Bone infection due to a species of *Pseudomonas* is being reported in drug addicts and in patients with debilitating disease or who are immunosuppressed. Involvement of bone is usually secondary to that of an adjacent joint or to an abscess or focus of infection contiguous to bone. Local bone trauma may also be a factor. The spine is the most common site of involvement, particularly in addicts. The roentgen findings are not specific, but usually bone destruction along

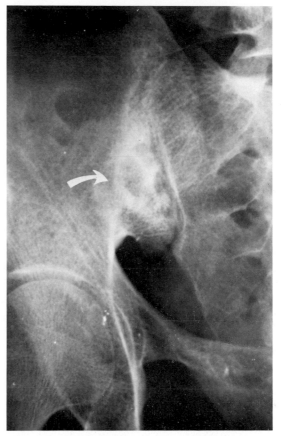

Fig. 6-19. Coccidioidomycosis of the ilium. Small irregular abscess cavities are surrounded by considerable sclerosis **(arrow).**

with some sclerosis and periosteal reaction are noted. There is a tendency toward involvement of the intervertebral disc when the adjacent vertebral body is infected.

ASPERGILLOSIS

Aspergillosis of bone also is found in immunosuppressed patients. The organism responsible, which ordinarily is a saprophyte, may cause osteomyelitis with bone destruction also.

ECHINOCOCCOSIS

In *echinococcosis*, hydatid cysts are formed in the liver or lung. Occasionally there is rib involvement which may extend to include an adjacent vertebral body. The disease tends to destroy bone and may encroach on the spinal canal and cord when it involves a vertebral body.

SYPHILIS

The incidence of osseous syphilis has increased somewhat in the past few years. In general, syphilis has a tendency to form multiple lesions when it involves the bones. No age period is exempt. The lesions are both destructive and proliferative and often the proliferative phase is much more pronounced than the destructive. Syphilis is usually a disease of

the shafts of the bones and it rarely involves the epiphyses or the joints.

CONGENITAL SYPHILIS

Extensive periosteal calcification is a feature of congenital syphilis.[3] The calcium is laid down parallel to the shafts, forming a thin, shell-like shadow surrounding them (Fig. 6-20). To be of significance for the diagnosis of congenital syphilis, periostitis must be widespread throughout the skeleton and involve the bones in a symmetrical manner. Unilateral periostitis or disease confined to one or two bones is

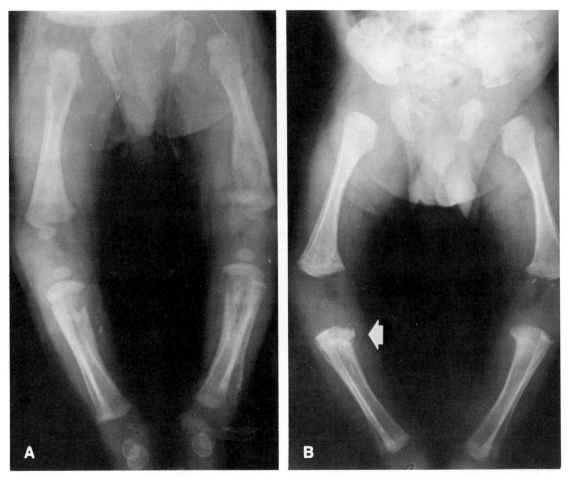

Fig. 6-20. Congenital syphilis. **A.** There is periosteal calcification involving all of the long bones depicted. Focal areas of destruction indicate osteomyelitis in the medial aspects of the upper ends of the tibias and the distal end of the femur. **B.** In this newborn infant, stripelike shadows of periosteal calcification are seen along the cortical margins. **Arrow** indicates an area of more localized bone involvement in the proximal tibia.

most often not caused by congenital syphilis. In infantile rickets the deposition of a large amount of uncalcified osteoid beneath the periosteum may simulate the appearance of periostitis. In this disease the other findings characteristic of rickets will orginarily be quite obvious.

Syphilitic osteomyelitis may develop in localized areas and cause irregular defects in the shafts. Foci of osteomyelitis often are symmetrical in location and one of the favorite sites is along the medial side of the upper end of the tibia. This is seen as a localized area of bone destruction involving cortex and extending into the medullary canal (see Fig. 6-20). Pathologic fracture may occur through such an area because of the amount of bone destroyed.

The metaphyses of the long bones may be serrated or irregular and occasionally considerable destruction may be present in these areas. In some cases there is a band of increased density crossing the metaphyses with an adjacent zone of lessened density on the shaft side, which resembles rather closely the changes found in scurvy. However, in congenital syphilis these findings are usually much less pronounced than they are in scurvy, the ring contour of the epiphyseal centers is not present, and the ground-glass demineralization of the bones is not as apparent. Some authors believe that the widespread, symmetrical bone lesions are more suggestive of a disturbance of endochondral and periosteal bone formation, that is, a metaphyseal dystrophy rather than an inflammatory process.

The cranial bones may show areas of patchy destruction or localized areas of thickening, which in themselves are not specific of the disease.

Differential Diagnosis

Rickets. Cupping, flaring, and fraying of the metaphyses are characteristic of infantile rickets. The serrated ends of the shafts seen in syphilis lack the fine frayed appearance noted in rickets. There are no focal areas of destruction in rickets but bowing is a prominent feature in the weight-bearing bones. Rickets is uncommon before the age of 6 months while congenital syphilis usually is evident at birth or shortly thereafter.

Scurvy. Ground-glass demineralization of the bones with thin cortices is a significant finding in scurvy. The ring contour of the epiphyses, the dense zones of provisional calcification with transverse bands of rarefaction, and the epiphyseal separations are characteristic of scurvy. Scurvy does not develop during the

first 6 months of life, while syphilitic changes may be present at birth. Subperiosteal hemorrhages are not found in syphilis but are very frequent in scurvy.

Osteomyelitis. The individual lesions of pyogenic osteomyelitis are more localized than the changes encountered in congenital syphilis. Extensive periostitis in multiple bones is absent. Sequestration is common in pyogenic osteomyelitis and it is one of the diagnostic features of this disease.

LATENT CONGENITAL SYPHILIS

Latent congenital syphilis is manifested by a chronic periostitis and osteitis and is most frequently seen in the tibia. (Fig. 6–21). The bone changes are often discovered during late childhood or even during adult life. The affected bone becomes thickened as a result of the chronic periostitis. This is more intense on the anterior aspect and in the tibia leads to a "saber-shin" deformity. Characteristically in this lesion the epiphyses remain normal (Fig. 6-22).

In juvenile syphilis there is also joint involvement in which there appears to be a synovitis with soft-tissue swelling and involvement of cartilage with resultant irregularity and erosion of articular surface, usually of the knee joints. Cartilage may actually ulcerate; if ulceration becomes extensive, ankylosis may result.

ACQUIRED SYPHILIS

Acquired syphilis assumes a wide variety of roentgen appearances. Generally it occurs in the form of a chronic osteitis and periostitis, and multiplicity of lesions is the rule. The periosteal calcification is characterized by its unusual density, which approaches that of normal cortex. The chronic osteitis is manifested by irregular sclerosis of the medullary cavity. Localized areas of destruction simulating a pyogenic osteomyelitis are frequent, usually indicative of gumma formation. Occasionally syphilitic periostitis is seen as a coarsely trabeculated periosteal shadow described as "lacelike." The typical sequestra common to pyogenic osteomyelitis usually are not found in syphilis.

There is a wide variation in the time of appearance of bone disease in acquired syphilis. It has been reported as early as 6 weeks following the appearance of the primary chancre and as late as 14 months after the secondary skin eruption. Although there may be a considerable amount of bone destruction in the gumma, there are few symptoms.

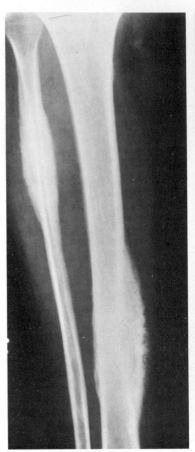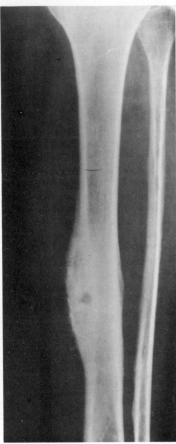

Fig. 6-21. Syphilitic osteitis and periostitis noted bilaterally in an adult with tertiary disease.

LYMPHOGRANULOMA INGUINALE

This disease, sometimes termed "donovanosis," is caused by a gram-negative bacillus which may produce osteomyelitis. The bone lesions are metaphyseal and cause destruction of cancellous bone with little tendency to involve cortical bone. There is some sclerotic reaction including periosteal reaction late in the disease. No sequestration is observed.

INFECTIONS AFTER LOWER URINARY TRACT AND OTHER SURGERY

OSTEITIS PUBIS

"Osteitis pubis" is the term given to an inflammatory condition involving the pubic bones, which seems to develop chiefly after operations on the lower urinary tract, usually suprapubic or retropubic prostatec-

tomy. The disease begins some weeks after the operation with severe pain in the region of the pubis, which is aggravated by motion. A few weeks later, roentgenograms reveal beginning rarefaction of the margins of the pubic bones. The affected bone has a washed-out appearance at first; later, complete dissolution occurs in the region of the symphysis (Fig. 6-23). The process may remain confined to this area or it may spread into the pubic rami. After a variable length of time, which usually is at least 3 or 4 months, there is a gradual recalcification of the rarefied or destroyed bone. In patients with slight involvement the bone may return to a fairly normal appearance. In other patients healing is shown by the development of sclerosis; the normal cartilaginous space in the symphysis becomes thin. In patients with the most severe involvement there will be a permanent loss of bone substance in the body of the pubis adjacent to the symphysis, the margin of the defect being bounded by a zone of sclerosis (Fig. 6-

24). The cause of osteitis pubis is unknown, but the infectious theory has received considerable support. This presupposes trauma to the periosteum or to the nutrient vessels of the pubic bones and subsequent infection of the injured tissue caused by a spread of urine or infected material from the wound. Steinbach[18] found distended venous channels in the area that produced hyperemia and this, in turn, led to bone resorption with localized thrombophlebitis. He considered these changes to be responsible for the alterations noted in the roentgenogram.

Sclerotic lesions in the pubis with narrowing of the symphysis are fairly common in women who have borne children. Usually these women are asymptomatic and the lesions are found by chance. We prefer to call the lesion *osteitis condensans pubii* (see Ch. 9 in the section entitled "Osteitis Condensans Ilii") because of its similarity to *osteitis condensans ilii,* which, also, usually is seen in women who have borne children and both the pubic and the iliac lesions may be seen in the same individual. The changes most likely represent a reaction of the bone to chronic stress.

VERTEBRAL OSTEOMYELITIS

Vertebral osteomyelitis is an infrequent complication of prostatic surgery. The spread of infection from the prostatic area evidently is by way of the plexus of vertebral veins described by Batson. These are in direct communication with the prostatic veins. In one study, pain in the back was the primary complaint and it began on the average 4 weeks after the operation. Fever and leukocytosis were present. The pain invariably was severe and was aggravated by motion. The average time required for the appearance of bone changes in roentgenograms was 9 weeks after operation. A similar type of vertebral osteomyelitis may develop after genitourinary tract infection. Also, operative procedures on the spine, or even a simple spinal puncture, may be followed by a very similar type of lesion. Many investigators consider this lesion to be a very low-grade inflammatory process although proof of this is lacking in some cases.

The earliest roentgen evidence in this form of vertebral osteomyelitis consists of narrowing of the intervertebral disc space indicative of cartilage destruction. In most patients there soon develops destruction of adjacent vertebral surfaces, usually along an anterolateral margin (see Fig. 6-14). This is followed by a dense sclerosis in the affected portion of the bodies. A paravertebral soft-tissue shadow represen-

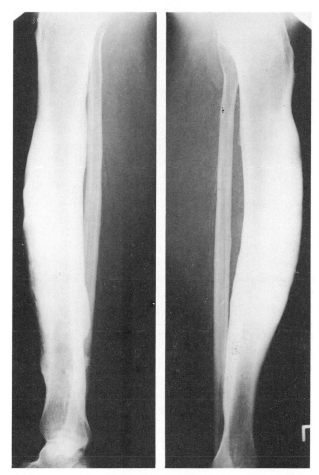

Fig. 6-22. Chronic syphilitic osteoperiostitis of the tibia causing bilateral saber-shin deformity.

tative of abscess formation is not seen very often. Any part of the spine may be affected, but the most common location is in the region of the thoracolumbar junction. The disease runs a self-limited course. With the milder degrees of involvement, little residual deformity persists except for some thinning of the disc space and some sclerosis in the vertebra. With more severe involvement, narrowing of the disc may progress to complete loss and this is usually followed by bony ankylosis of the vertebrae. Immobilization of the spine by means of a plaster jacket combined with antibiotic therapy has been recommended as the most satisfactory method of treatment. For other aspects of vertebral osteomyelitis and nonspecific spondylitis see section on "Osteomyelitis in Special Areas."

SARCOIDOSIS

Sarcoidosis is a chronic, often widely disseminated disease, the cause of which remains unknown. While originally considered to represent a form of tuberculosis of a low degree of virulence, the tuberculous nature of the disease has never been established with any certainty. The opinion has been expressed that sarcoidosis is a nonspecific response of the body tissues to a variety of inflammatory and toxic agents of which the tubercle bacillus may be one. The characteristic histologic lesion of sarcoid in the ''hard'' tubercle composed of epithelioid cells, giant cells of the Langhans' type, often with central necrosis but without the caseation typical of tuberculosis.

Of interest roentgenologically is the fact that sarcoidosis not only involves the viscera frequently but occasionally the osseous system as well. Osseous lesions are usually associated with involvement of the skin but this is not a necessary prerequisite. The incidence of bone lesions in patients with cutaneous or visceral sarcoidosis is difficult to determine but has been reported to occur in approximately 15% of cases. The high incidence of osseous involvement in blacks who have the disease is noteworthy and figures dealing with the incidence of the lesions are probably influenced by this fact. Sarcoidosis is generally a more severe disease in the black race than in the white.

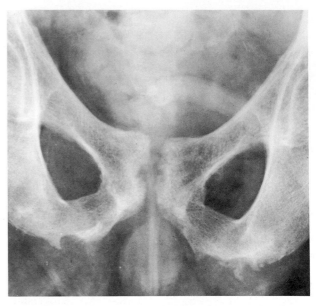

Fig. 6-23. Osteitis pubis following a suprapubic prostatic resection. There is irregular loss of bone adjacent to the symphysis pubis and irregular periosteal proliferation along the inferior margins of the inferior pubic rami.

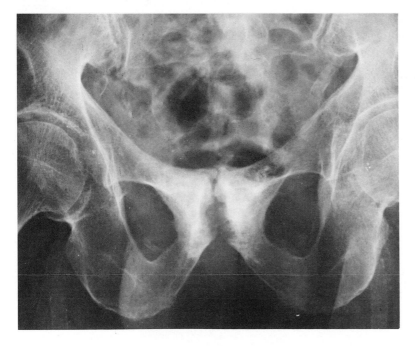

Fig. 6-24. Osteitis pubis in a patient in whom the lesion had become quiescent. There is considerable irregularity of bone adjacent to the symphysis and marked sclerosis in both pubic bones.

The bones most frequently involved are those of the hands and feet, although the lesions have been found in practically all parts of the skeleton. In the hands and feet the distal and middle phalanges are affected somewhat more frequently than the others. There may be single or multiple lesions and they are almost always associated with clinical evidence of pain and swelling. Two types of lesions have been described. In one, the lesion is seen as a sharply marginated cystlike area of rarefaction. A more frequent and more characteristic lesion appears as an area of destruction, having a lacelike pattern (Fig. 6-25). The margins often are not sharply defined and coarse trabeculae remain in the area. In some, there is a fine granular stippled rarefaction involving cancellous and cortical bone. There is no periosteal reaction associated with the lesions of sarcoid and they do not extend across the joint to involve adjacent bone.

A few cases have been reported in which the skull was involved by lytic lesions that were poorly defined and appeared to have no reactive bone at the periphery of the multiple lytic areas. Also a few patients have been reported in whom destructive lesions with considerable amount of marginal sclerosis were observed involving the vertebrae. No disc involvement appears to be present, but some of the destructive lesions extend out to produce a soft-tissue mass in the paraspinal areas, and the posterior elements of the vertebrae may occasionally be involved. Also, densely sclerotic lesions have been noted in the pelvis, spine, and ribs of a few patients. Because the sclerotic lesions are very unusual, the diagnosis must be confirmed by biopsy.

In differential diagnosis one must be careful to exclude the small cystlike areas commonly found in the metacarpal heads or in some of the carpal bones. Some of these follow previous trauma but in many cases these small defects are believed to represent only developmental ossification defects and to have no clinical significance. The marginal erosions of rheumatoid arthritis and the defects caused by gouty tophi usually can be distinguished without difficulty. Such defects occur in or along the joint margins and the other manifestations of these diseases should be present. A rare disorder in which numerous xanthomatous tumors develop in and along the tendon sheaths and known as *xanthoma tuberosa* has caused difficulty because these tumors may erode underlying bone and the type of rarefaction is somewhat suggestive of that seen in sarcoidosis.

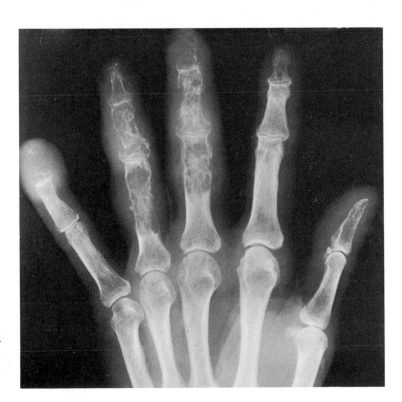

Fig. 6-25. Sarcoidosis involving the phalanges. The lacelike destruction with rather minimal cortical expansion is fairly characteristic when present. There is associated swelling of soft tissue.

VIRAL INFECTIONS

Bone lesions have been reported as occurring in association with a number of epidemics of smallpox.[17] Disturbances of bone growth, deformity, and ankylosis have been described. The lesions seem to have a predilection for areas of active bone growth. There may be an initial joint lesion with spread to the adjacent bone. The rogentgen findings consist in metaphyseal destruction, and osteoporosis and periostitis that often involve the entire shaft of the affected bone. There may be a residual diaphyseal sclerosis. Occasional bone lesions have also been reported to occur in association with vaccinia and cat-scratch fever, but the diagnosis is extremely difficult to confirm in these situations.

LEPROSY

Bone changes in leprosy are found most frequently in the neural type of the disease. The other main clinical form of leprosy, the lepromatous (also known as the cutaneous or nodular), is not often associated with bone changes. The lesions occurring in neural leprosy are similar to those found in a number of other diseases, including scleroderma, Raynaud's disease, syringomyelia, and tabes dorsalis. Occasionally the lesions resemble those of a chronic infection such as is seen in diabetic patients. In some cases of longstanding chronic rheumatoid arthritis the appearance resemble in many ways the absorptive changes that are found in leprosy.

As reported by Faget and Mayoral,[9] the neurotrophic changes of neural leprosy are found in the hands and feet. In the former the changes begin in the distal phalanges with a slowly progressive absorption of bone. The terminal tufts disappear, leading to a "collar-stud" appearance, followed by a gradual disappearance of the bone. The proximal phalanges are the last to disappear. Rarely, the metacarpals are affected but the process does not ascend higher than this. In the feet the absorption of bone begins in the metatarsal heads or in the proximal phalanges. There is a gradual thinning of the shafts and the ends become pointed. Eventually the involved bone may completely disappear. In some of the joints a painless arthropathy resembling the Charcot joint of tabes dorsalis develops with gross disorganization of the articular ends of the bones.

The granulomatous lesions[8] produce focal areas of destruction and, when they heal, small, punched-out rarefied areas ranging from 2–6 mm in diameter can be observed in the area of previous involvement. When the disease occurs in the epiphysis, there may be flattening of the adjacent articular surface. The anterior nasal spine and adjacent alveolar process as well as the nasal bones are sometimes involved by a destructive process, but this may be caused by secondary infection. The granulomatous lesions also tend to involve the hands and feet where they produce a honeycomb or cystlike appearance associated with soft-tissue swelling. These cysts have sclerotic margins. Periostitis has been described involving the tibia and fibula, presumably caused by the presence of the organism rather than change secondary to involvement of the nervous system.

REFERENCES AND SELECTED READINGS

1. ALEXANDER CJ: The aetiology of juvenile spondylarthritis (discitis). Clin Radiol 21: 178, 1970
2. CAPITANIO MA, KIRKPATRICK JA: Early roentgen observations in acute osteomyelitis. Am J Roentgenol 108: 488, 1970
3. CREMIN BJ, FISCHER RM: The lesions of congenital syphilis. Br J Radiol 43: 333, 1970
4. DALINKA MK, DINNENBERG S, GREENDYKE W et al: Roentgenographic features of osseous coccidioiodomycosis and differential diagnosis. J Bone Joint Surg [A] 53: 1157, 1971
5. DALINKA MK, GREENDYKE WH: Spinal manifestations of coccidioidomycosis. J Can Assoc Radiol 22: 93, 1971
6. DAVIS LA: Antibiotic modified osteomyelitis. Am J Roentgenol 103: 608, 1968
7. DOYLE JR: Narrowing of the intervertebral disc space in children: presumably infectious lesion of disc. J Bone Joint Surg [A] 42: 1191, 1960
8. ENNA CD, JACOBSON RR, RAUSCH RO: Bone changes in leprosy. Radiology 100: 295, 1971
9. FAGET GH, MAYORAL A: Bone changes in leprosy: a clinical and roentgenologic study of 505 cases. Radiology 42: 1, 1944
10. FELDMAN F, AUERBACH R, JOHNSTON A: Tuberculous dactylitis in the adult. Am J Roentgenol 112: 460, 1971
11. GOLD RH, DOUGLAS SD, PREGER L et al: Roentgenographic features of the neutrophil dysfunction syndromes. Radiology 92: 1045, 1969
12. GRUNOW OH: Radiating spicules, a nonspecific sign of bone disease. Radiology 65: 200, 1955
13. HOLT JF, OWENS WI: Osseous lesions of sarcoidosis. Radiology 53: 11, 1949
14. LOWMAN RL, ROBINSON F: Progressive vertebral changes following lumbar disc surgery. Am J Roentgenol 97: 664, 1966

15. MORTENSSON W, EKLOF O, JORULF H: Radiologic aspects of BCG osteomyelitis in infants and children. Acta Radiol [Suppl] (Stockh) 17 (6): 845, 1976

16. PAJEWSKI M, VURE E: Late manifestations of infantile cortical hyperostosis (Caffey's disease). Br J Radiol 40: 90, 1967

17. Silverman FN: Virus diseases of bone; do they exist? Am J Roentgenol 126: 677, 1976

18. STEINBACH HL: Infections of bone. Semin Roentgenol 1: 337, 1966

19. SUTCLIFFE J, CHRISPIN AR: Chronic granulomatous disease. Br J Radiol 43: 110, 1970

20. WILLIAMS JL, MOLLER GA, O'ROURKE TL: Pseudoinfections of the intervertebral disc and adjacent vertebrae. Am J Roentgenol 103: 611, 1968

21. WOLFSON JJ, KANE WJ, LAXDAL SD et al: Bone findings in chronic granulomatous disease of childhood. A genetic abnormality of leucocyte function. J Bone Joint Surg [A] 51: 1573, 1969

7

BONE TUMORS AND RELATED CONDITIONS

In the evaluation of any bone lesion, particularly tumors and tumorlike processes, certain features as listed below should be considered. As a result, the number of diagnostic possibilities often will be reduced to a relatively few or even to one.[23] These features are: (1) Age and sex, (2) Single or multiple, (3) The bone or bones involved, (4) Site within the bone (epiphysis, metaphysis, diaphysis), (5) Probable site of origin (medullary canal, cortex, periosteum), (6) Destructive, reactive, or mixed. If destructive, whether circumscribed or geographic, moth-eaten (patchy) or granular (permeative). If reactive, whether cancellous sclerosis, endosteal thickening, or periosteal calcification. (7) "Tumor bone" (only chondro- or osteogenic tumors), (8) Soft-tissue involvement.

The division of tumors into benign and malignant groups rather than according to cells of origin may be oversimplified since some benign tumors may become malignant. However, some pathologists believe that most tumors in the benign group were probably malignant initially and do not actually undergo a malignant transformation. In addition, there is some difference of opinion as to whether some of the tumors to be discussed are actually tumors since a number of them stop growing, often at the time of epiphyseal closure, and do not appear to have the potential for further growth. Others appear to be a reactive process, probably reactive to some form of trauma. Since there is considerable disagreement among pathologists regarding these lesions, our discussions will deal principally with radiographic features. In the text to follow, the term "tumor" is used even though the lesions described may not be true neoplasms.

As a rule, routine clinical use of angiographic methods for the study of bone tumors and tumorlike lesions is not indicated. However, in selected cases, arteriography may add important information as to the extent of the tumor. This may assist in the selection of the best site for biopsy and may aid the radiotherapist, should radiotherapy be indicated.

BENIGN BONE LESIONS

ENCHONDROMA; CENTRAL CHONDROMA

A chondroma is a benign cartilaginous tumor that arises from cartilage cell rests. It is found chiefly in young adults. The major locations for these tumors are in the small bones of the hands and feet, less frequently in the long tubular bones and in the ribs. Chondroma is one of the most frequent tumors found in the bones of the hands. When this tumor occurs in the hands or feet, it is rarely malignant, but in the flat bones, such as the ribs and ilium, and in the long bones of the extremities, malignancy is always a pos-

sibility in a solitary mass that has the appearance of enchondroma. Changes indicating malignancy include blurring or loss of marginal definition, cortical disruption, local periosteal reaction, and growth of a previously defined enchondroma. Clinically, the patient may experience pain in the area.

Roentgen Features. Chondroma is a central lesion originating within the medullary canal, usually at or near the epiphysis. It grows slowly and as it enlarges it expands the bone locally, thins the cortex, and eventually weakens the bone to a point where fracture may result from very slight trauma (Fig. 7-1). The inner surface of the cortex has a scalloped appearance and the radiolucent mass usually is clearly

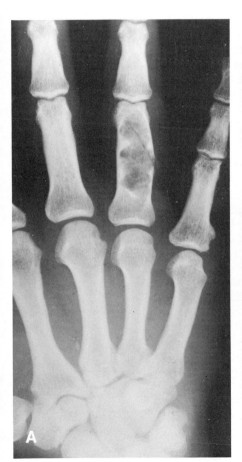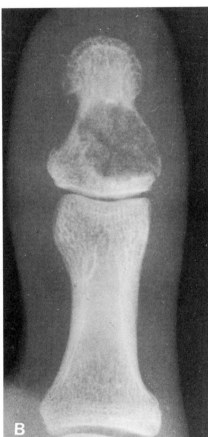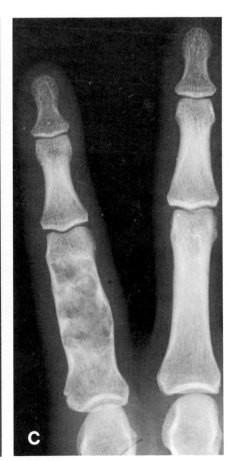

Fig. 7-1. A. Enchondroma of the proximal phalanx of the fourth finger. The fracture following minimal trauma caused the first symptoms. **B.** Pathologic fractures through the enchondroma involving the distal phalanx of the thumb. **C.** Enchondroma of the proximal phalanx of the fifth digit. Note small calcifications distally; these are typical in cartilaginous tumors.

outlined by a thin margin of reactive bone. There is no soft-tissue involvement and no periosteal reaction except for callus after fracture. In the long tubular bones these lesions may undergo partial calcification, giving them a mottled appearance (see Fig. 8-17). Tiny rounded areas of lucent cartilage observed within the calcified lesion are characteristic. Ollier's disease is a congenital osseous dysplasia characterized by the occurrence of multiple enchondromas at the ends of the long bones and very commonly in the hands, often in one extremity only or in the extremities on one side of the body. When this condition is associated with multiple cavernous hemangiomas, the rare combination is termed "Maffucci's syndrome" (see Ch. 2).

OSTEOCHONDROMA, EXOSTOSIS

Osteochondroma is a benign tumor composed of cartilage, calcified cartilage, and bone in variable amounts. The term "exostosis" is more or less synonymous with osteochondroma. The lesion most likely represents local dysplasia of cartilage at the epiphyseal growth plate; it retains a cartilage cap that often is so thin as to be unrecognizable roentgenographically. Occasionally, osteochondromas arise in flat bones, such as ribs, ilia, and scapulae, and in the posterior elements of vertebrae where they may produce compression of the cord or nerve root. These tumors begin during early childhood; growth is slow and usually ceases when skeletal growth is complete. Single lesions may appear in any part of the skeleton preformed in cartilage; they occur most frequently in the distal ends of the long tubular bones, particularly the lower end of the femur and the upper and lower ends of the tibia. When multiple, practically all the bones will be involved; this condition is known as "osteochondromatosis" or "hereditary multiple exostoses." It is discussed in Chapter 2. As a rule, single lesions are asymptomatic unless the mass becomes large enough to interfere with the function of the part. Any osteochondroma is capable of becoming malignant, developing into an osteochondrosarcoma. When an osteochondroma, after a period of stationary size, begins to enlarge and become painful, malignant degeneration should be suspected. This has been reported to occur in approximately 15% of cases.[3]

Roentgen Features. The tumor arises from the cortex and grows outward, pointing away from the nearest joint. It usually is pedunculated and cauliflower-shaped, the pedicle merging smoothly with the nor-

mal cortex of the bone (Fig. 7-2). The borders of the pedicle are formed of cortical bone; the center has a cancellous texture which merges with the spongiosa of the involved bone. The peripheral part of the mass has an irregular density since it is composed of cartilage, calcified cartilage, and bone. The outer margin of the tumor is distinct and usually bounded by a thin rim of calcification or bone. Indistinctness of margin and poor demarcation between the tumor and the contiguous soft tissues always raises the question of sarcomatous degeneration. Occasionally, instead of a pedunculated appearance, the lesion is flat and broad but has the other features of an osteochondroma.

Subungual Exostosis

This is a special type of exostosis that develops at or near the end of the terminal phalanx of a toe, usually the first, and grows upward beneath the nail. Because of its location, pain, swelling and elevation of the nail result. Trauma or chronic irritation probably is the cause and the lesion is found more often in females than in males. Clinically, it may be mistaken for an infected ingrown nail or even for a malignant tumor.

Osteoma

Osteomas are flat, bony growths having the density of cortical bone and thus appearing dense and structureless in roentgenograms. They arise from areas of membranous bone formation and probably are hamartomas. They usually occur in the skull, most often arising from the surface of the outer table in the posterior parietal or occipital area. Less frequently they arise from the inner table. A similar lesion is seen rather frequently in the nasal sinuses, chiefly in the frontal or ethmoid cells. These tumors show little tendency to enlarge and the small ones are probably of no clinical significance. Occasionally a sinus osteoma may enlarge sufficiently to cause bulging of the sinus wall or, by obstructing the orifice, lead to retention of secretions and the development of sinus infection. These complications are infrequent.

Juxtacortical (Periosteal) Chondroma

This type of chondroma has a distinctive roentgen appearance. The lesion develops in the periosteum or immediately contiguous tissues. The soft-tissue mass is characterized by the presence of multiple mottled calcareous deposits usually without the sharply marginated outer boundary common to the more fre-

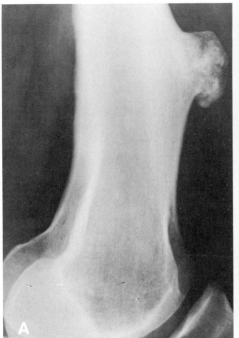

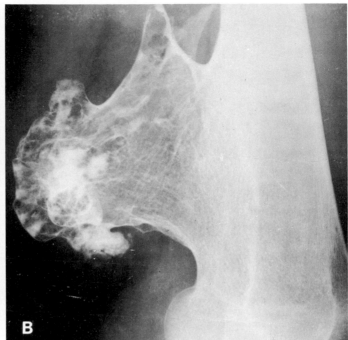

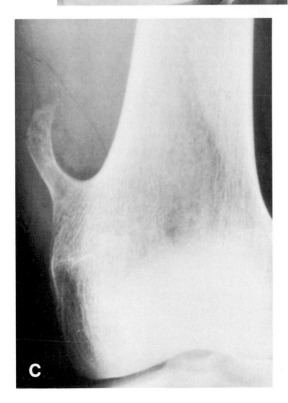

Fig. 7-2. Osteochondroma. **A.** Broad-based osteochondroma arising from the anterior cortex of the femur. The pedicle is composed of cortical bone which merges and is continuous with the normal femoral cortex. The irregular, mottled density is caused by islands of calcified cartilage in the periphery of the mass. **B.** Large osteochondroma arising from the posterior cortex of the lower femur. The periphery of the tumor is composed of a mixture of cartilage, calcified cartilage, and bone. **C.** Hornlike osteochondroma arising from the medial aspect of the distal femur. This tumor contains very little cartilage.

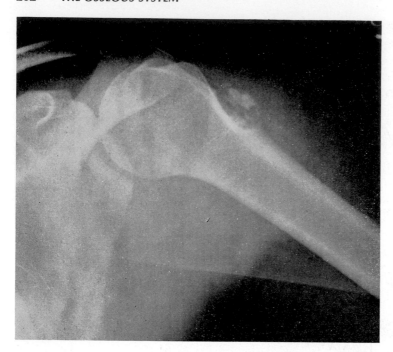

Fig. 7-3. Juxtacortical chondroma. There is mottled calcification within the mass. The base of the lesion is bounded by a zone of sclerosis. There is no pedicle as in the usual osteochondroma.

quent osteochondroma. The base of the lesion erodes the underlying cortex but is bounded by a sclerotic zone and the tumor does not invade the medullary cavity (Fig. 7-3). Ordinarily the lesion is relatively small, on the order of several centimeters in size. It produces a small saucerlike erosion of the underlying cortex with a rather dense rim of reactive bone beneath the erosion.[29] The most common site is in the phalanges of the hand, but it may occur at the ends of the long bones of the extremities and rarely in carpal and tarsal bones.

OSTEOID OSTEOMA

This is a benign osteoid-forming lesion that resembles, in many ways, a low-grade chronic bone abscess. Most investigators now consider it to be a reactive process, possibly inflammatory in origin, but its pathogenesis is unknown. About 75% of cases occur in persons between the ages of 11 and 26 years. It is more than twice as common in males as in females. The tibia and the femur are frequent sites of involvement, but the lesion may be found in any of the tubular bones as well as in the pelvis and vertebrae. The patient complains of pain, usually of a mild and intermittent character, worse at night, and relieved by acetylsalicylic acid. In some patients, pain may be severe and virtually intractable. The central nidus, ranging up to 2 cm in diameter, is made up of irregu-

lar masses of osteoid in a vascular fibrous matrix; some calcifications may be present. The histologic appearance is very similar to that of benign osteoblastoma (giant osteoid osteoma).

Roentgen Features. Osteoid osteoma is usually a lesion of the cortex but it may be periosteal and sometimes medullary or endosteal. Although usually solitary, rarely there may be two or even three small ovoid lesions in adjacent bones or in adjacent areas in the same bone. It is seen, roentgenologically, as a small lucent area or "cavity" surrounded by a dense sclerosis. The "cavity" is often no more than a few millimeters in diameter, Within it a small, central nidus of calcific density may be found at times. The translucent area is bounded by a zone of increased density forming a sclerotic wall. Usually the sclerotic reaction is intense and may be sufficient to obscure the cavity (Fig. 7-4). In the long bones a dense periosteal calcification commonly forms over the lesion and may almost surround the shaft at the level of the lesion. The periosteal reaction, the sclerotic wall, and the normal cortex tend to merge into one another without sharp demarcation. Tomography is a useful method for visualizing this lesion and often will demonstrate the cavity when routine exposures fail to show it. In the flat bones, such as the pelvis, a diffuse zone of sclerosis of variable width surrounds the cavity. Because the essential part of the tumor lies

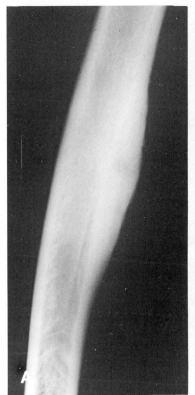
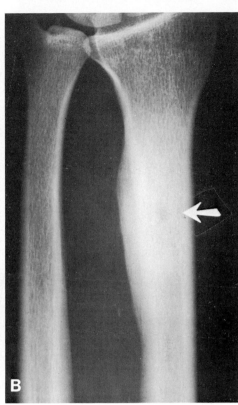

Fig. 7-4. A. Osteoid osteoma of the humerus. There is a small area of rarefaction within the anterior cortex. It is surrounded by a considerable amount of reactive bone resulting in thickening of the cortex. **B.** Osteoid osteoma in the distal radius. **Arrow** points to a small central nidus of rarefaction surrounded by a moderate amount of reactive bone.

within the rarefied area or "cavity," this must be removed completely at the time of surgical excision or the lesion will recur. It is not necessary to remove the reactive calcification even though this may form the major part of the lesion. Prompt surgical excision is of particular importance when the lesion is located in or near a joint in a young patient.[15] In this location it can produce synovitis as well as proliferative arthritis which may lead to premature osteoarthritis. Also these lesions are vascular, and hyperemia plus local muscle contractions may lead to significant deformity, particularly when the femoral neck is involved.

BONE CYSTS

A bone cyst is not a true neoplasm but it may resemble one roentgenologically and clinically and it must be considered in the differential diagnosis of bone tumors. There are a number of lesions that appear as "cysts" in roentgenograms, that is, as sharply outlined cavities in bone, but which are filled with solid tissue rather than fluid. The roentgenographic density of fluid and of the various soft tissues that may occupy such a cavity is the same. These "pseudo-cysts" are not included in the present discussion. Several varieties of bone cyst can be recognized, each having some fairly characteristic features.

Solitary (Unicameral) Bone Cyst

A solitary bone cyst is a lesion of childhood and adolescence. Most of these are located in the proximal end of the femur and humerus but have been reported to occur in the tibia, fibula, calcaneous, and in flat bones including the ribs and pelvis (usually ilium). Their incidence is greater in males than in females in a ratio of 2:1. The pathogenesis is unknown, although there is good evidence to suggest that many are post-traumatic and may follow intraosseous hematoma. The lesion is asymptomatic unless fracture occurs. Most are recognized only because of a fracture that may have followed a very slight injury. After fracture, some cysts will recalcify and heal; others do not and require surgical curettage and the placement of bone chips within the cavity. Because of the frequency of the lesion in children and its rarity in adults, it seems likely that spontaneous healing takes place in some cases.

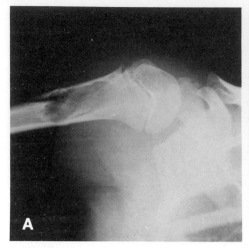
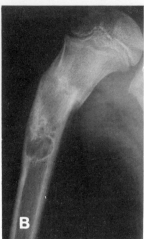

Fig. 7-5. Solitary bone cyst. **A.** The lesion was discovered because of a fracture occurring through it. There had been no symptoms referrable to the cyst prior to the injury. **B.** Same patient 1½ years later. The initial fracture has healed, but the cystic cavity has not been obliterated completely. A second fracture occurred more proximally. This has healed nearly completely with recalcification of the cyst in this region. The small residual cystic cavity in the shaft illustrates the apparent migration of a cyst into the shaft caused by bone growth at the metaphysis.

Roentgen Features. A solitary bone cyst forms an expansile, destructive, centrally situated lesion that appears as a cavity within the bone (Fig. 7-5). According to Lodwick the lesion does not actively expand the bone but it interferes with normal modeling; thus the greatest diameter of the cyst is no larger than that of the epiphyseal plate.[22] The margins of the lesion are well defined from the normal bone adjacent to it. There may be a thin, limiting border of sclerosis. The lesion gradually thins the cortex, and thus predisposes to fracture. It is located near the epiphysis but does not cross the epiphyseal plate to involve the epiphysis. Some cysts have a multilocular appearance as though composed of multiple communicating cavities. This is usually the result of ridges along the thinned cortex rather than actual bony septa within the cyst. With healing the expanded appearance of the bone remains for a time, but the rarefied appearance of the cyst is replaced gradually by calcium density and, eventually, this is transformed into bone. Because this takes some time and since skeletal growth is continuing, the healing cyst will appear to migrate toward the midshaft. Little or no "scar" remains after healing is complete.

Latent Bone Cyst

A latent bone cyst represents a cyst of childhood that has persisted into adult life, becoming inactive as far as increase in size is concerned, but with a cystic cavity remaining. During its active stage, the cyst is located near or adjacent to the epiphyseal plate. With growth of the bone it appears to migrate toward the midshaft; thus latent bone cysts are found within the shaft but some distance from the growth plate. An inactive or latent cyst usually has a thin, sclerotic border around the margin and the diameter of the bone is not appreciably increased at the site of the lesion. It is an uncommon cause of cystlike lesions in the adult skeleton.

Post-traumatic Bone Cyst

Small cystic areas are found with considerable frequency in the bones particularly of the wrist and hand and these may be caused by trauma. Such a cyst forms as a result of a localized area of hemorrhage within the bone. Multiple cysts of this type have been reported in workers using pneumatic air drills. Similar cystlike lesions also are found in persons without a history of previous injury. Some of these may be islands of cartilage that failed to ossify during the course of skeletal growth. A small round cavity or "cyst" of this type is a frequent finding in the neck of the femur; it has no clinical significance.

Aneurysmal Bone Cyst (Subperiosteal Giant Cell Tumor; Giant Cell Variant of Bone Cyst)

Aneurysmal bone cyst is not a true neoplasm and may have multiple causes. It consists of numerous blood-filled arteriovenous communications formed possibly secondary to injury, to intraosseous hemangioma, to hemorrhage into cancellous bone, or to other causes. Pathogenesis is not definitely known and it is possible that trauma in an area of abnormal bone is a factor in most cases. For example, some pathologists and radiologists have noted the occurrence of this lesion in some patients with giant cell tumor.[2]

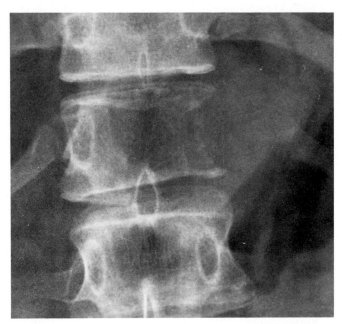

Fig. 7-6. Aneurysmal bone cyst. The lesion involves the left side of the body and arch of T12 and the adjacent part of the twelfth rib. Note absence of the left pedicle. The lesion is purely destructive.

From a roentgenologic point of view the lesion is important because it can be mistaken for a malignant bone tumor, while actually it is benign and curable by surgical excision or curettage. It occurs chiefly during childhood and adolescence, although it has been found during infancy and up to middle age. Its incidence is the same in both sexes. It involves the shaft rather than the epiphysis, a feature that aids in distinguishing it from giant cell tumor. It may extend into the epiphysis following closure, but rarely extends into a joint. It develops most commonly along the external cortical margin of a bone near the metaphysis. While practically any bone in the skeleton can be the site of this lesion, it occurs most frequently in the long bones and in the vertebrae (Fig. 7-6). The clavicle occasionally is involved. In the vertebrae the lesion usually involves the posterior elements (the arch and spinous process), producing an expanded ballooned-out mass which is characteristic. In the long bones the roentgen features are those of an expansile, cystlike lesion, often with a honeycomb or septate appearance, which involves the cortex and forms a visible mass external to the bone. The outer margin of the mass usually is bounded by a thin shell of periosteal bone. This may be incomplete radiographically, but a thin cortical layer is present histologically (Fig. 7-7). Thin layers of calcification may

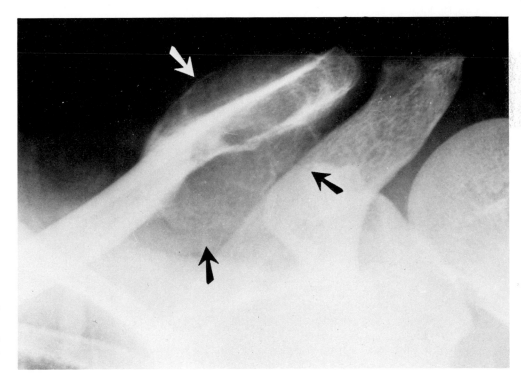

Fig. 7-7. Aneurysmal bone cyst of the clavicle. The thin shell marking the boundaries of the expanded lesion is indicated by the **arrows.**

be seen at the junction of the tumor and the normal cortex, somewhat similar to the onion-skin periosteal reaction found in Ewing's tumor. At times this lesion appears to arise subperiosteally, in an extraosseous location. There is often a definite history of trauma in this type. There is a tendency to erode the cortex locally, leaving a thin sclerotic margin. Symptoms of pain and swelling are noted clinically. Atypical examples of aneurysmal bone cyst are difficult to diagnose correctly on roentgen examination. Occasionally the lesion arises within the medullary cavity of the shaft near the metaphysis and causes an expanded rarefied area resembling a solitary bone cyst. In these cases, biopsy will be needed to establish the correct diagnosis.

GIANT CELL TUMOR

Giant cell tumor is a rather uncommon tumor of cancellous bone. It is apparent from the literature that its pathologic diagnosis is difficult to establish and that correlation with roentgen and clinical findings is essential in most cases. The tumor, characteristically, is limited to subjects who are between 20 and 35 years of age. It is essentially a lesion of early adult life. Its favorite locations are the proximal end of the tibia, distal end of the femur, and distal ends of the radius and ulna. It seldom develops in the vertebrae and most of those so diagnosed from biopsy specimens are probably aneurysmal bone cysts. Most of the reported giant cell tumors of the jaws and skull are probably reactive or reparative processes rather than true tumors. Pelvic bones, ribs, spine, clavicles, hands, and feet have also been reported as sites of the lesion. However, pathologic diagnosis is difficult and the incidence must be very low in these sites. As noted previously, aneurysmal bone cysts may coexist with giant cell tumors.

Roentgen Features. Giant cell tumor is an expansile destructive lesion situated in the end of a long bone after epiphyseal closure. Thus it is rarely found in a person younger than 17 years old and is uncommon in those older than 35. It arises at the site of the old epiphyseal plate and extends both into the metaphysis and the epiphysis, but particularly into the latter so that by the time of the initial examination the lesion often has reached the articular plate. Initially the lesion is usually eccentric in position, but may be central. As it enlarges it involves the entire end of the bone. The tumor extends to the articular surface of the bone but does not involve the joint. On the shaft side the destruction is fairly well demarcated from

normal bone but there is no sclerotic shell or border (Figs. 7-8 and 7-9). This finding is helpful in differentiating giant cell tumor from other benign tumors such as chondroblastoma and chondromyxoid fibroma of bone. The lesion may have a trabeculated appearance. There is no periosteal calcification unless there has been a fracture. With the larger lesions the cortex may be completely destroyed in areas—a finding that suggests the malignant nature of the tumor. Surgical curettage with placement of bone chips in the cavity is a favored method of treatment. It has the advantage in that biopsy specimens are available and the histologic nature of the lesion can be determined. Repeated recurrences or difficulties in obtaining a satisfactory response to the initial treatment are suggestive signs of malignancy. There is considerable controversy regarding the matter of benign versus malignant giant cell tumor. Many believe that all giant cell tumors are potentially malignant. Local recurrence following curettage is common. Pulmonary metastases are very rare and tend to be very indolent, with little apparent growth for years. The lack of a sclerotic boundary aids in differentiation from a chondroblastoma or chondromyxoid fibroma. The occurrence in an epiphysis and in an adult aids in distinguishing it from a simple bone cyst. It does not have the ballooned-out appearance characteristic of an aneurysmal bone cyst. The absence of periosteal reaction with periosteal spicules or Codman triangles is evidence against an osteolytic osteogenic sarcoma. The "brown tumor" of hyperparathyroidism may cause difficulty in diagnosis if it occurs at the end of a bone. However, other signs of the disease usually are present in the skeleton and there may be multiple tumors; giant cell tumor is a solitary lesion.

HEMANGIOMA OF BONE

Hemangiomas, primary in bone, are uncommon tumors except in the cranial bones and the vertebrae. They are benign lesions corresponding, histologically, to the more frequent hemangiomas of the skin and subcutaneous tissues. They are infrequently seen in children but are encountered in adults of all ages. Usually there are no symptoms. In the skull the tumor may cause a small palpable mass. In a vertebra it is usually found incidentally. Rarely, the tumor may cause collapse of a vertebral body and result in clinical signs and symptoms of vertebral compression. The rare tumors of the long tubular bones may cause symptoms because of growth of the tumor mass.

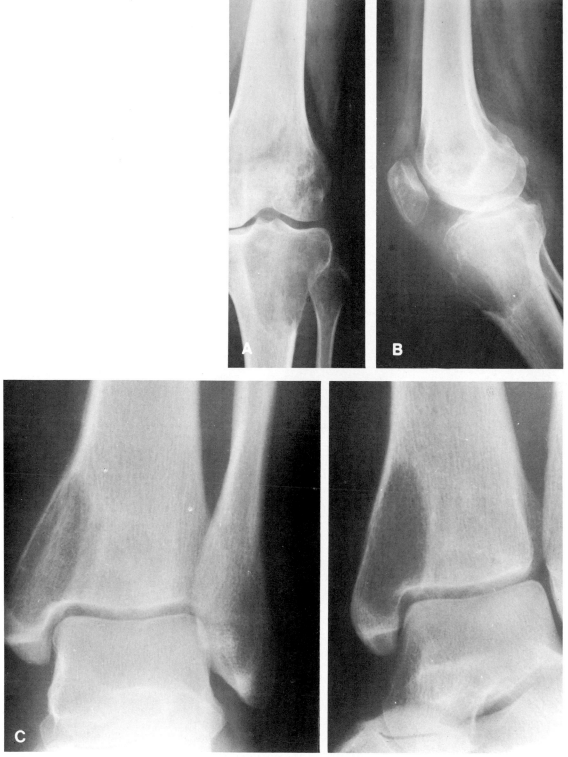

Fig. 7-8. Anteroposterior **(A)** and lateral **(B)** roentgenograms of giant cell tumor of the upper end of the tibia. **C.** Giant cell tumor of the lower end of the tibia. Note that the lesion extends to the joint surface, crosses the epiphyseal line, and is eccentric and lytic.

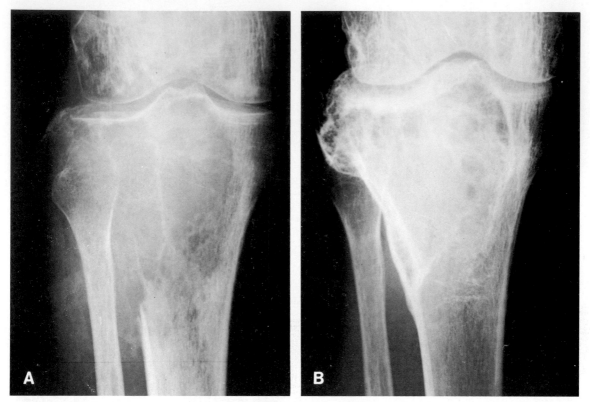

Fig. 7-9. Giant cell tumor of the tibia. **A.** Note the coarse trabecular appearance throughout the otherwise lytic tumor, the apparent loss of the lateral tibial cortex, and the eccentricity of the lesion which extends to the joint surface. **B.** Lesion shown in **A** after surgical curettage and insertion of bone chips. There has been partial recalcification but the bone remains abnormal in appearance.

Roentgen Features. In the skull the lesion appears as a round translucent area of small size and on the order of 1 to 2 cm in diameter. It is most common in the frontal area. The bone within the area has a fine granular appearance. When viewed on edge, the lesion is visualized as a smoothly convex bony mass protruding from the outer table and showing fine vertical striations. This is characteristic and almost diagnostic of this tumor (Fig. 7-10). In a vertebra, a hemangioma produces a coarse vertical striation within the vertebral body. The bony striae are separated by clear zones. The normal trabecular architecture is more or less completely replaced by these alternating vertical trabeculations and the clear spaces between them. Short horizontal striations may extend between two or more of the vertical trabeculations to produce a "honeycomb" appearance. The vertebral processes may or may not be affected, but they usually are not. Multiple lesions are common in the spine but not elsewhere. Rarely the posterior elements are involved, producing pedicle erosion and sometimes a paravertebral soft-tissue mass. In some persons a large number of vertebral bodies will show some features of this pattern, perhaps to only a slight degree. In these the changes represent hardly more than an anatomic variation. In the flat bones, such as the scapula and pelvis, hemangioma causes a sunburst appearance with radiating spicules of bone somewhat suggestive of an osteogenic sarcoma. The margin of the tumor usually is sharp and distinct, there is no evidence of soft-tissue invasion, and clinical symptoms are slight or entirely absent. In the long tubular bones the appearance of hemangioma is completely different from that of a hemangioma in other locations. Here the tumor has an expansile, multilocular appearance sometimes described as "soap-bubble." It may resemble giant cell tumor rather closely except that the trabeculations are coarser and

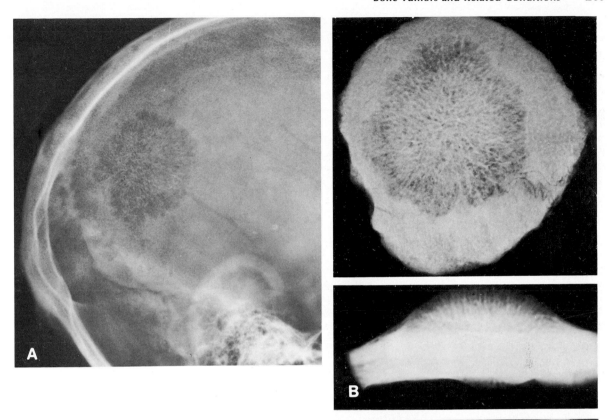

Fig. 7-10. A. Benign hemangioma of the skull. Note the somewhat granular appearance of the involved parietal bone lesion. **B.** Excised specimen of a benign hemangioma of the skull shown in two projections. The characteristic linear striation is noted in the tangential view. (Courtesy of Radiological Registry of the Armed Forces Institute of Pathology, Washington, D.C.) **C.** Benign hemangioma of a vertebral body. Note the palisadelike vertical striations that are characteristic of this lesion.

its location may be in the shaft rather than in the end of the bone.

DIFFUSE CYSTIC ANGIOMATOSIS (HEMANGIOMATOSIS AND LYMPHANGIOMATOSIS)

This rare condition is a congenital malformation[6] involving endothelial-lined vessels that may contain blood or lymph. Widespread skeletal involvement, including the skull, vertebrae, ribs, and long bones, produces numerous lucent lesions of varying sizes and shapes. The cortex may be eroded and expanded. The condition is usually discovered in an adolescent in whom a pathologic fracture leads to the diagnosis. Individual lesions are clearly defined and many have a thin sclerotic margin. Prognosis is usually good unless the condition is associated with visceral involvement. Arteriography is useful in establishing the presence of visceral lesions. Malignancy is always a possibility, with hemangiosarcoma usually rapidly fatal.

SPONTANEOUS OSTEOLYSIS (DISAPPEARING BONE)

There are a number of syndromes associated with osteolysis that can be differentiated clinically and radiographically.[4, 21] These are: (*1*) *Idiopathic hereditary osteolysis.* This is inherited as an autosomal dominant trait. It is manifest in early childhood with pain that may resemble that due to arthritis. The carpal and tarsal bones are involved first and the bone destruction may extend to involve adjacent long bones. There is no angiomatosis, no renal disease, and no threat to life. (*2*) *Autosomal recessive, carpal and tarsal osteolysis.* Several syndromes have been described in which there is progressive and extensive destruction of carpals and tarsals. Elbows may also be involved. (*3*) *Idiopathic osteolysis with nephropathy.* This also involves the carpal, tarsal, and adjacent tubular bones of young children. These patients develop azotemia and usually die in early adult life. (*4*) *Massive osteolysis of Gorham.* This is a painless condition, usually affecting the proximal skeleton and is usually unifocal. There is complete destruction of all or part of involved bone by angiomatous tissue which may spread to adjacent bones and soft tissues. This syndrome occurs in children and young adults and is not life threatening unless vital structures are encroached upon. Some of these patients recover spontaneously, often with some residual deformity.

A number of other rare syndromes resulting in osteolysis have been reported. Classification is very difficult because their pathophysiology and etiology are poorly understood. The radiologic features are those of bone destruction without evidence of callus formation or sclerosis in adjacent bone or bones.

BENIGN FIBROUS CORTICAL DEFECT

A fibrous cortical defect is not a true neoplasm but represents only a localized defect in bone growth. It is found in children and tends to disappear as growth proceeds. Usually there are no symptoms referable to the lesion and it is found incidentally during an examination performed for other reasons. It has been estimated that from 30% to 40% of all children will develop one or more such defects during the period of ossification. Favorite locations are the upper or lower third of a long bone. The lower shaft of the femur is a common site and the condition generally occurs more frequently in the lower than in the upper extremities. Usually no treatment is required.

The lesion is seen as a small area of rarefaction, sharply marginated, and bounded by a thin rim of sclerosis. It often has a scalloped border and may appear multilocular. It is found in or directly beneath the cortex and may involve the cortex with a slight localized bulging of the thin cortical plate that remains over the defect (Fig. 7-11). Sometimes it appears as a small dished-out defect involving the outer surface of the cortex.

In children, local cortical irregularity may coexist in association with a benign fibrous cortical defect in the distal femur or may occur as a solitary lesion. Roentgenographically it appears as an irregularity of the cortex of the distal shaft or metaphysis which may be prominent enough to raise concern as to the possibility of malignancy. The iregularity may be medial, lateral, or posterior in location. It usually decreases significantly or disappears at the time of epiphyseal closure. It is a common lesion that can usually be recognized as being benign.

NONOSTEOGENIC FIBROMA (NONOSSIFYING FIBROMA)

According to Jaffe, this represents essentially a benign fibrous cortical defect that continues to enlarge instead of regressing and eventually may reach considerable size. As it does so it may be a cause of clinical complaints including pathologic fracture. It has been termed "xanthoma" or "xanthofibroma" in the past. However, it probably is best to consider benign fibrous cortical defect and nonosteogenic fibroma as

Fig. 7-11. Benign fibrous cortical defect of the tibia. The lesion is radiolucent but is limited by a thin sclerotic shell of bone that clearly defines it. This defect was an incidental finding.

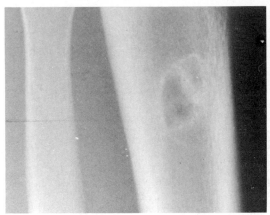

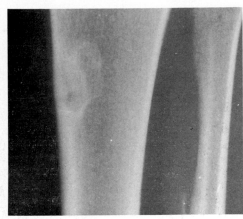

essentially the same lesion, differing chiefly in size. Thus the lesion is not considered to be a true tumor, in spite of its name, but rather represents a fault in ossification. Most of these lesions occur in adolescents, but they may be found in adults. The most frequent sites are the ends of the long bones of the lower extremities on the shaft side of the epiphyseal line, but occasionally the flat bones are implicated. Roentgenologically a nonosteogenic fibroma is seen as a sharply marginated area of translucency bounded by a thin sclerotic shell. It does not differ appreciably in appearance from that of a benign cortical defect except for its size. There may be a slight cortical bulge but no periosteal reaction unless fracture occurs. The defect may extend completely across the shaft (Fig. 7-12).

CHONDROBLASTOMA

Chondroblastoma[9, 24] is a rare benign tumor of bone representing a variety of chondroma arising in or near the region of the epiphyseal cartilage. It is an essentially epiphyseal lesion although the epiphysis may have fused by the time the tumor is first discovered. The cells making up this tumor are not mature cartilage cells as in chondroma and thus may be confused with chondrosarcoma by pathologists who may not be familiar with the lesion. The age period for the appearance of this tumor lies between 5 and 25 years. The usual locations are the upper end of the humerus, lower femur or upper tibia, lower tibia, and upper femur, in that order of frequency. About 60% occur in the lower extremities. A few have been reported in the tarsal bones, metatarsals, sternum, spine, carpals, mandible, and calvarium.

Roentgen Features. A chondroblastoma consists of a well-defined area of rarefaction with a fuzzy or mottled appearance produced by flocculent calcification.

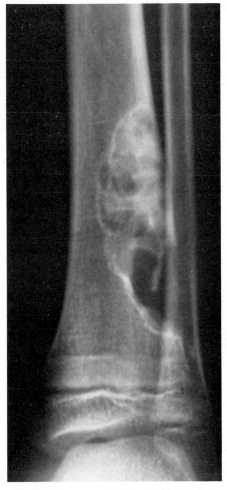

Fig. 7-12. Nonossifying (nonosteogenic) fibroma of bone. The lesion resembles a benign fibrous cortical defect except for its larger size. (The defect in the inferior aspect of the lateral tibial cortex is due to a biopsy performed previously.)

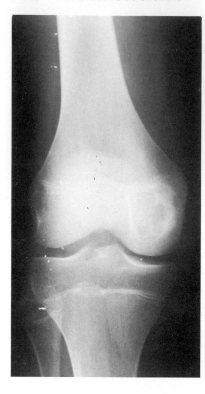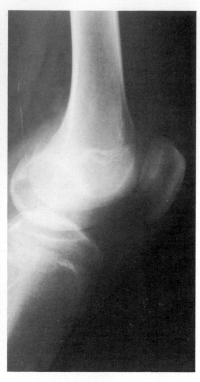

Fig. 7-13. Chondroblastoma of the femur. Note this lesion's location in the epiphysis and its scalloped, well-circumscribed eccentric appearance.

Its usual location is in the epiphysis, but, as it enlarges, it may extend into the metaphysis. The lesion is often small and located eccentrically. It sometimes has a scalloped appearance. There may be some expansion of the cortex, but periosteal reaction is unusual. The margins of the lesion are well defined and limited by a thin zone of sclerosis. The tumor often extends to the articular surface but does not invade the joint. Occasionally there is some sclerosis extending beyond the thin dense rim of the lesion (Fig. 7-13).

CHONDROMYXOID FIBROMA

Chondromyxoid fibroma is a relatively rare benign tumor of bone first described by Jaffe and Lichtenstein in 1948. It is found chiefly in young adults with a lesser incidence in older people and children. The tibia is its most common site, but the femur, fibula, metatarsals, or calcaneus may be involved. Occasional tumors are found in the humerus, ribs, ilium, clavicle, patella, vertebra, or skull. Pain is the most frequent symptom.

The tumor most frequently involves the metaphysis of a long bone and occasionally crosses the epiphyseal plate, if this is still present. Except in the smaller bones, the lesion does not extend completely across the width of the shaft.

Roentgenologically the tumor is seen as a sharply marginated area of rarefaction of rounded or oval shape which causes local bulging and thinning of the overlying cortex. In some of the patients the cortex may be completely destroyed over the tumor but the lesion usually is contained by a shell of cortex. Internally the lesion has a clear-cut margin with a thin sclerotic shell separating it from adjacent normal bone (Figs. 7-14 and 7-15). There is usually no periosteal reaction. The tumor is oval or round and in long bones its axis is oriented along the long axis of the bone. Its margin may be scalloped and the sclerotic margin may vary in thickness and density in different areas of the lesion.

Differentiation from a simple bone cyst may be difficult in some subjects. Location in the upper end of the humeral shaft is a characteristic of a simple bone cyst and there usually is no sclerotic boundary. Giant cell tumor usually occurs at a later age and involves the epiphyseal end of a bone. It does not have a sclerotic margin separating the tumor from normal bone. Other lesions such as enchondroma, benign chondroblastoma, nonosteogenic fibroma, and aneurysmal bone cyst enter into the differential diagnosis.

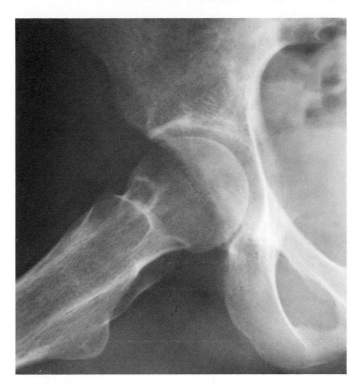

Fig. 7-14. Chondromyxoid fibroma. Lesion is visualized as a cystlike defect in the neck of the femur with a sclerotic boundary zone outlining it.

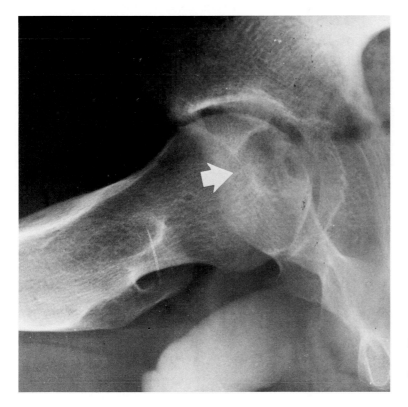

Fig. 7-15. Chondromyxoid fibroma in the head of the femur **(arrow).** The thin sclerotic rim is somewhat indistinct in this patient.

OSTEOBLASTOMA (GIANT OSTEOID OSTEOMA)

This is a relatively rare tumor which occurs chiefly in persons in the 10- to 20-year age group.[25] It is found most frequently in the vertebral column, involving the neural arch and pedicles. Involvement of the femur and tibia is next in frequency and, rarely, the ribs, hands, feet, facial bones, skull, patella, scapula, or ilium may be implicated. In the long bones, in about three-fourths of the cases the diaphysis is involved and in the remainder the metaphysis. This tumor is considered by pathologists to represent the reaction of bone to some type of injury and thus not to represent a true neoplasm. Most of the lesions are cortical. In some cases they are sclerotic and more or less uniformly radiopaque. In others they are seen as lytic areas which tend to expand the overlying cortex and to be bounded by a sclerotic rim. Stippled calcified deposits often are present within the lesion. When this tumor occurs in the posterior elements of the spine with an area of destruction, some expansion, and minimal sclerosis, the appearance is highly suggestive of osteosarcoma from which it must be differentiated. There is a tendency for an osteoblastoma to expand the cortex and break through it, producing a soft-tissue component, often circumscribed by a thin calcific shell. The lytic type of lesion may be difficult to distinguish from an aneurysmal bone cyst. Osteoblastoma must also be differentiated from giant cell tumor, chondroblastoma, and chondrosarcoma. The typical location in a neural arch and the stippled calcification within the lesion are helpful distinguishing features.

MALIGNANT BONE TUMORS

OSTEOSARCOMA

Osteosarcoma is one of the most frequently encountered primary malignant tumors of bone, apparently arising from the primitive bone-forming mesenchyme. It is more common in males than in females. Its greatest incidence is in persons between 10 and 25 years of age. Thus it is essentially a lesion of late childhood and early adult life. Occasional examples are seen in persons older than 25 (Fig. 7-16). Some of these originate in bone involved by Paget's disease, especially in persons beyond the age of 40. However, the lesion occasionally does occur as a primary disease in older adults. Osteosarcoma also may arise from a preexisting osteochondroma. It has also been found as a rare complication of fibrous dysplasia, often the polyostotic form. Chondrosarcoma and fi-

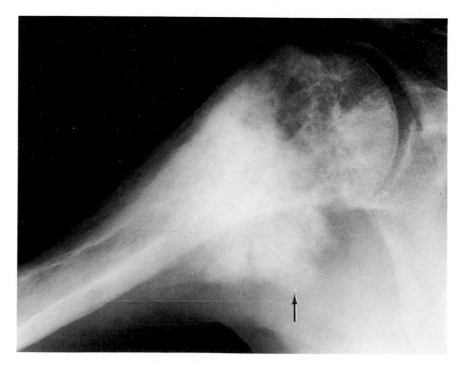

Fig. 7-16. Osteosarcoma developing in a patient with Paget's disease of the humerus. Note the thickened cortex of the proximal humerus indicative of Paget's disease. The tumor is largely sclerotic with tumor bone extending into the soft tissues **(arrow).**

brosarcoma are also found but are rarer than osteosarcoma in this situation. Heavy doses of roentgen radiation to an area has been followed by the development of osteosarcoma usually following a long latent period ranging up to 30 years after irradiation. Prognosis is better than in patients with "spontaneous" osteosarcoma. Osteosarcoma has been reported as occurring in persons working with luminous watch dials who had ingested radium and mesothorium in excessive amounts.

The most frequent locations are the lower end of the femur, the upper end of the tibia, and the upper end of the humerus. The tumor is less common in the upper fibula, the iliac bones, the vertebrae, and the mandible. It originates in the end of the shaft near the epiphyseal line. Pain and local swelling are the usual presenting complaints.

If the tumor is growing rapidly there may be weight loss and a secondary anemia. Pulmonary metastases may develop early and a chest roentgenogram should be obtained when osteosarcoma is a diagnostic consideration. The prognosis is generally poor, particularly when the tumor arises in childhood.

Although osteosarcoma is essentially a solitary lesion, a few examples of multiple tumors in a single individual have been reported. These have been of the sclerotic type. It is undetermined whether these represent multiple primary lesions or metastases from a single primary one.

For roentgenographic descriptive purposes three forms of osteosarcoma may be recognized, depending upon the presence or absence of new bone formation within the tumor and the periosteal reaction about it.

Osteolytic Form

The lesion begins in the metaphyseal end of a long bone as a central area of destruction with little or no new bone formation or periosteal reaction. The margins of the lesion are poorly defined and ragged. The cortex is involved early and is destroyed. Extension of the tumor into the soft tissues occurs relatively early and swelling of the soft tissues, sometimes with a well-defined mass, can often be recognized. Where the periosteum is being elevated at the margins of the rapidly growing tumor, triangular shadows of calcification may appear. These are called Codman's triangles. They are highly suggestive of a malignant tumor whenever encountered in a lesion of bone, although a similar periosteal reaction may be found occasionally with other lesions, mainly infections.

Sclerosing Form

The sclerosing form of osteosarcoma also arises within the medullary canal as a rule. Early, there is seen a hazy area of mottled sclerosis. As the cortex becomes involved its outline becomes lost; the sclerotic reaction of the tumor and the dense new bone formation completely cover it. The lesion soon extends into the soft tissues, forming dense spicules of bone. These tend to form at right angles to the surface of the bone. A characteristic of this type of osteogenic sarcoma is the amount and density of the bone formed by the tumor; when the lesion is well developed it produces an irregular dense mass surrounding the shaft. While there is always a destructive aspect, it is largely obscured by the proliferative reaction. There is a tendency for this form to metastasize to other bones as well as to the lungs, forming dense masses of metastatic tumor. Occasionally, several dense bone lesions are found at the time of the original examination, making it difficult or impossible to determine the site of the primary tumor. This type of tumor is usually found in children and its course is usually rapidly fatal.

Mixed Form

This roentgenologic type of osteosarcoma is the most frequent; it is characterized by a mixture of bone destruction and bone production. One or the other may predominate, but in most examples the destructive aspect overshadows the productive. The bone destruction is characteristically ragged and uneven. The tumor extends into the soft tissues early in its development. Codman's triangles are frequently seen at the edges of the tumor where it is elevating the periosteum, stripping it away from the cortex. Spicules of tumor bone or calcification are present throughout the mass, often arranged at right angles to the cortex, giving what has been described as sunburst appearance. Right-angle spiculation is not pathognomonic of a malignant bone tumor but it is seen infrequently with other lesions. In some cases there are irregular masses of mottled calcification or bone formation scattered throughout the tumor mass (Figs. 7-17 and 7-18).

Metastases

Osteosarcoma shows a great tendency to metastasize to the lungs and roentgenograms of the chest should always be obtained when this lesion is a diagnostic consideration. The pulmonary lesions are visualized

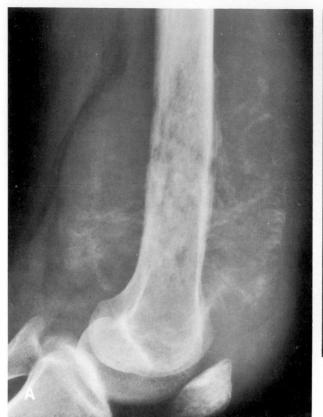

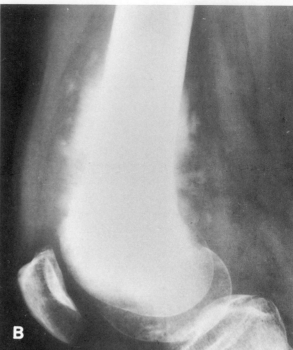

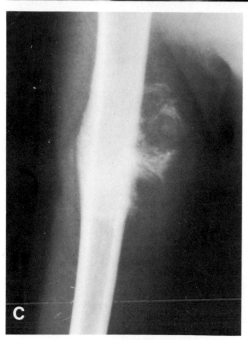

Fig. 7-17. Osteosarcoma **A.** In this tumor, note the extensive permeative type of destruction in the lower femur along with a few areas of sclerosis and the parallel layers of periosteal calcification anteriorly with the large soft-tissue mass and tumor bone extending into it. **B.** This sarcoma is much more sclerotic than that shown in **A.** It has a sunburst appearance noted best anteriorly. **C.** This lesion within the bone is largely sclerotic, but there is a sizable soft-tissue mass into which tumor bone projects.

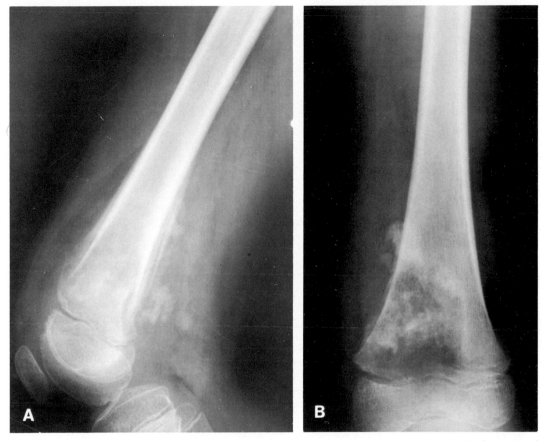

Fig. 7-18. Lateral **(A)** and frontal **(B)** projections of an osteosarcoma of the lower end of the femur. The area of irregular destruction is seen best in the frontal projection. Laminated periosteal calcification is noted particularly well posteriorly, and there is also some tumor bone within the medullary canal as well as extension into the soft tissues of the lower thigh.

in roentgenograms as discrete, round nodules of variable size, usually multiple, and sometimes partially calcified or ossified.

PAROSTEAL SARCOMA

This lesion has been known as parosteal osteoma and juxtacortical osteosarcoma. Most authorities now believe that it is a malignant neoplasm and thus the terms *parosteal* or *juxtacortical osteosarcoma* are used. The tendency now is to drop the "osteo" from the name and call the tumor *parosteal sarcoma* because various mesenchymal tissue types may be found in histologic sections.[2]

The lesion is found in a somewhat older age group than is osteosarcoma, that is, in persons between the ages of 15 and 55 years. About half of the patients are over the age of 30. It is an uncommon tumor. It is most frequently found in the distal end of the femur in the region of the popliteal space (Fig. 7-19). Its growth is slow, but it has a pronounced tendency to recur after local excision and, later, to metastasize, especially to the lungs. It appears, roentgenologically, as a broadbased, juxtacortical, densely ossified mass. The periphery is somewhat less dense than the base, but is usually sharply demarcated from the surrounding soft tissues and may be somewhat lobulated. The mass is attached to the cortex along a part of its base and its tends to encircle the shaft, leaving a narrow clear zone between the tumor and the cortex. Although growth is slow initially, the lesion eventually progresses to cortical destruction and medul-

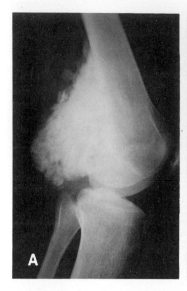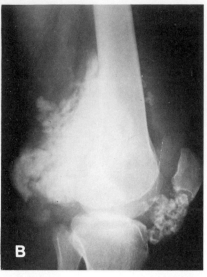

Fig. 7-19. Osteosarcoma, parosteal type. **A.** The large, dense mass protruding from the posterior aspect of the lower femur represents the bulk of the tumor with relatively little intramedullary involvement. There is no evidence of bone destruction. **B.** Extensive recurrence of lesion shown in **A** following local resection. The tumor is within the knee joint space and, in addition to the large recurrent posterior mass, extends anterior to the lower end of the femur.

lary invasion. After excision, recurrences are manifested by the development of densely calcified masses in the soft tissues and recurrence of the tumor where it was attached to bone. Histologically the lesion in its early stages is said to resemble myositis ossificans, but the roentgenologic features are usually sufficiently characteristic that a diagnosis can be made on this basis.

In differential diagnosis the possibility of *myositis ossificans* usually can be excluded if progress studies are done. The lesion follows trauma or paralysis, and the ossification becomes discrete and laminated with the passage of time. In an *ossifying subperiosteal hematoma,* the lesion follows trauma and is more likely to involve the central shaft of the bone. *Osteochondroma* is attached to the cortex by a broad or narrow pedicle which has the features of normal bone, that is, cortex and medullary cavity. The periphery of the lesion is characteristically mottled, owing to islands of calcified cartilage. *Osteosarcoma* is characterized by rapid growth, pain, and a systemic reaction. Codman triangles and periosteal spiculation often at right angles to the cortex are characteristic.

CHONDROSARCOMA

Chondrosarcoma is about half as common as osteosarcoma. It develops at a later age period, is more slowly growing, and metastasizes later. The age range is between 11 and 66 years with a median age of 45. Over half the patients are over 40 years old and most of the remainder are between 20 and 40. There

is a preponderance of males over females in most reported series.

Chondrosarcoma may be either primary or secondary. In the former instance the tumor originates without a preexisting lesion. In the latter type the tumor develops on the basis of a preexisting lesion, usually an enchondroma or osteochondroma. The tumor also can be classified as central or peripheral, depending on its location in the bone. Central chondrosarcomas are found most commonly in the bones of the trunk and the proximal parts of the humerus and femur. Peripheral tumors are somewhat more frequent in the bones of the extremities but also occur in flat bones, such as pelvis, ribs, scapula, and sternum.[2] The bones of the hands and feet are uncommon sites and tumors that develop here usually begin in preexisting enchondromas. Both peripheral and central types may be either primary or secondary.

Central Chondrosarcoma

Many of these tumors arise from enchondromas but by the time the lesion is first examined the original lesion may have been so distorted or obscured as to be unrecognizable. Chondrosarcoma is reported to occur in about 10% of patients with hereditary multiple exostoses. Solitary enchondromas may become malignant, the potentiality for this change decreasing from the hip or shoulder areas distally to the fingers or toes.[2] Thus the tumor is very uncommon in the small bones of the hands and feet. If examined early the change from benign to malignant tumor may be difficult to recognize. Any enchondroma or osteochondroma that becomes painful or begins to enlarge should be viewed with considerable suspicion.

The average central chondrosarcoma of a tubular bone appears as a radiolucent area of bone destruction within the cancellous bone of the diaphysis and is rather poorly marginated from normal bone at either end. It may be situated near the metaphysis or towards the midshaft. The internal surface of the cortex overlying the lesion often is eroded. This combined with external reactive periosteal new bone formation gives an appearance of local expansion (Fig. 7-20). One of the characteristics of chondrosarcoma is the presence of numerous spotty, or stippled foci or streaks of dense calcification within the tumor. This type of calcification, however, also is seen in benign cartilaginous tumors (i.e., in enchondroma and osteochondroma) and is not specific for malignancy. Eventually, the tumor erodes through the cortex and forms a soft-tissue mass adjacent to the bone lesion. This mass also may show foci of calcification which may be quite extensive (Fig. 7-21).

Any change in the radiographic appearance of an enchondroma should be viewed with suspicion, since early findings of chondrosarcoma may be subtle. In a few of our cases the early lesion was seen as a small, rather uneven, area of sclerosis in the medullary canal. The cortex appeared thickened over the lesion owing to reactive periosteal new bone formation and a small soft-tissue mass was present. Evidence of bone destruction was minimal. In the pelvis, large bulky masses containing spotty or streaky calcification, along with variable amounts of bone destruction, are common, the lesion probably arising from an osteochondroma.

At times the extension into the soft parts seems to result from a pathologic fracture through the weakened bone.

Peripheral Chondrosarcoma

This type of chondrosarcoma arises adjacent to the external surface of the bone. It probably began, in most cases, in an osteochondroma and, if examined early, remnants of the original lesion may still be present. However, in many, if there was a preexisting lesion it has been destroyed by the malignant tumor when first examined. Most of these tumors arise in patients with multiple hereditary exostoses. Chondrosarcoma is a rare complication of a solitary osteochondroma. A soft-tissue mass, often large and bulky, forms adjacent to the bone. The characteristic spotty

and streaky calcifications are usually present in the mass. The underlying cortex may be intact or show erosion of its external surface. Eventually the cortex is destroyed beneath the mass and the tumor then invades the medullary canal. The large mass may displace soft-tissue planes, fat, and muscle early and then invade and obliterate these planes.

OTHER PRIMARY MALIGNANT TUMORS
Fibrosarcoma of Bone

This is a rare tumor and is not to be confused with the more common fibrosarcoma of the periosteum or other soft tissues which may eventually erode the contiguous bone. This tumor begins within the interior of the medullary cavity. It produces a fairly well-circumscribed area of radiolucency as the tumor destroys bone. It eventually thins the cortex, often causing periosteal new bone formation as it extends into the surrounding soft tissue. The diagnosis of fibrosarcoma is very difficult to make on the basis of roentgen examination, but radiographic findings are those of a malignant tumor. The lesions we have seen have mimicked a central lytic type of chondrosarcoma or other lytic tumor. The age of these patients is variable but most of these lesions occur in the older group; growth usually is slow. The prognosis somewhat better than in osteosarcoma.

Malignant Hemangioendothelioma of Bone (Angiosarcoma)

This is another rare tumor of bone that reveals itself mainly as a localized destructive lesion. A diagnosis based on roentgen evidence usually cannot be made. Multiple sites of involvement in a number of bones are common as in the benign lesion, cystic angiomatosis of bone. There is no tendency to produce sclerosis or calcification. The periphery of the individual areas of bone destruction produced by the tumor is poorly defined. Periosteal new bone formation may occur when the lesion breaks through the cortex. There are relatively few cases on record and knowledge of the lesion is relatively limited.

Ewing's Tumor

Ewing's tumor is a primary malignant tumor arising in the bone marrow. Some investigators believe that it is closely related to plasma cell myeloma and reticulum cell sarcoma. The clinical symptoms of pain, fever, and leukocytosis may suggest osteomyelitis. Ewing's tumor is most frequently found in persons

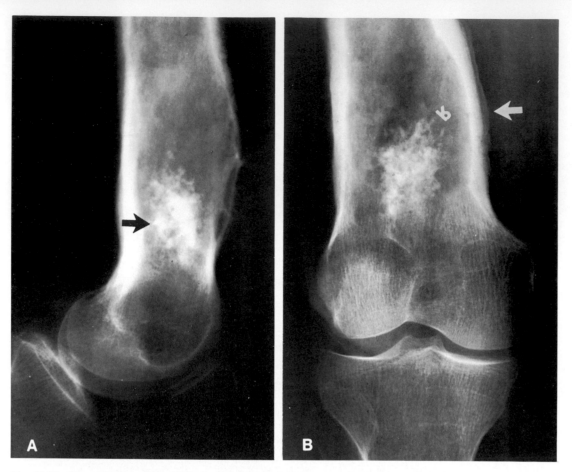

Fig. 7-20. Chondrosarcoma. This is a central chondrosarcoma that probably developed from the enchondroma in the medullary canal designated by the **arrow** in **A.** There has been expansion and thinning of the cortex with minimal periosteal calcification designated by the **white arrow** in **B.**

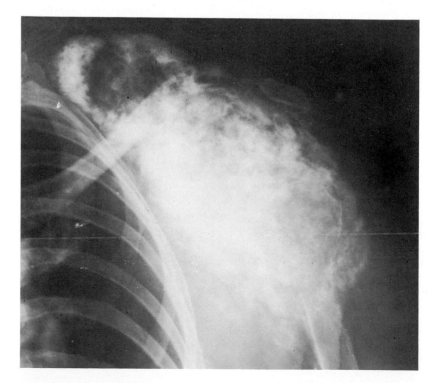

Fig. 7-21. Massive chondrosarcoma which arose in the scapula and distorted the entire shoulder. Its superior aspect contains a number of rounded lucent areas that are typical of cartilaginous tumors.

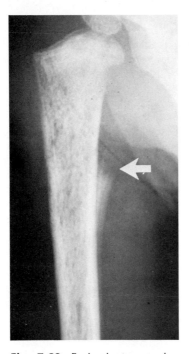

Fig. 7-22. Ewing's tumor involving the proximal shaft of the humerus. There is a permeative type of rarefaction of the bone and a well-defined laminated Codman triangle **(arrow).**

between the ages of 5 and 25 years and rarely occurs in those over 30; males are affected more frequently than females in the ratio of 2:1. Favorite sites of involvement are the long bones of the extremities, the femur being most frequently affected with the tibia second. It also is found in the pelvis, ribs, and scapulae. It is relatively common in the vertebrae and in the bones of the foot, particularly the os calcis. In patients over 20 years of age, the incidence is higher in the flat bones than in the long bones.

This tumor shows a distinct tendency to metastasize to other bones and thus multiple lesions may be present at the time of the initial study.

Roentgen Features. When Ewing's tumor occurs in a long bone the lesion usually involves a considerable length of the shaft (Figs. 7-22 and 7-23). It begins as an area of central destruction. A variable amount of sclerosis may be present intermingled with the osteolysis. When the tumor perforates the cortex it elevates the periosteum stimulating it to deposit calcium. This often forms in multiple layers, and results in the so-called "onionskin" appearance. This type of

periosteal calcification is always suggestive of Ewing's tumor but is not specific for it (see Fig. 7-22). The lesion may have a coarsely mottled appearance because of intermixed destruction and sclerosis. In other instances it is primarily destructive or there may be radiating spicules of bone in the soft tissues resembling those seen in osteosarcoma. At times the tumor may present as a small area of cortical destruction without periosteal reaction, quite unlike the more common picture of a large lytic or permeative lesion with periosteal new bone formation. In

Fig. 7-23. Ewing's tumor involving the midshaft of the femur in a young adult. Laminated periosteal calcification extends for a considerable distance. This type of lesion may be difficult to distinguish from inflammation. The poor definition of the outer border of the periosteal calcification is a helpful sign in addition to the lamination.

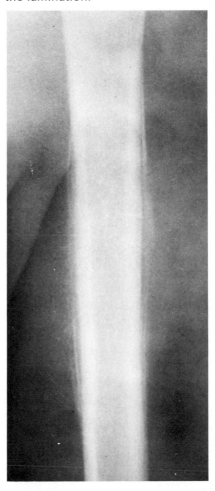

vertebral involvement, the appearance may vary from that of uniform sclerosis of the vertebral body, and sometimes of some of the posterior elements, to that of an almost completely lytic destructive process. A soft-tissue mass is often present around the lesion. In the pelvis the tumor often causes a mixture of osteolysis and sclerosis, resulting in a mottled shadow without sharply defined margins. In the vertebrae, mixed destruction and sclerosis may be present and one or the other may predominate. The differentiation of Ewing's tumor from osteomyelitis may be very difficult and biopsy should be performed if there is the slightest doubt concerning the diagnosis. Ewing's tumor may also mimic other malignant tumors and requires biopsy for differentiation. Most of these tumors are radiosensitive but this cannot be relied upon as a diagnostic test since other tumors may respond as well. The occurrence of a malignant-appearing lesion in the shaft of a long bone in a patient under the age of 30 should make Ewing's tumor the most likely diagnosis.

METASTATIC CARCINOMA

While any carcinoma may metastasize to bone, the common primary sites are the breast, prostate, kidney, thyroid, and lung. Because of their frequency, cancers of the breast and prostate result in the majority of bone metastases. Spread to the bones from carcinomas of the gastrointestinal tract and the pelvic organs is relatively infrequent. Favorite sites for the appearance of metastatic foci are the red marrow bones, i.e., the spine, pelvis, ribs, skull, and upper ends of humerus and femur. Metastatic lesions below the elbow and knee are infrequent but do occur, especially with bronchogenic tumors.

As indicated, any malignant tumor may metastasize to bone; the tumors mentioned in the following metastasize infrequently but vary somewhat in the type of lesion produced. Colonic metastases are often blastic but may be lytic. Carcinoma of the esophagus usually produces lytic metastases; the same is true of malignant melanoma, which also has a tendency to break through the cortex and extend into adjacent soft tissues. Medulloblastoma tends to produce a mixed lytic-blastic disseminated or local lesion resembling breast metastases. Retinoblastoma produces similar lesions. Basal cell carcinoma of the skin will produce local bone invasion if neglected, but rarely may also cause lytic disseminated lesions, usually after the tumor has been untreated for years. Bone metastases usually occur late in the tumors mentioned above and indicate a very poor prognosis.

Any of them may also cause subperiosteal new bone formation if they break through the cortex.

Detection of skeletal metastases is not always possible on radiographic examination, since areas of bone destruction may not be visible until approximately one-half of the mineral content has been lost. Therefore, it is useful to employ skeletal scanning, with one of the bone-seeking radionuclides in the detection of early metastases. This becomes especially important when the therapy modality to be used is heavily dependent upon the presence or absence of osseous metastases. Brady and Croll[5] suggest the use of ^{99m}Tc-labeled methylene diphosphonate since toxicity is low and there is a relatively short (2 hours) interval between injection of the radionuclide and obtaining the scan. Then the positive or suspicious areas can be radiographed for better anatomic delineation of the area(s) in question. Texts and articles on radionuclide scanning should be consulted for further details that are beyond the scope of this volume.

Roentgen Features

Osteolytic Type. The lesion begins in the medullary canal. The bone is destroyed as the tumor grows; it eventually involves the cortex, thus predisposing to pathologic fracture (Fig. 7-24). The margins of the defect are ragged and frayed, seldom sharp and smooth. In some instances the lesion causes only a granular mottled appearance. There is usually no periosteal reaction and no sclerosis around the margins (Fig. 7-25). The most common sources for this type of metastasis are the breast, kidney, and thyroid. Tumors of the kidney are prone to cause a large and apparently single metastatic focus; metastases from breast carcinoma are more often multiple when first seen. Occasionally, metastatic foci from the thyroid result in an expansile trabeculated lesion somewhat resembling a giant cell tumor.

In the spine there is a tendency for involvement not only of the vertebral bodies, but of the pedicles and neural arches also. In some cases loss of outline of one or more pedicles may be the only or the earliest sign of involvement (Fig. 7-26).

The disease most commonly considered in differential diagnosis is multiple myeloma. At times the differentiation cannot be made on roentgen evidence. In the spine, myeloma is less likely to involve a pedicle; an associated soft-tissue mass is more common than in metastatic carcinoma. In the skull the lesions of myeloma are more sharply defined. Also, in myeloma the bones generally may appear quite osteo-

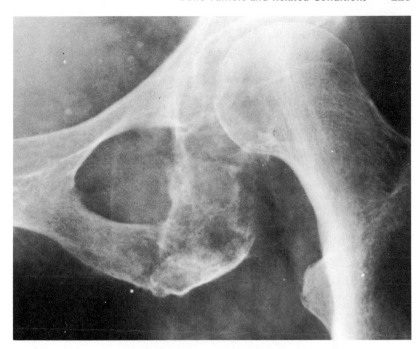

Fig. 7-24. Osteolytic metastasis to the inferior ischial ramus in a patient with breast carcinoma. In addition to the bone destruction there is a little increase in density medially, probably the result of pathologic fracture with some healing.

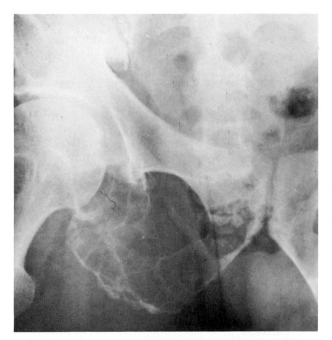

Fig. 7-25. Osteolytic metastasis of the inferior ischio-pubic ramus which shows the cortex to be expanded, but the thin outer layer is preserved. The patient had carcinoma of the thyroid gland; this may produce these expansile lesions.

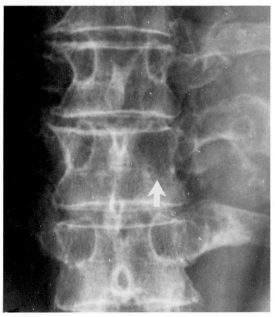

Fig. 7-26. Metastasis to the left pedicle **(arrow)** of a thoracic vertebra from carcinoma of the breast. Note absence of the normal ovoid "ring" shadow of the pedicle. There are also destructive lesions in the ribs.

porotic; in metastatic carcinoma they often are of normal density except for the foci of disease.

As a rule, when a solitary osteolytic lesion is observed in patients over 50 years of age, metastatic carcinoma and plasma cell myeloma are the major considerations and the possibility of their presence must be ruled out in every instance.

Osteoblastic Type (Sclerotic). Sclerotic metastatic foci are characterized by their pronounced density. They may occur as more or less isolated rounded foci of sclerotic density or as a diffuse sclerosis involving a large area in the bone and in multiple bones (Figs. 7-27, 7-28, and 7-29). Within the involved region the normal architecture is lost and the lesion shows a fairly uniform density similar to that of cortical bone.

In males this type of metastasis usually is secondary to a primary carcinoma in the prostate gland. An increase in the acid phosphatase in the blood serum, often to very high levels, is observed frequently in the presence of prostatic metastases. In females, sclerotic metastasis usually is secondary to carcinoma of the breast. Sclerotic metastases also have been observed from primary carcinoma of the gastrointestinal tract, particularly from the pancreas.

Mixed Form. In the mixed type of metastasis there is a combination of destruction and sclerosis, usually with destruction predominating. The affected bone has a mottled appearance with intermixed areas of rarefaction and increased density. Periosteal calcification sometimes is seen over the lesion. Following

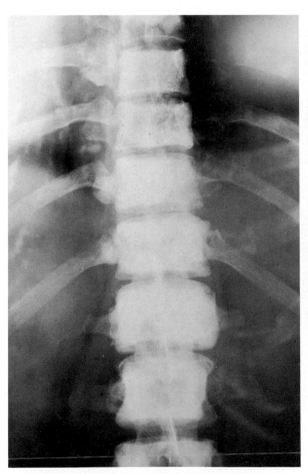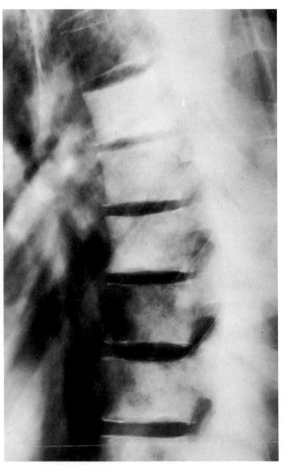

Fig. 7-27. Sclerotic metastases. The areas of involvement are manifested by a dense sclerosis that tends to obliterate the normal architecture. All of the vertebrae included show some degree of involvement.

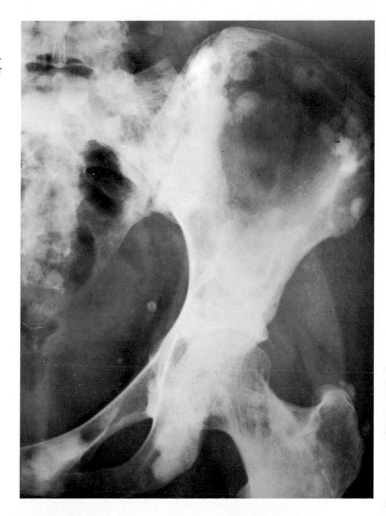

Fig. 7-28. Sclerotic metastasis involving the pelvis. The lesions are very dense and discrete with a number of uninvolved areas noted in the left hemipelvis.

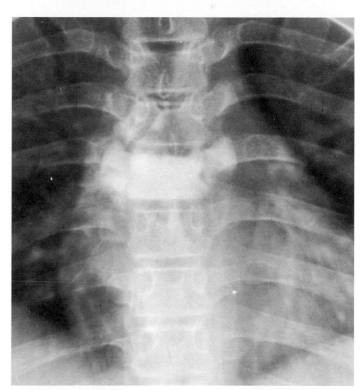

Fig. 7-29. Osteoblastic metastasis to a thoracic vertebra, including its transverse processes, in a child with sclerotic type of osteosarcoma.

roentgen irradiation, destructive metastatic lesions often develop varying degrees of sclerosis, sometimes with complete recalcification of the area. The same response is seen in metastatic carcinoma of the breast after roentgen or surgical sterilization and following hormonal therapy or chemotherapy.

METASTATIC NEUROBLASTOMA

Neuroblastoma is a highly malignant tumor arising from the sympathetic nervous tissue and often from the adrenal gland. The tumor is encountered mainly in infants and young children. A palpable mass in the abdomen may be the first evidence of the primary tumor. Calcification in the form of fine granular deposits may be visible within the primary tumor. The shadow of the mass and evidence of downward displacement of the kidney are other roentgen signs of the lesion in the abdomen. The tumor shows a pronounced tendency to metastasize to the skeletal system.

Roentgen Features

1. In the skull, neuroblastoma produces rather characteristic changes. The cranial sutures are spread, owing to plaques of tumor tissue growing along the surface of the brain. There are poorly defined areas of spotty rarefaction causing a finely granular type of osteoporosis. Thin, whiskerlike calci-

fications are frequently present, extending outward and inward from the tables of the skull. The combination of these findings is highly suggestive of the diagnosis of metastatic neuroblastoma (Fig. 7-30).

2. In the long tubular bones, foci of fine granular rarefaction may be seen. The cortex may be eroded in some areas. Such zones of cortical erosion frequently are symmetrical and it is common to find them along the medial surfaces of the proximal metaphyses of the humeri and the distal metaphyses of the femurs (Fig. 7-31). The periosteum may be elevated by tumor tissue and result in hazy shadows of periosteal calcification either parallel to the cortex or, as in the skull, forming whiskerlike spiculations at right angles to the cortex.

TUMORS AND ALLIED LESIONS OF BONE MARROW, LYMPHATIC TISSUE, ETC.

MULTIPLE MYELOMA (PLASMA CELL MYELOMA)

Myeloma is a tumor that appears to arise from the bone marrow cells, but the precise cell of origin is not clear.[26] Occasionally it develops in extraskeletal tissues. It is made up of plasma cells and is the most common primary tumor arising within bone. It is as-

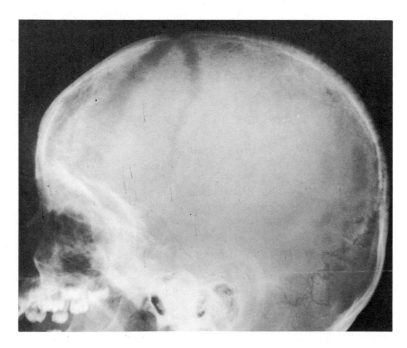

Fig. 7-30. Metastasis to the skull from neuroblastoma. There is an area of mixed sclerotic and lytic involvement in the frontal bone. The coronal suture is widened, indicating increased intracranial pressure secondary to metastasis.

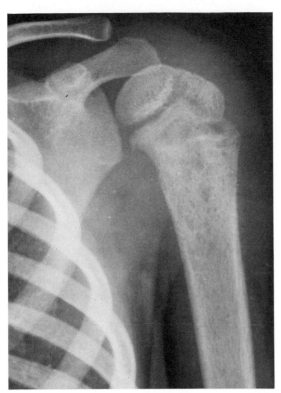

Fig. 7-31. Metastasis to the upper humeral shaft from adrenal neuroblastoma. This is a somewhat permeative type of destruction which was also present in the opposite humerus and the femurs.

sociated with abnormal gamma globulins and with an abnormal substance, Bence Jones protein, in the urine. It is often associated with, or accompanied by, amyloidosis. Masses of amyloid may produce various neuropathies which may be the presenting complaint in patients with myeloma. Myelofibrosis has also been associated with multiple myelomas but is rare. Abnormal gamma globulins can be found in patients with malignant tumors of epithelial, mesodermal, or lymphatic origin and with chronic inflammatory disease of the lung, kidney, and liver.[7] Therefore, a definite diagnosis of multiple myeloma cannot always be made from one or all of the standard criteria, and a bone biopsy is necessary.

Myeloma is found chiefly in persons between 40 and 70 years of age. It is somewhat more frequent in males than in females. The bones involved by myeloma are the same as noted in metastatic carcinoma—the spine, ribs, pelvis, skull, proximal ends of the humerus and femur.

Roentgen Features. The lesions of myeloma are, typically, multiple, round, clean-cut areas of destruction with no surrounding sclerosis. In the flat bones, such as the pelvis and skull, the individual lesions can be seen to best advantage, appearing as numerous, small, punched-out defects (Fig. 7-32). As a rule the lytic lesions in the skull are smaller than those of metastatic carcinoma, but occasionally large lesions are observed. Rarely, there is an extensive local thickening of the calvarium with spiculation and soft-tissue mass resembling changes sometimes observed in parasagittal or convexity meningioma. In some of the patients the lesions in the skull may be very small, producing a porous appearance somewhat similar to that observed in severe hyperparathyroidism. In the long bones (Fig. 7-33) the lesions may enlarge, coalesce, and lead to pathologic fracture; this is of frequent occurrence in the ribs. Occasionally a myeloma may cause expansion of the cortex or even appear trabeculated or honeycombed. Extension to the surrounding soft tissues is frequent and, in the ribs, these tumor masses may produce soft-tissue shadows that bulge into the lung fields. Associated soft-tissue masses are more common in myeloma than in metastatic carcinoma. In perhaps one-fourth of the cases of multiple myeloma the typical circumscribed defects may be absent during the early phase of the disease. In some patients the bones may be essentially normal. In others there is only a generalized decalcification which, in the spine, may lead to compression of the vertebral bodies similar to that seen in senile or postmenopausal osteoporosis. Bone biopsy or other studies may be necessary to establish the diagnosis in a case of this type.

Rarely, in myeloma, one or more vertebrae will appear unusually translucent, forming a "negative" density as contrasted with the surrounding soft tissues. This is probably caused by extensive deposition of fat in the marrow, since, of the body tissues, only fat is more translucent than water. Also, rare examples of myeloma have been reported in which the foci of disease were sclerotic rather than lytic. The sclerotic lesions may be solitary or diffuse, the latter simulating osteoblastic metastases observed in prostatic metastases. Also, occasionally an osteolytic lesion may have thin sclerotic margins. These manifestations must be considered as distinctly unusual. Involvement of para-aortic nodes may cause concavity of anterior margins of one or more vertebrae; this appears to be a pressure phenomenon because the anterior cortex remains intact. This is also an uncommon finding.

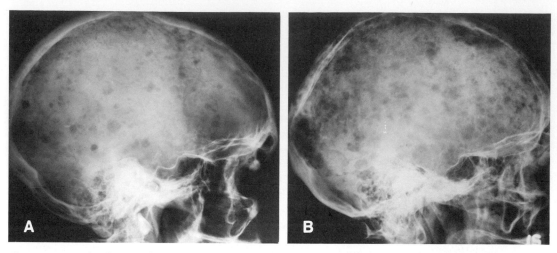

Fig. 7-32. Multiple myeloma in two patients. Multiple lytic areas are scattered throughout the calvarium. Note that the lesions tend to coalesce when widespread.

SOLITARY MYELOMA

Infrequently, myeloma occurs as an apparently solitary lesion. Some of these pursue a relatively benign course, remaining as single lesions for years. In the majority of cases, however, the tumor eventually becomes widespread throughout the skeleton and develops into typical multiple myeloma. The average age of patients when solitary myeloma is first detected is 45 years. The tumor is more frequent in males than in females. The favorite sites for it are the spine, upper end of the femur, pelvis, and upper humerus.

Roentgen Features. In the long bones, solitary myeloma causes a central area of destruction, usually in the shaft. Expansion and some trabeculation are common with little or no periosteal reaction. The lesion resembles giant cell tumor but the location in the shaft rather than in the epiphysis and the age of the patient are important differences. In the pelvis, expansile trabeculated tumors are the rule. In the spine, some lesions show expansion and trabeculation; others are purely destructive, causing collapse of the affected body. A soft-tissue mass surrounding the vertebra is common. The tumor has a tendency to extend around the intervertebral discs to involve contiguous vertebrae. Extension into the vertebral processes is frequent.

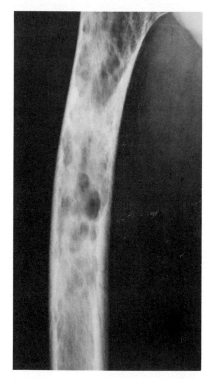

Fig. 7-33. Multiple myeloma. The midfemoral shaft is involved by a number of lytic lesions that appear to be largely within the medullary canal but extend to destroy part of the inner cortex in several areas.

LYMPHOSARCOMA

Involvement of bone by lymphosarcoma is not common and when it does happen the lesions usually are of destructive type and resemble metastatic carcinoma of osteolytic form. Rarely the bone lesions are sclerotic, and occasionally they are mixed.

HODGKIN'S DISEASE

Hodgkin's disease affects bone more frequently than does lymphosarcoma. In many instances the lesions resemble those of metastatic carcinoma very closely and the diagnosis of Hodgkin's disease cannot be made from the roentgen appearance (Fig. 7-34). Sometimes the lesions are purely destructive; at other times they are of mixed destructive and sclerotic type; in still other cases, they are mainly sclerotic. About two-thirds are mixed lytic and sclerotic; a few are lytic, and the remainder (about 10% to 15%) are sclerotic. Sclerotic lesions tend to be confined to the vertebrae ("ivory vertebrae") which are frequent sites of the disease. In some cases there is erosion of the anterior surfaces of one or several contiguous bodies, suggesting that the tumor invaded the bone by direct extension from adjacent lymph nodes. At times there may be preservation of the cortex, suggesting a form of pressure atrophy rather than invasion of the vertebra. As would be expected, the greatest incidence occurs in the upper lumbar and lower thoracic regions corresponding to the sites of prevertebral nodes. In the pelvis the lesions are of mixed osteolytic and osteoblastic type. Multiple lesions are the rule. In children, bone involvement usually indicates a poor prognosis, but in adults this is not necessarily the case.

RETICULUM CELL SARCOMA OF BONE

This infrequent tumor now is recognized as a distinct entity. In the past, most cases of reticulum cell sarcoma probably were diagnosed as Ewing's tumor, which it resembles closely. In contrast to Ewing's tumor it occurs mainly in older persons, the average age of these patients being about 40 years; it is more common in males than in females, the ratio being

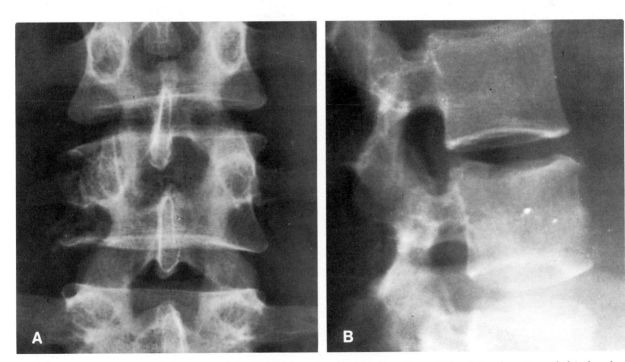

Fig. 7-34. Hodgkin's disease. **A.** Note destruction of the lateral cortex of this lumbar vertebra on one side. In the lateral view **(B)** the anterior cortex of the involved body is not clearly defined inferiorly and there appears to be a little sclerosis, indicating a mixed lytic and sclerotic type of lesion.

3:1. In about 80% of the cases the lesion involves a long tubular bone and its most frequent site is near the knee. In the upper extremities the proximal humerus is the most common site. The lesion causes ragged destruction of bone; it arises in the medullary cavity but soon involves the cortex. Periosteal proliferation is a variable finding, being absent in some cases, minimal in others, and fairly pronounced in a small percentage. Reactive bone may also appear at the tumor site. In some cases the bone lesion is associated with a large soft-tissue mass which does not contain calcium. Pathologic fracture may be the presenting complaint and is quite common. Since reticulum cell sarcoma resembles, in some cases, osteosarcoma and, in others, Ewing's tumor, it usually is impossible to make a definitive diagnosis from roentgenograms and about all that can be said is that one is dealing with a malignant bone tumor.

ACUTE LEUKEMIA

In the acute leukemias of infants and young children, changes in the bones are very common. Occasionally, bone lesions will precede the typical findings in the peripheral blood and roentgen examination may be of considerable value in suggesting the correct diagnosis. One of the early changes consists in the appearance of transverse zones of diminished density crossing the shafts of the long bones adjacent to the metaphyses (Fig. 7-35). These are somewhat similar to the "scurvy zones" seen in infantile scurvy. Fracture may occur through such a weakened area. Similar zones of demineralization are sometimes seen as a manifestation of osteoporosis. Thus, while not specific, especially during early infancy, this finding always suggests the possibility of leukemia, particularly in patients over the age of 2 years.

Another change is the development of areas of fine, patchy, bone destruction. These may be found in any bone and are often symmetric in distribution. Periosteal calcification is frequent (see Fig. 7-35). Large areas of destruction and thickening or transverse striations of the ends of the shafts may be seen. Metastatic neuroblastoma may cause similar findings, but transverse zones of rarefaction are not usual. The fine granular foci of bone destruction often are quite similar; at times they tend to be more distinct and to involve both cortical and medullary bone. Periosteal reaction is common either as calcified shadows parallel to the cortex or as fine, whisker-like striations perpendicular to the cortex. In the skull, spreading of the sutures, patchy bone destruc-

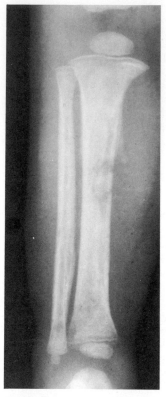

Fig. 7-35. Leukemia involving the tibia. There are poorly defined areas of destruction as well as periosteal calcification forming a Codman's triangle on the medial aspect of the tibia. Note the thin, translucent band crossing the upper and lower metaphyses of the tibia and, to a lesser extent, of the fibula.

tion, and fine vertical spicules along the surfaces of the tables are seen in neuroblastoma but also can occur at times in leukemia.

CHRONIC MYELOID LEUKEMIA

While involvement of the bone marrow is frequent in myelogenous leukemia, the disease rarely causes distinct roentgen changes other than, perhaps, a nonspecific osteoporosis. Osteosclerosis has been described as occurring in this disease. However, it seems likely that most cases so diagnosed are actually examples of myelofibrosis which terminate with a leukemoid blood picture (see next paragraph). It is not to be expected, therefore, that roentgen examination of the skeleton will yield any significant information in most patients having this disease.

MYELOFIBROSIS WITH OSTEOSCLEROSIS

This is now recognized by most investigators as a separate disease entity, closely related to myeloid leukemia, but not a variant of it. Myelofibrosis runs a relatively benign course and in approximately half of the patients osteosclerosis will develop. The disease is also known as nonleukemic myelosis, agnogenic myeloid metaplasia, osteosclerotic anemia, and leukoerythroblastic anemia, to mention only a few. It may be of the idiopathic variety, which is the most common, or be secondary to some other disease such as polycythemia vera. It is estimated that from 10% to 20% of cases of polycythemia vera terminate with the picture of myelofibrosis. Clinically there are anemia; a normal, lowered, or moderately elevated white blood cell count; the constant presence of immature red and white cells in the peripheral blood; and significant enlargement of the spleen and often of the liver. When osteosclerosis is present it is often widely distributed throughout the bones of the trunk and some of the bones of the extremities, particularly the humerus and femur. In smaller bones such as the ribs there may be a uniform increase in density with loss of much of the trabecular architecture. In larger bones such as the femur the sclerosis is more mottled and patchy in distribution (Fig. 7-36). In the femur the earliest changes can often be recognized in the distal end. When diffuse increase in density of the skeleton is encountered in an adult, one should think first of the possibility of this disease being present. Osteoblastic metastasis is rarely distributed as uniformly. Osteopetrosis (marble bones) is essentially a disease of the young.

GAUCHER'S DISEASE AND NIEMANN–PICK DISEASE

Gaucher's disease is not a tumor but a metabolic disorder characterized by the abnormal deposition of cerebrosides in the reticuloendothelial cells of the spleen, liver, and bone marrow. These develop a characteristic histologic appearance and are known as *Gaucher's cells.* Replacement of the bone marrow by these cells may lead to patchy areas of destruction which may simulate tumors such as myeloma. In some cases there is only a rather generalized demineralization. If the disease has existed for some time, expansion of the lower end of the femur may occur resulting in the so-called "Erlenmeyer flask" appearance. This is suggestive but not diagnostic of Gaucher's disease. In children the disease may cause changes of ischemic necrosis in the femoral head,

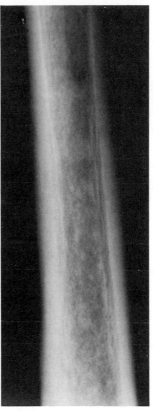

Fig. 7-36. Myelofibrosis with osteosclerosis. Anteroposterior roentgenogram of a portion of the femur of a patient with myelofibrosis. There is a mottled sclerotic increase in density distributed throughout the medullary canal. The cortex is thickened, and there are linear stripelike areas of increased density along the internal cortical margins which are characteristic.

most likely the result of infarction. In the adult, ischemic necrosis of the head of the femur is less comon unless manifestations of the disease date back to childhood. Involvement of the vertebrae may lead to collapse of one or more bodies. In the long bones there may be numerous sharply circumscribed osteolytic defects resembling, to some extent, the lesions of metastatic carcinoma or even multiple myeloma. The cortex is thinned and scalloped internally and there may be periosteal calcification over the involved area. Occasionally, sclerotic areas are present. The skull is rarely affected, and the same is true of the hands and feet. A very large spleen and a moderately enlarged liver are clinical features of this disease and roentgen evidence, particularly of the splenomegaly, will be present.

Niemann–Pick disease apparently is a very rare variant of Gaucher's disease occurring in families of whom about 50% are Jews. It, too, is a form of lipid reticulosis, the lipid at fault being sphingomyelin. The effect on the bones is similar to that of Gaucher's disease, but it occurs in infants (under 18 months of age) and is usually fatal within a year of its onset.

AMYLOIDOSIS

Bone lesions are occasionally found in primary amyloidosis. The upper part of the humerus and the proximal femur are the most frequent sites. The lesions are caused by replacement of bone by large deposits of amyloid and appear, roentgenologically, as well-demarcated areas of destruction. This appearance is not specific and the diagnosis is made on other grounds such as the abnormal serum protein patterns.

According to Weinfeld, Stern, and Marx,[34] amyloid lesions may occur in two forms: (*1*) In the first type large deposits of amyloid may occur in and around the major joints; these are visualized roentgenologically as soft-tissue swellings. The masses may invade contiguous bones causing multiple small erosions. (*2*) In the second form there is diffuse infiltration of the marrow causing generalized demineralization with collapse of vertebral bodies, resembling multiple myeloma or other diseases causing diffuse demineralization. Or, there may be more localized areas of bone lysis as noted above. Weinfeld and associates also found ischemic necrosis of the femoral head in one patient caused by the deposition of amyloid in and around the blood vessels of the bone marrow. Subluxation may be caused by pressure of a deposit of amyloid within a joint, but there is usually no involvement of articular bone.

HISTIOCYTOSIS X

The terms "reticuloendotheliosis," "reticulosis," and "histiocytosis X" are synonymous and include Letterer–Siwe disease (nonlipid reticulosis), Hand–Schüller–Christian disease (xanthomatosis), and eosinophilic granuloma, since many investigators believe that these three conditions represent various manifestations of the same disorder. The basic change is a granulomatous proliferation of the reticulum cells in various parts of the body.

In Letterer-Siwe disease the lesions are widely disseminated throughout the body. It is a disease of infants and young children. The course is rapid and death occurs so early that roentgen changes often are not present even though the bone marrow may be extensively involved. There are splenomegaly, hepatomegaly, generalized lymphadenopathy, localized tumors over the bones, a tendency to hemorrhage, and a secondary anemia.

Hand–Schüller–Christian disease is a much more benign process and is characterized by the development of destructive lesions, mainly in the skull and other flat bones. It develops during late childhood, adolescence, or even during early adult life. There may be diabetes insipidus and exophthalmos (depending upon the presence of lesions involving the orbital walls and the sella). The clinical course may extend over a period of years. The bones most frequently involved are the skull, pelvis, and scapulae.

Eosinophilic granuloma is the most benign lesion of the group, usually occurring as a solitary process that may respond well to curettage or to steroid therapy. Spontaneous regression is not unknown. Eosinophilic granuloma is a lesion of childhood or of young adult life. In location, it is widely distributed throughout the skeleton but is most frequent in the skull (including the mandible), pelvis, femur, and ribs in that order of frequency. Lesions are infrequent below the knee and the elbow.

Roentgen Features. There are solitary or multiple areas of bone destruction. The edges of the individual lesion are sharply marginated, often slightly scalloped or irregular, and with no boundary zone of sclerosis. When Hand–Schüller–Christian disease involves the skull the lesions may become very large and "maplike" (Fig. 7-37). The lesions of eosinophilic granuloma tend to be small, on the order of 1 to 2 cm in diameter. In the skull, characteristically, the lesion usually involves the diploë and one or both tables, causing a sharply outlined, slightly irregular, translucent defect. A beveled appearance is common and is caused by unequal destruction of the inner and outer table. The lack of a sclerotic boundary is noteworthy (Fig. 7-38). Rarely, a small fragment of bone may remain in the cavity, resembling a sequestrum. In the long tubular bones, eosinophilic granuloma causes a somewhat different picture. An area of bone destruction is present but the lesion also may cause local expansion of the bone and there may be considerable periosteal calcification about it, forming a laminated shadow around the shaft. Thus it may resemble a bone abscess or even a Ewing's tumor (Fig. 7-39). In the mandible the lesions of histiocytosis cause destruction of bone without any sclerotic

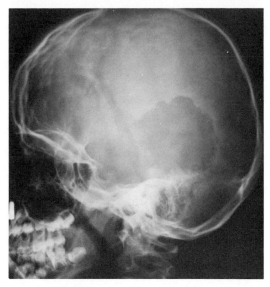

Fig. 7-37. Hand–Schüller–Christian disease. Lateral roentgenogram of the skull of a child. There is a large area of destruction in the posterior inferior parietal area. The margins of the lesions are scalloped, but there is no reactive sclerosis.

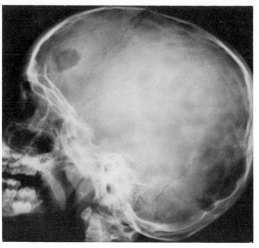

Fig. 7-38. Eosinophilic granuloma of the skull manifested by a sharply outlined destructive lesion in the frontal area.

Fig. 7-39. Eosinophilic granuloma of the lower tibial shaft. In addition to the irregular area of destruction, there is a considerable amount of surrounding sclerosis which occurs not infrequently in lesions involving weight-bearing bones.

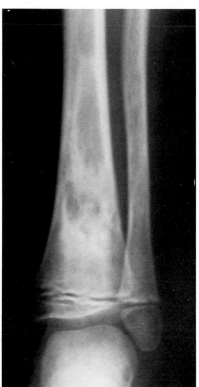

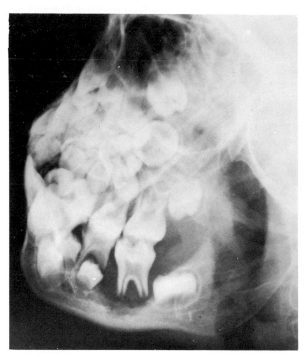

Fig. 7-40. Hand–Schüller–Christian disease. The lytic lesion in the left mandible in the region of the lower teeth results in the so-called "floating" tooth. It is surrounded by the tumor mass of soft tissue rather than by bone.

reaction. The bone may completely disappear around one or more of the teeth, causing them to appear as if they were "floating," the soft tissues that retain them not being visualized readily (Fig. 7-40). This is a highly significant finding. In the ribs the lesions may appear somewhat expansile with a slight periosteal reaction. In the vertebrae, eosinophilic granuloma may cause extensive destruction of one vertebral body leading to uniform collapse so that the body appears as a thin, "waferlike" shadow in lateral roentgenograms (Fig. 7-41). Thus this lesion is probably the most frequent cause of *vertebra plana* or *Calve's disease* (see Chapter 8). Visible and palpable soft-tissue masses may be noted in association with the bone lesions. The lesions of eosinophilic granuloma often are tender to pressure. In weight-bearing long bones, there may be some sclerosis at the site of the destructive lesion; pathologic fracture and periosteal new bone formation may also be observed. (see Fig. 7-39). Pulmonary involvement occasionally is seen in the form of fine nodular shadows with reticulation scattered throughout the parenchyma.

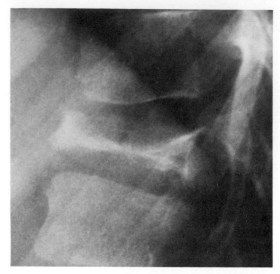

Fig. 7-41. Eosinophilic granuloma involving a vertebral body. The vertebra is considerably compressed but may in time become even thinner and more waferlike in appearance.

MISCELLANEOUS TUMORS
NEUROFIBROMA

The condition "neurofibromatosis" or "von Recklinghausen's disease" has been discussed in Chapter 2. Neurofibroma occurring as a solitary lesion without the other stigmata of von Recklinghausen's disease is a moderately common lesion. As it involves bone, the roentgen findings are generally similar to those seen in the multiple form of the disease. Neurofibroma of an intercostal nerve causes a soft-tissue mass adjacent to a rib and often with pressure erosion of the cortex of the rib. The rib interspace may be locally widened if the mass is of appreciable size. Tumors arising from a spinal nerve root often are of "dumbbell" type with intra- and extraspinal extensions. Erosion of vertebral pedicles adjacent to the mass is commonly seen and the intraspinal part of the mass may cause a concavity of the posterior surface of the vertebral body (Fig. 7-42). The extraspinal component can be visualized as a rounded, soft-tissue mass adjacent to the spine in the thoracic area. In the lumbar spine the extraspinal mass usually cannot be seen unless very large, when it may cause a lateral bulge of the psoas muscle margin. Neurofibroma of a long tubular bone may cause a localized cystlike translucency in the shaft. Occa-

sionally it is seen as a small excavation in the cortex of the bone, described as a "pit" or "cave" defect. Neurofibromas of the cranial nerves often cause enlargement of the corresponding foramen. The acoustic nerve is the most frequent site of the tumor within the skull.

FIBROSARCOMA

Fibrosarcoma of the soft tissues has a great tendency to invade the bone by direct extension. This tumor may arise from the outer layer of the periosteum, which does not have osteogenic properties, or it may arise from tendon sheaths or other fibrous tissue. At first only the roentgen density of the soft-tissue mass is present. Occasionally flecks or larger deposits of calcium are noted within the mass. Later, evidence of invasion of the adjacent bone is seen. This is characterized by local erosion of the outer surface of the cortex at first, and later, by extension of the destruction into the medullary canal. This may become severe enough to cause pathologic fracture. When the destruction of bone is this far advanced it may be impossible to determine whether the lesion originated within the bone or extrinsic to it. Rarely, a fibrosarcoma arises within a bone, causing a local destructive

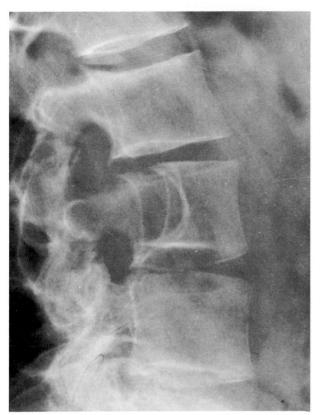

Fig. 7-42. Neurofibroma. A large neurofibroma arising from a lumbar nerve root has resulted in pressure erosion of the posterior aspect of the vertebral body and also of the posterior elements at the site of the lesion.

lesion that cannot be distinguished from other malignant tumors, particularly metastatic carcinoma.

MALIGNANT FIBROUS HISTIOCYTOMA OF BONE

There is a benign as well as a malignant form of this rare disease, sometimes termed "fibrous xanthoma."[13] The soft tissues tend to be involved more often than bone and, in this situation, direct extension into bone may occur. However, the disease may originate in bone producing an osteolytic lesion that may destroy the cortex or expand bone, particularly in ribs. Periosteal reaction may occur and pathologic fracture is common. Location is metaphyseal in long bones. In the spine, posterior elements are involved as frequently as vertebrae. The femur is the most commonly involved bone.

CHOLESTEATOMA (EPIDERMOID CYST)

A sharply marginated, cystic-appearing tumor is occasionally encountered in the cranial bones, usually in children or young adults, which, pathologically, shows a lining of squamous epithelium and with the cyst filled with a mushy, pearly colored material consisting of cholesterol and cellular debris. These are known as cholesteatomas or epidermoidomas. When the cyst is lined only by squamous epithelium, the term "epidermoid cyst" is used. When dermal structures (hair, teeth, etc.) also are included the lesion is known as a dermoid cyst.

In the skull, epidermoid cysts usually are of congenital origin arising from epidermoid inclusions at the time of closure of the neural groove or of other epithelial fusion lines. A similar lesion is found in the hands, usually in a terminal phalanx; these are believed to be acquired owing to trauma with implantation of epidermoid cells at the time of injury. Epidermoid cysts also may follow a surgical procedure or a spinal puncture and thus have been found in episiotomy scars, in the cecum following appendectomy, and in the spinal canal.[27] In the skull the lesion arises in the diploic space and expands the tables and thins them (Fig. 7-43). Viewed *en face* it appears as a sharply outlined, rounded or ovoid area of bone deficit with a thin surrounding zone of sclerosis. The edge of the defect is often slightly scalloped in places, a rather characteristic finding. Viewed tangentially it will be seen that the tables have been expanded symmetrically. The tumor grows very slowly and at first may be asymptomatic except for the deformity caused by the mass. When large it may cause the signs and symptoms of brain tumor because of the intracranial portion of the mass. Those that develop in or near the base of the skull may cause symptoms of pressure on the contiguous cranial nerves plus the evidence of increased intracranial pressure.

The epidermoid inclusion cyst usually found in the distal phalanx of the hand is usually a sharply circumscribed, round or oval destructive lesion, often with a very clearly defined border or a thin sclerotic rim marking the border between it and the adjacent bone.

TERATOMA

A teratoma is, fundamentally, an attempt at formation of a new individual within the tissues of another. A malignant tumor, either carcinoma or sarcoma, may develop within a teratoma and the lesion then is

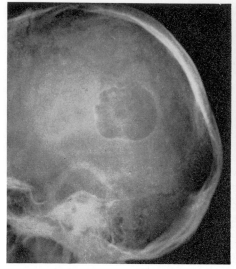
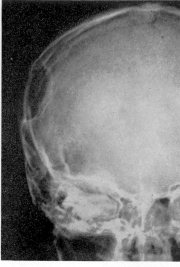

Fig. 7-43. Cholesteatoma of the cranial vault. There is an area of rarefaction surrounded by a thin zone of dense bone that is somewhat scalloped in appearance. On the original film the frontal projection showed expansion of the tables, a characteristic of this lesion.

commonly referred to as a malignant teratoma. There are two sites where external teratomatous malformations are most frequently encountered—the upper jaw and the sacrococcygeal area. In either location a mass of tissue, usually composed of all germinal layers, projects from the body. Because practically all teratomas contain bone or calcified cartilage, the nature of the mass can be recognized by roentgen examination. The characteristic locations, the presence of the mass at birth, and the finding of bone or calcification within it are reliable diagnostic signs (7-44). The normal structure, jaw or sacrum, to which the teratoma is attached, often shows abnormal ossification and may be grossly distorted.

Other sacrococcygeal masses include meningocele and myelomeningocele, chordoma, neurofibroma, hemangioma, ependymoma, and glomus tumor. Meningoceles are usually more proximal than teratoma, and are associated with defects in the spine; the others tend to be more internal in that they tend to lie within the pelvis.

CHORDOMA

Chordoma is an infrequent tumor that arises from remnants of the fetal notochord. This is discussed in Chapter 3. The two common sites for chordoma are at the cervico-occipital junction and in the sacral or sacrococcygeal area. It is in these locations that notochordal remnants most frequently occur. The tumor is a rather slowly growing one, of a low degree of malignancy, that spreads by infiltration, metastasizing only in the late stages of growth. Roentgenologically,

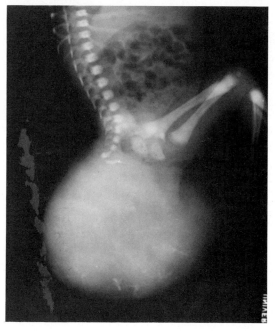

Fig. 7-44. Sacrococcygeal teratoma. This large mass found in a newborn infant contains scattered areas of calcification and bone. The lower sacrum and coccyx are deformed.

chordoma causes localized destruction of bone and evidence of a soft-tissue mass. In the cervico-occipital lesions, destruction of the clivus, the margins of the foramen magnum, or portions of the upper cervical vertebrae may be found and there may be flocculent calcification posterior to the clivus at the site of the tumor mass. The mass may project into the retropharyngeal space and cause a demonstrable thickening of the soft tissues. In the sacral region, the lesion usually causes a sharply marginated area of destruction, often involving a large part of the sacrum. The mass displaces the rectum forward and may compress it. There is usually very little in the appearance of the lesion to establish the diagnosis from roentgen findings alone, but whenever localized bone destruction is found in either of these two characteristic regions, one should consider the possibility of a chordoma.

INTRAOSSEOUS GANGLION

This rare lesion[12] is believed to arise from intramedullary fibroplasia followed by secondary degenerative and cystic changes. Its most frequent site is in the tubular bones of the lower extremities. It usually arises in the epiphysis or adjacent metaphysis. Roentgen findings are those of an eccentric, lytic, sharply circumscirbed defect at the end of a long bone. Most of these lesions are unilocular, about one-third have sclerotic margins; expansion of bone and cortical thinning are uncommon. Intraosseous ganglion must be differentiated from a number of local lytic bone lesions occurring at the ends of long tubular bones.

REFERENCES AND SELECTED READINGS

1. AAKUS T, EID O, STOKKE T: Parosteal osteogenic sarcoma. Acta Radiol [Suppl] (Stockh) 54: 29, 1960
2. AEGERTER E, KIRKPATRICK JA JR: Orthopedic Diseases, 4th ed. Philadelphia, Saunders, 1975
3. AMSTUTZ HC, CAREY EJ: Skeletal manifestations and treatment of Gaucher's disease. Review of twenty cases. J Bone Joint Surg [A] 48: 670, 1966
4. BEALS RK, BIRD CB: Carpal and tarsal osteolysis. J Bone Joint Surg [A] 57: 681, 1975
5. BRADY LW, CROLL MN: Clinical uses of bone scanning. Skeletal Radiol 1: 161, 1977
6. BROWER AC, CULVER JE JR, KEATS TE: Diffuse cystic angiomatosis of bone. Am J Roentgenol 118: 456, 1973
7. BUONOCORE E, SOLOMON A, KERLEY HE: Pseudomyeloma. Radiology 95: 41, 1970
8. CAMPBELL CJ, HARKESS J: Fibrous metaphyseal defect of bone. Surg Gynecol Obstet 104: 329, 1957
9. DAHLIN AC, IVINS JC: Benign chondroblastoma: a study of 125 cases. Cancer 30: 401, 1972
10. FALK S, ALPERT M: The clinical and roentgen aspects of Ewing's sarcoma. Am J Med Sci 250: 492, 1965
11. FELDMAN F, HECHT HL, JOHNSTON AD: Chondromyxoid fibroma of bone. Radiology 94: 249, 1970
12. FELDMAN F, JOHNSTON A: Intra-osseous ganglion. Am J Roentgenol 118: 328, 1973
13. FELDMAN F, LATTES R: Primary malignant fibrous histiocytoma (fibrous xanthoma) of bone. Skeletal Radiol 1: 145, 1977
14. FREIBERGER RH, LOITMAN BS, HELPERN M et al: Osteoid osteoma. A report of 80 cases. Am J Roentgenol 82: 194, 1959
15. GIUSTRA PE, FREIBERGER RH: Severe growth disturbance with osteoid osteoma. Radiology 96: 285, 1970
16. Goldenberg RR, Campbell CJ, Bonfiglio M: Giant cell tumor: an analysis of two hundred and eighteen cases. J Bone Joint Surg [A] 52: 619, 1970
17. GREENFIELD GB: Bone changes in chronic adult Gaucher's disease. Am J Roentgenol 110: 800, 1970
18. GROSSMAN RE, HENSLEY GT: Bone lesions in primary amyloidosis. Am J Roentgenol 101: 872, 1967
19. HUNT JC, PUGH DG: Skeletal lesions in neurofibromatosis. Radiology 76: 1, 1961
20. JOHNSON PM, MCCLURE JG: Observations on massive osteolysis: a review of the literature and report of a case. Radiology 71: 28, 1958
21. KOHLER E, BABBITT D, HUIZENGA B et al: Hereditary osteolysis. Radiology 108: 99, 1973
22. LODWICK GS: In Hodes PH (ed): Atlas of Tumor Radiology: The Bones and Joints, Vol 4. Chicago, Year Book Medical, 1971
23. McGAVRAN MH, SPADY HA: Eosinophilic granuloma of bone. J Bone Joint Surg [A] 42: 979, 1960
24. McLEOD RA, BEABOUT JW: Roentgenographic features of chondroblastoma. Am J Roentgenol 118: 464, 1973
25. McLEOD RA, DAHLIN DC, BEABOUT JW: Spectrum of osteoblastoma. Am J Roentgenol 126: 321, 1976
26. MESCAROS WT: The many facets of multiple myeloma. Semin Roentgenol 9: 219, 1974
27. PEAR BL: Epidermoid and dermoid sequestration cysts. Am J Roentgenol 110: 148, 1970
28. REYNOLDS J: The "fallen fragment sign" in the diagnosis of unicameral bone cysts. Radiology 92: 949, 1969
29. ROCKWELL MA, SAITER ET, ENNEKING WF: Periosteal chondroma. J Bone Joint Surg [A] 54: 102, 1972
30. SHERMAN RS, SOONG KY: A roentgen study of osteogenic sarcoma developing in Paget's disease. Radiology 63: 48, 1954

31. TILLMAN BP, DAHLIN DC, LIPSCOMB PR et al: Aneurysmal bone cyst: an analysis of ninety-five cases. Mayo Clin Proc 43: 415, 1967

32. TURCOTTE B, PUGH DG, DAHLIN DC: The roentgenologic aspects of chondromyxoid fibroma of bone. Am J Roentgenol 87: 1085, 1962

33. VAN DER HUEL RO, VON RONNEN JR: Juxtacortical osteosarcoma. J Bone Joint Surg [A] 49: 415, 1967

34. WEINFELD A, STERN MH, MARX LH: Amyloid lesions of bone. Am J Roentgenol 108: 799, 1970

8

MISCELLANEOUS CONDITIONS

ISCHEMIC NECROSIS; OSTEOCHONDROSIS

The *osteochondroses* or *ischemic necroses* comprise a group of lesions, usually involving an epiphyseal ossification center or one of the small bones of the hand or foot of a child or adolescent. It is becoming apparent that these terms have been used in the past to designate two essentially different conditions. In the one group, the *ischemic necroses,* occlusion of blood vessels supplying a portion of the bone will lead to death of the bone supplied by the vessels. In the other group, the *osteochondroses,* trauma is being stressed as a causative factor, either as an avulsion injury or as a chronic stress type of fracture. A few of the entities are difficult to classify because the pathogenesis still is uncertain. At one time or another practically every epiphyseal ossification center in the body has been described as the site of osteochondrosis or ischemic necrosis and an eponym has been attached to each. It now is recognized that some of these represent only variations in normal ossification and that others should more properly be classified as a form of injury (Table 8-1). Some of the eponyms have become firmly established in the literature and it is difficult to eliminate them.

EPIPHYSEAL AND SMALL BONE LESIONS IN CHILDREN

Capital Femoral Epiphysis

Ischemic necrosis of the proximal epiphysis of the femur is more commonly known as *Perthes' disease* or *Legg–Calvé–Perthes' disease.* Other names applied to this lesion include *osteochondritis deformans* and *coxa plana.* The etiology of Perthes' disease has been debatable. Some authors have classified it as the idiopathic type of ischemic necrosis based on study of resected specimens even though occlusion of major arteries often cannot be demonstrated. The pathology is one of degeneration and necrosis followed by eventual replacement of the necrotic osseous tissue when revascularization occurs. Trauma or repeated microtrauma has often been considered as a cause with injury to the vessels supplying the epiphysis. Caffey[1] has presented evidence which he believes indicates that the early lesion is a form of chronic stress or fa-

239

Table 8-1. Ischemic Necrosis; Osteochondrosis

I. Epiphyseal and Small Bone Lesions in Children
  A. Capital Femoral Epiphysis
  B. Other Areas
      1. Tarsal scaphoid
      2. Tibial tuberosity
      3. Vertebral epiphyses
      4. Second matatarsal head
      5. Apophysis of os calcis
      6. Osteochondritis dissecans
      7. Epiphyseolysis
      8. Others
II. Epiphyseal Ischemic Necrosis Secondary to Other Diseases
III. Ischemic Necrosis of the Ends of the Bones in Adults
  A. The head of the femur
  B. Other areas
IV. Bone Infarction of the Diaphyses

tigue fracture, the ischemic necrosis being a later manifestation and secondary to the fracture. His findings again emphasize the role of trauma in the so-called osteochondroses.

Perthes' disease is a benign condition that runs a self-limited course with eventual healing. Because this takes several years or longer, the epiphyseal ossification center and femoral neck undergo change in shape; permanent deformity usually follows and often leads to the early development of degenerative joint disease. It is a disease of childhood and is more frequent in boys than in girls. It is bilateral in about 10% of its subjects.

The relationship of skeletal maturation and the development of Perthes' disease has been evaluated by Girdany and Osman,[7] who found that, among boys, skeletal age was below normal in most and that in none was the value for skeletal maturation above the mean for the age. This observation did not hold true for girls.

The early roentgen findings in Perthes' disease are largely in the soft tissues of the joint. The joint capsule is distended with fluid and the joint space may be widened slightly. Also, a slight lateral displacement of the head of the femur is commonly present owing to hyperemia of the synovium and subsynovial tissues (Fig. 8-1). These changes often are subtle and require careful observation for detection. If the hip is put at rest at this stage, often the signs and symptoms will disappear and the joint will return to normal. Some consider changes of this nature, with disappearance after a period of rest leaving little or no residuals, as indicative of the entity known as *transient synovitis of the hip*. In a review of cases by Nachemson and Scheller,[18] 6% of patients initially thought to have transient synovitis of the hip later developed Perthes' disease. In the remainder the condition almost completely cleared with only minor residual changes in a small percentage (slight increase in size of the femoral head on the affected side, a few cortical cysts, and dense spots in the femoral neck). Since there may be a relationship between transient synovitis and ischemic necrosis, these patients

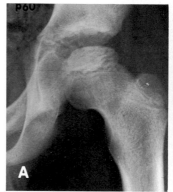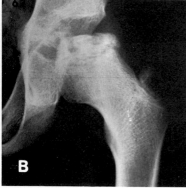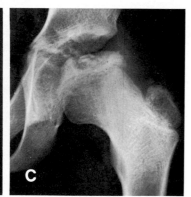

Fig. 8-1. Perthes' disease. **A.** Early film showing slight uniform increase in density of the femoral head, several thin, irregular fissures within it, and widening of the joint space as compared to the opposite, normal hip. **B.** Film obtained 10 months later shows more flattening of the femoral head and increased density with lucent areas of bone resorption as well. **C.** In the film obtained 5 months following that shown in **B** the central fragment appears to lie within a cavity and is fragmented. Elsewhere the density is more normal, but the flattening persists.

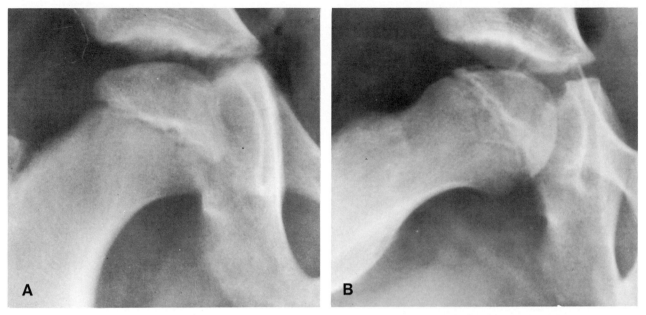

Fig. 8-2. Perthes' disease. **A.** In the anteroposterior projection the superior aspect of the capital epiphysis appears slightly flattened, but the density is normal. **B.** In the lateral projection a thin, translucent zone is noted in the subchondral bone superiorly. This is considered to represent a stress fracture through necrotic bone. It is often the earliest sign of Perthes' disease.

should be followed until signs and symptoms have disappeared.

The first change in the femoral head in Perthes' disease usually is a thin arclike translucent zone which develops in the subchondral bone close to the bony articular surface along the anterosuperior aspect of the epiphyseal ossification center. This has been considered to represent a stress fracture occurring through the necrotic bone (Fig. 8-2). Caffey[2] has described the occurrence in some patients of a thin, dark line adjacent to the fracture which he believes is a fissure in the bone filled with gas from the blood or tissue fluids. Martel and Poznanski[16] and others have demonstrated an increased lucency of the radiolucent crescent line in ischemic necrosis of the femoral head in adults when traction was applied to the leg and which they believe is caused by release of gas secondary to the vacuum caused by the traction. Intra-epiphyseal gas has also been reported in the humeral capitellum in patients with ischemic necrosis, usually when some traction is exerted. In other patients there is a slight flattening of the center and irregularity of its superior articular surface (see Fig. 8-1). At times, during this early stage, the entire center will show a slight uniform increase in density.

This is more apparent than real owing to disuse osteoporosis in the viable bone immediately adjacent (*e.g.,* the acetabulum and femoral neck). The head, having lost its blood supply, maintains the density of normal bone and it keeps this density until revascularization takes place.

The next well-defined stage is represented by crushing and fragmentation of the epiphysis or a portion of it (Figs. 8-3 and 8-4). The extent of involvement of the epiphysis varies among patients. In some the entire center is affected; in others the changes are limited to an area of subchondral bone along the superior aspect of the head. Once revascularization has taken place, dead bone can be removed. In some patients this happens before much new bone has been formed and large areas of the epiphysis will be absorbed. In other patients, reossification occurs before dead bone has been removed, the new bone being laid down on the scaffolding formed by the dead trabeculae. The increased thickness of the trabeculae causes increased density of the epiphysis and this is probably the major cause of the increased density of the head or its fragments at this stage of the disease. Compression of the bone causes impaction of trabeculae and this may add to the increased radi-

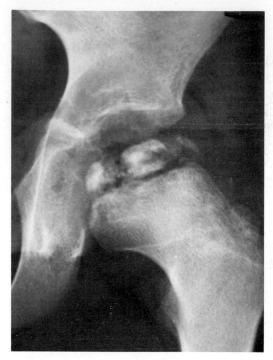

Fig. 8-3. Perthes' disease. Advanced disease showing marked flattening of the femoral epiphysis, several dense, white fragments, and areas of absorption. The joint space is wide. The neck of the femur is broad, and the epiphyseal line is wider than normal.

opacity. At this stage the revascularization process is well advanced and reossification is taking place. Eventually the dead trabeculae are removed and the center returns to a normal density. However, in some cases, the old trabeculae may never be removed and the increased radiopacity of the head persists after healing is complete.[5] Reossification begins adjacent to the epiphyseal plate and the subchondral bone next to the articular surface is the last to ossify. Healing is a slow process and may require several years or longer.

During the active stage of the disease there often is a slight widening of the epiphyseal line. (The epiphyseal cartilage derives its blood supply from the same vessels that supply the head). The surface of the metaphysis becomes irregular, sometimes with small cystic areas, and the femoral neck broadened and foreshortened (see Fig. 8-3). The acetabulum is not involved in Perthes' disease but, because of disuse, ossification of it lags behind that of the opposite hip and it develops a wavy contour.

The major late complication of ischemic necrosis of the femoral head in children is premature degenerative disease of the hip joint which is generally directly proportional to the amount of residual deformity of the femoral head. Another late complication is an increase in the incidence of osteochondritis dissecans of the femoral head in patients who have had juvenile Perthes' disease. In one study the average interval between the diagnosis of ischemic necrosis and the appearance of osteochondritis was found to be 8.8 years. The site is usually the superior lateral aspect of the femoral head. Separation of the bony fragment from its bed is uncommon in these patients. Discomfort in a hip previously affected by Perthes' disease should suggest the possibility of osteochondritis dissecans.

Other Areas

Some of the more common sites where osteochondrosis has been said to occur are described in the following paragraphs. As noted previously, some of these now are recognized as being either avulsion

Fig. 8-4. Perthes' disease. The capital epiphysis is flattened, fragmented, and irregular in density.

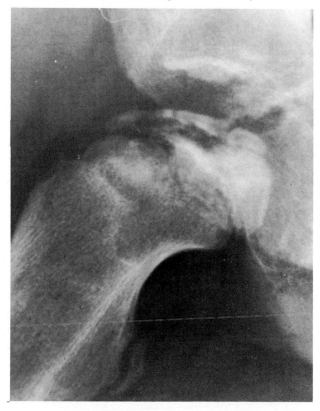

fractures or chronic fatigue fractures instead of primary ischemic necrosis.

The Tarsal Scaphoid (Köhler's Disease). Infrequently the tarsal scaphoid may be involved by a process similar to Perthes' disease (Fig. 8-5). It occurs during childhood and the roentgen findings consist of flattening and crushing, increased density, and a tendency for fragmentation of the bone. In some patients the lesion has been asymptomatic.

The Tibial Tuberosity (Osgood–Schlatter Disease). The tibial tuberosity develops as a tonguelike extension on the anterior aspect of the proximal tibial epiphysis. While the major part of this epiphysis begins to ossify at or shortly before birth, the tuberosity remains cartilaginous until late childhood. When it does begin to ossify it frequently does so from one or more centers; these fuse to the major part of the epiphysis within a relatively short time and subsequently the entire epiphysis fuses to the shaft. The tuberosity serves for the attachment of the patellar tendon and thus is readily subjected to injury. Most investigators believe that this lesion represents either a fracture of the tuberosity or the sequelae of previous fracture. The lesion also may represent a stress or fatigue type of fracture of the tuberosity rather than an ischemic necrosis. It is more frequent in boys than in girls and is more common during adolescence (*i.e.*, 13 to 15 years). When the lesion develops the ossified portion of the tuberosity becomes ragged in outline, it often fragments, and it may develop irregular increase in density (Fig. 8-6). The inferior portion often is elevated slightly from its normal position. Localized swelling of the soft tissues over the tuberosity can be visualized. The roentgen diagnosis of osteochondrosis of the tibial tuberosity should be made with caution and the findings correlated with clinical symptoms and signs. There is considerable variation in the appearance of the normal tuberosity during the process of ossification. It may ossify from several centers and its inferior portion may be elevated. The appearance may resemble rather closely that seen in osteochondrosis. Visualization of soft-tissue swelling over the tuberosity plus the clinical signs of pain and local tenderness should be present before the diagnosis of Osgood–Schlatter disease is made. As a sequela to healing, some of the fragmented portions may not unite but remain as small, round or ovoid bony shadows.

Vertebral Epiphyses (Scheuermann's Disease). At about the ages of 13 to 15 there appear narrow ring-like epiphyses along the upper and lower margins of the vertebral bodies. These may be involved by an osteochondrosis, particularly those in the midthoracic area. Pain is often present, particularly early in the development of the condition. The epiphyseal plates lose their sharp outlines and regular appearances; they often become fragmented and somewhat sclerotic. The adjacent border of the vertebral body becomes irregular. Probably because of disturbance in growth, such vertebrae tend to become wedge-shaped with decrease in height anteriorly and this in turn leads to a dorsal kyphosis (Fig. 8-7). While involvement of several or many vertebral bodies is the rule, occasionally the disease may be confined to only one or two. After the disease has healed, some irregularity of the disc surfaces persists and the anterior wedging and kyphotic deformity continue throughout life. Deficiency of the anterior portions of the epiphyseal plates may cause a notchlike defect along the anterior corners of the bodies. Schmorl's nodes also are common. These are seen as small, concave defects on the disc surfaces of one or more vertebrae. They are said to be caused by the softness of the vertebral body, allowing protrusion of disc material into it. However, their presence also suggests that the fault is a defect in ossification of the vertebral endplate allowing herniation of the nucleus pulposis of the disc into the body and that the process is one of faulty ossification. Some investigators have expressed doubt that the vertebral epiphyses are ever affected by ischemic necrosis; rather, they believe that the irregularities in contour, anterior wedge deformities, and the dorsal kyphosis represent the effects of faulty ossification.

Second Metatarsal Head (Köhler–Freiberg Infraction). This lesion is found in the head of the second metatarsal, less commonly in the third and the first. Although originally considered by Köhler to be a form of aseptic necrosis it now is generally considered to represent an infraction or a stress type of fracture involving the metatarsal head. It is found during late adolescence. The articular end of the bone becomes flattened, sometimes concave, and irregular. With healing the neck of the metatarsal becomes thickened and sclerotic (Fig. 8-8). Tiny fragments of bone may become separated from the articular surface and remain as small ossicles after healing is complete. Degenerative joint disease is commonly a late complication.

Apophysis of Os Calcis. The apophysis of the os calcis is an epiphyseal plate that develops along the posterior border of the bone. It has been reported as

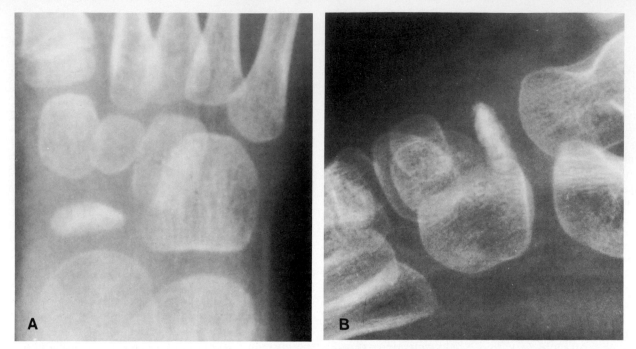

Fig. 8-5. Osteochondritis of the tarsal scaphoid in frontal **(A)** and lateral **(B)** positions. Note the dense, flat bone characteristic of this lesion (Köhler's disease).

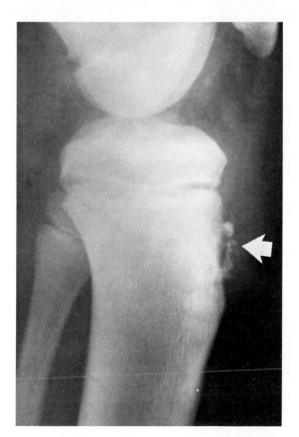

Fig. 8-6. Osgood–Schlatter disease of the tibial tuberosity. The epiphysis is fragmented (arrow), and local soft-tissue swelling was observed on the original film.

made with caution and is seldom justified on roentgenologic grounds alone.

Osteochondritis Dissecans. This lesion is a form of ischemic necrosis but one that involves only a small portion of bone, usually the articular surface of the medial condyle of the femur. It occurs in young adults after epiphyseal closure, chiefly in males, and is characterized by the gradual separation of a button-shaped fragment of bone and cartilage from the condylar surface (Fig. 8-9). It is bilateral in about 20% of these patients. The disease shows an unusual tendency for involving this particular site for reasons that are not clear. The fragment may separate completely from its bed and become a loose body within the joint cavity, leaving a shallow defect in the articular surface of the femur. If it does not become completely separated the button of bone may remain within its cavity either becoming absorbed or eventually developing a new blood supply and becoming revitalized. Less frequently, this lesion is found in

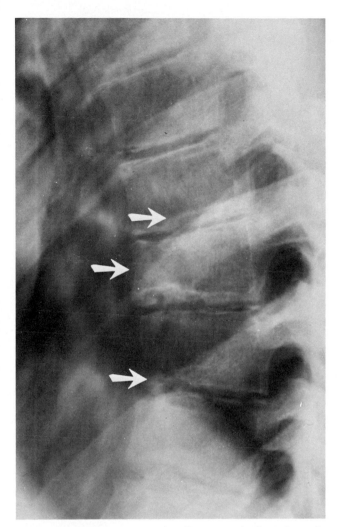

Fig. 8-7. Scheuermann's disease of the thoracic spine. One of the vertebrae **(central arrow)** is wedge-shaped and its disc surface is irregular. The latter change appears to be caused by fragmentation of the ring epiphyses, particularly the inferior. There is minor involvement with Schmorl-node defects in several of the other bodies **(upper and lower arrows).**

the site of an osteochondrosis with the apophysis becoming dense and sclerotic and undergoing fragmentation. It has been considered to be a frequent cause for painful heels in children. This apophysis normally varies a great deal in density and in many normal children it has a uniform chalky white appearance; it may ossify from several centers. The diagnosis of osteochondrosis involving it should be

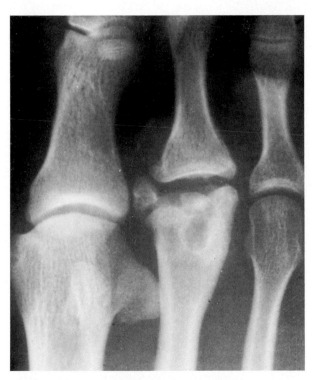

Fig. 8-8. Köhler–Freiberg infraction of the head of the second metatarsal. The distal end shows an irregular, concave articular surface, and the head and neck are generally thickened. This is a characteristic appearance of this lesion.

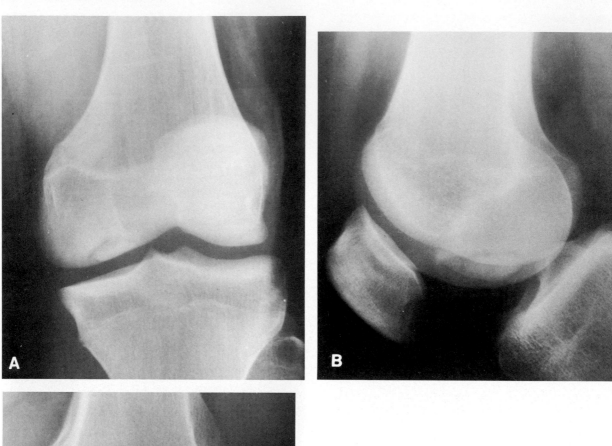

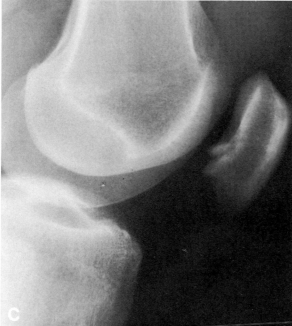

Fig. 8-9. A and **B.** Osteochondritis dissecans of the medial condyle of the femur. In **A,** the buttonlike fragment of bone lies surrounded by an area of radiolucency. The fragment is denser than the remainder of the bone. In the lateral view **(B)** the fragment is quite clearly outlined along the surface of he medial femoral condyle. **C.** Osteochondritis dissecans of the patella. Note the resemblance between this smaller area of necrotic bone and the one in **A** and **B.**

other areas, particularly in the head of the femur, the astragalus, the elbow, the shoulder, and the patella.

Epiphysiolysis (Slipping of the Capital Femoral Epiphysis). This lesion has been classified by some as an ischemic necrosis affecting the epiphyseal plate of the proximal end of the femur; the head of the femur does not become avascular. Most writers, however, believe that the lesion is most likely caused by trauma, either in the form of an acute injury or, more often, a stress type of injury. Before epiphyseal closure, the periosteum is thinned and weakened and the normal cortical thickness has not been attained, making the epiphysis more susceptible to stress than at any other time. The lesion develops during adolescence (10 to 18 years) and is most frequent in overweight boys of the Froelich type. There is an increased incidence of epiphysiolysis in renal osteodystrophy. The lesion is a gradual slipping of the femoral head on the neck or, more correctly, of the neck on the head as the head remains in the acetabulum. There is upward displacement, external rotation, and adduction of the neck on the head, so that the head is displaced posteriorly and downward. The early deformity is seen to best advantage in a lateral or "frog" view of the hip (Fig. 8-10). In straight anteroposterior views the displacement may not be apparent. There is widening of the epiphyseal line and

irregularity of the surface of the metaphysis. The lesion progresses slowly over a period of several years. Since growth is proceeding during this time the neck of the femur is remodeled to some extent. It develops a convex superior surface instead of the normal concavity; the characteristic appearance is seen in straight anteroposterior views (Fig. 8-11). When the epiphysis fuses the lesion stops progressing but any deformity that has occurred will be permanent. As with Perthes' disease, the early development of degenerative joint disease in the hip is a frequent complication.

In addition to the foregoing, many other epiphyseal centers have been reported as sites of osteochondrosis. Thus the disease has been described as occurring in the epiphyseal plates along the lateral margins of the sacrum, in the carpal scaphoid, and in other locations. An example of one of the rare lesions is *Calvé's vertebra plana.* In this lesion a single vertebral body undergoes a uniform compression and flattening until it comes to resemble a thin disc. A number of cases have been reported in which this configuration has been found to result from involvement of the vertebral body by an *eosinophilic granuloma.* It has also been seen in Hand–Schüller–Christian disease. When this type of lesion is encountered in a child, the diagnosis of histiocytosis usually is justified. These observations again emphasize the need for

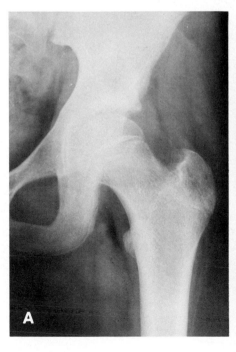
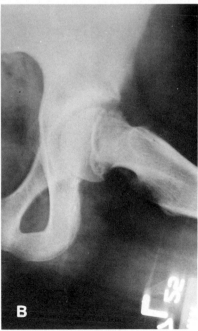

Fig. 8-10. Epiphysiolysis. **A.** No definite abnormality is observed in this projection. **B.** Lateral roentgenogram of the same hip obtained at the same time as the frontal one shows the displacement of the epiphysis and the irregularity of the metaphysis which was not as well seen on the frontal projection. A lateral roentgenogram is necessary to make the diagnosis early.

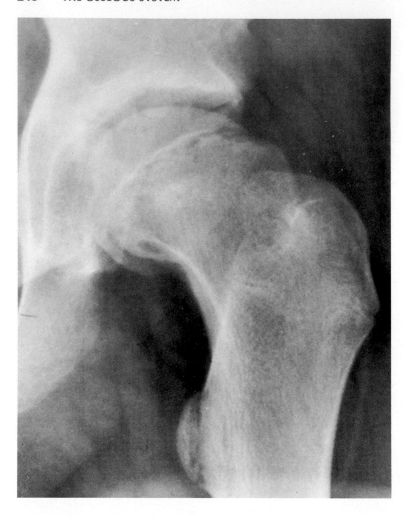

Fig. 8-11. Epiphysiolysis. Note the medial position of capital epiphysis on the femoral neck which is broad. There is a little irregularity of the epiphyseal line, and there is convexity of the upper femoral neck in contrast to the concavity in this area observed in the normal femur.

caution whenever the diagnosis of osteochondrosis is a consideration in the growing skeleton.

EPIPHYSEAL ISCHEMIC NECROSIS SECONDARY TO OTHER DISEASE

There are several generalized diseases and toxic agents that can cause ischemic necrosis of an epiphysis, particularly that for the head of the femur, by occlusion of the vessels supplying the epiphysis. The causes of ischemic necrosis in adults are listed in the section on "Ischemic Necrosis of the Ends of Bones in the Adult"; some of these will also be found in children. In sickle cell anemia, thrombosis is considered to be the cause of the occlusion. In Gaucher's disease the medullary spaces are filled with Gaucher's cells and the vessels are occluded by

pressure. A similar situation may exist in the histiocytoses. In still other entities the mechanism of vascular compromise has not been entirely clarified. Repeated trauma or microtrauma may be responsible in some of these patients in whom the bone and joint structures may have been rendered less sensitive or insensitive to pain.

When the capital femoral epiphysis is the site of the lesion, the roentgen appearance resembles that of Perthes' disease. However, the metaphysis may not be involved as it is in Perthes' disease and the lesion often develops at a later age period. Also, other areas of ischemic necrosis may be found not only in epiphyses but also as infarcts involving the shafts of the long and short tubular bones or the vertebrae and the causative disease may have been identified previously.

ISCHEMIC NECROSIS OF THE ENDS OF BONES IN THE ADULT

Changes in the articular ends of the bones in adults that suggest ischemic necrosis are relatively common. The head of the femur is most frequently involved but other bones may be the sites of the disease. As in the child, these changes appear to have two major causes: (1) trauma and, (2) vascular occlusion. Posttraumatic changes may follow a single, acute injury or be the result of repeated episodes of trauma or microtrauma. A list of the diseases or toxic agents that may cause ischemic necrosis and that have been mentioned in the literature follows.

1. Acute trauma—fracture or dislocation
2. Caisson disease
3. Steroid therapy
4. Cushing's disease
5. Gaucher's disease
6. Histiocytosis
7. Sickle cell anemia
8. Radiation therapy
9. Pain-relieving drugs other than steroids
10. Chronic alcoholism
11. Chronic pancreatitis
12. Arteriosclerosis
13. Gout
14. Systemic lupus erythematosis
15. Pregnancy (rare)
16. Idiopathic

In several of these diseases there is diminished quantity or quality of bone, making the bone more susceptible to stresses; this may lead to trabecular fractures followed by osteonecrosis. Multiple lesions are often observed in many of the conditions.

The Head of the Femur

Following acute injury, either a fracture of the femoral neck or a dislocation of the femoral head, there may be sufficient disruption of the blood supply to the femoral head so that a portion of it undergoes ischemic necrosis.

The area of femoral head involved usually is the superior portion where weight-bearing stress is greatest. The lesion may not develop until some time after healing of the fracture, particularly if operative procedures on the hip have been performed, or it may begin immediately after the injury. During the early stage the area of devitalized bone usually appears denser than the adjacent viable bone and may be separated from it by a thin lucent zone. The increased density in this early stage is most likely owing to osteoporosis in the adjacent viable bone. The dead bone, having no blood supply, cannot change density and thus maintains the appearance of normal bone until revascularization has taken place. The dead fragment often has a triangular shape with the apex pointing toward the femoral neck. Later, the fragment undergoes compression, causing flattening of the articular surface of the head and it may separate into several pieces. The lucent zone becomes more distinct and a dense sclerotic reaction develops in the viable bone adjacent to the dead fragment (Fig. 8-12). Healing is a slow process with revascularization followed by removal of dead bone and the deposition of new bone.

A similar lesion may develop from a variety of other causes as listed in the preceding section. In many of these the early appearance resembles Perthes' disease with the presence of a thin, curved or arclike translucent zone separating a narrow fragment of subchondral bone from the articular surface. Fragmentation and crushing of the subchondral bone develop and further progress is similar to that seen in Perthes' disease. This appearance is frequent when ischemic necrosis develops after steroid therapy (Fig. 8-13) or in Cushing's disease. It may be rapidly destructive in patients with renal transplantation on steroid therapy, particularly if the renal transplant fails. Rarely, ischemic necrosis of the femoral head in adults may present as a lytic lesion with a sclerotic rim resembling chondroblastoma.[8] It is usually a round or oval lesion which occurs in adolescents and young adults. In older adults the border of the lesion is partially angular or straight. In caisson disease and in sickle cell anemia there often are associated shaft infarctions that are visible roentgenologically. In some patients no causative lesion is apparent and this is known as the idiopathic form of the disease. Many of these hips also show evidence of well-marked degenerative joint disease.

The pathogenesis of ischemic necrosis developing in chronic alcoholics and in persons with chronic pancreatitis is uncertain although several theories have been proposed including that of fat embolism. However, the high incidence of trauma, often unremembered, in chronic alcoholics is well known. The frequency of chronic subdural hematoma in these individuals is noteworthy. The same factors may be operative in the causation of ischemic necrosis of bone. Many patients with chronic pancreatitis also suffer from chronic alcoholism and the relationship may be significant. In acute pancreatitis, multiple lytic bone

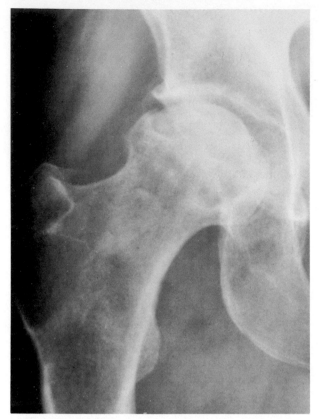

Fig. 8-12. Ischemic necrosis of the femoral head in an adult. The dense femoral head is somewhat impacted with the poorly defined linear lucency noted laterally at the demarcation between normal and ischemic bone.

lesions have been reported; these progress rapidly (in a period of 10 days or so), destroying cortical and cancellous bone with little, if any, periosteal reaction. This is thought to be caused by metastatic fat necrosis.

Other Areas

Either as a result of a single injury or following repeated minor traumas, the carpal lunate may develop changes suggesting ischemic necrosis. This lesion has been known as *Kienbock's malacia.* The bone becomes flattened in contour, increased in density, and may fragment (Fig. 8-14). The proximal fragment of a fractured carpal navicular may develop a similar type of change. Normally, the blood supply to this part of the bone is poor.

Spontaneous ischemic necrosis of the medial fem-

oral condyle that differs from osteochondritis dissecans has been reported.[27] This occurs in the elderly and is associated with much more pain and no antecedent trauma, in contrast to the usual form of osteochondritis dissecans of the medial femoral condyle. The pain precedes roentgenographic evidence of disease, often by months. Eventually, flattening and irregularity of the medial femoral condyle, followed by a semilunar break in the condylar margin surrounded by irregular sclerosis, are noted on the roentgenogram. The sequestrum formed is usually not detached and the lesion tends to be larger than those in young patients.

A fracture through the neck of the astragalus very often is followed by ischemic necrosis of the articular portion of the bone.

Ischemia is manifested by relative density when surrounding bone becomes osteoporotic (Fig. 8-15). Evidence of revascularization consists of diffuse and irregular mottled areas of opacity and lucency within

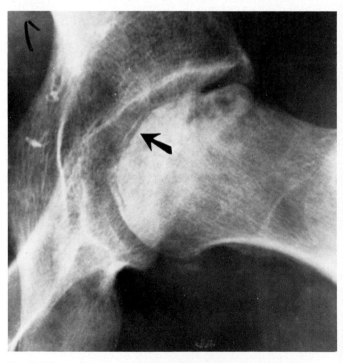

Fig. 8-13. Ischemic necrosis of the head of the femur after steroid therapy. Note the thin, lucent crescent separating the narrow fragment of subchondral bone **(arrow).** The head is moderately flattened and generally sclerotic except for areas of absorption superiorly. The acetabulum and joint space are not involved.

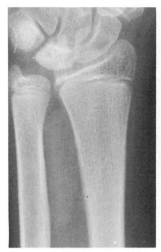
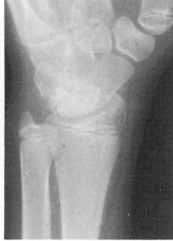
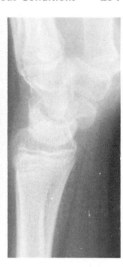

Fig. 8-14. Ischemia of the carpal lunate (Kienböck's). Note the density of the lunate as compared to that in the remaining carpal bones in this child.

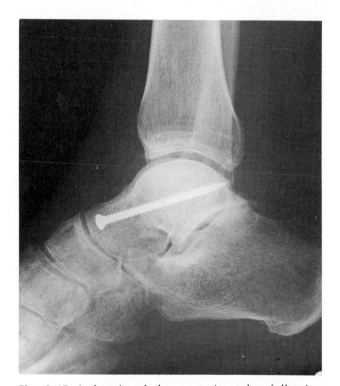

Fig. 8-15. Ischemia of the posterior talus following fracture. This examination, made 4 weeks after open reduction of the fracture, shows the posterior fragment to be much denser, and therefore ischemic, as compared to the anterior fragment. The actual fracture line is not visible because of the close apposition of fragments.

the involved bone; this may take months or years to develop.

Kümmel's disease has been considered to be an avascular necrosis of a vertebral body that develops after an injury, with no roentgen evidence of fracture immediately after the injury. The lesion, however, may very well be an unrecognized fracture with compression of the vertebral body occurring later because of continued weight bearing. It occurs infrequently and some authors have expressed doubt of its existence.

BONE INFARCTION OF THE DIAPHYSIS

In addition to infarcts in the subchondral areas of bone, infarction may involve an area in the shaft and with a different roentgen appearance. In some diseases, such as sickle cell anemia and caisson disease, infarction may occur in both areas. Also in sickle cell anemia, infarction of one or more of the short tubular bones may occur (*i.e.,* the "hand–foot syndrome"). At other times only shaft infarction is seen. Not infrequently bone infarction is completely asymptomatic and roentgen changes are found by chance on examination for some other reason. The role of arteriosclerosis in causation of the infarction in these cases is difficult to assess.

During the acute stage of an infarct of the diaphysis there are no roentgen changes. Infarcted bone does not undergo change in density because there are no vessels to carry minerals away or bring new minerals in. Not until revascularization takes place does the density of the infarcted area change. Then the dead bone is gradually removed and the area becomes irregularly calcified. Usually there is a thin rim of sclerosis bounding the lesion (Fig. 8-16). The "scar" of the infarct apparently remains throughout the rest of the life of the individual. Infarction of the shafts of the short tubular bones in the hands and feet in sickle cell anemia has a different appearance and resembles osteomyelitis very closely. Both infarction and infection may be present in the same patient. Sclerotic areas—sclerotic bone islands and cysts—are not positive evidence of osteonecrosis, however, because these variations may be found in normal subjects who have had no barotrauma and have no systemic disease capable of producing bone infarcts.

Irregular calcification of cartilage islands that have failed to ossify during the course of bone growth may lead to a rather similar appearance in the long bones.

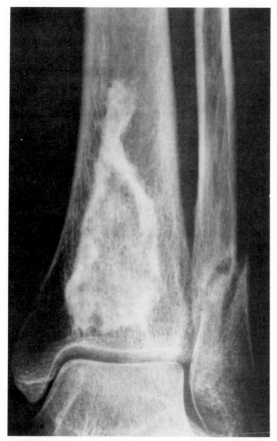

Fig. 8-16. Bone infarct. The "scar" of the infarct remains as a triangular area of sclerosis bounded by a sclerotic rim. Examination was performed because of the fracture noted in the lateral malleolus.

These have been termed *calcified enchondromas* or *calcified medullary defects* (Fig. 8-17). Differentiation from a healed bone infarct may be difficult and probably is unnecessary in most instances. Calcified enchondromas are likely to be more mottled in appearance and without a rim of density marking off the boundary as is noted in infarction.

CHEMICAL POISONING
LEAD POISONING

While lead is deposited in the bones of adults, it produces no recognizable alteration in the roentgen shadows of the osseous system and roentgen examination cannot be expected to yield any important information. If lead poisoning occurs before endochondral bone growth is completed, however, changes do occur that may be of considerable value in arriving at the correct diagnosis. The significant alteration is the appearance of dense transverse bands extending across the metaphyses of the long bones and along the margins of the flat bones, such as the iliac crest (Fig. 8-18). The width of the "lead line" varies and depends upon the amount of lead ingested and the length of time it has been taken. It has been shown that the increased density is not caused by lead alone but also by increased calcium content. This results from a failure of proper absorption of calcium from the zones of provisional calcification. Approximately 3 months after inhalation of lead and 6 months after ingestion of lead, the "lead line" can be observed in growing bone. Except for the development of these transverse zones of density, the bones and epiphyses remain normal. Because ingested lead shot may cause lead poisoning, abdominal films should be obtained as a part of the investigation in persons suspected of having lead poisoning. Also, when children have unexplained cerebral symptoms that may be caused by lead, a roentgenogram of the knee is indicated, since nearly all children with lead encephalopathy will demonstrate definite bony "lead lines." After the intake of lead has been discontinued, normal bone forms on the epiphyseal side of the metaphysis and the lead line appears to migrate into the shaft. It usually becomes wider and less dense for a time and then gradually disappears. In normal active infants the metaphyses of the long bones often show an unusual whiteness and appear wider than one might expect. This should not be confused with lead poisoning. The incidence of lead poisoning in infants is low except in children living in "inner-core" areas of large cities.

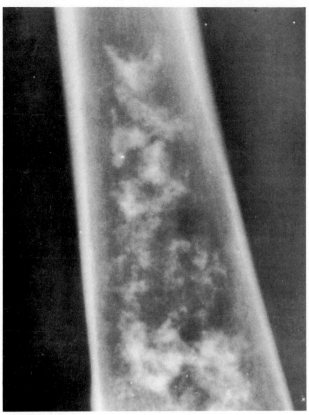

Fig. 8-17. Calcified enchondroma. This close-up view of the lower femur shows the characteristic mottled calcification within the medullary canal. Note the lack of a boundary rim of sclerosis and the small rounded areas of lucency representing islands of uncalcified cartilage. This figure should be compared with Figure 8-16, since infarcts and enchondromas may be similar in some instances.

PHOSPHORUS POISONING

At one time, phosphorus poisoning was a serious health hazard during infancy but this is no longer the case. The possibilities for obtaining yellow phosphorus are negligible at the present time. The ingestion of this substance in sufficient amounts produces changes that are indistinguishable from those resulting from the ingestion of lead.

BISMUTH POISONING

Poisoning from bismuth usually has followed the administration of large doses of this substance for the treatment of congenital syphilis. Bismuth produces changes exactly like those caused by lead and, as with phosphorus, cannot be differentiated from lead poisoning on the basis of roentgen examination (Fig. 8-19).

FLUORINE INTOXICATION

Fluorine poisoning is a rare cause of abnormal bones and is found mainly in adults, either as a result of exposure to high concentrations of fluorides as an occupational hazard or from drinking water containing a high concentration of these substances. There are only a few areas in the United States where such concentrations occur in the drinking water and these are chiefly in certain parts of Texas. In industry the mining and conversion of phosphate rock into fertilizer and the use of fluorides in the smelting of metals offer possible sources for poisoning. The major alteration in the skeleton is a diffuse increase in density. The bones appear abnormally white. The trabecular architecture is accentuated. The cortices become thickened. Calcific spurs may form at the sites of ligament attachments and calcification may be observed in the interosseous membrane of the forearm. Coarse sclerosis of the spine and pelvis is usually present. In spite of rather marked alteration in the bones, there usually are few symptoms referable to the condition and the patients may be surprisingly healthy. Fluoride poisoning must be considered as an unusual cause of generalized increase in density of the bones in this country.

HYPERVITAMINOSIS D

Excessive intake of vitamin D may lead to changes demonstrable by roentgenographic examination. Hypervitaminosis D in adults has been seen most frequently in patients with rheumatoid arthritis who were treated with large doses of vitamin D. It has also been found in children to whom excessive doses or errors in dosage have occurred. The serum calcium is elevated and the urine calcium is high. On roentgen examination of adults there may be found: (*1*) Deposition of calcium in the soft tissues, particularly around the joints. These deposits have an amorphous puttylike appearance. Calcification of the arteries may be noted even in the young. Renal calcification often occurs. (*2*) Chronic decalcification of the skeleton is frequent. Since many of these patients have rheumatoid arthritis and this disease usually is accompanied by skeletal decalcification, this finding may be difficult to evaluate.

In infancy, hypervitaminosis D usually follows

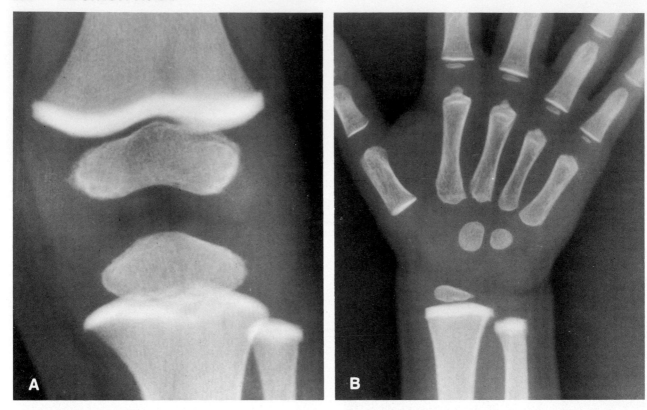

Fig. 8-18. Lead poisoning. The dense metaphyses of the femur, tibia, and fibula are shown in **A.** In **B,** similar densities are noted in the distal radius and ulna and to a lesser extent in the metaphyses of the long bones of the hand. The marked density is characteristic of heavy metal poisoning.

errors in dosage. It results in metastatic calcification in the media of the blood vessels, kidneys, heart, gastric wall, falx cerebri, tentorium, and adrenals. In the tubular bones there is widening of the zones of provisional calcification, causing dense bands extending across the metaphyses similar to those noted in lead poisoning. Later, there may be cortical thickening. Also, in the later stages there may be alternating bands of increased and decreased density crossing the ends of the shafts and an overall osteoporosis.

IDIOPATHIC HYPERCALCEMIA

In this rare disorder there is an abnormally high level of calcium in the blood, causing an osteosclerosis similar to that seen in some patients with osteopetrosis (marble bone disease) and in infants with hypervitaminosis D. The cause is obscure, but it has been suggested that the disease may represent an unusual sensitivity to vitamin D. According to Aegerter and Kirkpatrick, the disease has been more prevalent in England than in the United States and in the past the amounts of vitamin D supplement in foods were not well regulated in Britain. It has been suggested that some infants may have ingested excessive amounts of vitamin in food and as a result developed vitamin D poisoning. More recently, stricter controls and limits have been put into effect and the incidence of the disease has decreased considerably. The clinical observations mirror the effects of the hypercalcemia and include muscular weakness and hypotonia, anorexia, vomiting, and failure of the infant to thrive and to develop properly. There is mental as well as physical retardation. The roentgen findings are essentially the same as those found in hypervitaminosis D (Fig. 8-20). The most specific sign in both is the demonstration of calcium in the falx, tentorium, and gastric wall during infancy.

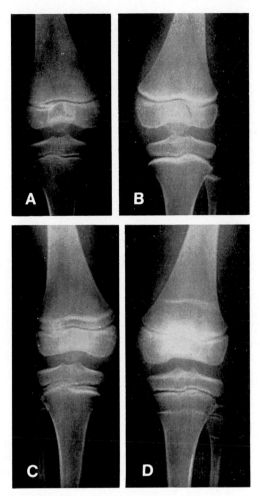

Fig. 8-19. Bismuth lines. This child was treated with bismuth preparations for treatment of congenital syphilis. **A.** The knee before administration of bismuth. **B.** Note the metaphyseal density shortly after completion of the bismuth therapy. **C.** Several months later the bismuth lines have migrated into the shafts of the femur and tibia. **D.** One year after treatment further migration of the bismuth line into the shaft is noted. This is indicative of further growth. The density, however, has diminished.

HYPERVITAMINOSIS A

Vitamin A poisoning from excessive administration is seen most frequently in the young infant as a result of errors in dosage. Clinically there are anorexia, failure to gain weight, pruritus, pain and swelling over the long bones, and hepato- and splenomegaly. The serum alkaline phosphatase may be increased and the serum proteins lowered. The level of vitamin A in the blood serum is high. On roentgen examination one may find periosteal calcification, mainly around the central shafts of some of the long bones. The bones most frequently affected are the ulna and clavicle; next in frequency are the femur and tibia. The periosteal calcification is the greatest near the center of the shaft and tapers toward the ends.

Hypervitaminosis A must be distinguished chiefly from infantile cortical hyperostosis (see the following section). In this latter disease the mandible is almost always affected and is usually the first bone to be in-

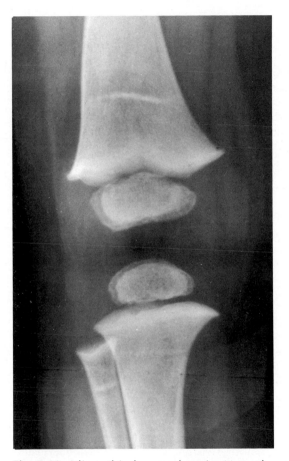

Fig. 8-20. Idiopathic hypercalcemia. Note the poorly demarcated dense zones extending across the metaphyses; remnants of similar zones are noted in the shafts. Several of these dense bands may be observed in some of these patients. The changes resemble those of heavy metal poisoning and are similar to those found in association with hypervitaminosis D.

volved. Both diseases are accompanied by fever and the other signs of infection. Infantile cortical hyperostosis develops early in life within the first few weeks or months; vitamin A poisoning usually occurs somewhat later, rarely before the child is 1 year old. The final diagnosis rests upon the history of the administration of excessive amounts of vitamin A and the determination of the level of vitamin A in the serum.

INFANTILE CORTICAL HYPEROSTOSIS (CAFFEY'S DISEASE)

This is an uncommon disease of early infancy, the cause of which is unknown. In many respects it behaves like an infection, but there is no proof of this. However, an unidentified virus may be responsible. The disease has its onset within the first few weeks of life in most cases. Occasionally it has been encountered in older children up to the age of 4½. Clinically, there is swelling of the soft tissues overlying the affected bone. The skin, however, is neither hot nor red. There are fever, irritability, and other signs suggesting an infection.

Soft-tissue edema may be observed roentgenographically when the disease is active. Histologic study reveals chronic inflammatory cells, chiefly lymphocytes, in the area of periosteal involvement and also in the medullary cavity. There is also an increase in fibrous tissue. No response to antibiotics has been reported, but there is usually a prompt clinical response to corticosteroids. A few cases have been reported in which the process reappears up to age 10 to 12 years in those who have had the disease in infancy.[25] Although the disease tends to show remissions and exacerbations, eventually recovery takes place after a period of weeks, months. The favorite sites for the development of the lesions are the mandible and the clavicles. Less frequently the ulna, radius, ribs, tibia, and fibula are affected. Apparently the mandible is nearly always involved, regardless of what other bones are affected, and this seems to be one of the characteristics of the disease. On roentgen examination there is noted a laminated subperiosteal calcification surrounding the bone. This may involve only a short segment at first but eventually may extend throughout the entire shaft of a long bone (Fig. 8-21). Not all bones are affected at the same time; some appear to be healing or improving while in others the disease becomes active or is reactivated. In the jaw the major portion of the mandible may be affected. At first the subperiosteal new bone formation

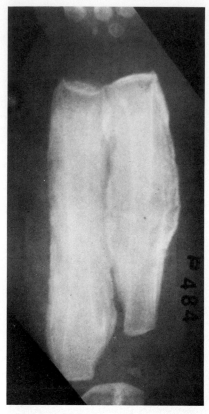

Fig. 8-21. Infantile cortical hyperostosis of the radius and ulna. There is extensive periosteal calcification surrounding the shafts of these bones. The original cortex can be faintly seen through the dense calcification.

is less dense than the cortex beneath it, but eventually the density increases and the two shadows merge (Fig. 8-22). The outer margin may be rather irregular and wavy or it may be smooth. As healing takes place, there is a gradual resorption of the subperiosteal bone formation and the bone gradually returns to a normal or nearly normal appearance. Neuhauser[19] reported a 10-week-old boy in whom osteolytic lesions were present in the skull in addition to typical hyperostosis of the clavicle and mandible. The lesions disappeared spontaneously in a few months. Lytic lesions in the skull are very rare, however. Infantile cortical hyperostosis must be differentiated from hypervitaminosis A; the history and clinical findings are very helpful in this regard. The possibility of the progressive diaphyseal sclerosis of Engelmann and Ribbing may be very difficult to exclude when making the differential diagnosis.

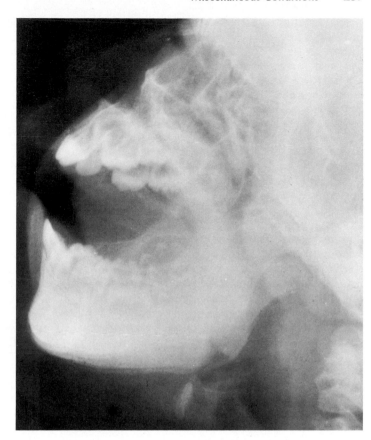

Fig. 8-22. Infantile cortical hyperostosis. This roentgenogram of the jaw of a 5-month-old male infant who had symptoms for 3 months demonstrates the characteristic appearance of cortical hyperostosis in an infant. The mandible is thick and dense, and there is a thin shell of periosteal calcification along the inferior surface.

THE EFFECTS OF FROSTBITE ON BONE

Severe frostbite causes soft-tissue swelling[26] followed by infection. When gas-forming organisms are involved, amputation is usually required. The first bone change is osteoporosis; this may be observed in 4 to 10 weeks following the incident and may persist for months. Other bone changes usually develop late—from 6 months to several years after injury. Often there is soft-tissue atrophy followed by the appearance of small areas of increased density at the ends of the involved bones, in many instances the phalanges. These late bone changes are usually noted within 12 months following frostbite and presumably represent bone infarcts. In some of these patients, small punched-out areas evolve along the articular surfaces of the involved bones; usually from 15 to 24 months are required for their development. Resorption of the terminal tuft and distal phalangeal ends is usually the result of infection but may occur in the absence of any detectable infection. When changes of the joint surfaces are severe, bony fusion may result. This is more common in children than in adults. In children, there may be fragmentation of unfused epiphyseal ossification centers leading to deformity and premature fusion along a part or all of the epiphyseal line.

EFFECTS OF RADIATION ON BONE

Damage to bone can result from heavy doses of roentgen radiation. It seems probable that the effects of the radiation are largely upon the blood vessels supplying the bone. Initially there may be hyperemia, leading to osteoporosis. In a later stage, disintegration of the bone with ischemic necrosis and pathologic fracture may result. The effects can be seen in any bone that has received a sufficient amount of radiation. Fracture of the femoral neck following pelvic irradiation for carcinoma in the female is an occasional complication of the treatment. The bone may appear surprisingly normal to roentgen examination except for the fracture. As a rule, femoral neck fractures tend to occur within a year after treatment, but there may be a delay of 5 years or more. Acetabular fractures may also result from pelvic irradiation. They are generally painless in contrast to painful femoral neck fractures. Nonunion and pseudoarthrosis are common. Areas of mixed sclerosis with zones of focal radiolucency are often observed in the sacrum and adjacent ilium. Fractures of the ribs with focal areas of absorption have been seen after repeated treatment given to the chest wall following mastectomy performed for treatment of carcinoma of the breast. These have been asymptomatic as a rule (Fig. 8-23).

Sarcoma is a very rare complication of radiation therapy. Although there is a considerable amount of evidence to show a real relationship of sarcoma to previous irradiation, there is no absolute proof of it. Osteosarcoma and fibrosarcoma are somewhat more commonly observed than chondrosarcoma in sites of previous irradiation.

Injury to the growing skeleton can be produced by heavy doses of radiation given for the treatment of a malignant lesion. Damage to the active centers of bone growth will lead to retardation or cessation of growth and consequent skeletal deformity. Changes include sclerosis and fraying of the metaphysis and widening of the epiphyseal plate, resembling the changes seen in rickets. Later, a broad band of increased metaphyseal density develops. When these signs are absent, this may indicate destruction of cartilage cells which results in a significant limb short-ening. An increased incidence of epiphysiolysis of the femoral head is also reported as a complication of pelvic irradiation, probably secondary to diminution or arrest of chondrogenesis in the metaphysis.[4]

PAGET'S DISEASE (OSTEITIS DEFORMANS)

The cause of Paget's disease is unknown. Pathologically it is characterized by destruction of bone, followed eventually by attempts at repair. The destructive phase may predominate, but most frequently there is a combination of destruction and repair. In the pelvis and the weight-bearing bones of the lower extremities, the reparative process may begin early and be a prominent feature. When widely disseminated, elevation of the serum alkaline phosphatase is present and the values may be very high. Renal calculi (or nephrocalcinosis) may develop from the hypercalciuria.

The average age of onset is between 50 and 55 years. It is increasingly rare below the age of 50 and its occurrence in young persons and children is disputed. Its incidence in men predominates over that in women in the ratio of 2:1. There are a number of reports of Paget's disease occurring in multiple members of the same family. Rosenbaum and Hanson[22] have commented on the marked difference in incidence of the disease in different geographic areas.

Paget's disease may involve any bone in the body.

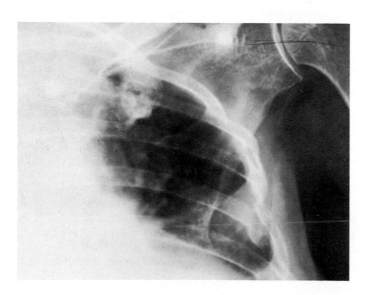

Fig. 8-23. Radiation osteitis of the ribs. This patient, who had breast carcinoma, had received intensive radiation therapy to the chest several years earlier. Note an area of absorption in the lateral arc of the fifth rib with pathologic fractures of several of the ribs, some of which have healed.

It may affect a single bone and never extend to others. It may begin in one bone with others becoming involved at a later date. At times it is widely distributed throughout the skeleton when first discovered. Its slow spread over a period of years has been observed frequently, but this does not always happen. In the order of frequency the following bones are affected: pelvis, femur, skull, tibia, vertebrae, clavicle, humerus, and ribs. Rarely, the sternum, calcaneous. talus, phalanges, metatarsals, mandible, and patella may be involved.

Roentgen Features. The roentgen appearance depends upon the extent of the reparative process that has developed. If repair (recalcification) is limited, the destructive phase predominates. This is common in the skull and is known as *osteoporosis circumscripta,* But it is also seen in other bones (Fig. 8-24). It is represented by a sharply demarcated area of decalcification within which the architecture of the bone is poorly defined. The bone also may be thickened. Characteristically, the junction between the rarefied bone and normal bone is very sharp. This lesion may enlarge slowly and later, when repair begins, islands of sclerosis develop, giving the lesion a mottled appearance. In the skull the bone becomes thickened, usually only outward, and this may be very great so that the bone measures 3 cm or more in thickness. In severe involvement of the skull, basilar invagination may result in compression of the brain stem, sometimes necessitating surgical decompression.

In the weight-bearing bones of the lower extremities a combined destructive and reparative type of the disease is the most frequent. The bones become bowed because of their softness, the femur outward and the tibia anteriorly. The cortex is thickened but of lessened density and may be mottled as is seen in the skull. The trabeculae that remain are coarse and thickened and extend in the direction required to strengthen the bone for its weight-bearing purposes. Between the coarsened trabeculae, cystlike spaces may be present. The cortex of involved bone is thickened, resulting in an increase in its diameter. The disease typically extends to one end of the long bone and may involve the entire bone. Most of the reparative abnormal new bone is periosteal, so that the medullary cavity is preserved. In severe disease, however, there may be encroachment of dense cortical bone into the cancellous bone of the medullary cavity. Although the early active osteolytic phase is not observed in long bones as frequently as in the skull, the appearance is similar. There is a clearly demarcated zone of bone destruction extending from the end of a long bone for a varying distance into the diaphysis. The periphery of the destructive lesion is clearly de-

Fig. 8-24. Paget's disease of the skull (osteoporosis circumscripta). **A.** This lateral roentgenogram of the skull shows the characteristic appearance of a large area of decreased density sharply demarcated from the normal bone above it. **B.** This lateral roentgenogram of the skull of another patient shows osteoporosis circumscripta involving the anterior and inferior portions of the skull with more normal bone above it. In the occipital area, there is more florid evidence of Paget's disease with coarse appearance of the bone, and marked thickening of bone and flattening of the basal angle.

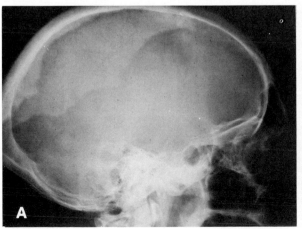
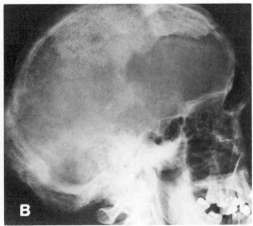

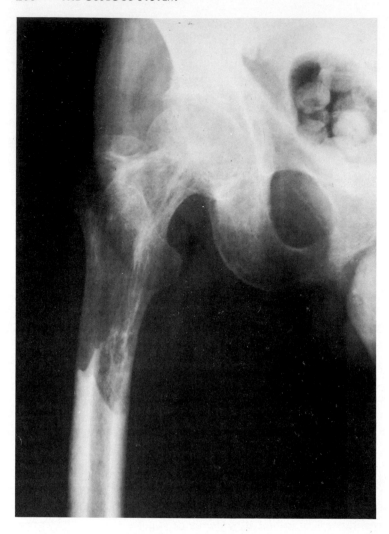

Fig. 8-25. Paget's disease of the upper femur. Note the sharply demarcated, somewhat flame-shaped edge of the lytic phase of Paget's disease projecting downward into the normal femoral cortex. Above this there is severe osteopenia. When present, this sharply defined appearance is characteristic.

marcated and often is flame-shaped (V-shaped Fig. 8-25). Inactivity such as bedrest or immobilization in a cast tends to accentuate the bone destruction. Pseudofractures (see Ch. 5) are common along the convex side of the bowed bone (Fig. 8-26). These begin as incomplete transverse fissures and they often are multiple; they may extend completely through the bone and with minor trauma a complete fracture with displacement of fragments may result. Fractures in bones involved by Paget's disease are, characteristically, transverse rather than spiral as they are in ordinary traumatic fracture.

In the pelvis a combination of destruction and repair is most frequent. Coarsening of the trabeculae is present and is best seen, early, along the iliac margins. The sacrum may be the first or the only bone

involved and the coarse trabeculation causes a distinctive cross-hatched appearance. Areas of decalcification are common in the central portions of the iliac bones, similar to those found in the skull. The reparative process occasionally predominates so that the affected bone is very dense and somewhat enlarged. The resemblance to osteoblastic metastasis is striking, but careful observation will usually show areas with the typical coarse trabeculation, which is not encountered in metastasis (Fig. 8-27). Because of softening there may be intrapelvic protrusion of the acetabular cavities. When the pelvis and femur are involved, there may be narrowing of the hip joint which is either concentric or medial, unlike the narrowing observed in degenerative disease which is on the superior or weight-bearing surface of the joint.

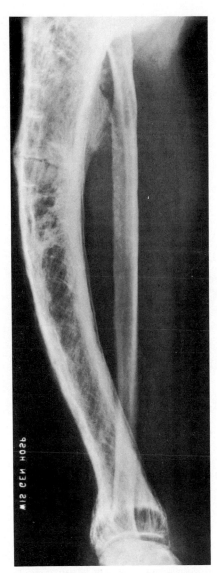

Fig. 8-26. Paget's disease of the tibia showing anterior bowing, some irregular thickening of the posterior cortex, and a number of pseudofractures of the anterior cortex. Coarse trabeculations intermingled with areas of decreased density are also observed.

Hypertrophic spurring is uncommon in Paget's disease of the hip.

In the vertebrae the disease usually affects multiple bodies but rarely all of them. Coarse trabeculation is prominent along the edges so that the margin of the body is emphasized. The general texture is coarse. The vertebra is usually enlarged. Compression fractures are frequent because of the soft-ness of the bones. Compression of the spinal cord is an occasional complication of vertebral involvement caused by increased size and compression of the vertebra with posterior protrusion of the body into the spinal canal.

In the ribs it is common to find only one or a few affected. The bone is thickened, the general density is increased, but the trabecular structure is typically coarse. The same pattern occurs in the clavicle. Osteogenic sarcoma may develop in an area of Paget's disease. Its incidence is difficult to ascertain, but in one review of 1298 patients with Paget's disease of the hip[3] there were 6 with osteosarcoma, an incidence of four- to five-tenths of 1%. Nevertheless, Paget's disease accounts for many of the cases of osteogenic sarcoma that develop in persons beyond the age of 50 years (see Fig. 7-16).

Recently, Kadir and associates[12] reported the occurrence of extramedullary hematopoiesis in two patients with Paget's disease. One had a paraspinal mass adjacent to vertebral bodies involved with Paget's disease and the other had a pelvic mass of hematopoietic tissue attached to the lateral pelvic wall which was involved with Paget's disease. The authors believe the extramedullary hematopoiesis to be secondary to pathologic fracture leading to extrusion of marrow which caused a soft-tissue mass.

CHRONIC ANEMIAS

There are a number of congenital hemolytic anemias, most of them uncommon, that can cause changes in the skeletal system. The three that are best known, roentgenologically, are: (1) Cooley's anemia, (2) sickle cell anemia, and (3) hereditary spherocytosis (familial hemolytic anemia). In addition, variants of these three and other rare hemolytic anemias can cause similar changes, although usually much milder. Also, changes in the skull similar to those of the congenital anemias have been found in chronic iron deficiency anemia, cyanotic congenital heart disease, and polycythemia vera in childhood.

The skeletal alterations are caused by erythroid hyperplasia of the bone marrow which fills and expands the cancellous bone and disturbs the trabecular architecture.

COOLEY'S ANEMIA (THALASSEMIA)

Cooley's anemia is also known as thalassemia major and Mediterranean anemia. It occurs predominately in persons inhabiting areas along the Mediterranean

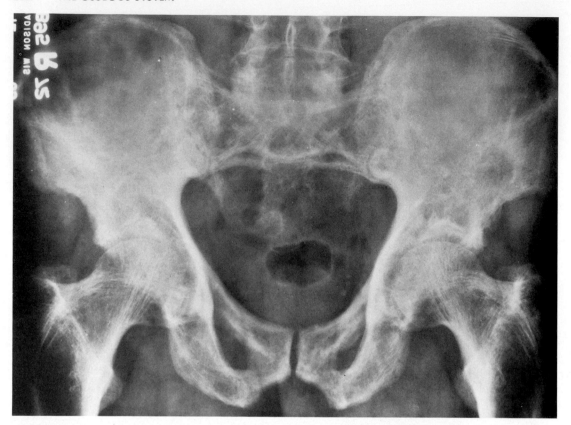

Fig. 8-27. Paget's disease of the pelvis. Note the general prominence of the trabecular pattern involving all of the bones of the pelvis, including the sacrum and the upper femurs. Minimal protrusio acetabuli is observed on the left with thickening of cortical bone medial to the acetabulum. The thickening is slightly greater than that on the right.

Sea (*i.e.,* Greeks and Italians). The disease occurs occasionally in persons of other nationalities. Cooley's anemia is the homozygous form of thalassemia inherited from both parents. The heterozygous form, thallasemia minor, is inherited from one parent. The latter usually have no skeletal stigmas and mild anemia. In adult life, there may be some vertebral osteoporosis and minimal diploic widening in the skull.

In a patient with Cooley's anemia the peripheral parts of the skeleton show roentgen changes consisting in widening of the shafts so that bones such as the metacarpals, metatarsals, and phalanges have a rectangular appearance, the normal concavity of the shafts being lost. The cortices are thinned. The medullary cavities have a spongy, mottled appearance. The trabecular pattern of the bone is coarsened (Fig. 8-28A). At times thin transverse bands of increased density, the so-called growth lines, can be seen crossing the shafts. In the skull, characteristically, there is a widening of the diploic space, particularly in the frontal and parietal regions (Fig. 8-28B). The occipital squamosa usually is not affected. The outer table is thinned and may become deficient in areas so that marrow can protrude into the subperiosteal space. Frequently there are radiating trabeculae of bone extending at right angles to the inner and outer tables giving a "hair-on-end" appearance.

In severe cases there is retardation of skeletal growth. In older patients the changes in the small bones of the hands and feet become less striking and may disappear completely by the time puberty is reached. Changes in the skull, spine, and pelvis, where red marrow persists, may become more pronounced after puberty. The paranasal sinuses may be poorly developed, particularly the maxillary sinuses. Encroachment on the sinus air spaces is caused by

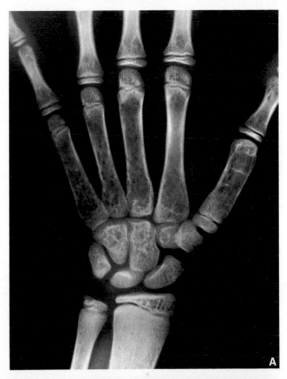

Fig. 8-28. Cooley's anemia. **A.** The phalanges are less involved than are the metacarpals. There is thinning of the
cortex with decrease in normal constriction of the midshafts.
Normal trabeculation is not observed in the areas of mottled
radiolucency. **B.** Lateral view of the skull illustrates marked
thickening of bone in the frontal area. (Courtesy of Dr. M. P.
Neal, Jr., and Dr. T. R. Howell, Richmond, Virginia)

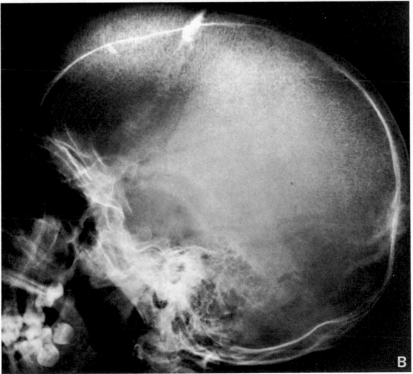

thickening of the bony walls owing to marrow hyperplasia; it does not affect the ethmoid cells because of a lack of red marrow here. Enlargement of the maxilla may lead to malocclusion and overbite on the mandible. Pathologic fracture may occur through weakened bone, although it is not common. Occasionally masses of extramedullary hematopoiesis are noted in the mediastinum. These appear as multiple, bilateral, smoothly outlined, soft-tissue masses projecting laterally in the posterior mediastinum. Apparently they arise from the bone marrow of the ribs and vertebrae that is extruded through the cortex following lysis by the expanding mass of hematopoietic tissue. Gallstones also occur as a complication of Cooley's anemia, often in young patients.

SICKLE CELL ANEMIA

This disease occurs in members of the black race as a result of an abnormal hemoglobin (hemoglobin S); it is transmitted by heredity as a dominant gene. Those who are heterozygous for the hemoglobin S gene have what is referred to as the *sickle cell trait*. Those who are homozygous for the gene, inheriting one such gene from each parent, develop sickle cell anemia.

In general the roentgen findings are similar to those in Cooley's anemia (Fig. 8-29A). Loss of bone due to marrow hyperplasia, the most common finding, results in decreased bone density. The trabecular pattern is often sparse, with wide separation resulting in a wire-mesh pattern. In addition, bone infarction is common (Fig. 8-29B). During infancy the infarcts tend to involve the small bones of the hands and feet producing a dactylitis (the "hand–foot syndrome"). This appears as an irregular area of destruction with overlying periosteal calcification resembling an inflammatory process. Since both infarction and infection may be present in the same bone differentiation is extremely difficult in many instances because both may cause rarefaction, periosteal new bone formation, and sequestration. In older children bone infarction is more common in the epiphyses. This may cause an appearance quite similar to that of Perthes' disease. There is local rarefaction of bone followed by impaction of the weight-bearing surface. Increase in subchondral bone density especially in the heads of the femur and humerus, apparently owing to previous multiple small infarctions, may be seen. The appearance of a "bone within a bone" also has been described, again probably the result of previous infarction. Osteomy-

elitis also is a complication of sickle cell anemia and may develop in any bone. Infection with *Salmonella* is frequent. Pathologic fracture is relatively common, often symmetrical, a complication of the thin bones and of infarction and infection.

In the vertebrae, osteoporosis may be quite severe, leading to compression deformities. The disc surfaces become concave as the discs expand into the softened vertebrae. Reynolds[21] believes that the vertebral contour in sickle cell anemia is characteristic, consisting of localized central depressions of the disc surfaces owing to a disturbance in growth from local ischemia rather than the biconcave contours seen in vertebral collapse of other causes. In adults with long-standing sickle cell anemia a diffuse sclerosis of the bones may be seen, resembling that found in myelofibrosis. The vertebrae, in spite of a sclerotic appearance, are softer than normal and develop biconcave disc surfaces (Fig. 8-30). This, combined with the sclerotic appearance is distinctive for sickle cell anemia in the older child or adult.

The hair-on-end appearance of the skull is infrequent, but there may be widening of the diploic space. Mottled strandlike areas of sclerosis are common in long bones. Bone-within-a-bone appearance due to medullary infarcts parallel to the endosteal cortex is found occasionally. The incidence of infarcts in the long bone tends to increase with age. However, when infarcts occur during childhood, growth disturbances may result. These consist of cupped metaphyses and triangular epiphyses, and there may be widening of the diaphysis near the metaphysis, usually in the lower femur, as a result of lack of modeling.

A sign recently reported, a tibiotalar slant, consists of a slant from above and laterally, downward and medially. This results in a high lateral aspect of the talus and adjacent tibial joint surface which conforms to the shape of the talus and is probably a growth disturbance secondary to alteration in blood supply.[21] It may be unilateral or bilateral and is not pathognomonic, since it has been reported in association with hemophilia, Still's disease, and epiphyseal dysplasia multiplex.

In addition to the bone changes there frequently is considerable cardiac enlargement and hepato- and splenomegaly. Cholelithiasis is fairly frequent and may be found in young individuals.

Sickle cell β-thalassemia is a doubly heterozygous condition in which the hemoglobin S gene is inherited from one parent and the β-thalassemia gene from the other. Bone changes are similar to those in sickle cell anemia (hemoglobin SS disease).

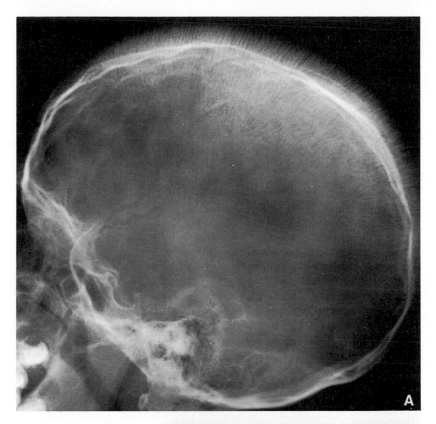

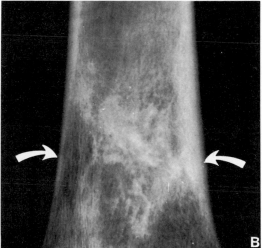

Fig. 8-29. Sickle cell anemia. **A.** Lateral view of the skull illustrating thickening of the bones of the cranial vault, particularly in the frontoparietal area where there are characteristic perpendicular striations. The outer table is indistinct in some areas and absent in others. There is also premature fusion of the sutures. **B.** An infarct of the distal shaft of the femur is observed as an irregularly calcified area **(arrows).** A similar lesion was noted in the opposite femur. (Courtesy of Dr. M. P. Neal, Jr., and Dr. T. R. Howell, Richmond, Virginia)

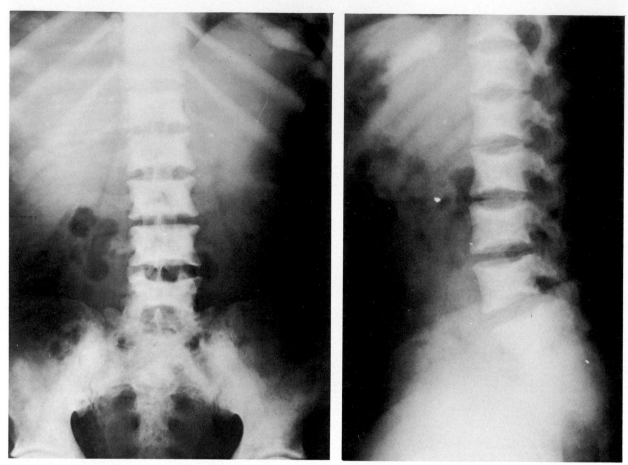

Fig. 8-30. Sickle cell anemia in an adult. The bones are increased in density, have a somewhat mottled appearance, and there is biconcavity caused by expansion of the intervertebral disc into the disc surfaces. (Courtesy of Dr. J. E. Miller, Dallas, Texas)

OTHER ANEMIAS

HEREDITARY SPHEROCYTOSIS

In hereditary spherocytosis the bones frequently are entirely normal. When changes are present they resemble those seen in Cooley's anemia, except that they are of a lesser degree and may be limited to the skull.

CHRONIC IRON-DEFICIENCY ANEMIA

Cases of iron-deficiency anemia have been reported in which skull changes occur that are quite similar to those of Cooley's anemia; we have had similar experience. There is widening of the diplöe and perpendicular trabeculation in the frontal and parietal areas. Changes in other bones, however, are less striking and these bones may be essentially normal or, at most, slightly osteoporotic, even when well-marked skull changes are present. When long and short tubular bone changes are present they resemble the findings in Cooley's anemia except that there are no facial bone changes as in Cooley's anemia.

SYSTEMIC MASTOCYTOSIS

While this disorder was originally thought to be a disease only of the skin, and known as *urticaria pigmentosa*, it is now recognized that there may be involvement of multiple systems, including the skin, lymph nodes, spleen, liver, and other organs, and the bone marrow. It is characterized by an increased number of connective-tissue mast cells in the involved tissue. The disease is of interest roentgenologically because it can cause an osteosclerosis of the skeleton. In the patients whom we have seen the osteosclerosis was in the form of generalized increase in density of the bones of the skull, thorax, spine, and pelvis. The appearance may closely resemble that seen in patients having myelofibrosis with osteosclerosis. Others have reported cases in which the changes consisted in scattered, well-defined foci of sclerosis. In still other cases, radiolucent zones have been found associated with areas of decreased density resembling mixed osteolytic and blastic metastases from which the systemic mastocytosis may be difficult to differentiate.

Systemic mastocytosis is a rare cause of osteosclerosis.

THE RUBELLA SYNDROME

During a virulent epidemic of rubella that occurred in a number of large cities in the United States in 1964, infants born of mothers who had had the disease during the first trimester of pregnancy were found to have a syndrome of anomalies affecting chiefly the cardiovascular system (congenital heart disease), the abdomen (hepatosplenomegaly), and the skeletal system.[23] The last is of importance to the present discussion.

In the skull, the anterior fontanelle is unusually large, often extending into the metopic suture. The sutures are not spread but there is deficient mineralization of the margins of the cranial bones. In the long bones, changes occur in the metaphyses, best demonstrated at the knees. The zones of provisional calcification are poorly defined and irregular. The most striking characteristic is the presence of alternating lucent and sclerotic striations extending perpendicular to the epiphyseal plate and parallel to the long axis of the bone (Fig. 8-31). These fade into normal-appearing bone in the shafts. Transverse lucent metaphyseal bands are also seen. The bone changes improve rapidly in those infants who thrive and the zones of provisional calcification regain normal smoothness and density. In those infants who do not do well clinically the abnormal trabecular pattern persists but the zones of provisional calcification show increased density.

Some delay in skeletal maturation is noted at birth or in the newborn period. This is manifested by decrease in the width of the medullary portion of the femur expressed as a percentage of the total diameter of the shaft. It is usually corrected in a few weeks.

Failure of normal modelling associated with the metaphyseal striations previously mentioned also is occasionally noted.

The most frequent cardiac lesion is a patent ductus arteriosus followed by pulmonary artery branch stenosis. Additional abnormalities include growth retardation, thrombocytopenic purpura, eye defects, and deafness. Similar skeletal changes have been reported in a patient having cytomegalic inclusion disease, therefore such changes may represent a nonspecific response to intrauterine viral infections.[17] Lack of intracranial calcifications in the rubella syndrome has been cited as a differential diagnostic feature in distinguishing this syndrome from cytomegalic inclusion disease, but recently intracranial calcifications have also been reported as occurring in patients with the rubella syndrome.

SCOLIOSIS

Scoliosis consists of a lateral curvature of the spine and rotation of the vertebrae around the long axis of the spine. The ribs on the convex side of the curve become prominent. The vertebral bodies rotate toward the convex side and the spinous processes rotate toward the concave side of the curve. Eventually the disc spaces on the concave side are narrowed, and on the convex side the discs are widened.

Scoliosis may be divided into the idiopathic form (about 70%) and scoliosis for which a cause can be found. The latter is often congenital and is due to hemivertebra, fused vertebra, neuromuscular disorders, neurofibromatosis, or any of a number of bone dysplasias. The idiopathic type is not only more common but it is often amenable to treatment. There are a number of curve patterns, but the most common is the right thoracic which extends from about T4 down to the upper lumbar spine. The thoracolumbar curve is longer and extends from T4 to L4. The lumbar curve usually runs from T11 or T12 to L5. The double major curve consists of two curves of almost equal prominence, such as a right thoracic and a left lumbar which is the most frequent of the double curves.

Radiologic evaluation of scoliosis requires upright films of the entire spine in frontal and lateral projections. If surgery is contemplated, side-bending films are taken to determine flexibility. The angle of the curve can be measured on the film. The Cobb method is used in our institution. In this method a horizontal line is drawn at the superior border of the vertebra that is at the upper end of the curve and a second horizontal line is drawn parallel to the inferior

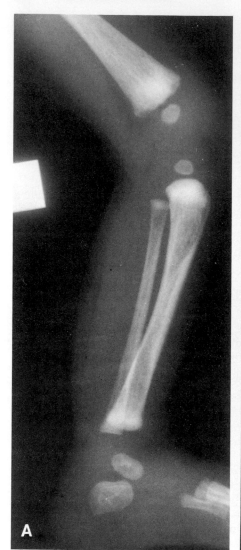
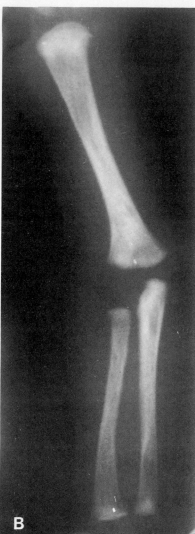

Fig. 8-31. Rubella syndrome. **A.** Note the density in the ends of the tibia and femur and to a lesser extent in the fibula with suggestion of vertical striations noted particularly in the lower end of the femur. **B.** Upper extremity of the newborn whose lower extremity was shown in **A.** There is a lesser amount of density in the zones of provisional calcification, but they are poorly defined as in the lower extremity. No transverse lucent metaphyseal bands are noted in this child.

border of the vertebra that is at the lower end of the curve. Perpendicular lines are then drawn from each of the horizontal lines, and the intersecting angles are measured. This measurement is then repeated as necessary following treatment to determine the treatment's effectiveness.

REFERENCES AND SELECTED READINGS

1. CAFFEY J: Chronic poisoning due to excess of vitamin A. Description of the clinical and roentgen manifestations in seven infants and young children. Am J Roentgenol 65: 12, 1951

2. CAFFEY J: The early roentgenographic changes in essential coxa plana: their significance in pathogenesis. Am J Roentgenol 103: 620, 1968

3. DETENBECK LC, SIM FH, JOHNSON EW: Symptomatic Paget's disease of the hip. JAMA 224: 213, 1973

4. DESMET AA, KUHNS LR, FAYOS JV et al: Effects of radiation therapy on growing long bone. Am J Roentgenol 127: 935, 1976

5. EDEIKEN J, HODES PJ, LIPSHITZ HI et al: Bone ischemia. Radiol Clin North Am 5: 515, 1967

6. GERLE RD, WALKER LA, ACHORD JL et al: Osseous changes in chronic pancreatitis. Radiology 85: 330, 1965

7. GIRDANY BR, OSMAN MZ: Longitudinal growth and skel-

etal maturation in Perthes' disease. Radiol Clin North Am 6: 245, 1968

8. GOHEL VK, DALINKA MK, EDEIKEN J: Ischemic necrosis of the femoral head simulating chondroblastoma. Radiology 107: 545, 1973

9. HOLMAN CB: Roentgenologic manifestations of vitamin D intoxication. Radiology 59: 805, 1952

10. JACOBS P: Intra-epiphyseal gas in osteochondritis. Clin Radiol 21: 318, 1970

11. JEREMY R: Nontraumatic aseptic necrosis of the femoral head. Med J Aust 1: 323, 1967

12. KADIR S, KALISHER L, SCHILLER AL: Extramedullary hematopoiesis in Paget's disease of bone. Am J Roentgenol 129: 493, 1977

13. LANZKOWSKY P: Radiological features of iron deficiency anemia. Am J Dis Child 116: 16, 1968

14. LEONE AJ JR: On lead lines. Am J Roentgenol 103: 165, 1968

15. LEONE NC, STEVENSON CA, HILBISH TF et al: Study of human population exposed to high fluoride domestic water: a ten year study. Am J Roentgenol 74: 874, 1955

16. MARTEL W, POZNANSKI AK: The effect of traction on the hip in osteonecrosis. Radiology 94: 505, 1970

17. MERTON DF, GOODING CA: Skeletal manifestations of cytomegalic inclusion disease. Radiology 94: 333, 1970

18. NACHEMSON A, SCHELLER S: A clinical and radiological follow-up study of transient synovitis of the hip. Acta Orthop Scand 40: 479, 1969

19. NEUHAUSER EBD: Infantile cortical hyperostosis and skull defects. Postgrad Med 48: 57, 1970

20. NEUHAUSER EBD, REYERSBACH GC, SOBEL EH: Hypophosphatasia. Am J Roentgenol 78: 392, 1957

21. REYNOLDS J: Radiologic manifestations of sickle cell hemoglobinopathy. JAMA 238: 247, 1977

22. ROSENBAUM HD, HANSON DJ: Geographic variation in the prevalence of Paget's disease of bone. Radiology 92: 959, 1969

23. SINGLETON EB, RUDOLPH AJ, ROSENBERG HS et al: The roentgenographic manifestations of the rubella syndrome in newborn infants. Am J Roentgenol 97: 82, 1966

24. STAHELI LT, CHURCH CC, WARD BH: Infantile cortical hyperostosis (Caffey's disease). JAMA 203: 384, 1968

25. SWERDLOFF BA, OZONOFF MB, GYEPES MT: Late recurrence of infantile cortical hyperostosis (Caffey's disease). Am J Roentgenol 108: 461, 1970

26. TISHLER JM: Soft tissue and bone changes in frostbite injury. Radiology 102: 511, 1972

27. WILLIAMS JL, CLIFF MM, BONAKDARPOUR A: Spontaneous osteonecrosis of the knee. Radiology 107: 15, 1973

9

DISEASES OF THE JOINTS

In a roentgenogram of a normal joint the ends of the bones are seen to be separated by an apparent space; this space is occupied by the articular cartilage and the small amount of synovial fluid normally present. For roentgen descriptive purposes this apparent space is commonly referred to as the "joint space." Cartilage and synovial fluid are of approximately the same degree of radiopacity and resemble the soft tissues in this respect. The opposing ends of the articular cartilages capping the bones forming a joint cannot ordinarily be identified (see section on "The Vacuum Phenomenon; Gas in the Joints"). Hyaline cartilage, once destroyed, does not regenerate to any degree and loss of articular cartilage is characterized in the roentgenogram as a diminution in the joint space. The synovial membrane cannot be visualized as a structure in roentgenograms. When the joint capsule is distended by fluid, its outer limits often can be seen if there is any fat in the periarticular tissues to offer contrast, but in the normal joint the capsule is often an indistinct structure in the roentgenogram. Periarticular edema or hemorrhage tends to obliterate the fat and tissue planes, and joint fluid distending the capsule may displace periarticular fat. Therefore, close observation of periarticular soft tissues in good quality roentgenograms will often permit detection of early signs of inflammatory disease in the joint or adjacent structures. Elbow, wrist, hand, foot, ankle, knee, and shoulder injuries also may cause similar changes. In adults the tissue planes about the hip may be difficult to define.

CLASSIFICATION OF JOINT DISEASE

I. Infectious Arthritis
  A. Acute infectious arthritis (pyogenic arthritis; septic arthritis)
  B. Chronic infectious arthritis
    1. Chronic pyogenic arthritis
    2. Tuberculous arthritis
    3. Others
II. Rheumatoid Arthritis
  A. Rheumatoid arthritis of the peripheral joints
  B. Rheumatoid arthritis of the spine
  C. Arthritis associated with scleroderma and psoriasis
  D. Still's disease and Felty's syndrome

III. Degenerative Joint Disease (osteoarthritis; osteoarthrosis, etc.)
IV. Gouty Arthritis
V. Neurotrophic Arthropathy
VI. Periarticular Disease (bursitis; tendinitis; fibrositis)
VII. Miscellaneous
    A. Hemophiliac arthropathy
    B. Pigmented villonodular synovitis
    C. Xanthomatous tumors of tendons and joints
    D. Synovioma
    E. Chondromatous tumors
        1. Osteochondromatosis
    F. Loose bodies
    G. Other conditions

INFECTIOUS ARTHRITIS

ACUTE AND CHRONIC PYOGENIC ARTHRITIS

Involvement of a joint by pyogenic organisms may be caused by a blood-stream infection, by direct extension into a joint from a focus of osteomyelitis adjacent to it, from surgical procedures on the joint, or may follow compound injuries. The clinical pattern of the disease may vary considerably. In some cases the lesion represents a relatively mild synovial inflammation that subsides and heals; it may become a purulent infection causing a pyarthrosis with rapid destruction of joint cartilages; it may follow a comparatively chronic course from the outset.

Unusual sites of pyogenic infection may be observed in patients abusing intravenous drugs, such as heroin. These include sternoclavicular and sternochondral articulations. Septic arthritis may also complicate intra-articular injection of steroids, such as in patients with rheumatoid arthritis.

Roentgen Observations

Soft-Tissue Swelling. For the first few days and perhaps for a week the only changes to be observed roentgenologically are those of soft-tissue swelling and distention of the joint capsule by fluid. This causes an increase in soft-tissue density about the joint. Periarticular edema tends to obliterate the tissue planes about the joint and may extend into the subcutaneous fat in some instances. In the absence of trauma, such findings, particularly in a febrile child with pain and/or tenderness in the area, strongly suggest the diagnosis of septic arthritis. Soft-tissue changes of this type are, of course, not specific and, at this stage of the disease, needle aspiration should be performed promptly to establish the

diagnosis or exclude the possibility of infectious arthritis as the cause of the findings.

Joint Space Narrowing. If the inflammation progresses into a purulent type with pyarthrosis, there soon develops destruction of the articular cartilages and this in turn causes a diminution in the roentgen joint space (Fig. 9-1). In this more virulent type of infection the evidence of joint space narrowing usually becomes apparent after a week or 10 days following the onset of the disease. If the disease is untreated or inadequately treated, this narrowing progresses rapidly and the joint space may have disappeared to a large extent within several weeks. Since these changes occur within a short period, there may not be sufficient time for osteoporosis to develop and the bones maintain a normal density, for a week or so. This is an important roentgen observation in determining the acute nature of the lesion since osteoporosis may be recognizable in a week and increase quickly in acute disease. It indicates the rapidly progressive nature of the infection.

Bone Destruction. This is manifested by irregularity of the subchrondral bone. The destruction may be focal at first; later, it may be more extensive. Since bone destruction isn't usually evident on roentgenograms secured before 8 to 10 days following onset of the infection, this sign is of no value in the early diagnosis.

Ankylosis. If the articular cartilages are completely destroyed, bony ankylosis usually follows. Eventually, bony trabeculae form across the ends of the bones and in time all evidence of the joint disappears.

Variations. The descriptions given in the foregoing refer mainly to an untreated or inadequately treated infection of great virulence. With present-day therapeutic measures, most cases of acute pyogenic joint infection can be brought under control before appreciable damage to the joint structures occurs. When antibiotic treatment is ineffective or is discontinued too quickly the acute infection may be transformed into a chronic indolent one with a slowly progressive course extending over a period of months. In a case of this type there is a gradual decrease in the joint space, the articular ends of the bones become roughened, and sequestra may separate from them. In time, as the infection subsides, reactive spurs form along the joint edges, the bones gradually regain density, there may be bony ankylosis, and, if not, fibrous ankylosis is likely with little or no joint motion possible (Fig. 9-2). Rarely, periarticular calcifica-

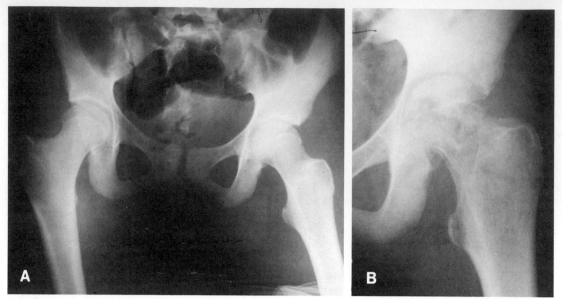

Fig. 9-1. Acute infectious arthritis of the left hip secondary to osteomyelitis. **A.** The left thigh is held in abduction and external rotation, the usual position when the hip is involved by acute inflammation. There is soft-tissue swelling which can be recognized in the upper thigh. **B.** Same hip 2½ months later. There is irregular destruction of bone in the head and neck of the femur, thinning of the joint space, and poor definition of bony articular margins.

Fig. 9-2. Chronic infectious arthritis of the knee. **A.** At the time of the patient's admission to the hospital, some erosion of bony articular surfaces medially, as well as some thinning of the joint space, is evident. **B.** Further destruction of bone and the virtual absence of joint space, indicating cartilage destruction, are evidenced 4 months later. **C.** Nine months after the onset, the infection has subsided and there is early bony ankylosis. Note that the osteoporosis secondary to the disease has persisted.

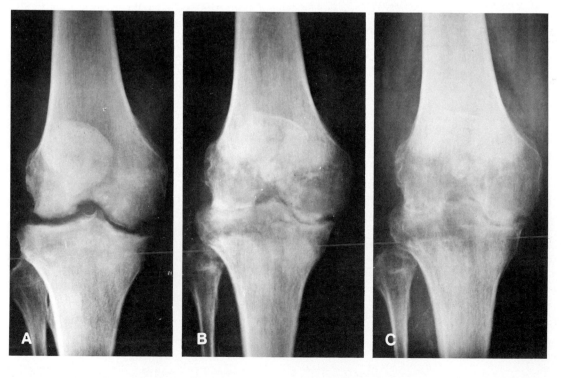

tions may be observed as a late finding, probably the result of extension of infection into the soft tissues following rupture of the capsule.

PYOGENIC ARTHRITIS IN SPECIFIC AREAS AND SITUATIONS

Intervertebral Discs

The earliest roentgen sign is a decrease in height of the disc space. Symptoms may antedate this finding by several weeks. Depending upon the virulence of the infection, there may be progressive sclerosis of subchrondral bone preceded, accompanied, or followed by evidence of bone destruction beginning with irregularity of the subchrondral margin. The sclerosis may become so extensive as to simulate ballooning of the disc. Paraspinal abscess is uncommon.

Sacroiliac Joints

Roentgen findings are variable, but there is usually some bone destruction and reactive sclerosis. These are rare but must be considered in patients with unilateral sacroiliac disease, particularly if they have staphylococcal infection elsewhere. If the infection is neglected, an accumulation of pus may cause rupture of the anterior capsule and extend into the iliac fossa, the upper thigh, the buttocks, or into the low lumbar region.

Neonatal Infections

Septic arthritis occasionally occurs in patients who have had catheterization of umbilical vessels, and also in neonates who have had femoral venipuncture. In the latter, the hip is usually involved. Lateral displacement of the upper femur is an early finding along with enlargement of soft tissues around it. This displacement can be simulated by osteomyelitis involving the epiphyseal–metaphyseal junction which causes an epiphyseal slip. Therefore, when the hip is aspirated, it is wise to inject some contrast medium into the joint (arthrogram) to make the differentiation and to be certain that the material is from the joint.

TUBERCULOUS ARTHRITIS

TUBERCULOSIS OF THE PERIPHERAL JOINTS

Tuberculosis of the joints is a chronic, indolent infection having an insidious onset and a slowly progressive course. It usually affects a single joint or, at the most, only a few joints in an individual case.

The joint disease may result from a hematogenous dissemination to the synovial membrane or be secondary to a tuberculous abscess in neighboring bone. The latter is rather common in childhood tuberculosis of joints. Pathologically, tuberculosis usually begins as a synovitis. Proliferation of inflammatory granulation tissue, known as pannus, begins at the perichondrium and spreads over the joint surfaces. It interferes with nutrition of the cartilage, resulting in degeneration and destruction. In weight-bearing joints and, to a lesser degree in the nonweight-bearing joints, there is a tendency for preservation of the joint cartilages at the sites of maximum weight bearing or close apposition of cartilage. This is in contrast to pyogenic infections in which the joint exudate contains proteolytic enzymes that destroy cartilage rapidly throughout the joint surfaces. Thus, a fairly normal joint space may persist for a considerable period of time.

The incidence of tuberculous arthritis has decreased considerably in the past few years.

Roentgen Observations

Joint Effusion (*Fig. 9-3*). The earliest evidence of tuberculous arthritis of a peripheral joint is that of joint effusion secondary to the synovitis. This can be detected without much difficulty in roentgenograms of the knee, ankle, wrist, and elbow joints but may be more difficult to visualize in the shoulder and hip. Since fluid within a joint may result from a number of causes, this single roentgen observation does not establish the diagnosis.

Decalcification of the Bones. With the passage of time, often a matter of several months, the bones adjacent to the joint undergo a gradual decrease in density representing osteoporosis. The bony trabeculae disappear uniformly causing a washed-out appearance. The degree of osteoporosis often is severe and probably is caused by hyperemia plus disuse of the part.

Cartilage and Bone Destruction. The disease may remain in the stage just described for some time but more often there develops gradually the evidence of destruction of articular cartilages and of bone. In the weight-bearing joints, particularly in the knee, there is a tendency for preservation of cartilage at the points of maximum weight-bearing. (Fig. 9-4). Thus narrowing of the roentgen joint space may be delayed for a long time, even for several years.

The earliest evidence of bone destruction usually is seen at the margins of the articular ends of the bones. Here marginal erosion becomes apparent. The de-

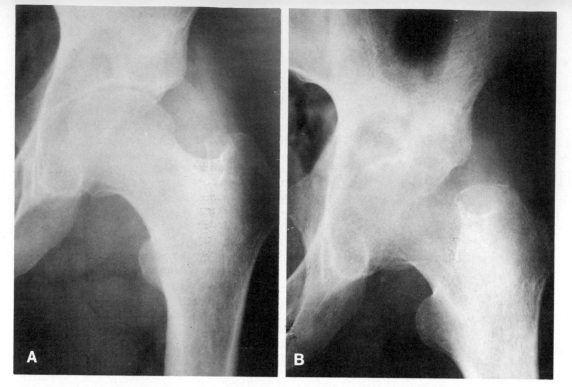

Fig. 9-3. Tuberculous arthritis of the hip in an adult. **A.** The joint capsule is distended with fluid, and there is thinning of the joint space. **B.** Three months later the cartilage destruction is seen to have progressed to complete loss of joint space, and there is now considerable osteopenia of adjacent bone.

Fig. 9-4. Tuberculosis of the knee. The appearance of the knee in three different patients shows different degrees of involvement. **A.** In this patient the joint space is intact but there are marginal erosions along the inner side of the tibia and femur and a radiolucency representing a tuberculous abscess in the upper end of the tibia below the tibial spine. **B.** The disease is more advanced in this patient than in the one shown in **A.** Erosion of articular surfaces on both sides of the femur and loss of joint space, indicating cartilage destruction, are noted. **C.** Advanced disease is evident in this patient. There are multiple sequestra producing the dense, white fragments and considerable destruction of bone, particularly in the lateral tibial plateau which is now concave.

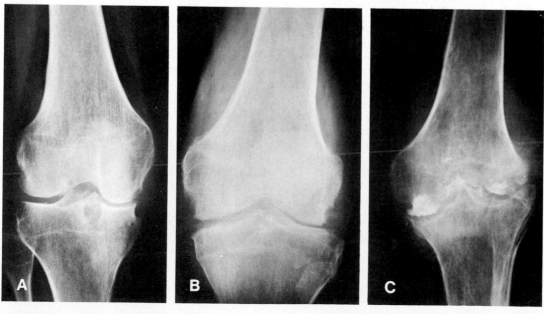

fects may be punched out and sharply circumscribed and thus resemble very closely those seen in rheumatoid arthritis. In addition to marginal erosion, the infection often burrows beneath the articular cartilage or extends through it to involve the articular ends of the bones. Thus these ends become ragged in outline and frank abscess cavities may appear (Fig. 9-4A).

Disorganization of the Joint. With further progression of the disease, gross disorganization of joint structures may result. The articular cartilage disappears, ragged destruction of the articular ends of the bones is noted, and separation of dead fragments (sequestra) is common (Fig. 9-4C), often involving opposing surfaces (kissing sequestra). Very little reactive sclerosis is observed in patients with untreated tuberculosis.

Caries Sicca. Caries sicca is a relatively uncommon form of tuberculosis characterized by a very chronic and indolent course with an absence of joint effusion. Except for the lack of fluid and the associated swelling of soft tissues, there is little difference in the roentgen findings in this type of the disease from those described in the foregoing. This lesion occurs most frequently in the shoulder.

Differential Diagnosis

Acute Pyogenic Arthritis. This disease has an acute onset and, if the patient is not treated or is inadequately treated articular cartilage is destroyed rapidly. With a tuberculous joint, on the other hand, by the time the joint space has decreased as a result of cartilage destruction, chronic osteoporosis, soft-tissue atrophy, and the other signs of chronic disease are clearly apparent.

Chronic Pyogenic Arthritis. Chronic pyogenic infection may subside into a slowly progressive course, particularly if the patient is not treated properly; then it may rather closely resemble tuberculosis. In other instances the disease is chronic from the beginning. There are several differences between it and tuberculosis. In chronic pyogenic arthritis the loss of articular cartilage is more severe for the duration of the disease and there is no tendency for preservation of cartilage at the points of maximum weight-bearing in the joints of the lower extremities as is noted in tuberculosis. With chronicity, reactive spurs may form along the edges of the bones and sclerotic changes are frequent. Marginal erosion is slight or absent in chronic pyogenic arthritis while in tuberculosis this

is a common observation. Bony ankylosis frequently develops after destruction of articular cartilages in chronic pyogenic infection. In tuberculosis there is little tendency for spontaneous healing and bony ankylosis seldom develops without surgical aid.

Rheumatoid Arthritis. This disease is characterized by multiplicity of joint involvement affecting the proximal interphalangeal and metacarpophalangeal joints of the hands. Loss of articular cartilage is uniform; marginal erosion is prominent in the small joints but is usually minimal when the large joints are involved. Sequestra do not form in rheumatoid arthritis. Serial observations may reveal evidence of spontaneous remissions. When rheumatoid arthritis involves a single joint as it does occasionally, the appearance is very similar to that of tuberculosis and correlation with the clinical and laboratory findings is important.

TUBERCULOSIS OF THE SPINE

Spinal involvement is present in approximately two-thirds of patients with bone and joint tuberculosis. Depending largely upon the location of the initial focus of infection, three main roentgenologic patterns are encountered in tuberculosis of the spine: the intervertebral, the central, and the anterior.

Intervertebral Type. In the intervertebral form of the disease the lesion begins in a vertebral body adjacent to the intervertebral disc. There is early extension of the infection into the disc and destruction of cartilage. In turn this results in a thinning of the intervertebral disc space in roentgenograms. The lesion in the bone becomes visualized as a poorly marginated focus of bone destruction. Accumulation of purulent material with abscess formation around the affected area is readily visualized in the dorsal spine as a fusiform soft-tissue shadow surrounding the vertebra (Fig. 9-5). The abscess shadow is present along both sides of the spine but often is larger on one side than on the other (Fig. 9-6). In the lumbar spine, abscess formation is more difficult to demonstrate but its presence may be demonstrated by an outward bulging of the psoas muscle shadow.

With further progression of the disease, the intervertebral disc space undergoes further thinning and may disappear. The destruction of the vertebral body also progresses and the infection extends across the disc to involve the adjacent vertebra. Since the arches and articular processes are not affected as a rule, col-

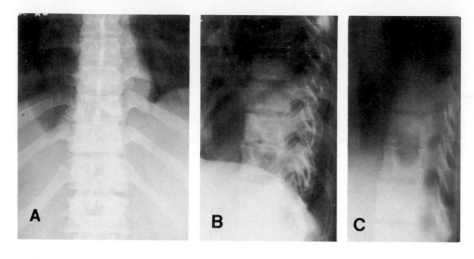

Fig. 9-5. Tuberculosis of the spine. **A.** Note the paraspinal soft-tissue mass on the left. Bone involvement is not clearly identified in this projection. **B.** Lateral view showing thinning of the disc and central bone destruction which is much better outlined in **C,** a tomogram of the same area.

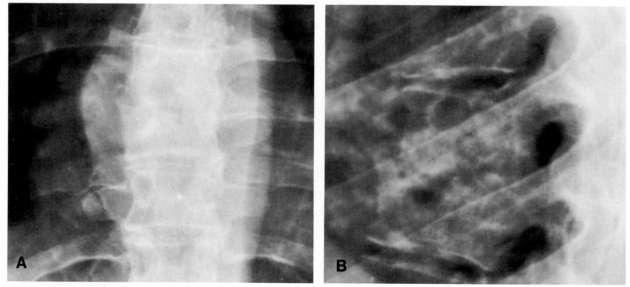

Fig. 9-6. Tuberculosis of the spine. **A.** Note the paraspinal mass that is more localized on the right than on the left. There is also loss of the disc and evidence of destruction of adjacent bone. **B.** In the lateral projection the bone destruction is more readily outlined, and there is virtual complete loss of the cortical end-plates of the vertebral bodies as well as loss of the disc space.

lapse of the vertebral body occurs anteriorly to a large extent. This leads to a sharp angular kyphosis or gibbus. Lateral angulation or scoliotic deformities are less frequent in tuberculosis. Periosteal reaction along the margins of the vertebral body involved by tuberculosis is uncommon and little if any sclerotic response is seen.

Central Type. The primary focus of the infection in the central type occurs within the vertebral body rather than along a margin and it develops as an abscess cavity (Fig. 9-7). The intervertebral discs are not involved as early as in the intervertebral form and some collapse of the vertebra may occur before disc changes are obvious. Paravertebral abscess formation

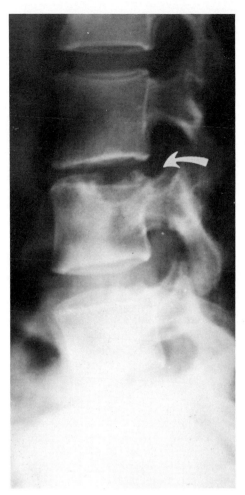

Fig. 9-7. Tuberculosis of the spine. There is some thinning of the intervertebral disc **(arrow)** and an abscess cavity in the upper part of the fourth lumbar vertebra.

likewise may be less apparent in the early stages. The central type of the infection is much less common than the intervertebral. It actually represents tuberculous osteomyelitis, with subsequent spread to the disc.

Anterior Type. The anterior type of the disease usually results from extension of the infection from a focus above or below. The infection burrows upward or downward, bathing previously unaffected vertebrae in pus and eventually extending into one or more of the bodies. Roentgenologically, this is seen as an irregular erosion of the anterior border of the vertebral body, or as a smooth saucerized defect. There

is little or no vertebral collapse and the disc intervals may be preserved. In long-standing cases of tuberculosis of the spine, very extensive involvement of this type may be present because of the tendency of the disease to extend by sinus formation and by burrowing along fascial planes.

Other Roentgen Observations. 1. In very chronic disease, calcium may be deposited in the paravertebral abscess, giving it a mottled appearance. Such calcified or partially calcified abscesses will remain throughout life.

2. In very old cases several contiguous vertebrae may have been destroyed to such an extent that their individual outlines are no longer recognizable and all evidence of an intervertebral disc space has disappeared.

3. With quiescence and healing of the disease the bones regain a more normal density and sharpness of outline. Areas of destruction tend partially to recalcify and bony ankylosis may ensue. Paravertebral abscess shadows diminish in size but seldom disappear completely without treatment.

Differential Diagnosis

Compression Fracture. There is no destruction of bone, only compression of it. The compressed zone is denser than normal. The intervertebral disc space often is narrowed but not completely absent. The superior surface of the vertebral body usually is concave because of infraction of it and expansion of the disc into the injured bone. Hemorrhage around the involved vertebra may cause a slight thickening of the paravertebral soft-tissue shadow but this seldom is a prominent feature. Lateral angulation often is present in addition to a gibbus deformity.

Tumor. A neoplasm of the vertebra may cause a paravertebral soft-tissue mass that may mimic an abscess shadow very closely. Tumors, however, rarely affect disc cartilage and narrowing of the intervertebral disc space does not develop. Collapse of the vertebral body often is uniform so that the posterior part may be affected as much as the anterior. This is unusual in tuberculosis. Gibbus formation, therefore, may not develop even in the presence of an extensive lesion.

Pyogenic Osteomyelitis. In pyogenic infections, sclerosis is more pronounced and periosteal calcification usually is a noticeable feature. The disease has an acute onet and is more rapid in its development than tuberculosis.

Fungal Infections. Involvement of the spine is moderately frequent in actinomycosis, blastomycosis, and coccidioidomycosis. The roentgen appearances usually are not distinctive except for the tendency for the development of sinus tracts which may be extensive. Most lesions in the spine resemble tuberculosis and roentgen diagnosis usually is not possible.

OTHER CHRONIC INFECTIONS OF JOINTS

BRUCELLOSIS

Brucella arthritis is very rare. Roentgen findings of synovial swelling, effusion, and subarticular erosions are similar to those in tuberculosis and rheumatoid arthritis. Biopsy or culture is necessary to make the diagnosis.

FUNGAL INFECTIONS

Joint involvement is rare in fungal infections; however, blastomycosis, histoplasmosis, actinomycosis, coccidioidomycosis, and cryptococcosis joint infections are occasionally observed. As a rule, these tend to cause more destruction of bone than does tuberculosis. Periarticular extension with abscesses and sinus tracts is often present. Diagnosis must be based on recovery of the causative organism.

SYPHILIS OF THE JOINTS

Joint disease is observed very rarely in patients with congenital syphilis. When it does occur it is usually manifest in the post-infantile or juvenile period, probably representing a secondary or tertiary form of the disease. There is a synovial form that occurs mainly in children; soft-tissue swelling is the only radiologic feature of this form. Clinically the involved joints are warm and painful. A second type of syphilitic arthropathy is characterized by irregularity due to erosion of subchondral bone. This also occurs in juveniles. The process may go on to an ulcerating chondroarthritis (von Gies joint) and eventually may ankylose.[9]

RHEUMATOID ARTHRITIS

While the clinical pattern of rheumatoid arthritis varies, most cases begin insidiously and run either a protracted and progressive course or undergo remissions of variable length. In many cases the disease eventually leads to more or less crippling deformity of the affected joints. In the typical case it begins in the peripheral joints, usually the proximal interphalangeal and metacarpophalangeal of the hand and the ulnocarpal of the wrist. There is a tendency for symmetrical distribution in the two hands. In the feet, metatarsophalangeal joint involvement of one or more toes is common. As the disease progresses it affects the more proximal joints advancing toward the trunk in all extremities, until finally practically every joint in the body may be involved. The disease may become arrested at any stage. If this happens before much structural change has been caused, the joint may return to a normal or almost normal appearance. A curious feature of the disease is the frequent sparing of the terminal joints of the fingers. Females are affected much more frequently than males.

Pathologically, rheumatoid arthritis begins as a synovitis and in the early stages there is edema and inflammation of the synovium and the subsynovial tissues. Joint effusion also is frequent. If the disease advances, the synovium becomes greatly thickened with enlargement of the synovial villi. This is followed by a proliferation of fibrous connective tissue in the region of the perichondrium. This vascular connective tissue is known as pannus; it grows over the surface of the articular cartilage, interfering with its normal nutrition and resulting in cartilage degeneration. In advanced disease the joint becomes filled with pannus, articular cartilages disappear, and a fibrous ankylosis results. Frequently this is followed in time by bony ankylosis. As these changes are occurring in the joint, the bone adjacent undergoes osteoporosis and the muscles atrophy from disuse. Foci of inflammatory cells often accumulate in the bone adjacent to the joint.

Roentgen Observations

Soft-Tissue Swelling. The earliest roentgen evidence of the disease is a diffuse swelling of soft tissues around the joint, leading to a fusiform enlargement (Fig. 9-8). This is easily seen when the proximal interphalangeal joints are affected but can also be observed in some of the other joints, particularly in the knee and ankle. Since the disease tends to attack the proximal interphalangeal and metacarpophalangeal joints first, these should be observed carefully for such evidence of synovitis. The third area often affected early is the inner aspect of the wrist, where soft-tissue swelling may be observed readily. The swelling observed roentgenologically is caused by joints of the hands and feet commonly affected by this disease.

Marginal Erosions. After an interval of time, which varies greatly among patients, marginal erosions become apparent. These are seen as small foci of destruction along the margins of the articular ends of the bones. They are caused by the development of granulation tissue at the perichondrium and indicate the early stage of pannus. These erosions may be very minute but they represent one of the significant roentgenologic observations of the disease (Figs. 9-8, 9-9, and 9-10). The use of a magnifying lens is helpful when searching for the smallest erosions. The most common sites are the distal first, second, and third metacarpals on the radial side; the radiocarpal joint; the distal ends of the proximal third and fourth phalanges; and the radial aspect of the ulnar styloid as well as the adjacent margins of the radioulnar joint. Other joints of the hands and wrists, except the distal interphalangeal joints, are often involved. In the knee they are seen chiefly along the medial edge of the tibia and the posterior aspects of the tibia and femur. Erosions occasionally occur at the sites of tendinous attachments such as the Achilles tendon and the plantar attachment on the os calcis.

Thinning of the Joint Space. Narrowing of the joint space results from degeneration of the articular cartilages as pannus spreads across the joint surfaces. Typically, this diminution in space is uniform throughout the joint (see Fig. 9-12A). It may progress gradually until the ends of the bones impinge against one another. The articular ends may remain smooth. Often, however, they become roughened. In some joints a deep excavation may form in the base of one bone with the end of the opposing bone projecting into the cavity. This is seen in severe cases and is common in the metacarpophalangeal joints where the rounded or pointed head of the metacarpal lies within an eroded cavity in the adjacent base of the phalanx. In advanced cases there may be a striking loss of bone substance at the outer end of the clavicles, with widening of the acromioclavicular joint space. It resembles the erosion seen in hyperparathyroidism, but the other joint changes are absent in this latter disease. In some patients, again with advanced disease, marked destruction of the articulating ends of the bones may be found (Fig. 9-11). Thus the ends of the metatarsals, metacarpals, and phalanges may be sharpened almost to a point.

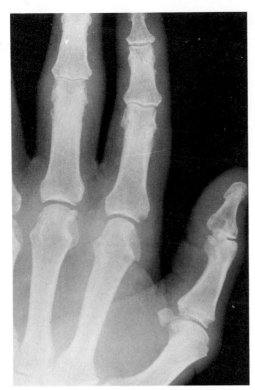

Fig. 9-8. Rheumatoid arthritis. Fusiform swelling is noted around the proximal interphalangeal joint of the third finger. The joint space is thin, and there are small marginal erosions in the heads of the first and second metacarpals and the adjacent proximal phalanges.

joint effusion and also by edema of the subsynovial tissues.

Subarticular Osteoporosis; Periostitis. Another early sign of the disease is local demineralization of bone adjacent to an involved joint. This is seen as a thinning of the cortex in the end of the bone and a decrease in number of trabeculae. It is often seen to good advantage in the metacarpal heads when there is involvement of one or more metacarpophalangeal joints. Associated with this a thin layer of periosteal calcification around the contiguous portion of the shaft frequently occurs. The subperiosteal calcification is usually transient and may disappear very quickly. These early changes—soft-tissue swelling, subarticular demineralization, and periostitis—are highly suggestive, if not characteristic, of rheumatoid arthritis particularly when they are found in the

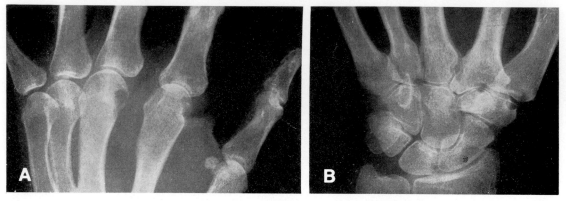

Fig. 9-9. Rheumatoid arthritis. **A.** Marginal erosions are apparent on the distal ends of the second, third, and fifth metacarpals. There is also thinning of the joint space at the second metacarpal–phalangeal level. **B.** Marginal erosions are seen in the hamate and in the proximal ends of several of the metacarpals.

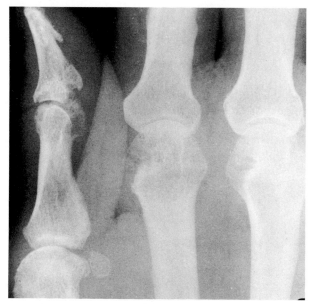

Fig. 9-10. Rheumatoid arthritis illustrating characteristic marginal erosions in the heads of the second and third metacarpals and in the terminal phalanx of the thumb.

When extensive destruction of the articular ends of the bones in the hands, wrists, and feet occurs, the disease has been termed *"arthritis mutilans."* Some authors consider this to be a separate entity although its similarity to rheumatoid arthritis in many of its aspects is to be noted.

In the hip, thinning of the central aspect of the joint space causes displacement of the femur (Fig. 9-12). The femoral head tends to move in the plane of the femoral neck (upward and inward) in contrast to osteoarthritis in which the femoral head tends to migrate superiorly in about three-fourths and medially in about one-fourth of patients.[27] The acetabular cavity becomes deepened and eventually may lead to the characteristic changes of *protrusio acetabuli* (Otto's pelvis) (see section on "Intrapelvic Prostrusion of Acetabulum" and Figs. 9-12 and 9-46). Rheumatoid arthritis is one of the common causes of this condition.

Generalized Osteoporosis. If the disease has become fairly generalized and sufficient to cause limitation of bodily activity, generalized disuse osteoporosis will develop. The bones will become demineralized throughout the skeleton. If the disease remains confined to the peripheral joints, only the bones in these areas will show appreciable demineralization.

Clavicular Changes. Resorption of the distal end of the clavicle is common in severe to moderately severe rheumatoid arthritis. It can often be detected on a chest roentgenogram which may confirm or suggest the diagnosis. Other causes of bony absorption of the distal clavicles include hyperparathyroidism, scleroderma, traumatic osteolysis, and spontaneous massive osteolysis of unknown cause. A lesser-known finding in rheumatoid arthritis[31] is an elongated erosion on the undersurface of the distal clavicle at the attachment of the coracoclavicular ligament. This

Fig. 9-11. Rheumatoid arthritis of the hand and wrist. The disease is moderately destructive with considerable erosion of the bone ends at the first metacarpal–phalangeal joint and a concave erosion of the proximal end of the proximal phalanx of the third digit. Smaller erosions are noted elsewhere in the wrist and hand.

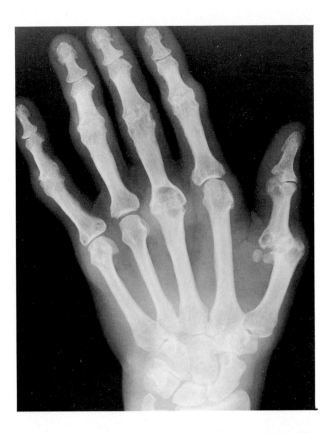

also occurs in ankylosing spondylitis and often is associated with bony proliferation at the attachments of the ligament to both the clavicle and coracoid process.

Cartilage Calcification. Calcium deposition in the articular cartilages (chondrocalcinosis) is seen occasionally but is more frequent in other entities.

Subluxations and Contractures. In the later stages of the disease, soft-tissue contractions and subluxations are common. By this time the joint will have been damaged to the point where little or no articular cartilage remains and fibrous ankylosis is present.

Bony Ankylosis. In other joints, destruction of articular cartilages leads to the development of bony ankylosis. This is particularly frequent in the intercarpal and radiocarpal joints of the wrist. After all cartilage

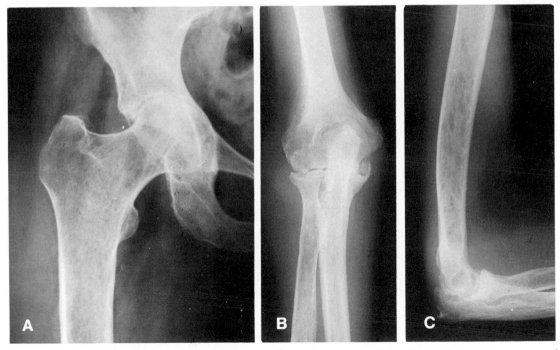

Fig. 9-12. Rheumatoid arthritis. **A.** There is uniform thinning of the joint space and deepening of the acetabular cavity causing a moderate degree of protrusio acetabuli. **B.** and **C.** Note the destructive lesions of the joint surfaces of the radius and ulna along with joint thinning, local soft-tissue swelling, and spotty osteoporosis of the distal humerus.

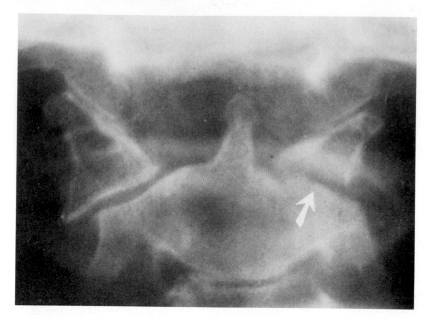

Fig. 9-13. Rheumatoid arthritis of the upper cervical spine showing erosion and thinning of the odontoid process and lateral subluxation of C1 on C2 as well as involvement of the joint on the left side where there is loss of subchondral bone **(arrow).**

has been destroyed, bony trabeculae form across the previous joint space and the end result is a complete obliteration of the joint cavity and formation of a solid bony ankylosis. Bony ankylosis seldom develops if there has been much destruction of the articular ends of the bones or if there has been any appreciable degree of subluxation.

The Spine. Involvement of the spine, particularly the cervical area, may occur especially in long-standing disease.[23] One of the characteristic changes is erosion of the odontoid process of the second cervical vertebra (Fig. 9-13). At times the dens is almost completely destroyed. Erosions and malalignment of the facet joints particularly of the atlantoaxial and atlanto-occipital joints may develop. The attachments of the transverse ligament, which holds the odontoid in position immediately posterior to the anterior arch of C1, may be loosened by the disease. This may lead to forward subluxation of the first cervical on the second (Fig. 9-14). Normally the distance between the posterior aspect of C1 and the dens is no more than 2.5 mm. It remains constant in flexion. In these patients the distance may be normal on extension or even in the neutral position, but may increase greatly on flexion.

There may also be upward displacement of C2, so that the dens may impinge on the upper cervical cord or medulla. Either of the displacements may cause an acute neurologic syndrome requiring immediate

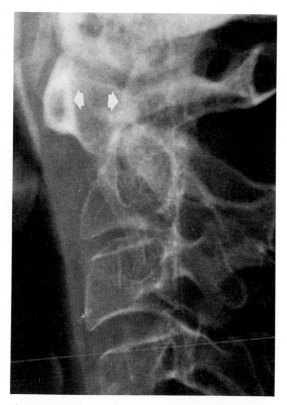

Fig. 9-14. Rheumatoid arthritis. Note the anterior subluxation of C1 on C2 **(arrows).** The odontoid process is thinned.

traction or decompression. Arterial compression (vertebral or basilar) has also been reported in severe involvement of C1 and C2. Therefore, it is imperative that adequate roentgen examination including tomography of this area be carried out in patients with rheumatoid arthritis who complain of neck pain or have neurologic symptoms suggesting cord or vascular compression.

There may also be involvement of facet joints elsewhere allowing subluxation at one or more levels. Erosive changes in the vertebral end plates may result in either a localized area of destruction or involvement of the end-plate in which the cortex is eroded, and the disc is often narrowed. With time, extensive sclerosis may occur with uniform density extending from the irregular end-plate for varying distances into the vertebral body. When both vertebral end-plates are involved, the entire body may become sclerotic. Occasionally, the spinous processes are involved. In some of these patients there is bone destruction resulting in a small, pointed, posterior process. In others, there may be pressure deformities when involvement of the apophyseal joints has permitted subluxations at several levels. In late stages, ankylosis of these facet joints usually occurs (see Fig. 9-15).

UNUSUAL MANIFESTATIONS OF RHEUMATOID ARTHRITIS

Giant Bone Cysts. Subarticular bone "cysts" or geodes are uncommon, but not rare.[4] They may become 8 to 10 cm or more in diameter, usually occur in a subarticular position, and may expand the cortex and lead to pathologic fracture. Apparently they may be caused by synovial fluid under pressure extending into the subarticular bone by way of a defect in the articular surface, particularly in the upper tibia. Some authors have reported the geodes (not true cysts) to contain rheumatoid granulation tissue which may be an extension of pannus through an articular surface defect. There is some controversy regarding this, but in certain instances geodes may be caused by intramedullary rheumatoid nodules.

Rheumatoid Synovial Cysts. Increased intra-articular pressure may enlarge a joint capsule and produce cystlike extensions. Alteration in connective tissue of the capsule may also be a factor. This has been reported adjacent to a number of different joints in rheumatoid arthritis. Cysts about the knee are the most common. Popliteal cysts may dissect into the calf where they may present clinical signs resembling

those of deep vein thrombosis. Arthrography is used to make the diagnosis. Such cysts may occur in a number of other diseases associated with joint effusion. They are rare in children with Still's disease.

Intrasynovial Masses. Intra-articular rheumatoid nodules and fatty masses may produce mechanical disabilities causing joint instability and limitation of motion as well as a "click." Arthrography is necessary to outline the mass. Relief of symptoms may be obtained by surgical excision.

"Unilateral" Rheumatoid Arthritis. Neurologic deficits caused by central or peripheral damage in patients with rheumatoid arthritis may lead to a sparing of the paralyzed side. The degree of protection tends to be directly proportional to the amount of paraplegia. The cause is not clear.

Peripheral Gangrene. This rare complication of rheumatoid arthritis is caused by a necrotizing vasculitis resulting in vascular occlusions.

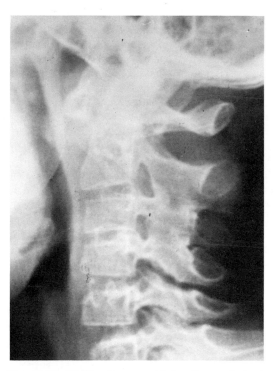

Fig. 9-15. Still's disease. Note the ankylosis of the apophyseal joints between C2, C3, and C4 secondary to long-standing disease.

Reparative Changes. Since, in many cases, remissions and exacerbations of the disease have occurred, reparative changes may be apparent. Marginal spurs similar to those seen in degenerative disease are frequent along the articulating ends of the bones. There also may be a considerable amount of sclerotic density along the articular surfaces. It may be difficult to determine whether these changes are caused by a combination of rheumatoid arthritis and degenerative joint disease or by rheumatoid disease alone. In weight-bearing joints, such as the hip, knee, and ankle, degenerative changes are common after middle age and combinations of the two diseases may be seen.

JUVENILE RHEUMATOID ARTHRITIS

The terminology for chronic arthritis in children is confusing since the term "Still's disease" is used by some to indicate all forms of rheumatoid disease in children.[34] Others reserve the designation of Still's disease to the form that often begins in infancy with systemic symptoms of fever and rash and findings of hepatosplenomegaly and lymphadenopathy, often with pericarditis, muscle wasting, and ultimate dwarfism. This designation will be used in the current discussion of the roentgen findings. All other forms will then be designated "juvenile rheumatoid arthritis."

As a rule, systemic manifestations are more severe in the juvenile than in the adult form of rheumatoid arthritis, and there is often a period of 2 or more years in which systemic symptoms are present before the roentgen features of joint space narrowing and marginal erosions are observed radiographically. Peripheral joints are usually involved first, and, if spondylitis occurs, it involves the cervical spine most often. In Still's disease there may not be much destruction of articular cartilage or bone, and there is a tendency to involve large joints such as knees, ankles, and wrists (Figs. 9-15 and 9-16). Periosteal calcification is much more common and severe than in the adult form of the disease. Muscle wasting may be prominent so that the overall appearance of the joints is that of fusiform enlargement with soft-tissue swelling, often with contractures and sometimes subluxation. Cervical spine involvement, including bony ankylosis and atlanto-axial subluxation, may occur. In adults, a systemic disease resembling Still's produces similar symptoms leading to a presumptive diagnosis of leukemia or lymphoma in some instances. In the report of over 700 patients with this form of the disease,[19] bony ankylosis was observed in the intercarpal and carpo-metacarpal articulations relatively early. This does not ordinarily occur early in the course of the adult form of rheumatoid arthritis. In juvenile rheumatoid arthritis the findings are similar to those in the adult form of the disease except for the late manifestation of joint-space narrowing and articular erosion. There may be some interference with skeletal development, sometimes manifested as accelerated bone growth and at other times as retarded growth. Spondylitis is somewhat more frequent than in patients with the adult form. There are variations in juvenile rheumatoid arthritis; some patients have a typical polyarthritis while others have a few large joints involved. Occasionally isolated finger and toe joints may be involved, and the same is true with the wrist and cervical spine.

Felty's syndrome is a term applied to rheumatoid arthritis associated with splenomegaly which may be massive. Also present is leukopenia involving the neutrophils more than other cells. This is a very rare condition.

ANKYLOSING SPONDYLITIS (MARIE–STRÜMPELL DISEASE)

Ankylosing spondylitis is a rheumatoid variant in which the rheumatoid factor is usually not present in the serum. If differs in some important respects from rheumatoid arthritis of the peripheral joints in that it affects young adult males predominantly, in the ratio of about 15 to 1, while the disease affecting the peripheral joints is more common in females and the age of onset generally is later in life. It frequently remains confined to the joints of the spine and the sacroiliacs, although about 30% of patients with the spinal disease develop subsequent manifestations in peripheral joints. The lesions are similar pathologically.

The earliest clinical manifestation is usually persistent low back pain of insidious onset. The disease involves the synovial joints of the spine. These include the apophyseal joints between the articulating facets of the vertebrae, the costovertebral joints, and the sacroiliac joints. While the disease may begin in any of these areas. roentgen visualization of the small joints is difficult and thus the sacroiliacs often show the earliest signs of the disease.

Juvenile onset ankylosing spondylitis differs somewhat from the usual form which begins in young adults. Most of these cases present with complaints of pain in appendicular joints: hips, knees, or shoulders; the more distal joints are affected in decreasing frequency. Soft-tissue swelling caused by synovitis

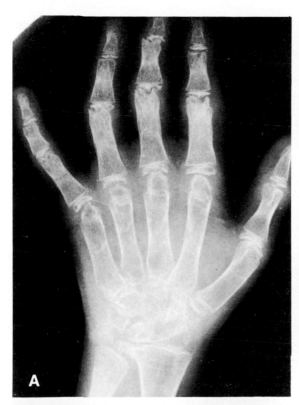

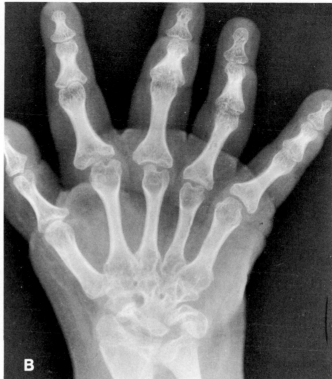

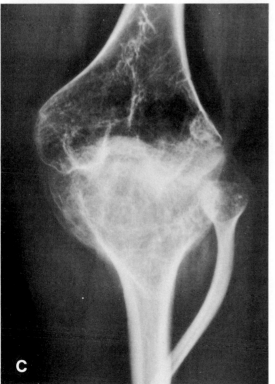

Fig. 9-16. Still's disease. **A.** Erosion of the articular surfaces in most of the joints of the hand and wrist as well as severe osteoporosis is manifest. **B.** In this older patient, residuals of Still's disease have resulted in marked deformity of the carpal bones and to a lesser extent of the metacarpals and phalanges. **C.** Chronic Still's disease of the knee with club-shaped bone ends, loss of joint space, irregularity of joint surfaces, and abnormal growth in length of the fibula, which is extensively bowed.

and effusion may be the only roentgen sign present for a long time. In some of these patients, this swelling subsides without further damage and in others the findings of joint narrowing, erosions, and osteoporosis resemble those of rheumatoid arthritis, indicating progression of the process.

Roentgen Observations. 1. The articular surfaces of the affected joints become blurred and the joint spaces are irregular in width. The blurring of the sacroiliac joints is caused by loss of subchondral cortex and the joints may appear irregularly widened. At times, the earliest sign in the sacroiliac joints appears to be sclerosis, but the onset is often insidious so that it is difficult to ascertain the true duration of the disease. (Fig. 9-17). Usually this involves both the iliac and the sacral side of the joint, although it may be more severe on one side or the other. In the apophyseal joints it is infrequent to find uniform involvement of all the joints at the same time. More often one or several joints are more severely affected than others, and some may appear fairly normal during the early stages. The same is true of the costovertebral joints. The findings in these apophyseal joints consist of loss of subchondral cortex, often resulting in a somewhat granular irregularity of the joint surface. Also, there is loss of joint space.

2. One of the characteristic features of rheumatoid arthritis of the spine is the tendency for bony ankylosis to develop in the affected joints. This is seen in the sacroiliac, the apophyseal or facet joints, and the costovertebral joints and represents the end stage of the disease.

3. Squaring of the anterior surfaces of the involved vertebrae is a relatively early sign. This appears to be caused by an erosive process involving the anterior, superior, and inferior vertebral edges or corners. In the lateral view the superior and inferior edges of the vertebral body appear unusually square and sharp instead of smoothly rounded as is normal. Later, a shell-like calcification of the soft tissues surrounding and between the vertebrae develops. Still later the paraspinal ligaments calcify and ossify to form the fixed ankylosed "bamboo" spine (Fig. 9-18).

4. Generalized skeletal osteoporosis is a frequently associated finding in this disease with the decalcification generally more intense in the vertebrae than elsewhere. It is produced, to a large extent, by the in-

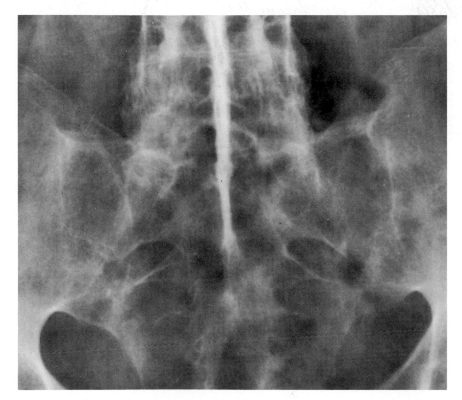

Fig. 9-17. Ankylosing spondylitis. This view of the upper pelvis shows complete bony ankylosis of the sacroiliac joints and calcification and ossification of the interspinous ligaments in the low lumbar area as well as ankylosis of the lower apophyseal joints.

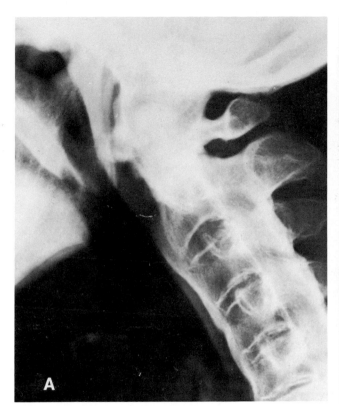

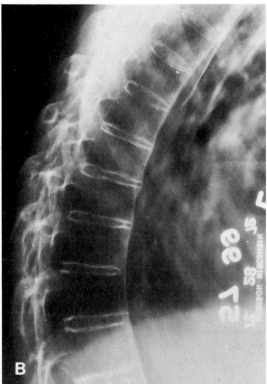

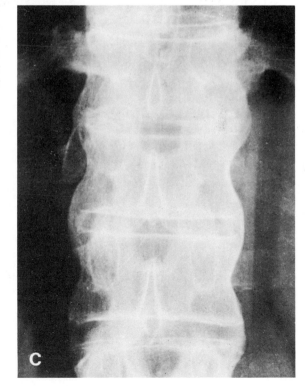

Fig. 9-18. Ankylosing spondylitis. **A.** Note the complete ankylosis of apophyseal joints and dense ossification and calcification of the anterior spinal ligament. **B.** Typical ossification and calcification of the anterior spinal ligament in the thoracic spine resulting in ankylosis there. **C.** Similar changes are noted on this anteroposterior view of the lower thoracic and the upper lumbar spine.

activity or limited activity caused by the disease. It may be the earliest sign recognizable radiographically.

5. Infrequently, the disease causes a localized destruction of a single intervertebral disc and margins of the adjacent vertebral bodies. The vertebral destruction is more apparent along the anterior margins, but may affect the entire disc surface. The lesion tends to undergo slow repair, with the development of sclerosis. This lesion is usually found in patients showing rheumatoid disease of long duration, with extensive ankylosis of the spine. It is probably caused by trauma, either a stress fracture or an acute process. Motion at the site is probably the cause of the extensive sclerosis often observed to develop in these patients, since this is the only unstable site in the entire ankylosed spine.

6. Erosion and periosteal calcification may be noted in areas such as the ischial tuberosities, femoral trochanters, and at other sites of ligamentous or muscular attachments. Erosive changes also may occur at the symphysis pubis and the manubriosternal joint in patients with advanced rheumatoid spondylitis.

7. Peripheral joint disease[28] is also observed in ankylosing spondylitis. As a rule it is not as symmetrical as in rheumatoid arthritis. Joint spaces are not as narrow and osteoporosis is not as severe. Large joints, including hip, shoulder, knee, elbow, and ankle, tend to be involved. Small joints of the extremities are not as frequently involved as in rheumatoid arthritis. There is more periostitis, subchondral sclerosis, and osteophyte formation than in rheumatoid arthritis. Protrusio acetabuli with migration of the femoral head may occur when the hip is affected. Temporomandibular joint involvement has also been reported. There is more tendency to bony ankylosis of large central joints than in rheumatoid arthritis. Subchondral cysts are not as large or as frequent as in rheumatoid arthritis. Also subluxations and peripheral joint deformity are less frequent than in rheumatoid arthritis.

ARTHRITIS ASSOCIATED WITH PSORIASIS (PSORIATIC ARTHRITIS)

Some patients with psoriasis have rheumatoid arthritis, but occasionally a patient with psoriasis will develop an arthritis that resembles rheumatoid arthritis, a rheumatoid variant in which the serum is negative for rheumatoid factor. This disease is characterized by the following: (*1*) A destructive process involving predominantly the distal interphalangeal joints of the hands and toes (Fig. 9-19). (2) A tendency for bony ankylosis of some of the interphalangeal joints (in rheumatoid arthritis, ankylosis is more common in the intercarpal joints). (3) Abnormally wide joint spaces with sharply demarcated bony surfaces. (4) Destructive arthritis of the interphalangeal

Fig. 9-19. Psoriatic arthritis. Note involvement of the distal interphalangeal joints of the fingers and the interphalangeal involvement of the great toe. There is also involvement of the proximal and distal joints of the fourth and fifth toes.

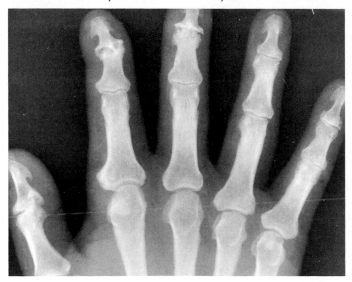
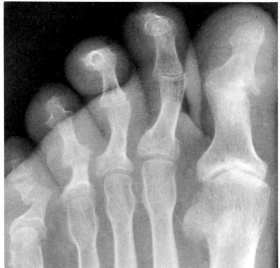

joint of the great toe. (5) Resorption of the terminal tufts of the terminal phalanges. (6) Less osteoporosis than rheumatoid arthritis. At times no osteoporosis can be detected on roentgenograms. (7) Sacroiliac involvement. This is fairly common; it may be unilateral and consist of erosions, sclerosis, and sometimes ankylosis. (8) Bony proliferation at sites of erosion, subchondral sclerosis, and proliferation of the distal ends of the distal phalanges resulting in ivorylike density in some instances.[29] (9) Periostitis. This is more common than in rheumatoid arthritis. (10) Paravertebral ossification that is separated from the vertebral body so that it does not appear to be a marginal syndesmophyte which extends from the surface of one vertebral body to that of another. This may appear before any other roentgen change in psoriatic arthritis. (11) Erosive changes of the sternal synchondrosis. These are common.[12] (12) Osteolysis of the ends of the distal phalanges and the diaphyses of metacarpal and metatarsals which may result in "arthritis mutilans."

ARTHRITIS ASSOCIATED WITH SCLERODERMA AND OTHER CONNECTIVE-TISSUE DISEASE

Some patients with scleroderma develop a rheumatoidlike disease in the joints of the hands. In addition to the arthritic changes certain other findings caused by the scleroderma may be observed in roentgenograms (see Fig. 10-13):

1. Atrophy of the soft tissues in the tips of the fingers, giving them a tapered appearance.
2. Loss of bone substance in the terminal tufts of the distal phalanges, resulting in a pointed or rounded end.
3. Small punctate calcific deposits in the soft tissues, especially in the ends of the fingers.
4. Osteoporosis may be present, and varies from minimal to severe.
5. Joint narrowing usually involving the intercarpal and radiocarpal joints.[26] The interphalangeal joints may be involved in a random, asymmetric manner.
6. Rarely, intra-articular calcification.

When the above changes are observed the diagnosis of scleroderma can be made with considerable certainty.

Other collagen diseases may have an associated joint disease similar to rheumatoid arthritis except for a tendency toward a milder course in most cases.

In *dermatomyositis* and *disseminated lupus erythematosis* a rheumatoidlike arthritis is frequent. Similar joint changes may be found in *ulcerative colitis*, occasionally in *Crohn's disease, Behcet's syndrome*, following *jejunoiliac* or *jejunocolic bypass*, and in *Whipple's disease*. Sacroiliac joints are the most common site of involvement in ulcerative colitis and Crohn's disease, but the course of the joint disease does not parallel that of the bowel inflammation, and the arthritis usually does not progress to the classical ankylosing stage. There are also peripheral joint manifestations in the form of migratory pain and soft-tissue swelling that does follow the course of the bowel inflammation.

MIXED CONNECTIVE-TISSUE DISEASE

Mixed connective-tissue disease[41] combines some features of scleroderma, systemic lupus erythematosis, polymyositis, and rheumatoid arthritis. Radiographic features are varied, consisting of diffuse and periarticular osteoporosis, soft-tissue swelling, erosive changes, narrow joint space, terminal tuft resorption, soft-tissue atrophy, and, occasionally, subluxations. There is much clinical variation ranging from no symptoms to features of scleroderma or rheumatoid arthritis.

REITER'S SYNDROME

Reiter's syndrome is characterized by urethritis, conjunctivitis, and mucocutaneous lesions in the oropharynx, tongue, glans penis, and skin as well as arthritis. The lesions do not usually appear simultaneously so that the diagnosis is often difficult to determine. This is probably a postinfectious syndrome following certain enteric or venereal infection and therefore it is a reactive type of arthritis. There is a tendency for asymmetrical involvement of the sacroiliac joints with some bony destruction along the joint edges that results in irregularity and loss of cortical outlines. Later, sclerosis may develop. In other joints the findings are similar to those in other inflammatory diseases and consist of joint effusion, destructive lesions in the periarticular area, and loss of articular cartilage. The most characteristic finding is exuberant, fluffy, or whiskerlike periostitis at the site of tendon insertions, most frequently at the attachment of the plantar fascia to the calcaneus. Periostitis is also found in the metatarsal shafts and in the distal tibia and fibula. There is sometimes involvement of the metatarsophalangeal and proximal interphalangeal joints of the feet (Fig. 9-20). Joint effusions may occur in other joints of the fingers, toes, ankles, and

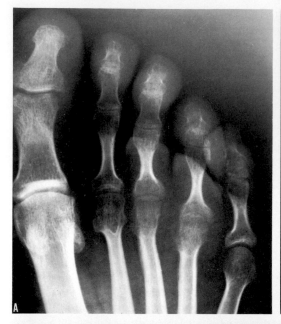
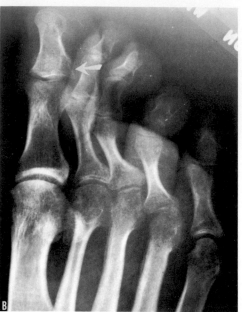
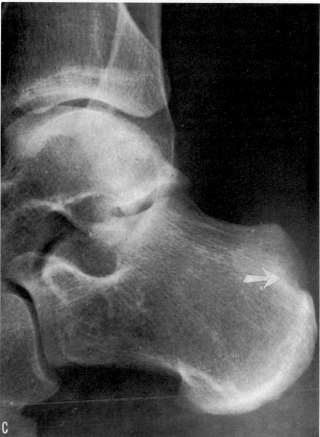

Fig. 9-20. Reiter's syndrome. Anterior **(A)** and **(B)** oblique views of the forefoot. There is involvement of the interphalangeal joint of the great toe with marginal erosion **(arrow).** There is also involvement of the metatarsal phalangeal joints with the most severe changes involving the fourth joint, where there is thinning of the joint space, local osteoporosis, and irregular joint surfaces. In the lateral view of the heel **(C),** cortical erosion of the os calcis **(arrow),** sclerosis along the posterior surface of the os calcis, and some spur formation inferiorly at the attachment of the plantar fascia are noted.

knees. Tendonitis is also relatively common, manifested by soft-tissue swelling, often in the Achilles tendon adjacent to the calcaneus.

The asymmetry and tendency to involve the feet and not the hands helps to differentiate Reiter's syndrome from rheumatoid and psoriatic arthritis. Paravertebral ossification similar to that noted in psoriatic arthritis is occasionally observed in Reiter's disease and may antedate other radiographic findings.

DEGENERATIVE JOINT DISEASE (OSTEOARTHRITIS)

The term "degenerative joint disease" is used to designate the condition also known as osteoarthritis, osteoarthrosis, or hypertrophic arthritis.

Degenerative joint disease is characterized pathologically by degeneration of the articular cartilages and of the other tissues comprising the joint. It is not an inflammatory lesion and the term "arthritis" is really a misnomer, but its use is widely accepted. It is a disease mainly of older individuals affecting the weight-bearing joints (spine, hip, knee, ankle) and the interphalangeal joints of the fingers. It is convenient to think of degenerative joint disease as occurring in two major forms, primary and secondary. The primary form may be a generalized disease affecting the weight-bearing joints, the spine, and the terminal interphalangeal joints of the fingers, the cause of which is unknown. The disease often appears to be the result of the aging process, representing the effects of wear and tear, to which may be added the factor of abnormal weight-bearing stresses and strains. Aging and trauma in one form or another, therefore, are common predisposing factors. The secondary form of the disease develops in a joint that has been subjected to abnormal stresses and strains over a period of time or one that has been traumatized repeatedly. In the hip it often follows congenital abnormalities in the shape and form of the acetabulum or of the femoral head, Legg–Perthes' disease, epiphysiolysis, etc., or it may develop as a result of abnormal weight-bearing such as follows a shortening of one leg or a scoliotic deformity of the spine. The roentgen signs and pathologic changes are similar in the two forms and the dividing line between them often is not distinct. Degenerative joint disease of the fingers (Heberden's nodes) represents a separate clinical entity. It seems to have little relationship to trauma, it may develop in fairly young individuals, is not necessarily associated with disease in other joints, and appears to have a distinct hereditary tendency.

Roentgen Observations

Spurring. One of the earliest changes in the development of small bony spurs or osteophytes along the articular edges of the bones. This is sometimes referred to as lipping. The osteophytes may become large, particularly in the spine, but rarely form ossified bridges between the bones along the joint edges (Fig. 9-21).

Eburnation. Increased density of the articular ends of the bones is another relatively early finding. This is noted particularly on the joint edges where the maximum weight-bearing stresses and strains occur.

Thinning of the Joint Space. Sometimes as an early manifestation and at other times occurring later in the course of the disease, thinning of the joint space develops. In contrast to rheumatoid arthritis, thin-

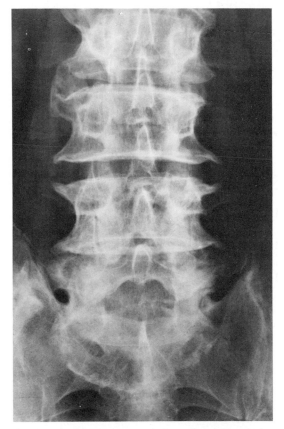

Fig. 9-21. Degenerative joint disease manifested by osteophytes on the vertebral margins in the lumbar spine.

ning of the roentgen joint space in this condition is almost invariably uneven. It is more pronounced in the part of the joint where weight-bearing strains are greatest and is caused by degeneration of the articular cartilages. In extreme cases the cartilage may be completely destroyed in areas and the articular ends of the bones then form the apposing joint surfaces. The greater the thinning of the joint space, the more severe the sclerosis of the articular ends and the more intensive the spurring is likely to be. These findings, however, do not always follow one another in severity and at times considerable thinning of the joint space may be seen with relatively little marginal osteophyte formation.

Cysts. In certain joints, notably the hip, cystlike rarefactions frequently develop along the articular borders. Occasionally these are an early manifestation of the disease in the hip joint (Fig. 9-22). More often they are seen only after the other findings enumerated in preceding paragraphs have become definite. Cystic cavities vary in size but in the hip may reach a diameter of several centimeters. They are bounded by a dense wall of sclerosis. They extend to the bony articular surface and sometimes are more prominent on one side of the joint than on the other. They may communicate with the joint cavity.

Subluxation. As a manifestation of late disease subluxation is frequent. Relaxation of the joint capsule and the other ligament structures around the area may allow a certain amount of displacement of one bone upon the other. When this happens the joint becomes even more unstable and thus more subject to trauma and aggravation of the existing disease.

Intra-articular and Periarticular Ossification. In some joints, particularly the knee, formation of calcific or ossified loose bodies is common. These may represent osteophytes that were broken off and became loose bodies, but more often they represent fragments of cartilage that have been detached and have undergone calcification. In other instances the loose body may be formed by the synovium. Not infrequently, dense masses that have the characteristics of bone are noted along the joint margins, usually in the tendons and not free within the joint. Again, these are particularly common in the knee.

SPECIAL AREAS
Joints of the Fingers

The disease affects primarily the terminal interphalangeal joints but need not be limited to these areas. The early findings consist of tiny marginal spurs or

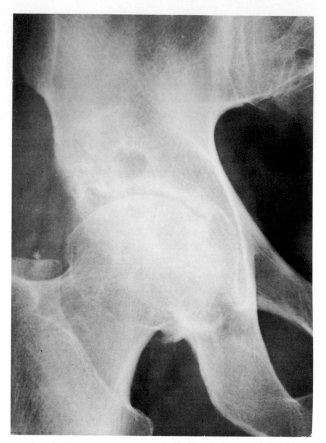

Fig. 9-22. Degenerative joint disease of the hip showing a pseudocyst above the acetabulum, some marginal spurring, and minimal eburnation as well as a little narrowing of the superior aspect of the hip joint space.

small calcific flakes along the bases of the distal phalanges. These spurs enlarge gradually to form well-defined bony protuberances that cause an irregular knobby thickening, palpable and visible, representing the well-known *Heberden's nodes*, one of the significant clinical diagnostic features of the disease. The largest spurs form on the dorsal edges of the articular ends of the bones and thus are best demonstrated in lateral roentgenograms. In more severely affected joints, narrowing of the joint space is present and the bony articular surfaces become irregular. The appearance is somewhat similar to that seen in rheumatoid arthritis. There are, however, no areas of marginal erosion and decalcification of the articular ends of the bones is not present. The bony trabeculae remain sharp and the cortical margin is apparent. The terminal phalanx becomes flexed on the middle and the finger cannot be completely straightened. Lateral angulation of the distal on the middle phalanx is common. Partial subluxations may occur but bony ankylosis does not develop. In some patients small cystic cavities form in the ends of the bones, but eburnation of the articulating ends of the bones seldom is striking (Fig. 9-23).

Erosive Osteoarthritis of the Hands[24]

This is an inflammatory form of osteoarthritis that is usually confined to the interphalangeal joints of the hand in middle-aged women. Typical osteophytes develop in the distal interphalageal joints; one or more of the joints then becomes acutely inflamed to variable degree for several months to years. Erosive changes are observed radiographically and there is an acute synovitis noted pathologically that cannot be differentiated from rheumatoid arthritis. The radiographic appearance may also resemble rheumatoid disease. The involved joints may undergo bony ankylosis. Classical osteoarthritis rarely results in ankylosis, but a few cases have been reported.

Hip Joint

In the hip the early signs of this disease are variable. In some subjects, the first evidence consists of increased density along the superior acetabular rim. In others, marginal spurring is the earliest feature, but, in most, narrowing of the joint space is the most significant finding (see Fig. 9-21). In contrast to rheumatoid arthritis, decrease in joint space in degenerative disease is characterized by its asymmetry and is related closely to the distribution of weight-bearing in the joint. In the hip this affects the superior portion almost exclusively, since this is the area that receives the thrust of the femoral head in weight-bearing. The joint space narrowing progresses to complete loss of the joint space but without bony ankylosis. This asymmetrical narrowing of the space leads to varying degrees of subluxation or lateral wandering of the femoral head and, if accompanied by a wearing away of the superior portion of the acetabular fossa, may result in notable deformity. The femoral head may also migrate superiorly and/or medially in contrast to its axial (along the axis of the femoral neck) migration in rheumatoid arthritis. Marginal osteophytes of large size may be present. As the head moves upward and laterally in the enlarged acetabular cavity, considerable amounts of calcium may be laid down along the undersurface as if to fill more completely the enlarged cavity. The joint surfaces, particularly the acetabular, show increased density or eburnation (Fig.

9-24). Cystic-appearing cavities develop as sharply outlined rarefactions surrounded by dense sclerotic walls. In some cases the cysts appear early. The cysts may communicate with the joint cavity. Infrequently, degenerative disease in the hip may lead to a general deepening and inward bulging of the acetabular cavity and at least some cases of intrapelvic protrusion of the acetabulum seem to result from this disease.

Knee Joint

Degenerative joint disease is the most common chronic joint affection encountered in the knee. Usually the early changes consist in the development of small spurs along the joint margins, on the tibial spine, along the borders of the intercondylar fossa of the femur, and on the edges of the patella. Hypertrophic excrescences may develop on the joint surface of the tibia, particularly at the attachments of the cruciate ligaments. As in the hip, narrowing of the joint space usually appears early and may be the first sign. It is almost always asymmetrical with the medial aspect undergoing the most severe change (Fig. 9-25). Occasionally the outer side of the joint narrows first. Increased density of the bony articular surfaces also is most pronounced along the site of greatest joint-space narrowing. Because of the uneven narrowing of the space and the consequent disturbance of weight-bearing alignment, some degree of lateral subluxation of the tibia on the femur is common in advanced lesions and a varus deformity is frequent. "Weight-bearing films" often demonstrate joint-space narrowing and varus or valgus deformity that is not evident on films exposed with the patient in the prone position.

In contrast to the hip, formation of cystic cavities in the articular ends of the bones is infrequent. However, a common feature of the disease in this joint is the development of calcific or bony loose bodies within the joint. The fabella, if present, may be enlarged and roughened. Joint effusion is not infrequently seen in roentgenograms and usually results from either the mechanical irritation of intra-articular loose bodies or because of trauma to a joint rendered unstable by the disease.

Joints of the Spine

The same process that involves the peripheral joints may also affect the spine but because of anatomic structures peculiar to this region it requires separate discussion. The most common finding almost universally present in patients above middle age is hypertrophic spurring along the anterior and lateral mar-

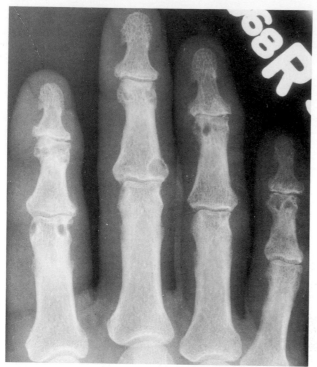

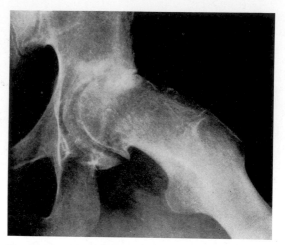

Fig. 9-24. Characteristic joint thinning and spurring in this patient with degenerative hip joint disease.

Fig. 9-23. Degenerative joint disease involving the distal interphalangeal joints where there is thinning and irregularity of joint margins. There are also numerous pseudocysts which may accompany the degenerative disease and are believed to be post-traumatic.

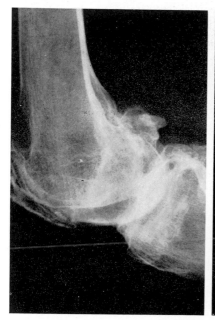

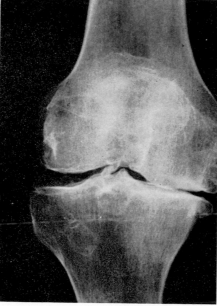

Fig. 9-25. Degenerative disease of the knee joint. There is thinning of the medial aspect of the joint space, lateral subluxation of the tibia on the femur, some tibia vara, and extensive spurring along the articular margins as well as some eburnation of bony surfaces.

gins of the vertebral bodies (Fig. 9-26). These marginal osteophytes are particularly prone to develop in the lower cervical, lower dorsal, and lower lumbar areas. When the process begins in younger persons below the age of 50 the lower cervical vertebrae often are affected primarily. In addition to the spurs, small calcific or bony deposits may form in the spinal ligaments, especially the anterior, without any attachment to the adjacent bodies. Bony proliferation along the margins of the spinous processes often is present, as is marginal spurring of the costovertebral joints. In more severe forms of the disease, some degree of thinning of the intervertebral discs is found. This is particularly likely to occur in the lower cervical region and at the lumbosacral joint, but other disc

Fig. 9-26. Degenerative joint disease of the lower cervical spine. Note the large marginal osteophytes and thinning of the intervertebral discs at the C5–6 and C6–7 levels.

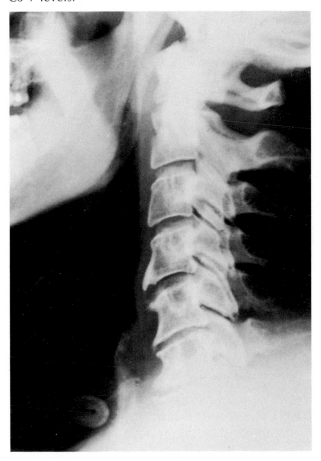

Fig. 9-27. Degenerative joint disease of the thoracic spine. Anterior spurs of varying sizes as well as ligament calcification of the type that occurs in diffuse idiopathic skeletal hyperostosis (DISH) are present.

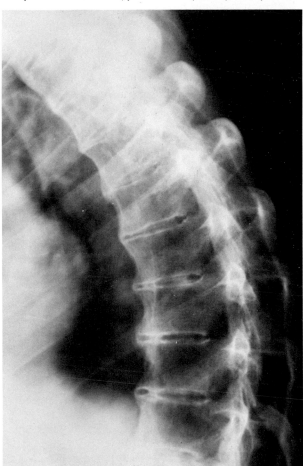

spaces may be affected (see Fig. 9-26). Narrowing of the disc space usually is uniform except in the dorsal region, where it is more pronounced along the anterior borders (Fig. 9-27). In the presence of scoliosis these changes are more severe along the concave side of the curvature. Because this disease is found chiefly in the older age period, senile decalcification of bone usually is present although the cortical margins of the vertebrae remain distinct and actually may show increased density. The small apophyseal joints may or may not be involved. The changes consist in thinning of the joint space, marginal spurring, increased density of bony articular surfaces, and some degree of subluxation, the uppermost facets slipping forward on the ones below. These combined with the thinning of the adjacent intervertebral disc may result in a distinct narrowing of the corresponding spinal foramina and lead to the production of clinical symptoms. The forward displacement of one vertebra on the one below is called spondylolisthesis and a minor degree of this is common in degenerative joint disease (also see p. 84). Marginal spurs are not infrequent on the posterior margins of the vertebrae in the lower cervical and lower lumbar areas. These are more significant from a clinical standpoint than spurs on the other surfaces because of the close association with spinal nerve roots. Occasionally a thin, waferlike, translucent space is visualized within one or more of the discs severely involved by degenerative disease. This is called a *phantom disc* (see p. 313) and is seen mainly in the lower lumbar area (Fig. 9-28).

DIFFUSE IDIOPATHIC SKELETAL HYPEROSTOSIS (DISH, FORRESTIER'S DISEASE)

This is characterized by extensive hyperostoses or massive ossification of the paraspinal ligaments anteriorly and laterally (right more than left in lower thoracic spine).[30] It tends to be more severe in the lower cervical and thoracic spine than elsewhere. The ossifications are large and result in a corrugated appearance of the spine. Bony bridging is common and may be continuous throughout the portion of the spine involved or there may be areas of lesser involvement with no bridging across an intervening vertebra. The appearance is very irregular and unlike that of the thin, vertical syndesmophytes representing ossification of the peripheral portion of the annulus fibrosis which produce the relatively smooth bamboolike bony bridging in ankylosing spondylitis. This condition is also characterized by a tendency to hyperostoses elsewhere in the body with irregular outgrowths or whiskering of the iliac crest, ischial tuberosities, greater trochanters, acetabular margins, and sacroiliac and symphysis pubis margins.[34] Ossifications may also occur in the iliolumbar and sacrotuberous ligaments and at almost any muscular or ligamentous attachment to bone. This process may not represent a disease but rather may be an exaggerated response to stimuli that produce minimal to moderate formation of new bone in healthy persons. In addition to the greater irregularity of the spine, the absence of change in the lumbosacral spine and sacroiliac joints tends to differentiate this condition from ankylosing spondylitis.

TRAUMATIC ARTHRITIS

The term "traumatic arthritis" should be reserved to designate that form of degenerative joint disease in which the process is initiated by acute trauma, either as a single episode or as the result of repeated injuries. Thus, traumatic arthritis may develop in a joint following a fracture that extended into the joint; after a hemorrhagic effusion following trauma; as a result of a severe sprain or recurrent injuries to the supporting structures of the joint. Because the diagnosis of traumatic arthritis may have medicolegal implications and because it may be a compensable disease, it is not wise to use this term unless it can be established with reasonable certainty that the joint was normal prior to the trauma and that following the injury the arthritic changes became evident. In general the roentgen findings are similar to those of degenerative joint disease and the pathologic alterations are similar.

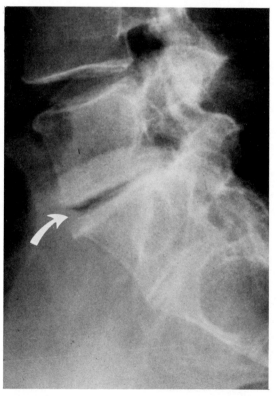

Fig. 9-28. Phantom disc. There is severe thinning of the lumbosacral disc with a dark, translucent space within it **(arrow).**

GOUTY ARTHRITIS

Gout is a metabolic disturbance of unknown cause. It is characterized by the occurrence of acute attacks of arthritis in certain joints with freedom of symptoms between the attacks; by elevation of the uric acid in the blood serum and the body fluids; by the deposition of sodium urate in various body tissues (joints, bones, periarticular tissues); and by the development of degenerative changes, particularly in the blood vessels of the kidneys. The most common joint to be affected is the first metatarsophalangeal, where the disease is clinically known as *podagra*. Other joints commonly involved are the ankle, knee, and the joints of the hands and wrists and the elbow. Roentgen changes are not likely to be present unless the disease has existed for some time and until after there have been several attacks of the disease. Thus, a negative roentgenogram does not necessarily exclude the possibility of gout. The disease affects males predominantly.

Roentgen Features

Early Changes.[42] The joint may appear entirely normal or there may be soft-tissue swelling during the acute exacerbation of the disease. A variable amount of disuse osteoporosis may be present, depending upon the length of the attack and the amount of disuse associated with it. Osteoporosis is not a prominent feature of this disease, however, and may not be present even though extensive bone and joint involvement is observed.

Later Changes. After several attacks of the disease, localized soft-tissue swellings appear. These are irregular and lumpy in appearance, representing accumulations of monosodium urate monohydrate crystals and are known as tophi. Similar deposits occur in the articular cartilages and in the bones adjacent to the joint. As they enlarge, these deposits result in localized punched-out defects in the ends of the bones. These not infrequently have the appearance of cysts with a fairly well defined cavity which may develop a thin sclerotic wall (Figs. 9-29 and 9-30). The cyst may lie completely within the bone or be marginal and cause some destruction of cortex. When marginal, the partially eroded cortex may form a characteristic spurlike projection. Involvement of bursae, particularly the olecranon bursa, is common. Involvement of soft tissues at and adjacent to the Achilles tendon is also common.

Advanced Changes. After the disease has existed for many years the roentgen findings usually become typical. There are large marginal erosions and cavities in and along the ends of the bones. There are, in association with these, large, lumpy, soft-tissue swellings representing gouty tophi (Fig. 9-31). The joint spaces may be somewhat thinned as a result of degeneration of articular cartilages but usually this is not particularly severe. Bony ankylosis does not occur but fibrous ankylosis may develop as a late manifestation. The bones often maintain a surprisingly good density because disuse osteoporosis does not develop since the patients are relatively free of symptoms between the acute exacerbations. Periosteal new bone formation is unusual but may occur at the base of an overhanging marginal area of cortex near a large area of destruction. At times, periosteal new bone may be extensive. Tophi consisting only of sodium urate are radiolucent. Calcification of gouty tophi occurs occasionally, particularly in more advanced disease and usually in para-articular tophi. Sacroiliac joint involvement is unusual, but not rare. Destruction of bone resulting in an irregularity of the joint margins and cystlike areas with thin, sclerotic rims are characteristic. The lower one-third of the joint is the most frequent site of the changes, which are unilateral in about half of the cases. Occasionally, large popliteal cysts resembling those observed in rheumatoid arthritis are observed.

Differential Diagnosis. The diagnosis of gouty arthritis is largely a clinical one in the early stages of the disease although this condition may be suspected roentgenologically because of the typical joint or joints involved and the character of the soft-tissue swelling caused by the tophi. However, confusion with rheumatoid arthritis is entirely possible since both of these diseases cause marginal erosions and soft-tissue swelling. The distribution of the disease is significant. In rheumatoid arthritis, characteristically, the proximal interphalangeal, metacarpophalangeal, and ulnocarpal joints are affected early. It is here that one expects to find the more characteristic changes. In gouty arthritis the first metatarsophalangeal joint is the one most frequently involved. This is not commonly involved by rheumatoid arthritis unless the disease is generalized.

CHONDROCALCINOSIS AND THE PSEUDOGOUT SYNDROME

Calcium pyrophosphate dihydrate deposition disease (CPPD) or chondrocalcinosis is defined as the pres-

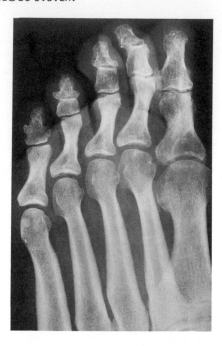

Fig. 9-29. Gouty arthritis. Note the cystlike rarefaction in the proximal end of the proximal phalanx of the great toe. This represents a gouty tophus containing urate crystals.

Fig. 9-30. Gouty arthritis showing cystlike erosion in the middle phalanx and some erosion of the distal phalanx along with lumpy soft-tissue swelling.

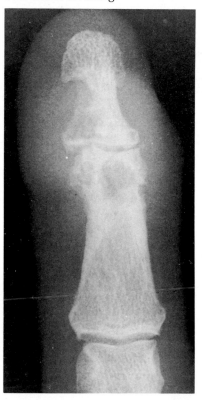

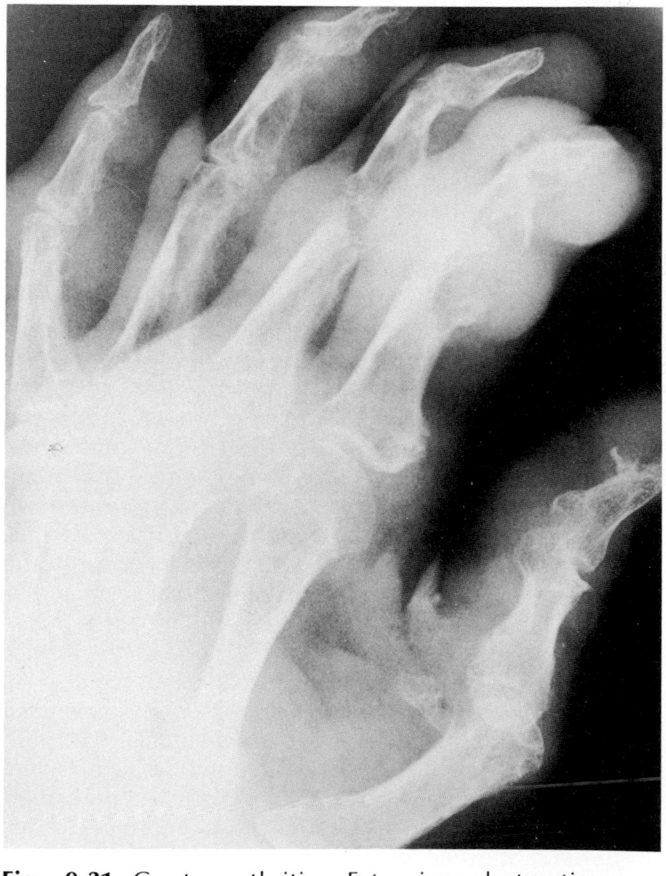

Fig. 9-31. Gouty arthritis. Extensive destruction, lumpy soft-tissue swellings, and a characteristic spur-like projection of bone of the distal end of the distal phalanx of the thumb.

ence of intra-articular calcium-containing salts within hyaline and fibrocartilage.[32] It occurs in association with hyperparathyroidism, hemochromatosis, ochronosis, gout, and rheumatoid arthritis. It also occurs in asymptomatic elderly individuals as well as in the idiopathic form, to be described here, which usually is first manifest in the sixth and seventh decades of life. When the crystals are present within a joint, an acute synovitis is produced causing joint effusion and pain. The clinical spectrum of pseudogout includes: (*1*) intermittent acute attacks of arthritic pain that subside completely; (*2*) continuous acute attacks of arthritic pain; (*3*) progressive, chronic arthritic pain with acute exacerbations; and (*4*) progressive chronic arthritic pain without acute episodes. The acute disease predominates in men and the chronic in women. In some instances, degenerative changes precede chondrocalcinosis and attacks of pain may be present without radiographically visible cartilage calcifications. The severity of symptoms is not directly related to radiologic changes of arthritis. The most commonly involved joints are the metacarpophalangeal, shoulder, elbow, wrist, ankle, and knee. In addition to calcification in joint cartilage (Fig. 9-32), roentgen findings include subchondral cyst formation, thinning of articular cartilage with subchondral sclerosis, marginal spurs, and para-articular tendon and bursal calcifications. Chondrocalcinosis differs from osteoarthritis[32] in that joints unusually involved in osteoarthritis, such as the radiocarpal, wrist, elbow, and shoulder, may be implicated. Also, subchondral cyst formation may be severe, leading to bony collapse and fragmentation, with loose body formation. These changes may be so severe as to resemble those in neuropathic arthropathy. The diagnosis is made by identification of the calcium pyrophosphate crystals in the synovial fluid.

NEUROTROPHIC ARTHROPATHY

Any disease that impairs sensation in the joint structures renders it susceptible to repeated trauma and may lead to severe disorganization of the joint. Included among such diseases are tabes dorsalis, syringomyelia, diabetic neuropathy, leprosy, transection of the spinal cord, and peripheral nerve injury. The resulting arthropathy is known as a *Charcot joint.* The weight-bearing joints of the lower extremities are the most frequently affected in tabes dorsalis. Less common is involvement of the spine, usually the lower part of the lumbar. Neurotrophic arthropathy in the joints of the upper extremities is much less common and in these ares syringomyelia is the usual cause

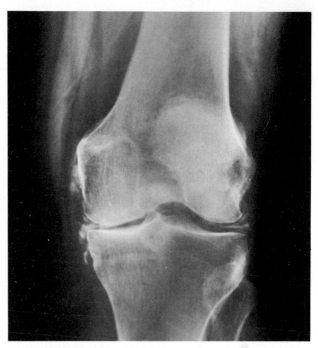

Fig. 9-32. Chondrocalcinosis. Note the extensive calcification of cartilage in this patient with chondrocalcinosis.

(see Fig. 9-33B). Diabetic arthropathy predominantly affects the foot (see Fig. 9-35).

Roentgen Features. Pathologically the lesion is one of repeated infractions, often of minor degree, but, with summation of these injuries, considerable breakdown and fragmentation of the articular cartilages and articulating ends of the bones result. Hemorrhage in the soft tissues may also occur. In the early stages the roentgen findings are usually limited to soft-tissue swelling, in most instances the result of joint effusion. Then there develops a condensation of bone in the articular ends, producing an eburnated appearance of the articular surfaces and some loss of the joint space. There is a tendency for subluxation to occur rather early. These changes are followed by breakdown of bone structures and eventually considerable disorganization of the joint results. Once the breakdown begins it may progress very rapidly. In the hip the acetabular cavity becomes enlarged, the head of the femur undergoes fragmentation and absorption, often with increase in density of the bone (Fig. 9-33A). In the knee, similar changes take place. Wearing away of the condylar surfaces occurs, particularly on the medial side. Fragmentation and generalized disorganization develop. Soft-tissue swelling is

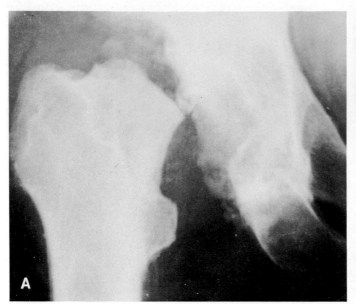
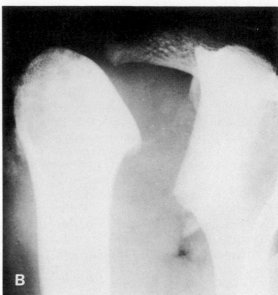

Fig. 9-33. Neurotrophic arthropathy (Charcot joint). **A.** Note gross disorganization of the hip joint with fragmentation of the head and dislocation in this patient with tabes dorsalis. Bone density is somewhat greater than normal, and there is a considerable amount of fragmented bone within the joint space. **B.** This patient had syringomyelia. Note gross distortion of the joint and severe eburnation of bone.

pronounced; multiple calcified and osseous fragments are found in and around the joint. The pattern of soft-tissue calcification[10] indicates that the debris may break out of the joint capsule and dissect along muscle planes. This may produce local pain, swelling, and heat. The calcifications may then resorb and the clinical signs regress. The changes are similar in other large joints that may be affected. The frequency of subluxation is to be noted and instability of the joint is one of the prominent clinical signs. In the spine the affected vertebral bodies develop increased density; they tend to undergo some degree of compression and fragmentation, and alteration in alignment (Fig. 9-34). Thinning or disappearance of the intervertebral discs accompanies these changes in the vertebral bodies. The rapidity of development of these changes is variable but in some cases relatively advanced disease has been reported as occurring in from 9 days to 6 weeks after roentgenograms had shown a normal joint.

Diabetic osteoarthropathy differs somewhat from the other neurotrophic arthropathies. It is confined almost exclusively to the ankle and foot (Fig. 9-35); rarely it involves the hands, femur, and tibia. Trauma is an important initiating event, with incomplete fractures and dislocations leading to fragmentation,

osteolysis, and periosteal reaction. At times, destructive changes are extensive, leading to absorption of distal ends of the metatarsals with pencil-point narrowing and "arthritis mutilans." The role of infection in the destructive process is not clear, but sequestration occurs and in some instances infection must play an important part. There is a tendency to heal, even though destruction may have been extensive. Bony ankylosis may occur as part of the healing process.

PERIARTICULAR DISEASE

The various tissues around a joint, such as bursae, tendons, and muscles, may become involved by acute or chronic inflammatory changes. Involvement of the tendons and bursae is common, particularly in the shoulder, and results in limitation of motion and considerable disability. This is referred to variously as periarthritis, periarticular disease, bursitis, fibrositis, tendinitis, and the like. It is the most frequent cause of shoulder disability. Roentgenologically, in addition to disuse osteoporosis, amorphous calcium depositions frequently are seen in the tendons of the shoulder cuff (Fig. 9-36). These usually occur in the tendon of the supraspinatus and are found directly above

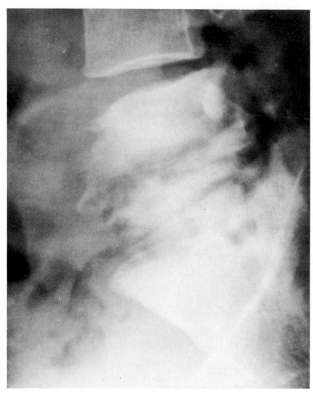

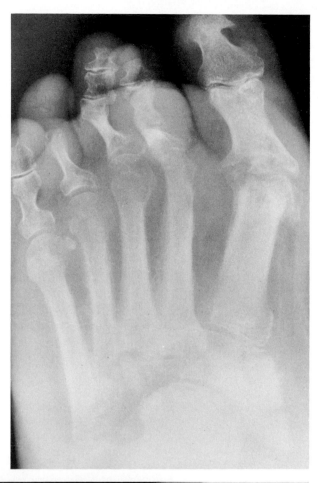

Fig. 9-34. Neurotrophic arthropathy in the lower lumbar spine in a patient with tabes dorsalis. Note extensive bone destruction with fragmentation, malalignment, and dense sclerosis.

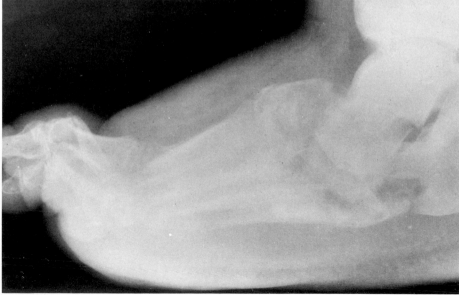

Fig. 9-35. Diabetic arthropathy involving the anterior tarsal bones as well as the great toe and the fourth toe. Bone destruction, marked distortion of the distal tarsals, and soft-tissue swelling are evident. Also a considerable amount of periosteal calcification involving the phalanges is seen. This process is most likely caused by infection in a patient with diabetic neuropathy.

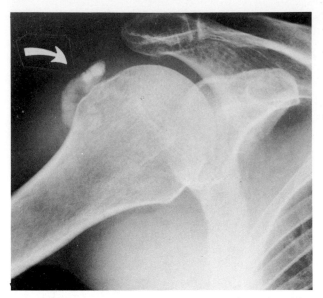

Fig. 9-36. Calcifying tendinitis of the shoulder **(arrow).**

the greater tuberosity of the humerus. Less common are similar deposits in the tendons of the subscapularis, infraspinatus, and teres minor. Such deposits in the tendons often are associated with inflammation of an overlying bursa, hence the clinical designation of a painful shoulder as "bursitis" or "subacromial bursitis." Rupture of a mass of calcium into a bursa may occur, but as a rule the calcification occurs within the tendon and not in the overlying bursa. Approximately 50% of patients with complaints of pain and disability in the shoulder will show demonstrable calcification on roentgen examination. In the remainder there will be noted only the evidence of disuse osteoporosis if the disability has been present for any appreciable time and if limited motion is demonstrated when films are exposed with the patient's arm in abduction and rotation. It is not at all infrequent to find calcium deposits in the tendinous cuff of the shoulder in patients who have no complaints, or at least none at the time of the examination. Thus the mere presence of demonstrable calcium does not indicate the existence of an active inflammatory process. In addition to the shoulder area, similar calcifications sometimes are found in association with the trochanteric bursa that overlies the greater trochanter of the femur. They also are encountered in the periarticular tissues around the elbow, especially on the radial side; at the wrist; along the interphalangeal joints; or in any location where bursae are present with ten-

dons overlying them. Such deposits should be searched for in patients complaining of acute inflammatory changes in any of the joints.

MISCELLANEOUS

HEMOPHILIAC ARTHROPATHY

In hemophilia, recurrent hemorrhages into the joints are of frequent occurrence. The knee and elbow are somewhat more vulnerable to repeated injuries than are the other joints, but any joint may be involved. As a result of the repeated hemorrhages and the irritating effect of the blood within the joint, a chronic synovitis develops. It is estimated that permanent joint changes will develop if more than two bleeding episodes occur into the joint. There is degeneration of articular cartilages and erosion of bony surfaces. The soft tissues become thickened. If there has been recent injury the joint capsule may be distended with fresh blood, and the signs of joint effusion will be present. In chronic cases the deposition of iron pigment in the tissues may lead to areas of cloudy increase in density resembling calcification (Fig. 9-37). Cartilage degeneration is shown by narrowing of the joint space. Hemorrhage into the articular ends of the bones may cause them to appear eroded and irregular in the subchondral area. In some instances the cartilage collapses into the small cystic subchrondral areas, resulting in a false impression of loss of cartilage in these regions. In the knee, enlargement of the intercondylar fossa of the femur may be apparent. Occasionally, hemorrhage may occur within the bone at a distance from the joint and result in a cystlike cavity (Fig. 9-38). The ilium has been reported as an occasional site of this lesion, which may expand and destroy a rather large area of bone. It is well to be acquainted with this fact so that a biopsy will not be undertaken, a very dangerous procedure in patients with hemophilia. The lesion has been called a *pseudotumor of hemophilia*. Acceleration of epiphyseal growth from chronic irritation leads to club-shaped enlargement of the ends of the bones. This is noted in other chronic inflammatory lesions such as Still's disease and tuberculosis. The differential diagnosis of hemophiliac arthropathy may be difficult from roentgen examination alone but it should be considered as a possibility when a destructive arthritis is encountered in a child. An arthropathy similar to that in hemophilia may occur in patients with synovial hemangiomas which bleed into the joint.

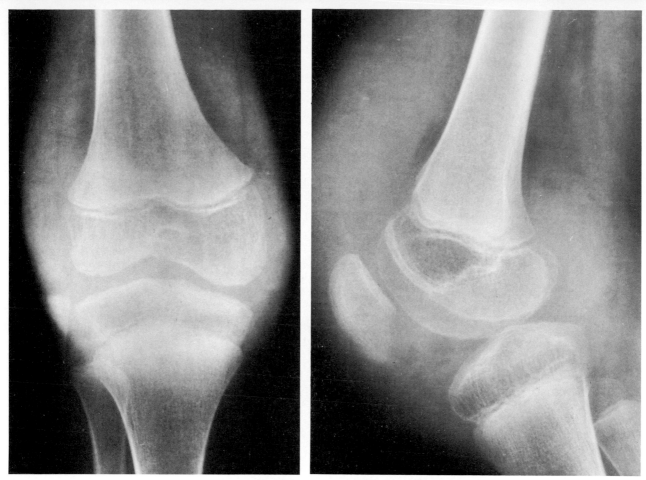

Fig. 9-37. Hemophiliac arthropathy. This child had repeated episodes of hemarthrosis. Note the massive, dense, joint effusion caused by accumulation of iron in the joint. There is a little loss of joint space and a slight granular irregularity of joint surfaces.

Fig. 9-38. Note the large, expanding, cystlike cavity in the os calcis in this patient with hemophilia (pseudotumor).

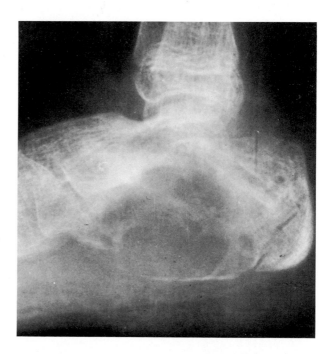

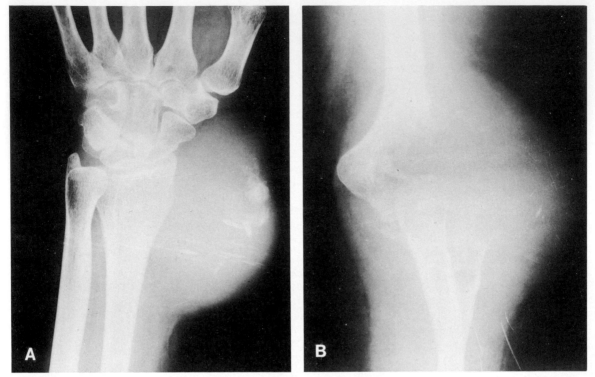

Fig. 9-39. Synovial sarcoma. **A.** Synovial sarcoma in the wrist. The tumor is in the soft tissues adjacent to the distal radius. There does not appear to be any involvement of the bone in this patient. Note calcification within the soft-tissue mass. **B.** Synovial sarcoma of the elbow in which there is extensive involvement of the adjacent bones and very little soft-tissue calcification.

TUMORS AND RELATED LESIONS

Because of the diversity of the tissues entering into the formation of a joint, a wide variety of tumors and tumorlike lesions may develop. Most of these are uncommon but of sufficient importance to warrant some discussion. The ones described in the following are considered to be the most significant from a roentgenologic point of view.

Synovioma (Synovial Sarcoma)

Synovioma (synovial sarcoma) is an uncommon but important tumor. It is unusual for synovial sarcoma to arise from the synovial lining of a joint. However, it usually begins in the vicinity of a large joint, starting in the para-articular soft tissues just beyond the confines of the capsule. Occasionally it is found at some distance from a joint. It is most frequent in young adults. The knee area is a favorite site. It is generally considered that the tumor must be classed with the malignant neoplasms, although the degree of malignancy may vary from case to case. The lesion is visualized in roentgenograms as a mass of soft-tissue density, adjacent to a joint. Usually the outer margin of the mass is fairly well demarcated from the adjacent soft tissues. Calcification of portions of the tumor occurs rather frequently. This may be in the form of hazy, punctate deposits or linear streaks (Fig. 9-39). During the early development of the tumor the bone beneath it remains normal. Sooner or later the lesion begins to invade the bone and destroy it. At first this is seen as a ragged erosion of the cortex directly beneath the tumor. Subsequently, destruction of the cancellous bone develops (Fig. 9-39). The type of bone destruction is similar to that caused by fibrosarcoma arising in the soft tissues and invading bone. The location of the lesion within or close to the joint is presumptive evidence of synovial origin (Fig. 9-40). Calcium deposition also occurs in fibrosar-

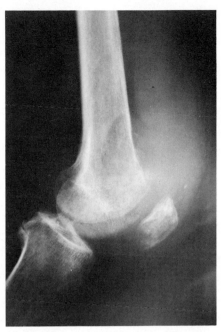

Fig. 9-40. Synovial sarcoma of the knee. Note the large, soft-tissue, tumor mass invading the anterior aspect of the femur.

coma but is less frequent. Before the stage of bone invasion has been reached, and in the absence of calcification within the mass, accurate roentgen diagnosis usually is impossible. Biopsy is therefore necessary for making the diagnosis.

Pigmented Villonodular Synovitis

The cause of pigmented villonodular synovitis is unknown, but most investigators have considered it to be of inflammatory rather than of neoplastic origin. In some cases there is a history of trauma, but in the majority there is none. Usually the symptoms are mild and of long duration, often extending over a period of years. Two major pathologic types are recognized, the localized and the diffuse.[5] In the former, roentgenograms reveal the outlines of a soft-tissue mass within the joint but not distending the entire joint pouch. The mass may have a nodular outline but more often is smooth. In this form the fingers are the common sites; rarely, multiple joints are involved. In the diffuse form there is a generalized swelling of soft tissues of the joint indicative of a synovitis. Usually there is very little in the appearance of this swelling to indicate the nature of the lesion. In the

diffuse form, the knee, hip, ankle, subtalar, elbow, shoulder, and carpal are the joints involved most often. Since the disease does not cause much disability, disuse osteoporosis is not a prominent feature and may be lacking entirely. Narrowing of the joint space also is seen infrequently. If the disease has been present for some time, deposition of iron pigment in the tissues may cause a cloudy increase in density very similar to that found in some patients with hemophiliac arthropathy. In chronic lesions, local pressure erosions or actual invasion may develop along the margin or within medullary cavity. This results in cystlike areas of rarefaction that vary greatly in size, usually have a very thin, sclerotic margin, and may be solitary or multiple, usually the latter. Accurate diagnosis from roentgen examination alone is difficult and often impossible. Significant features include the presence of a chronic lesion in a young adult characterized by synovitis and causing very little disability, slight or no changes in the joint space, and, occasionally, cloudy areas of density in the soft tissues. Some observers[5] think that the localized nodular form is a reactive process or a true neoplasm and that the diffuse, villonodular form represents a vascular anomaly, even though histologic differentiation of the two is not always possible. Surgical exploration and the examination of tissue usually are required to establish the diagnosis with certainty and are indicated in most cases in order to differentiate the lesion from synovial sarcoma.

Giant Cell and Xanthomatous Tumors

There is a group of tumors or tumorlike lesions of the tendon sheaths and joints that have been difficult to classify. Following the investigations of Jaffe, Lichtenstein, and Sutro, many pathologists now consider most of these, if not all, to be closely related to pigmented villonodular synovitis. Evidence has been presented to show that these "tumors" are linked rather closely and probably represent only stages in the development of the same disease. Nevertheless, agreement on the subject is not complete and there are certain clinical and roentgen features that tend to separate some of them from pigmented villonodular synovitis, at least from the diffuse form of the disease. The xanthomas and giant cell tumors are prone to develop in the tendon sheaths and are found most frequently in the hands and feet. In roentgenograms they are visualized as discrete masses of soft-tissue density but with no specific features by which their histologic nature can be recognized. In some cases the mass may cause a smooth, pressure type of erosion of the bone beneath it. In an occasional patient the tumor appears to grow directly into the bone, forming an irregular cystlike cavity. A peculiar variant is the disease known as *xanthoma tuberosa*. In this condition, multiple nodular masses form along the tendons and synovial membranes in the hands and feet; these cause very little clinical disability. The bones may be perfectly normal and the joint spaces preserved. In some cases, however, erosion and destruction of the bone beneath one or more of the masses may occur. The resulting appearance resembles that of gout very closely (Fig. 9-41). To avoid confusion it is preferable to consider the single xanthomas as lesions distinct from xanthoma tuberosa. The former are apparently related closely to the giant cell tumor of the tendon sheaths and to pigmented villonodular synovitis. Xanthoma tuberosa, on the other hand, has no such relationship. Instead, it may be one of the manifestations of hypercholesterolemia.

Cartilaginous Tumors

Cartilaginous tumors, either benign chondroma or chondrosarcoma, may arise from the articular cartilages, but they are uncommon lesions. Because the tumor forms a hard mass within the joint, symptoms of joint dysfunction may appear early. In other cases the mass has grown chiefly outside the joint cavity and thus has reached a large size before removal became necessary (Fig. 9-42). Cartilaginous tumors are prone to calcify no matter where they may originate and those developing within a joint are no exception to the rule. Typically, the calcium occurs in the form of multiple, very dense, discrete foci, resulting in a mottled appearance. If the calcified areas are few in number it may be impossible to distinguish between a chondroma and a synovioma from the roentgen appearances.

Synovial Chondromatosis (Osteochondromatosis). Probably initiated by trauma, the synovial villi may hypertrophy and, by cellular metaplasia, form cartilaginous masses. These become calcified or even ossified in part and often become detached to lie free within the joint cavity. This condition is known as synovial chondromatosis (Fig. 9-43). Usually there are multiple bodies but at times only one or a few are present. Calcification or ossification of the bodies usually is irregular and often has a laminated appearance. The presence of the masses within the joint causes a chronic synovitis with generalized thickening of the synovium and joint effusion. Degenerative

changes in the form of joint space narrowing, eburnation of articular surfaces, and marginal osteophytes are common and may be severe. Occasionally, pressure erosions of bone by the loose bodies may cause a clearly defined defect, usually at the joint margin. Osteochondromatosis is seen most frequently in the knee, occasionally in the elbow and the hip. Involvement of other joints is rare.

Hemangioma

Hemangiomas involving the articular and periarticular tissues are moderately common lesions. As is true when this tumor develops elsewhere in the body, calcified thrombi may be present and give a clue concerning the nature of the lesion. A calcified thrombus within a vein appears as a small round or ovoid shadow and is called a phlebolith. Frequently these are ringlike with a dense outer rim and a less dense center, or else the shadow is laminated. Unless such phleboliths are visualized there usually is nothing specific about the appearance of a hemangioma of a joint that will allow its recognition in roentgenograms. If the intra-articular synovial hemangioma bleeds into the joint, an arthropathy similar to that in hemophilia may develop. The presence of cutaneous hemangiomas aids in the diagnosis. The lesions are usually found in the knee in a child or young adult. The vascular nature of the tumor may be demonstrated by arteriography and an intra-articular mass is visible on arthrography.

Loose Bodies

Intra-articular loose bodies may arise from multiple causes. Among these are (1) intra-articular fracture with separation of a fragment of cartilage, (2) rupture and fragmentation of a meniscus cartilage in the knee, (3) osteochondritis dissecans, (4) synovial chondromatosis, (5) degenerative joint disease (see page 292). Injury accounts for the majority of loose bodies and they occur most frequently in the knee. If composed only of cartilage, the fragment cannot be visualized in roentgenograms. Many cartilaginous bodies calcify, becoming radiopaque and thus easily demonstrable in roentgenograms. Such calcified cartilage masses may arise from the synovial membrane as a result of metaplasia and are seen in synovial chondromatosis. Similar calcified bodies may be formed in degenerative joint disease as a result of fragmentation of articular cartilage or as a sequela to chronic synovial irritation in a joint rendered unstable by the disease.

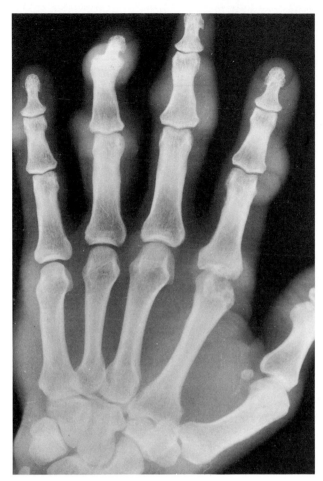

Fig. 9-41. Xanthoma tuberosa. Note the multiple, lumpy, soft-tissue swellings in the hand. There is erosion in the head of the second metacarpal. Similar bone involvement occurs with solitary xanthoma.

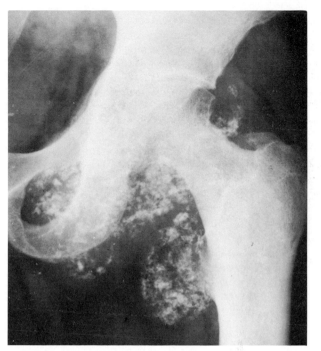

Fig. 9-42. Synovial osteochondromatosis of the hip joint manifested by large masses of partially calcified cartilage in and around the joint associated with some erosion of the superior aspect of the femoral neck and adjacent head.

OTHER CONDITIONS

Ochronosis. This is a rare disorder of metabolism in which there is an abnormal accumulation of homogentisic acid in the blood and urine due to a lack of homogentisic acid oxidase. The urine is either very dark on voiding or becomes black after standing or after it is alkalinized. The deposition of homogentisic acid (alkapton) in the articular cartilages results in their degeneration. The significant roentgen observation is the extensive deposit of calcium that occurs in the articular cartilages. This is seen most frequently in the spine where there is extensive calcification of the discs. In addition to calcification of the disc cartilages, the intervertebral disc spaces become

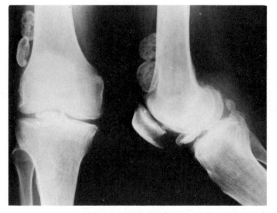

Fig. 9-43. Osteochondromatosis of the knee joint.

thinned as a result of degeneration. Because many patients are in the older age group, senile osteoporosis and marginal spurring also may be present. Calcification of the articular cartilages of the peripheral joints is rather frequent as a simple degenerative process and may occur in association with ochronosis; in the spine, however, extensive calcification of the discs should arouse the suspicion of ochronosis. The cartilages in the ears may be extensively calcified.

In the peripheral joints a severe degenerative type of arthritis may develop, with thinning of the articular cartilages and even destructive changes in the bony articular surfaces. Calcifications may form in the synovium and periarticular tissues, such as ligaments and tendons. Peripheral joint involvement usually follows that in the spine and is symptomatic, unlike the spinal disease which is often asymptomatic. The shoulders are often affected, much more severely than is usual in osteoarthritis.

Idiopathic Hemochromatosis.[40] Idiopathic hemochromatosis is frequently associated with an arthropathy which may antedate the signs of cirrhosis, diabetes, and brown pigmentation of the skin. Involvement of the second and third metacarpophalangeal joints is characteristic, but there may be involvement of the other metacarpophalangeal joints; and proximal interphalangeal, wrist, shoulder, hip, and knee joints may also be affected. Narrowing of the joint space, subchrondral erosion of bone, cyst formation, sclerosis, and osteophyte formation are common in the hands. In other joints, osteophyte formation is somewhat less than in osteoarthritis which idiopathic hemochromatosis resembles. Chrondrocalcinosis is very common and tends to involve hyaline cartilage more than fibrocartilage in contrast to the pseudogout syndrome.

Jacoud's Arthropathy[21] (*Chronic Post-rheumatic fever arthritis*). This is a migratory polyarthritis in which there is an insidious painless onset of joint deformity after resolution of the active polyarthritis of acute rheumatic fever. These patients have rheumatic valvular heart disease. The joint deformities consist of ulnar deviation, flexion deformity, or subluxations of the metacarpophalangeal joints which are reducible early but later become fixed. The proximal interphalangeal joints are hyperextended. The toes may be involved with hallux valgus and subluxation of the great toe. Roentgenograms showing changes of severe deformity with minimal, if any, bone destruction should suggest the diagnosis in a patient with a history of rheumatic fever.

Wilson's Disease (*Hepatolenticular Degeneration*). This is an autosomal recessive disorder characterized by rentention of copper in excess amounts.

Bone and joint involvement is unusal except for demineralization of bone which occurs in about 50% of these patients. Joint manifestations include subarticular cysts and fragmentation of subchrondral bone, chiefly in hands, wrists, feet, and ankles. The fragments are small, corticated, and resemble accessory ossifications. The cysts are small and occur mainly in small joints of hands, feet, wrists, and ankles. Other findings include osteochondritis dissecans, irregularity of subchondral vertebral bone suggesting osteochondritis, unusually tall vertebral bodies, and thoracolumbar scoliosis.

Hyperparathyroidism. Hyperparathyroidism is accompanied by erosive arthritis of the hands and wrists. Roentgen findings include: (*1*) erosive changes involving the radial aspects of phalanges and metacarpals; (2) predilection for radiocarpal, inferior radioulnar, and metacarpophalangeal joints and the interphalangeal joint of the thumb; (3) tendency to spare proximal interphalangeal joints; (4) "whiskering" at margins of involved joints; (5) little or no joint space narrowing; (6) chondrocalcinosis and capsular or periosteal calcifications; (7) no narrowing of joint space; and (8) occasional involvement of temporomandibular joints.

Primary Amyloidosis. Primary amyloidosis may involve bone and when the bone at joint surfaces is affected, joint changes are manifest. Multiple lytic bone lesions are usually distributed about large joints, particularly the shoulder. They are poorly marginated and have no active sclerosis but may expand the cortex. The joint space tends to be increased in diameter.

Tietze's Syndrome. This is characterized by involvement of the sternoclavicular and the first two chondrosternal junctions. Roentgen findings include hypotrophic or hypertrophic medial clavicular changes, sometimes with osteosclerosis, and chondrosternal and periarticular calcifications.

Lipoid Dermatoarthritis (Multicentric Reticulohistiocytosis). This is a rare disorder, affecting skin and synovium, that causes an erosive polyarthritis. Roentgen findings include: striking symmetry of clearly defined erosive changes, spreading from joint margins to the articular surfaces; interphalangeal joint predominance; early and severe atlantoaxial disease; minimal or no periosteal reaction; minimal osteoporosis; and soft-tissue nodules in skin, subcutaneous tissues, and tendon sheaths. The joint involvement often progresses rapidly resulting in crippling deformity of the hands. Symptoms are disproportionately mild.

Relapsing Polychondritis. Relapsing polychondritis is an intense inflammatory and degenerative process which may result from altered immunity or hypersensitivity. Joints of the hands, wrists, and feet are involved by erosion of articular surfaces accompanied by soft-tissue swelling. Sacroiliac joints may also show erosive change resulting in irregularity of joint space and partial obliteration of the space in some areas. Also, bony end-plates of vertebral bodies may show areas of erosion with sclerosis of adjacent bone. Cartilage dissolution in the ear, nose, trachea, and bronchi may also occur, leading to saddle nose and to respiratory disease and death. Calcifications may appear in the ear cartilage.

Cartilage Atrophy. This may occur in patients with flaccid paralysis, leading to narrowing of the hip-joint space. It is probably caused by a decreased production of synovial fluid which results in altered nutrition of cartilage.

Idiopathic Chondrolysis of the Hip.[17] This is a rare condition in young girls characterized by radiologic evidence of loss of joint space of one hip preceded by pain and periarticular osteoporosis. Later, some erosion of cortex at the weight-bearing areas is observed. Rheumatoid factor is negative, and there is no joint effusion or evidence of rheumatoid disease on biopsy. The cause is unknown.

Synovitis. Synovitis may be caused by a number of factors including joint injury due to penetration of a joint by a plant thorn, resulting in a low-grade granulomatous synovitis. Transient synovitis of the hip occurs in children and leaves no sequelae. A lymphofollicular synovitis has been reported associated with intra-articular osteoid osteoma. All of these conditions are accompanied by pain and there may be enough effusion to be demonstrated radiographically.

CYSTS CONNECTED WITH THE JOINTS

Distended Bursae. Any bursa adjacent to a joint may become distended with fluid and present as a cystic mass. Common examples are the prepatellar and olecranon bursae. Trauma is the most common cause for distention of these bursae. Some of the bursae around the major joints may communicate with the joint and become distended whenever joint effusion develops. Bursitis may be a complication of gout, particularly when the inflammation involves the olecranon bursa. Extensive distention of bursae associated with the hip joint has been found in rheumatoid arthritis of the hip by Melamed, Bauer, and Johnson.[18] The distended bursae bulged into the pelvis and caused pressure on the rectum and bladder suggesting a tumor mass. Similar large, fluid-distended bursae may be found near other large joints involved by rheumatoid arthritis.

Baker's Cyst. Baker's cyst or popliteal cyst is caused by a herniation of synovial membrane through an opening in the posterior part of the joint capsule of the knee. The cause is not definitely known but it has been considered to be a congenital lesion, at least as far as predisposing factors are concerned. There is nothing characteristic about the roentgen appearance of the cyst and it cannot be differentiated from other soft-tissue masses that may occur in the popliteal space (synovioma, aneurysm of the popliteal artery, fibrosarcoma, etc.).

Cyst of the Semilunar Cartilage of the Knee. This is not a very common lesion. There often is a history of antecedent trauma but some investigators have considered the cyst to be of developmental nature. The external semilunar cartilage is involved most frequently and the lesion is seen in roentgenograms of the knee as a small soft-tissue bulge along the outer side of the joint.

OSTEITIS CONDENSANS ILII

This condition is found almost exclusively in females during the childbearing period and it almost always follows one or more pregnancies. It consists in a zone of dense sclerosis that develops along the iliac side of the sacroiliac joint. It is usually bilateral and symmetrical although some variation in intensity sometimes is observed between the two sides. The joint space is not affected and the sacrum is normal (Fig. 9-44). The area of sclerosis may be slight and fade off into normal bone or it may be several centimeters in width and be rather sharply demarcated from adjacent normal bone. The cause of this condition is unknown, but, because it does seem to be related to pregnancy, it may represent the reaction to the abnormal stress to which this area is subjected during pregnancy and delivery. In many cases the lesion is discovered during roentgenography of the pelvis performed because of some other condition. In other cases the patient complains of pain in the lower back and in the sacroiliac region. The lesion probably disappears spontaneously in most subjects. This is borne out by observations of some of these patients carried out over a period of years and by the fact that sclerotic changes of this type are found very infrequently in older women. A similar type of sclerotic reaction is observed in the pubic bones adjacent to the symphysis (Fig. 9-45). This too is seen almost exclusively in women who have borne children and both the pubic and the iliac sclerosis have been seen in the same individual. This lesion is termed *osteitis con-*

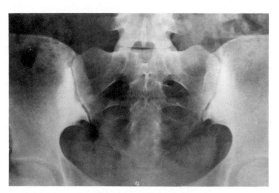

Fig. 9-44. *Osteitis condensans ilii.* The areas of sclerosis are typically on the iliac sides of the joints. The joint spaces are intact.

densans pubii. Osteitis condensans ilii must be differentiated from rheumatoid arthritis of the sacroiliac joints. The latter disease affects the joint space and the articular surfaces of the bones on both sides of the joint although the iliac changes may be more noticeable than the sacral. Characteristically, the joint margins become blurred and eventually ankylosed. This disease affects young males predominantly and is relatively uncommon in females (approximate ratio of males to females is 15:1).

INTRAPELVIC PROTRUSION OF ACETABULUM (OTTO'S PELVIS; PROTRUSIO ACETABULI)

In this condition there is a deepening of the acetabular cavity, the head of the femur is deeply seated in the acetabulum, and the floor may bulge into the pelvis (Fig. 9-46). The condition may be classified into primary and secondary groups. Primary acetabular protrusion does not have an obvious cause. The secondary group is the result of a recognized disease process. In this group, protrusio acetabuli may arise from a number of causes. In a unilateral lesion, deepening of the acetabulum may have resulted from a destructive arthritis, particularly tuberculosis. Trauma with fracture of the acetabulum and with the head of the femur driven into the acetabular cavity is

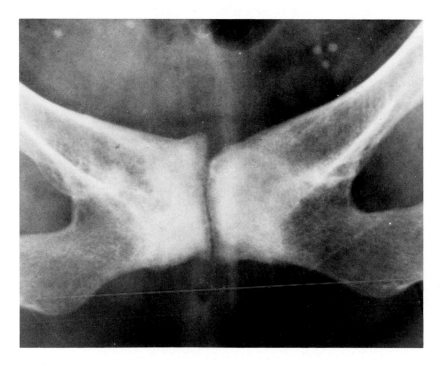

Fig. 9-45. *Osteitis condensans pubii.* The symphysis is thinned with considerable sclerosis of the adjacent pubic bones.

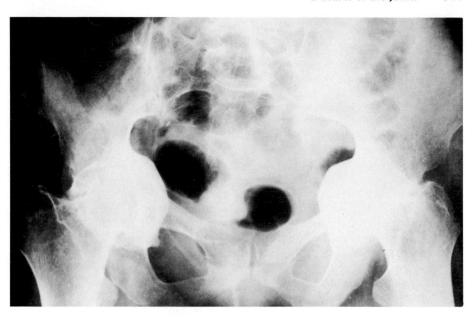

Fig. 9-46. Intrapelvic protrusion of the acetabulum in a 50-year-old patient with rheumatoid arthritis. Note the thinning of the joint spaces in addition to the severe inward protrusion.

another cause. Bilateral lesions occur rather frequently as a result of rheumatoid arthritis. When the pelvic bones are involved by severe osteomalacia, Paget's disease, or any other condition that causes the bones to be abnormally soft, the weight-bearing thrust of the femur may, over a period of time, cause a deepening of the acetabula and the development of a form of intrapelvic protrusion. Severe osteomalacia, in particular, often causes a general inward bending of the pelvic sidewalls which resembles that due to protrusio acetabuli. In some cases the cause is obscure, but it seems probable that, barring the presence of a joint disease such as rheumatoid arthritis, bilateral intrapelvic protrusion of the acetabula depends upon softening of the bones.

The radiologic criteria for diagnosis of protrusio acetabuli are somewhat arbitrary since there is a gradation from obvious medial protrusion of the femoral head to a normal configuration. The "teardrop" seen on the anteroposterior radiographs of the pelvis is formed by the acetabular floor laterally and the pelvic wall medially. Distortion of the pattern involves narrowing or actual crossing of the medial and lateral components. The crossing of these components has been designated arbitrarily as the criterion for the diagnosis of acetabular protrusion. In primary acetabular protrusion there must be an abnormally soft acetabulum but biochemical studies have revealed no positive factor. In some instances there is a strong familial tendency to protrusio acetabuli and to deep acetabuli.

CALCIFICATION OF INTERVERTEBRAL DISCS IN CHILDHOOD; JUVENILE SPONDYLARTHRITIS (JUVENILE DISKITIS)

Calcification of one or more intervertebral discs in childhood is a rare disorder.[11] The patients are usually in the 2- to 11-year age range, with a predominance of boys. The patients usually complain of pain, with limitation of motion, muscle spasm, tenderness, and torticollis. Roentgenograms show calcification in one or more intervertebral discs, usually in the cervical area. The disease tends to be self-limited and the calcifications gradually disappear over a period of several months. It has been regarded as an infection by some observers. However, there is evidence to indicate that some cases, if not all, are of traumatic origin. The cartilaginous epiphysis covers the vertebral body like a cap. The junction between the epiphysis and metaphysis is weak and susceptible to traumatic disruption followed by disc narrowing and erosion. It is possible that disc calcification results in some instances. It is also possible that some cases are infectious and others traumatic in origin. Calcification within the discs of adult patients, usually in the thoracic area, is common and appears to be a different entity and related to the aging process, with degenerative changes responsible.

HYPERTROPHIC OSTEOARTHROPATHY

As a result of certain diseases, usually intrathoracic, subperiosteal calcification develops in the bones of the hands and feet and, in many cases, in the other long tubular bones. This condition is known as *hypertrophic osteoarthropathy*. In the past the term "hypertrophic pulmonary osteoarthropathy" was used. However it now is known that diseases involving systems other than the lungs or cardiovascular system can cause similar changes so that it is preferable to delete the "pulmonary" part of the term. In association with the periosteal changes there may be synovial thickening and arthralgia. A related condition is even more common clinically and is referred to as *clubbing of the digits*. Clubbing consists of thickening of the soft tissues of the ends of the fingers. Clubbing may exist without the periosteal changes of osteoarthropathy or the two may be found together. Likewise periosteal calcification may be seen occasionally without soft-tissue clubbing. Current opinion indicates that clubbing and hypertrophic osteoarthropathy are closely related; that clubbing follows chronic pulmonary disease, particularly suppurative lesions such as bronchiectasis and lung abscess, and congenital cardiovascular disease; that osteoarthropathy, on the other hand, occurs more often as a result of intrathoracic neoplasms, especially mesothelioma of the pleura and bronchogenic carcinoma, is more rapid in its onset and development, and may recede promptly after removal of the tumor. Rarely, gastrointestinal diseases such as ulcerative colitis and Crohn's disease may be associated with hypertrophic osteoarthropathy.

In soft-tissue clubbing, roentgenograms of the hands and feet reveal the enlarged soft tissues but the bones may be entirely normal. When hypertrophic osteoarthropathy is present the changes are those of subperiosteal calcification (Fig. 9-47). During the early stages this is seen as thin pencil-line stripes of increased density along the outer surfaces of the bones. Multiple bones are involved although some may be unaffected or show only slight changes. The radius and ulna and the tibia and fibula are the bones most frequently affected. In the hands and feet the metacarpals and metatarsals are more often involved than the phalanges and the terminal phalanges may escape altogether. Later, the periosteal calcification becomes thicker and denser and may become nearly as dense as normal cortical bone. The outer surface also becomes wavy. In the adult there usually is little difficulty in diagnosis if multiple areas, such as both hands and feet, are examined. No other condition is as likely to cause this type of periosteal calcification involving multiple bones of the hands and feet with the underlying bone structure perfectly normal. In the legs a very similar type of periosteal

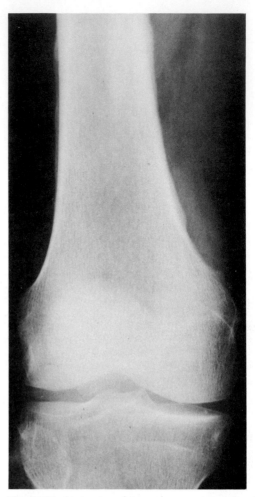

Fig. 9-47. Hypertrophic pulmonary osteoarthropathy. Note the irregular periosteal calcification along the cortical borders of the lower femur.

calcification is seen in association with chronic venous stasis but the involvement is limited to the tibia and fibula and does not affect the upper extremities. During childhood there are a number of causes for periosteal calcification that may be a source of difficulty in diagnosis. These are considered in Chapter 10.

Rarely, an idiopathic type of hypertrophic osteoarthropathy is encountered in which no cause for the periosteal changes is apparent. In some patients there is an associated thickening of the skin of the forehead and face with prominent creases and folds (*pachydermoperiostosis*). This idiopathic form shows essentially the same roentgen features as have just been described except for more diffuse soft-tissue enlargement of hands and feet. This is a familial condition transmitted as an autosomal dominant trait with variable penetrance. Bone (periosteal) changes may be minimal in form fruste and the appearance is then much like that of acromegaly.

CAISSON DISEASE

Caisson disease affects those who have worked under increased atmospheric pressure and is caused by too rapid decompression. It is more familiarly known as "the bends." It is the result of liberation of bubbles of nitrogen from the blood after the body has absorbed an excess of the gas while under compression. The bone and joint changes that may develop are the result of infarction. When infarcts have involved the articular ends of the bones, ischemic necrosis results and the bones become softened. Eventually joint changes develop that resemble those of degenerative joint disease. The joints most frequently affected are those of the lower extremities and the shoulder. In the hip the head of the femur becomes flattened, the superior portion often undergoes fragmentation or compression, and reactive spurring and sclerosis ensue. While the bone and joint changes are not particularly specific, the presence of areas of irregular calcification in the medullary cavities of the bones adjacent to the joints should raise the suspicion of caisson disease since these calcified areas may represent healed bone infarcts. In aviators a rapid ascent to high altitudes may cause aeroembolism similar to that found in caisson disease. In this instance the condition is due to a rapid reduction in atmospheric pressure. Bone and joint changes similar to those found in caisson disease also have been described in these individuals.

THE VACUUM PHENOMENON; GAS IN THE JOINTS

The normal joint space is only a potential one and ordinarily cannot be identified in roentgenograms. What is called the "joint space" in the description of roentgenograms refers to the relatively clear or translucent space between the ends of the bones that is occupied by the articular cartilages and what little synovial fluid is present. Under certain circumstances an actual space can be visualized in roentgenograms as a thin, translucent, dark line or space between the articular cartilages. In certain joints the potential joint space can be made into a real one by proper traction exerted during the exposure. Manual traction[16] of 30 to 50 pounds applied to the hip usually

results in production of a "vacuum phenomenon"; gas in the joint outlines the cartilage of the femoral head. If the traction produces an increase in the joint space and no gas is visible, joint effusion is likely. Conversely, if a "vacuum phenomenon" is produced by traction with the patient in the supine position, no significant effusion is present. Administration of a muscle relaxant before this examination may be helpful. This phenomenon is most frequently visible in the shoulder, often on chest roentgenograms obtained with the humerus internally rotated. It is not entirely clear whether this space represents a vacuum or whether it becomes filled with gas liberated from the blood. Most authors writing on the subject consider it to be filled with gas and that the term "vacuum phenomenon," is a misnomer.

In other areas more persistent "spaces" will occasionally be demonstrated. For example, in the lumbar spine in association with severe degenerative disease of one or more of the discs, there may be seen a waferlike dark space within the disc. This has been called a "phantom disc." (See Fig. 9-28) A similar appearance has been noted with considerable frequency in the symphysis pubis of women during pregnancy. In these cases it is assumed that the space becomes filled with gas derived from the blood or tissue fluids rather than being a persisting vacuum (Fig. 9-48).

ARTHROGRAPHY

Arthrography consists of the injection of a contrast substance into a joint and obtaining a series of roentgenograms to visualize the internal structures of the joint. While the procedure has been practiced for a number of years it has become a common procedure only in recent years. While any of the peripheral joints can be examined by this means, the knee is the joint most often studied because of the frequency of injuries to this joint and its supporting structures. Either a radiolucent substance such as room air or, more frequently, a water-soluble radiopaque material can be used as the contrast agent. Some writers have expressed a preference for double-contrast arthrography, that is, combining a gas with an opaque substance. Our own preference is for a water-soluble, radiopaque contrast agent such as Renografin 60.

After suitable preparation of the skin and the injection of a local anesthetic, from 10.0 to 15.0 ml of Renografin 60 are injected with a 20-gauge needle and with the puncture made on the lateral side of the patella. If fluid is present in the joint it is aspirated before the contrast material is injected. The tech-

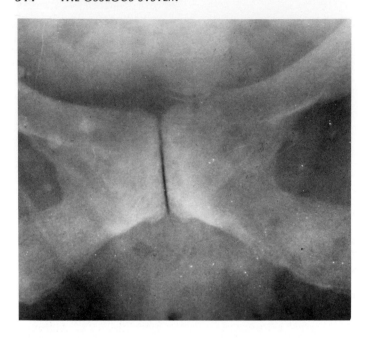

Fig. 9-48. Vacuum phenomenon in the symphysis pubis. There is thinning of the symphysis. The vertical translucent stripe indicates the presence of gas rather than a vacuum. This phenomenon usually indicates degeneration of the cartilage.

nique should be performed meticulously to prevent infection. The patient's leg is flexed and extended a number of times to distribute the contrast agent throughout the joint. If the examination is being performed because of the possibility of injury to the internal structures of the joint, an Ace bandage is wrapped tightly around the lower thigh to the level of the joint space to obliterate the suprapatellar pouch and prevent dissemination of the material away from the joint space. Multiple films are exposed (usually "spot-films" under fluoroscopic guidance) promptly after injection as the material is absorbed rather rapidly.

By this method tears of the menisci can be visualized. Also ruptures of the collateral ligaments can be recognized by the extravasation of contrast material beyond the confines of the joint cavity. Ruptures of the cruciate ligaments and nonopaque, cartilaginous loose bodies are other conditions that often can be identified. If the entire joint pouch is examined, synovial abnormalities such as villonodular synovitis often can be recognized. With experience on the part of the examiner the accuracy of the method is very good and it has proved extremely useful in detailing the anatomy of the knee-joint structures in cases of acute injury when the results of clinical examination may be equivocal. For details of the technique and its interpretation, references are appended.[13, 22, 39] Among other uses, arthrography has been recommended for the study of injuries to the supporting structures of the shoulder joint and in congenital dislocation of the hip in infants.

TOTAL HIP PROSTHESIS AND ITS COMPLICATIONS

Even though the artificial hip[8] can withstand considerable stress, fractures may occur in the vicinity of the prosthesis. Stress fractures of the pubis related to increased activity have been reported, as have fractures of the acetabulum and femur following minimal to moderate trauma.

Complications of the hip replacement itself may occur, the two most common being infection and loosening. On plain films, often a thin lucent line is seen at the interface between the cement and bone. This appears to be about 1 mm wide in most instances. When it becomes 2 mm or more in width, loosening is strongly suggested in a patient with pain even though a line this wide may be present without loosening. Arthrography has been used in evaluating pain after total hip replacement, but it appears that the dense fibrous tissue surrounding the prosthesis may be permeable to contrast agents so that the opaque material may be seen at the bone–cement interface in patients without symptoms. Gross loosening can be evaluated by push–pull or abduction films. Since infection can also cause similar widening, this is very difficult to detect radiographically unless there are gross changes of irregular periostitis or areas of bone destruction. Hip aspiration for culture is necessary even though a negative culture does not completely exclude the possibility of infection.

REFERENCES AND SELECTED READINGS

1. ALEXANDER CJ: The etiology of juvenile spondylarthritis (discitis). Clin Radiol 21: 78, 1970

2. BOCHER J, MANKIN HJ, BERK RN et al: Prevalence of calcified meniscal cartilages in elderly persons. N Engl J Med 272: 1093, 1965

3. CAMIEL MR, AARON JB: The gas or vacuum phenomenon in the symphysis during pregnancy. Radiology 66: 548, 1956

4. CARTER AR, LIYANAGE SP: Large subarticular cysts "geodes" adjacent to the knee joint in rheumatoid arthritis. Clin Radiol 26: 535, 1975

5. CAVANAGH RC, SCHWAMM HH: Localized nodular synovitis. Radiology 100: 409, 1971

6. CRAIG RM, PUGH DG, SOULE EH: The roentgenologic manifestations of synovial sarcoma. Radiology 65: 837, 1955

7. DETENBECK LC, YOUNG HH, UNDERDAHL LO: Ochronotic arthropathy. Arch Surg 100: 215, 1970

8. DuSAULT RG, GOLDMAN AB, GHELMAN B: Radiologic diagnosis of loosening and infection in hip prostheses. J Can Assoc Radiol 28: 199, 1977

9. FISCHER RM: The lesions of congenital syphilis. Br J Radiol 43: 333, 1970

10. HARRISON RB: Charcot's joint: two new observations. Am J Roentgenol 128: 807, 1977

11. HENRY MJ, GRIMES HA, LANE JW: Intervertebral disc calcification in childhood. Radiology 89: 81, 1969

12. KORMANO M, KARVONEN J, LASSUS A: Psoriatic lesion of the sternal synchondrosis. Acta Radiol [Diagn] (Stockh) 16: 463, 1975

13. LINDBLOOM K: Arthrography of the knee: a roentgenographic and anatomical study. Acta Radiol [Suppl] (Stockh) 74: 1–112, 1948

14. MARTEL W: The pattern of rheumatoid arthritis of the hand and wrist. Radiol Clin North Am 2:221, 1964

15. MARTEL W, CHAMPION CK, THOMPSON GR et al: A roentgenologically distinctive arthropathy in some patients with the pseudogout syndrome. Am J Roentgenol 109: 587, 1970

16. MARTELL W, POZNANSKI AK, KUHNS LR: Further observations on the value of traction during roentgenography of the hip. Invest Radiol 6: 1, 1971

17. MEDSGER TA JR, CHRISTY WC: Carpal arthritis with ankylosis in late-onset Still's disease. Arthritis Rheum 19: 232, 1976

18. MELAMED A, BAUER CA, JOHNSON JH: Iliopsoas bursal extension of arthritic disease of the hip. Radiology 89: 54, 1967

19. MOSKOWITZ RW, KATZ D: Chondrocalcinosis and chondrocalsynovitis (Pseudogout syndrome). Analysis of twenty-four cases. Am J Med 43: 322, 1967

20. MOULE NJ, GOLDING JSR: Idiopathic chondrolysis of the hip. Clin Radiol 25: 247, 1974

21. MURPHY WA, STAPLE TW: Jaccoud's arthropathy reviewed. Am J Roentgenol 118: 300, 1973

22. NICHOLAS JA, FREIBERGER RH, KILLORAN PJ: Double-contrast arthrography of the knee: its value in the management of two hundred and twenty-five knee derangements. J Bone Joint Surg [A] 52: 203, 1970

23. PARK WM, O'NEILL M, McCALL IW: The radiology of rheumatoid involvement of the cervical spine. Skeletal Radiol 4: 1, 1979

24. PETER JB, PEARSON CM, MARMOR L: Erosive osteoarthritis of the hands. Arthritis Rheum 9: 365, 1966

25. POGONOWSKA MJ, COLLINS LC, DOBSON HL: Diabetic osteopathy. Radiology 89: 265, 1967

26. RABINOWITZ JG, TWERSKY T, GUTTADURIA M: Similar bone manifestations of scleroderma and rheumatoid arthritis. Am J Roentgenol 121: 35, 1974

27. RESNICK D: Patterns of peripheral joint disease in ankylosing spondylitis. Radiology 110: 523, 1974

28. RESNICK D: Patterns of migration of the femoral head in osteoarthritis of the hip. Roentgenographic-pathologic correlation and comparison with rheumatoid arthritis. Am J Roentgenol 124: 62, 1975

29. RESNICK D, BRODERICK TW: Bony proliferation of the terminal toe phalanges in psoriasis: the ivory phalanx. J Can Assoc Radiol 28: 187, 1977

30. RESNICK D, NIWAYAMA G: Radiographic and pathologic features of spinal involvement in diffuse idiopathic skeletal hyperostosis (DISH). Radiology 119: 559, 1976

31. RESNICK D, NIWAYAMA G: Resorption of the undersurface of the distal clavicle in rheumatoid arthritis. Radiology 120: 75, 1976

32. RESNICK D, NIWAYAMA G, GOERGEN TG et al: Clinical radiographic and pathologic abnormalities in calcium pyrophosphate dihydrate deposition disease (CPPD)—Pseudogout. Radiology 122: 1, 1977

33. RESNICK D, SHAUL SR, ROBINS JM: Diffuse idiopathic skeletal hyperostosis (DISH). Forrestier's disease with extraspinal manifestations. Radiology 115: 513, 1975

34. SCHALLER J, WEDGWOOD RJ: Juvenile rheumatoid arthritis: a review. Pediatrics 50: 940, 1972

35. SEAMAN WB, WELLS J: Destructive lesions of the vertebral bodies in rheumatoid disease. Am J Roentgenol 86: 241, 1961

36. SEGAL G, KELLOGG DS: Osteitis condensans ilii. Am J Roentgenol 71: 643, 1954

37. SHOLKOFF SD, GLICKMAN MG, STEINBACH HL: Roentgenology of Reiter's syndrome. Radiology 97: 497, 1970

38. SMITH JH, PUGH DG: Roentgenographic aspects of articular pigmented villonodular synovitis. Am J Roentgenol 87: 1146, 1962

39. TURNER AF, BUDIN E: Arthrography of the knee. A simplified technique. Radiology 97: 505, 1970

40. TWERSKY J: Joint changes in idiopathic hemochromatosis. Am J Roentgenol 124: 139, 1975

41. UDOFF EJ, GENANT HK, KOZIN F et al: Mixed connective tissue disease: the spectrum of radiographic manifestations. Radiology 124: 613, 1977

42. WATT RI, MIDDLEMISS H: The radiology of gout. Clin Radiol 26: 27, 1975

10

THE SUPERFICIAL SOFT TISSUES

Because the soft parts are much less radiopaque than the bones they may be overlooked when an average roentgenogram, obtained primarily to bring out bone detail, is being examined. Nevertheless the soft tissues, even in a heavily exposed film, exert a distinct influence on the appearance of the bones that they cover. One has only to compare the difference in density of a part of a bone over which there is a loss of soft-tissue because of ulceration, traumatic avulsion, or surgical removal, with that of the adjacent uninvolved part to appreciate how much radiation is absorbed by the soft tissues. Conversely, a small, localized, soft-tissue enlargement such as a wart or a mole in close contact with the film cassette or Bucky table can cause a sharply marginated increase in density that may be mistaken for a pathologic process within the tissues. For example, a mole on the surface of the chest wall may produce a round density that can be mistaken for a nodule within the lung and a similar lesion of the soft tissues of the lower back may suggest a renal or gallbladder calculus (see Fig. 10-21). The nipples are a common source of difficulty in the interpretation of chest roentgenograms. If one breast is pressed more firmly against the film cassette than the other the nipple on one side may form a sharply outlined round density while the other may be invisible. Absence of one breast following a radical mastectomy causes one lung field to be more translucent than the other. After amputation of one upper extremity and the consequent unilateral disuse atrophy of the pectoral muscles in the male, similar increased translucency in the lung field often is observed. These are but a few examples of the influence of the peripheral soft tissues on the radiographic density of the deeper structures.

The soft tissues can be visualized in practically every roentgenogram, even those that have been heavily exposed, by viewing the film with a strong beam of light. Some type of spotlight should always be available in addition to the usual illuminators for the scrutiny of overexposed roentgenograms and particularly for the study of the soft-tissue coverings.

When specifically indicated, a suitable selection of exposure factors ranging from 26 to 40 kV with relatively low filtration (*e.g.,* 0.5 mm Al) will produce a roentgenogram of high quality in which the soft-tissue outlines are preserved and good differentiation of the soft-tissue densities is obtained. This type of roentgenogram is useful when the examination is made primarily for soft-tissue visualization. These factors have been emphasized for some time in mammography. With the advent of newer types of special equipment for low-voltage soft-tissue radiography, more attention is now being given to soft-tissue techniques in other areas. Xeroradiography is also being used by many for examination of soft tissues. The use of high kilovoltages (80 to 125 kV) in diagnostic roentgenology tends to produce a roentgenogram with considerable latitude in density so that the soft-tissue outlines are preserved even though good penetration of the bone is obtained. Such an "all purpose" roentgenogram can be used as a routine type of exposure and will eliminate the need for special soft-tissue studies except in particular circumstances (Fig. 10-1).

While the specific gravity of the soft tissues as a whole is close to that of water, there is enough difference between fat and other tissues to make the subcutaneous fat zone distinctly visible in roentgenograms as a more translucent area beneath the skin. The fat zone also makes the outer surface of the muscles stand out clearly. Localized accumulations of fat near the joints aid in recognizing joint effusion because of their displacement when the joint capsule is distended. When there has been wasting from disease with consequent loss of fat, the soft parts have a very homogenous density. Fat, therefore, is very important in giving texture to the soft tissues. The importance of the perirenal fat in enabling visualization of the kidneys has been indicated elsewhere and the value of intra-abdominal fat for soft-tissue differentiation is considerable.

XERORADIOGRAPHY

Xeroradiography is now widely used in mammography, in the study of soft tissues of the cervical area, including the pharynx and larynx, and in study of soft-tissue disease, bone disease, and fractures of the extremities.

The process depends on the discharge of electrostatic charges placed on a plate coated with vitreous selenium, a photoconductor. The plate is charged to a potential of 1000 to 1600 volts. Low-voltage x-rays are used to expose the plate which is placed in conventional relationship to the part being examined. Each segment of the plate is discharged in direct proportion to the number of photons penetrating the patient to strike the plate. Thus, a pattern of electrostatic

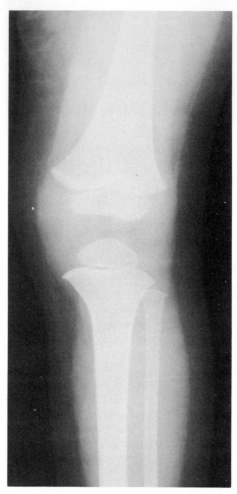

Fig. 10-1. Normal soft tissues. This demonstrates the difference in density of muscles and fat. The more radiolucent subcutaneous fat causes the muscles to stand out clearly.

charge is produced corresponding to the variations in relative radiographic density of the part examined.

The pattern is made visible by exposing the plate to a blue, finely divided, charged plastic powder (toner), thus producing an image. Depending on the charge (negative or positive), the thick parts may be produced in white (light blue) or blue (darker).[17] The powder image is then transferred by electrostatic means from the plate to paper to provide a permanent record. Heat is then applied to fix the image on the paper.

There are certain image characteristics that make the process useful in mammography and other soft-tissue imaging. One is edge enhancement which tends to accentuate the image of a mass in soft tissue and to clearly define it; this occurs whenever there is an abrupt difference in density of tissue or object examined. Another is the relatively wide latitude of structures recorded on one image. Also, microcalcifications seem to be more easily identified on xerograms than on films. Resolution is very good. Positive and negative mode can be used; in our experience, calcifications are more readily identified on the positive and small masses on the negative xerogram. Underexposure is more of a problem in the negative mode than in the positive; this is probably the reason that one feels more comfortable with the positive xerogram in identification of microcalcifications. Because of the many problems presented by xerotomography we have not used it recently.

THE DISORDERS OF MUSCLE

Muscle disorders usually result in an increase or a decrease in muscle mass that is not directly correlated with the diameter of the part being studied since the amount of fat present may vary greatly. The relative amounts of muscle and fat and their distribution are usually apparent on the roentgenogram. Gay and Weens[9] suggest the following system for roentgen evaluation of muscle disorders: (1) definition of the muscle margin at its junction with the subcutaneous fat; (2) general muscle size; (3) local swelling or tumor within muscle; (4) amount of fat within muscles; (5) thickness of subcutaneous fat relative to muscle; (6) presence of calcification or ossification in soft tissues; (7) bone structure, *e.g.*, presence of osteoporosis, dysplasia, periostitis,and the like; (8) presence of joint abnormality; and (9) abnormal vascular structures.

MUSCULAR DYSTROPHIES

The replacement of muscle by fat in the muscular dystrophies results in a fairly characteristic appearance in roentgenograms of the extremities. The muscles do not shrink appreciably in size, but the extensive accumulations of fat within the remaining muscle bundles gives them a fine striated or striped appearance. In later stages most of the muscle tissue is replaced by fat, the fascial sheath bounding the muscle standing out as a thin shadow of increased density as it is visualized on edge (Fig. 10-2). One of the clinical subgroups is known as *pseudohypertrophic muscular dystrophy* (Duchenne). It is characterized by the enlargement of certain muscle groups,

usually those of the calves and of the shoulder girdles. The appearance clinically is that of a very muscular individual but actually the strength is extremely weak. In addition to the extensive replacement by fat in this type of dystrophy the muscles are enlarged. This is the only condition in which the combination of large muscles interlaced with fat is found (Fig. 10-3). Another sign of this disease consists of an unusual widening of the shaft of the fibula in its anteroposterior diameter. This can be noted, for example, in Figure 10-3, in which the midshaft of the fibula is seen to be nearly as wide as the narrowest part of the tibial shaft. There are several other types of muscular dystrophy that may exhibit pseudohypertrophy of some muscle groups, but they are rare.

In patients with long-standing paralysis of one or more extremities from causes other than muscular dystrophy, including such conditions as poliomyelitis, spinal-cord injuries, and cerebral vascular accidents, muscles may contain stripes of fat but the affected muscle groups are decreased in size while the subcutaneous fat layer may be thick. When complete paralysis of an extremity has existed for a long time the muscle bundles may be almost completely absent, with subcutaneous fat making up most of the soft tissues surrounding the bones.

The increase in intramuscular fat in obesity does not pose a differential problem because of an associated increase in subcutaneous fat. In some elderly persons, there tends to be an increase in intramuscular fat, but this is not nearly as marked as in those with pseudohypertrophic muscular dystrophy.

MUSCLE ATROPHY

In addition to primary muscle conditions there are numerous diseases involving the nervous system in which muscle atrophy may be present. Differentiation by means of roentgen examination is usually not possible since the appearance is similar in many of them. The major radiographic finding is a decrease in muscle mass. There may be an increase in fat between muscle groups or in the subcutaneous area. In some acquired conditions (*e.g.,* poliomyelitis), specific muscle groups may be atrophic; of course, there is a wide variation in distribution in such instances.

MUSCLE HYPERTROPHY

Hypertrophy of muscles may occur in a number of diseases and may also result from use, as in certain conditioning programs. The only roentgen finding is

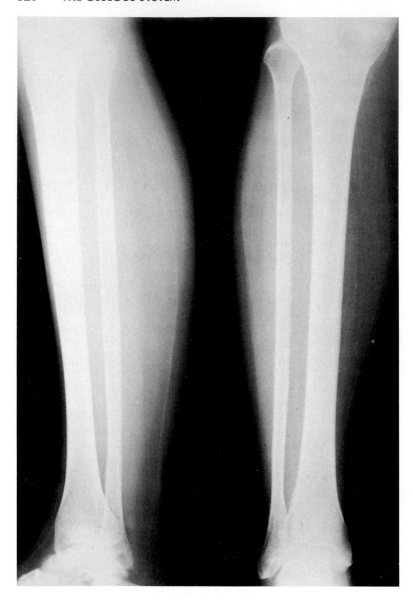

Fig. 10-2. Muscular dystrophy. The muscles are not decreased in size but have been replaced to a large extent by fat. The thin stripes of density noted best in the lateral view represent the outer fascial boundaries of muscles, with subcutaneous fat on the external side and the fat in muscle within the stripes.

disproportionate muscle thickness in comparison to subcutaneous fat.

EDEMA AND HEMORRHAGE

Subcutaneous edema or hemorrhage causes a diffuse increase in density that as a rule is not sharply demarcated. The fluid obliterates the normal distinct boundary between the muscles and overlying fat. The subcutaneous space develops a fine striated or, occasionally, a slightly mottled appearance. The margins fade off gradually into normal density. When the accumulation of fluid is within the muscles or be-neath them it causes only a uniform swelling of the part; if small it may be entirely unnoticed. Hemorrhage under the periosteum is invisible until the periosteum reacts to the irritation by depositing calcium. This requires a week or more before sufficient calcium is present to be visible in roentgenograms. Calcification develops more rapidly in the very young than it does in older individuals. In general the type of fluid within the tissues cannot be determined from the roentgen appearances and there is not enough difference in specific gravity of the various fluids to cause an appreciable variation in radiographic density.

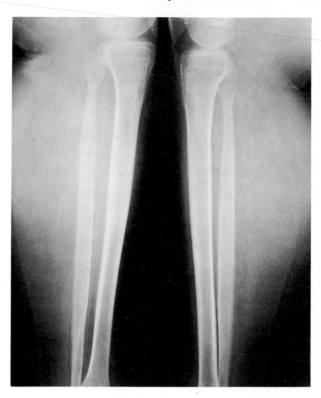

Fig. 10-3. Pseudohypertrophic muscular dystrophy. The muscles of the calves are very large but are streaked with fat producing streaks of radiolucency within the muscles. Note the wide fibular shafts.

CALCIFICATION IN THE SOFT TISSUES

ARTERIAL CALCIFICATION

Calcification in the walls of the larger arteries of the abdomen and of the extremities is a frequent observation in roentgenograms of individuals of middle age or over. Of the three major pathologic types of arteriosclerosis, diffuse arteriolar sclerosis is not included in the present discussion; the small size of the vessels involved precludes roentgen visualization even if the vessels should be calcified. The other two types have certain roentgen characteristics by means of which they often can be identified.

Mönckeberg's Medial Arteriosclerosis

This type of arteriosclerosis is characterized by the formation of calcific plaques in the medial layer of the blood vessel wall. These plaques do not narrow the vessel lumen and they cause no interference with the circulation. Mönckeberg's arteriosclerosis is an almost constant finding in elderly individuals and it is not at all infrequent in persons of the 35- to 50-year-old age group, particularly in diabetics. The vessels

most often affected are the femoral, popliteal, and radial arteries. This type of arteriosclerosis has the following roentgenologic features:

1. The calcification occurs in the form of closely spaced, fine concentric rings. These may be complete or incomplete but the process generally is diffuse, involving long segments of a vessel and multiple vessels (see Fig. 10-4C).

2. The characteristic changes are seen to best advantage in the femoral, popliteal, and tibial arteries but often can be identified in other moderate-sized vessels, such as the radial and the dorsalis pedis.

Intimal Arteriosclerosis (Atherosclerosis)

Intimal arteriosclerosis is characterized pathologically by the formation of atheromatous plaques in the thickened intima of the arteries. The lumen of the vessel is narrowed, thrombosis may develop, and complete occlusion may result. This is the type of arteriosclerosis that leads to the clinical signs and symptoms of arterial insufficiency. The atheromatous plaques may not be calcified. When they are, the calcification is seen as irregular plaquelike areas of variable size, from small flecks to larger areas a centimeter or more in length. They may be elongated or somewhat triangular, with a considerable variation in shape. They seldom completely encircle the lumen of the vessel and are distributed irregularly along the course of the vessel without any specific arrangement (Fig. 10-4A and B). The amount of visible calcification bears no relationship to the severity of the vascular occlusion; complete obstruction may exist with no visible calcification.

Mixed Types

Combined medial and intimal arteriosclerosis is common and when much medial calcification is present the intimal plaques may be hidden. In the feet it usually is difficult to determine the type of disease that may be present; the small vessels often are heavily calcified and combined forms are frequent. Calcified plaques are very frequently seen in the abdominal aorta and the iliac vessels. The typical ringlike calcification of medial arteriosclerosis is not seen in a vessel the size of the aorta and the type of arteriosclerosis cannot be determined from the roentgen appearances of the calcification. The most frequent type of aortic arteriosclerosis, however, is a form of medial arteriosclerosis that weakens the vessel wall and predisposes to the development of aneurysm. There is usually enough calcification in aortic aneurysms to make them visible in abdominal roentgenograms. Rupture with hematoma dissecting into the retroperitoneal fat may simulate interstitial emphysema because of the difference in density between fat and blood.[20] This finding may be helpful in confirming the presence of retroperitoneal hemorrhage.

Generalized Arterial Calcification in Infancy

More than 50 cases of idiopathic arterial calcification in infants have been reported, but diagnosis was made in only two infants during life when the calcification was observed radiologically.[21] Roentgen findings include calcification in coronary arteries, the aorta, the iliac arteries, and the femoral artery and its branches down to the ankles, as well as calcification in the arteries of the upper extremities and of the carotids in the neck. This rare condition most likely represents a congenital abnormality of connective tissue with fibroblastic proliferation in the intima and degenerative change in the elastic tissue with calcium deposition. The two infants in whom the diagnosis was made during life both had hypertension.

CALCIFICATION OF THE VEINS

Normal blood vessels are visualized only as they course through the subcutaneous fat and only the larger vessels, chiefly the veins, can be seen readily. When the superficial veins in the leg become enlarged, they are easily identified as tortuous linear shadows representing varicosities. Changes in the deep veins are not visible as a rule because they have a density similar to that of the muscles surrounding them. Calcification associated with the superficial or deep veins occurs in one of the following forms.

Phleboliths

A phlebolith is a calcified thrombus within a vein. Phleboliths are found very frequently in the pelvic veins (see Ch. 13) and most adults will have a few of them. They occur in the form of small round or slightly ovoid calcified shadows of variable size from very tiny ones up to those that measure on the order of 0.5 cm in diameter. They may be of homogeneous density, be laminated, or have a ringlike appearance. Phleboliths are common in varicose veins of the lower extremities. They frequently form in the dilated venous spaces of a cavernous hemangioma and result in one of the characteristic roentgen signs of this lesion. When a number of small, rounded calcifications are visualized in a localized area of the superficial soft tissues one should think of the possibility of a cavernous hemangioma (Fig. 10-5). The phleboliths in a hemangioma very often have a ringlike appearance.

Calcification of Larger Thrombi

Occasionally a long thrombus within a vein will calcify and be visible as an elongated, somewhat irregular, calcification following the course of one of the larger veins.

Calcification Associated with Venous Stasis

In the presence of venous stasis of long duration, usually secondary to varicosities and thrombosis, thin stripelike shadows of calcification may be seen in the subcutaneous tissues. These usually are visualized as double parallel stripes or with distinctly tubular and branching characteristics. Additionally there often are plaquelike calcifications in the subcutaneous tissues throughout the legs (Fig. 10-6) or as a more localized process in the neighborhood of a varicose ulcer. The calcification in some of these patients resembles very closely that seen in patients with diffuse

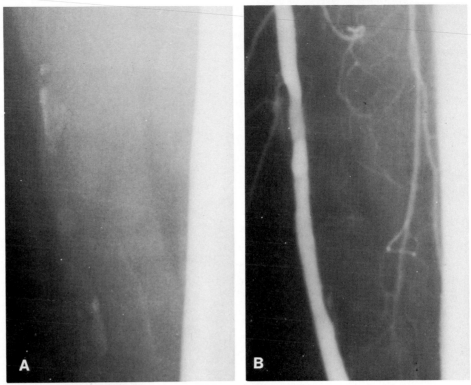

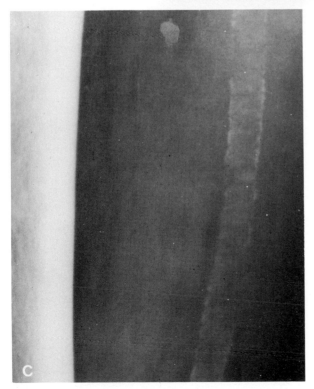

Fig. 10-4. A. Several irregular plaques are visible in the femoral artery in the thigh. The femur is at the right. **B.** Femoral arteriogram on the patient shown in **A.** The uppermost plaque has caused narrowing of the arterial lumen, with lesser narrowing at the lower sites. **C.** In this patient there is calcification in the femoral artery of the type usually found in association with involvement of the media.

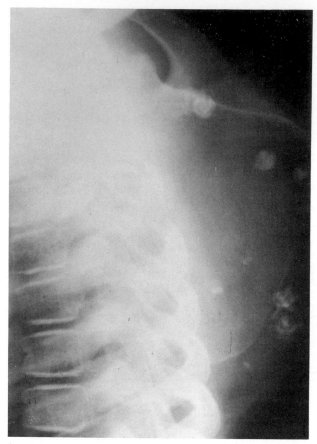

Fig. 10-5. Phleboliths in a cavernous hemangioma beneath the scapula. The multiple, round, ringlike and laminated densities are characteristic of phleboliths.

scleroderma or dermatomyositis except that it is localized to the leg. The calcification is not in the walls of the vessels but rather in the subcutaneous tissues. Phleboliths are often seen in association with the plaques. Periosteal calcification along the tibial and fibular shafts also is common (see Fig. 10-16) and there are often stasis ulcers and marked induration of skin and subcutaneous tissues as well as discoloration of the skin.

PARASITIC CALCIFICATION

Cysticerosis. The encysted larvae of the pork tapeworm (*Taenia solium*), known as *Cysticerus cellulosae,* occasionally form in the brain, meninges, muscles, and other structures. Normally the pig is the intermediary host and human infestation occurs from eating improperly cooked pork. The eggs may be

swallowed as a result of self-infection, with the larvae subsequently entering the tissues and becoming encysted, man thus acting as the intermediate host. The parasites may become calcified, making them visible roentgenologically. When calcified, the larvae form small round or slightly elongated masses from 1 to several millimeters in diameter or length, which may be widely disseminated throughout the muscles (Fig. 10-7) or the brain and its coverings. The small size of the calcifications and the wide dissemination of them should suggest the proper diagnosis.

Trichiniasis. The encysted embryos of *Trichina spiralis* are said to undergo calcification very fre-

Fig. 10-6. Subcutaneous calcification in a patient with long-standing venous stasis.

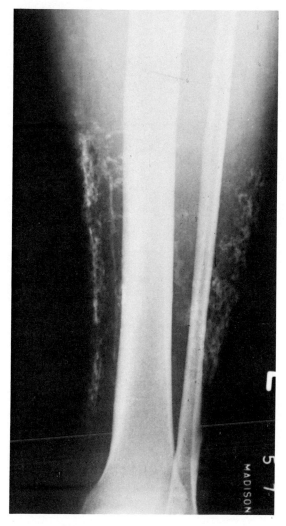

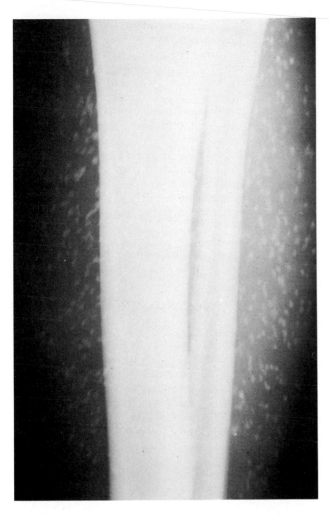

Fig. 10-7. Cysticercosis. Numerous tiny round and oval calcifications in the muscles of the leg. The patient had eaten a considerable amount of raw pork while a Japanese prisoner during World War II. (Courtesy of Dr. Margaret Winston)

quently but the parasite is so small that it cannot be visualized readily in roentgenograms and the diagnosis of trichiniasis usually cannot be made from roentgen examination.

Hydatid Disease. This is due to infection with hydatid cysts, the larval forms of an ecchinococcal tapeworm. These cysts are usually found in visceral organs of the thorax and abdomen. Rarely they occur in soft tissues of the extremities. They tend to be small and fragmented in contrast to large visceral cysts. Therefore, the appearance is not characteristic,

and the calcifications may present a variety of bizarre patterns.

TROPICAL PARASITIC DISEASES

Dracunculiasis (Guinea Worm Infestation). This infestation may be manifest in roentgenograms when fibrositis or myositis develops around a dead female guinea worm that migrates to subcutaneous tissues before discharging eggs. The worm may calcify, particularly if it remains deep in the tissues. It appears as a long, stringlike calcification, usually in the lower limbs, and may be as long as 10 to 12 cm.

Loiasis. This is caused by the filarial nematode *Loa loa,* or African eye worm. When dead worms calcify, they may resemble a thick thread of cotton that may be coiled to form a lacy or filamentous calcification several millimeters in length. At times, only tiny rods or dots of calcium are present. In some instances they produce thicker calcific densities, 1 mm in width, with beadlike lobulated contours.

MYOSITIS OSSIFICANS

Calcification or ossification often follows trauma to the deep tissues of the extremities. So-called calcified hematomas involving the muscles of the thigh are observed frequently in athletes, particularly football players, but may follow any local injury sufficient to cause bruising of the muscle or a frank hemorrhage within it. An injury of this nature severe enough to cause a deep muscle bruise often traumatizes the periosteum as well and there may be hemorrhage beneath it; this also frequently undergoes calcification. Calcification within a muscle that follows trauma is called *traumatic myositis ossificans* because the condition progresses to actual bone formation in most cases. This form of myositis ossificans should not be confused with the disease known as *progressive myositis ossificans (Vide infra).*

The calcified hematoma may become visible as a hazy shadow of increased density within a few weeks after the initiating trauma (Fig. 10-8). Over a period of several weeks this gradually becomes denser and finally it develops the appearance of actual bone. The mass has a laminated character caused by the hemorrhage dissecting along the muscle and fascial planes (Fig. 10-9). Usually, after a period of time, the ossification gradually decreases in size; smaller masses may disappear completely. Cases have been reported in which osteogenic sarcoma has developed in an area of traumatic myositis ossificans but this appears

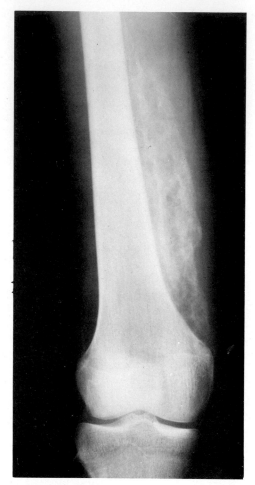

Fig. 10-8. Traumatic myositis ossificans. There is calcification in a large hematoma on the inner aspect of the thigh.

to be a rare lesion. Calcification or bone formation within a laparotomy scar is occasionally seen; this represents a form of traumatic myositis ossificans. Myositis ossificans is a very rare complication of tetanus, evidently caused by hemorrhage secondary to severe tetanic extensor spasms. The calcification and ossification are observed in 4 to 7 weeks after onset of the convulsions.

Myositis Ossificans Circumscripta

The term "myositis ossificans circumscripta" is used to designate a localized area of active myositis ossificans that occurs without a history of trauma. Goldman[12] classifies these lesions as follows: (1) extraos-

seous lesions arising in the muscle not in continuity to bone; (2) periosteal lesions that produce a layer or a sunburst periosteal reaction sometimes called "ossifying subperiosteal hematomas"; and (3) lesions arising in the immediate proximity of bone sometimes termed "parosteal myositis ossificans." The lesions may also be associated with periosteal reaction. Radiographically and clinically, a soft-tissue mass may be noted to be present initially; then flocculent calcification is observed in 10 to 40 days. The lesion must be differentiated from a malignant one. Roentgen signs favoring a benign lesion include a lucent zone between the lesion and adjacent bone, intact underlying cortex, diaphyseal location, dense calcification at the periphery, and the loss of volume or decrease in size with time. In addition, the most dense calcification is peripheral in this lesion as opposed to the dense central calcification in most tumors.

PROGRESSIVE MYOSITIS OSSIFICANS

Progressive myositis ossificans is a rare disorder of unknown cause. It appears to be a congenital dysplasia. It begins in early childhood with the development of doughy and often painful swellings, chiefly in the muscles of the neck and back. As these swellings subside, a diffuse fibrosis is left and this, in turn, is followed by the development of platelike masses of bone (Fig. 10-10). There is a slow progression of the

Fig. 10-9. Post-traumatic myositis ossificans. A lateral roentgenogram of the midthigh shows typical laminated calcification of an intramuscular hematoma.

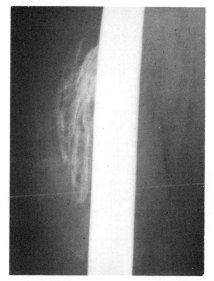

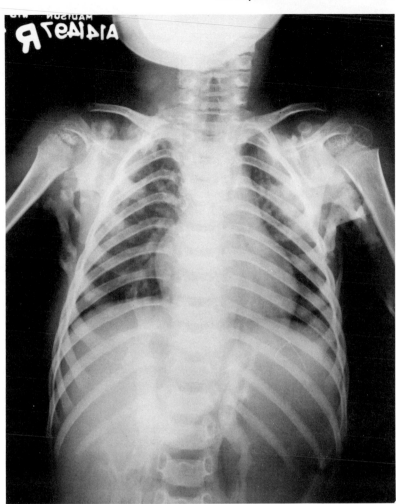

Fig. 10-10. Progressive myositis ossificans. Extensive ossifications of back and shoulder muscles are evident in this child. Irregular bony plaques can be seen along the lower thoracic and upper lumbar spine as well as around the shoulders.

disease with periods of remission and exacerbation, but eventually a widespread fixation of the muscles occurs until the body becomes immobile and death ensues. The patient may have considerable limitation of motion in the affected areas before much bone has been formed. The amount of bone demonstrated roentgenographically does not give a true indication of the extent of the process. The abnormal ossifications are often observed first in the muscles of the neck and back. Initially, these ossifications are relatively hazy and somewhat difficult to identify. In time, irregular, elongated bony plates are observed extending along the long axis of the involved muscle. In later stages, numerous muscles become extensively ossified and the joints become virtually immobile. There is no relationship between this condition and the myositis ossificans that is due to trauma and

is described in a foregoing section of this chapter. Associated anomalies of the skeleton are found in almost all of the patients. These include microdactyly of the first toe, with ankylosis of the interphalangeal joint and of the metatarsophalangeal joint, hallux valgus, and hypoplasia of the first metacarpals and of some of the phalanges. Occasionally, there is hypoplasia of the middle phalanges of the fifth digits of the hands. The changes in the feet are more frequent than those in the hands.

THE EHLERS–DANLOS SYNDROME

The Ehlers–Danlos syndrome is a rare cause of disseminated subcutaneous calcifications. It is characterized by an unusual hyperelasticity and fragility of the skin and blood vessels, hypermobility of the joints, pseudotumors over the bony prominences, and disseminated movable subcutaneous nodules. In addition, other congenital defects have been noted frequently and the disease is considered to be a congenital dystrophy with hereditary and familial influences. The syndrome is of interest roentgenologically because the subcutaneous nodules may calcify. The nodules appear as round, discrete densities, usually ringlike with a central zone of translucency ranging from 2 to 10 mm in diameter. They occur most frequently over the bony prominences of the forearms and legs. Additional findings include a variety of thoracic deformities among which are scoliosis, kyphosis, pectus excavatum, subluxation of the sternoclavicular joints, and abnormal costochondral junctions. Other anomalies that have been observed in patients with this syndrome include areas of stenosis in the pulmonary arteries, and a number of minor anomalies of the small bones of the extremities. There is also a tendency for the development of osteoarthritis, particularly in weight–bearing joints. Occasionally, megaduodenum is observed along with multiple duodenal and jejunal diverticula that may result in malabsorption ("blind-loop syndrome").

CALCIFICATION IN TUMORS

Calcification is not a specific finding for any single type of tumor of the soft tissues with the exception of hemangioma. As indicated earlier in this chapter, calcification in the form of phleboliths is a frequent finding in cavernous hemangioma and is often diagnostic of this tumor. In other tumors, calcification results usually because of a deficient blood supply with subsequent necrosis within a solid, slowly growing neoplasm. Deposits of calcium occur in lipomas, liposarcomas, fibrosarcomas, and synovial sarcomas, to mention the most common. Calcification may also occur in leiomyoma and leiomyosarcoma of the soft tissues. These tumors are uncommon in the soft tissues and probably arise from smooth muscle of arteries. Very rarely, calcification is found in rhabdomyosarcoma. *Pseudosarcomatous fasciitis,* which is considered by some to be malignant, may be diffusely calcified.[3] Rarely, calcification may also be found in soft tissues adjacent to a basal cell carcinoma, as well as in the carcinoma in the nevoid basal cell carcinoma syndrome. *Xanthoma* in tendons and fascia may occasionally contain calcium deposits. There is often nothing characteristic about the appearance of the calcification to aid in identifying the type of tumor. Rarely, *osteosarcoma* has been found arising

in the soft tissues, apparently as a result of cellular metaplasia.

CALCIFICATION AFTER SPINAL CORD INJURY

The development of masses of calcium or bone in the extremities of paraplegics or quadriplegics is one of the interesting and rather poorly understood complications of spinal cord injury. In some patients the calcification appears to follow decubitus ulcers and chronic infection of the deep tissues overlying the bony prominences, particularly the greater trochanters and the ischial tuberosities. In others, extensive calcification or ossification develops along the shafts of the bones and within the muscles of the paralyzed extremities. The calcification and ossification may occur as early as 3 to 4 weeks following the injury that caused the paraplegia. This may represent a traumatic myositis ossificans (*q.v.*) since the lack of pain sensation predisposes to repeated injuries with intramuscular and subperiosteal hemorrhages and subsequent calcification. However, in some cases this explanation does not seem correct and the exact mechanism at times remains obscure (Fig. 10-11). The patients who develop ossification often have an elevated serum alkaline phosphatase, while paraplegics who do not develop myositis ossificans tend to have a normal alkaline phosphatase.

Because of the severe disuse osteoporosis in these patients the bones fracture easily and the injury may go undetected for a time. Exuberant callus is common around such a fracture because of the lack of proper immobilization. Dislocation may also occur and not be recognized for some time.

INTERSTITIAL CALCINOSIS

Interstitial calcinosis is an uncommon although not a rare disease in which there is either a localized or a widely disseminated deposition of calcium in the skin, subcutaneous tissues, muscles, and tendons. Calcinosis often is associated with and apparently a part of the collagen diseases, scleroderma, and dermatomyositis. However, it can exist in a relatively asymptomatic form with no signs of any associated disorder. The cause of interstitial calcinosis, therefore, is unknown but the process is generally considered to represent tissue calcification secondary to some type of injury and thus to fall in the general group of dystrophic calcifications. The following types of calcinosis can be recognized.

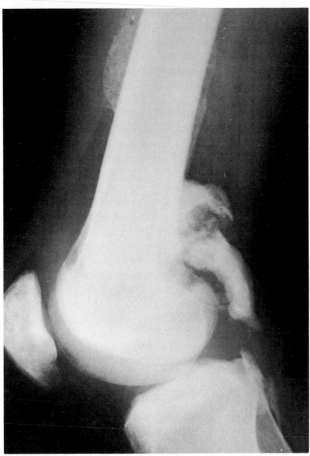

Fig. 10-11. Periosteal and soft-tissue calcification in a paraplegic patient. Large masses of calcium have formed in the popliteal area, and there is some subperiosteal calcification along the shaft of the femur.

Calcinosis Universalis (Diffuse Calcinosis)

Calcinosis universalis is characterized by the wide dissemination of thin calcific plaques of various sizes throughout the soft tissues, chiefly in the subcutaneous layer, occasionally within the muscles and tendons. From a clinical point of view there are several types of diffuse calcinosis:

1. Asymptomatic. This has been reported but in our experience it is a rare lesion.
2. Diffuse calcinosis associated with generalized scleroderma. *Werner's syndrome,*[24] in which scleroderma is associated with premature senility, cataracts, extensive Mönckeberg's arteriosclerosis, and an erosive arthritis, is also accom-

panied by subcutaneous interstitial calcinosis and calcifications in ligaments about the knee, ankle, and foot.
3. Diffuse calcinosis associated with dermatomyositis (Fig. 10-12).

The diseases "scleroderma" and "dermatomyositis" are closely related, both being considered to belong to the group of collagen-vascular or connective tissue diseases. The calcification occurs in the form of thin plaques. In scleroderma they are limited to the skin and immediate subcutaneous tissues; in dermatomyositis, calcification also occurs in the muscles. In addition to the plaques there is a general loss of soft-tissue differentiation with the subcutane-

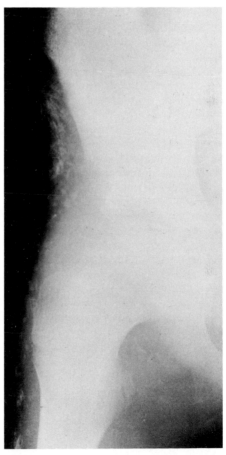

Fig. 10-12. Diffuse interstitial calcinosis in a patient with dermatomyositis. There are extensive plaques of calcification in the tissues of the upper thigh and buttocks along with a loss of normal differentiation of soft tissue.

ous fat layer becoming very scanty or disappearing altogether.

Subcutaneous Fat Necrosis in Infants. This is a rare condition[25] in which extensive subcutaneous calcification is present in the newborn. The cause is obscure but it may be related to intrauterine anoxia. At times, the mottled calcifications may be focal rather than general. The prognosis is good, since the calcification regresses gradually in a year or two. This condition must be differentiated from calcinosis universalis and congenital fibromatosis.

Calcinosis Circumscripta

In the localized type of calcinosis the calcifications occur in the form of small rounded foci having an amorphous appearance. These foci are found chiefly in the tips of the fingers and along the margins of the joints in the hands and feet. The changes are noted more frequently in the hands than in the feet and when present in both areas are usually more intense in the hands. As is true with the diffuse form of calcinosis, the localized type occurs in several different clinical manifestations:

Without Associated Skin or Vasospastic Phenomena. The lesions appear most frequently in elderly persons and are more common in women than in men. There may be some aching in the joints of the affected areas or the calcifications may be found by chance. The foci may be numerous and some may be sufficiently large to cause visible swellings (Fig. 10-13). In some of these patients, ulceration of the skin occurs over the larger lumps, followed by extrusion of cheesy, whitish material and subsequent healing. Because of the physical similarity to gout, the condition has been termed *chalk gout*. This is not good usage and should be discontinued because the disease has no relationship to gout. Gouty tophi, being composed of urates, are radiolucent and of a density comparable to the soft tissues. However, gouty tophi may calcify occasionally but the other bone and joint changes of gout are usually present to aid in diagnosis.

Associated with Scleroderma. Calcinosis is of frequent occurrence when scleroderma affects the fingers and hands. The calcification may be in the form of a few tiny rounded subcutaneous nodules or occur as larger masses. These are found commonly in the terminal phalanges or along the margins of the joints. Other roentgen signs of scleroderma often are present, including (*1*) diminution in the amount of soft tissues in the tips of the fingers so that these digits develop a tapered or almost pointed appearance, (*2*) uniform density of the subcutaneous tissues with loss of normal soft-tissue architecture, and (*3*) absorption of bone. The latter begins in the terminal tufts of the distal phalanges of the affected fingers so that these tufts disappear and the shaft of the phalanx becomes pointed. The absorption may extend to involve the shaft and can be sufficiently severe so that most of the bone disappears or fragments (Fig. 10-14).

Associated with Raynaud's Phenomenon and Secondary Scleroderma. These patients usually are women; the disease may begin during adolescence or later. The early symptoms are those of intermittent arteriolar spasm with the scleroderma appearing either contemporaneously or at a variable time afterward. The scleroderma may progress and involve extensive areas of the body. In other cases it is limited to the face and neck, the fingers and hands, with progressive decrease to the elbows; less marked changes may be present in the feet and toes. This more limited disease goes by the name of *acrosclerosis*. The roentgen findings are no different from those described for scleroderma alone.

Subcutaneous and Intramuscular Calcification in Calcium Gluconate Therapy

When calcium gluconate is administered intramuscularly to infants or when it extravasates on intravenous injection, a tissue reaction occurs. This results in hazy amorphous calcification in muscle and subcutaneous tissues which is not produced by the administered calcium since no roentgen findings are present early. Erythema and induration develop and produce a hard mass that begins to calcify in a few days, is then visible radiographically, and increases in size for about 2 weeks. Then there is a gradual decrease followed by eventual disappearance of the calcium deposition. If large subcutaneous doses are administered, ulceration and extrusion of the calcium may occur. Calcification may also be observed in vessels in the area of extravasation.

PERIOSTEAL CALCIFICATION

The periosteum, although intimately related to bone and bone formation, has the same "water density" as other soft tissues. Regardless of cause, irritation of it usually is followed by reactive calcification. The appearance of this often gives a valuable clue to the na-

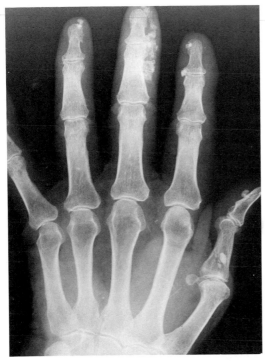

Fig. 10-13. Localized interstitial calcinosis. Deposits of calcareous material are noted in the soft tissues of the first four digits.

ture of the underlying bone disease. The following list of types of periosteal calcification indicates how this information can be used in diagnosis:

I. Continuous layer (mostly benign lesions)
  A. Uniform density (hazy [early]; dense [older])
    1. Parallel surface (infections; hemorrhage; callus)
    2. Wavy surface (osteoarthropathy; venous stasis; tuberous sclerosis)
    3. Convex surface (hemorrhage; benign tumors; callus)
  B. Laminated (some active infections or other process causing rapid production of periosteal new bone)
  C. Spiculated (anemias; acropachy; hemangioma)
II. Interrupted layer (many are malignant)
  A. Uniform density
  B. Laminated (multiple layers) (Ewing's)
    1. Codman triangles (usually primary malignancy)
  C. Spiculated (malignant tumors)

The most frequent causes include: (*1*) fracture (callus), (*2*) infection, (*3*) metabolic, (*4*) tumors, (*5*) melorheostosis, (*6*) infantile cortical hyperostosis, (*7*) vitamin A poisoning, (*8*) hypertrophic osteoarthropathy, (*9*) subperiosteal hemorrhage, (*10*) tuberous sclerosis, (*11*) others (see following).

Chronic Vascular Stasis. In the presence of chronic venous stasis in the legs occurring as a result of long-standing varicosities and venous thrombosis, chronic periosteal calcification along the tibial and fibular shafts is frequent (Fig. 10-15). The appearance resembles closely that found in hypertrophic os-

Fig. 10-14. Scleroderma with associated interstitial calcinosis. Note the punctate calcifications in the soft tissues of the thumb and index finger. There is also absorption of the terminal tufts, giving the phalanges a pointed shape. There is also some decrease in the amount of soft tissue at the fingertips. The latter two findings are particularly evident in the fourth and fifth digits.

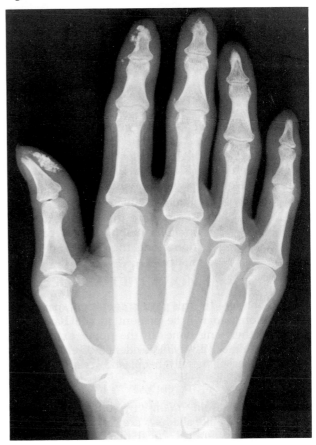

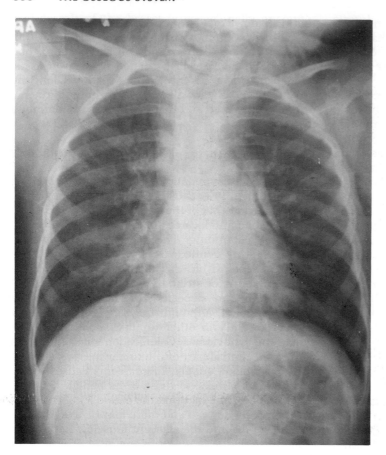

Fig. 10-19. Subcutaneous and mediastinal emphysema. There is air in the soft tissues of the neck, left axilla, and left side of the mediastinum noted as linear radiolucent streaks in these areas. This condition followed an injury to the upper thorax.

The mass of the tumor usually is fairly well defined unless it is completely within the major muscle bundles of the extremity. The density of a fibrosarcoma is similar to that of muscle. If the tumor lies largely in the subcutaneous tissues, the normal fat may allow the margin of the tumor to be visualized clearly so that a fairly good estimate of its size and shape can be obtained. Deep tumors result only in a diffuse enlargement of the part. Calcification is fairly common in fibrosarcomas, occurring as mottled shadows, usually near the center of the mass. Deep-seated fibrosarcomas show a definite tendency to invade contiguous bone. This is seen as a ragged loss of the external cortical surface of the bone. Periosteal reaction at the limits of the erosion is not present very often. The tendency for fibrosarcoma to recur after local excision is noteworthy and roentgenograms of soft tissue may be useful in demonstrating the recurrent tumor mass. Of greater importance, perhaps, is the use of roentgenograms to determine if a recurrent tumor has begun to invade bone; the result of this de-

termination may influence the method of treatment to a considerable degree.

Fibrosarcomas metastasize to the regional nodes and also to the lungs. Roentgenograms of the chest should be obtained in all cases and whenever the patient returns for periodic checkup examinations.

OTHER TUMORS

Tumors of the joints have been considered in Chapter 9 and will not be discussed further in this section. A variety of other tumors of soft-tissue nature may develop in the extremities but with nothing characteristic in their roentgen appearances. Mention has been made earlier, in the section dealing with subcutaneous calcification, of the roentgen findings in *cavernous hemangiomas*. In addition to the visualization of calcified thrombi, the tortuous shadows of dilated vessels may be visible in such a tumor if it extends to involve the subcutaneous fatty layer. The tumor may cause either cortical thickening or erosion of the

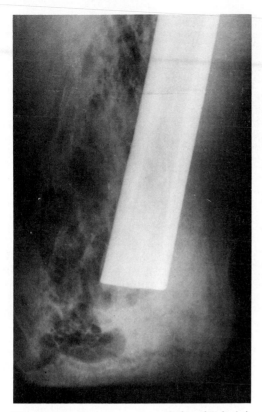

Fig. 10-20. Gas gangrene of the thigh following amputation. The gas forms irregular streaks and rounded translucent areas in the soft tissues of the thigh.

SOFT-TISSUE TRAUMA

Burns. Heterotopic soft-tissue calcifications occur in about one-fourth of patients with severe burns. They tend to be flocculent and poorly defined and occur more commonly in children than in adults. Some spontaneous regression is the rule unless tissues adjacent to and surrounding a joint are involved. In the latter instance, a bony bridge may form resulting in immobilization of the joint involved.

Hypothermia and Frostbite. Severe hypothermia in infants may produce fat necrosis leading to extensive subcutaneous calcification. The calcification regresses and disappears in a few months. Frostbite is followed quickly by soft-tissue swelling. When the injury is severe, infection by gas-forming organisms at the site of the injury is common. It is manifested by interstitial gas in the soft tissues of the affected extremity which appears 2 to 6 days following the injury. This is a poor prognostic sign, since amputation is almost always necessary when it is observed. Soft-tissue atrophy may develop when the injury is severe, resulting in tapering of the distal digits involved. Bone changes are described in Chapter 8.

Fig. 10-21. A mole on the skin of the back was responsible for the round density **(arrow)** seen in this film of the abdomen.

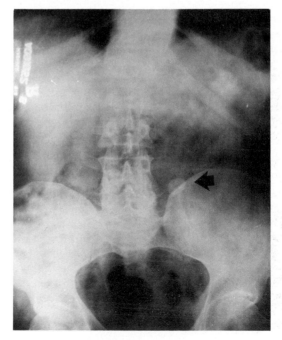

bone immediately adjacent if it is deeply situated. Otherwise the lesion causes only a diffuse increase in density.

Smooth muscle tumors (*leiomyomas* and *leiomyosarcomas*) are rare in soft tissues and present as masses of varying size with no distinctive roentgen features. Calcification may be present. *Rhabdomyosarcoma* (the others are liposarcoma and fibrosarcoma) is one of the most common soft-tissue sarcomas. These sarcomas arise in deep soft tissues and present as poorly defined soft-tissue masses that may be very large. Fine punctate calcification occurs rarely.

Giant cell tumors may also arise in soft tissues and tend to be more malignant than those arising in bone. There are no characteristic roentgen features. Angiography may be helpful in that neovascularity indicates that the mass is malignant but this does not differentiate it from other soft-tissue sarcomas.

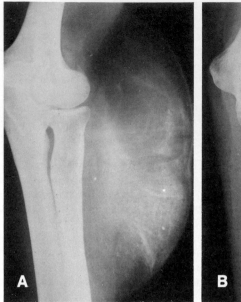
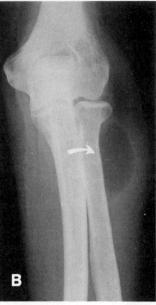

Fig. 10-22. Lipoma of the subcutaneous tissues. **A.** Large lipoma of the forearm. The radiolucent areas are due to fat and the striations are due to fibrous tissue and vessels within the mass of fat. **B.** Small lipoma of the forearm **(arrow)**. The mass of fat is clearly outlined because it is surrounded by muscle.

Mechanical Soft-Tissue Trauma. Severe trauma to soft tissues may separate subcutaneous tissues from deeper tissues, allowing hemorrhage to create a space that may persist and become chronic. A fibrous lining may result, preventing closure of the space, which then remains as a posttraumatic cyst.

MAMMOGRAPHY

Mammography is soft-tissue radiography of the female breast which is now and has been widely used for detection of breast tumors.[7, 32, 33] Conventional soft-tissue radiography or xeroradiography may be used. As a general rule, the dose in xeromammography is slightly higher than that in conventional radiography, but constant improvements are being made to reduce the radiation dosage.

The use of mammography as a screening method for breast cancer has been very controversial recently, but there is little question of its value in the study of women beyond the age of 50 years. A group of younger women who are at higher risk than the general population may also be candidates for mammography. These include: (*1*) those who have a family history of breast cancer, particularly if the mother had bilateral breast cancer or had the disease before the menopause; (*2*) those who had previous pre-malignant breast disease; (*3*) those with a suspicious breast mass found on physical examination; (*4*) those having adenocarcinoma found on biopsy when the primary site is unknown; (*5*) those having physical findings indicating or suggesting mammary dysplasia (fibrocystic disease); (*6*) those having nipple discharge or retraction; (*7*) those having skin thickening or dimpling; (*8*) those who had a late (after age 28) first pregnancy; (*9*) nulliparas; (*10*) those having adverse hormonal (estrogen and progesterone) milieu as related to parity; and (*11*) those with cancer in the opposite breast. When mammograms have been obtained, the patient can be placed in high- or low-risk categories, depending on the mammographic patterns. Wolfe[31] has described several risk patterns based on mammographic appearances. These are: N–1, fatty breast; P–1, prominent ducts in less than one-fourth of the breast; P–2, prominent ducts in over one-fourth of the breast, particularly when the ducts are somewhat nodular; D–Y, severe involvement with dysplasia (adenosis and fibrocystic disease) that may obscure prominent ducts. N–1 and P–1 are the low-risk patterns, while P–2 and D–Y constitute a higher-risk group.

The following guidelines have been issued by the National Cancer Institute/National Institutes of Health for asymptomatic females: (*1*) In women over 50 years of age, mammography and physical examination are useful adjuncts to cancer screening. (*2*) Asymptomatic women 40 to 49 years old should have mammography screening only if they have a personal history of breast cancer or there has been breast cancer in a mother or sibling. (3) Asymptomatic women 35 to 39 years old should have mammography screening only if they have a personal history of breast cancer.

Technology continues to improve, resulting in better studies with lower radiation doses. In the future, ultrasound and dedicated computerized tomographic scanners may prove to be better methods than the current ones. Magnification techniques have been developed in which tubes with a small focal spot are employed; these also improve the diagnostic quality of the examination.

MALIGNANT BREAST NEOPLASMS

Primary signs of breast cancer[33] in film or revealed by xeroradiography are as follows:

1. Subtle signs of breast cancer:
   a. Asymmetry of breasts should always arouse suspicion unless explained by previous biopsy, trauma, or infection.
   b. Densities which increase in size or opacity.
   c. Solitary dilated ducts, particularly when unilateral.
   d. Intraductal calcifications, thin and rod-shaped or Y-shaped.
   e. Intralobular calcifications that are in a solitary cluster and not very smooth and not rounded or oval. Tightly grouped clusters of calcifications are found in adenosis; these are usually multiple clusters and individual calcifications are smoothly rounded or oval in contrast to thin linear calcifications found in intraductal carcinoma. When there is any doubt, however, biopsy should be recommended.
2. *Breast mass*—ranging from large, obvious, spiculated scirrhous lesions to a subtle, asymmetric density in one breast. The masses may be characterized as:
   a. *Scirrhous*—spicules radiating in straight lines from a central mass of varying size (Figs. 10-23 and 10-24B).
   b. *Nodular*—a mass with an irregular or "knobby" border (Fig. 10-23A).
   c. *Lobulated*—a minimal and rather smooth lobulation; often with only a small, poorly defined local irregularity or indistinct border to differentiate it from fibroadenoma.
   d. *Smooth*—may be round or oval.
   e. *Diffuse*—mass without definable limits; an area of increased density as compared to the

opposite breast. This pattern may be observed in "inflammatory" cancer with associated edema of skin and enlarged axillary nodes.
3. *Calcifications*—tumor calcifications usually have some or all of the following characteristics:
   a. *Size:* Small—0.1 to 2.0 mm in diameter.
   b. *Shape*—round, rodlike or lacy.
   c. *Contour*—irregular.
   d. *Number*—usually 15 to 20 more; occasionally only 2 or 3.
   e. *Location*—in a group or groups; in comedocarcinoma, along the course of ducts or in radiating or rosette formation with no definite mass. There may be several clusters, scattered in several areas of the breast.
4. *Duct patterns:*
   a. *Asymmetrical* collection of ducts on one side and not on the other. Ducts tend to be localized, tortuous, and somewhat discontinuous.
   b. *Segmental duct prominence*—begin in subareolar area and extend posteriorly; large, tortuous, and asymmetrical. Occasionally a solitary, very prominent duct indicates cancer.

Secondary signs of breast cancer:

1. *Vascularity*—an increase in size and/or number of veins in the affected areas; this sign is often of little help in making a diagnosis.
2. *Skin thickening* over the site of malignancy—may be very helpful in calling attention to a small, poorly defined mass.
3. *Skin retraction* resulting in straightening or concavity of normal contour. Spicules extending to skin may be observed (Fig. 10-23B).
4. *Nipple retraction*—may be normal, but when associated with spicules or prominent ducts, it is an important sign.
5. *Axillary lymph nodes,* when large, dense, and mottled or closely packed.

BENIGN BREAST NEOPLASMS

Benign breast neoplasms have certain characteristics that usually permit accurate roentgenographic or xeroradiographic diagnosis.

Fibroadenoma is the most common and is the usual cause of a breast mass in teenage girls. Its radiographic characteristics are those of a dense, oval or lobulated mass with sharp, well-defined borders that is often surrounded by a halo of fat. Calcification is observed when the tumor degenerates. The calcifications tend to be large, somewhat irregular and

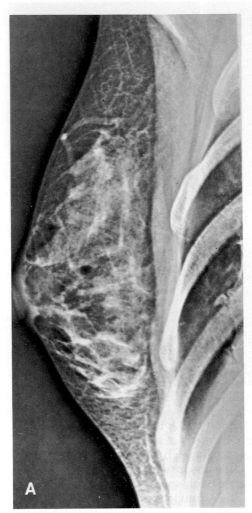

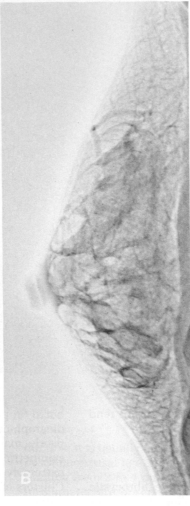

Fig. 10-25. Mammary dysplasia. Xerogram in the positive mode **(A)** and negative mode **(B)** showing mammary dysplasia consisting predominantly of fibrocystic disease. (Courtesy of Dr. R. H. Matallana)

tients who have had dysplasia earlier in life. It consists of a mass of collagen surrounding ducts making them appear beaded and tortuous radiographically. This tends to extend from the subareolar area posteriorly into the central breast and posterolaterally toward the axilla. It may involve only the retroareolar area or be so extensive as to involve most of the breasts. Since collagenosis tends to be associated with a high incidence of malignancy, any asymmetry should be viewed with suspicion.

INFLAMMATORY DISEASE OF THE BREAST

In acute inflammation, there is a local increase in density, the area of which depends on the size of the inflammatory reaction. This is associated with thickening of the skin produced by edema. In chronic in-

flammatory disease of the breast, abscess is usually present. It is usually subareolar or anterior in location and is very difficult to differentiate from carcinoma on mammography, particularly when the lesion is viewed *"en face."* The history and clinical findings are important in differentiation.

BREAST TRAUMA

Blunt trauma to the breast may produce hemorrhage and edema, including edema of the skin. This produces a mass-like density on mammography which is very difficult to differentiate from malignancy. History is helpful and follow-up study will show regression of the post-traumatic changes. Similar changes may occur in the post-operative period following breast biopsy, and later on there may be scarring which may simulate neoplasm since local skin thickening may persist for some time. Therefore, an accurate history plus physical examination is important in these instances.

OTHER PROCEDURES FOR BREAST EXAMINATION

Other procedures in examination of the breast include *galactography* (injection of opaque medium into the ducts), which is beyond the scope of this volume, and *tumor localization* as well as *cyst puncture.* Cyst puncture is used to confirm the diagnosis of cyst in a patient in whom the presence of this lesion is strongly suspected. The cyst is usually palpable and can be punctured readily. Fluid is aspirated for cytologic study. If there is suspicion of malignancy, Renografin or other organic iodide may be injected into the cyst to outline the contour of the cystlike space or may be added for double contrast study. Ultrasonography is very useful in differentiating a cyst from a solid mass. Tumor localization is usually performed immediately before biopsy. A needle is placed with the tip as close to the suspected lesion as possible. Films are then obtained to note the relationship of the needle tip to the lesion. A small amount of dye (*e.g.*, 0.1 cc, Evans blue), plus organic iodide, is injected before the needle is removed to mark the site of its tip; then biopsy is accomplished.

VENOGRAPHY

Venography consists in the injection of an aqueous radiopaque substance into one of the peripheral veins of an extremity and the making of one or several roentgenograms. Venography has its greatest use in the examination of the veins of the lower extremities for the detection of thrombosis of the deep veins. In the upper extremity the method can be used for the study of obstructions of the axillary and subclavian veins or of the superior vena cava. The value of venography for the determination of deep venous thrombosis in the lower extremities has been disputed. While many reports have indicated enthusiasm for the method, in others doubt has been raised concerning its value. In our experience it is difficult to fill all the veins in the normal extremity. The interpretation of venograms is often difficult and at times the decision cannot be made whether a given vein is pathologically obstructed or did not fill merely as a normal variant. Contrast material injected into one of the small tributaries in the foot, which is the usual site of injection, finds its way into the larger veins of the thigh by the most direct route as a rule and it is unusual to be able to fill all of the medium-sized or larger veins.

TECHNIQUE

Many technical variations have been introduced to improve the value of venography but, essentially, all of them depend upon the rather slow injection of an aqueous contrast substance such as Hypaque (50%) into one of the small veins on the dorsum of the foot or in the region of the ankle.* In general, we have followed the method outlined by DeBakey, Schroeder, and Ochsner. A tourniquet is placed on the thigh as high as possible and tightened sufficiently so that the superficial veins are occluded and the blood is shunted into the deeper veins. If desired, a blood pressure cuff can be inflated to no more than 25 to 30 mmHg and used in place of the rubber tourniquet but this is not essential. Any vein on the dorsum of the foot can be used for the venipuncture. If none can be found easily, the lesser saphenous vein can be used. This is constantly present directly behind the external malleolus and if necessary a cutdown on this vessel can be performed to locate it. If only the veins of the leg are to be examined, a 14- by 17-inch cassette is placed beneath the leg and 20 cc of the contrast solution are injected at the rate of about 1 cc per second. The film is exposed 20 seconds after the injection is completed. If both the leg and the thigh are to be examined, 25 cc of the contrast solution are used. A film of the leg is exposed 20 seconds after the injection is completed; another film is placed beneath the thigh and it is exposed as soon as possible, usually within another 20 to 30 seconds. We usually have the patient in a semi-erect position. The progress of the opaque medium can be followed fluoroscopically and spot films obtained as needed. Some prefer this method to overhead filming.

ROENTGEN OBSERVATIONS

The anatomy of the veins of the lower extremity is shown in Figure 10-26. As mentioned previously, failure to visualize any given vein does not necessarily indicate that it is obstructed by a thrombus. If there are no signs of collateral vessels around the nonvisualized vein and if the filled veins have a normal

---

* See Chapter 20 for a discussion of the contrast substances available for intravenous and intra-arterial injections, with particular reference to the possible dangers, the use of sensitivity tests, and the treatment of drug reactions when they occur.

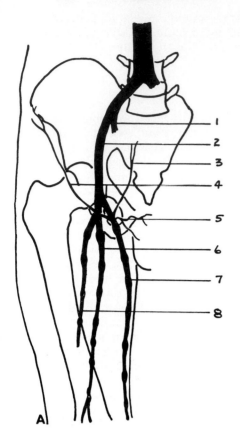

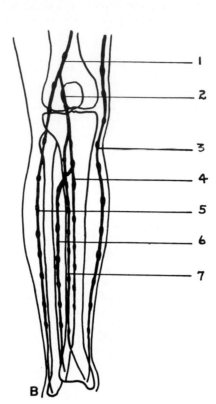

Fig. 10-26. Diagram of veins of lower extremity. **A.** Veins of the thigh: **(1)** hypogastric; **(2)** external iliac; **(3)** superficial epigastric; **(4)** superficial circumflex iliac; **(5)** superficial external pudendal; **(6)** femoral; **(7)** greater saphenous; **(8)** deep femoral. **B.** Veins of the leg: **(1)** femoral; **(2)** popliteal; **(3)** greater saphenous; **(4)** posterior tibial; **(5)** lesser saphenous; **(6)** peroneal; **(7)** anterior tibial.

caliber and follow a normal direction, the likelihood of deep venous obstruction is remote. On the other hand, visualization of one of the deep veins up to a certain point with failure of contrast material to outline it any higher, the presence of dilated and tortuous vessels in the region, and filling of other deep or superficial veins at a higher level in the extremity are valuable observations. In some cases of partial obstruction the thrombus may be outlined. Often it will be found necessary to repeat the examination to determine if a given finding is constant. At other times the evidence of obstruction and its exact site will be reasonably definite.

Most venographic examinations in the upper extremity are performed for study of obstruction of the axillary or subclavian veins. The contrast material can be injected into a branch of the basilic vein at the elbow. One exposure is made at the completion of the injection and another 20 to 30 seconds later. If the clinical evidence of obstruction is definite a third exposure can be made as rapidly as film cassettes can be changed. These serial roentgenograms serve to demonstrate the site of obstruction and the collateral circulation around it. It is preferable to use a large-sized film so that the entire shoulder area and the upper mediastinum can be included in one view.

ARTERIOGRAPHY

The arteries of the lower extremities can be visualized following injection of contrast material into the femoral artery in the upper thigh or after puncture of the abdominal aorta. The latter procedure, known as abdominal aortography, is discussed in Chapter 20. Direct aortic puncture has been replaced to a great extent by the Seldinger catheter technique or a modification of it. If the aorta or femoral artery is obstructed the catheter can be introduced into the axillary artery or other major vessel and passed to the upper abdominal aorta and the contrast material injected to outline the site of obstruction. Injection of the contrast material into the abdominal aorta has the advantage that both extremities can be visualized

Fig. 10-27. Diagram of the arteries of the pelvis, thigh, and leg. **A.** Arteries of the pelvis and thigh: **(1)** iliolumbar; **(2)** inferior epigastric; **(3)** external iliac; **(4)** hypogastric; **(5)** superior gluteal; **(6)** deep circumflex iliac; **(7)** inferior gluteal; **(8)** internal pudendal; **(9)** obturator; **(10)** medial femoral circumflex; **(11)** lateral femoral circumflex; **(12)** femoral; **(13)** perforating branch; **(14)** deep femoral (profunda). **B.** Arteries of the lower thigh and leg: **(1)** femoral; **(2)** popliteal; **(3)** lateral superior genicular; **(4)** medial superior genicular; **(5)** lateral inferior genicular; **(6)** medial inferior genicular; **(7)** posterior tibial; **(8)** anterior tibial; **(9)** peroneal (Based on Morton S and Byrne R: Radiology 69: 63, 1957)

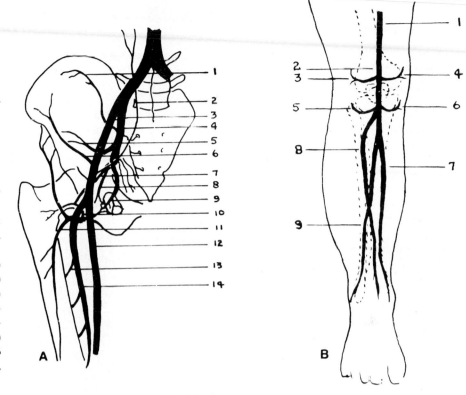

with one injection and information may be obtained concerning the lower part of the aorta and iliac vessels (Fig. 10-27). For localized disease, such as aneurysm, arteriovenous fistula, and occlusive disease, and for study of the vascularity of neoplasms, it is advisable to inject the contrast material into the femoral artery. This can be done after surgical exposure of the vessel, but most frequently is performed by percutaneous puncture. The contrast material used is similar to that for venography except that there is an advantage in the use of more concentrated solutions. The blood flow is so much faster in the arteries than in the veins that the medium becomes diluted even when injected rapidly. The contrast solution is injected as quickly as possible. For the examination of a lesion such as an aneurysm the site of which is known, the film cassette is placed beneath the region and the exposure made immediately at the completion of injection. When the vessels in both the thigh and the leg are to be examined by means of abdominal aortic injection the technical difficulties increase. Usually this examination is made possible by utilizing multiple films, suitable cones, and shielding to

expose two roentgenograms in rapid succession so that the pelvis, thighs, and upper parts of the legs can be visualized. For descriptions of special radiographic techniques the current literature should be consulted.

ROENTGEN OBSERVATIONS

The visualization of an aneurysm usually is accomplished without difficulty. The appearances of the aneurysm are characteristic. Occasionally an aneurysm will be partially filled with an old thrombus that may have become canalized and the channel, as visualized when filled with the contrast material, may give an entirely erroneous impression of the actual size of the vessel. In some cases the vessel may appear to be fairly normal. Therefore, one should be aware that the apparent size of the aneurysmal sac as visualized following contrast filling may not be the actual size of the aneurysm. Arteriovenous fistulae, usually caused by penetrating wounds, give unequivocal signs when examined by means of arteriography. The extension of the contrast material through the fistula into the

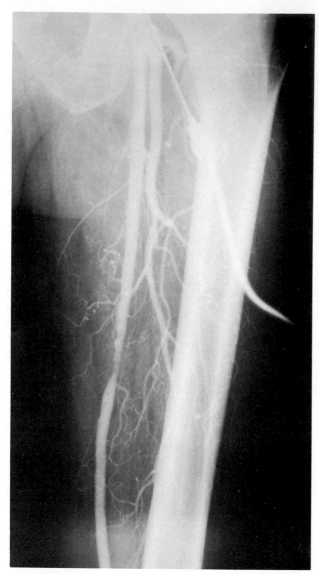

Fig. 10-28. Femoral arteriogram. Arteriosclerotic plaque narrows the lumen in the middle third of the thigh; elsewhere the superficial femoral artery appears normal.

communicating veins can be clearly demonstrated. The abnormal veins are greatly dilated and tortuous and they fill extensively in the region of the fistula.

The most frequent use of arteriography of the peripheral vessels is in the study of occlusive disease. Intimal arteriosclerotic plaques cause areas of irregular narrowing of the vessel (Fig. 10-28) or, if severe, complete occlusion of it. The lumen may be slightly dilated between areas of constriction. When complete occlusion has taken place as a result of thrombosis the contrast ends with a sharp cutoff. One or more collateral vessels usually can be visualized arising just above the level of obstruction. Frequently these can be followed down to the point where they join the vessel again below the level of the occlusion (Fig. 10-29). If a satisfactory set of roentgenograms can be obtained, arteriography offers a valuable means of identifying the presence and location of arterial occlusion and the extent of disease that may be present in the vessels.

Fig. 10-29. Segmental occlusion of the femoral artery **(arrow).** Refilling below the site of occlusion is by way of collaterals, several of which are faintly outlined.

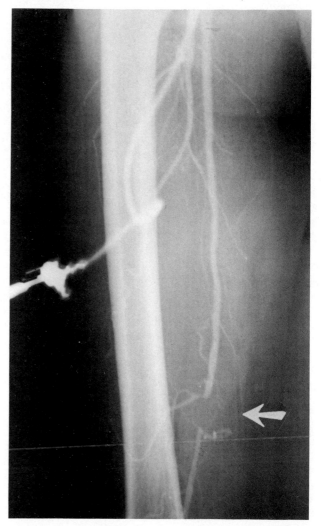

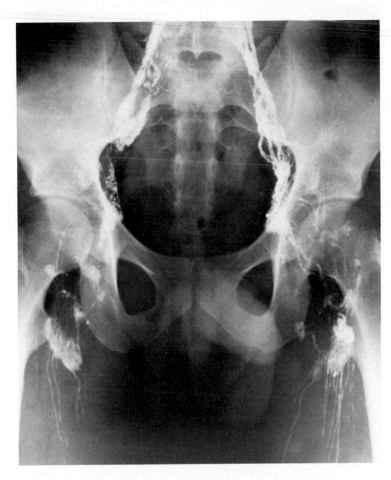

Fig. 10-30. Normal lymphangiogram. Vascular phase showing filling of lymphatic vessels in the upper thighs and pelvis. A few nodes are opacified.

LYMPHANGIOGRAPHY

Lymphangiography is used as a method for opacifying the lymphatic channels and lymph nodes.

TECHNIQUE

Staining of lymphatic channels in the feet is done by intradermal injection of a mixture of 1% xylocaine (1 cc) and 4% direct sky blue (3 to 4 cc) or a similar dye between the first three toes of each foot. In 15 to 30 minutes the subcutaneous lymphatic vessels are stained. With the area locally anesthetized a 1-inch skin incision is then made over a selected channel in the dorsum of each foot. The vessel is freed from its fibrous sheath for 1½ to 2 cm on each side. It is then stabilized with a small hairclip. A 30-gauge cannula especially designed for the purpose is then inserted with the aid of magnifying lens or glasses. Once the cannula is fixed, 6 to 8 cc of ethiodol are injected in each foot. We use a gravity injector designed by Arts. Scout films of the upper thighs and abdomen are obtained and when the contrast material reaches the level of L3 or L4, the injection is discontinued. Films of the abdomen, pelvis, and upper femurs demonstrate the vascular phase. A second set of films is obtained in 24 hours to demonstrate nodal filling.

Lymphography is indicated: (*1*) to evaluate edema of an extremity of unknown cause; (*2*) to evaluate the extent of adenopathy and staging of lymphomas; (*3*) for localization of nodes for treatment planning, either surgical or radiotherapeutic; (*4*) for evaluation of the nature of intra-abdominal masses when biopsy material is not readily available; (*5*) to search for metastasis in patients with suspected intra-abdominal nodal disease; and (*6*) for localization of lymph fistulas in chylothorax, etc.

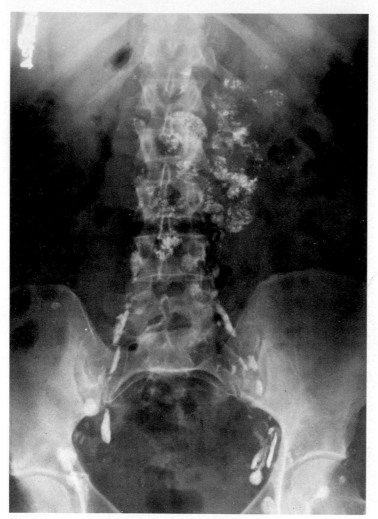

Fig. 10-31. Lymphangiogram of a patient with Hodgkin's disease. This 24-hour film shows a number of midabdominal para-aortic nodes that are enlarged and appear foamy. Pelvic and iliac nodes are normal.

Contraindications include known iodine hypersensitivity, severe pulmonary insufficiency, cardiac disease, and advanced renal or hepatic disease.

Complications in the main are related to embolization of the contrast material into the lungs which diminishes pulmonary function temporarily and in some patients may produce a lipid pneumonia. Extravasation is a complication that usually does not cause any clinically significant changes.

Normally the initial films show filling of the lymphatic channels in the thigh, pelvis, and abdomen. Some of the nodes are filled at this time (Fig. 10-30). In the 24-hour film, the lymph channels are no longer visible in the normal person and the lymph nodes are filled (Fig. 10-31). Interpretation of lymphangiograms is difficult and there are limitations in that nodes completely replaced by neoplasm may not take up contrast material while nodes involved by inflammatory disease may sometimes show a pattern similar to that observed in lymphoma (Fig. 10-32). Detailed lymphangiographic interpretation is beyond the scope of this book.

Body C-T scanning is also used to identify masses of lymph nodes. It is likely that it will supplement lymphangiography in many instances, but may replace it in others.

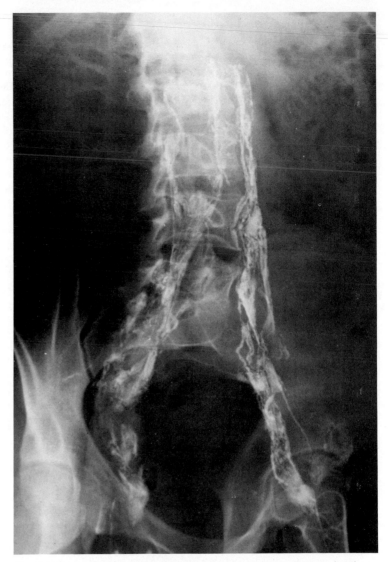

Fig. 10-32. Lymphangiogram. The vascular phase shows displacement of channels by large nodes that are not opacified.

REFERENCES AND SELECTED READINGS

1. ARTS V: An injection apparatus for lymphangiography. Am J Roentgenol 100: 466, 1967

2. BEIGHTON P, THOMAS ML: The radiology of Ehlers-Danlos syndrome. Clin Radiol 20: 354, 1969

3. BRODER MS, LEONIDAS JC, MITTY IIA: Pseudosarcomatous fasciitis: an unusual cause of soft tissue calcification. Radiology 107: 173, 1973

4. CARLIN RA, AMPLATZ K: Downstream aortography. Am J Roentgenol 109: 536, 1970

5. CRISPEN JF, JEFFRIES PF: Lymphangiography. A simple method of dye infusion. JAMA 182: 872, 1962

6. DICHIRO G, NELSON KB: Soft tissue radiography of extremities in neuromuscular disease with histologic correlations. Acta Radiol [Diag] (Stockh) 3: 65, 1965

7. EGAN RL: Mammography. Springfield, IL, C Thomas, 1964

8. FISHER HW, ZIMMERMAN GR: Roentgenographic visual-

ization of lymph nodes and lymphatic channels. Am J Roentgenol 81: 517, 1961

9. GAY BB, WEENS HS: Roentgenologic evaluation of disorders of muscle. Semin Roentgenol 8: 25, 1973

10. GAYLER BW, BROGDEN BD: Soft tissue calcification in systemic disease. Am J Med Sci 249: 590, 1965

11. GERSHON-COHEN J, BERGER SM: Breast cancer with microcalcifications: diagnostic difficulties. Radiology 87: 612, 1966

12. GOLDMAN AB: Myositis ossificans circumscripta. A benign lesion with a malignant differential diagnosis. Am J Roentgenol 126: 32, 1976

13. HASSOCK DW, KING A: Neurogenic heterotopic ossification. Med J Aust 1: 326, 1967

14. JAMES AE JR, EATON SB, BLAZEK JV ET AL: Roentgen findings in pseudoxanthoma elasticum. Radiology 106: 642, 1969

15. JAMES WB, IRVINE RW: Mammography in management of breast lesions. Br Med J 4: 655, 1969

16. LIBERSON M: Soft tissue calcifications in cord lesions. JAMA 152: 1010, 1953.

17. MATALLANA RH: Negative technique in xeroradiography of the breast. Cancer 39: 112, 1977

18. MEZAROS WT: The regional manifestations of scleroderma. Radiology 70: 313, 1958

19. MOULE B, GRANT MC, BOYLE IT et al: Thyroid acropachy. Clin Radiol 21: 329, 1970

20. NICHOLS GB, SCHILLING PJ: Pseudoretroperitoneal gas and rupture of aneurysm of the abdominal aorta. Am J Roentgenol 125: 134, 1975

21. PALMER PES: Tumoural calcinosis. Br J Radiol 39: 518, 1966

22. PARKER RJ, SMITH EH, STONEMANN ER: Generalized arterial calcification of infancy. Clin Radiol 22: 69, 1971

23. REEDER MM: Tropical diseases of the soft tissues. Semin Roentgenol 8: 47, 1973

24. ROSEN RS, CIMINI R, COBLANTZ D: Werner's syndrome. Br J Radiol 43: 193, 1970

25. SHACKELFORD GD, BARTON LL, McALISTER WH: Calcified subcutaneous fat necrosis in infancy. J Can Assoc Radiol 26: 203, 1974

26. SHOPFNER CE: Periosteal bone growth in normal infants: preliminary report. Am J Roentgenol 97: 154, 1966

27. SINGLETON EB, HOLT JF: Myositis ossificans progressiva. Radiology 62: 47, 1954

28. TORRES-REYES E, STAPLE TW: Roentgenographic appearance of thyroid acropachy. Clin Radiol 21: 95, 1970

29. WALLACE S, JACKSON L, DODD GD et al: Lymphangiographic interpretation. Radiol Clin North Am 3: 467, 1965

30. WHEELER CE, CURTIS AC, CAWLEY EP et al: Soft tissue calcification with special reference to its occurrence in "collagen diseases." Ann Intern Med 36: 1050, 1952

31. WOLFE JN: Risk patterns in breast carcinoma. Am J Roentgenol 126: 1130, 1976

32. WOLFE JN: Xeroradiography of the Breast. Springfield, IL, C Thomas, 1972

33. WOLFE JN: Xeroradiography, Breast Calcification. Springfield, IL, C Thomas, 1977

SECTION II

THE BRAIN AND SPINAL CORD

11

INTRACRANIAL DISEASES

THE NORMAL SKULL

Fractures, infections, congenital dysplasias, and primary tumors involving the cranial bones have been discussed in the appropriate chapters dealing with these conditions as they affect the general skeletal system. In the present chapter, attention will be given to changes in the cranial bones caused by intracranial disease and the examination of the skull undertaken primarily for the detection of intracranial abnormalities. Other specialized methods for study of the intracranial structures will be discussed, including pneumoencephalography, ventriculography, cerebral arteriography, tomography, and computerized tomography.

Roentgen examination of the skull consists in obtaining multiple exposures with the patient in different positions. As a minimum, posteroanterior and lateral roentgenograms are required. There is a difference of opinion regarding the use of stereoscopic views. They are particularly valuable in examination of the base of the skull in the axial projection and in examination of facial bones and sinuses in the half-axial and Waters projections. Many prefer to examine the skull by using single views in several planes.[41] Stereoscopic films are then employed only when some problem arises in the initial projections. In many instances other projections are needed, since the shape of the skull and the density of the basal structures make it impossible to visualize all parts of the cranial bones if only two positions are used. It is good practice to supplement the frontal and lateral views with additional projections, depending upon the problem at hand. Thus special positions are available to show the basal structures and the important foramina, the pars petrosa of the temporal bones and internal auditory canals, the sphenoid wings, etc. Figures 11-1 and 11-2 show two of the standard projections and the major anatomic features that can be demonstrated in each.

In the study of skull roentgenograms it is well for the beginner to adopt a plan of observation, since there are many anatomic structures that must be scrutinized. It is easy to have one's attention attracted by some apparently significant alteration from the normal only to miss a more important but less readily visualized abnormality. Any method of

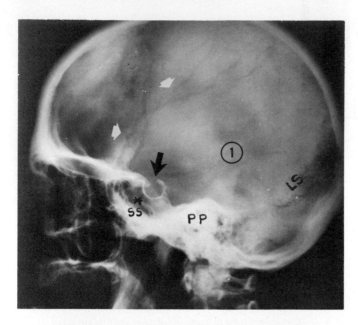

Fig. 11-1. Lateral roentgenogram of the normal skull. **1** indicates position of pineal gland. **Black arrow** points to sella turcica. **Short white arrows** indicate branches of middle meningeal artery. **SS,** sphenoid sinus; **PP,** petrous pyramids; **LS,** lambdoidal suture.

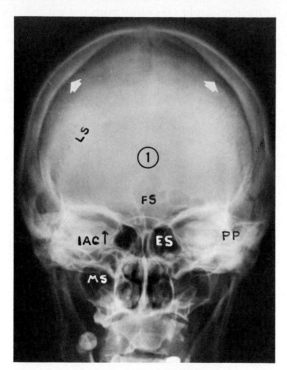

Fig. 11-2. Posteroanterior roentgenogram of normal skull. Figures and lettering are the same as for Figure 11-1. In addition, **IAC,** internal auditory canal; **FS,** frontal sinus; **ES,** ethmoid sinuses; **MS,** maxillary sinuses.

observation is satisfactory as long as it allows an orderly review of all the structures depicted.

BLOOD VESSEL MARKINGS

The pattern of the blood vessel grooves should be observed closely. The middle meningeal artery, a branch of the external carotid, enters the cranial cavity through the foramen spinosum. It courses upward, branching fairly extensively, and the branches lie on the internal surface of the skull within sharply defined grooves that indent the inner table. These grooves usually are visible in roentgenograms as they extend upward to the vertex parallel with and posterior to the coronal suture. The posterior branch of the middle meningeal artery sometimes is unusually straight and extends directly upward through the temporal squamosa, mimicking a linear fracture. Careful observation of stereoscopic views or of right and left lateral roentgenograms will usually show the same line on the opposite side and help to distinguish it from a fracture line.

A certain amount of difference in the size of the right and left middle meningeal vessels is found occasionally as a normal variant. If the vessels on one side are appreciably larger than those on the opposite side, the possibility of an underlying meningioma must be considered. This tumor derives most of its blood supply from the middle meningeal artery and it

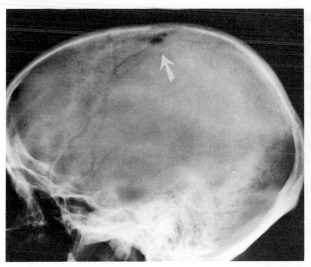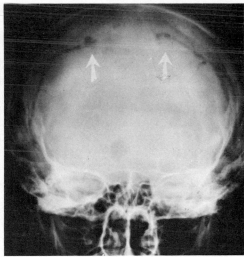

Fig. 11-3. Vascular lakes. Branches of the middle meningeal vessels end in vascular spaces near the vertex **(arrows).**

may cause considerable dilatation of the vessels supplying it. When unilateral vascular prominence is encountered, the appearance of the bone near the vertex should be closely scrutinzed. If a meningioma is responsible for the dilated vessels, the bone may appear to be slightly moth-eaten over the site of the tumor. At other times a localized thickening or hyperostosis may be visible and be a clue to the nature of the lesion. The dilated vessels tend to form an irregular network at the point of attachment of the tumor to the dura.

Of some significance is the anatomic finding that the branches of the middle meningeal artery are accompanied by venous channels (middle meningeal veins). Thus some grooves contain both arteries and veins. Arterial grooves tend to decrease slightly in size as they extend toward the vertex of the skull. Venous grooves or channels change very little in caliber. The most common is the bregmatic groove which roughly parallels the coronal suture. At their terminations the venous channels enlarge into lakes (lacuna lateralis) within which dangle the cauliflowerlike masses of arachnoid granulations, the pacchionian bodies. The arachnoid granulations are not present at birth but develop in the second to fourth decades of life. Most are found in the posterior frontal bone and anterior two-thirds of the parietal bones. The impressions often are large enough to form distinct, sharply outlined areas of rarefaction in roentgenograms. Characteristically, a vessel groove is seen entering and terminating in the lake and this appearance is helpful in distinguishing lakes from foci of destruction caused by disease (Fig. 11-3). Also, if viewed tangentially, a venous lake will be seen to lie within the diploe with intact tables overlying it. The lakes drain into the superior sagittal sinus by means of small venous channels. Some veins drain directly into the superior sagittal sinus and do not end in venous lakes.

The *diploic veins* or *veins of Breschet* lie within the

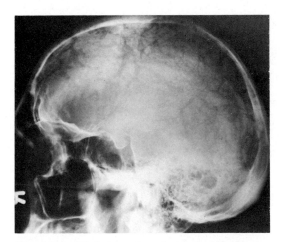

Fig. 11-4. Diploic veins. Lateral roentgenogram of a skull shows a rich network of diploic veins throughout the vault. This is not abnormal, but the vascularity is more than is usual.

diploë of the skull and thus cannot be seen in anatomic specimens unless one of the tables has been removed. However, these can be visualized in roentgenograms of most normal skulls. The size and number of these veins is extremely variable (Fig. 11-4). Anatomically the diploic veins may form plexuses in the frontal, temporal, and anterior and posterior parietal areas, but distribution is often random and is quite variable. They are most prominent, as a rule, in the posterior parietal region, where they assume a stellate radiation. The venous channels are more tortuous and irregular than the middle meningeal arterial grooves. They often show localized enlargements or lakes. These venous channels may stand out so prominently in roentgenograms as to suggest strongly that they are abnormal. The bilateral nature is always good evidence that such prominent veins are only a variation of the normal and little attention need be paid to them providing they are equally prominent or nearly so on both sides. The condition has been termed *phlebectasia*. The only significance is when craniotomy is to be performed. Then the surgeon may encounter brisk bleeding from the bone and he should be forewarned of this possibility. Unilateral enlargement of the diploic veins has less significance than unilateral enlargement of the middle meningeal artery (there are no accompanying diploic arteries; the meningeal and pericranial arteries supply the blood to the diploë).

PHYSIOLOGIC INTRACRANIAL CALCIFICATION

Certain structures within the skull are found to contain calcium deposits with considerable frequency. Such calcification is, as far as is known, without clinical significance. An outline listing the major causes of normal and abnormal intracranial calcification follows.

Causes of Intracranial Calcification

   I. Physiologic Causes
      A. Pineal gland
      B. Habenular commissure
      C. Choroid plexus
      D. D. Dura
      E. Pacchionian bodies
  II. Abnormal Findings
      A. Traumatic lesions
         1. Subdural hematoma
         2. Epidural hematoma
         3. Intracerebral hematoma
      B. Parasitic lesions
         1. Cysticercosis
         2. Trichinosis
         3. Toxoplasmosis
         4. Echinococcosis
      C. Vascular lesions
         1. Arteriosclerosis
         2. Aneurysms
         3. Arteriovenous malformations
         4. Capillary and venous angiomas (Sturge-Weber syndrome)
      D. Tuberous sclerosis
      E. Inflammatory and other lesions
         1. Tuberculosis
         2. Viral (cytomegalic inclusion disease)
         3. Other infections
            a. Old abscesses
            b. Nontuberculous granulomas
            c. Torulosis
      F. Degenerative and atrophic lesions
         1. Congenital atrophy or hypoplasia (lissencephaly)
      G. Symmetric calcification of basal ganglia
         1. Hypoparathyroidism
         2. Pseudohypoparathyroidism
         3. Idiopathic disease
      H. Neoplasms
         1. Gliomas
         2. Craniopharyngiomas
         3. Dermoids, teratomas, and epidermoids
         4. Meningiomas
         5. Lipomas
         6. Pituitary adenomas
         7. Metastatic tumors
      I. Toxicosis
         1. Hypervitaminosis D
         2. Idiopathic hypercalcemia
      J. Other causes
         1. Lead poisoning
         2. Fahr's disease

The Pineal Gland

The pineal gland, known also as the pineal body, is found to contain sufficient calcium to be visible in roentgenogram in from 33% to 76% of adult skulls. Rarely, it is found in the very young, and the frequency of its visualization increases with advancing age. Calcification is usually in the form of a cluster of amorphous, irregular densities but may be solitary.

The size of the calcification ranges up to 10 or 12 mm in the greatest diameter but is usually between 3 and 5 mm. When calcifications over 1 cm in diameter are observed, the question of abnormality such as the presence of a pinealoma or a calcified arteriovenous malformation should be raised. Since the calcified gland is a midline structure and its position in the lateral view can be plotted with a fair degree of accuracy, displacement from its normal position may be a valuable clue in indicating the presence of an intracranial lesion (Fig. 11-5). Space-taking lesions such as tumors, hematomas, and abscesses displace the gland away from the mass; atrophic lesions cause displacement toward the side of the abnormality. In general, masses are more apt to cause significant displacement than are atrophic processes. Because many skulls are slightly asymmetric when viewed frontally, a slight apparent shift of the pineal gland from the midline may be a normal finding. Ordinarily a variation of from 1 to 2 mm from the midline is allowable as being within the range of normal. Measurement of the position of the pineal gland in posteroanterior roentgenograms must be made only when the skull has been positioned carefully so that the midsagittal plane is at a right angle with the film. At times the calcification is so small that it is visible only in the lateral film. Tomography in the frontal projection may then identify the calcification, and very small amounts of calcium can be identified on the CT scan. The position of the calcified pineal gland can be determined in the lateral view by measuring its distance from the most distant point on (1) the inner table of the frontal bone, (2) the inner table of the occiput, (3) the inner table of the vault at the vertex, and (4) the inner table of the occiput. Using the charts prepared by Vastine and Kinney[51] (Fig. 11-6), measurement 1 is plotted as the abscissa and the sum of measurements 1 and 2 as the ordinate. In like manner measurement 3 is plotted as the ordinate and the sum of measurements 3 and 4 as the abscissa. By this means forward, upward, downward, or posterior displacement of the gland can be identified. These charts are satisfactory only when the skull is reasonably normal in shape. If it is of abnormal shape, false results may be obtained and such measurements cannot be relied upon. Lack of obvious displacement, of course, does not exclude the possibility of a space-filling mass since the amount of shift may not be enough to cause the pineal to fall outside the range of normal in the charts; or the lesion may be too small to cause appreciable displacement.

Habenular Calcification

Calcification in the habenular commissure (actually in the choroid plexus of the third ventricle where it attaches to the commissure) has a characteristic shape. It resembles the letter "C," opens posteriorly, and lies 4 to 6 mm anterior to the pineal gland. Displacements are similar in significance to those of the pineal gland.

The Choroid Plexus of the Lateral Ventricles

The choroid plexus lies along the floor of the lateral ventricles, its function being to elaborate cerebrospinal fluid. The glomus of the choroid plexus is a localized enlargement found along the posterior part of the floor of the ventricle just in front of the point of origin of the occipital horn. Calcification of the glomus occurs in about 10% of normal adult skulls. Such calcification is seen infrequently in young children. Usually the glomus of each lateral ventricle calcifies and the position of these structures and their relation to the midline of the skull can be determined. The calcification tends to be mottled, amorphous, and somewhat oval in shape but may be ring-like. It is from 10 to 15 mm in diameter. The glomera lie above the posterolateral to the pineal gland. Any appreciable shift of one glomus in relation to the other or to the midline suggests the presence of either a space-filling mass on one side or an atrophic lesion on the other side (Fig. 11-7). Displacement of a calcified glomus has less significance than a corresponding amount of displacement of the pineal gland. This is because the positions of the glomera may vary somewhat on the two sides or different parts may calcify and lead to visible asymmetry of the resulting shadows. Also, the positions may shift somewhat with positional change. When only one glomus is calcified little information can be obtained, since its position cannot be determined too accurately and one must see the opposite one for comparison. Recognition of unilateral calcification is important because the shadow may be mistaken for a displaced pineal gland or for some other important lesion such as calcification within a tumor.

Calcification of the Dura

Plaquelike areas of calcification are common in the dura, particularly in the falx and along the margins of the superior sagittal sinus. The calcified plaques are often very dense and tend to be larger and occur

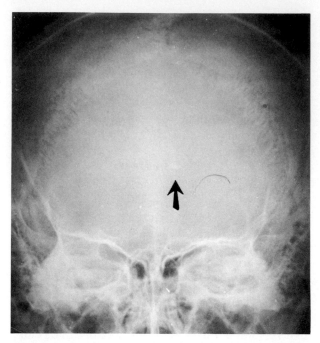

Fig. 11-5. Displacement of calcified pineal body towards the left side **(arrow)** by a tumor in the right cerebral hemisphere.

more frequently anteriorly than elsewhere. No significance can be attached to the finding of such plaques, so far as is known. Calcification is frequent in the free edges of the tentorium posterior to the sella in the so-called petroclinoid ligaments. These are formed by the margins of the tentorium as it extends from the petrous ridges of the temporal bones to the posterior clinoids projecting from the dorsum sellae. The calcifications are seen as spurlike projections extending posteriorly and downward from the dorsum (see Fig. 11-8C). Calcification in other parts of the tentorium is less common but may occur at the free margins near the posterior margin of the incisura which is posterior to the pineal. In the lateral view, calcifications there produce a curvilinear density posterior to the pineal gland. In the Towne projection, they appear as an inverted "V" which is characteristic.

Calcification of Pacchionian Bodies

The pacchionian granules or bodies are small localized enlargements of the pia arachnoid that lie in the vertex of the skull, as depressions of the inner table in the posterior frontal and anterior parietal areas near the superior sagittal sinus. Histologically, these granules are said to contain calcium often but they are not observed frequently in roentgenograms. When visible they are seen as small punctate calcified shadows immediately adjacent to the inner table. More often only the small depressions or lakes within which the bodies are situated are visualized.

THE SELLA TURCICA (Fig. 11-8)

The importance of the sella turcica in the interpretation of skull roentgenograms can hardly be overemphasized. Not only does it harbor an important structure, the pituitary gland, but changes in the thin bony walls and processes of the sella are among the prominent roentgen signs of increased intracranial pressure. This is discussed more fully in the section on "Intracranial Tumors." As visualized in the lateral view of the skull, the normal sella is usually of a flat, oval shape and represents a central depression in the sphenoid bone. Anteriorly, the planum and limbus sphenoidale represent an extension of bone posterior to the cribiform plate, ending at the limbus. As viewed in the frontal projection, the planum is the dense bone connecting the lesser sphenoid wings. The chiasmatic sulcus is a depression that extends from one optic canal to the other at their posterior or cranial openings. It may be deep and concave or shallow and straight; if there is extensive pneumatization of the sphenoid sinus, it may be convex. It is usually horizontal but may be nearly vertical and extends from the limbus to the tuberculum sellae. The latter is a transverse ridge forming the posterior margin of the chiasmatic sulcus and the anterior margin of the pituitary fossa. The anterior clinoid processes are posteromedial extensions of the lesser sphenoid wings. The floor of the sella includes the anterior and posterior walls of the pituitary fossa and is lined by cortical bone, the lamina dura. In the frontal projection, the floor is usually flat or slightly concave. The lateral angles are usually rounded but may be sharp when the floor is more concave. There may be a slight slope of 6 to 8 degrees to one side or the other. When this is present, there will be a slight depression of the floor on one side noted in the lateral projection. Slight thinning of the lamina dura has been observed in the normal individual, thus minor alterations may be present simulating pituitary enlargement. This makes interpretation of the film very difficult in some instances. The dorsum sellae is the posterior vertical portion of the sella. The posterior clinoids are small, lateral and superior extensions of the dorsum. Normally, the central aspect of the dorsum is posterior to

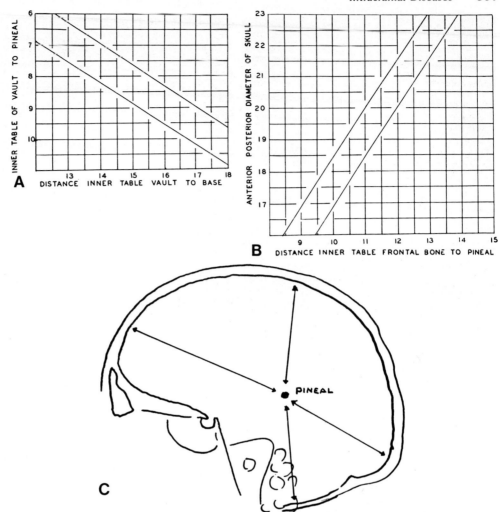

Fig. 11-6. Vastine–Kinney charts for determining displacement of the pineal body in the lateral roentgenogram. **A.** Chart for determining if pineal body is displaced up or down from its normal position. The distance in centimeters from the inner table of the vault to the pineal body is plotted against the total distance from the inner table of the vault to the base. If normal, the position will fall between the two diagonal lines. **B.** To determine displacement forward or backward, the distance in centimeters between the inner tables of the frontal and occipital bones is plotted against the distance from the inner table of the frontal bone to the pineal body. The normal range will lie between the two diagonal lines. (Modified by Dyke, C.) **C.** Tracing of lateral roentgenogram of skull showing method of measurement.

the lateral portions, making the anterior aspect concave.

The normal measurements of the sella turcica are given as a maximum of 16 to 17 mm in the anteroposterior diameter, measured from the tuberculum to the dorsum sellae on a film exposed at a 40-inch focal-film distance. A measurement from a line drawn from the tuberculum to the top of the dorsum should be no more than 13 mm in depth. The width varies from 10 to 15 mm with an upward limit of 19 mm. Area and volume can also be measured, but alterations in sellar walls and configuration are often much

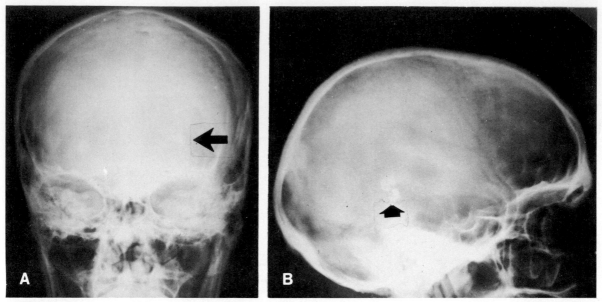

Fig. 11-7. Displacement of calcified glomus of choroid plexus. **A.** In the posteroanterior view the glomus on the right side is elevated because of an abscess beneath it. **Arrow** points to the elevated glomus. **B.** The lateral view shows the two calcified glomera lying above one another **(arrow).**

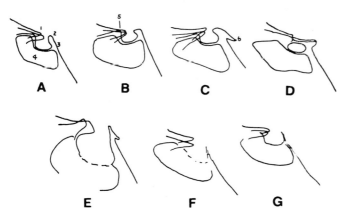

Fig. 11-8. Diagrams of the sella turcica. **A–D.** Normal sella and variations: **(1)** anterior clinoids; **(2)** posterior clinoids (the two are superimposed in the lateral view); **(3)** dorsum sellae; **(4)** sphenoid sinus; **(5)** tuberculum sellae; **(6)** calcific spur along posterior edge of dorsum occurring at attachment of tentorium (petroclinoid ligament). In **D,** bony bridging is shown between the anterior and posterior clinoids. **E.** Enlarged sella caused by chromophobe adenoma of the pituitary gland. **F–G.** Decalcification of posterior clinoids, dorsum, and floor secondary to increased intracranial pressure.

more important than measurements. The shape of the sella can vary considerably within normal limits from a flattened oval to a rounded or an upright oval contour. The clinical significance of the "small sella" is somewhat doubtful. There is some evidence that a small sella is found in many patients with idiopathic hypopituitary dwarfism, apparently secondary to the small size of the pituitary gland in this condition. In most cases, however, sellar sizes less than those listed above can be disregarded. The sphenoid sinus lies directly below the sella and is separated from the pituitary fossa by only a thin bony wall. The dorsum of the sella is of variable thickness, usually measuring on the order of 2 to 3 mm. At times a large sphenoid sinus will extend into the dorsum. The posterior clinoid processes form the upper limit of the dorsum in the lateral view and often are superimposed upon one another in this projection. They are best demonstrated, individually, in anteroposterior views. The anterior clinoid processes form the upper anterior boundary of the sella and are seen as pointed bony projections. They, too, tend to be superimposed one upon the other in lateral views, although it usually is possible to visualize them independently in stereoscopic roentgenograms. At times there appears to be a bony bridging between the anterior and posterior clinoid processes as viewed in the lateral projection, either on one or on both sides (Fig. 11-8D). This may be a true bony bridge or only a pseudobridging because long clinoid processes overlap one another. In any event, bony bridging is not believed to be of any clinical significance. The extension of the dura that is attached to the clinoid processes and forms a membranous cover over the sella (the diaphragm or diaphragma sellae) may be partially calcified. The walls of the normal sella are composed of cortical bone and thus appear sharp and dense. Loss of this normal density and sharpness may be an early sign of decalcification due to increased intracranial pressure (Fig. 11-9). In elderly individuals and in others showing evidence of skeletal demineralization, the margins of the sella may become indistinct as a result of osteoporosis. Some degree of osteoporosis is common in persons over 60 years of age but may be seen in younger individuals. Tomograms are useful in evaluating the sella in the presence of osteoporosis and usually resolve the question as to the presence or absence of pathologic erosion. In addition to senile osteoporosis, demineralization of the sella can occur in any condition that causes generalized skeletal demineralization such as hyperparathyroidism, Cushing's disease, or following steroid therapy.

THE CRANIAL FORAMINA

Most of the important foramina of the skull cannot be seen in the standard lateral and posteroanterior views and require special projections for demonstration. Such views are available and it is possible to visualize clearly the optic and internal auditory canals; the foramen ovale, spinosum, and rotundum; the jugular foramina; and the foramen magnum, as well as other smaller openings in the skull base. These projections are utilized when the clinical problem indicates the need for them.

ABNORMAL INTRACRANIAL CALCIFICATION

TRAUMATIC LESIONS

At times, a *subdural hematoma* that has not been recognized and treated surgically may undergo calcification in later life and appear as a dense, plaquelike,

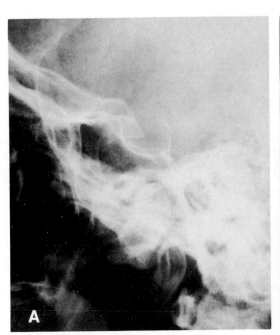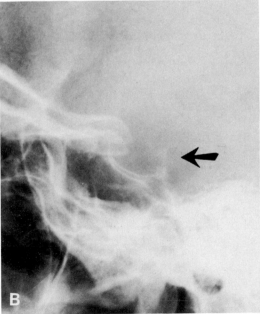

Fig. 11-9. Erosion of sella turcica secondary to increased intracranial pressure. The initial study **(A)** was made 6 months before the second one **(B)**. The latter illustrates loss of cortical outlines of the floor and dorsum **(arrow)** of the sella.

calcified mass overlying the cerebral hemisphere. These hematomas often are small and thin, occurring as a sheetlike calcification directly beneath the inner table. Occasionally a rather extensive calcified hematoma will be encountered. The usual location is over the superior parietal area but it may be found elsewhere, even in the posterior fossa. In like manner an *intracerebral hematoma* may calcify and be visualized as a dense mass of calcium within the brain. There usually is little in the roentgen appearance of such a calcified mass to determine its nature and, in such instances, a history of previous trauma is important. At times it may be necessary to explore and remove surgically such a mass, either because the diagnosis cannot be made otherwise or because it is probable that the calcified scar is causing significant symptoms. Linear and punctate calcifications may occur in the needle track of patients who have had ventricular puncture.

PARASITIC LESIONS

Calcified Cysticercus Cysts

Cysticercosis is an uncommon disease in the United States. The encysted larvae may calcify and be visualized in roentgenograms of the muscles and the brain. These form small calcified masses from 1 to 2 mm in length, either rounded or of an elongated shape, somewhat resembling a small grain of rice. When disseminated small calcifications of this type are found within the brain, the diagnosis of cysticercosis can be suggested. Small, ring-contoured and small nodular calcifications have been noted; these tend to be more common in the brain than do the elongated calcifications observed in muscles. If similar calcified lesions are found widely distributed in the skeletal muscles, the roentgen diagnosis becomes more certain (see Fig. 10-7).

Trichinosis

Calcified encysted larvae in the brain and muscles are frequent, pathologically, in persons having trichinosis, but they are uncommon roentgen observations. The small size of the lesions makes them difficult to detect and probably explains the lack of positive roentgen evidence.

Toxoplasmosis

Toxoplasmic encephalitis is an infection caused by a protozoan parasite. The infection may develop in the fetus and be manifest at birth or shortly thereafter. In the congenital or infantile form of toxoplasmic encephalitis, dense nodules of calcification may form (Fig. 11-10). Often these are widely distributed throughout the brain. The foci are variable in size in the individual case and some of the nodules may measure a centimeter or more in diameter. When the basal ganglia are involved the calcification may be more linear or curvilinear in shape. Calcified deposits also have been found in the meninges, choroid plexuses, and the ependyma of the ventricles. The incidence of associated hydrocephalus during infancy is high (reported to occur in 80% of patients). Microcephaly also has been noted as a sequela of the infantile form of the disease and is a later manifestation representing the effects of scarring and shrinkage in volume of brain tissue. Toxoplasmosis should be considered as a diagnostic possibility when widely disseminated calcified nodules of variable sizes are found within the brain. If there is evidence of either hydrocephalus or microcephaly, this diagnostic possibility is enhanced. Clinically, these patients show the signs of brain injury with convulsions, and mental retardation. The incidence of chorioretinitis is high. Neutralizing antibodies will be found in the blood serum of the infants and in a high percentage of the mothers. Roentgen differential diagnosis includes tuberous sclerosis and cytomegalic inclusion disease. Skin lesions are usually present in tuberous sclerosis and there is a tendency for lesions to form along the ventricular walls. The patients are usually older when the lesions are first discovered.

Other Parasitic Diseases

Paragonimiasis, caused by the oriental lung fluke *Paragonimus westermani*, involves the brain in about 25% of those infested. Calcification occurs in about 40% of these. Involvement is usually in the posterior parietal and occipital lobes where punctate or amorphous calcifications, along with spherical clusters of calcified cysts, appear; the calcification may be extensive. Calcifications in *Echinococcosis* are rare and usually are found in children. The calcification is manifest as a linear density in the walls of the cyst.

BACTERIAL AND VIRAL DISEASES

Pyogenic infection causing meningitis and brain abscess is not uncommon, but calcification is very rare. It may occur as a late sequela in brain abscess and

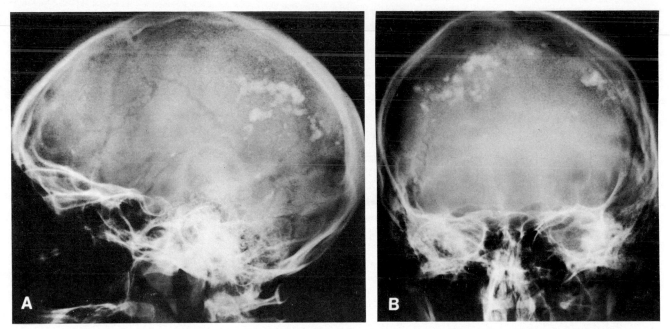

Fig. 11-10. Toxoplasmosis. Lateral and frontal projections showing calcified areas in the brain following the infantile form of the disease.

has been reported following meningitis. *Tuberculomas* of the brain have been reported as showing the presence of calcification in a small (6%) percentage of cases. Pathologically, multiple lesions are the rule, but calcification usually occurs in a single lesion. The calcified tuberculoma has an irregular outline with a crenated margin. Calcifications in tuberculous meningitis usually occur in children. They are seen at the base in the region of the basal cisterns above the sella or behind the posterior clinoid processes in the form of small punctate deposits or as calcified plaques. Calcification in the meninges and adjacent cerebral cortex has been reported as a complication of *Pseudomonas* meningitis. Calcification has also been reported in disseminated *coccidioidomycosis* but is extremely rare. The same is true in *cryptococcosis.*

Calcified plaques along the walls of the lateral ventricles have been reported in *cytomegalic inclusion disease.* At times these form a nearly complete cast of the ventricles. A similar type of calcification has been noted in some cases of toxoplasmosis so that it is not pathognomonic of cytomegalic inclusion disease. Calcified deposits have also been found in the cerebral cortex and in the subcortical white matter in the latter disease. Massive calcification in both hemi-

spheres has been reported in the *rubella syndrome. Herpes simplex encephalitis* may also be followed or accompanied by diffuse calcification.

VASCULAR LESIONS

Calcified Arteriosclerotic Plaques

Calcifications in the walls of the intracranial portions of the internal carotid arteries are common in elderly individuals and are occasionally seen in younger persons suffering from vascular disease. In lateral roentgenograms the calcifications are seen as thin, curved calcific shadows alongside the sella (see Fig. 11-11). At times the entire circumference of the vessel will be calcified and it will appear as a ring-contoured shadow when viewed end-on in posteroanterior views. This type of calcification indicates a medial or Mönckeberg form of arteriosclerosis. Intimal plaques tend to be smaller and irregular and usually do not completely encircle the lumen. Because intimal plaques may encroach upon the lumen of the vessel and interfere with bloodflow through it, it is of some importance to be able to determine from the roentgen appearance whether medial or intimal calcification is present. This is not always possible, but in many

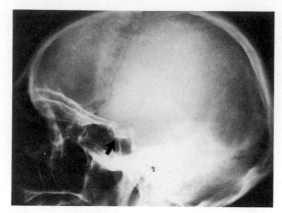

Fig. 11-11. Calcified internal carotid arteries in the circle of Willis. Note the tubular calcified shadow overlying the sella turcica **(arrow).**

Fig. 11-12. Calcification in the wall of an aneurysm above the sella **(arrow).**

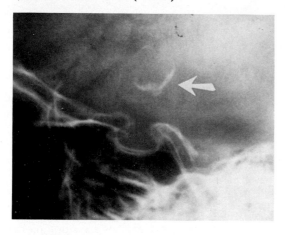

cases the differentiation can be made. Usually the calcifications lie below the level of the clinoid processes. Calcification above this level may be in the wall of an aneurysm, if plaquelike or circular in nature, or indicate the presence of a tumor or other significant lesion.

Calcification of Aneurysms

Aneurysms of the internal carotids or of the other components of the circle of Willis and the larger branches arising from the circle are common lesions. In most cases, roentgenograms of the skull will reveal no abnormality. Occasionally calcification in the wall of the aneurysmal sac will be seen (Fig. 11-12).

While it is unusual for the entire sac to be calcified, even small plaques may give a valuable clue as to the presence of the lesion. In contrast to simple arteriosclerotic plaques that seldom extend above the upper border of the sella, those in the wall of an aneurysm usually lie above the level of the clinoid processes. The shape of the curve also may indicate the approximate diameter of the sac even though the entire wall is not visualized. Of importance in the diagnosis of these lesions is the occasional finding of unilateral erosion of the sella from pressure. The combination of unilateral sellar destruction and curvilinear shadows of calcification in the immediate parasellar area forms a highly reliable diagnostic sign complex for this lesion. In the absence of these findings, internal carotid arteriography (see section on "Arteriography") is the method of choice for the roentgen demonstration of these lesions.

Arteriovenous Malformations

Calcified plaques may form in the walls of the dilated vessels making up a congenital vascular malformation. There may be only a few small linear shadows or a fairly extensive calcification. The calcific shadows are linear and curved when viewed from the side and circular or tubular when viewed end-on, corresponding to the lumen of the vessel. Usually the nature of the calcification is such that one can recognize its vascular nature without too much difficulty. As with the true neoplasms, the extent of calcification rarely indicates the actual size of the lesion and, as a rule, the malformation will be found to be much more extensive than the calcified areas would suggest. Arteriography is the roentgen method of choice for the diagnosis and study of these lesions.

Capillary and Venous Angiomas

In association with cutaneous angiomas or nevi, often showing a distribution corresponding to that of the trigeminal nerve, an area of abnormal calcification may be found within the cerebral cortex on the ipsilateral side. The lesion is most frequent in the posterior parietal area. It appears as a collection of wavy, curved plaques simulating the convolutions of the brain but lying 1 or 2 cm beneath the inner table (Fig. 11-13). Histologically, the calcium is found in the second and third layers of the cortex, occasionally in the basal ganglia. It is deposited in the perivascular tissues in the cortex rather than in the walls of blood vessels. This combination of cerebral and cutaneous

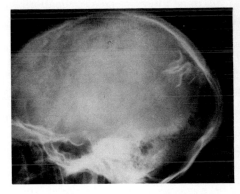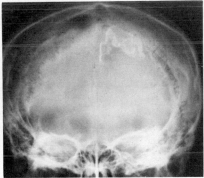

Fig. 11-13. Capillary angioma in the parieto-occipital area as viewed in lateral and frontal projections.

angiomatosis is known as the *Sturge-Weber syndrome;* there may be associated visual defects, contralateral hemiplegia, migraine, epilepsy, and, often, mental deficiency. The cerebral lesion may exist without the facial nevus. Because similar calcifications have been described in patients with no other findings, evidently there is an idiopathic form. Similar but more extensive calcifications have been found bilaterally in patients with childhood leukemia following chemotherapy with several drugs and radiotherapy. Methotrexate appears to be involved somewhat more frequently than other antimetabolites.[31]

TUBEROUS SCLEROSIS

Tuberous sclerosis is one of the developmental neurocutaneous syndromes (others include von Recklinghausen's neurofibromatosis and the Sturge–Weber syndrome). Clinically this syndrome is characterized by sebaceous, warty adenomas distributed in a butterfly fashion over the nose and cheeks, mental deficiency, and epilepsy. Other malformations may be present including spina bifida, cleft palate, nodulation of the skin and retina, and polydactyly. A characteristic skin lesion, the shagreen patch, is usually found on the trunk as a slightly elevated area of variable size and having an "orange-peel" appearance. Other abnormalities that may be present include premature graying of the hair, café au lait spots, and hemangiomas. In the central nervous system, hard tumorlike nodules are found scattered widely in the hemispheres. Of significance to the roentgenologist is the fact that these nodules are prone to calcify and thus become visible in skull roentgenograms. The calcified nodules vary greatly in size from very tiny ones up to those measuring a centimeter or more in diameter. There is a

distinct tendency for them to develop along the ventricular margins. Thus, even when uncalcified, they may be visualized, on CT scans or pneumoencephalograms, as nodules projecting into the ventricular cavities. The large lesions may obstruct the ventricular foramina or the aqueduct of Sylvius and lead to an obstructive hydrocephalus and the roentgen signs of increased intracranial pressure (Fig. 11-14). Children are less likely to have calcification in the lesions than adults. The incidence of calcification seems to increase with age. There may also be calcification in the basal ganglia in this condition. CT scanning is the method of choice to outline the calcification and de-

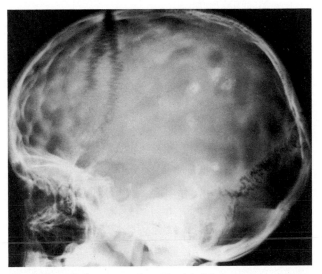

Fig. 11-14. Tuberous sclerosis. Multiple areas of mottled calcification in the brain. The sutures are spread, indicating increased intracranial pressure. A large mass was found occluding the foramen of Monro.

tect the subependymal tumors; it appears to be more accurate than pneumoencephalography in the diagnosis of tuberous sclerosis and localizing the masses.

A second roentgen sign of tuberous sclerosis is the occurrence of dense sclerotic islands in the bones of the cranial vault. This seems to be fairly common in adults but is rare in children. A combination of such sclerotic foci and scattered areas of intracranial calcification is highly reliable evidence of the disease. Similar sclerotic islands have been found in the spine and pelvis in many cases and probably can occur in any bone. Localization of the sclerosis to the posterior portions of the vertebrae has been reported.

An additional roentgen finding is the occurrence of cystlike defects in the phalanges, especially of the hands, and a wavy periosteal calcification along the shafts of the metatarsals and metacarpals. As with other syndromes, not all these findings need be present in the individual patient. Central nervous system lesions may occur without the typical skin lesions and other parts of the syndrome may be lacking at times.

Tuberous sclerosis of the brain is accompanied by a high incidence of renal masses. The renal tumors are of various connective tissue types, or hamartomas. One of the lesions, known as an angiomyolipoma, may contain enough fat to be visualized in plain roentgenograms. Similar tumors also may be found less frequently in the heart, spleen, lungs, and gastrointestinal tract.

DEGENERATIVE LESIONS

Occasionally there is seen a fairly extensive area of calcification of wavy, tortuous form, resembling closely the more restricted calcification seen in the Sturge–Weber syndrome but without the other stigmata of this disease. The calcification may involve much of one hemisphere and tends to form an outline of the cortical convolutions although separated somewhat from the inner table. Histologically, the calcium is found to be deposited in the perivascular spaces, similar to that in the Sturge–Weber lesion. There may be a more stippled calcification in the basal ganglia. In most cases the lesion probably is one of congenital atrophy or hypoplasia of the brain and the skull may be smaller in size and the calvarium thickened on the side of the lesion to compensate for the atrophic cortex. Bilateral lesions have been observed.

Fahr's disease, or *idiopathic familial cerebrovascular ferrocalcinosis,* is a rare cause of intracranial calcification.[3] The disease has a familial occurrence and shows the clinical manifestations of severe growth disorder and progressive mental deterioration. The intracranial deposition of iron and calcium causes widespread, irregular, punctate and dustlike densities in the brain. Its cause is not definitely known but it has been thought to be a genetically determined metabolic or vascular disorder.

Lissencephaly, congenital absence of gyri and sulci, may be associated with local calcification in the roof of the cavum septi pellucidi posterior to the foramen of Monro.[54] *Cockayne's* syndrome and other conditions in which microcephaly is a feature may be accompanied by calcification, usually in the basal ganglia, but also in the retrosellar area and tentorium. Calcification rarely may occur in the pituitary fossa (pituitary stones), probably caused by a degenerative process similar to that sometimes observed in other glands. Craniopharyngioma and pituitary adenoma must be considered first when an intrasellar calcification is observed.

SYMMETRIC CALCIFICATION OF THE BASAL GANGLIA

In the presence of parathyroid insufficiency, usually the result of surgical removal or injury to the parathyroid glands, fine granular calcifications have been noted in the regions of the basal ganglia on either side of the midline. Occasionally such calcification is more extensive, and wavy calcification in the deeper layers of the cerebral cortex may also be found (Figs. 11-15 and 11-16). Cerebellar calcification of similar type can occur. The calcium is found chiefly in the perivascular spaces of the finer cerebral vessels. The fact that the calcification is bilateral and symmetric and its location in the basal ganglia are helpful in distinguishing this lesion from the cerebral angiomas of the Sturge–Weber syndrome and from the atrophic degenerations described in the previous section of this chapter. The same type of calcification has been found in patients with *pseudohypoparathyroidism.* Of all patients with basal ganglion calcification, 50% have hypoparathyroidism, 15% have pseudohypoparathyroidism, and in 35% the calcification appears to be idiopathic, although a few patients have been reported in whom it followed irradiation to the area. A few cases of unilateral calcification of the basal ganglia have been reported. Some of these patients had no signs referable to the central nervous system and others had contralateral extrapyramidal symptoms.

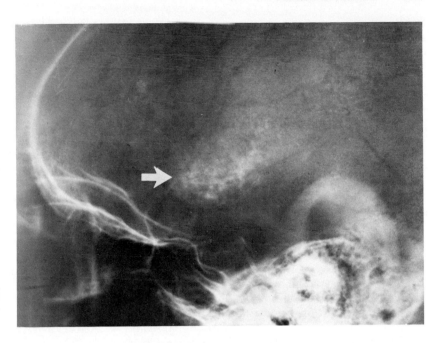

Fig. 11-15. Calcification in the basal ganglia **(arrow)** in a patient with hypoparathyroidism.

Fig. 11-16. Frontal view of the patient shown in Figure 11-15 showing the bilateral, symmetrical, basal ganglion calcifications **(arrows).**

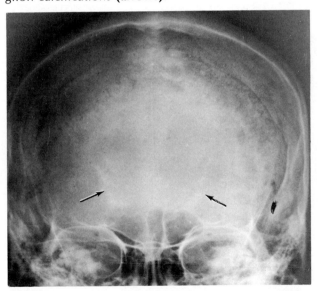

CALCIFICATION IN NEOPLASMS

Calcification within a tumor offers one of the certain roentgen signs of the presence of a lesion. The site and character of the calcification may suggest the histologic type of tumor, but little reliance can be placed on this finding alone. In general, the more slowly growing and benign a lesion may be, the more likely it will calcify. Thus, among the gliomas, the slowly growing oligodendrogliomas usually show extensive calcification when first recognized. Astrocytomas are more likely to show calcification than the more malignant and rapidly growing glioblastoma multiforme. Other tumors that are prone to calcify include the craniopharyngiomas (about 80%), ependymomas, dermoids, teratomas, and rarely, meningiomas. For further discussion see the section dealing with "Intracranial Tumors."

HYPEROSTOSIS FRONTALIS INTERNA

Hyperostosis frontalis interna is a peculiar overgrowth of bone developing on the inner table of the frontal bone. The hyperostosis usually is bilateral and symmetric and is found chiefly in females over the age of 35. The abnormal bony proliferation is confined to the internal surface of the inner table; the diploë and external table are not affected. It forms a dense, irregular thickening that surrounds the venous sinuses but does not obliterate them. As a result these sinuses stand out as prominent translucent zones, the superior sagittal sinus and the veins draining into it forming a recognizable pattern (Fig. 11-17). The extent of the thickening varies considerably among patients, but the hyperostosis may measure 1 cm or more in thickness. The process spreads upward and laterally from the midline of the frontal area for a variable distance. The external limits may be abrupt, or the process may fade gradually into normal bone at the periphery. While usually limited to the frontal area, occasionally it extends into the parietal bones and over the orbital roofs. As a variant of hyperostosis frontalis interna there may be a more diffuse thickening of the vault involving both tables with a poorly defined or absent diploë; the term *hyperostosis calvariae diffusa* has been applied to this condition.

The significance of hyperostosis frontalis interna from a clinical standpoint has been disputed. By some it has been considered to be a part of a syndrome indicative of endocrine dysfunction and variously called *metabolic craniopathy*, the *Morgagni syndrome*, and the *Stewart–Morel syndrome*. There is now general agreement that it is of no clinical significance in females. Roentgenogenographic study reveals irregular cortical thickening in the frontal area, sparing the areas occupied by the superior sagittal sinus and venous channels. Usually there is no problem in making the diagnosis.

HYPERVITAMINOSIS D AND IDIOPATHIC HYPERCALCEMIA

During infancy, calcification of the falx and tentorium has been observed in association with *hypervitaminosis D* and also in *idiopathic hypercalcemia*. In children, there is also marked increase in density of the calvarium. The occurrence of such calcification during the first year or two of life is almost certain evidence for either of these diseases (see Ch. 8, under "Hypervitaminosis D" and "Idiopathic Hypercalcemia"). Dural calcification usually has no significance during adult life since calcified plaques are common, especially in the falx, without clinical signs or symptoms.

ABNORMALITIES OF THE SKULL

Congenital anomalies and changes in the skull caused by hematologic and metabolic disorders have been discussed in previous chapters devoted to

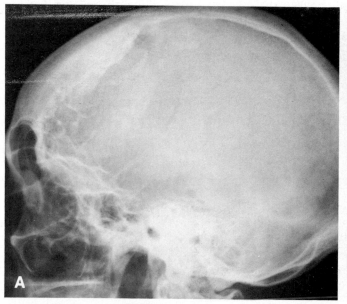
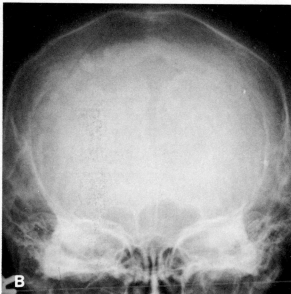

Fig. 11-17. *Hyperostosis frontalis interna.* There is heavy, wavy calcification on the inner table of the frontal bone **(A).** The hyperostosis does not form over the superior sagittal sinus, accounting for the midline translucent area noted in the frontal projection **(B).**

those conditions. Discussion of a few miscellaneous general and local lesions will be presented here.

Thickening of the skull, either local or general, may result from lack of development or contraction of the cerebral hemispheres secondary to trauma or disease occurring early in life. For example, inward growth of the inner table appears to be a physiologic response to diminution of intracranial content in children following *shunting procedures* performed because of hydrocephalus. There is also thickening in the mentally defective in whom the brain is small. Local thickening may occur secondary to cortical loss or growth failure in trauma. Long-term *dilantin medication* (3 years or more)[23] may also cause thickening, manifested mainly by widening of the diploic space. There may also be gradual increase in width of the tables of the skull and a slight increase in cranial vault size with *advancing age.* The enlargement involves the paranasal sinuses and sella turcica as well.[16] Local thickening of the skull is found in *fibrous dysplasia* which may cause massive thickening, often involving the paranasal sinuses and the skull base, encroaching on foramina, causing proptosis and often facial deformity.

Thinning of the skull or loss of mineral content is usually associated with metabolic disorders. *Massive osteolysis* has been reported in the skull but is extremely rare in this site. The etiologic background is still in question, but the osteolysis may be a form of angiomatosis. *Aneurysmal bone cyst* also causes rarefaction even though there is local widening of the tables. This is rare in the calvarium; it produces an irregular radiolucent area with faint marginal sclerosis. The tables are separated and thinned; there may be a local depression of the inner table causing pressure on the cortex as well as a palpable external mass. *Plasmacytoma* of the calvarium is also rare but may occur as a solitary lytic lesion with no marginal sclerosis. *Leptomeningeal cysts* are most likely secondary to childhood trauma; presumably the dura is torn and the arachnoid herniates through the dural tear into an overlying fracture. Pulsating arachnoid ultimately erodes bone, enlarging the fracture to produce a radiolucency which gradually enlarges—the *growing skull fracture,* usually found in children. Cerebral cortex may also protrude through the defect. When this occurs in the occipital bone, an intraosseous cyst may be formed with erosion of the inner table, the outer table remaining intact.[18] More important than the cyst is the communicating hydrocephalus which often accompanies it.

The *"button" defect or sequestrum* is another local lucent defect of the calvarium, but it contains a central bony density. It may be solitary, but is often multiple. A number of lesions can cause this defect. They include meningioma, eosinophilic granuloma, osteomyelitis, tuberculous osteitis, radiation necrosis, hemangioma, and metastatic carcinoma. Therefore, biopsy is often necessary to identify the lesion.

INTRACRANIAL TUMORS

The roentgenology of intracranial tumors can be considered under four main divisions: (*1*) Changes produced in the cranial bones and demonstrable in plain roentgenograms of the skull. (*2*) Changes observed on computerized tomographic (CT) scanning including enhancement by contrast media containing organic iodides. (*3*) Changes in the fluid pathways and the ventricular system demonstrated after injection of air or oxygen into the subarachnoid space (encephalography) or directly into the ventricles (ventriculography). This examination has been largely replaced by CT scanning. (*4*) Changes in the intracranial vascular system demonstrated by angiography.

Since this is a general text, plain skull film findings will be emphasized and the findings in the special procedures presented in a general manner. Using the special neuroradiologic procedures, it is possible to localize accurately almost all intracranial tumors and in many the histologic type can be predicted with considerable accuracy.

CHANGES IN THE CRANIAL BONES

Signs of Increased Intracranial Pressure

The roentgen signs of increased intracranial pressure are, of course, not specific for tumors. Other conditions can cause obstructive hydrocephalus by interfering with the free flow of cerebrospinal fluid from within the ventricles where it is formed to the arachnoid granulations over the superior aspects of the cerebral hemispheres where it is absorbed. Inflammatory adhesions and congenital defects are examples of such nonneoplastic obstructive processes. Other mass lesions such as abscesses or hematomas may occupy sufficient space within the skull to cause the signs and symptoms of increased intracranial pressure. The changes described in the following, therefore, indicate only that a space-taking mass is present within the cranial cavity or that something is obstructing or increasing the flow or interfering with the absorption of cerebrospinal fluid.

Widening of the Cranial Sutures. In children and occasionally in young adults, increase in intracranial pressure will cause a spreading of the vault sutures. This widening may amount to as much as several centimeters and it is a very reliable sign of increased pressure (see Figs. 11-14 and 11-32). This sign is not found in adults because the bones are held tightly together and in persons above the age of 35 the sutures often are completely fused. Widening of the sutures is prevalent in the presence of tumors within the posterior fossa of the skull since these lesions are prone to obstruct the aqueduct of Sylvius or the fourth ventricle and thus cause an obstructive hydrocephalus. In the infant, sutural spread can develop rapidly if there is a sudden increase in intracranial pressure. In the older child or adolescent the sutures are not as likely to spread unless the pressure rises considerably or unless it has existed for some time. It follows that the younger the child the more valuable the sign becomes. In children with slowly developing increased intracranial pressure the sutures may not be spread to any appreciable degree but the digitations along the suture edges become lengthened. This is because the bone adjacent to the suture has time to grow. When the increase in pressure is sudden or rapid, the sutures become widened, often very quickly. As a rule, in children over 3 years of age, if there is a spread of more than 2 mm, the sutures are considered to be abnormally wide. Occasionally some widening of the sutures is observed in normal, healthy neonates who have a normal head circumference and normal intracranial pressure. Although this may be idiopathic, it is wise to make certain that no disease associated with sutural prominence is present.

Bulging at the fontanels. In normal infants, soft-tissue contour at the fontanels is smooth, but when the intracranial pressure is increased a local bulging of the soft tissues is observed, most commonly in the region of the anterior fontanel. Minimal bulging may also be seen when the child is crying or straining when the film is being exposed.

Enlargement of the cranium. An increase in head size in infants and children can easily be measured clinically. Roentgen measurements can also be made and a comparison between size of the calvarium and the facial bones may also indicate cranial enlargement.

Enlargement of Occipital Emissary Foramen. This is a small opening in or near the midline of the occipital bone through which an emissary vein passes. This rare foramen usually measures no more than 2 mm in diameter. It has been reported as increasing in size with increased intracranial pressure, but a large foramen is of doubtful significance since it may occur in persons who do not have increased intracranial pressure. It is likely that in some instances the emissary vein does enlarge in the presence of increased intracranial pressure.

Decalcification and Erosion of the Sella Turcica. Loss of density and sharpness of outline of the walls and processes of the sella turcica can develop as a result of chronic increase in intracranial pressure. The time lag between the onset of increased pressure and the detection of changes in the sellar walls in roentgenograms will vary depending upon the degree of increased pressure and its constancy. However, in most cases it is probable that several months must elapse before roentgen evidence becomes distinct. When the ventricular system has been obstructed by a lesion in the posterior fossa there is a resulting dilatation of the lateral and third ventricles; the latter ventricle then projects downward over the sella and may actually bulge into it. Constant pressure from a greatly dilated third ventricle may cause erosion of the posterior clinoid processes and the dorsum of the sella, leaving the rest of the sellar walls intact. The dorsum then becomes short. The early change is one of loss of the normal sharp cortical margin of the anterior surface of the base of the dorsum. The floor of the sella becomes thinned and the margins of the sella undergo a general loss of density. The sharp cortical bone that normally forms the borders of the cavity becomes lost and the edges become ill defined (see Fig. 11-9). This type of change is noticeable particularly in the floor of the sella when the sphenoid sinus is well developed. In such a case the sinus is separated from the intracranial cavity only by the thin floor of the sella and this may undergo decalcification or even actual loss of bony substance. The anterior clinoid processes and the tuberculum sellae are the last to show effects from increased intracranial pressure. Enlargement of the sellar cavity may or may not occur. It is particularly likely to develop if the dilated third ventricle is responsible for pressure erosion. This ventricle may, as indicated previously, actually bulge into the cavity of the sella and thus enlarge it. Such enlargement may be in all directions and resemble very closely that produced by a pituitary adenoma. At times it may be very difficult to be certain from the contour of the sella whether it has been enlarged as a result of a distant lesion or by an expanding tumor within the confines of the sella. Because pituitary adenomas rarely produce other signs of increased intracranial pressure, the presence or absence of these other findings is of considerable value in differentiation. Thus the presence of widened sutures in the child or prominent convolutional impressions on the inner table in the adult is valuable evidence that the lesion responsible for the sellar enlargement is actually at a distance from the sella. Likewise displacement of the calcified pineal or evidence of calcification within the tumor mass itself may be an important sign of the nature of the lesion. In determining whether or not a given sella turcica is abnormal, attention must be paid to the density of the bony walls since the early signs of pressure often are manifested in this way. Enlargement of the sella is a later sign and a less valuable one from the standpoint of extrasellar tumors. Multidirectional tomography is necessary to examine the sella satisfactorily when the presence of a small intrasellar tumor is suspected.

Increased Convolutional Impressions. Pressure from the developing gyri of the brain causes a variable amount of waviness of the inner table of the skull and in roentgenograms the variation in thickness of the bones produced by these impressions can be visualized as alternating areas of lessened and increased density (while the visualized impressions may not actually correspond to the convolutions of the brain anatomically, the term has received wide usage). In general the infant skull does not show evidence of these convolutional impressions. They are more prominent during late childhood and early adolescence. The adult skull frequently shows little evidence of them. In the presence of increased intracranial pressure an increase in prominence of these convolutional impressions may develop. If this becomes at all marked the appearance of the skull is striking and has been likened to that of beaten silver. If, in the infant or child, the sutures are not fused prematurely, increase in pressure will cause them to spread before it will produce much change in the convolutional impressions. Thus this sign is seldom encountered in the child unless there is abnormal fusion of the cranial sutures (see Fig. 3-6). Even in the adult it is not too reliable a sign of increased intracranial pressure. The existence of increased pressure over a considerable period of time is required to produce these changes, at least of a degree sufficient that they can be recognized from the normal variation. Occasionally, in an adult who has had a low-grade increase in intracranial pressure dating back to childhood which was caused by some type of benign lesion such as inflammatory adhesions or congenital stenosis of the aqueduct, this beaten-silver appear-ance will be a striking manifestation of the chronic increase in intracranial pressure. The pressure in these patients may have existed for such a length of time and have been of relatively mild degree that sutural spread is not apparent. In practically all patients, however, the sella turcica will be abnormal if the convolutional impressions are increased as a result of pressure. The same pressure is more likely to affect the thin walls and processes of the sella and produce decalcification or erosion. Thus in borderline cases where there is some question as to the presence or absence of abnormal convolutional impressions the appearance of the sella may be helpful in deciding whether abnormality exists or not.

Localizing Evidence of Tumor

Displacement of Calcified Pineal Gland. In previous paragraphs the importance of displacement of the calcified pineal gland and methods for determining its position have been discussed. The significance of pineal displacement is emphasized by the fact that Vastine and Kinney found it occurring in 39% of all patients having tumor of the brain. Frequently the shift of the pineal only indicates the existence of a mass in the contralateral hemisphere and does not localize the lesion more closely (see Fig. 11-5). Occasionally the pineal will be shifted in two planes, laterally from the midline and in one other direction. Such a shift is of value in localizing the site of the mass lesion responsible for it. In general, tumors of the frontal lobe displace the pineal backward and toward the contralateral side. Lesions of the temporal lobe produce a shift away from the side of the lesion with little or no other displacement. Parietal lobe tumors are likely to cause a downward displacement of the pineal and some degree of lateral shift. Occipital lobe tumors displace it forward and in some subtentorial tumors an upward displacement will be noted. Other space-taking masses such as subdural hematomas and intracerebral abscesses may also cause pineal displacement. Unilateral atrophic lesions may cause a shift toward the side of the lesion but the amount is seldom very large. As has been noted previously, a variation of 1 to 2 mm from the midline as viewed in the frontal position should be allowed as a normal variation before a diagnosis of lateral shift of the pineal is made. In the lateral view, as the charts of Vastine and Kinney[51] indicate, there is a range of normal variation in the position of the pineal and small degrees of shift may not be apparent when the position of the pineal is plotted on these charts. In general, minimal degrees of pineal shift are more accurately recognized in the frontal view than they are in the lateral projection.

Displacement of Calcified Choroid Plexus. This has been discussed in the section on "The Choroid Plexus of the Lateral Ventricles." Displacement of the calcified glomus of a choroid plexus is a less significant finding than is a corresponding degree of pineal displacement. These structures may be asymmetric in position in a normal skull since the glomus may not be at similar levels in the two lateral ventricles or different parts of it may calcify on the two sides. Thus minor asymmetry in position of the glomera can be a normal finding. If asymmetry of the glomera is encountered, the appearance of the sella should be carefully observed, the position of the calcified pineal should be determined, and special observation for other possible signs of intracranial disease as enumerated in previous paragraphs should be carried out.

Calcification of the Tumor. Calcification within an intracranial tumor forms one of the significant roentgen signs of intracranial disease. Roentgen evidence of calcification is found in about 15% of all intracranial tumors. Certain tumors show a very high incidence of calcification while others rarely if ever calcify. Thus, in individual lesions the incidence of calcification may be high. Among the tumors that frequently show calcification are the oligodendrogliomas, astrocytomas, craniopharyngiomas, and ependymomas. Mention will be made of these lesions in more detail in the summaries of brain tumors in the following sections.

Local Changes in the Cranial Bones. Change in the bone overlying a meningioma is a common finding but is rare in other types of tumor. Infrequently, local thinning and outward bulging of the bone directly overlying a tumor is seen. This is more common in the temporal area in children and the lesion usually is a slowly growing or expanding process. Unilateral expansion and thinning may occur when the foramen of Monro is obstructed on one side. The meningioma shows a tendency to invade the overlying bone and may actually extend through it to form a visible and palpable soft-tissue mass on the outer side of the calvarium. The changes described in the following, therefore, refer largely to meningiomas.

INCREASED VASCULARITY. The blood supply to meningioma is frequently from the middle meningeal artery. Dilatation of this artery and its branches and of the accompanying veins causes a widening and tortuosity of the bony vascular grooves when the meningioma arises from the vertex of the skull (Figs. 11-18 and 11-19). When the tumor is situated close to the coronal suture and near the midline, a network of dilated vascular grooves may develop in and around the area of attachment of the tumor to the dura. The bone may have a fine moth-eaten appearance because of the numerous small vascular channels. Since there normally can be some variation in the prominence of the middle meningeal grooves, this finding must be interpreted with caution and with correlation of other roentgen and clinical findings. It is not unusual to find one or more branches of a middle meningeal artery on one side ending in a well-defined vascular lake with no similar change on the opposite side. This is usually a normal variation. Pathologic dilatation of these vessels is likely to form a much more irregular network of vascular spaces. When the tumor lies more posteriorly or lower down over the convexity, only one or several dilated vessels may be visualized extending to the region of the tumor (Fig. 11-18A).

LOCALIZED EROSION OF BONE. The bone directly overlying a meningioma may be invaded by the tumor with resulting dissolution of bone structure (Fig. 11-18B). This varies widely from a fine moth-eaten appearance to an occasional instance in which the bone is completely destroyed over the tumor and the mass protrudes into the soft tissues of the scalp.

PROLIFERATIVE RESPONSE. Meningiomas also tend to invoke a hyperostotic response in the bone directly overlying them. In some cases this is manifested by a local hyperostosis producing an elevated area of cortical bony density on the inner table (see Fig. 11-19). At other times the tumor may extend through the bone and cause a dense hyperostotic reaction on the outer table, with resulting external swelling. In other instances there is a mixture of bone destruction and proliferation (see Fig. 11-18B). Variations in meningiomas and the effects on the overlying bone are remarkable and one must allow a wide range of roentgen changes in the bone to cover all possible variations that can be produced by this tumor.

SPECIAL PROCEDURES

Computerized Tomography (CT)

Computerized tomography has been a major breakthrough in the examination of the central nervous system, particularly the brain; it has significantly al-

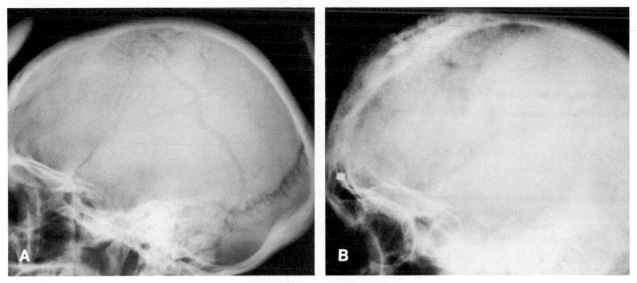

Fig. 11-18. A. Convexity meningioma with increased vascularity. Note the dilated, tortuous vascular groove extending to the vertex. There is a loss of outline of the floor and dorsum of the sella indicative of increased intracranial pressure. **B.** Meningioma of the frontal area causing an extensive change in bone. There is a mixture of destruction and proliferation with the latter predominating. The result is a thickened bone with fine spiculation extending outward from the outer table.

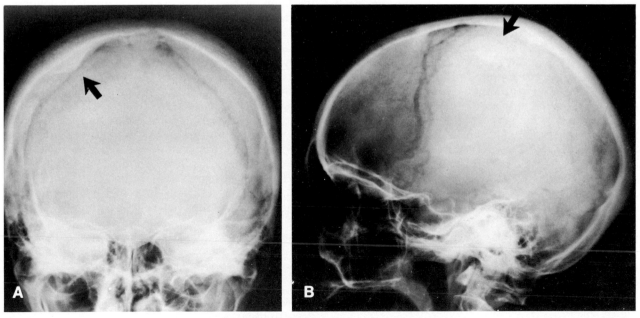

Fig. 11-19. Convexity meningioma causing a localized hyperostosis on the inner table at the site of its attachment to the dura. Arrows indicate the location of the hyperostosis in the frontal **(A)** and lateral **(B)** views.

tered the diagnostic approach to a number of intra-cranial diseases.[2, 21, 40] Although preceded by much basic work, Hounsfield designed and built the first clinically usable computerized tomographic unit. The components of the system are an x-ray gantry which supports the x-ray tube or tubes, the detectors and the patient. The x-ray beam is narrow, usually a centimeter in width. In the newer units a fan-shaped beam about 30 degrees in aperture and a large number of xenon or solid state detectors are used. The source of radiation and the detectors rotate around the patient with a scanning time of about 5 seconds. In the early units a narrow beam which needed more exposures to obtain the required data was employed and the scanning time was much longer. Each detector contributes to the imaging of each point within the part examined. The prototype of a new device with a large number of fixed detectors and a rotating tube is being tested. The data are stored and are subsequently utilized for reconstruction of the tomographic section by the application of the proper algorithm. The reconstructed section can then be displayed as a numerical printout or in an analog form as an anatomic image. The image can then be processed to obtain potentially diagnostic information. The output then is representative of the x-ray attenuation properties of the transverse section examined. Sections are usually about 10 mm, although thinner sections can be selected. Numerical scales are used for representing the attenuation properties of tissues. Most widely used is the Hounsfield unit which spans the range of 2000. The attenuation of air is −1000, that of water is 0, and that of dense bone is +1000. Therefore, 10 of these units represent a 1% change of attenuation. The equipment is so devised that the range to be examined can be selected. Most tissues are in the middle of the spectrum. For example, cerebrospinal fluid is +15, blood is in the range of +40 to +50 and fat is −80. One of the largest problems, that of motion, has been solved to a considerable extent by the newer 5-second scanners. The contrast resolution has reached the point of being able to distinguish gray from white matter in the brain. Any further increase requires that much higher dose of radiation would be received by the patient.

The clinical use of CT scans in neuroradiology is now extensive. Contrast enhancement is used extensively. Optimal dosage appears to be in the range of 28 to 42 gm of iodine, although some institutions use higher doses. The iodine is given rapidly intravenously in the form of Hypaque 60 (methylglucamine diatrizoate) or Reno–M 60 (diatrizoate meglumine). Other workers use diatrizoate meglumine (30%) or meglumine iothalamate (Conray 30). Some believe that contrast-enhanced scanning should be used alone in brain tumor suspects, believing that diagnostic accuracy is not improved by a preliminary, noncontrast study. There are a number of advantages in contrast enhancement: (1) Detectability of many lesions including tumors and arterovenous malformations is increased. (2) A lesion adjacent to the skull, such as a chromophobe adenoma, may become obvious. (3) Equivocal lesions may become obvious. (4) Optimal tumor biopsy area may become evident. (5) The presence and pattern of enhancement may assist in the differential diagnosis. (6) A second lesion as a metastatic disease may become apparent. (7) Suprasellar extension of a tumor may be detected. (8) Enhancement may clearly detect a rapidly changing process even though its nature may not be evident.

CT scans are used in the preliminary examination of tumor suspects, patients with head trauma, patients with hydrocephalus or suspected hydrocephalus or evidence of increased intracranial pressure, those having subarachnoid hemorrhage, those with cerebrovascular lesions, and those having suspected atrophy or degenerative diseases (Fig. 11-20 and 11-21). This examination is also very useful in patients with diseases of the orbit and in patients with lesions of the paranasal sinuses or nasopharynx.

There are some limitations. These include: the problem of motion artifacts in uncooperative patients; isodensity of a pathologic lesion and the brain; inability to make a definite tissue diagnosis although the scan gives positive indication of disease; and the possibility that small lesions may be missed or obscured by adjoining structures such as the skull. There has been a considerable dispute about efficacy as far as health costs are concerned. It appears that the examination is cost effective in patients with trauma and brain tumors but not in those with cerebrovascular disease. The frequency of negative cerebral angiograms has been reduced, but the increase in detection of occult disease by CT scanning has kept the total level of cerebral angiograms comparable to that of the time before CT scanning was used. The necessity for pneumoencephalography has been reduced markedly. Since CT scanning is noninvasive, it carries no risk except that of radiation which is a considerable advantage to the patient.[4, 14]

Pneumoencephalography and Ventriculography

Ventriculography is a surgical procedure in which a needle is inserted through a trephine opening or drill hole directly into one of the lateral ventricles, the

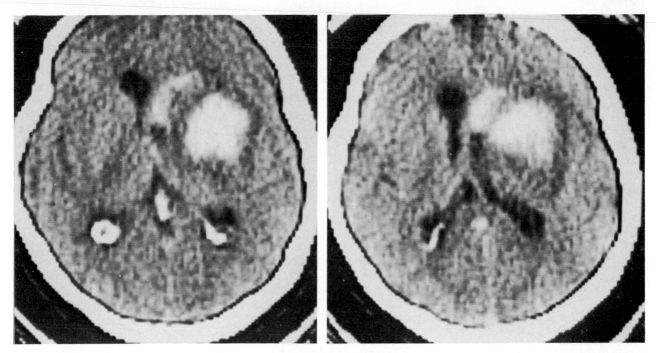

Fig. 11-20. CT scan of hypertensive patient with a 1-week-old intracapsular hemorrhage. Note that the blood, which is denser than the brain tissue, is in the left lateral ventricle as well as in the adjacent brain. The dark area surrounding the blood represents edema. (Courtesy of Drs. JE Sackett and CM Strother).

fluid is withdrawn and substituted by air or oxygen, the roentgenograms are made. The ventricular system thus is made visible because of the contrast between the density of the gas and the surrounding brain tissue. In pneumoencephalography the gas is introduced into the lumbar subarachnoid space after lumbar puncture. The cerebrospinal fluid is removed in small increments and replaced by gas, and this can be continued until the major portion of the fluid has been drained from the system. However, attempted complete drainage is seldom necessary and usually unwise. Small amounts of gas, *e.g.,* 20 to 30 cc, generally will allow satisfactory visualization if multiple projections are used. In pneumoencephalograms, in addition to visualization of the ventricles, the subarachnoid fluid pathways over the hemispheres and the basal cisterns can be demonstrated (Figs. 11-22 and 11-23). If there is increase in intracranial pressure, herniation of the cerebellar tonsils through the foramen magnum may occur so that pneumoencephalography carries some risk in this situation. It should be carried out only when neurosurgical personnel and facilities are available to tap the ventricles and relieve the pressure. The neurosurgeons with

whom we are associated prefer doing a ventricular tap, in these circumstances, through drill holes through the posterior parietal areas. With this method reduction of intraventricular pressure can be accomplished in a matter of minutes if the situation is critical. Pneumoencephalography is particularly useful in showing small masses that may encroach upon the basal cisterns and in posterior fossa lesions; in most other situations, it has been replaced by CT scanning, which is noninvasive and carries no risk except for that of radiation exposure. Tomography is often used in these problem cases when basal cisterns, parasellar areas, and the brain stem are being examined. Ventriculography has a limited field of usefulness because the subarachnoid spaces and cisterns are not demonstrated and it often is impossible to fill the third and fourth ventricles even though the ventricular system is patent. Pantopaque has been used occasionally when there are problems in the third or fourth ventricles, but metrizamide is replacing it as an opaque medium because of its water solubility. Tomography may be used in conjunction with the opaque medium to demonstrate intraventricular detail.

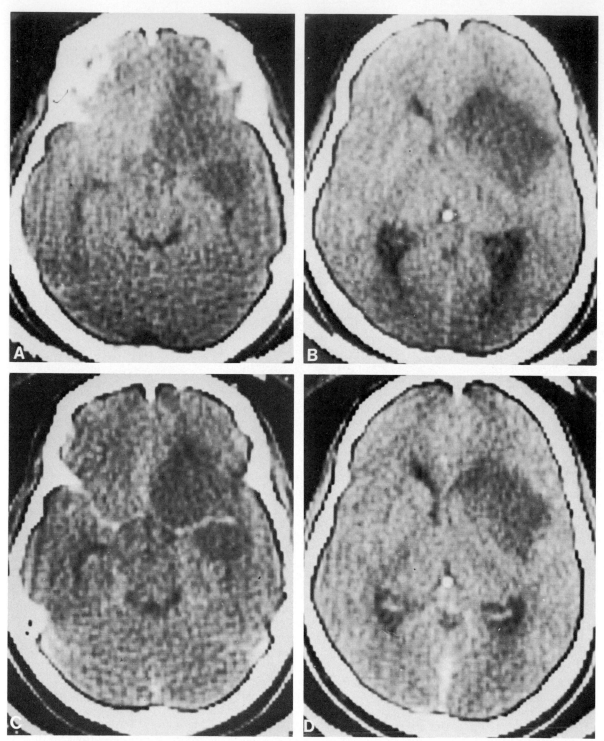

Fig. 11-21. CT scan of a patient with right hemiplegia who has a low-density mass in the deep left frontotemporal area. **A** and **B** show the mass with minimal ventricular distortion. **C** and **D** show no enhancement following intravenous Conray. The tumor was a low-grade glioma. (Courtesy of Drs. JE Sackett and CM Strother)

The complicated pneumographic diagnosis of brain tumors is briefly summarized here. Generally speaking, cerebral neoplasms show evidence of their presence by deformities in the outline of the adjacent ventricle and displacement of the ventricular system away from the tumor. Tumors of the third ventricle reveal absence of filling of this cavity or a portion of it and a bilateral and symmetrical dilatation of the lateral ventricles if the lesion is large enough to obstruct the foramina of Monro. Tumors of the cerebellum and adjacent structures are likely to obstruct the ventricular system, resulting in dilatation of the third ventricle and a symmetrical enlargement of the lateral ventricles. When in the midline, deformity or absence of filling of the fourth ventricle is the rule. When the tumor is in a cerebellar hemisphere, the fourth ventricle will be shifted away from the side of the lesion. Many of these tumors, however, are large enough to prevent filling of the fourth ventricle. In these cases the aqueduct usually fills, and a sharp forward angulation of the lower on the proximal portion can be identified in lateral views (see Fig. 11-39). Tumors arising within a lateral ventricle or very close to it cause a localized filling defect in the ventricular cavity in addition to the evidence of displacement of the system away from the mass. The effect of a neoplastic mass on the ventricular system, therefore, will depend to a considerable extent upon its position, its size, and to some degree on its cellular

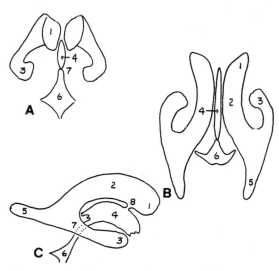

Fig. 11-22. The normal ventricular system. Diagrams show the appearances of ventricles as viewed from different directions. Anteroposterior view **(A)**; appearance as viewed from above **(B)**; and lateral view **(C)**. Lateral ventricle: anterior horn **(1)**; body **(2)**; temporal horn **(3)**; and occipital horn **(5)**. Third ventricle **(4)**; fourth ventricle **(6)**; aqueduct of Sylvius **(7)**; foramen of Monro **(8)**.

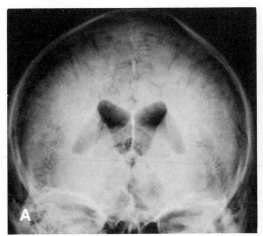
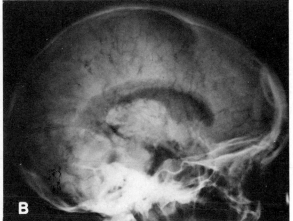

Fig. 11-23. Normal encephalogram. **A.** Upright posteroanterior view. **B.** Lateral view. Compare with diagrams of normal ventricular system shown in Figure 11-22. Multiple projections are used to shift the fluid and gas so that all parts of the ventricular system can be outlined. In this patient the basal cisterns around the sella are well outlined and there is reasonably good filling of subarachnoid spaces over the hemispheres.

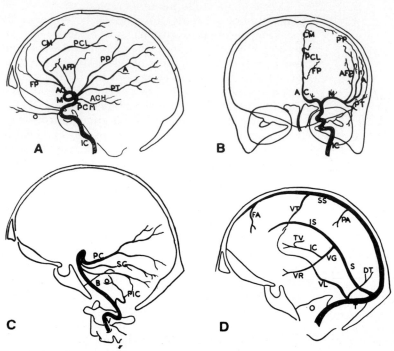

Fig. 11-24. The normal arterial and venous systems. **A.** Lateral internal carotid arteriogram: **IC,** internal carotid artery; **M,** middle cerebral artery; **AC,** anterior cerebral artery; **FP,** frontopolar artery; **CM,** callosomarginal artery; **PCL,** pericallosal artery; **AFP,** ascending frontoparietal artery; **PP,** posterior parietal artery; **A,** angular artery; **PT,** posterior temporal artery; **ACH,** anterior choroidal artery; **PCM,** posterior communicating; **O,** ophthalmic. **B.** Frontal internal carotid arteriogram (same lettering as **A**). **C.** Lateral vertebral arteriogram: **PC,** posterior cerebral artery; **SC,** superior cerebellar artery; **B,** basilar artery; **V,** vertebral artery; **PIC,** posterior inferior cerebellar artery. **D.** Lateral view of venous drainage: **FA,** frontal ascending vein; **SS,** superior sagittal sinus; **IS,** inferior sagittal sinus; **VT,** anastomotic vein of Trolard; **PA,** parietal ascending vein; **IC,** internal cerebral vein; **VG,** vein of Galen; **S,** straight sinus; **VR,** basal vein of Rosenthal; **VL,** anastomotic vein of Labbe; **T,** transverse sinus. The site of the foramen of Monro is indicated by the location of a small angular vein, the thalamostriate **(TV),** entering the internal cerebral vein.

characteristics. The most pronounced shift and deformity of the ventricular system often is encountered in glioblastoma multiforme because of the invasive characteristics of this tumor and the associated edema that may be present. In contrast, a small globular-shaped meningioma along the surface of a hemisphere may cause only a slight displacement of the ventricular system and very focal indentation of the roof of the lateral ventricle directly beneath the mass. Lesions in the posterior fossa are prone to cause obstructive hydrocephalus, and even a small tumor mass situated in or close to the fourth ventricle may readily obstruct the aqueduct of Sylvius and produce a high-grade dilatation of the ventricular system above the level of the aqueduct. These changes are also observed on CT scans which have the added advantages of differentiation of density and augmentation of density by the use of intravenous contrast agents. Pneumoencephalography may be useful in the study of tumors of the pituitary gland and those

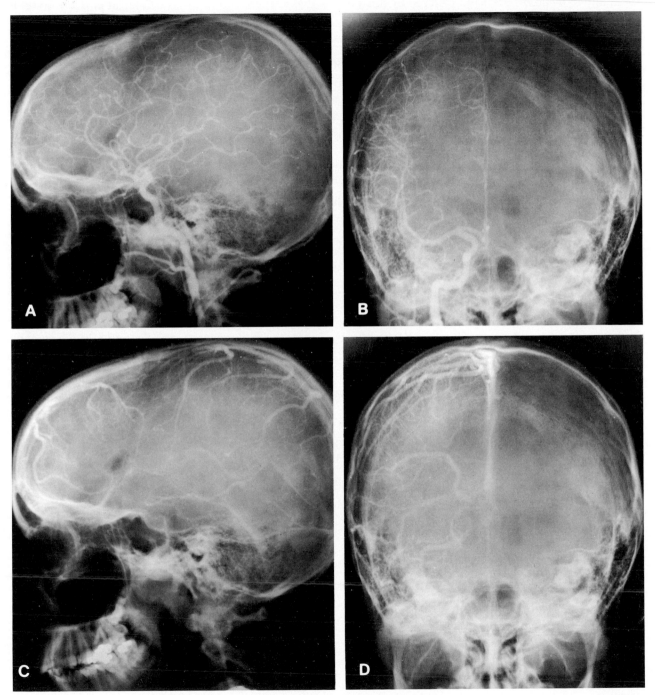

Fig. 11-25. Normal internal carotid arteriogram and venogram. Lateral **(A)** and frontal **(B)** roentgenograms during the arterial phase. (Compare with Figure 11-24.) Lateral **(C)** and frontal **(D)** roentgenograms during the venous phase.

arising in the immediate parasellar region because of the ability to visualize the basal cisterns by this procedure. These tumors tend to encroach into the cavities of the basal cisterns and the outline of the tumor often is clearly seen when it is surrounded by gas.

Angiography

Intracranial angiography consists in the rapid injection of an iodine-containing substance, such as Hypaque 60, Reno–M 60, or Conray 60, into the carotid artery in the neck or into the vertebral artery and obtaining a series of roentgenograms in rapid sequence while the material is passing through the vasculature of the brain. Angiography has received wide acceptance and is used extensively but has been replaced as a screening technique by CT scanning. By means of angiography not only can space-taking masses be identified, but at times a specific diagnosis can be made. For vascular lesions such as aneurysms, arteriovenous malformation, and occlusive disease it is the method of choice. Most neuroradiologists prefer the Seldinger method of inserting the catheter into the femoral artery and guiding it to the desired area in the carotid system. Direct carotid puncture and brachial artery catheterization are used in special situations. By this means multiple vessels can be outlined with one injection or individual vessels may be catheterized selectively allowing better opacification of the vessel and its smaller branches. It is possible to visualize clearly the cerebral vessels and, as the contrast material is followed in the series of roentgenograms, sequential filling of the arteries, capillaries, and veins is obtained. Usually it is advisable to obtain roentgenograms in both lateral and frontal positions so that the vessels can be studied in two different planes (Figs. 11-24 and 11-25). With biplane equipment this can be done with one injection of contrast substance. In the absence of such equipment, two separate injections are made. The amount of contrast material injected should be kept as small as possible and from 6 to 10 cc or less usually is sufficient for each injection. Subtraction and magnification techniques are used extensively to improve visualization of small vascular changes. Details of the technique are beyond the scope of this volume. There are risks that must be explained to the patient in order to obtain valid informed consent.

The angiographic findings in brain tumors depend upon (1) stretching or displacement of vessels by the mass, (2) the demonstration of tumor vessels or a diffuse "blush" or "stain" with the lesion, (3) early or delayed filling of veins draining the lesion, and (4) the visualization of an avascular area if the mass is cystic, necrotic, or otherwise has little circulation within it. In glioblastoma multiforme, for example, multiple small, tortuous vessels may be identified. In some tumors, particularly the more vascular meningiomas, a deep tumor stain develops during the phase of late arterial or capillary filling (see Fig. 11-36). This tends to persist after visualization of the major arteries and veins has disappeared. In some cases of metastatic carcinoma, "tumor vessels" may become opacified clearly outlining the mass; in others a dense blush or tumor stain develops; in still others there is only displacement of vessels away from the lesion. Intracranial angiography is particularly useful when, for one reason or another, CT scan has been unsatisfactory or cannot be performed. It also is useful in giving some indication of the histologic nature of the tumor in some cases, as has been noted. It is valuable in the study of vascular malformations and aneurysms. Arteriography also is a worthwhile procedure in the diagnosis of subdural hematomas, although it may not be necessary if a satisfactory CT scan is obtained.

In occlusive disease, arteriography is the method of choice for the study of the intracranial vessels, the carotids in the neck, and the vertebrals, particularly if Doppler ultrasonography has suggested a significant obstructive lesion. Arteriosclerotic plaques are visualized as areas of narrowing of the vessel lumen. With complete obstruction there is a sharp cutoff of the column of contrast material. The accompanying illustrations demonstrate some of the more characteristic changes that may be found in the presence of vascular lesions by means of angiography (Figs. 11-26 through 11-28).

SPECIFIC TUMORS—INTRODUCTION

A brief résumé of the findings in specific tumors will be given in the following section. Special emphasis will be paid to the roentgen findings on plain-film examination. The findings on CT scans, arteriograms, and pneumoencephalograms, when pertinent, will be briefly presented. From a clinical point of view it is customary to consider brain tumors, according to location in relation to the tentorium, as being either supratentorial or infratentorial. The tumors are further subdivided into intra- and extra-axial types. The location of the lesion is important not only from the aspects of symptomatology and clinical signs but also because of differences in surgical approach. Roent-

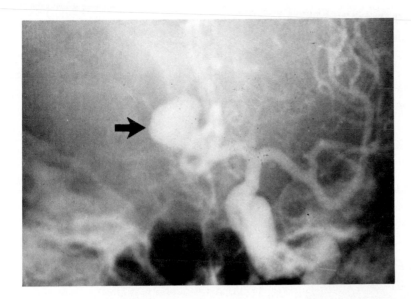

Fig. 11-26. Aneurysm of anterior communicating artery fills from a left-sided carotid injection but projects to the right. This is the same patient as in Figure 11-12.

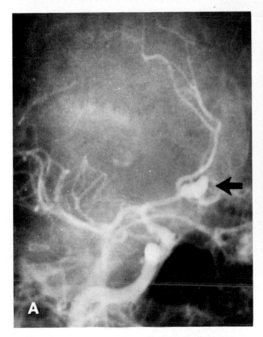

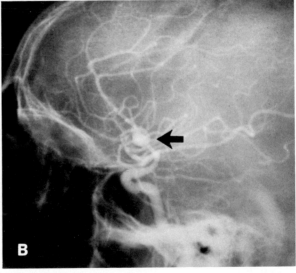

Fig. 11-27. Aneurysm of the anterior cerebral artery **(arrows).** It is best demonstrated on the oblique view **(A).**

gen findings are also best considered in the same way because the location of a tumor in its relation to the tentorium may alter the roentgen findings considerably. Only the pertinent roentgen observations will be given here, chiefly to indicate to the student the ways in which roentgen diagnosis can be used in the study of intracranial neoplasms and to illustrate the more frequently encountered signs of various lesions. The incidence of various intracranial tumors as listed by Potts[41] is as follows: Gliomas, 43%; meningiomas, 15%; pituitary adenomas, 13%; acoustic neuromas, 6.5%; metastatic tumors, 6.5%; congenital tumors, 4%; blood vessel tumors, 3%; and miscellaneous, 9%.

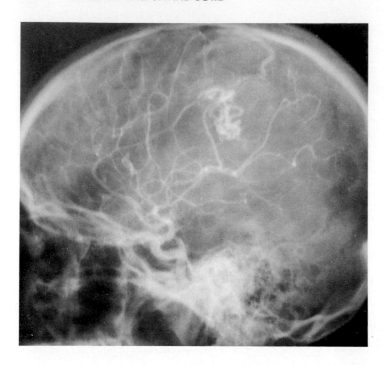

Fig. 11-28. Arteriovenous malformation in the right parietal area. The lesion originates from a branch of the middle cerebral artery and consists of a tangled mass of dilated vessels.

SUPRATENTORIAL TUMORS

Gliomas

Glioblastoma Multiforme (Astrocytoma, Grades III and IV). Glioblastoma multiforme is an invasive, locally malignant tumor and it the most common of the gliomas occurring above the tentorium, forming about 40% of all such tumors. The tumor is most frequent in persons between the ages of 40 and 60 years. The duration of symptoms usually is short and averages about 6 months prior to the initial examination. However, in many cases the symptoms are of very short duration, sometimes only a matter of days. The tumor may occur anywhere in the brain, it is characterized by its infiltrating nature and its ability to spread rapidly.

Roentgenograms of the skull frequently reveal nothing abnormal because of the short duration of the tumor. This is true in spite of the clinical signs of severe increase in intracranial pressure. Calcification sufficient to be visible in roentgenograms occurs infrequently because of the rapid growth of the lesion. Some decalcification of the sella, especially of the dorsum, may be seen if the tumor has been present for several months or longer. If calcified, the pineal body will usually be found to be displaced from its normal position and a pronounced lateral shift is frequent. Occasionally the tumor destroys brain tissue as it grows, so that the mass effect of the tumor is not apparent and the pineal body may remain in the normal location. Absence of pineal displacement, therefore, does not rule out the possibility of an infiltrating glioblastoma.

CT scans may show a low density mass representing a vascular tumor surrounded by lower density caused by edema (Fig. 11-29). There is usually great contrast enhancement because of neovascularity and blood–brain-barrier damage. Some displacement of the ventricular system away from the lesion is usual. Temporal-lobe tumors displace the temporal horn of the lateral ventricle or compress it. Often there is gross distortion of the ventricle on the side of the lesion. When the tumor involves a frontal lobe, it is prone to extend across the midline beneath the falx or by way of involvement of the corpus callosum so that some deformity of the opposite ventricle may be visualized.

Angiographic findings are varied, but typically the tumor is very vascular with a bizarre pattern of irregularly dilated arteries and early filling of dilated veins. The tumor may be well circumscribed, and vascularity may vary from one area to another. Avascular areas caused by necrosis and/or cyst formation may be seen. In some cases the tumor may be relatively avascular and in others there is very little hypervascularity. Displacement of the vessels away from the area of the lesion with stretching and straightening of their branches is a common observation. In

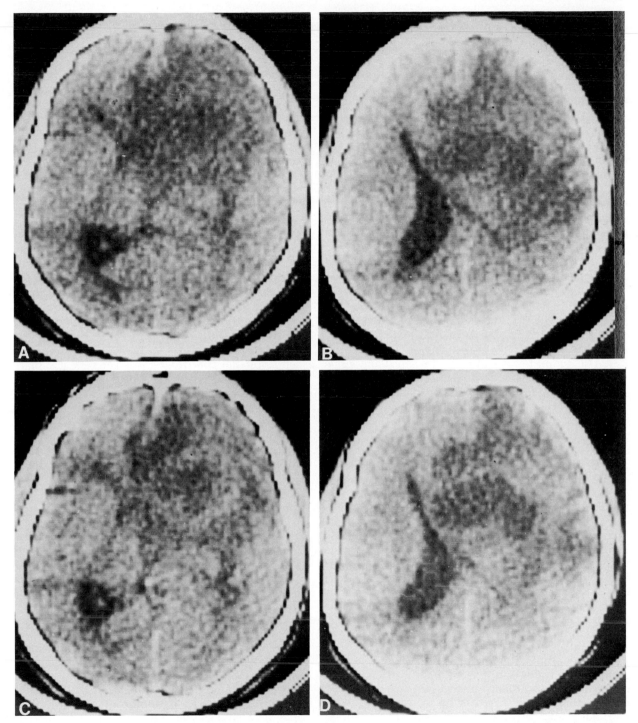

Fig. 11-29. Glioblastoma. This CT scan shows a low-density, left frontal mass causing virtual obliteration of the left lateral ventricle and some obstruction with dilatation of the right ventricle. There is a little enhancement noted, particularly in **C** centrally. **D** is also an enhanced study. (Courtesy of Drs. JE Sackett and CM Strother)

some cases a stain or blush develops during the late arterial or capillary phase (Figs. 11-30 and 11-31). During the venous phase, displacement of veins may be seen.

Contrast-enhanced CT scanning is now the primary method for investigating suspected supratentorial tumors of the brain.

Astrocytoma. Astrocytoma (grades I and II) is the second most common glioma occurring above the tentorium, representing approximately 32% of gliomas in this area. The duration of symptoms averages 3 years. The tumor may involve any part of the brain. Large cysts commonly form in astrocytomas and the cystic element may predominate in the pathologic appearance of the lesion.

Roentgenograms of the skull may reveal calcification and this finding is reported to occur in 13% of astrocytomas (Fig. 11-32). The calcium frequently is seen in the form of coarse, strandlike densities with intermixed small punctate shadows. At times, in a predominantly cystic lesion, a nodule of tumor tissue along the wall of the cyst will calcify and appear as a more or less rounded calcific density (see Fig. 11-32). The amount of calcium often is small and by no means indicates the extent of the tumor. Only occasionally when a lesion is cystic and calcium is deposited in the wall of the cyst does the calcium shadow indicate reasonably well the extent of the lesion. Because of the duration of this lesion prior to its recognition, roentgen signs of increased intracranial pressure often are noted. Decalcification and erosion of the sella are frequently observed. Displacement of the calcified pineal body is frequent in this tumor.

CT scans may show the mass effect, with displacement, distortion, or compression of the ventricular system, but in some of the slowly growing lesions there is very little mass effect. The tumor itself may be difficult to detect on CT scans. Contrast enhancement may demonstrate inherent hypervascularity (neovascularity) or blood–brain-barrier damage so that the tumor is then outlined. Abnormal enhancement is much less common than in grades III and IV astrocytomas.

On angiography the findings are similar to those of glioblastoma multiforme except that there tends to be fewer and shorter tumor vessels. If the mass is largely cystic, an avascular area will be seen together with stretching and displacement of vessels adjacent to the mass. Contralateral shift of the anterior cerebral artery will be present, the amount of shift depending upon the size of the mass. A tumor stain may be present at times in the nodular component of the lesion or if the entire mass is solid but is not very intense. It

tends to occur later (in the venous phase) than the stain in glioblastoma which is usually observed in the arterial phase.

Oligodendroglioma. This tumor comprises about 7% of the supratentorial gliomas. The average age of the patients is 35 years. The duration of symptoms is long and it is the most slowly growing and benign of the supratentorial gliomas; the average duration of symptoms is given as 11 years. This tumor is predominantly one of the cerebral hemispheres.

Because of its slow growth, calcification within the tumor occurs very frequently. The calcium usually is distributed in the form of coarse, irregular strands (Figs. 11-33 and 11-34). As in astrocytoma, other types of calcification may occur including a rather conglomerate dense mass and a mass made up of fine punctate densities. As with the other gliomas, the extent of calcification rarely indicates the actual extent of the tumor. Roentgen signs of increased intracranial pressure are frequent, with evidence of sellar erosion and decalcification, and displacement of the pineal body if it is calcified.

CT scans are similar to those in low-grade astrocytomas in that the tumors are not very vascular but may enhance slightly. The presence of calcification may provide some clue as to the nature of the lesion.

Arteriography will show displacement of vessels away from the mass, with stretching of smaller vessels and occlusion of some. The interior of the tumor usually does not develop a tumor stain during the capillary phase.

Ependymoma. This tumor comprises about 5% of the supratentorial gliomas. The average age of appearance is reported to be 30 years. The duration of symptoms is relatively short, usually less than 1 year. Most of these tumors which develop above the tentorium, arise from and lie within a lateral ventricle.

The tumor frequently contains small, scattered, punctate, calcified deposits. Otherwise it shows only the roentgen findings of increased intracranial pressure which are not specific. CT scans may show the tumor in a ventricle outlined by fluid. In this situation, it is readily detected without enhancement. Fourth ventricle ependymomas may also be detected without enhancement. The tumor may cause obstructive hydrocephalus by obstructing the outlets of the fourth ventricle. In supratentorial tumors, there may be a shift of the ventricular system away from the side of the mass. If the tumor blocks the foramen of Monro it may cause a pronounced dilatation of the ipsilateral ventricle. There is usually some contrast enhancement and there may be calcification within the tumor which tends to exclude the possibility of

(*Text continues on p. 391.*)

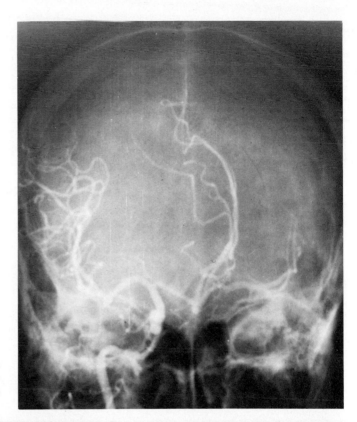

Fig. 11-30. Frontal lobe glioblastoma multiforme. This internal carotid arteriogram shows displacement of the anterior cerebral artery to the opposite side.

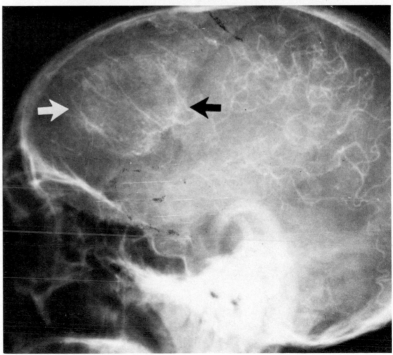

Fig. 11-31. Lateral view of frontal lobe glioblastoma multiforme shown in Figure 11-30. During the late arterial and capillary phase the lesion shows a tumor blush **(arrows).**

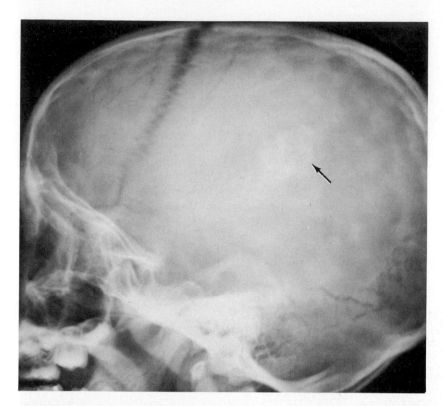

Fig. 11-32. Astrocytoma of the parietal lobe. A mottled calcified area is demonstrated in the parietal lobe **(arrow).** The spreading of the sutures, particularly the coronal, indicates increased intracranial pressure.

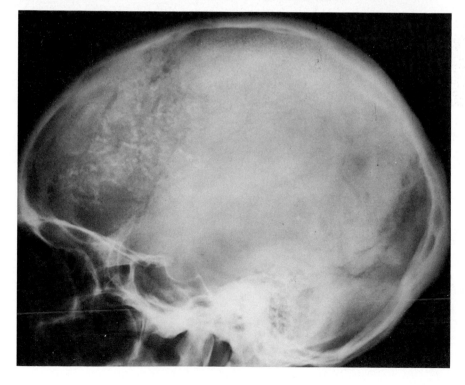

Fig. 11-33. Oligodendroglioma of the frontal lobe. There is extensive calcification within the tumor that involves nearly the entire lobe. The floor of the sella is decalcified and the dorsum and posterior clinoid processes are almost completely destroyed, indicating a chronic increase in intracranial pressure. Note the posterior displacement of the calcified pineal body.

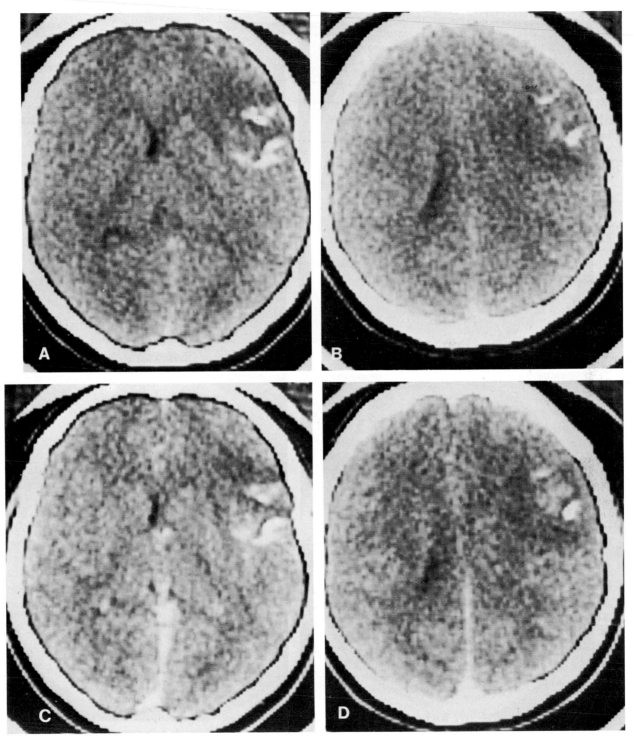

Fig. 11-34. Left frontal oligodendroglioma. **A.** and **B** show calcification in the left posterior frontal area. **C** and **D** show very slight enhancement of the tumor. (Courtesy of Drs. JE Sackett and CM Strother)

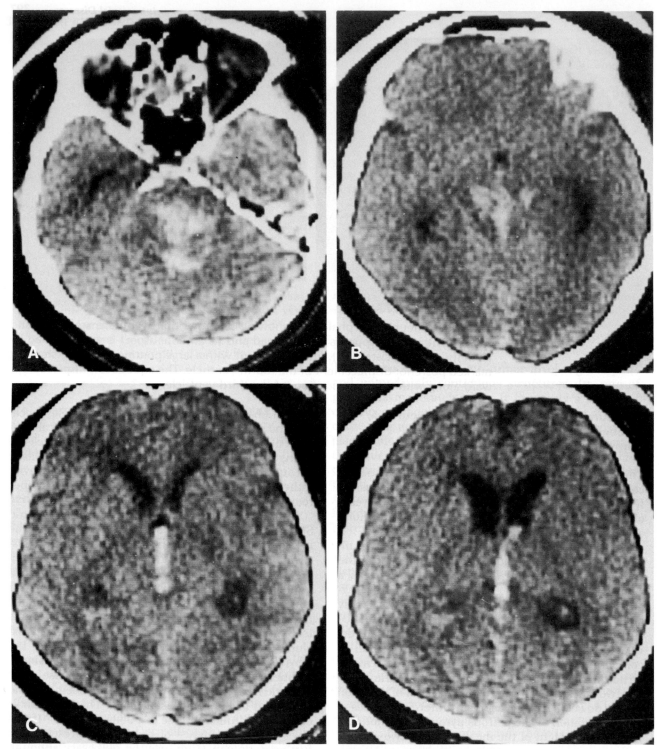

Fig. 11-41. Pontine hemorrhage. Density representing blood in the pons is shown best in **A.** Blood in the third ventricle is shown in **B, C,** and **D.** There is a little ventricular dilatation, indicating some obstruction caused by the hemorrhage. (Courtesy of Drs. JE Sackett and CM Strother)

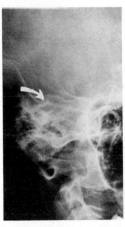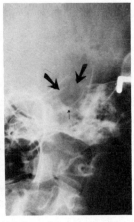

Fig. 11-42. Acoustic neuroma. Stenver's views of the temporal bones show a normal internal auditory canal on the right **(white arrow)** and an enlarged canal and internal meatus on the left **(black arrows).**

order to exclude tumor, the internal auditory meatus should be filled and the cerebellopontine angles clearly demonstrated. This method is being replaced by metrizamide CT scanning, however. The contrast material used for positive contrast cisternography is Pantopaque, the same as used for myelography. The procedure is carried out the same as myelography except that the contrast medium is allowed to flow into the posterior fossa. By proper positioning of the patient's head it can be displaced into one or both cerebellopontine cisterns and thus outline the tumor as a filling defect. If other methods of examination do not demonstrate the tumor, positive-contrast visualization should be done in most cases.

Abnormalities of the canals may cause problems in the differential diagnosis. In neurofibromatosis, the canals may be enlarged by the dural ectasia in the absence of tumor. Occasionally, large air cells in the petrous apex may distort the internal auditory canals or displace them. Tomography usually permits the correct diagnosis.

OTHER TUMORS
Choroid Plexus Papilloma

This tumor is usually found in children and is usually benign. It occurs in one of the lateral ventricles or in the fourth ventricle. It is often pedunculated, giving it some mobility. Often the most significant finding is hydrocephalus which is caused by obstruction or overproduction of cerebrospinal fluid. On CT scan, the mass is visible within a ventricle, often seen clearly enough to detect the irregular margins. Since the tumor is very vascular and is outside the blood–brain barrier, contrast enhancement is marked. Angiography also demonstrates the lesion and outlines the blood supply, which is from the choroidal arteries.

Chordoma

This tumor arises from remnants of the fetal notochord and its common locations are at the cervico-occipital junction and in the sacrococcygeal area of the spine. It is a slowly growing tumor that results in bone destruction. The cervico-occipital lesion, therefore, leads to destruction in the base of the occiput or the clivus together with evidence of a soft-tissue mass in the retropharyngeal soft tissues and occasionally some destruction of the first or second cervical vertebral body. Extensive destruction of the coccyx and lower part of the sacrum is found in lesions of the lower end of the spine.

Metastatic Tumors

Metastasis to the brain from distant primary tumor is common. Carcinomas of the lung, breast, and kidney frequently metastasize to the brain. While multiple metastatic foci may be present, usually the clinical and roentgen signs point toward the presence of a solitary lesion. The roentgen findings of intracranial metastasis do not differ significantly from those described for other brain tumors, particularly the gliomas. The mass of the tumor causes displacement of normal structures away from it. Displacement of a calcified pineal gland is frequent. CT scan is very useful in detecting metastases.[12] Some are isodense, others may be more or less dense than normal brain. If the lesion is isodense, there is usually a lucent area of edema around it. Also, displacement and distortion of the ventricular system can be detected. Even though some lesions are isodense and have no edema, most show enhancement after contrast. Multiple metastases must be differentiated from multifocal gliomas and multiple abscesses. Solitary metastases may be impossible to differentiate from a malignant glioblastoma on CT scan. Characteristics of posterior fossa (cerebellar) metastases are similar on CT scans. Most show contrast enhancement, some homogeneous, other ringlike. On arteriography the vessels will be displaced away from the lesion and those in proximity appear stretched. With the more vascular lesions, increased vascularity may be seen and a distinct tumor stain may occur during the capillary phase of filling. Evidence of increased intracranial pressure in plain roentgenograms of the skull is usually absent since the duration of the disease is relatively short. *Every patient suspected of harboring a brain tumor should have routine roentgen examination of the chest;* this may demonstrate an otherwise silent bronchogenic tumor or perhaps evidence of pulmonary metastasis from some other primary site. Tumors which metastasize to the brain less frequently include melanoma, lymphoma, osteosarcoma, colon carcinoma, chorionic carcinoma, and nasopharyngeal carcinoma.

OTHER CONDITIONS

BRAIN ATROPHY

The causes of atrophy of the brain are numerous and include arteriosclerosis and hypertensive disease leading to encephalomalacia, certain degenerative diseases such as Pick's disease and Alzheimer's disease, multiple sclerosis, trauma, and local vascular occlusion and rupture.

When brain atrophy is generalized it is practically impossible to state the cause from roentgen examination alone because there is nothing specific in the findings. As a matter of fact, it is usually impossible to distinguish between a congenital hypoplasia of the brain and an acquired atrophy. When the atrophy is localized or focal the causes are few in number. Focal atrophy most often is caused either by trauma or by occlusion or rupture of a blood vessel.

The CT signs of brain atrophy are essentially those of increased size of the subarachnoid cisterns, the surface subarachnoid pathways or channels, and the ventricles. In some cases there is a dilatation of all these spaces or cavities also observed on pneumoencephalography (Fig. 11-43); the diagnosis of atrophy then is obvious. In others, the dilatation is limited either to the ventricular system or the superficial subarachnoid spaces. The term "cortical atrophy" often is used when the dilatation is limited to the superficial channels, with the ventricular system reasonably normal. This term may not be anatomically correct even under these circumstances, and it is preferable to speak of cerebral atrophy rather than cortical atrophy. Occasionally the atrophy is limited to or is more severe in the cerebellum than in the cerebrum. This is shown by an enlarged fourth ventricle, increased accumulations of gas over the surface of the cerebellar hemispheres, and enlargement of the cisterns, especially the cisterna magna.

Focal atrophy or cicatrix formation is recognized by a localized dilatation of one ventricle or a portion of a ventricle nearest the site of scarring, a retraction of structures toward the side of the atrophy, and by a local enlargement of the subarachnoid pathways over the site of the lesion (Fig. 11-44). Brain trauma may be followed by such changes which also are readily demonstrated on CT scans.

Multifocal Leukoencephalopathy. This is a progressive, asymmetric or focal disorder characterized by multiple demyelinating lesions in the white matter of the cerebral hemispheres. It usually occurs in patients with lymphoproliferative disorders and altered immune response and may be associated with lymphoma, leukemia, viral disease, sarcoidosis, or tuberculosis. On CT scans, decreased density is noted in the areas involved by the demyelinating lesions. There is no enhancement and no mass effect.

Porencephaly. Porencephaly and porencephalic cyst are terms used to indicate a cystlike space in the brain which may communicate with the subarachnoid space or ventricular system and sometimes with both. Various insults such as infarction, intracerebral hemorrhage, abscess, or various types of trauma including surgery may be involved in the formation of these atrophic areas. In some of these patients, no definite cause can be determined. Porencephaly may be associated with leptomeningeal cyst (growing fracture) in children. CT scanning is the method of choice for the study of these patients. The cystlike spaces have the density of cerebrospinal fluid and do not change on contrast enhancement.

Subarachnoid Cysts. These are usually associated with some loss of brain tissue and are found in the region of the sylvian fissure, in the interhemispheric fissure, in the posterior fossa, or in the region of the basal cisterns, or sometimes over the convexity.[52] They may or may not communicate with the subarachnoid space. They usually occur in children. There is often a history of trauma. The most common site is the sylvian fissure. When a cyst in this area is large, plain film may show a temporal bulge and an elevation of the lesser wing of the sphenoid as well as an anterior displacement of the greater sphenoid wing. There is usually associated atrophy or hypoplasia of the temporal lobe and sometimes of the adjacent frontal lobe. As in porencephaly, because these cysts have the density of cerebrospinal fluid and do not enhance they are best studied by CT scans.

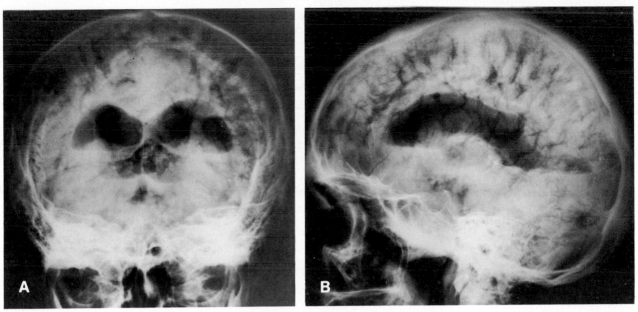

Fig. 11-43. Generalized cerebral atrophy. Frontal **(A)** and lateral **(B)** pneumoen-cephalograms show ventricular dilatation, chiefly involving the lateral ventricles, and dilatation of subarachnoid channels over the hemispheres.

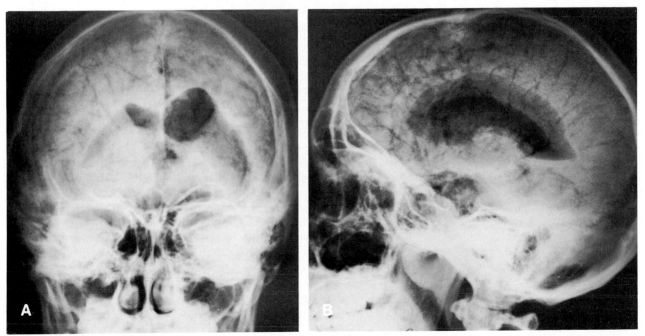

Fig. 11-44. Unilateral cerebral atrophy following birth injury. Frontal **(A)** and lateral **(B)** encephalogram showing a decrease in volume of the left cerebral hemisphere with a shift of midline structures to that side and dilatation of the homolateral ventricle.

SUBDURAL HEMATOMA AND HYGROMA

Bleeding into the subdural space is a frequent complication of head injuries and results in the formation of a subdural hematoma. The most common location is over the superior parietal area but the lesion may develop at some other site; we have observed it infrequently in the posterior fossa. The roentgen findings are essentially those of an intracranial mass. A fracture may or may not be present; most frequently a fracture is not demonstrated. There is some difference in the roentgen findings, depending upon whether the hematoma is an acute or a chronic one. Acute subdural hematomas give the clinical and roentgen signs of an intracranial mass with increase in intracranial pressure (Fig. 11-45). Hematomas of more than 4 weeks' duration are usually designated as chronic. Shift of the calcified pineal is frequent in these cases. In very chronic cases, in which the hematoma has been present for months or longer, there often is associated atrophy of the brain beneath the hematoma and there may be little evidence of a mass, the atrophy compensating for the space occupied by the hematoma (Fig. 11-46). With acute unilateral hematomas, displacement of the pineal, if it is calcified, is demonstrable. Bilateral hematomas are not uncommon (approximately 20% of patients) (Fig. 11-47). Absence of pineal shift may not be reliable in excluding the possibility of hematoma.

CT scanning is now widely used in the study of patients with suspected subdural hematoma.[58] In acute hematoma, the attenuation of the hematoma is greater than brain tissue and the lesion appears light; later, there is a period, usually from 15 to 90 days after the bleeding, in which the hematoma is isodense. Then the attenuation may decrease when the fluid loses its protein content. The most difficult problem in the CT diagnosis is in patients with bilateral isodense hematomas. Infusion scan may identify a cortical vein displaced away from the inner table or the sulci may be identifiable extending to the inner table, which makes or excludes the diagnosis. Most hematomas have a concave or straight inner margin, but large subdural hematomas are often biconvex. The shape does not differentiate acute from chronic hematoma accurately. When the diagnosis is not certain on CT scan, arteriography or radionuclide scan may be indicated.

Arteriography is a very useful procedure in the diagnosis of subdural hematoma. When the internal carotid and its branches have been opacified by the injection of contrast substance, a subdural hematoma will cause an inward displacement of the branches of the middle cerebral artery easily seen in anteroposterior arteriograms (Fig. 11-48). On the other hand, if the vessels are seen to be closely apposed to the inner table, the possibility of a convexity hematoma can be excluded with assurance.

With a unilateral hematoma the anterior cerebral artery is displaced toward the contralateral side. Absence of displacement of this vessel or minor degrees of shift in the presence of characteristic shift of the middle cerebral vessels are highly suggestive of the presence of a hematoma on the contralateral side and warrant carotid arteriography on the opposite side. Displacement of the deep veins (internal cerebral vein) has the same significance as shift of the anterior cerebral artery, and, in the absence of filling of this latter vessel, the position of the internal cerebral vein may be the deciding factor as to the presence or absence of a contralateral hematoma. If the hematoma is small there may be little or no shift of the anterior cerebral artery and, in the presence of such a small lesion, it may be necessary to perform arteriography on the opposite side to rule out the possibility of a hematoma there.

Subdural Hygroma (Subdural Effusion; External Hydrocephalus)

In a subdural hygroma there is an accumulation of fluid in the subdural space; the fluid may be either loculated or freely movable. A limiting membrane as in subdural hematoma may or may not be demonstrable and the fluid is either clear or slightly xanthochromic. Some subdural hygromas, particularly those that are limited by adhesions, undoubtedly represent the effects of trauma and some appear to be the residues of previous subdural hematomas. In other cases, however, the cause is obscure. Roentgenologically an encapsulated subdural hygroma gives findings identical with those of a subdural hematoma. Free effusions behave somewhat differently. The fluid accumulations usually are bilateral because there is, normally, free communication between the subdural spaces over both hemispheres. Thus little or no ventricular shift is apparent.

EPIDURAL HEMATOMA

An epidural hematoma results from laceration of a branch of the middle meningeal artery, these vessels coursing in grooves on the inner table of the skull. Less frequently the bleeding is caused by rupture of a vein. The tear often occurs secondary to a fracture and the fracture can be identified in skull roentgeno-

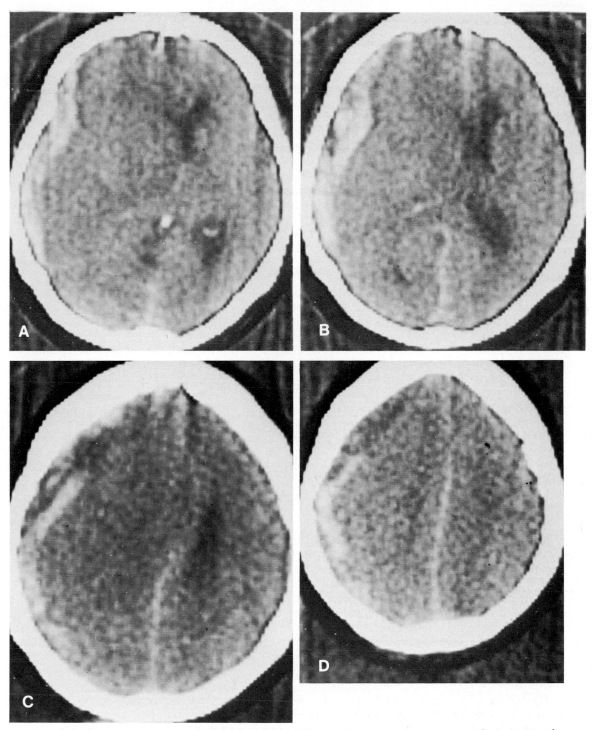

Fig. 11-45. Acute subdural hematoma. The patient was comatose on admission to the hospital following an accident. The hemorrhage is noted on the right side on all sections. Note the marked shift of the ventricular system. (Courtesy of Drs. JE Sackett and CM Strother)

grams. The diagnosis of an epidural hematoma is often made from the clinical examination. The history is that of an individual who suffers a head injury that is followed after a period of time, usually several hours, by progressive stupor and other signs of increased intracranial pressure. At times the clinical course is not characteristic and the diagnosis may be in doubt. The roentgen demonstration of a fracture extending across a meningeal arterial vascular groove is important and suggests the diagnosis in a patient who deteriorates rapidly after head trauma. The roentgen signs on CT scanning are those of a mass lesion, usually in the frontoparietal or temporal area, which has the high attenuation coefficient of blood. The contour is usually biconvex. When the diagnosis is in doubt, the next radiographic examination is carotid arteriography. The inward displacement of the branches of the middle cerebral artery away from the inner table of the skull as seen in anteroposterior arteriograms is diagnostic of either a subdural or an epidural hematoma. The latter are more localized than subdural hematomas because of the normal adherence of the dura to the skull. The subdural space, on the other hand, is potentially a free one and hemorrhage within it can spread over a wide area. In some epidural hematomas, extravasation outlines the site of bleeding. Other angiographic signs include displacement of meningeal arteries and sometimes displacement of dural venous sinuses from the inner table of the skull. If the CT scan gives positive evidence of the hematoma, arteriography may be omitted in some cases since the condition often represents an acute surgical emergency.[7]

OTHER BRAIN TRAUMA

Computed tomography has had a significant impact on the management of patients with acute head trauma. The more rapid CT scanners will decrease motion artifacts and make the examination even more useful. A number of abnormalities can be demonstrated on CT scans in addition to epidural and subdural hematomas. These include intracerebral hematomas, intraventricular hemorrhage, both general and local cerebral edema, cerebral contusion, foreign bodies, and depressed skull fractures. In a series of 286 patients, CT scanning reduced the use of arteriography by 84%, skull radiography by 24%, and surgical intervention by 58%. Intracerebral and intraventricular hematomas are radiodense on CT scan and are usually readily recognized in the acute stage. In cerebral contusion without the formation of a hematoma, small petechial hemorrhages may be pres-

ent, but the accompanying edema may be outlined as an area of decreased attenuation on the CT scan. The same is true of general cerebral edema and swelling. The majority of foreign bodies are readily identified and localized as are fragments of bone in patients with depressed skull fractures. This noninvasive method can also be used to follow the course of the patient with head trauma.

BRAIN ABSCESS

The roentgen signs of brain abscess are usually nonspecific and consist only of the evidence of a mass lesion. In most patients, plain roentgenograms of the skull will reveal an essentially normal state. If the pineal is calcified it may be displaced from its normal position; displacement of a calcified choroid plexus is observed occasionally. During childhood, spreading of the cranial sutures may be demonstrable. These findings only indicate the existence of a mass lesion or the presence of increased intracranial pressure. In a few patients we have observed gas within an abscess cavity when the lesion followed a fracture through the frontal or ethmoid sinuses. In such cases it is impossible to state, from roentgen findings alone, whether one is dealing with an abscess caused by anaerobic gas-forming organisms or whether the gas represents air introduced through the fracture (traumatic pneumocephalus). For all practical purposes, therefore, the roentgen signs of brain abscess are only those of a space-occupying mass. When the clinical findings point to the possibility of a brain abscess, roentgen examination of the nasal accessory sinuses and mastoids may reveal evidence of infection and thus indicate that a potential source for intracranial abscess exists. CT scanning is very useful in the detection and subsequent follow-up of a brain abscess. Often the abscess cannot be diagnosed without the intravenous injection of a contrast medium. This will reveal a typical ringlike enhancement that probably represents the abscess capsule. The capsule tends to be smooth and uniform in thickness. There usually is no enhancement within the cavity. Detectable cerebral edema may be present surrounding the abscess. The CT scan cannot differentiate chronic pyogenic abscess from cavitation caused by fungi or by tuberculosis. Multiple abscesses may be present and can be detected and followed by means of CT scanning. Cerebral metastases or cystic glioma may simulate abscess, but, compared with abscess, both tend to be more irregular and on enhancement the capsule of each is less uniform in thickness. Also, the history and clinical findings are valuable in the differentiation.

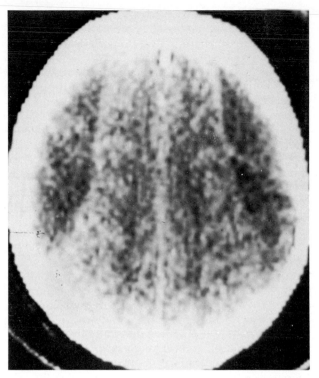

Fig. 11-46. Chronic subdural hematoma. Note the bilateral, bi-concave lucencies along the lateral aspect of the calvarium on both sides. (Courtesy of Drs. JE Sackett and CM Strother)

HYDROCEPHALUS

Hydrocephalus means an increased amount of cerebrospinal fluid within the cranial cavity, usually associated with dilatation of the ventricles. It may be either congenital or acquired. Hydrocephalus may be further subdivided into the following:

I. Obstructive hydrocephalus
   1. Communicating (normal pressure hydrocephalus): The ventricular system is patent, but there is obstruction to the flow of cerebrospinal fluid either in the basal cisterns, the subarachnoid pathways over the surface of the brain, or in the arachnoidal villi.
   2. Noncommunicating: The obstruction is in the ventricular system or at the outlets of the fourth ventricle.
II. Nonobstructive hydrocephalus (overproduction of cerebrospinal fluid)
   1. Excess secretion of cerebrospinal fluid. This is uncommon and usually results from a choroid plexus tumor (papilloma).

It is generally accepted that the cerebrospinal fluid is formed by the choroid plexuses within the ventricles. From the ventricles the fluid passes through the outlets of the fourth ventricle, the foramina of Luschka and Magendie, into the subarachnoid cisterns around the base of the brain. It then flows up-

Fig. 11-47. Bilateral subdural hematoma. Frontal **(A)** and lateral **(B)** pneumoencephalograms demonstrate the marked displacement of subarachnoid channels away from the inner table by subdural hematomas of approximately equal size. Note the extensive parieto-occipital fracture in the lateral view. Increased pressure has resulted in separation of the fracture.

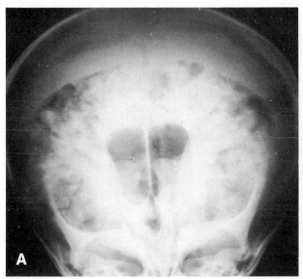
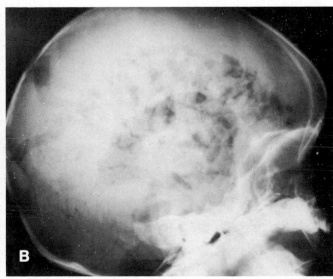

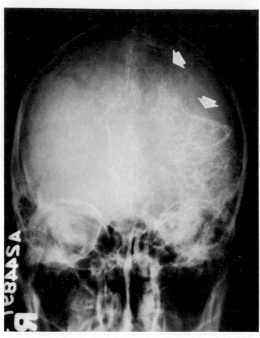

Fig. 11-48. Subdural hematoma demonstrated by internal carotid arteriography. The anterior and middle cerebral branches of the internal carotid artery are filled. **Arrows** outline inward displacement of the vessels by a large subdural hematoma. The anterior cerebral artery is displaced toward the right which tends to exclude the possibility of a hematoma on that side.

ward over the convexities of the cerebral hemispheres to the arachnoid villi where it is absorbed.

Acquired Hydrocephalus

It is possible to have an obstruction develop anywhere along the cerebrospinal fluid pathway from the foramina of Monro, the openings between the lateral ventricles and the third ventricle, to the points of absorption along the superior surface of the brain. Tumors and adhesive processes may block the flow of fluid at any of these sites and the roentgen findings are those of the causative lesion as described in previous sections of this chapter.

Congenital Hydrocephalus

The cause of congenital hydrocephalus is not completely understood but it is the belief of many investigators that the fault often lies in some defect in the

absorbing mechanism so that the cerebrospinal fluid, which continues to be elaborated by the choroid plexuses, cannot be removed properly from the subarachnoid space. Many cases of congenital hydrocephalus are of the communicating type.

The clinical diagnosis of congenital hydrocephalus is usually made without difficulty but roentgen examination, particularly CT scanning, is utilized frequently to confirm the diagnosis, to establish the severity of ventricular dilatation, and to follow the progress of treatment. Plain roentgenograms of the skull reveal the large size of the head and demonstrate spreading of the sutures. In the infant, the cranial bones often are poorly ossified and their margins are indistinct. The anterior fontanelle is large. If the condition becomes arrested the bones ossify and, with growth, fill in the defects caused by the previous spreading of the sutures.

Pneumoencephalography may be used to determine whether the hydrocephalus is of the communicating or noncommunicating type. In the former, the gas will ascend and enter the dilated ventricles. If the ventricular system is obstructed, only the subarachnoid space will fill and CT scans or direct ventricular puncture will be necessary if information concerning them is wanted (Fig. 11-49). The removal of 50 cc or less of fluid and replacement with gas will give sufficient information in most of these pateints if pneumoencephalography is carried out. Radionuclide cisternography is useful in some instances; this consists of intrathecal injection of radioactive [111]Indium or [169]ytterbium-labeled DTPA by way of lumbar puncture. If the subarachnoid spaces are patent, radioactivity will be observed over the hemispheres in 24 hours; if not, the radioactivity will be concentrated in the ventricular system. Normally, none of the labeled material is detected in the ventricles at 48 hours.

Normal Pressure Hydrocephalus

The term "normal pressure hydrocephalus" has been used to identify the syndrome of dementia, gait disturbances, and urinary incontinence in patients with hydrocephalus and normal cerebrospinal fluid pressure.[5] In some patients with these clinical findings and normal pressure hydrocephalus there is free communication with easy flow to the cortical subarachnoid channels. In others the isotope scans show most, if not all, of the activity to be at the cranial base and in the ventricular system. There is some debate as to whether both of these varieties should be considered as the same anomaly. In any event, those with the clinical triad just described and normal pressure hydrocephalus appear to benefit from cere-

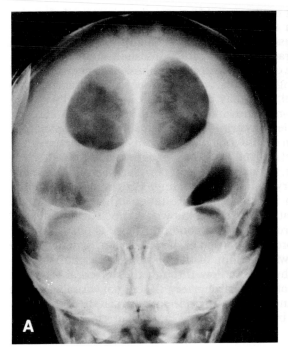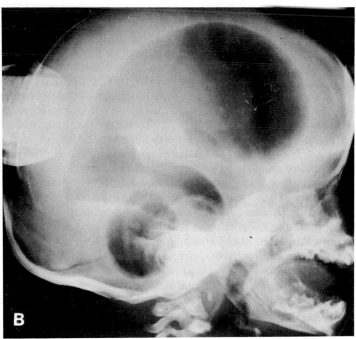

Fig. 11-49. Obstructive hydrocephalus following meningitis. Frontal **(A)** and lateral **(B)** roentgenograms after ventricular puncture (ventriculogram). All of the ventricles are greatly dilated. The obstruction was caused by adhesions blocking the outlets of the fourth ventricle.

brospinal fluid shunting procedures. The amount of cerebrospinal fluid present initially in the cranial cavity and any changes following surgery are readily detected on CT scans. The changes in ventricular size postoperatively do not necessarily correlate with the clinical status of the patient.

ADHESIVE ARACHNOIDITIS

Adhesions involving the arachnoid may arise from a number of causes, including inflammatory disease, subarachnoid hemorrhage following rupture of an aneurysm or other vascular malformation, and trauma. Roentgen diagnosis is difficult. The ability to fill the normal subarachnoid space with gas during pneumoencephalography is variable and lack of complete visualization is usual. When filling of the subarachnoid pathways is poor, not too much emphasis can be placed upon the finding providing the rest of the examination reveals no abnormality. Presumably any extensive obliteration of the subarachnoid space by adhesions will obstruct the flow of cerebrospinal fluid and result in ventricular dilatation. Scattered adhesions or the involvement of relatively localized areas may exist, however, with a perfectly normal

ventricular system. Radionuclide cisternography may be helpful in some of these patients.

Arachnoidal adhesions around the base of the brain, particularly if the process involves the region of the cisterna magna, give more definite signs than when the condition exists over the surfaces of the cerebral hemispheres. This is because of the greater likelihood of the flow of fluid being obstructed with resulting internal hydrocephalus. Posterior fossa adhesions of rather limited extent may obstruct the outlets of the fourth ventricle completely and lead to severe signs of increased intracranial pressure (See Fig. 11-49).

EXTRACRANIAL OCCLUSIVE VASCULAR DISEASE

As mentioned earlier in this chapter, arteriography is the method of choice for the identification and study of occlusive disease of the vessels supplying the brain. However, there is now an accurate means of screening the extracranial carotid system for stenotic lesions. In one study of 100 patients examined by the Doppler ultrasound method, there was a 90% agreement rate with carotid arteriography and a significant

Intracranial Aneurysms

Most intracranial aneurysms arise in or near the circle of Willis, the three most common sites being: (1) the posterior communicating artery at its anterior end; (2) the junction of the anterior cerebral and anterior communicating arteries; and (3) the proximal middle cerebral artery. They occur at points of branching or at junction points of arteries. The major danger is rupture, although large aneurysms may exert enough pressure on adjacent structures to produce neurologic signs. The majority rupture into the subarachnoid space causing bloody cerebrospinal fluid. Bleeding into the subdural space is unusual. The distal anterior cerebral and middle cerebral aneurysms often rupture into the brain substance with hemorrhage there; occasionally they may rupture into the ventricular system. Angiography is the method of choice used in the detection of aneurysm (Fig. 11-51). Multiple projections are often necessary to outline the aneurysm completely and determine its site of origin as well as its relationship to surrounding vessels. Changes related to spasm and to adjacent hematoma may also be observed on the arteriogram. The use of CT scanning is limited, but large aneurysms can be detected if they contain calcium or they may enhance after contrast. Hematoma adjacent to the aneurysm can be identified and occasionally a completely clotted aneurysm that does not fill at angiography can be identified on CT scans.

Arteriovenous Malformations

Arteriovenous malformations are the most common vascular anomalies within the calvarium. They may contain calcium and therefore are visible on plain films. Also there may be displacement of the calcified pineal body or choroid plexus in some instances. There may be prominent arterial or venous grooves, depending on the blood supply and venous return. Arteriography is the definitive examination which identifies the lesion and its blood supply. As in intracranial aneurysm, CT scanning plays a secondary role in the study of hemorrhage secondary to the lesion.

REFERENCES AND SELECTED READINGS

1. ALLEN JH, RILEY HD JR: Generalized cytomegalic inclusion disease, with emphasis on roentgen diagnosis. Radiology 71: 257, 1958

2. AMBROSE J: Computerized transverse axial scanning (tomography). Part II. Clinical application. Br J Radiol 46: 1023, 1973

3. BABBITT DP, TANG T, DOBBS J et al: Idiopathic familial cerebral vascular ferrocalcinosis (Fahr's disease) and review of differential diagnosis of intracranial calcification in children. Radiology 105: 352, 1969

4. BAHR AL, HODGES FJ III: Efficacy of computed tomography of the head in changing patient care and health costs: a retrospective study. Am J Roentgenol 131: 45, 1978

5. BENSON DF, LEMAY M, PATTEN DH et al: Diagnosis of normal pressure hydrocephalus. N Engl J Med 282: 609, 1970

6. CAMP JD: Pathologic non-neoplastic intracranial calcification. JAMA 137: 1023, 1948

7. CLAVERIA LE, DUBOULAY GH, MOSELEY IF: Intracranial infections: investigation by computerized axial tomography. Neuroradiology 12: 59, 1976

8. CLAVERIA LE, SUTTON D, TRESS BM: The radiological diagnosis of meningiomas, the impact of EMI scanning. Br J Radiol 50: 15, 1977

9. CORNELL SH, GRAF CJ, DOLAN KD: Fat-fluid levels in intracranial epidermoid cysts. Am J Roentgenol 128: 502, 1977

10. CRONQVIST S: Total angiography in evaluation of cerebrovascular disease: correlative study of aortocervical and selective cerebral angiography. Br J Radiol 39: 805, 1966

11. CRUMMY AB, ZWIEBEL WJ, BARRIGA P et al: Doppler evaluation of extracranial cerebrovascular disease. Am J Roentgenol 132: 91, 1979

12. DECK MDF, MESSINA AV, SACKETT JF: Computed tomography in metastatic disease of the brain. Radiology 119: 115, 1976

13. DUBOIS PJ, DRAYER BP, BANK WO et al: An evaluation of current diagnostic modalities in the investigation of acoustic neurilemmomas. Radiology 126: 173, 1978

14. EVENS RG, RUJANAVECH N, MIKHAEL MA: Utilization, reliability and cost-effectiveness of cranial computed tomography in evaluating pseudotumor cerebri. Am J Roentgenol 129: 263, 1977

15. FELSON B (ed): A primer on cerebral angiography. Semin Radiol 6: 1, 1971

16. FINBY N, KRAFT E: The aging skull: comparative roentgen study, 25–34 year interval. Clin Radiol 23: 410, 1972

17. GOLD LHA, KIEFFER SA, PETERSON HO: Intracranial meningiomas. A retrospective analysis of the diagnostic value of plain skull films. Neurology (Minneap) 19: 873, 1969

18. HILLMAN RSL, KIEFFER SA, ORTIZ H et al: Intraosseous leptomeningeal cysts of the posterior cranial fossa. Radiology 116: 655, 1975

19. HINCK VC, DOTTER CT: Appraisal of current techniques

for cerebral angiography. Am J Roentgenol 107: 626, 1969

20. HOLT JF, DICKERSON WW: The osseous lesions of tuberous sclerosis. Radiology 58: 1, 1952

21. HOUNSFIELD GN: Computerized transverse axial scanning (tomography). Part I. Description of system. Br J Radiol 46: 1016, 1973

22. KALAN C, BURROWS EH: Calcification in intracranial gliomata. Br J Radiol 35: 589, 1962

23. KATTEN KR: Calvarial thickening after dilantin medication. Am J Roentgenol 110: 102, 1970

24. KOMAR NN, GABRIELSEN TO, HOLT JF: Roentgenographic appearance of lumbo-sacral spine and pelvis in tuberous sclerosis. Radiology 89: 701, 1967

25. LAGOS JC, HOLMAN CB, GOMEZ MR: Tuberous sclerosis. Neuroroentgenologic observations. Am J Roentgenol 104: 171, 1968

26. LAPAYOWKER MS, CLIFF MN. Bone changes in acoustic neuromas. Am J Roentgenol 107: 652, 1969

27. LEMAY M: The radiologic diagnosis of pituitary disease. Radiol Clin North Am 5: 303, 1967

28. LOFSTROM JE, WEBSTER JE, GURDJIAN ES: Angiography in the evaluation of intracranial trauma. Radiology 65: 847, 1955

29. MADDISON FE, MOORE WS: Ulcerated atheromata of the carotid artery. Arteriographic appearance. Am J Roentgenol 107: 530, 1969

30. MARAVILLA KR: Intraventricular fat-fluid levels secondary to rupture of an intracranial dermoid cyst. Am J Roentgenol 128: 500, 1977

31. MUELLER S, BELL W, SEIBERT J: Cerebral calcifications associated with intrathecal methotrexate therapy in acute lymphocytic leukemia. J Pediatr 88: 650, 1976

32. MUENTER MD, WHISNANT JP: Basal ganglia calcification, hypoparathyroidism and extrapyramidal manifestations. Neurology (Minneap) 18: 1075, 1968

33. MUSSBICHLER H: Radiologic study of intracranial calcification in congenital toxoplasmosis. Acta Radiol [Diagn] (Stockh) 7: 369, 1968

34. NATHAN MH, COLLINS VP, COLLINS LC: Premature unilateral synostosis of the coronal suture. Am J Roentgenol 86: 433, 1961

35. NEW PFJ, WEINER MA: The radiological investigation of hydrocephalus. Radiol Clin North Am 9: 117, 1971

36. NEWTON GH, POTTS DG: Radiology of the Skull and Brain, 4 Vols. St. Louis, CV Mosby, 1978*

37. NORTON GA, KISHORE PRS, LIN J: CT contrast enhancement in cerebral infarction. Am J Roentgenol 131: 881, 1978

38. OH SJ: Roentgen findings in cerebral paragonimiasis. Radiology 90: 292, 1968

* These books comprise a comprehensive reference to virtually all aspects of intracranial disease

39. PEAR BL: Epidermoid and dermoid sequestration cysts. Am J Roentgenol 110: 148, 1970

40. PERRY BJ, BRIDGES C: Computerized transverse axial scanning (tomography). Part III. Radiation dose considerations. Br J Radiol 46: 1048, 1973

41. POTTS DG: Brain tumors: radiologic localization and diagnosis. Radiol Clin North Am 3: 511, 1965

42. POTTS DG: A system of skull radiography. Radiology 94: 25, 1970

43. ROZARIO R, HAMMERSCHLAG SB, POST KD et al: Diagnosis of empty sella with CT scan. Neuroradiology 13: 85, 1977

44. SACKETT JF, MESSINA AV, PETITO CK: Computed tomography and magnification vertebral angiotomography in the diagnosis of colloid cysts of the third ventricle. Radiology 116: 95, 1975

45. SALMI A, VOUTILAINEN A, HOLSTI LR et al: Hyperostosis cranii in a normal population. Am J Roentgenol 87: 1032, 1962

46. SANTIN G, VARGAS J: Roentgen study of cysticercosis of the central nervous system. Radiology 86: 520, 1966

47. SCOTT WG, SIMRIL WA, SEAMAN WB: Intracerebral arteriovenous malformations; their diagnosis and angiographic demonstration. Am J Roentgenol 71: 762, 1954

48. SOTER CS, GILMORE JH: Roentgenologic study of the vascular markings of the skull. Am J Roentgenol 82: 823, 1959

49. STEINBERG I, HALPERN M: Roentgen manifestations of the subclavian steal syndrome. Am J Roentgenol 90: 528, 1963

50. TAVERAS JM, WOOD EH: Diagnostic Neuroradiology. Baltimore, Williams & Wilkins, 1976*

51. VASTINE JH, KINNEY KK: The pineal shadow as an aid in the localization of brain tumors. Am J Roentgenol 17: 320, 1927

52. WEINBERG PE, FLOM RA: Intracranial subarachnoid cysts. Radiology 106: 329, 1973

53. WESCOTT JL, CHYNN KY, STEINBERG I: Percutaneous transfemoral selective arteriography of the brachiocephalic vessels. Am J Roentgenol 90: 554, 1963

54. WESENBERG RL, JUHL JH, DAUBE JR: Radiological findings in lissencephaly (congenital agyria). Radiology 87: 436, 1966

55. WILSON M: Angiography in cerebrovascular occlusive disease. Am J Med Sci 250: 554, 1965

56. WOLPERT SM: The neuroradiology of hemangioblastomas of the cerebellum. Am J Roentgenol 110: 56, 1970

57. YUHL ET, SCHMITZ AL: The occipital emissary foramen and increased intracranial pressure. Acta Radiol [Diag] (Stockh) 9: 124, 1969

58. ZIMMERMAN RA, BILANIUK LT, GENNARELLI T et al: Cranial computed tomography in diagnosis and management of acute head trauma. Am J Roentgenol 131: 27, 1978

12

THE SPINAL CORD AND RELATED STRUCTURES

The roentgen diagnosis of tumors of the spinal cord and its coverings and herniation of intervertebral discs will be considered in this chapter. Also brief reference to the findings in certain inflammatory lesions and vascular malformations will be included. Roentgen examination for the detection of these conditions will be discussed under two main headings: (*1*) plain roentgenograms of the spine without the use of contrast media and (*2*) myelography, or contrast examination, of the spinal canal.

METHODS OF EXAMINATION

PLAIN ROENTGENOGRAMS

Roentgenograms of the spinal column should always be obtained as the first step whenever a lesion of the cord or of the intervertebral discs is suspected. Not only will these roentgenograms reveal positive evidence of considerable value in many cord tumors, but also they are useful in excluding or in demonstrating infections, tumors, degenerative changes, and injuries involving the vertebrae. In many cases the examination can be limited to a single anteroposterior and a lateral view. In others it may be necessary to use multiple projections, including oblique views or roentgenograms obtained with the patient flexing or extending the spine.

Variations in size of the spinal canal are very important in determining the likelihood of spinal cord compression due to small defects produced by bony ridges or spurs, small intervertebral disk herniations, or tumors. Developmental narrowing or stenosis usually occurs in the cervical and lumbar areas and may involve several segments. Although single vertebral involvement occurs rarely, it may cause significant local stenosis. Normal measurements are listed in Lusted and Keats.[17a]

As is true with other anatomic parts, when observing roentgenograms of the vertebral column the student should develop an orderly system of viewing the structures so that small changes from the normal will not be overlooked. It makes little difference how one proceeds as long as all parts are observed carefully.

MYELOGRAPHY

Myelography consists in the introduction of a contrast substance into the spinal subarachnoid space to render it visible in roentgenograms. It is used to confirm the presence of a lesion that is strongly suspected clinically; to identify the lesion's extent, size, and level; and to find, or exclude the possibility of, multiple lesions. It is also of value in the study of patients with suspected degenerative lesions of the cord. Postsurgical (laminectomy) complications or persistent pain may also be studied, but the presence of arachnoiditis may preclude accurate interpretation in some of these patients. Either a gas such as air or oxygen, which is less opaque than the cerebrospinal fluid, or a material such as an iodized oil, which is more radiopaque than the fluid, can be used as the contrast substance. The major contraindication to the use of iodine-containing compounds in myelography is a documented history of the patient's adverse reaction to iodine in the past. Blood in the spinal canal is an absolute contraindication to the use of Pantopaque as the contrast medium since there is evidence to indicate that the presence of blood potentiates the irritating effect of this material. Metrizamide (Amipaque), a water-soluble medium, can be used in the presence of blood, however. The main advantage of air or oxygen is that either one is absorbed rapidly from the subarachnoid space and leaves no residues. Disadvantages include: (1) The contrast between the gas and the soft tissues is not very high and visualization often is poor. (2) It is difficult to control the gas once it has been introduced and it will ascend rapidly into the cerebral ventricles and other intracranial spaces if the patient's head and thorax are elevated unless the head is in full extension; (3) In the cervical region, air in the trachea interferes with visualization when the patient is in the anteroposterior position. If gas is used, tomography is essential to improve visualization and help eliminate objectionable shadows. In addition to tomography, it is also necessary to have fluoroscopy available and to be able to tilt the table as an aid to keeping the gas in the spinal subarachnoid space and out of the intracranial spaces and ventricular system. Although the use of air myelography is limited, indications for it include iodine sensitivity, cervical disc herniation or spondylotic myelopathy, hydromyelia, intramedullary tumors, cervical trauma, and congenital anomalies. It is preferable to the use of large-volume Pantopaque in these situations because it will reveal small changes in the contour and caliber of the cord which may be obscured by Pantopaque.

Water-soluble contrast materials have been used more extensively in the Scandinavian and other European countries than in the United States. Prior to the development of metrizamide, all of these materials have been more irritating than oily media and adverse side effects have prevented their wide acceptance in this country. Furthermore, the agents used until recently required spinal anesthesia. Adhesive arachnoiditis, which occurs as a late complication of myelography, is severe enough to diminish markedly the diagnostic value of subsequent myelographic study. Meglumine (methylglucamine) iocarmate (Dimer-X) is less irritating than agents used earlier and does not require spinal anesthesia, but because it may cause clonic spasm, its use is restricted to the lumbar spinal canal.

The new water-soluble contrast agent, metrizamide, has less acute and chronic neurotoxicity than other agents available have, and no instance of post-myelography adhesive arachnoiditis has been reported following its use in humans. Currently, it appears to be the water-soluble agent of choice for myelography. The advantages are: it is absorbed and need not be removed; with it the subarachnoid space can be examined and visualized in greater detail than with Pantopaque; it is the only water-soluble medium now available that can be used for examination of the spinal cord and related structures above the lumbar area.

Oil Myelography

Oil myelography consists in the injection of radiopaque oil into the spinal subarachnoid space, usually by way of lumbar puncture. Early investigations of the spinal canal by this method were carried out with an iodized poppyseed oil known as Lipiodol. This material has been supplanted by iodophenylundecylic acid (Pantopaque). This is an oily substance that depends upon its iodine content for radiopacity. It produces a very opaque shadow in roentgenograms, is visualized easily during fluoroscopy, and can be removed after the examination is completed. Pantopaque is not miscible with the cerebrospinal fluid. It is heavier than the fluid and can be displaced up or down the spinal canal by means of gravity. For this reason the examination is performed with the patient on a tilting fluoroscopic table that can be changed from vertical to at least a 60-degree Trendelenberg position; a 90-degree tilt in both directions is preferred, however.

Pantopaque is slightly irritating and, if allowed to remain in the subarachnoid space, will cause a temporary pleocytosis. There has been some difference of opinion concerning the long-term effects of the oil on the arachnoid membrane when it is left in contact over a period of time. However, experience with Pantopaque now extends over many years, and a great many thousands of examinations and numerous reports affirm that significant reactions from its use are uncommon. While in some departments the oil is left in place after the examination is completed we prefer to remove it if possible.

Technique. The injection usually is made in the lumbar area. The preferred site of lumbar puncture varies and depends to a large extent upon the clinical findings. If the examination is being performed because herniation of a lumbar intervertebral disc is suspected the puncture should be made at the second or third lumbar interspace. Because the majority of herniated lumbar discs are found at the fourth and fifth interspaces it is better that the puncture be made at a site other than at the level of the lesion. If the clinical signs and symptoms indicate that the lesion may be at a higher level, the puncture should be made in one of the lower lumbar interspaces. Venous extravasation is a rare occurrence in myelography, but in two-thirds of the cases reported the puncture was performed at the lumbosacral junction. Furthermore, this interspace is the most frequent site of a herniated disc and should not be used for lumbar puncture if possible. It is important, particularly when investigating for a possible disc herniation, to make the needle puncture with the patient in a prone position, being careful to see that the needle enters directly in the midline. This can be checked by fluoroscopy and by spot roentgenograms if necessary. A direct midline puncture lessens the chance for injection of the material into the subdural or epidural spaces, and makes it much easier to aspirate the oil when the examination has been completed. Should the point of the needle enter the subarachnoid space to one side of the midline, the bevel of the needle may only partially penetrate the arachnoid and part of the oil may be injected directly into the subdural space. A satisfactory study cannot be done if much of the oil is extraarachnoidal. An offset needle also makes it difficult to aspirate the oil.

The amount of oil to be injected varies from 12 to 15 ml for lumbar and cervical myelography in the average adult. For the thoracic area, larger amounts, ranging from 25 to 30 ml, usually suffice. Occasionally it is advisable to fill the spinal canal with amounts of Pantopaque ranging up to 90 ml (large-volume myelography); this is especially useful in evaluating patients with scoliosis when an organic cause is suspected. However, gas or the water-soluble agent metrizamide is superior for evaluation in these circumstances.

After the oil has been injected into the subarachnoid space, the needle is left in place while fluoroscopy is carried out and the oil displaced throughout the region of interest. The examiner watches for defects in the oil column and obstructions to its free flow. Spot roentgenograms are made during fluoroscopy of the various parts of the canal and particularly of any defects or suspicious areas. Lateral decubitus views (horizontal beam) are useful in detecting laterally placed lesions, in eliminating flow defects, particularly in the thoracic region, in demonstrating that apparent block is not complete, and in obtaining satisfactory studies in patients with scoliosis. Oblique and cross-table lateral views are obtained in addition to anteroposterior views to include each level in lumbar myelography. For cervical myelography the head of the table is lowered gradually and the oil moved over the dorsal curvature. By keeping the patient's head in extreme extension it is usually possible to prevent the oil from entering the cranial cavity. In patients with acute cervical and thoracic trauma, it is sometimes preferable to introduce Pantopaque by way of a lateral puncture at the C1-2 level so that it will not be necessary to extent the upper cervical spine to keep the oil out of the cranium. Furthermore, maintenance of cervical traction is very difficult if the head must be hyperextended. Air myelography is preferable when cord atrophy secondary to trauma is suspected. As soon as the oil has accumulated in the upper cervical region the table is brought to the horizontal position and the oil then will remain in the dependent part of the cervical curve so that by slight changes in the level of the table the entire cervical canal can be inspected without much chance of the oil escaping into the intracranial cisterns. Oil that has entered the cranial cavity is difficult to dislodge and most of it will remain there. At times it is necessary to examine the upper part of the cervical canal, including the cisterna magna. By proper tilting and positioning of the head it is usually possible to carry the oil into the cranial cavity overlying the clivus almost to the level of the dorsum sellae. In these cases some of the oil may spill into the cisterns and cannot be removed. Anteroposterior views to include the entire cervical area are obtained in addition to horizontal-beam lateral projections. Occasionally oblique views may be indicated.

In thoracic myelography, horizontal-beam anteroposterior views plus vertical-beam lateral views are obtained with the patient in right and left lateral positions in addition to anteroposterior prone and horizontal-beam lateral projections. For complete evaluation of the thoracic area, it is necessary to use either a high-volume technique so that the spinal cord is surrounded by contrast medium or to turn the patient supine. The latter may be done without removal of the needle if adequate bolsters are available.

When the examination has been completed, the oil column is brought under the point of the needle by fluoroscopic control and it then is aspirated. If a satisfactory placement of the spinal puncture needle was accomplished, complete removal of the oil usually is possible with the exception of a few small drops or streaks that may be caught around the nerve roots. If a poorly placed needle is responsible for difficulty, sometimes it is advisable to perform another puncture at a different level.

The rate of absorption of Pantopaque that may have been left in the subarachnoid space is extremely slow and has been estimated to be about 1 cc per year or less. The oil tends to remain freely movable and can be displaced by gravity for a long time after the injection. It is common to find small droplets of oil in the basal cisterns of the skull in patients who have had an oil myelogram without complete removal of the oil. Should an individual with oil in the spinal canal stoop over or assume a position in which the head and trunk are lower than the buttocks the oil can move rapidly into the cranial cavity and, once there, may become lodged. The chance for harm from oil lodged in the intracranial subarachnoid space is remote. Myelography should be performed only when there are sufficient clinical indications for it and it should not be looked upon as a screening procedure.

Normal Results. The appearance of myelograms with normal findings is shown in the accompanying illustrations (Figs. 12-1 through 12-4). In the lumbar region there usually are small triangular projections on either side of the oil column at each vertebral level. These are known as axillary pouches or root pouches and they represent extensions of the arachnoid along the inferior edges of the nerve roots. Except for these projections, the normal canal is smooth along its lateral borders. The distal end of the thecal sac generally extends below the level of the lumbosacral joint, sometimes as far as the second sacral segment. As an anatomic variant, occasionally a shortened lumbosacral cul-de-sac is present that does not extend below the lumbosacral joint level. This anomaly prevents adequate myelography of the lumbosacral junction.

When viewed from the side there occasionally is seen a smooth anterior bulging of the oil column at the level of each vertebral body, apparently caused by an anatomic variation in the shape of the vertebrae, which have more concave indentations of their posterior surfaces than is usual. This particular configuration may be sufficient to cause the oil to pool at each vertebral body level when the patient is placed in the prone position. It is difficult to examine the discs adequately in these patients and a larger amount of oil than usual may be necessary to form a continuous column. In the thoracic region, axillary pouches are not present except for the upper two or three roots; they are found in the cervical part of the canal and form distinct notchlike shadows at each nerve exit.

In general, examination of the midthoracic part of the canal is unsatisfactory unless a large volume of Pantopaque is used or there is an obstruction present. It is difficult to keep the oil in a solid column when the head of the table is tilted so that the oil will flow over the dorsal curvature.

A series of examples of metrizamide myelography are included (Fig. 12-5 through 12-12) to show the value of this medium in outlining detail.

Artifacts

Needle Defects. A traumatic spinal puncture with laceration of a blood vessel may lead to the formation of a hematoma at the site of puncture. This is more likely to happen when difficulty has been encountered in attempting to enter the subarachnoid space or when the needle is laterally situated and does not enter the dural sac in or close to the midline. A needle defect interferes with interpretation because it resembles a herniated disc. As a rule it can be recognized as an artifact because the needle will be centrally situated within the area of the filling defect and the upper and lower borders taper smoothly and gradually (Fig. 12-13). It is possible, of course, to have a herniated disc and a needle defect at the same location; if the clinical signs point to a lesion at the same level and on the same side, it is almost impossible to determine the true state of affairs. For this reason, as recommended in the paragraphs dealing with technique, when a herniated lumbar intervertebral disc is suspected clinically, the needle puncture should be carried out at a level other than where the clinical localization indicates the hernia to be. The preferred sites are at the second and third lumbar interspaces. When a needle defect causes difficulty in interpretation it is advisable to discontinue the examination, aspirate as much of the oil as possible, and repeat the

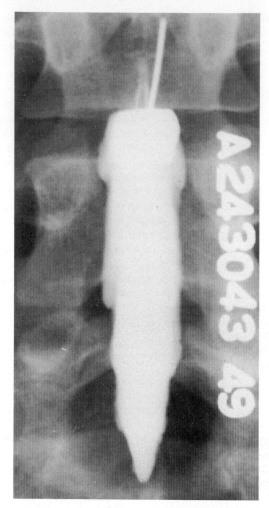

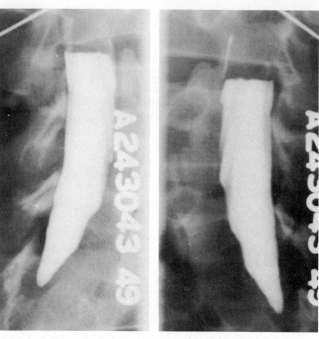

Fig. 12-2. Lumbar myelogram—normal findings. Oblique views with the subject upright. The nerve roots are visible as linear radiolucencies. The upper end of the oil column is flat, indicating that the subject is in a vertical position.

Fig. **12-1.** Lumbar myelogram—normal findings. The typical cone-shaped configuration of the sacral cul-de-sac is shown. The axillary root pouches vary slightly on the two sides. This does not necessarily signify abnormality.

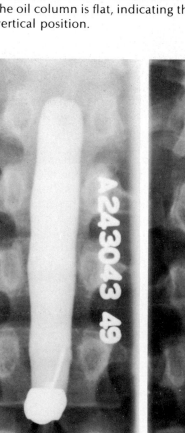

Fig. 12-3. Myelogram of the lower thoracic and upper lumbar region—normal findings.

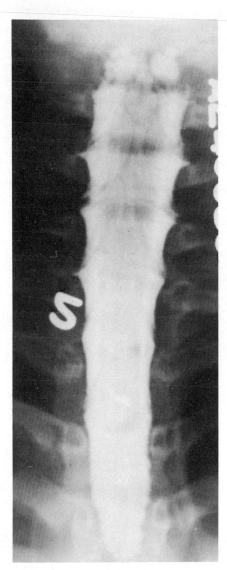

Fig. 12-4. Cervicothoracic myelogram—normal findings. In the cervical canal the axillary pouches and nerve roots are quite well seen, and in the thoracic region there are only slight projections at the sites of the nerve exits. The cord forms a distinct translucent central area surrounded by the radiopaque oil.

study at a later date, preferably after an interval of a week or 10 days.

Globule Formation. At times the oil breaks up into multiple drops or globules during injection or globule formation occurs while the examintion is in progress (Fig. 12-14). Slow or intermittent injection of the oil

favors globule formation. The contrast substance should be injected in a steady stream so that it flows from the needle in a solid column rather than in drops. In displacing the oil into the cervical region it sometimes breaks up into globules as it passes over the thoracic curvature. Proper tilting of the table helps to prevent this but in some cases it cannot be avoided. Fortunately, globule formation often disappears during the examination, so that by the time roentgenograms are to be made the oil has become a solid mass.

Subdural Oil. Improper placement of the needle so that the bevel is only part way through the arachnoid membrane may lead to a partial injection of the oil into the subdural rather than into the subarachnoid space. Difficulty in doing the spinal puncture with repeated attempts to enter the subarachnoid space may result in a laceration of the filmy arachnoid and allow escape of the oil. If the myelography is performed within a week or 10 days after a spinal puncture, there is some chance for leakage of oil. It is preferable not to precede oil myelography by another spinal puncture or, if a puncture has been done, to wait a week or longer before doing the myelography. Oil in the subdural space can be recognized by the sluggish way that it moves when the table is tilted and by the characteristic tapered ends of the oil accumulations. Also the oil does not assume a dependent position on the cross-table lateral projection. An example of subdural oil is shown in Figure 12-14B. It is very important to recognize that the oil is in the subdural space because the contours of such oil masses simulate filling defects when none actually exist. The subdural space rarely fills completely and the spaces that remain suggest the presence of tumor or disc herniation. Typically these defects do not remain constant during tilting of the table. Inconstancy of a filling defect during fluoroscopy should alert the examiner to the possibility that the oil is subdural rather than subarachnoid in location. When oil has entered the subdural space an attempt should be made to aspirate it. If this is not possible, it may be necessary to discontinue the examination and wait until the oil has become more widely dispersed. This may require several weeks or even longer.

Epidural Injection. Oil that has been injected or that extravasates extradurally accumulates in the form of streaky shadows along the spinal canal and extends for some distance along the nerve roots. A characteristic example of epidural oil is shown in Figure 12-4C. The presence of extradural oil interferes greatly with

(*Text continues on p. 422.*)

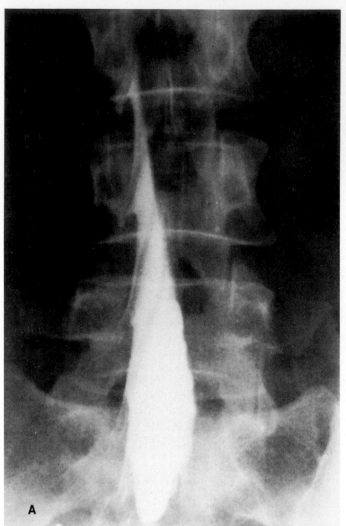

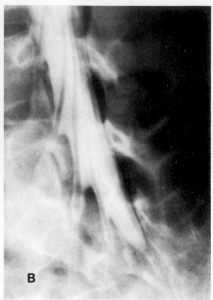

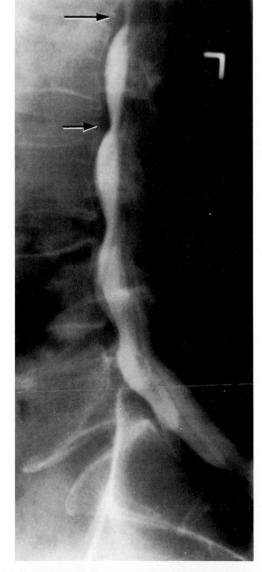

Fig. 12-5. A. Horizontal beam anteroposterior projection showing the normal relationships of the thecal sac and spinal nerves to the vertebral column. **B.** The normal relationships of the spinal nerves to the pedicles and posterior bony elements are shown in the oblique projection. (Sackett JF, Strother CM: New Techniques in Myelography. Hagerstown, Harper & Row, 1979)

Fig. 12-6. Metrizamide myelogram. Slight indentations in the contrast column are seen at L1, L2, and L2–3 interspace **(arrows).** These may be normal. (Sackett JF, Strother CM: New Techniques in Myelography. Hagerstown, Harper & Row, 1979)

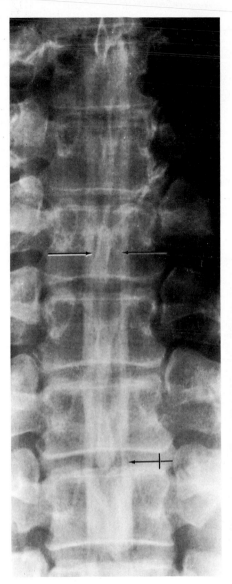

Fig. 12-7. Metrizamide myelogram. Dilute contrast medium in the thoracic subarachnoid space following lumbar myelography (270 mgI/ml). The spinal cord is outlined between arrows. Thoracic nerve root exiting **(crossed arrow).** (Sackett JF, Strother CM: New Techniques in Myelography. Hagerstown, Harper & Row, 1979)

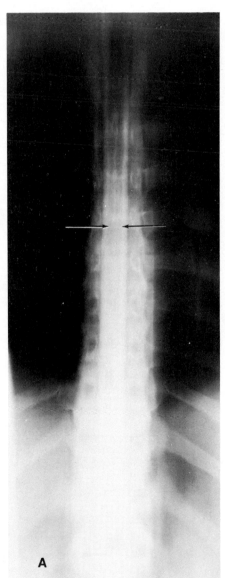

Fig. 12-8. Metrizamide myelogram. **A.** Frontal tomogram. Thoracic spinal cord between **arrows. B.** Midsagittal tomogram. Thoracic spinal cord between **arrows.** (Sackett JF, Strother CM: New Techniques in Myelography, Hagerstown, Harper & Row, 1979)

Fig. 12-9. Smooth filling of posterior thoracic sub-arachnoid space with metrizamide **(arrow).** (Sackett JF, Strother CM: New Techniques in Myelography. Hagerstown, Harper & Row, 1979)

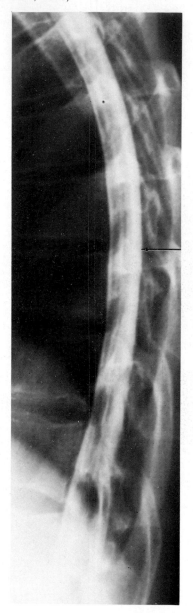

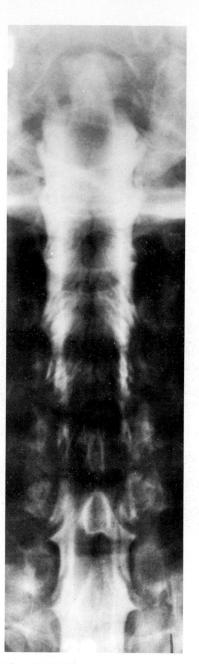

Fig. 12-10. Posteroanterior cervical metrizamide myelogram. The first cervical roots pass horizontally through the subarachnoid space. Below this level the nerve roots have increasingly progressive downward inclination within the subarachnoid space. The diameter of the spinal cord is maximal between C3 and C5. This represents a normal cervical enlargement. Extradural defects are present at the C5–6 level bilaterally. (Sackett JF, Strother CM: New Techniques in Myelography. Hagerstown, Harper & Row, 1979)

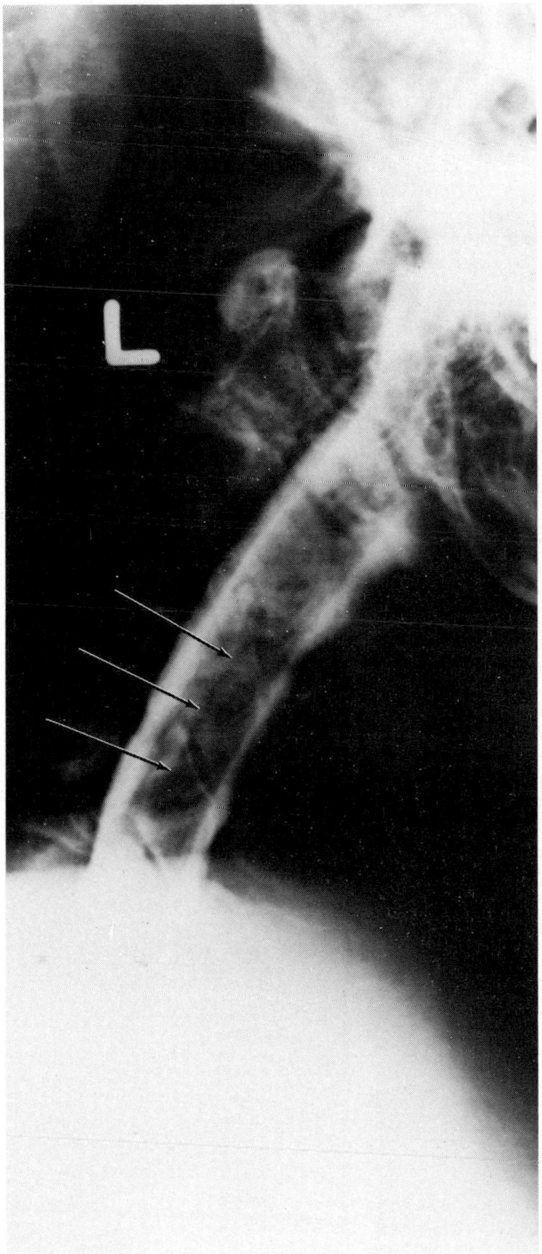

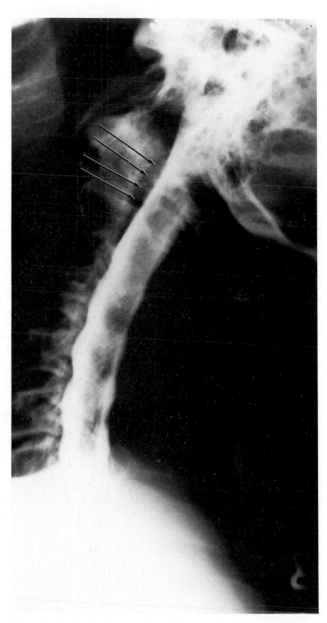

Fig. 12-11. Lateral metrizamide cervical myelogram. The dentate ligament is well visualized **(arrows).** The multiple interlacing defects seen posteriorly represent posterior nerve roots. (Sackett JF, Strother CM: New Techniques in Myelography. Hagerstown, Harper & Row, 1979)

Fig. 12-12. Lateral metrizamide cervical myelogram. The widening of the epidural space adjacent to the odontoid process is normal **(arrows).** This should not be confused with a ventral epidural mass. Minimal ventral bulges at the level of the intervertebral disc below this level also represent normal findings. (Sackett JF, Strother CM: New Techniques in Myelography. Hagerstown, Harper & Row, 1979)

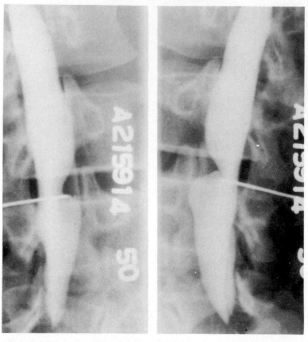

Fig. 12-13. Needle defect. Oblique lumbar myelograms show a deep indentation directly beneath the point of the needle.

the examination and it usually is necessary to defer further study for several weeks, until the material has become dispersed or partially absorbed.

DISCOGRAPHY

Discography consists in the direct injection of a water-soluble contrast material, such as Conray–60, into the intervertebral disc and the making of suitable roentgenograms. The contrast material is injected through a needle that has been inserted by way of lumbar puncture through the posterior annulus fibrosis into the disc substance. First introduced by Lindblom of Sweden in 1950, the method has received some acceptance in this country.[14] It has been recommended for use particularly in those patients complaining of low back pain with sciatic radiation, in whom standard contrast myelography has failed to reveal abnormality. Degenerative changes in the disc, anterior ruptures, and rupture into the vertebral body can be visualized. Many believe that discography is of little value in patients over 35 years of age.

Following injection of the Hypaque or Conray into the disc, anteroposterior, lateral, and oblique views are obtained. Normally the disc can hold no more than 0.25 to 0.5 ml of contrast medium. When the disc is ruptured or degenerated, 2.5 ml or more may

Fig. 12-14. A. Globule formation in a lumbar oil myelogram. **B.** Extra-arachnoid subdural oil injection. The oil separates into masses of irregular shape but with tapered ends. **C.** Epidural oil injection.

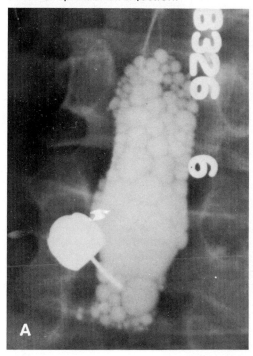
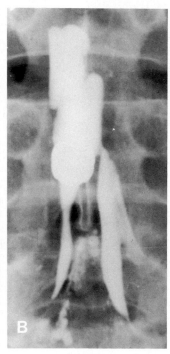
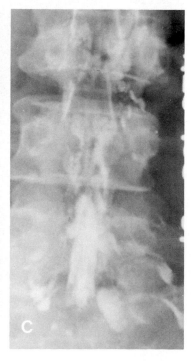

be injected, often reproducing the patient's pain. A leak of the opaque medium out of the area of the normal disc indicates rupture, but not necessarily a symptomatic disc rupture.

Discography does not replace oil myelography for the detection of herniated disc and, in our experience, has a limited field of usefulness, usually in patients with atypical symptoms and myelographic findings.

LUMBAR EPIDURAL VENOGRAPHY

This is a method[10] used in recent years to opacify the epidural venous plexus by selective catheterization of the ascending lumbar and/or internal iliac veins. In patients with lateral disc herniation at the L5-S1 level, a compression or occlusion of an epidural and/or radicular vein at the disc level indicates protrusion. The examination may be useful in patients with normal or equivocal myelographic findings with strong clinical evidence to suggest compression of the root of a lumbar nerve which could be caused by a herniated intervertebral disc. It is of limited usefulness in the postoperative patient, however.[18]

ARTERIOGRAPHY OF THE SPINAL CORD

This examination requires bilateral selective catheterization of vertebral and costocervical trunks to outline the vascular supply at the cervical and high thoracic levels of the cord.[7] Selective bilateral intercostal and lumbar arteriography from T8 to L2 will identify the great anterior radicular artery of Adamkiewicz. The upper and midthoracic blood supply is from small radicular feeding arteries. At times, there are segmental cutaneous angiomas on the back which may indicate the site of an anterovenous malformation of the spinal cord. Bentson and Crandall[1] use a Fogarty balloon catheter in performing a preoperative test for possible cord ischemia prior to ligation of a feeding vessel. A 2-hour period of balloon inflation resulted in obliteration by clotting in one of their patients. Percutaneous embolization has been used successfully in treatment of these vascular malformations; steel pellets, gelfoam, and muscle fragments have been employed to induce clotting. This is a valuable alternative when surgical excision is not feasible.

Arteriovenous malformation of the cord is the major indication for spinal arteriography. Of the tumors involving the cord, hemangioblastoma and hypervascular glioma show the most striking findings of tumor vessels and stain, as well as displacement of the anterior spinal artery and rapid arteriovenous shunting. Arteriography may also be used in the study of posttraumatic paraplegia in which it is helpful in determining the extent of vascular damage. Some authors suggest its use in the study of scoliosis prior to surgery so that the site of major cord feeders is identified and can be protected during surgical corrective procedures.

POSTERIOR HERNIATION OF INTERVERTEBRAL DISC

Rupture of an intervertebral disc with extrusion of disc material into a vertebral body has been considered in Chapter 3. When the rupture occurs along the posterior or posterolateral surface of the disc, the mass of herniated disc material projects into the spinal canal or an intervertebral foramen. It may impinge upon a nerve root and is a frequent cause of low back pain with sciatic radiation. The clinical aspects of herniated intervertebral disc have been treated extensively in the literature and pertinent references are given at the end of this chapter. The diagnosis of a herniated intervertebral disc often can be made with considerable assurance from the clinical history and physical findings. However, many clinicians believe that the diagnosis should be confirmed by myelography in most cases. Clinical localization may not always be possible or completely reliable, the diagnosis may be in doubt, and other lesions can give rise to clinical findings, resembling those of a herniated disc. The indications for the procedure must be definite, however; the possible dangers have been mentioned previously.

The majority of herniated discs occur in the lumbar spine and most of these affect either the fourth or fifth disc. Only a small percentage of lumbar disc herniations are found above the fourth interspace level. The lesion is uncommon in the thoracic area except for an occasional case encountered in the lower thoracic disc interspaces. Posterior disc herniation in the cervical area is not infrequent, although less common than in the lumbar spine.

The varied terminology used in discussions concerning herniated discs is somewhat confusing; in order to avoid misunderstanding, in the present discussion the following usage is implied:

1. *Posterior disc herniation* and *ruptured intervertebral disc* are terms used synonymously to denote a rupture of the posterior part of the annulus fibrosus with extrusion of a mass of disc substance that projects into the spinal canal.

2. *Posterior disc protrusion* or *ridging* is a condition in which the annulus fibrosus is intact but there is a smooth, ridgelike bulging of the disc posteriorly. This condition is usually associated with and a part of degenerative disease affecting the spine. In association with a weakened annulus and a posterior bulging of the disc there frequently is hypertrophic bony spurring or osteophyte formation along the posterior or posterolateral edges of the adjacent vertebral bodies, resulting in a bony ledge projecting into the canal.

PLAIN ROENTGENOGRAMS OF THE SPINE

Roentgenograms of the spine may reveal no abnormality when a herniated intervertebral disc is present. More often there are one or more abnormal findings which, in the main, while suggestive of the presence of disc degeneration, are not specific for this condition. A combination of these signs is more significant than any one alone. These include:

Straightening or Reversal of the Lumbar Lordotic Curve. This abnormality is usually the result of muscle spasm. Because there are many causes for spasm of the low-back muscles, it is of limited value as an isolated observation.

Listing of the Lumbar Spine to One Side. This finding also is the result of muscle spasm. The list may be toward the side of the hernia or away from it.

Narrowing of the Disc Interspace. The amount of disc material that has been extruded is seldom enough to cause a discernible thinning of the intervertebral disc space as seen in roentgenograms. When thinning of the interspace is present in association with a disc hernia it is an indication of degenerative disease of the disc. This may have preceded the herniation or it may have followed it. Because localized thinning of an intervertebral disc, usually the fourth or the fifth lumbar, is a very frequent observation in this area without an associated hernia, thinning cannot be relied upon as a good diagnostic sign. It is not at all infrequent to find a thinned disc at one lumbar interspace and to demonstrate, by myelography and at subsequent surgery, a herniation at a different level where the height of the disc space was normal.

Posterior Offset of the Fifth Lumbar Vertebra on the Sacrum. Associated with a reversal of the lumbar lordotic curvature, the posterior surface of the fifth lumbar vertebra may appear to lie slightly behind the corresponding surface of the upper sacrum (reverse spondylolisthesis). This finding too is not specific for a herniated disc but when combined with some of the other observations as has been noted it becomes of greater significance.

Calcification of the Extruded Disc Material. This is a very reliable sign but is not observed very often. Calcified disc material in the spinal canal is found in a higher percentage of thoracic than lumbar disc ruptures. Thoracic protrusions are uncommon and are usually central or slightly eccentric; lateral protrusion occurs rarely.

Posterior Osteophytes on the Vertebral Bodies. Spurs or osteophytes may be found along the posterior or posterolateral edges of the vertebrae contiguous to a disc hernia. The presence of such spurs is positive evidence that at least a posterior bulging or protrusion of the disc is present, but they do not indicate whether there has been an actual rupture of the annulus fibrosus with extrusion of disc material. These osteophytes are a manifestation of degenerative disease (Fig. 12-15).

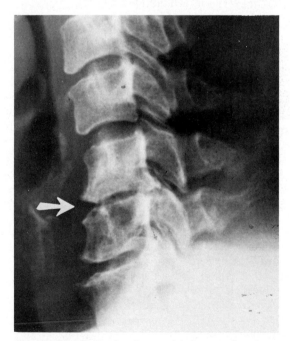

Fig. 12-15. Posterior bony ridging at the C5–6 level. The intervening disc is thin **(arrow).** There is slight backward offset of C5 on C6 in addition to the posterior spurs.

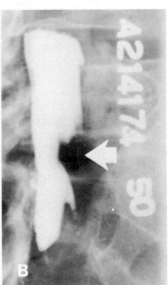

Fig. 12-16. Lumbar intervertebral disc herniation. **A.** Large herniated disc on the right at the fourth interspace. The notchlike filling defect is characteristic. **B.** Herniated disc on the right side of the L4–5 interspace **(arrow). C.** Small defect on the left caused by herniated disc at the lumbosacral interspace.

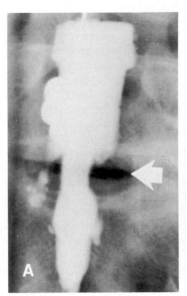
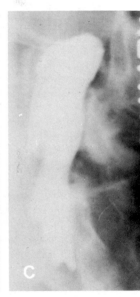

Fig. 12-17. Lumbar intervertebral disc herniation. Anteroposterior **(A)**, left **(B)**, and right **(C)** oblique views. There is a bilateral defect, but it is much larger on the right **(arrows)** than on the left side.

OIL MYELOGRAPHY

Because a herniated disc is a space-taking mass that encroaches upon the subarachnoid space it will cause a filling defect when radiopaque oil is injected into the space. Characteristically the defect is seen as a sharply outlined, smooth, unilateral indentation or notch in the oil shadow along the anterolateral aspect of the spinal canal. The axillary root pouch is either obliterated at the site of the defect or else it is displaced or distorted. Oblique views often bring out the defect to best advantage because they show it tangentially. Lateral decubitus views are valuable in detecting the more laterally placed lesions. Some typical examples of lumbar disc hernias are shown in Figures 12-16 and 12-17. Herniation at the fourth lumbar interspace usually causes a clear-cut and characteristic defect because the meninges are closely approximated to the anterior and lateral bony walls of the spinal canal, and encroachment upon the space by the hernia readily deforms the oil column. Because the lumbosacral cul-de-sac narrows gradually to a smooth rounded or pointed termination, there may be considerable space in the canal outside the dural sac at the level of the lumbosacral disc. The defect of a hernia often is less obvious at this interspace than when a mass of similar size has herniated at the level of the fourth disc. At times a lumbosacral defect is quite inconspicuous, being limited to a slight anterolateral indentation on the oil column with slight elevation of the axillary root pouch. Even a minor defect of this nature at this interspace must be viewed with considerable suspicion, especially when clinical findings indicate nerve root compression on that side and level. In itself a unilateral failure of filling of an axillary root pouch is not sufficient to indicate the existence of herniation since this is not infrequent as a normal variation. There must be some evidence of encroachment upon the contrast column even though this be very slight. It is in these cases that oblique views are particularly helpful. If the cul-de-sac is unusually short and terminates at or above the level of the lumbosacral disc, it is possible to have a rather large hernia without myelographic evidence of its presence.

Occasionally a very large herniation will completely or almost completely obstruct the canal and may mimic a tumor very closely. In fact a herniated disc, being an extradural mass, can cause myelographic changes similar to those of a tumor such as a small neurofibroma. It is chiefly the characteristic location of the lesion that is significant in diagnosis. At other times the extruded cartilage will become separated completely from the disc and lie free in the subarachnoid space. It may be displaced from its site of origin. In these cases the defect may be found behind a vertebral body rather than at a disc interspace and in rare instances it will be found along the posterior aspect of the canal rather than the anterior. It may be impossible to exclude the possibility of a neoplasm as a cause for such a defect.

In the cervical region, disc hernias are found most frequently at the fifth and sixth interspaces. The defect caused by the herniation may be large and notchlike and resemble that of a lumbar herniation. In other patients the herniation is small and laterally placed and produces a unilateral small, rounded or triangular defect that obliterates the root sleeve at the affected level. In some cases, the chief manifestation is a deformity of the axillary root pouch (Fig. 12-18). Because the hernia projects into a spinal foramen, the clinical signs of nerve root impingement may be severe; the small size of a myelographic defect does not necessarily indicate a clinically insignificant lesion.

Further Observations

Transverse Disc Ridging. Posterior bulging of a disc without actual herniation of disc material is known as "posterior disc protrusion" or "ridging." The lesion is a frequent accompaniment of degenerative joint disease of the spine. Also, hypertrophy of the ligamenta flava is frequently associated. As a result of these changes, pressure on a spinal nerve root may cause signs and symptoms suggestive of a herniated disc. The lesion may be found in any part of the spine but is infrequent in the thoracic area. In the cervical and lumbar areas, multiple disc ridging often is present. Neurosurgeons frequently speak of ridging as a "hard disc" in contrast to the "soft disc" of a true herniation. The bony marginal osteophytes are particularly prone to encroach upon the contiguous spinal foramen.

Roentgen Findings. Disc-space thinning and posterior or posterolateral spurs may be noted on plain roentgenograms (see Fig. 12-15). However, disc ridging can occur without significant plain-film findings although this is unusual. Often one can postulate the presence of the lesion from these plain-film findings. On myelography, disc ridging causes a transverse lucent defect in the oil column. If lateral cross-table views are obtained with the patient prone, a smooth, anterior indentation on the oil column will be seen at the affected disc level. In posteroanterior views the ridge may cause a transverse bandlike lucency (Fig. 12-19). Also bilateral indentations may be seen causing an hourglass type of deformity. If there is associated hypertrophy of the ligamenta flava these defects are accentuated (Fig. 12-20). Herniated disc may be present at the same level as the ridge but more often it exists alone. It accentuates the filling defect on the side of the herniation, and elevates and compresses the corresponding nerve root more than is seen with ridging alone. At times it is difficult to determine if both conditions are present or not.

The significance of such ridging is difficult to determine. In the cervical region, it is related to the anteroposterior diameter of the spinal canal. If this diameter is reduced to 13 mm or less there are often signs of cord compression and the lesion is significant. In the lumbar region as well the clinical symptoms determine the significance of the ridging, therefore history and physical findings must be correlated with myelographic findings in these cases.

The Postoperative Myelogram. The interpretation of myelograms performed after laminectomy and surgical removal of a herniated disc is difficult and often unsatisfactory. In many patients there is irregularity and deformity of the oil column at the level of the previous surgery, which are only the result of adhesions in the subarachnoid space. In some cases a filling defect resembling a herniated disc is found but at reoperation there is no evidence of recurrent hernia. In patients with the most severe deformity there may be a complete obstruction to the flow of oil at the level of the previous hernia and laminectomy. In general, slight to moderate irregularities in filling that do not show the characteristic notch defect of a herniated disc are most likely the result of adhesions. If a defect that fulfills the criteria for a herniated disc is found, one is justified in interpreting it as evidence for recurrent disc herniation.

SPINAL CORD TUMORS

Primary tumors of the spinal cord and its coverings can be classified as intramedullary, extramedullary intradural, or extradural. Such a breakdown is important, not only from the standpoint of operability but because of differences in roentgen findings in the three groups. The histologic types of tumors in the order of frequency are as follows: neurofibroma, meningioma, ependymoma, astrocytoma, glioblastoma, and a miscellaneous group including infrequent and rare lesions such as dermoid and epidermoid cysts, epidural cysts, lipomas, and hemangiomas. In addition to the group of primary tumors, metastatic neoplasms cause compression of the cord very frequently. Metastasis may be from extension of a focus in a vertebral body or its arch; less frequently the metastasis is directly to the cord or the meninges. Any malignant tumor can metastasize in this way.

Myelographic findings usually permit differentiation between the three major types of masses observed within the spinal canal. The *intramedullary* tumor usually causes a fusiform enlargement of the cord (see Fig. 12-27) which usually does not cause complete block. The spinal canal may be uniformly widened. *Intradural–extramedullary* masses are usually eccentric and tend to displace the cord and widen the ipsilateral subarachnoid space between the cord and the dura above and below the tumor site. The subarachnoid space is narrowed contralaterally

at the level of the mass and to varying degrees above and below it as a result of cord displacement. Complete obliteration of the subarachnoid space associated with complete block is not infrequent. (See Fig. 12-23.) *Extradural* masses may surround the dura and produce complete block or they may be eccentric and cause partial or complete block. The dura, cord, and the surrounding subarachnoid space are displaced by the latter type of lesion in a rather typical manner (see Fig. 12-24). Below the cord, the major finding is an indentation of the thecal sac corresponding to the site and size of the extradural mass.

EXTRAMEDULLARY TUMORS

Neurofibroma

Neurofibroma is an extramedullary tumor that can be either intradural or extradural in location, with the majority lying beneath the dura. Neurofibromas arise from the spinal nerve roots. In the lumbar area the tumor often is completely within the dural sac. In the thoracic and cervical regions the lesion tends to be of dumbbell type with an intraspinal portion and an extraspinal extension through an intervertebral foramen. In the thoracic area the extraspinal portion of the tumor often is visible because of the contrast afforded by the air-filled lungs. In the cervical region a mass is rarely demonstrated. In the lumbar spine the extraspinal part of the tumor may, if very large, cause an outward bulge of the psoas muscle margin. The intraspinal part of the tumor leads to erosion of the pedicle on one or both sides. Normally the pedicles are seen end-on in anteroposterior roentgenograms as vertical ovoid ringlike shadows (Fig. 12-21). The inner surface usually is convex but may vary from a flattened surface to one slightly concave. Pressure erosion from a neurofibroma causes a thinning of the pedicle with or without a loss of its inner cortical margin. Because of the variations in the contour of normal pedicles, Elsberg and Dyke measured the difference between the inner surfaces of the two pedicles of each vertebra, called the interpediculate distance, and published the results in the form of a chart. Erosion from a neurofibroma usually is limited to one or two vertebrae and comparison of the pedicle shadows above and below the lesion will clearly indicate the presence of abnormality without the need for measurement in most cases. If very large, an intraspinal neurofibroma will cause a smooth, pressure type of erosion of the posterior surface of the vertebral body so that it will have a concave contour as seen in the lateral roentgenogram (Fig. 12-22). A

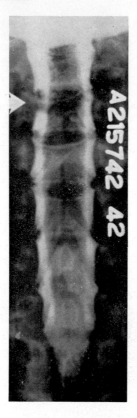

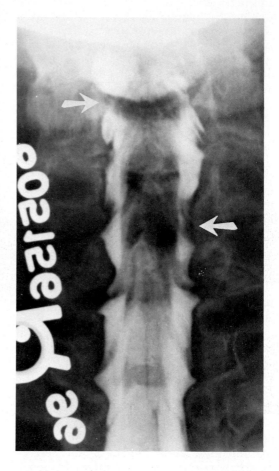

Fig. 12-18. Cervical intervertebral disc herniation. The defect is small **(arrow),** but there is lack of filling of the axillary pouch and a local indentation. Note the clear outline of the cord.

Fig. 12-19. Disc ridging in the cervical area. There is a transverse, translucent defect **(upper arrow)** indicative of a transverse ridge and the unilateral deformity on the left **(lower arrow)** due to posterolateral spurring.

dumbbell tumor will erode the upper and lower surfaces of the pedicles bounding an intervertebral foramen (see Fig. 12-21). Bone changes occur in about 20% of neurofibromas. In patients with neurofibromatosis, posterior scalloping of the vertebral bodies, with concavity resembling pressure erosion as has been described, may be present at several levels in the absence of tumor. There may be associated interpediculate widening, also in the absence of tumor. The changes are presumably caused by dural ectasia. Severe and sharply angulated scoliosis may also be present in these patients.

Neurofibroma as an intraspinal mass is rare in children, but neuroblastoma and ganglioma may pro-

duce an hourglass type of lesion with a paraspinal mass in addition to an extradural tumor compressing the cord. There may be bone changes, such as rib or vertebral erosion, producing pediculate thinning and posterior vertebral scalloping. Punctate calcification may be visible in these tumors.

Myelography. An intradural neurofibroma causes a sharply outlined, round or oval-shaped filling defect. Because the tumor often is large enough to block the canal completely, obstruction to the flow of oil is easily demonstrated and the end of the oil column has a sharp concave margin as it caps the end of the tumor (Fig. 12-23). Although this type of defect is not spe-

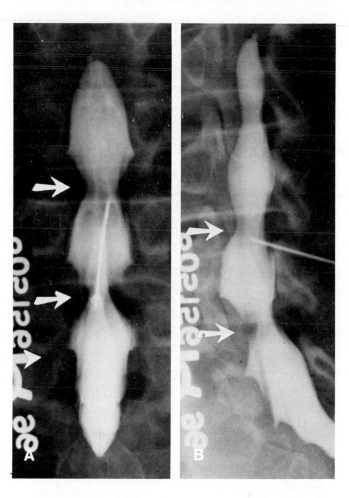

Fig. 12-20. Disc ridging in the lumbar area. **A.** In the posteroanterior view the deformities assume an hourglass configuration **(arrows). B.** The oblique view shows anterior indentations on the oil column **(arrows).**

cific for a neurofibroma, it is always most suggestive of this tumor and if erosive changes in the pedicles also are present the diagnosis is more certain. Sometimes it is important to know the upper limits of a neurofibroma that is above the level of lumbar oil injection. This can be obtained by injecting a small amount of the oil above the lesion, using a lateral puncture at the C1-2 level, and allowing the oil to drop down to the level of the lesion by gravity. Then it will cap the superior surface and the entire extent of the lesion can be established.

Meningioma

Meningiomas are second only to neurofibromas in frequency and are the most common tumor encountered in the thoracic region. Approximately 80% occur in women averaging 40 to 50 years of age. They are usually extramedullary–intradural in location, but occasionally may have an extradural component.

Meningiomas of the cord resemble their counterparts within the cranial cavity in being slowly growing tumors; symptoms usually extend over a period of several years or even longer before the diagnosis is established. Positive findings on plain roentgenograms of the spine are not common in meningiomas. While calcification in the tumor is common in pathologic specimens it is an infrequent finding in roentgenograms. This is due in part to the rather small amount of calcification and in part to the difficulty of visualizing small hazy calcific shadows within the thoracic portion of the spinal canal. If it is visible, calcification within the tumor is virtually pathognomonic of meningioma in the adult. Meningiomas do not erode pedicles or vertebral bodies very often and this sign, of great help in detecting neurofibromas, is not available. The roentgen diagnosis depends to a large extent upon myelography.

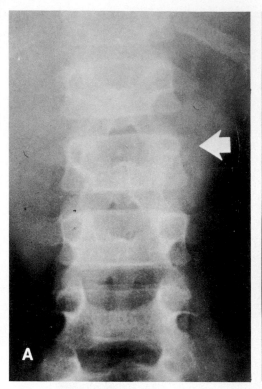
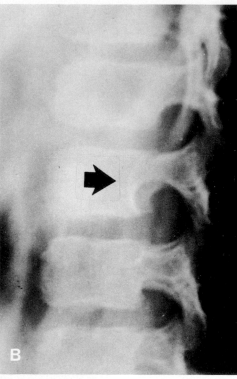

Fig. 12-21. Neurofibroma of the lumbar area. A dumbbell-type tumor protruded through the intervertebral foramen **(A)**, eroding the inner and inferior surface of the left pedicle of the second lumbar vertebra **(arrow)**. The pedicles are visualized as ringlike shadows because they are seen on end, the cortical margin forming the ring. In the lateral view **(B)**, the intraspinal part of the tumor is seen to have eroded the posterior surface of the vertebral body **(arrow)** and to have enlarged the intervertebral foramen.

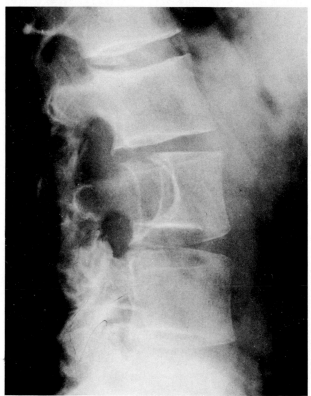

Fig. 12-22. Neurofibroma of the lumbar area. There is erosion of the posterior surface of the third lumbar vertebra. One pedicle is completely destroyed. The other one, which is intact, is clearly visualized.

Myelography. The tumor causes either partial or complete obstruction to the flow of oil. When the block is partial the oil column often narrows slightly just below the lesion and then ends with a fairly sharp cut-off (Fig. 12-24). In other cases the oil column is effaced more gradually. If the block is incomplete, the oil that passes by the defect does so along one side of the canal only and the column has the appearance of being squeezed off rather than sharply cut off as with a neurofibroma. The myelographic signs alone seldom are sufficiently characteristic to make a diagnosis of meningioma; when taken in conjunction with the clinical history and the thoracic location of the lesion the diagnosis is frequently possible. Tomography could be used as an aid in identifying calcification within the tumor, but, since surgery is indicated, tomography is not really necessary.

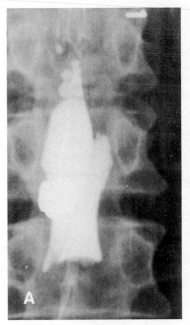
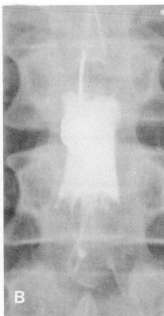

Fig. 12-23. Neurofibroma of a lumbar nerve root. The patient was partially upright in **A** and upright in **B**. The oil was injected at the upper cervical level and has descended to cap the superior surface of the tumor which almost completely obstructs the canal.

Fig. 12-24. Meningioma at the cervicothoracic junction. The oil flowed slowly around the tumor, which was outlined almost completely since it partially obstructed the canal.

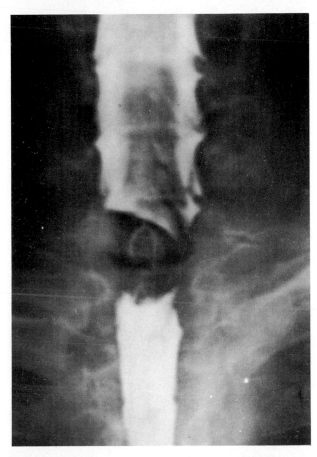

Other Extramedullary Tumors

Intraspinal *dermoid* or *epidermoid* tumors are very rare. Usually they are present in childhood and often are associated with spinal dysraphism. There may be pediculate erosion caused by the tumor. Epidural masses may compress the cord and produce myelographic changes that may be similar in a number of different lesions. These include *osteochondroma*, particularly in patients with hereditary multiple exostoses, which may be diagnosed on plain film study. Rarely, other cartilaginous tumors such as *enchondroma, chondromyxoid fibroma,* and *chondroblastoma* may project into the spinal canal as an extradural mass. Cervical chordoma may also compress the cord; it is usually associated with clearly defined erosion of the posterior aspect of the adjacent vertebrae, and may extend over several segments. Extramedullary hematopoiesis has also been reported as a very rare cause of extradural masses.

Lipoma. Intraspinal lipomas are rare but they produce fairly characteristic roentgen findings. Their

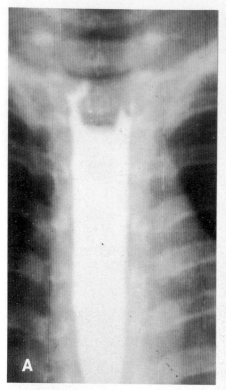

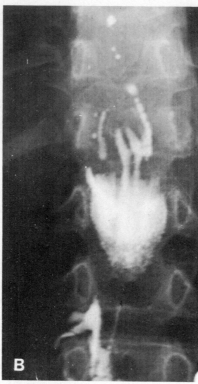

Fig. 12-25. A. Intramedullary tumor (ependymoma) at the level of the first thoracic vertebra. High-grade obstruction is produced by the tumor. **B.** Intramedullary tumor at the thoracolumbar level. Streaks of oil extend around the fusiform enlargement produced by the tumor. Obstruction is not complete.

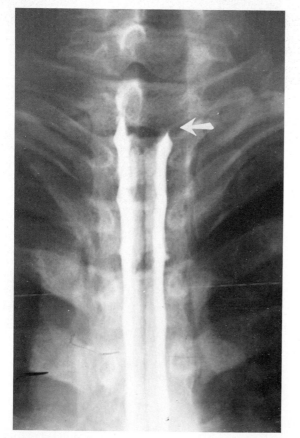

Fig. 12-26. Intramedullary lesion at the level of T1. Note the apparent widening of the central translucency represented by the expanded spinal cord which caused complete obstruction. The lesion was a hematoma.

most frequent site is the thoracic area but some involve the low cervical and thoracic areas and others may involve the low thoracic and lumbar areas. Erosion with thinning of the pedicles results in widening of the interpediculate distance at the level or levels of involvement. At times the lesion may extend over several segments. The pediculate erosion occurs in about one-half of these patients, and there may be some erosion of the posterior surface of the adjacent vertebral bodies resulting in widening of the anteroposterior diameter of the spinal canal. The tumors are often adherent to the cord surface, usually in the posterior position. Despite the size of the mass, complete subarachnoid block is not always evident on myelography. In some instances the tumor may be completely or partially extradural and may then be associated with spina bifida. Many of these tumors are associated with congenital anomalies of the spine; this suggests a developmental origin. Myelography is used to outline the extent of the lesion.

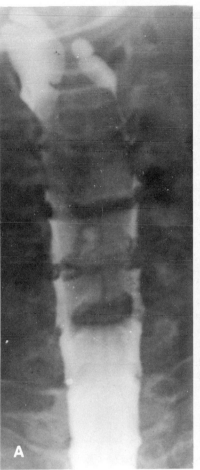 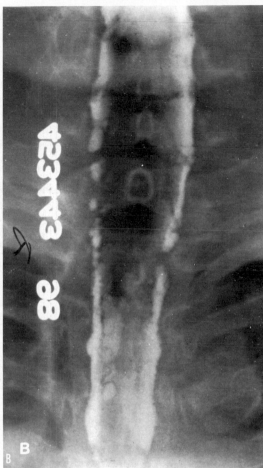

Fig. 12-27. A. Intramedullary astrocytoma involving the cervical cord. The lesion expands the cord but does not completely obstruct the canal. **B.** Syringomyelia. Note the fusiform expansion of the cord in the cervicothoracic area and its similarity to an intramedullary tumor.

Sarcoma. Sarcomas arising in the epidural area are rare. Plain films may show a paraspinal mass, particularly when the lesion is in the thoracic area. When it invades a vertebral body, irregular destruction may be observed, but this is usually a late manifestation. Myelography demonstrates the extradural lesion, which may partially or completely block the flow of oil. As with other epidural tumors, the final diagnosis depends on biopsy, usually performed at the time of surgical decompression and excision.

INTRAMEDULLARY TUMORS

As a group, the intramedullary tumors are uncommon lesions that resemble one another rather closely in their roentgen findings. Ependymomas are the most frequent. In the lumbar region they arise from the filum terminale. An ependymoma is more likely than the other lesions in this group to erode the vertebral pedicles and thus may cause roentgen findings

similar to those observed in neurofibroma. On myelography it may be impossible to distinguish between the lesions because an ependymoma of the filum terminale is usually a well-circumscribed mass and the myelographic defect may resemble that of an intradural neurofibroma (Fig. 12-25). Ependymoma of the filum terminale is intramedullary, but presents as an extramedullary–intradural mass on myelography. When the spinal cord is involved by any of the tumors of this group, the myelogram often is clearly indicative of the intramedullary location of the lesion (Fig. 12-26). Obstruction of the flow of oil may be either partial or complete. When partial, the oil column will be seen to widen out at the level of the tumor with thin streaks of it passing alongside the enlargement of the cord (Fig. 12-27). When the obstruction is complete, the oil shadow widens slightly and is effaced gradually without the sharp cut-off characteristic of an extramedullary intradural mass.

Other intramedullary tumors include astrocytoma,

hemangioblastoma, and oligodendroglioma. Intramedullary hematoma may simulate tumor. Sarcoidosis has also been reported as a rare cause of spinal cord widening.[16]

METASTATIC NEOPLASMS

Extradural metastatic tumors, usually metastatic carcinomas, are frequent lesions compressing the cord by extension from a focus in a vertebra or as an extension of a paravertebral tumor such as plasma cell myeloma and the round cell tumors of childhood.

Hematogenous metastases may result in the attachment of multiple small masses to the cord, the pia arachnoid, or the filum terminale and nerve roots. Carcinomatous and lymphomatous meningeal seeding by way of the cerebrospinal fluid may occur in patients even though they are on systemic chemotherapy. Multiple small filling defects which represent the tumor masses may be observed at myelography. Involvement of the nerve root may present as nodular or a fusiform thickening. More commonly, neurogenic tumors such as medulloblastoma and ependymoma, disseminate by way of the spinal fluid to form multiple nodules similar to those just described. Rarely, sarcoidosis may produce multiple intradural filling defects similar to those due to metastases. Roentgenograms of the spine may reveal the lesion as an area of destruction. Metastatic lesions that cause clinical signs of cord or nerve root compression often have developed in the vertebral arch and the roentgen findings may be minimal and difficult to visualize. A loss of outline of one pedicle sometimes is the only clue to the presence of the lesion.

Myelography. A metastatic lesion large enough to cause clinical signs and symptoms of cord compression will produce some degree of obstruction to the flow of radiopaque oil and in many cases this is complete. If the tumor is extradural, the oil column narrows slightly where the dura is being compressed by the mass. The end of the column tapers gradually (Fig. 12-28). If the block is only partial, droplets of oil may break off the main mass and flow upward on one side of the canal when the patient's head is lowered. Occasionally a metastatic nodule is intradural and extramedullary; rarely it is intramedullary in location. Unless there are associated signs in the vertebrae that clearly indicate the nature of the tumor, it usually is impossible from myelographic evidence to determine whether a given defect is caused by a metastatic tumor or a primary one.

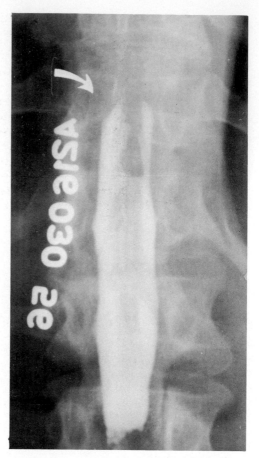

Fig. 12-28. Metastatic lymphosarcoma obstructing the spinal canal at the eleventh thoracic level **(arrow).** This film was exposed with the patient's head lowered about 45 degrees from the horizontal. The tumor is extradural and has surrounded the dura and obstructed the subarachnoid space.

OTHER CONDITIONS

ADHESIVE ARACHNOIDITIS

Arachnoidal adhesions arise from a number of causes, including inflammatory processes and chemical irritation. In some patients the cause remains obscure. The adhesive process can be localized or widespread. There are no plain-roentgen findings in adhesive arachnoiditis. If, during myelography, the adhesive process is localized, an obstruction to the flow of oil is encountered and may be complete. More often the block is incomplete and the oil passes through the region, outlining a rather tortuous channel with irregular filling defects. When the process is more diffuse it may be impossible to displace the oil to any extent after it has been injected into the subarachnoid space and it may accumulate in numerous linear and irregularly shaped cystlike pockets. Less extensive adhesions cause correspondingly less deformity. The diagnosis of adhesive arachnoiditis is a difficult one to make by myelography in some patients. One must be certain that the oil has been injected properly into the subarachnoid space rather than subdurally or epidurally. The latter injections cause artifacts and defects that may resemble those of arachnoid adhesions. One must also be certain that defects suggesting arachnoid adhesions are not merely associated findings secondary to some other lesion such as a herniated disc or a spinal cord tumor. A peculiar form of arachnoiditis has been described in which the only myelographic manifestation is failure of filling of the root sleeves. These blunted root sleeves are now believed to represent the mildest form of adhesive arachnoiditis.

HEMANGIOMA; ARTERIOVENOUS MALFORMATIONS

Hemangioma is a rather rare lesion involving the cord and meninges. A cavernous hemangioma causes irregular tortuous linear defects in oil filling at the site of the lesion (Fig. 12-29). There may be some interference with oil flow but seldom a complete obstruction. The symptoms of arteriovenous malformations appear to be caused by ischemia or recurrent hemorrhage. In hemangioblastoma, cord compression appears to produce the symptoms. As a complication of a cavernous hemangioma, there may be a sudden rupture of one of the vessels with the development of a subdural or epidural hematoma. This causes the rapidly progressive signs of pressure on the spinal cord. Myelography is useful in demonstrating the site of the hematoma.

Angiography is now utilized to demonstrate hemangiomas and other vascular lesions such as arteriovenous malformations and hemangioblastomas. Selective catheterization of the major feeder vessels is done to clearly define the lesion and its nature.

DiChiro and associates[5] describe three basic patterns of pathologic vessels as follows: Type I—a single coiled vessel fed by one artery. Type II—the glomus type in which there is a localized plexus of small coiled vessels confined to a short segment of cord and fed by a single artery; the flow is slow and draining vessels are seldom seen. Type III—the juvenile type found mainly in children, with multiple large feeding arteries supplying a tumorous malformation which may fill the spinal canal; the flow is rapid and draining veins are greatly dilated. These may be outlined myelographically but must also be studied angiographically if surgical removal is contemplated.

Arteriovenous malformations cause myelographic changes similar to those due to cavernous hemangiomas and differentiation may be impossible (see Fig. 12-29). Even on angiography it may be difficult to decide which of these lesions is present.

SPINAL EPIDURAL HEMATOMA

Spinal epidural hematoma may occur as a complication of arteriovenous malformations as indicated previously. Bleeding into the epidural space may also occur secondary to trauma, coagulopathy, anticoagulant therapy, or recent surgery, or it may be spontaneous with no apparent cause. Myelography shows varying degrees of block caused by an epidural mass, usually at the level of the spinal cord but occasionally lower at the level of the cauda equina. History of sudden onset of symptoms with rapid progression leading to paresis or paralysis suggests the cause, but hemorrhage into a tumor may also result in similar clinical findings.

PERINEURIAL CYSTS

As originally described by Tarlov,[20] perineurial root cysts consist of one or more cystlike spaces surrounding the nerve roots, usually in the sacral area. The cysts may or may not communicate with the subarachnoid space of the spinal canal. If they do not, roentgen diagnosis is not possible. With the larger cysts a rounded area of smooth erosion along one or more of the sacral foramina may be demonstrated. When the cysts communicate with the spinal subarachnoid space, they fill with oil during myelography, or subsequently, and then are visualized as rounded pockets close to the sacral cul-de-sac and contiguous to the sacral nerve roots (Fig. 12-30A). It has been our experience that these cysts are demonstrated most frequently when some of the radiopaque oil has been left in the canal and a reexamination of the spine is performed some weeks or months after myelography. Failure to demonstrate a root cyst during immediate myelographic examination does not exclude the possibility of its presence. Similar cystlike extensions of the arachnoid along the nerve roots have been found, rarely, in the lower cervical and upper thoracic regions. Most, if not all, cysts of this

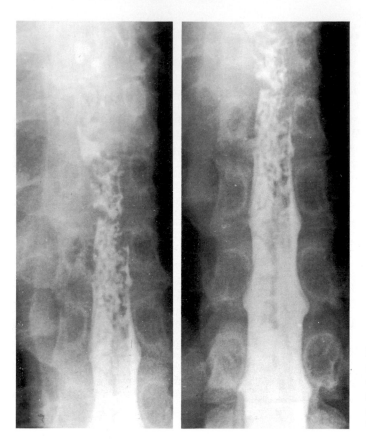

Fig. 12-29. Arteriovenous malformation or cavernous hemangioma in the thoracic area. Numerous tortuous filling defects caused by dilated vessels are observed. Angiography was somewhat equivocal, but arteriovenous malformation was the favored diagnosis.

type are asymptomatic and of no clinical significance. Occasionally they may cause nerve root compression resulting in pain, however.

MENINGEAL CYSTS AND MENINGOCELES

Intra-arachnoid cysts are usually found in the thoracic region and cause no symptoms. They may fill with contrast medium on myelography and produce a pouchlike defect that may retain the medium for a time or may empty with positional change. If not filled, they appear as radiolucent filling defects in the thoracic area. Rarely they become large enough to compress the cord and require surgical decompression.

An *epidural cyst* is a rare lesion found chiefly in the thoracic region. Here it results in the gradual development of a progressive spastic paraplegia. The patient usually is an adolescent and the history usually indicates a gradually progressive lesion. Erosion of the pedicles of multiple vertebrae is common. In some cases there have been findings indicative of a *vertebral epiphysitis of Scheuermann's type* with irregularity of disc surfaces, anterior wedging of the vertebra, and a kyphotic deformity in the spine. This has been thought to be due to disturbance of the blood supply to the vertebrae as a result of the cyst. Myelograms reveal obstruction of extradural type with compression of the oil column (Fig. 12-30B). Some epidural cysts communicate with the subarachnoid space and fill with contrast medium during myelography. Others do not and the myelographic signs then are those of an extradural mass.

Small *meningoceles* may present as a cystlike lesion in the lumbosacral area. We have observed patients in whom a small meningocele eroded the sacral laminae. Meningoceles are not to be confused with the perineurial cysts described in the preceding section. The sacral meningocele may fill with oil and its nature thus becomes apparent (Fig. 12-31).

In addition to the more common lumbar or lumbosacral meningocele usually associated with spinal dysraphism (spina bifida), a meningocele may appear as an intrathoracic posterior mediastinal mass.

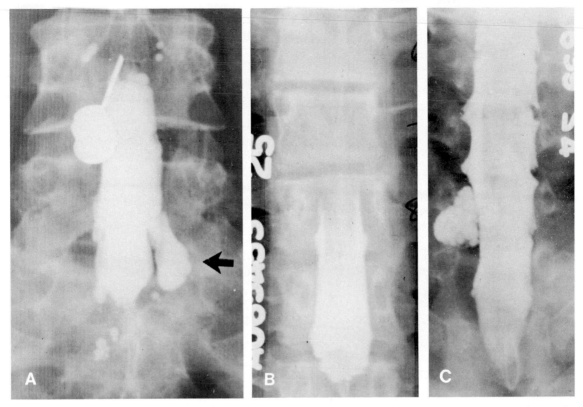

Fig. 12-30. A. Perineurial cyst of the sacral root filled with oil during myelography **(arrow). B.** Epidural cyst obstructing upward flow of the oil. The appearance suggests that the dura and cord are being compressed by an extrinsic mass. There is thinning of the pedicles at several levels above the block secondary to the expanding mass, which was of long duration. **C.** Traumatic avulsion of a cervical nerve root allowing the escape of oil. Because two axillary pouches above the rupture are enlarged there may have been partial avulsion there as well.

Most intrathoracic meningoceles occur in association with neurofibromatosis, are on the right side, may enlarge the intervertebral foramen, and, therefore, may resemble neurofibromas. Communication with the subarachnoid space demonstrated on myelography confirms the diagnosis. Rarely, anterior herniation through a sacral defect results in an anterior sacral meningocele. A pelvic mass in conjunction with partial or total sacral agenesis suggests the diagnosis, which is confirmed on myelography. Meningocele must be differentiated from teratoma in some instances.

AVULSION OF CERVICAL ROOTS

Traumatic arachnoid cysts or diverticula in the cervical and upper thoracic areas may result from brachial plexus avulsion or avulsion of cervical roots. When they occur intraspinally, compression of the cord may cause paresis or paralysis. Most of them extend out along the nerve roots to lie lateral to the spinal canal (see Fig. 12-30C). Myelography outlines the cysts which fill with contrast media. The injury and subsequent cyst formation are usually unilateral. We have observed similar small cystlike lesions in patients with no known antecedent trauma and no symptoms; these lesions are probably anatomic variants and may be bilateral. Rarely the same type of posttraumatic cyst is found in the lumbosacral area, but protection by the bony pelvis usually prevents root avulsion and meningeal tears in this region.

Pseudomeningoceles or diverticula have also been reported as relatively transient findings following

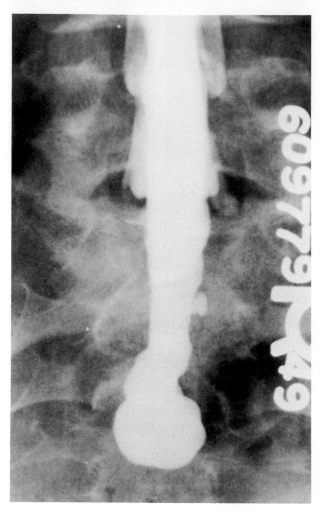

Fig. 12-31. Occult sacral meningocele. The spinal canal is elongated, extending to the third sacral segment and ending in a saclike dilatation representing the meningocele. (Courtesy of Dr. V. C. Hinck)

cervical laminectomy and section of dentate ligaments.[15]

HYDROMYELIA

This condition is usually a result of obstruction of the outlets of the fourth ventricle. The central canal serves to aid in decompression of the ventricular system. It dilates diffusely, widening the entire spinal cord in all diameters. This is often associated with the Arnold–Chiari malformation. Myelographic findings consist of uniform dilatation or widening of the entire cord.

SYRINGOMYELIA

Syringomyelia is a condition characterized by cavities considered to be a diverticula of the central canal; it may be caused by rupture of the canal within the cervical cord. Fluid dissects into the tissues producing the cavities which extend within the cord apart from the central canal. The cavity is lined by altered glial elements in contrast to hydromyelia in which the central canal is lined by ependyma. Syringomyelia is commonly observed in the cervical area where the myelographic findings resemble those of intramedullary tumor. Some workers have recommended cyst puncture to make the differentiation between syringomyelia and hydromyelia. Recently, computerized axial tomography has been used in conjunction with a water-soluble contrast agent to outline the cervical cord. Difference in density may provide an outline of the cavitation, but myelography is often necessary for complete evaluation.

THE TETHERED CONUS

This congenital anomaly[9] consists of low position of the conus which is held in a posterior position. External signs of spinal dysraphism including hypertrichosis, subcutaneous lipoma, dermoids, and sinus tracts are present in about one-half of these patients. Intradural abnormalities such as lipomas, dermoids, and widening of the dural sac were found in 10 of 24 patients reported by Fitz and Harwood–Nash.[9] Myelography performed with the patient supine shows the dorsally tethered conus in a low position as well as a small lipoma or cyst of the conus and a thick filum terminale. The widened dural sac, usually found when the conus is at the L4-5 level, is readily observed at myelography.

EPIDURAL ABSCESS

Epidural abscess may occur with any infection of the vertebrae or intervertebral discs. The most common cause of chronic epidural abscess or granuloma is tuberculosis. In addition to chronic lesions, an acute suppurative infection can develop in the epidural space, either by direct extension from an acute osteomyelitis of a vertebra or as a primary focus of infection in the epidural tissues. Because the lesion is a serious one that may compromise the blood supply of the cord, early diagnosis is imperative. The plain roentgenograms of the spine often are unrevealing. In the thoracic region one may see a widening of the soft-tissue paraspinal shadow indicative of the paraspinal abscess. If caused by an acute osteomyelitis it will be several weeks after the onset of symptoms before roentgen signs of the disease become evident in the vertebral body or disc. Myelography is an extremely valuable procedure in these cases because the clinical diagnosis may be in doubt. Myelograms reveal evidence of a block to the flow of oil. The nature of the obstruction often cannot be determined from the myelograms, but when correlated with the clinical signs a preoperative diagnosis of epidural abscess frequently is possible.

REFERENCES AND SELECTED READINGS

1. BENTSON JR, CRANDALL PH: Use of the Fogarty catheter in arteriovenous malformations of the spinal cord. Radiology 105: 65, 1972

2. BRIERRE JT, COLCLOUGH JA: Total myelography. Complete visualization of the spinal subarachnoid space. Radiology 64: 81, 1955

3. CRONQVIST S: The postoperative myelogram. Acta Radiol [Diagn] (Stockh) 52: 45, 1959

4. DAVIES ER, SUTTON D, BLIGH AS: Myelography in brachial plexus injury. Br J Radiol 39: 362, 1966

5. DICHIRO G, DOPPMAN JL, OMMAYA AK: Radiology of spinal cord arteriovenous malformations. Prog Neurol Surg 4: 329, 1971

6. DJINDJIAN R, HOUDART R, HURTH M: Angiography of the spinal cord. Acta Radiol [Diagn] (Stockh) 9: 707, 1969

7. DOPPMAN JL: Arteriography of the spinal cord. Semin Roentgenol 7: 231, 1972

8. EPSTEIN BS: Spinal canal mass lesions. Radiol Clin North Am 4: 185, 1966

9. FITZ CR, HARWOOD-NASH DC: The tethered conus. Am J Roentgenol 125: 515, 1975

10. CERGHATER R, HOLGATE RC: Lumbar epidural venography in the diagnosis of disc herniations. Am J Roentgenol 126: 992, 1976

11. HIRSCH C, ROSENCRANTZ M, WICKBOM I: Lumbar myelography with water-soluble media with special reference to the appearances of root pockets. Acta Radiol [Diagn] (Stockh) 8: 54, 1969

12. HOLMAN CB: The roentgenologic diagnosis of herniated intervertebral disc. Radiol Clin North Am 4: 171, 1966

13. JIROUT J: Pneumographic examination of lumbar disc lesions. Acta Radiol [Diagn] (Stockh) 9: 727, 1969

14. KECK C: Discography: technique and interpretation. Arch Surg 80: 580, 1960

15. KIM YW, UNGER JD, GRINSELL PJ: Postoperative pseudodiverticula (spurious meningoceles) of the cervical subarachnoid space. Acta Radiol [Diagn] (Stockh) 15: 16, 1974

16. KIRKS DR, NEWTON TH: Sarcoidosis: a rare cause of spinal cord widening. Radiology 102: 643, 1972

17. LILIEQUIST B: Gas myelography in the cervical region. Acta Radiol [Diagn] (Stockh) 4: 79, 1966

17a. LUSTED LB, KEATS TE: Atlas of Roentgenographic Measurement, 3 ed. Chicago, Year Book Medical Publishers, 1973

18. SACKETT JF, DAMM MG, JAVID MH: Unreliability of epidural venography in lumbar disc disease. Surg Neurol 7: 35, 1977

19. SACKETT JF, STROTHER CM: New Techniques in Myelography. Hagerstown, Harper & Row, 1979

20. TARLOV IM: Cysts (perineurial) of the sacral roots. JAMA 138: 740, 1948

21. TENG P, PAPATHEODOROU C: Myelographic findings in adhesive spinal arachnoiditis. Br J Radiol 40: 201, 1967

22. YOUNG IS, BRUWER AJ: The occult intrasacral meningocele. Am J Roentgenol 105: 390, 1969

SECTION 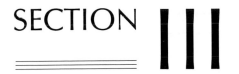 III

THE ABDOMEN
AND
GASTROINTESTINAL TRACT

13

The Abdomen

METHODS OF EXAMINATION

Roentgenograms of the abdomen produced without the use of contrast material serve many purposes. When limited to one or two, these sometimes are referred to as "scout roentgenograms." Such an examination frequently consists of a single roentgenogram obtained with the patient prone or supine. The addition of a lateral view or a roentgenogram obtained with the patient standing or sitting is desirable under certain circumstances. Another commonly used projection consists of a lateral decubitus view obtained with the patient lying on one side, the film cassette placed in front of the abdomen, and the roentgen-ray beam directed through the body in a horizontal plane. For example, in examining for the signs of bowel obstruction, recumbent, upright, and decubitus views are obtained more or less routinely. This becomes more than a simple scout examination but rather is a fairly detailed study of the soft tissues of the abdomen without the use of contrast media. As a preliminary step in the examination of the gastrointestinal tract, the gallbladder, or the urinary tract, it is customary to obtain a single scout roentgenogram of the abdomen for visualization of the soft tissues.

INDICATIONS FOR EXAMINATION

In addition to the use of a scout roentgenogram as a routine procedure prior to contrast visualization, roentgen examination of the abdomen without contrast media is useful in the study of the following:

1. Abnormal accumulations of gas within the intestinal tract
2. Calculi or other abnormal intra-abdominal calcifications
3. Size, shape, and position of the liver, spleen, and kidneys
4. Abnormal intra-abdominal masses
5. Free gas within the peritoneal cavity (pneumoperitoneum)
6. Ascites
7. Intra-abdominal abscesses
8. Radiopaque foreign bodies in the gastrointestinal tract or within the peritoneal cavity.

443

THE NORMAL ABDOMEN

The liver forms a homogeneous shadow in the right upper quadrant of the abdomen. Its upper border is limited by the right leaf of this diaphragm and thus is visualized easily because of the contrast afforded by the air-containing lung above it. The right lateral margin of the liver usually is separated from the density of the abdominal wall by a thin layer of fat. The lower edge (hepatic angle) of the right lobe of the liver usually is visualized in normal individuals and is seen to best advantage in the obese. The hepatic angle is probable outlined by omental and/or pericolic fat below the anteroinferior edge of the liver. On a film exposed with the patient supine, divergence of the roentgen beam places the most lateral part of the liver at about the anterior axillary line, which is at or near the anterior aspect of the hepatic angle. The omental and pericolic fat is often sufficient to outline the undersurface of the liver, and thus the radiographic inferior border is formed either by the anteroinferior edge or the more rounded protuberance of the posterior-facing inferior surface. This is dependent in part on the alignment of the inferior surface and the beam angle. However, there is a difference of opinion as to the portion of the right lobe of the liver (anterior or posterior) constituting the radiographic lower border.[22] It parallels the lower costal margin as a rule. In persons of asthenic habitus, however, the liver is more vertical in shape and the outer inferior edge of the right lobe may extend down almost to the same level as the posterior iliac crest. Gas in the hepatic flexure and the transverse portion of the colon also aids in determining position of the lower margin of the right lobe. When the liver is enlarged the hepatic flexure is displaced downward. The anterior aspect of the inferior surface of the liver may not be visible on the plain roentgenogram because it is not adjacent to the extraperitoneal fat. The same is true of the gallbladder which is not usually visible on plain films. The inferior margin of the left lobe is indistinct and is seldom seen clearly in the normal individual because it is anterior and there may be little adjacent fat.

The spleen or a part of it can be visualized in the normal individual as a rule. The inner surface and the inferior pole often can be outlined. The normal spleen is about 10 to 14 cm in length. Its anterior medial surface is not directly visualized, but is often outlined by gas in the adjacent stomach and splenic flexure of the colon. Posteriorly and inferiorly the spleen indents the extraperitoneal fat and is usually visible on plain films. Thus the medial surface is seen to best advantage when gas is present in the stomach and in the splenic flexure of the colon. In rare instances the spleen is unusually mobile and it may be found medial to the splenic flexure of the colon, below the body of the stomach, or above the gastric fundus. It may also be transverse, and, if the medial pole is large, renal displacement simulates that usually caused by adrenal masses. Accessory spleens are usually small and are not visible on plain films of the abdomen.

The kidneys are visualized on either side of the lumbar spine. They are more readily seen when an increased amount of perirenal fat is present. In emaciated persons the renal outlines may be completely lost. Fat is an important substance in rendering the margins distinct because of its relative radiolucency as compared to the density of the parenchymatous viscera. The extraperitoneal space around the kidney may be divided into the *perirenal space,* which is outside the renal capsule and within the renal fascia, and the *pararenal space,* which is outside the renal fascia. The space outside the fascia posterior to the kidney is termed the *posterior pararenal space* while that anterior to the kidney is known as the *anterior pararenal space.* The "flank stripe" is an extension of the posterior pararenal space into the lateral retroperitoneal area (*Vide infra*). The right kidney usually is at a slightly lower level than the left.

The pancreas cannot be visualized in the normal abdomen and even when enlarged the mass is seldom seen distinctly.

The outer margins of the psoas muscles form stripelike shadows on either side of the spine, extending from the level of the first lumbar vertebra down to the pelvis. The border becomes indistinct as the muscle passes over the midportion of the ilium. The integrity of the psoas muscle borders is important in excluding the possibility of retroperitoneal lesions of inflammatory or neoplastic nature. Retroperitoneal hemorrhage may also obliterate the psoas line. The muscles are normally symmetrical but scoliosis may cause one to stand out more prominently than the other. If the patient is rotated slightly, one shadow may be less distinct than the other; gas shadows in the bowel may blur the outline of one psoas margin while the other remains distinct. At times reexamination may be necessary in order to ascertain the condition of these muscle shadows; allowance must be made for the fact that, in the normal person, the muscle margins may be asymmetric, one standing out more clearly than the other. The outer margins of the quadratus lumborum also can be visualized in many individuals. This muscle lies lateral to the psoas and its lower border angles slightly more toward the lateral aspect of the ilium.

The lateral margins of the peritoneum often are bounded externally by thin layers of fat sufficient to cause a radiolucent stripe along the flanks. This is known as the extraperitoneal or properitoneal fat line (flank stripe) (Fig. 13-1). Obliteration of this line may occur in the presence of peritonitis when the infection involves the lateral aspect of the peritoneal cavity.

The urinary bladder usually is visible if it contains urine and its density may be increased considerably over that of adjacent structures if the specific gravity of the urine is high. Usually there is little difficulty in recognizing the urinary bladder because of its contour and its position behind and extending directly above the symphysis pubis. In women the shadow of the uterus often can be seen, especially if much intra-abdominal fat is present.

In roentgenograms of the abdomen obtained with the patient in the supine position, the fluid-filled gastric fundus may appear as a rounded mass in the left upper quadrant; this may be mistaken for a tumor, especially in obese patients. With the patient in the prone position the duodenal bulb likewise may appear as a round or avoid mass below the liver or overlying the kidney.

The appearance and distribution of gas in the intestinal tract and the types of intra-abdominal calcification often seen in the normal individual are discussed in the sections that follow.

GAS WITHIN THE INTESTINAL TRACT

Gas is present normally in the stomach and in the colon. Most of this is swallowed air, but some gas is produced by bacterial growth, and carbon dioxide may diffuse from the blood or may result from neutralization of bicarbonate within the bowel. Production of gas by bacteria depends upon the availability of fermentable material in the colon. Since carbon dioxide is rapidly absorbed, it probably contributes very little. Hydrogen sulfide and methane resulting from bacterial action in the colon are usually produced in relatively small quantity. Furthermore, hydrogen sulfide is rapidly absorbed. It is therefore likely that swallowed air is the main source of gas in the bowel and that bacterial metabolism may be a minor source, particularly in patients with prolonged colonic transit time. Small accumulations of gas may be found in the duodenum and the upper part of the jejunum resulting from swallowing air. In bedridden patients and in those who swallow large amounts of

air habitually, scattered bubbles of gas may be present throughout much of the small intestine (Fig. 13-2). These are seen as more or less individual bubbles or gas accumulations of rounded or ovoid shape. If a single loop of intestine can be recognized because of gas filling, the shadow is seldom more than 5 to 8 cm in length and the diameter of the lumen is not increased. More often, the gas does not form any specific loop pattern. When individual segments of small intestine can be recognized as such, are dilated, and of greater length than 8 to 10 cm, one should consider the possibility that the gas is abnormal. When patients are given an enema, colonic gas may be displaced in a retrograde manner through the ileocecal valve into the ileum. Therefore, some gas in the ileum in this circumstance is not abnormal. Colonic air-fluid levels may also be a result of an enema.

The intestinal gas pattern during infancy differs from that of the adult. Swallowed air can be visualized in the stomach immediately after the infant's birth. Within a few hours it will be found distributed throughout the intestinal tract, including the colon. The small intestine of the infant normally contains considerable amounts of swallowed air. Between the ages of 6 months and a year, as the infant gradually receives an adult diet and becomes ambulatory, the pattern of intestinal gas resembles more and more that of an adult. In feeble or premature infants or in those in whom there is severe respiratory distress, appearance of intestinal gas after birth may be delayed. Care should be taken not to interpret this as evidence of high intestinal obstruction in the newborn.

ACUTE OBSTRUCTION OF THE SMALL INTESTINE

METHOD OF EXAMINATION

Acute obstruction usually produces acute abdominal signs and symptoms, such as pain, distention, and alteration of bowel sounds, leading to the presumption of a possible surgical emergency. Since a number of acute abdominal conditions must be considered, a series of films should be obtained.[31] First, with the patient in the left lateral decubitus position (right side up) a film (horizontal beam) of the abdomen should be secured after the patient has been in this position for 5 to 10 minutes. Then an upright film of the abdomen and posteroanterior and lateral films of the chest should be obtained in patients who are able to stand or sit. The upright abdomen film should include the pelvis. The diaphragm often is not included in this

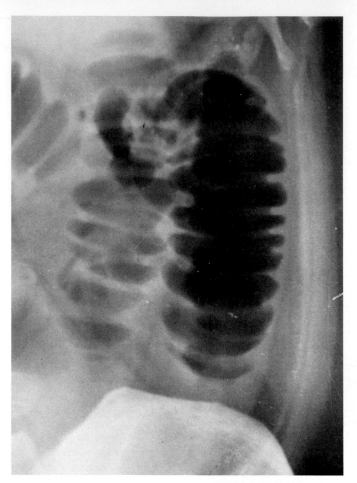

Fig. 13-1. Flank stripe. Note the translucent extraperitoneal fat line lateral to the loop of the gas-filled small intestine in this patient who had obstruction secondary to carcinoma of the cecum. The peritoneum parallels the outer walls of the intestine and the narrow distance of the bowel gas from the fat excludes the possibility of much ascitic fluid in this flank. There is also a thin layer of fat separating the lateral abdominal muscles in this patient.

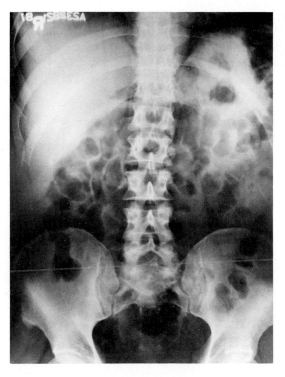

Fig. 13-2. Normal abdomen. Excess gas is noted in the small intestine because of air swallowing. The gas is seen in the form of multiple small accumulations of irregular size and shape. There are no long segments of bowel, and the caliber of the visible portions is normal.

film, but it is adequately visualized on the decubitus and chest films. The last film in the series is that of the abdomen with the patient recumbent; we prefer the prone position, making certain that the pelvic peritoneal cavity is included.

In examining for acute obstruction, roentgenograms of the abdomen without contrast media in the intestinal tract may be sufficient. Barium sulfate should not be given orally if bowel obstruction is a possibility until the colon can be eliminated as the site of the obstructing lesion. Should the obstruction be in the colon, the barium sulfate may become impacted above the lesion, absorption of water from the mixture follows, and the barium becomes a hard mass which may increase the severity of the obstruction. Masses of impacted barium sulfate also may cause difficulty for the surgeon when operating for the relief of an obstruction. Barium sulfate taken by mouth is not likely to cause harm if the obstruction is in the small intestine since the accumulation of fluid above the lesion keeps the barium from becoming inspissated. Furthermore, the water-soluble media available that are not absorbed by the gut are hypertonic, leading to so much dilution that the examination is of little diagnostic value.

If the obstruction is high in the small intestine, vomiting or the use of a negative suction apparatus may remove most of the gas and fluid that ordinarily would accumulate. Thus the typical findings described in the following paragraphs may not be apparent. In these cases a barium–water meal examination may be required to establish the diagnosis (Fig. 13-3). When the obstruction is in the lower part of the small intestine, the motility of the bowel usually is so impaired that it requires considerable time for the head of the opaque column to reach the site of block and reveal significant information about it. In these cases, plain roentgenograms can usually be depended upon to furnish adequate information.

If a double-lumen tube of the Miller–Abbott type has been introduced, it is often possible to obtain valuable information concerning the level of the obstruction and nature of the lesion causing it by injecting an opaque mixture through the tube under fluoroscopic control. After completion of the examination the barium mixture can be aspirated if desired.

SIMPLE OBSTRUCTION

In a simple obstruction the intestinal lumen is occluded at a single point without any significant interference with its blood supply. An example, and one of

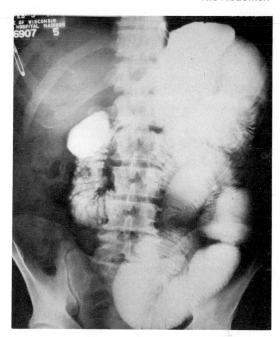

Fig. 13-3. Obstruction of the jejunum caused by an adhesive band. In this film, exposed after the patient had a barium meal, the jejunal loops are noted to be considerably dilated. The mucosal folds have not been obliterated even though there is distention and the appearance resembles that of stacked coins.

the common causes, of simple obstruction is a band of adhesions; another is the obstruction caused by an intraluminal tumor.[9, 49]

Roentgen Observations. Within 3 to 5 hours after the onset of an acute obstruction, gas and fluid accumulated above the lesion can generally be seen since distention of loops occurs quickly. The gas is swallowed air. It is visualized readily in recumbent view but the presence of the fluid may be observed only in upright or lateral decubitus views. In these positions the gas rises, overlying the fluid, and the interface between gas and fluid forms a straight horizontal margin. More than two air–fluid levels are generally considered as abnormal in the small intestine. (A fluid level is observed normally in the stomach because swallowed air is present almost invariably. A fluid level is frequent in the superior portion of the duodenum where air may be trapped temporarily when the patient assumes an upright position.)

The gas-filled loop or loops are increased in caliber over the normal. In an early stage of obstruction only a few such gas-distended segments may be visualized. The loop tends to form part of a circle, and, in the upright view, each end of the segment is limited by a fluid level. The fluid level in one limb of the loop may be at different height from the level in the other end. This does not necessarily differentiate mechanical obstruction from adynamic distention, however. When the air–fluid levels appear as a "string of beads," mechanical obstruction is almost always present.[28] With increasing distention more loops become visible; they may lie transversely one above the other forming a ladderlike arrangement (Figs. 13-4 and 13-5), or they may appear coiled and, at times, there is no particular pattern.

The gas-filled loops are recognized as small intestine rather than colon by:

1. Location of the loops in the central part of the abdomen rather than around the periphery.

2. Fine serrations along the margins caused by the mucosal folds, the valvulae conniventes (Fig. 13-6). These are finer and closer together than the colonic haustra. In the jejunum, simple distention, no matter how severe, will not efface the folds completely and in the obstructed segment they frequently show an appearance that has been likened to a stack of coins (it should be noted that edema and inflammatory changes may cause a diminution or absence of the folds or may cause thickening and resultant prominence). In the ileum the folds are fewer in number and the internal surface is much smoother. When the ileum is distended the folds disappear and the gas-filled loop has a smooth surface. This is an aid in distinguishing ileum from jejunum; often the site of obstruction can't be determined, however.

Where two gas-filled loops of bowel approximate one another the soft-tissue shadow between the gas represents a double thickness of bowel wall. Thus, information concerning the thickness of the intestinal wall is available. In simple obstruction such a double thickness seldom amounts to more than a few millimeters since the walls are thinned considerably by the distention. Inflammatory changes in the wall, exudate on the external surface, or fluid in the peritoneal cavity results in a thickening of this soft-tissue shadow. Abnormal thickening of the bowel wall is an important sign that the obstruction is no longer a simple one.

If the obstruction of the small intestine is complete, little or no gas will be found in the colon, a valuable differential point between mechanical obstruction and adynamic distention. Small amounts of gas or fecal accumulations may be present in the colon if the examination is performed within the first hours after the onset of symptoms (Fig. 13-7). In late obstruction the colon usually contains very little gas. When gas is found in the colon in the late stages of a completely obstructed small bowel it may be the result of putrefaction or it may be air introduced during the administration of an enema. If the small bowel obstruction is incomplete, some gas may pass through it and thus be visualized in the colon (Fig. 13-8). There will be a discrepancy, however, in the caliber of the distended small bowel and the colon, the latter being of normal or decreased width. This finding is useful in differentiating between a partial obstruction in the small bowel and one in the lower colon. In low colonic obstruction, the major distention affects the large intestine.

Early in the course of an obstruction it may not be possible to determine if abnormal gas accumulations are present or not. In such cases the value of serial observations is considerable. If the gas-visualized loops are the result of obstruction, the amount of gas will increase rapidly and often within a few hours the findings become more definite. Conversely, if the gas shadows are insignificant they may be absent at the second examination or at least not increased. Constancy in position of gas-filled loops and increasing distention in serial roentgenograms are valuable signs of a significant obstructive process. It is of vital importance to correlate clinical and radiographic findings in patients with acute abdominal disease, since obstruction and many other conditions require immediate or early surgery.

Gallstone Obstruction. Occasionally a large calculus in the gallbladder will ulcerate through the wall into an adherent duodenum and, because of its size, become impacted somewhere in the small intestine. In addition to the signs of simple bowel obstruction the stone may be partially calcified and thus be visible. More often it is nonopaque. A very significant finding in these cases is the frequent observation of gas outlining the common and hepatic ducts and forming a Y-shaped translucent gas shadow in the right upper quadrant. The demonstration of gas in the biliary duct system plus the signs of a simple obstruction is good evidence of gallstone obstruction with a fistulous communication between the gallbladder and the duodenum. The gallbladder may also be outlined by gas in these patients and it tends to be small in contrast to the distended gallbladder usually found in patients with emphysematous cholecystitis.

Obstruction Without Gas Distention. Rarely, in the presence of obstruction, the bowel above the lesion is

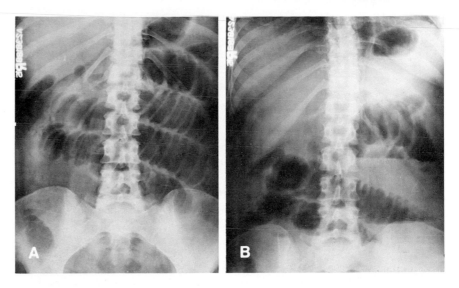

Fig. 13-4. Obstruction of the small bowel. Supine **(A)** and upright **(B)** views. Note the ladderlike arrangement of distended segments of dilated small bowel in the supine view. Gas-fluid levels are noted in the upright view. There is a little gas in the colon, which is not distended, and also in the stomach, which is normal in size.

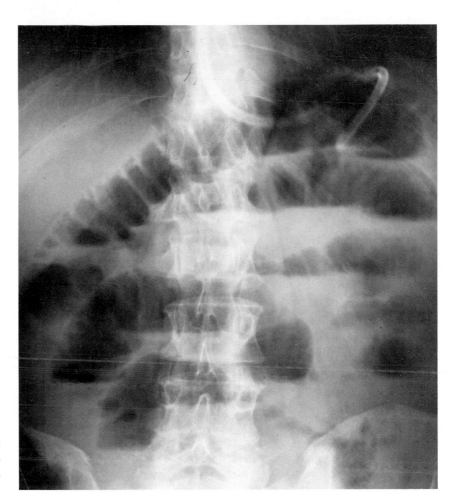

Fig. 13-5. Obstruction of the small intestine. Air-fluid levels are demonstrated in distended loops of small bowel.

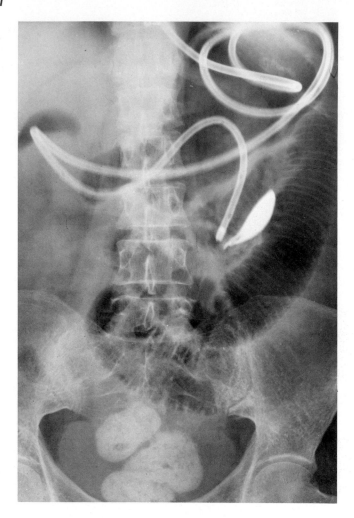

Fig. 13-6. Obstruction of the small bowel. Several loops of distended gas-filled small bowel are noted in the left side of the abdomen. The mucosal pattern resembling stacked coins is readily apparent. There is a little barium in the rectum—a residue from the previous examination.

filled with fluid but there is an absence of gas. The fluid-filled loops may form recognizable shadows in the abdomen, but sometimes they do not and the lack of gas may make it impossible to establish the diagnosis without the use of a barium–water meal (Fig. 13-9).

Strangulating obstruction may also be accompanied by very little or no gas in the bowel loops proximal to it, so there may be very few or no roentgen findings of obstruction.

Meconium Ileus. The absence of normal pancreatic and intestinal gland secretions during fetal life, the result of cystic fibrosis, leads to the formation of a thick, sticky, almost mucilagenous meconium that may cause bowel obstruction during the immediate postnatal period. The obstruction occurs in the distal ileum where the meconium may form into hard pel-

lets (Fig. 13-10 and 13-11). If a barium enema examination is performed the colon will be found to have a very small caliber since it has not been used during fetal life (*microcolon*). The caliber may be so narrow that an erroneous diagnosis of rectal obstruction may be made on the basis of a rectal examination or after attempts to pass a tube through the rectum. Plain-film findings suggest intestinal obstruction, but the roentgen signs are usually nonspecific. Uneven distension of intestinal loops, some of which may be markedly dilated, is the most frequent abnormality. It is difficult or impossible to differentiate small from large bowel loops in these newborns, however. The granular or bubbly pattern of intestinal gas (see Fig. 13-10) is not a reliable sign of meconium ileus since it may be noted in obstruction caused by imperforate anus, small bowel atresia, Hirschsprung's disease, or the meconium plug syndrome. Absence or paucity of

Fig. 13-7. Acute intestinal obstruction. This patient developed cramping abdominal pain about an hour prior to this examination. Note the dilated segment of jejunum **(arrows)** indicating obstruction with very little gas in the small bowel. The barium in the colon is a residual from previous examination of this structure.

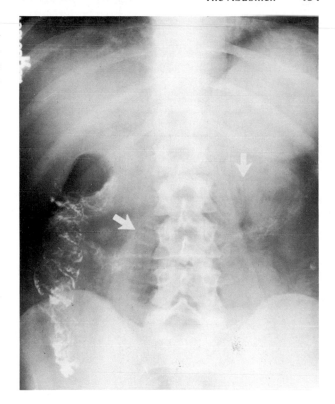

Fig. 13-8. Partial obstruction of the small intestine. Supine **(A)** and upright **(B)** projections show loops of dilated jejunum in the left side of the upper abdomen with air-fluid levels in the upright projection. There is a little gas and fecal material in the colon. This patient had long-standing obstruction.

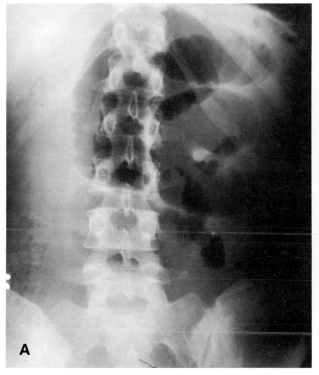

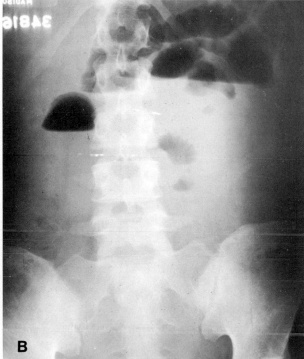

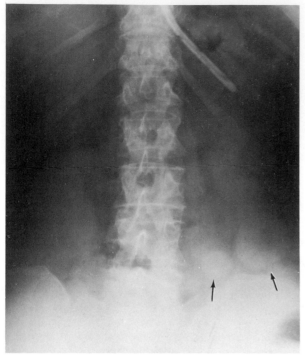

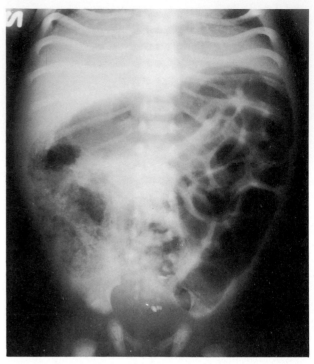

Fig. 13-9. Obstruction of the small intestine without much gas. This film, exposed with patient-in the recumbent position, shows some rounded soft-tissue masses in the left lower abdomen **(arrows)** caused by fluid-filled loops of bowel. This indicates that high-grade obstruction of the small intestine can be present without much gas and that fluid-filled loops of bowel may simulate abdominal masses.

Fig. 13-10. Meconium ileus in a newborn infant with clinical signs of bowel obstruction. There is a mottled shadow in the right lateral abdomen representing gas mixed wth solid material. At operation, this was found to be a mass of inspissated meconium.

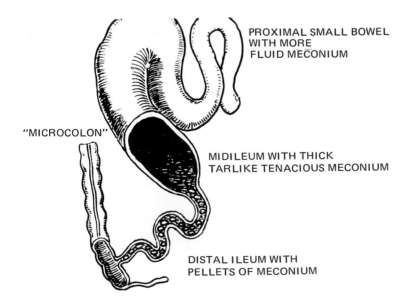

PROXIMAL SMALL BOWEL
WITH MORE
FLUID MECONIUM

"MICROCOLON"

MIDILEUM WITH THICK
TARLIKE TENACIOUS MECONIUM

DISTAL ILEUM WITH
PELLETS OF MECONIUM

Fig. 13-11. Meconum ileus. This diagram illustrates the pathologic findings. (Leonidas JC, Berdon WE, Baker DH, Santulli TV: Am J Roentgenol 108: 598, 1970).

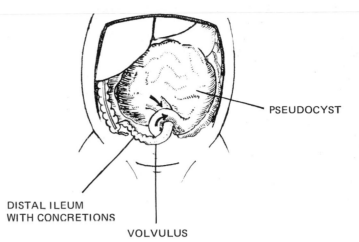

PSEUDOCYST

DISTAL ILEUM
WITH CONCRETIONS

VOLVULUS

Fig. 13-12. Meconium ileus. Diagram illustrates the formation of a pseudocyst secondary to volvulus in meconium ileus. (Leonidas JC, Berdon WE, Baker DH, Santulli TV: Am J Roentgenol, 108: 598, 1970).

air–fluid levels in upright or decubitus projections suggest the diagnosis, but may also be noted in obstruction of other types. Prominent air–fluid levels are rare, however, and if present should raise the possibility of complications such as volvulus, meconium peritonitis, and small bowel atresia.

One of the most frequent complications of meconium ileus both pre- and postnatally is volvulus (Fig 13-12). In prenatal volvulus, if the twist is of sufficient degree, the blood supply to the closed loop is compromised and it undergoes necrosis. It eventually may be absorbed, leaving an atresia of the bowel. In other patients the closed devitalized loop may lose its continuity with the bowel, become adherent, and form a "pseudocyst," again with resulting atresia of the intestine.[27] Single or multiple areas may be affected in this way. Rupture of the bowel may occur *in utero* and result in meconium peritonitis which may be recognized on plain roentgenograms, obtained shortly after the infant's birth, by the presence of scattered calcified deposits on the peritoneal surfaces (see under "Calcification in Fetal Meconium Peritonitis," in this chapter). Prenatal rupture of the bowel from any cause will result in this roentgen finding; therefore it is not specific for meconium ileus. In postnatal volvulus, a closed-loop obstruction is formed and gangrene and peritonitis may result. The closed loop may be visualized as a mass (*the pseudotumor sign*), but roentgen diagnosis generally is difficult. The demonstration of a mottled or granular collection of gas bubbles, the absence or paucity of air–fluid levels, the presence of the calcified deposits on the peritoneal surfaces, and the barium enema finding of a microcolon are signs to be looked for when meconium ileus is a diagnostic consideration.[27]

Intestinal obstruction occurring after the newborn period in children with cystic fibrosis, particularly in older children, and caused by inspissated material in the small intestine is termed *meconium ileus equivalent*. Inspissated material may also cause intussusception in the older child.

Meconium Plug Syndrome. In some infants without signs of cystic fibrosis there is difficulty in passing the first meconium stool and signs of intestinal obstruction develop. As soon as the meconium is passed the obstructive symptoms disappear. This entity has been called the *meconium plug syndrome.* It has been stressed that this diagnosis should not be made without first excluding the possibility of cystic fibrosis and of Hirschsprung's disease, either of which may present initially as a meconium plug syndrome.

In the meconium plug syndrome, a plain film will show (*1*) distention of the small bowel and proximal colon; (*2*) mottled and bulky colonic masses; (*3*) possibly, contracted distal colon if the meconium plug is proximal; (*4*) absence or paucity of air fluid levels, and (*5*) possibly, if the plug is distal, intracolonic soft-tissue (meconium) mass outlined by rectal gas on a lateral film of the sacral area. An enema consisting of an iodinated water-soluble contrast medium usually causes evacuation of the plug. Recently, Tween-80 and isotonic diatrizoate have been advocated.

Small Left Colon Syndrome. This condition results in signs and symptoms of low colonic obstruction.[15, 39] Mild to moderate abdominal distention, occasional vomiting, and failure to pass meconium are the common clinical manifestations. This condition is of frequent occurrence in offspring of diabetic mothers; it is not the meconium plug syndrome; and it can be differentiated from Hirschsprung's disease. Plain films show dilatation of the small bowel and colon to the level of the splenic flexure. Gastrografin enema, usually diluted 1:2 or 1:4, which is often curative, reveals a small left colon, dilated proximal colon, and the presence of some meconium but not necessarily a plug. Evacuation is usually normal in contrast to that in Hirschsprung's disease. The cause apparently is functional, since there is immaturity of elements of the neural plexus of the bowel. Perforation, usually of the cecum, may occur as a complication. If signs of obstruction persist, the possibility of Hirschsprung's disease should be reconsidered since the initial findings in this condition may be very similar to those in the small left colon syndrome.

Inspissated Milk Syndrome. This rare syndrome is usually found in premature babies who are fed on powdered milk.[19] The obstruction produced by the nonabsorbed inspissated milk is usually manifested as an acute process at least 5 days after passing altered stools and milk stools. The masses of inspissated milk causing small bowel obstruction are usually surrounded by gas in the dilated bowel. Bubbles of gas are not trapped in the masses. Contrast enema study shows the colonic caliber to be normal or slightly small. A high index of suspicion is essential in making the diagnosis, since findings may be somewhat similar to those in other causes of obstruction in premature infants. As in the small left colon syndrome, functional immaturity of the distal colon is probably a major factor in the etiologic background of this condition.

STRANGULATION OBSTRUCTION

Strangulation implies interference with the blood supply associated with the obstruction that may not necessarily be complete. It is often a closed-loop type of obstruction which refers to a closure of the lumen at two points, leaving a loop of bowel obstructed at both ends. Among the common causes are volvulus and incarcerated hernia. The significance of the lesion lies in the fact that the blood supply may be compromised. Serious interference with the blood supply may develop even though the loop of bowel is incompletely obstructed. Because the venous pressure is lower than the arterial, the veins are obstructed first and there often is extravasation of blood into the loop. If the lumen is not blocked completely, gas may enter it from above. In the colon, gas may

accumulate within a completely obstructed loop as a result of putrefaction. It is imperative to distinguish a closed-loop strangulation obstruction from a simple one as soon as possible, so that measures may be undertaken for its relief. The roentgen diagnosis is difficult and often impossible to make. Signs to be watched for are listed in the following paragraphs, but it always is important that these findings be considered in conjunction with the clinical observations. Even then there may be great difficulty in making the diagnosis of strangulating obstruction on plain film study.

Roentgen Observations

Gas within the Loop. During the early stage of a closed-loop obstruction the roentgen signs may be indistinguishable from those of a simple obstruction. In some patients, however, gas will be trapped within the obstructed loop, which may assume the form of two short segments of distended bowel lying parallel to one another and separated by the soft-tissue space of the thickened intestinal walls, the coffee-bean sign. When gas-distended bowel is also present above the obstructed loop this sign is difficult to recognize. In other patients the loop has the form of a U, usually inverted. This is a frequent observation in volvulus of the sigmoid colon (*q.v.*). Gas is almost always present in a closed-loop obstruction of the colon, probably the result of putrefaction. In the small intestine there may be nearly complete absence of gas above the obstruction.

Fluid within the Loop (Pseudotumor Sign). The closed loop may contain only fluid and result in a mass shadow similar to that of a solid tumor.[20] The outline of a pseudotumor shadow is easier to detect if there is gas distention of bowel above the obstruction (Fig. 13-13). It is more difficult to demonstrate when there are no gas-distended loops.

Fixation of Loop. Lack of movement of the closed obstructed loop may be demonstrable in roentgenograms obtained with the patient in recumbent, upright, and lateral decubitus positions.

Loss of Mucosal Markings. In simple obstruction the valvulae conniventes of the jejunum are not completely obliterated, even when the distention is severe; the valvulae conniventes cause the margins of the gas shadows to be serrated. When the blood supply of a closed-loop obstruction has been compromised, the folds tend to disappear and the margins of

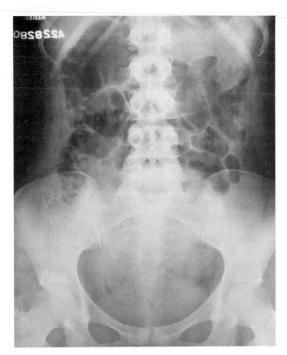

Fig. 13-13. Strangulated obstruction of the small intestine. There is a mass density in the lower central abdomen extending to the upper border of the fifth lumbar vertebra. Above it are several loops of dilated small bowel. At surgery the mass was found to be a fluid-filled distended loop of ileum. This is an example of the "pseudotumor sign" of strangulated obstruction.

the gas shadow become smooth. This sign is of value only if one can recognize the loop as being jejunum rather than ileum, since the folds disappear readily in the ileum under the effects of simple distention.

Signs of Peritonitis and Fluid in Peritoneal Cavity. In the later stages of a closed-loop obstruction the signs of exudate and free fluid in the peritoneal cavity appear. The soft-tissue spaces separating two adjacent loops of intestine become widened. Shifting fluid density may be demonstrable when roentgenograms are obtained with the patient in multiple positions. These are ominous signs although they do not necessarily indicate that the bowel has perforated. Bacteria may pass through the wall of an intact gut if the blood supply has been damaged and peritonitis may develop without frank rupture. If actual perforation does occur, free gas may be demonstrated in the peritoneal cavity in upright or lateral decubitus views.

The absence of gas proximal to a strangulating obstruction may result in a "normal" appearing abdomen on plain film. Therefore, a film of the abdomen showing no abnormality in a patient with clinical signs of obstruction should alert the examiner to look very closely for subtle signs of strangulation.

Bryk[9] suggested the use of two successive abdomen films exposed, with the patient supine, at a 5-minute interval to aid in evaluation of small bowel obstruction. He found that reduced activity in dilated loops was frequently associated with strangulation and other complications such as volvulus, perforation, hemorrhagic congestion, or peritonitis. Also, the presence of activity in dilated loops, as evidenced by changes in appearance in the two films, was a reliable sign of mechanical obstruction. A persistently narrow, rigid loop is a reliable sign of strangulation.

Intramural Gas. If necrosis develops, gas may be found within the wall of the involved bowel and seen as linear, lucent stripes paralleling the lumen. Gas enters the mesenteric venous system and extends into the portal venous system unless there is venous obstruction. Therefore, gas in the mesenteric system and not in the portal system suggests gangrene caused by volvulus, strangulated hernia, or other bowel obstruction associated with mesenteric venous obstruction.

INTESTINAL PSEUDO-OBSTRUCTION

The term "intestinal pseudo-obstruction"[10, 33, 50] is used to describe a condition in which clinical and roentgenographic signs of intestinal obstruction are present, with no apparent cause found at surgery. Any disease that alters motor function may cause pseudo-obstruction. The chronic conditions or diseases[33] that may be responsible include, among others, myxedema, scleroderma, hypo- and hyperparathyroidism, sprue, mesenteritis, amyloidosis, Chagas' disease, myotonia dystrophica, Hirschsprung's disease, and autonomic nervous system disorders. Transient pseudo-obstruction may be observed in association with renal failure, pancreatitis, pneumonia, congestive heart failure, spinal injury, and electrolyte imbalance. Various laboratory studies including biopsy may be necessary to determine the diagnosis or to exclude the possibility of these generalized diseases. Roentgen studies, at time with opaque media, are helpful in excluding mechanical obstruction and in providing diagnostic information in diseases such as sprue, scleroderma, amyloidosis, Chagas' disease, and Hirschsprung's disease. When all of the diseases mentioned have been excluded, a small group remains to which the term "idiopathic pseudo-obstruction" has been applied. This condition is very rare; usually the patients have been subjected to exploratory laparotomy on several occasions without the cause for the findings being determined. Occasionally, the distension is limited to the colon and simulates mechanical obstruction of the distal sigmoid or rectum.

In children with idiopathic pseudo-obstruction, there is motility disturbance, with delay in gastric emptying, duodenal dilatation, and poor contractions in the distal esophagus. Severe malnutrition is the usual result, so that supplemental nutriments given parenterally by catheter may be necessary.

OBSTRUCTION OF THE COLON

Roentgenograms of the abdomen may be sufficient for the diagnosis of colonic obstruction. The same type of film examination is used as described in the foregoing for small bowel obstruction. Because gas is present in the normal colon, the diagnosis of obstruction can be made only when the colon is found to be dilated from the cecum to the level of the lesion (Fig. 13-14). Usually the abnormal distention ends abruptly at the level of the lesion, with the colon distal to it being free of gas. The left lateral position is useful in patients with suspected low colonic obstruction because it facilitates the entry of air into the rectosigmoid and the rectum unless there is mechanical obstruction at or above the rectosigmoid. The rectum is therefore distended in adynamic ileus and collapsed in mechanical ileus. In case of doubt it is advisable to proceed immediately with a barium enema. This will determine either the presence of a lesion or the patency of the colonic lumen. Because the tissues at the site of an obstruction may be friable, care should be used to prevent undue pressure within the colon during the administration of the enema; palpation of the abdomen also should be done carefully.

As noted in the preceding section, colonic loops usually can be distinguished from the small intestine by the haustral sacculations and by the position of the loops, situated around the periphery of the abdomen. The haustra are deeper than the mucosal folds of the small intestine and the sacculations are considerably wider. When solid fecal matter is also present

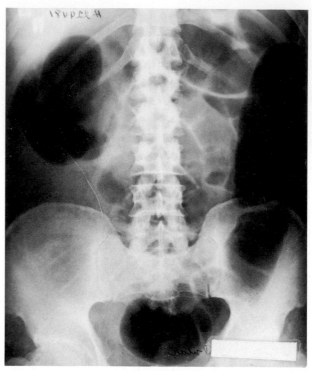

Fig. 13-14. Colonic obstruction caused by rectal carcinoma. The colon is distended wth gas. Several loops of distended, gas-filled small intestine are noted centrally. Since this pattern resembles that of adynamic ileus, a barium enema may be necessary to determine whether or not colonic obstruction is present.

in the colon the gas shadows often have a finely mottled appearance. This appearance is not seen in the small intestine except in some newborn infants with meconium ileus. As a rule, distension with gas plus particulate fecal material indicates early or incomplete obstruction; in more chronic obstruction, mottled fluid and gas are indicative of the condition. The amount of distension is related to the intraluminal pressure. Adherent secretions and fecal matter may cause the mucosal contour to appear ragged and the colonic septa to appear thickened. The latter may also be the result of edema and muscular hypertrophy.

If the ileocecal valve is incompetent, gas may back up into the small intestine and some degree of small bowel distention may be present. If the ileocecal valve is competent, small-bowel gas distention is slight or absent; instead, the colon becomes increasingly dilated. Because of its thinner walls the cecum undergoes the greatest distention and perforation is

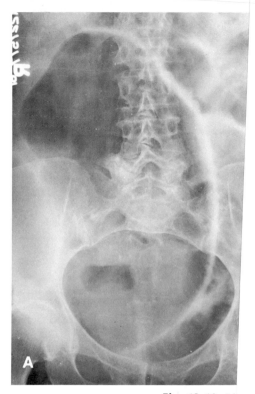

Fig. 13-18. V
tended cecun
to the right.
the abdomer
small bowel
cecum and i

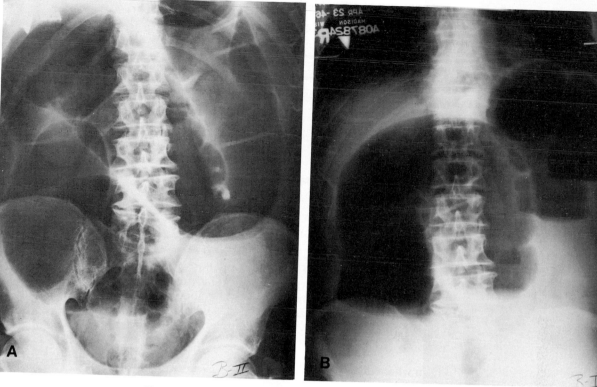

Fig. 13-15. A. Obstruction of the sigmoid colon. There is marked distention of the proximal colon to the region of the splenic flexure. No appreciable amount of gas is present in the small bowel, indicating a competent ileocecal valve. The obstruction in this patient was in the sigmoid. The end of the gas column shown on a single film of this type does not necessarily indicate the site of obstruction. In this patient the cecum is greatly distended; it ruptured shortly after this roentgenographic study was made. **B.** Upright film of the same patient shown in **A.**

volvulus, with the cecum undergoing
long axis. The cecum becomes greatly
gas and some degree of distention of
jejunum usually is present as well (Fi
colon distal to the volvulus will cont;
gas. Because of its mobility, the cecum
in almost any part of the abdominal ca
gas shadow of the distended cecum no
is found in the left upper quadrant of
or even in the left lower quadrant. W
or ovoid, gas-distended structure is vis
a location the possibility of a volvulus
should be entertained. When the cec
in this manner the long axis of the di
more horizontal than in its usual ve
Also there will be an absence of norn
shadows in the right lower quadrar
may see loops of gas filled-small bo\
mally the cecum should be. If the ile

most likely to occur here even when the obstruction
is in the distal part of the colon (Fig. 13-15). When
gas can back up into the ileum and jejunum there is
less likelihood of perforation. If the cecum distends to
more than 9 or 10 cm, perforation becomes a very
likely possibility. In some instances of intermittent or
chronic obstruction, however, the cecal wall may become hypertrophied and the diameter greatly exceeds 10 cm without perforation.

Fluid levels are of less significance in the diagnosis
of colonic obstruction than they are in the small
bowel. Patients frequently have had enemas prior to
roentgen examination and residual fluid from the
enema will lead to the formation of fluid levels. If
enemas have not been administered and fluid levels
are demonstrable in the colon they have the same significance as they do in the small intestine.

VOLVULUS OF THE SIGMOID COLON

A long redundant loop of sigmoid colon may undergo
a twist on its mesenteric axis and thus form a closed-
loop obstruction. Usually the loop of sigmoid becomes distended with gas forming an inverted U-
shaped shadow rising out of the pelvis and with the
limbs of the loop extending into or pointing toward
the pelvis (Fig. 13-16). Fluid levels (double) may be
revealed in the loop if an upright or a lateral decubitus view is obtained. Because of the obstruction the
colon proximal to the sigmoid also becomes abnormally distended with gas. It is not unusual to see
much more dilatation in the sigmoid than in the
colon proximal to it in these patients, however. A barium enema is needed if the diagnosis remains in
doubt and is ordinarily given in order to confirm the

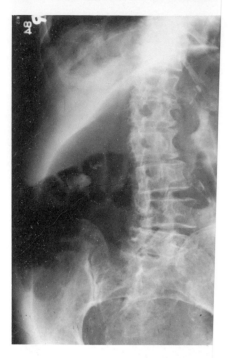

diagnosis, particularly in children, i
of the sigmoid is unusual and the ⎡
are often nonspecific. As the bariur
the sigmoid the end assumes a ⎡
form; the twisted or beaklike appe
cosal folds may be apparent. The o
incomplete and enough of the bar
pass through to outline clearly the
its nature (Fig. 13-17).

Ischemic colitis may result fron
and may complicate nonsurgical
colon. The resultant ulcerations m
rectal bleeding. Barium studies wi
cosal ulcerations, marginal fillin¦
printing), and transverse ridgi¦
served in ischemia. The developr
emic stricture is an uncommon c
cal correction is usually carried o
sigmoid volvulus unless the patier
candidate.

VOLVULUS OF THE CECUM

The ascending colon and cecun
mesentery as a fault of rotation
development of the gut; this conc

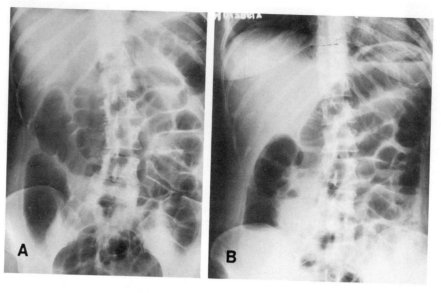

Fig. 13-19. Adynamic ileus. Recumbent **(A)** and upright **(B)** projections show a considerable amount of gas in the small bowel and colon. Fluid levels are inconspicuous except in the cecum. The small bowel loops are relatively short.

may develop in the presence of any severe infection such as pneumonia. (See previous discussion of intestinal pseudo-obstruction.)

Adynamic Distention without Peritonitis

In the absence of peritoneal inflammation, adynamic ileus (distention) usually results in generalized gas and fluid distention of the entire gastrointestinal tract. The colon often shows a relatively greater degree of distention than does the small intestine. The loops of small bowel usually are shorter than those seen in mechanical obstruction; also they are not as likely to form smoothly arched curves or appear to be under as much tension. Fluid levels will be seen, but they are not as prominent a feature as in mechanical obstruction (Fig. 13-19). In early cases, differentiation between the two conditions may be difficult, or impossible, on roentgen examination. Progressive examinations are helpful in such patients. In adynamic ileus the gas pattern does not change remarkably over a period of hours or even days, as it does in mechanical obstruction. Because the colon may be distended the question of an obstructive lesion in the distal part of the large bowel may arise. A barium enema is indicated in such a case and usually will determine the differential diagnosis.

Distention Secondary to Peritonitis

When peritonitis is present, in addition to the generalized distention as has been just noted, the signs of exudate or of free fluid in the peritoneal cavity will be seen. There is a widening of the soft-tissue spaces between contiguous gas-filled loops of bowel. In addition there may be shifting density demonstrated when upright or lateral decubitus views are obtained, to indicate the presence of free fluid. Evidence of apparent thickening of the bowel wall in the presence of distended bowel is a fairly reliable sign of an inflammatory process; simple distention causes a thinning of the wall.

Combined Dynamic Ileus and Adynamic Distention

Because certain lesions may cause both a mechanical block and a paralytic ileus (*e.g.*, some cases of appendiceal abscess), both conditions may be present at one time. It may be impossible to make an accurate estimate of the changes purely from roentgen examination. In general, it is important to remember that if the colon is gas-distended, a barium enema can be given to distinguish between a mechanical obstruction and a paralytic bowel. In small-bowel obstruction the colon will be free or almost free of gas. Adynamic ileus may occasionally be limited to the small bowel. When it is, serial observations are important and, of course, correlation with the clinical findings may be the deciding factor.

Acute Intermittent Porphyria

This is a familial metabolic disease characterized by attacks of severe colicky abdominal pain in association with obstipation. The character of the clinical symptoms and signs often leads to the erroneous diagnosis of bowel obstruction and many patients are operated upon for this reason. In some patients signs of central nervous system involvement are present, including an ascending Landry's type of paralysis, parasthesias, delirium and hallucinations, and coma. The diagnosis usually is made from the chance observation that the urine becomes dark on exposure to light or by the development of neurologic symptoms that may suggest the disease and lead to investigations for the presence of abnormal porphyrins in the urine and feces. The disease is of interest roentgenologically because of the signs and symptoms pointing toward bowel obstruction. Abnormal amounts of gas are present in the intestinal tract and the pattern is that of adynamic ileus rather than mechanical obstruction. Gas usually is present in both the small intestine and colon, but the distention may be more pronounced in the small bowel.

The distended segments are short, fluid levels are not particularly prominent in upright roentgenograms, and the gas pattern shifts from day to day in serial studies.

"Sentinel" Loop

In certain localized acute inflammatory processes within the abdomen a loop of bowel adjacent to the lesion may become distended with gas representing, in effect, a localized paralytic ileus (Fig. 13-20). This has been called a sentinel loop and it may offer a clue to the presence of the lesion. In acute pancreatitis the duodenum, the transverse colon, or a loop of jejunum may be visualized in this manner. In the presence of acute appendicitis, localized gas accumulation in loops of bowel in the ileocecal area is frequent. Acute cholecystitis may have an associated localized ileus in the right upper quadrant. While a sentinel loop is a valuable sign for such disease, it must be interpreted in relation to other findings and particularly to the clinical signs and symptoms in any given case, for the visualization of gas limited to a single segment of intestine often is a chance observation without significance. It has not been a very useful sign in our experience.

ACUTE MESENTERIC VASCULAR OCCLUSION

Acute mesenteric arterial occlusion may result from thrombosis in arteriosclerotic disease or from an embolus from the left side of the heart. The superior mesenteric artery is more frequently involved than the inferior and the arteries more frequently than the veins. Venous occlusion usually is secondary to some

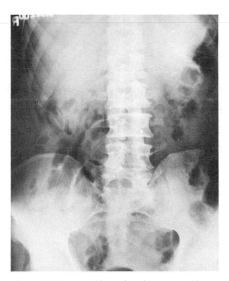

Fig. 13-20. Localized adynamic ileus (sentinel loops) in a patient with acute appendicitis. There are several segments of ileum in the right lateral portion of the abdomen that are slightly distended with gas. Elsewhere the gas pattern is normal.

disease that impairs venous flow. Unless there is an adequate collateral circulation, acute occlusion of a major vessel results in a severe, acute illness with infarction of the bowel, necrosis, peritonitis, and death. Venous occlusion causes thickening of the bowel wall which is visible on plain films in less than 50% of these patients. The specific findings are: (1) Thickening of the bowel wall and valvulae conniventes; the latter may be effaced as well as distinctly thickened. In arterial thrombosis and embolism resulting in infarction, bowel-wall thickening is not as great, and specific plain film changes tend to be infrequent and very subtle so that the diagnosis is very difficult to make, often depending upon close correlation of clinical and roentgen findings. (2) When sufficient air is present, intramural hemorrhage causing local enlargements simulating thumbprints may be visible in the small bowel as well as in the colon. (3) Bowel-wall gas is infrequent but is a specific finding when present. Nonspecific findings include: (1) An airless abdomen in a symptomatic patient. (2) Dilated small bowel and proximal colon (unusual). (3) Fluid-filled bowel with little or no gas. When there is gas distention of the small bowel and ascending and transverse portions of the colon, the cecum may be of smaller diameter than the transverse colon.[51]

When, on plain film, subtle deviations from normal or no abnormalities are observed in patients with clinical evidence suggesting bowel ischemia or infarction, angiography is usually indicated since gangrene followed by perforation, peritonitis, and death may result if the patient is not treated promptly. At best, the prognosis is poor in many instances. Selective mesenteric angiography is used to demonstrate the obstruction if the diagnosis is in doubt. Serial roentgenograms demonstrate the site of occlusion and the collateral blood supply, if present. The severity of any associated arteriosclerotic disease can be defined.

INTRA-ABDOMINAL CALCIFICATION

For a discussion of calculi in the biliary and urinary tracts and in the pancreas the appropriate sections dealing with these structures should be consulted. In addition to such calculi there are a number of other causes of intra-abdominal calcification including those listed in the following sections (see also Index).

CALCIFIED LYMPH NODES

Calcification of the mesenteric lymph nodes is observed most frequently in the right lower quadrant or in the lower central part of the abdomen and occasionally to the left of the midline. Calcification of these nodes represents the effects of previous infection, usually histoplasmosis and occasionally tuberculosis or other chronic granulomatous infection. The roentgen appearance of a calcified node is that of a mottled density seldom more than 1 to 1.5 cm in diameter (Fig. 13-21). Occasionally the shadow is more uniform in density. Often two or more nodes will be found in a cluster or within a relatively small area. In serial films or in those made with the patient in different positions such as recumbent and upright, the shadows of the calcified mesenteric nodes move over a fairly wide area. Such an observation is a useful one in differential diagnosis if there is doubt concerning the nature of the lesions. Calcification in other abdominal nodes occurs infrequently.

VASCULAR CALCIFICATION

Plaquelike areas of calcification in the aorta are common in persons beyond middle age. Such plaques may be seen occasionally in younger individuals, particularly in those suffering from diabetes. The plaques overlie the lumbar vertebrae in anteroposterior roentgenograms and are often seen to best ad-

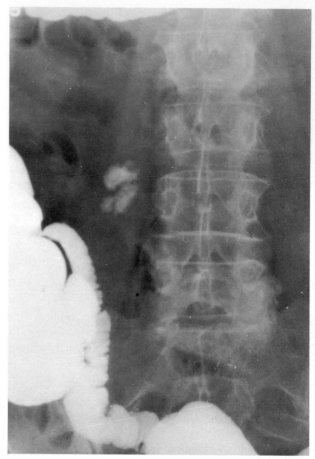

Fig. 13-21. Calcified mesenteric lymph nodes. Roentgenogram obtained following a barium enema demonstrates calcified nodes as mottled areas of density lateral to the right margin of the fourth lumbar vertebra.

vantage in left posterior oblique or lateral projections. In some cases, practically all the abdominal aorta will be visualized. Calcification of the arterial wall allows estimation of the diameter of the vessel. If aneurysmal dilatation is present, it can be recognized if there is sufficient calcification to delineate all or a part of the dilated segment.

In addition to the aorta, calcification occurs frequently in the iliac and splenic arteries. The splenic artery usually becomes tortuous and the calcification appears as one or more segments of tubular shape in the left upper quadrant. If the vessel turns so that it is seen end-on, the calcification appears as a thin-walled ring. Arteriosclerotic aneurysms of this artery can be demonstrated occasionally when the wall is

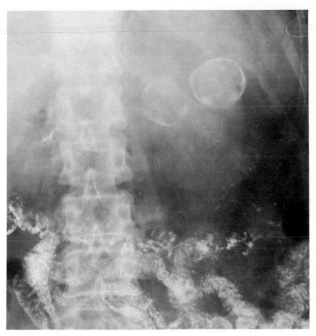

Fig. 13-22. Calcified aneurysms of the splenic artery discovered during a gastrointestinal examination. The aneurysms appear as calcified round masses in the left upper quadrant. (Courtesy of Dr. Wayne Rounds)

calcified (Fig. 13-22). Calcification in other branches of the celiac axis is less frequent and the same is true of the renal arteries. Visualization of crescentic or ringlike calcified shadows in the region of the kidney hilus should suggest the possibility of an aneurysm of a renal artery.

Calcification of the veins occurs mainly in thrombi and such calcified thrombi are called "phleboliths." These are observed very frequently in the pelvic veins and most adults have a few of them. Phleboliths are round or slightly oval in shape and vary in size from very tiny ones up to those that measure 0.5 cm or more in diameter. The small ones usually are evenly dense throughout; the larger ones tend to be ring-contoured or even laminated. They are found throughout the pelvis but are more frequent along the lateral aspects. It is easy to confuse a phlebolith with a calculus in the lower part of the ureter. A calculus often is irregular in shape and its long axis will lie parallel to the long axis of the ureter. Ureteral calculi seldom are found below the level of the ischial spine; phleboliths often occupy this position. At times it is impossible to determine the nature of the shadow until the ureter has been opacified by means of intravenous or retrograde pyelography. In a patient hav-

ing the symptoms of ureteral colic, a calcific density in the plane of the ureter must be looked upon as evidence of a ureteral calculus. Occasionally a long thrombus within a vein will calcify and be visualized as an elongated and somewhat irregular linear shadow of calcification. The location in the region of the larger pelvic veins helps to identify the nature of the shadow. Rarely, a calcified thrombus in the portal vein has been identified.

CALCIFIED FOCI IN THE SPLEEN AND LIVER

Small, round, dense foci of calcification are observed frequently in the spleen, occasionally in the liver. They may be extremely numerous and evenly distributed throughout these viscera. Usually they are considered to be the healed foci of previous widely disseminated infection, either tuberculosis or one of the fungi, such as histoplasmosis (Fig. 13-23). Recent observations suggest that histoplasmosis is responsible in most cases. Similar foci of calcification may be found in the lungs of some of these patients, distributed widely throughout the pulmonary parenchyma.

ENTEROLITHS AND APPENDICEAL FECALITHS

Enteroliths are uncommon causes for radiopaque objects in the abdomen, usually occurring in the colon. The enterolith may be primary or secondary. In the latter instance it forms usually after ingestion of foreign material such as a fruit pit, the pit serving as a nidus for the calcium salt deposition. In the primary type there is no predisposing foreign object to serve as a nidus. An enterolith may form within a Meckel's diverticulum or above a stenosing lesion of the small intestine such as regional enteritis. A large radiopaque gallstone may become lodged in the intestine after ulcerating through the duodenal wall.

Concretions within the lumen of the appendix may calcify (see Fig. 19-38). These are known as appendiceal fecaliths or coproliths. They are rounded or ovoid in shape and the calcium often is deposited in concentric laminations so that the shadow is not uniformly dense. Since they are located in or near the tip of the appendix, they may be found distributed over a fairly wide area in the right lower quadrant of the abdomen or below the brim of the pelvis. When inflammation of the appendix develops in the presence of a coprolith, gangrene and rupture are prone to follow. When examining roentgenograms of the abdomen in

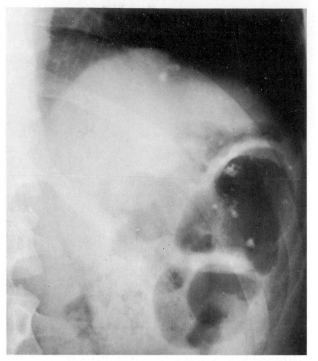

Fig. 13-23. Calcified splenic nodules due to chronic granulomatous disease. Note the variety of sizes and shapes of these calcifications.

a patient in whom an acute appendicitis or appendiceal abscess is a diagnostic possibility, search for evidence of a coprolith should be made. Because the shadow often overlies the ilium, it may be difficult to visualize unless this area is inspected with care.

CALCIFICATION IN THE ADRENAL GLANDS

Mottled shadows of calcification may be found in one or both adrenal glands when involved by tuberculosis and such an observation forms one of the positive roentgen signs of *Addison's disease,* occurring in about one-third of patients with this disease. (Fig. 13-24). The calcification is seen in the form of irregular mottling located directly over the superior pole of the kidney and sometimes forming almost a complete outline of the adrenal gland. Observation of the adrenal glands is facilitated if roentgenograms are obtained with the patient rotated slightly to the right and to the left of a supine position. Ordinarily a rotation of 15 degrees is sufficient. This degree of rotation will tend to displace any confusing calcified areas in the costal cartilages away from the adrenal region.

Occasionally, calcification is demonstrated in one or both adrenal glands of a patient who has none of the clinical signs of Addison's disease. Such calcifications have been observed in young infants and in children. In some of these patients, at least in infants, the calcification appears to have followed hemor-

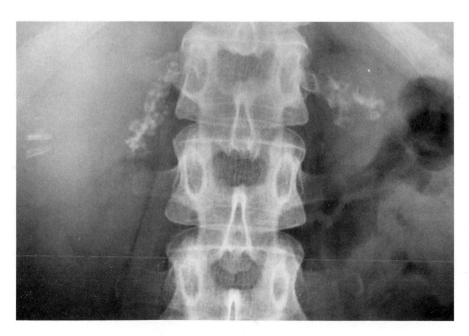

Fig. 13-24. Calcification in the adrenal glands is clearly defined on either side of the first lumbar vertebra.

rhage into the gland, but in others its cause remains obscure. In the latter group the calcification often is an incidental finding and does not seem to have any relationship to the patients' present complaints.

Calcification in the adrenal glands occurs in the lipidosis known as *Wolman's disease,* a rare familial xanthomatosis resulting in death early in infancy.[44] The adrenal glands are enlarged bilaterally and this, combined with the diffuse calcification, allows the diagnosis to be made (see Ch. 20).

CALCIFIED CYSTS

Calcification in the wall of an intra-abdominal cyst is seen occasionally and the cystic nature of the lesion can be surmised by the crescentic or ring-shaped form of the calcification. Such cysts may be found in the mesentery, spleen, kidney, or in the liver and rarely in the adrenal glands (Figs. 13-25 and 13-26). Usually they are simple cysts of congenital origin. Calcification is frequent in the wall of an appendiceal mucocele and cystlike calcification in the right lower quadrant may suggest this lesion (see Ch. 19).

Another type of intra-abdominal cyst that frequently calcifies is the echinococcus cyst (hydatid cyst). Echinococciasis is rare in the United States and particularly so in persons who have never lived outside this country. Echinococcus cysts in the abdomen may be found in the spleen or liver, occasionally elsewhere within the peritoneal cavity. Calcified echinococcus cysts usually have thicker walls than simple cysts and have somewhat less tendency for their entire walls to be calcified.

Dermoid cysts constitute about 10% of all ovarian cysts. The cyst may contain partially calcified or incompletely formed teeth, a characteristic feature of the lesion. Less frequently the wall of the cyst may be partially calcified. In addition to the presence of teeth, the interior of a dermoid cyst, being filled with a fatty material, is more translucent than the surrounding tissues and thus appears as a sharply circumscribed area of lessened density within the pelvis (fat is the most transparent of all the tissues). Even when the wall is not calcified, it may stand out as a thin ring surrounding the more radiolucent interior of the cyst (Fig. 13-27).

CALCIFICATION IN TUMORS

Uterine Leiomyoma

In women of middle age or older, roentgenograms of the lower abdomen frequently show the shadows of

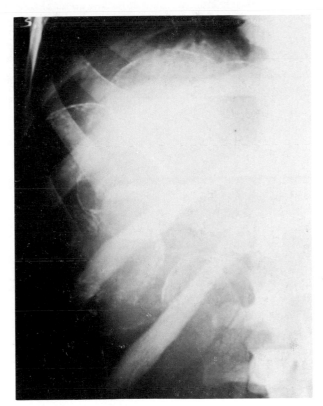

Fig. 13-25. Multiple calcified cysts in the liver. The rounded masses were distributed throughout the liver and were thought to represent congenital cysts.

calcified uterine fibroids. The calcification forms a mottled "mulberry type" of shadow in the midpelvis or close to the midline (Fig. 13-28). The size of the lesion, of course, may vary considerably and occasionally a very large calcified fibroid will be found that will occupy the entire pelvis or even extend out of the pelvis.

Cystadenocarcinoma of the Ovary

The papillary growths characteristic of this tumor frequently contain calcified deposits or psammoma bodies. These may be found not only in the primary tumor but also in its peritoneal implants and even in its more distant metastases. The calcification is seen as scattered, fine, amorphous shadows, hardly denser than the normal soft tissues, and therefore easily missed unless they are extensive. The hazy calcifications may be confused with semiopaque material in the gastrointestinal tract, such as a small residue of barium mixed with fecal material. This type of calci-

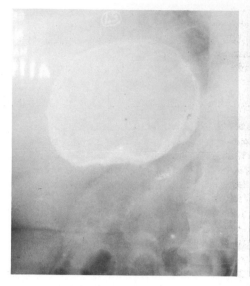
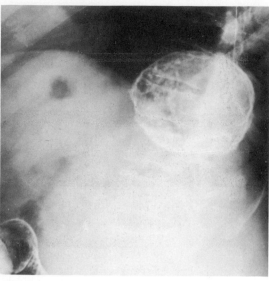

Fig. 13-26. Calcified cyst of the right adrenal gland. The large cyst with a densely calcified wall is noted to lie directly above the right kidney.

fication is almost characteristic of this tumor and when distributed in various parts of the abdominal cavity indicates the presence of peritoneal implants. In benign cystadenoma of the ovary, similar psammoma bodies may form, but there are, of course, no implants and the calcification is limited to the ovarian mass.

Neuroblastoma

Neuroblastoma, usually arising in the adrenal gland, is a rather uncommon tumor of childhood that very frequently shows the presence of calcification in the form of hazy granular deposits. Such calcification in a mass lying above the kidney in a young child is almost certain evidence of this tumor. Other malignant tumors of childhood occurring within the abdomen, such as Wilms' tumor of the kidney, infrequently calcify.

Renal Carcinoma

Calcification in a renal carcinoma is not unusual and is found in about 25% of these tumors. The calcification must be distinguished from renal calculi and other causes of renal calcification (see Ch. 20).

Gastrointestinal Carcinoma

As a rare finding in gastrointestinal carcinoma there may be small mottled or punctuate deposits of calcium. The tumors have invariably been of the mucinous type and the lesions have been found in the stomach or colon. The patients have generally been in the younger or middle-aged groups. Calcification in metastases to the liver from mucinous carcinomas of the gastrointestinal tract, particularly the colon, is more common than in primary mucinous colonic tumors. It tends to be finely stippled, producing cloudlike clusters of small calcified granules in the liver. Occasionally, similar calcification is observed in periaortic nodes in these patients.

Other Tumors

Calcified deposits occasionally are seen in carcinoma of the urinary bladder and in adrenal carcinoma. Rarely calcification has been reported in hepatic metastases from breast carcinoma, in renal metastases from osteosarcoma, in pheochromocytoma of the adrenal or para-aortic body (organ of Zuckerkandl), and in intra-abdominal teratoma, usually in infants or children.

CALCIFICATION IN FETAL MECONIUM PERITONITIS

Fetal meconium peritonitis has been defined as a chemical inflammation of the peritoneum caused by the escape of sterile meconium into the peritoneal cavity. The condition usually results from perforation *in utero*, secondary to a congenital stenosis or atresia of the bowel and in meconium ileus. The clinical manifestations of obstruction usually are recognizable at birth or shortly thereafter. Calcification of the cornified epithelial cells of the meconium occurs and may be visualized as small irregular calcifications widely distributed throughout the peritoneal cavity (Fig. 13-20). This is a very reliable sign of meconium peritonitis in the newborn when the calcification can be identified as being in the peritoneal cavity. Another finding that is seen occasionally in newborn males is the presence of calcified deposits in the scrotum. In one series this occurred in 20% of the infants.

Rarely, neonates with meconium peritonitis will present with abdominal distension caused by a giant calcified cyst. This condition has been termed *cystic meconium peritonitis.* In addition to calcification within the wall, calcification may be present outside of the cyst wall. The cause of the giant cyst is not definitely known. These cysts usually have no open communication with the intestinal lumen, but some of them may represent local duplication of the bowel.

If the amount of calcified material is small it may be impossible to determine whether or not it is within the intestinal tract. In patients with intramural calcification there often is an associated duplication of the bowel at the site of calcification. Wolfson and Engel[55] have described the occurrence of dense bands across the metaphyses of newborn infants as a significant finding in neonatal meconium peritonitis. They did not find similar bands in infants with intestinal obstruction without complicating meconium peritonitis.

MISCELLANEOUS CAUSES OF ABDOMINAL CALCIFICATION

Intramural intestinal calcification rarely may be observed in neonates with intestinal atresia. Intraluminal (in the meconium) calcification may also be observed in small-bowel stenosis and atresia, imperforate anus, Meckel's diverticulum, or blind rectal loop. Amputated appendices epiploica may calcify secondary to infarction or infection. They usually appear as small (1–2 cm) ring-contoured calcifications which may move within the peritoneal cavity. Calcification of the wall of the left colon has been reported in schistosomiasis; this is exceedingly rare. Calcifications are occasionally observed in autoamputation of the ovary.

PNEUMOPERITONEUM

The roentgen demonstration of free gas within the peritoneal cavity is a valuable sign in the diagnosis of perforation of the gastrointestinal tract. There are, however, other causes for pneumoperitoneum and the possible sources for such free gas in the peritoneal cavity are discussed in the following paragraphs. The method of plain-film examination in patients with suspected pneumoperitoneum is outlined in the section of this chapter entitled "Acute Obstruction of the Small Intestine."

CAUSES OF PNEUMOPERITONEUM

The most frequent cause of spontaneous pneumoperitoneum is rupture of a peptic ulcer, either gastric or duodenal. Other causes include perforation of a carcinoma of the stomach or colon, rupture of a colonic diverticulum, and traumatic rupture of the intestine or of the stomach. It is not observed very often following rupture of the small intestine other than of the duodenum because of the usual absence of gas in this part of the intestinal tract. The time interval following rupture and the appearance of sufficient gas to be visualized roentgenologically obviously will vary, depending upon the size of the rupture, the location of the lesion, and the amount of gas present within the lumen of the segment. It has been noted within an hour after rupture.

Pneumoperitoneum does not always follow rupture of a peptic ulcer and, in approximately 25% of these patients, free gas is not observed on roentgen examination. Failure to demonstrate such gas therefore is of no value in excluding the possibility of a perforated ulcer. Gastric perforation may be suggested when no gas is observed in the stomach, gas is present in the small and large bowel, and pneumoperitoneum is observed on the film exposed with the patient erect. Conversely, when there is a gastric air–fluid level, small bowel distention, and little, if any, colonic gas, colonic perforation may be suggested in a patient with pneumoperitoneum. These findings may be misleading, however, and therefore a firm diagnosis often cannot be made regarding the site of perforation.

Pneumoperitoneum may also occur following penetrating injuries of the abdominal wall and in blunt trauma when rupture of a hollow viscus may occur. Pneumomediastinum may dissect downward and rupture through the parietal peritoneum into the peritoneal cavity.

Septic infection of the peritoneal cavity from gas-forming organisms may result in the production of a considerable amount of gas and the roentgen demonstration of pneumoperitoneum. There is nothing characteristic in the appearance of this gas to identify its source except that other signs of peritonitis will be present, including the evidence of ileus and of fluid in the spaces between the loops of gas-distended bowel.

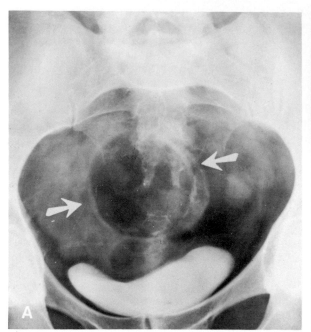
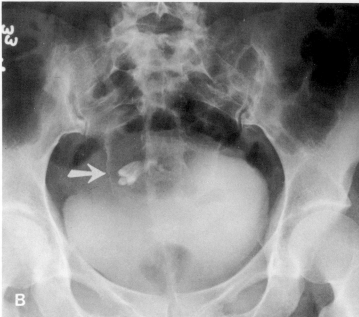

Fig. 13-27. Dermoid cyst of the ovary. **A.** This cyst has a translucent center indicating its fatty content. The wall is seen as a thin, circular density **(arrows)**. The bladder contains contrast material from a previous intravenous urogram. **B.** This cyst contains a cluster of teeth **(arrow)** and appears to indent the bladder somewhat.

Injection of Fallopian Tubes

Gas injected into the fallopian tubes as a part of the Rubin test for tubal patency may escape into the peritoneal cavity and be present in sufficient amounts to be visualized roentgenologically. Following vaginal lavage it has been reported that gas may enter the peritoneal cavity through the fallopian tubes in sufficient amounts to be demonstrable. Gas has also been observed in the peritoneal cavity of females who have had water-skiing accidents.

Postlaparotomy Air

Some air is almost always present within the abdominal cavity following laparotomy. Under ordinary circumstances sufficient air remains to be visualized roentgenologically for several days; occasionally it will persist for a week to 10 days and has been reported to remain visible at times for as long as 4 weeks after the laparotomy. Demonstration of pneumoperitoneum during the postoperative period is of no significance unless (1) the amount of gas is large, or (2) increasing gas is shown in serial roentgenograms. The latter observation is good evidence that the presence of gas is abnormal and may indicate

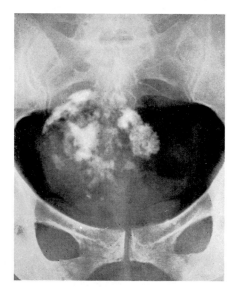

Fig. 13-28. Calcified uterine leiomyoma.

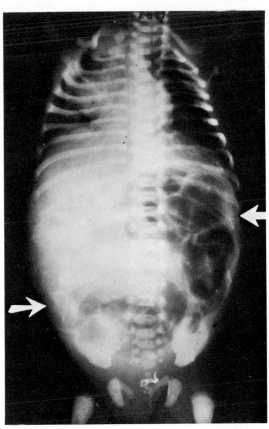

Fig. 13-29. Meconium peritonitis in a newborn. There are scattered, small, irregular calcifications along peritoneal surfaces **(arrows)**.

breakdown of a surgical anastomosis or other rupture of the intestinal tract. Occasionally a large amount of air is seen in the peritoneal cavity as a normal observation during the first day or two following laparotomy; however, such large accumulations should be viewed with suspicion and they warrant close observation for progress and a careful correlation with the clinical signs and symptoms.

Air frequently is introduced into the peritoneal cavity at the time of paracentesis for removal of fluid or during peritoneoscopy. The amount usually is small. Following peritoneal dialysis for chronic renal failure, a small amount of gas in the peritoneal cavity is common.

Diagnostic Pneumoperitoneum

In diagnostic pneumoperitoneum the source of the gas is obvious. The gas is introduced for diagnostic purposes such as: to aid in delineating the abdominal viscera, particularly the liver and spleen, to outline abdominal masses, and to demonstrate the undersurface of the diaphragm.

Idiopathic Spontaneous Pneumoperitoneum

In very rare instances, spontaneous pneumoperitoneum of unknown cause is encountered. It is generally considered that most if not all of these cases result from rupture of emphysematous gas cysts occurring as part of an otherwise unrecognized instance of pneumatosis cystoides. Pneumoperitoneum may also result from air arising in the mediastinum, a mediastinal emphysema. This, in turn, may follow an interstitial emphysema of the lung. We have observed it as a complication of pneumothorax.

ROENTGEN OBSERVATIONS

Free gas within the peritoneal cavity is best demonstrated in roentgenograms obtained with the patient upright, either sitting or standing. The gas ascends and accumulates beneath the summit of the diaphragm. It then can be visualized as a translucent zone limited by the thin, curved shadow of the diaphragm above and the density of the abdominal tissues beneath (Fig. 13-30). If the amount of gas is very small it forms a thin, curved, dark streak or a semilunar-shaped shadow, having a smoothly curved superior surface where the gas is bounded by the diaphragm and a horizontal flat inferior margin if fluid is also present. The gas may be found under one or both diaphragmatic domes. It is easier to recognize on the right side because of the homogeneous density of the liver. On the left the normal gas and fluid shadows present in the fundus of the stomach may be confusing (Fig. 13-31). Close observation, however, will usually show the presence of two shadows, one representing the normal gas–fluid level of the stomach and the other the abnormal gas in the subdiaphragmatic space.

If the patient is too ill to sit or stand, lateral decubitus views, as explained in previous paragraphs, must suffice. The gas will rise to the highest point in the flank and be visible as a horizontal translucent area. It is easier to recognize a small amount of gas when the patient is examined in a left lateral decubitus position because the right side of the abdomen is uppermost and the small gas accumulation will be found between the lateral surface of the liver and the abdominal wall; the homogeneous density of the liver again makes it readily apparent. Miller and Nelson[32] were able to demonstrate as little as 1 ml of air beneath the right hemidiaphragm by having the subject

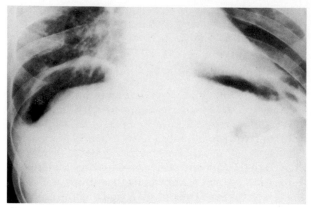

Fig. 13-30. Pneumoperitoneum following rupture of a peptic ulcer. Air beneath both hemidiaphragms is evident in this upright view of the lower thorax and upper abdomen.

assume the left lateral decubitus position for about 10 minutes prior to assuming the upright position for 10 more minutes. The air then accumulates in the right flank and moves readily upward beneath the right hemidiaphragm. The air is more easily observed in an upright film of the chest than in an upright film of the abdomen because the beam at the level of the dome of the diaphragm is more horizontal in the chest film than in the abdomen film, where it is tangential to the dome of the diaphragm. When large amounts of gas are present, other signs may be observed: (*1*) Both walls of an air-filled bowel loop are clearly visible. (2) With the patient supine, an oval-shaped lucent area may be observed in the upper abdomen; it may be bisected by the dense shadow of the falciform ligament, the "football" sign. This is more readily observed in infants but can be seen in adults. (3) The lateral and inferior margins of the liver and spleen are clearly visualized, particularly in a film exposed with the patient in the prone position. (4) In a critically ill patient a cross-table lateral film exposed with the patient supine, it is possible to detect free peritoneal gas which forms triangular lucent shadows with the base anteriorly and apex extending posteriorly between loops of bowel.

When an unusual amount of subserosal fat is present, the outer walls of the intestine may be visible, but not with the clarity noted in pneumoperitoneum (Fig. 13-32).

There are a number of infectious and obstructive causes for extraluminal, extraperitoneal collections of gas. Many of them are considered in sections dealing with the respective organs, but a brief review of

some of them seems pertinent here. Among the numerous causes are infections, obstruction, trauma, and unusual mucosal permeability. Examples of gas in the wall of various structures include emphysematous cholecystitis, gastritis, and cystitis. In patients with emphysematous cystitis, there may be gas within the urinary bladder and in upright films it may ascend into the renal collecting system. Pararenal, paracolic, and extraperitoneal abscesses may contain gas and gas may be observed in solid organs that are infected with a gas-forming organism. Intra-abdominal abscesses in various locations may also contain gas, either in a rounded or oval abscess cavity or sometimes scattered at random in an area of inflammation.

GIANT SIGMOID GAS CYST OR DIVERTICULUM

This is an unusual cause of a large, round, or oval collection of gas in the lower abdomen. The cysts may range up to 15 cm in diameter. Although most of the patients in whom they have been reported have diverticulosis, a communication between the diverticulum or gas cyst and the bowel lumen is not demonstrated. Some of the cysts have mucosa, submucosa, and muscularis while others have a wall comprised of granulation tissue and inflammatory cells. It is possible that some represent actual diverticula while

Fig. 13-31. Pneumoperitoneum secondary to rupture of a gastric ulcer. There is a small amount of gas beneath the right hemidiaphragm. Most of the gas on the left is in the stomach, but there is a very small amount of gas lateral to the gastric air bubble.

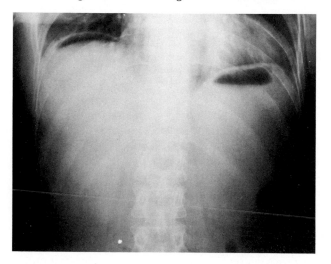

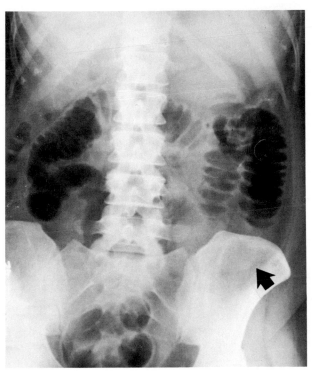

Fig. 13-32. Carcinoma of the cecum causing obstruction of the small bowel. The presence of intra-abdominal fat allows the outer surfaces of some of the segments of bowel to be visualized **(arrow).** Note also the retroperitoneal fat forming a radiolucent stripe along the lateral margin of the abdominal cavity.

others represent alterations secondary to diverticular disease or possibly a duplication communicating with the sigmoid or diverticulum of the sigmoid.

PNEUMATOSIS CYSTOIDES INTESTINALIS*

Gas "cysts" in the intestinal wall are found in the condition known as pneumatosis cystoides intestinalis. The intramural gas may be found in the small intestine or colon or in both. Gas in the wall of the stomach also has been reported. The entity is usually asymptomatic, but rupture of a gas cyst may cause pneumoperitoneum. The gas is visualized roentgenologically as small bubbles, or, less frequently, as linear streaks within the intestinal wall. The cause is

* Some authors prefer to use the term "pneumatosis cystoides intestinalis" to include all entities in which intramural gas is found. Others limit it to the idiopathic, usually asymptomatic form.

unknown but the condition usually clears spontaneously. Some investigators have expressed the opinion that the gas arises as a result of interstitial emphysema of the lungs brought about by forceful vomiting. It then extends to the mediastinum, from there along fascial planes to the retroperitoneal space, and from there to the subserosa of the bowel. In other instances the intramural gas has been found above an obstructing lesion such as a carcinoma of the colon. In these patients it is assumed that the increased intraluminal pressure above the obstruction, combined with the friable, ulcerated tissue sometimes seen above a carcinoma, is responsible for the entrance of gas into the wall (Fig. 13-33). Pneumatosis intestinalis also has been found in the small intestine when it is involved by scleroderma and, rarely, in patients with dermatomyositis and juvenile rheumatoid arthritis. A variety of gastrointestinal diseases may be accompanied by pneumatosis; these include chronic enteritis, esophageal stenosis, intestinal obstruction,

Fig. 13-33. Pneumatosis intestinalis in a patient with low colonic obstruction. The intramural gas is seen as thin, radiolucent stripes along the margins of the gas-distended bowel.

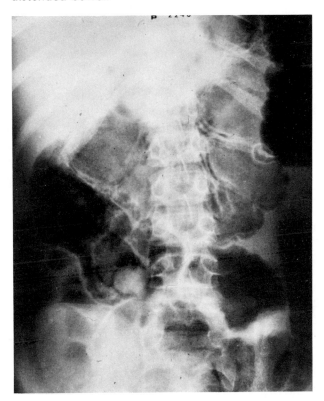

intestinal parasites, phlegmonous gastritis, pyloric stenosis, peptic ulcer, toxic megacolon, and Whipple's disease. Pneumatosis may complicate such procedures as gastroscopy, sigmoidoscopy, colonoscopy, and bowel surgery. It has also been reported in children on steroid therapy, in whom gas may persist for months.

The characteristic plain film findings are those of a collection of cystlike bubbles of gas that vary from a few millimeters to several centimeters in size. There may also be linear streaks of gas parallel to the bowel wall.

INTRAMURAL GAS

In addition to its occurrence in pneumatosis cystoides intestinalis, gas may be found within the wall of one or more loops of bowel in certain other diseases. These include: (1) necrotizing gastroenterocolitis, usually in infants; (2) mesenteric vascular thrombosis; (3) necrosis secondary to strangulated obstruction; (4) toxic ulcerative colitis; and (5) in ulcerative disease developing above an obstructing carcinoma of the colon. The pathogenesis may vary, but, in most instances, necrosis of a segment of intestine is present and the gas probably enters through a break or breaks in the mucosa of the involved segment. In patients with obstruction, the increase in intraluminal pressure above the lesion also may play a part. Infection with gas-forming organisms has been noted less frequently, but this can be a cause of intramural gas.

In patients with necrosis or impending necrosis, there may be a solitary abnormal segment of bowel or, at the most, several segments adjacent to one another. The segments contain an excessive amount of fluid, the mucosal folds are widened owing to edema, and there is thickening of the wall of the bowel. These changes can be determined if there also is gas within the lumen to outline the folds and two adjacent abnormal segments are found so that wall thickness can be estimated.

The intramural gas is seen as linear, stripelike translucencies paralleling the lumen of the intestine (see Fig. 13-33). If the segment is seen end-on, a ring-contoured translucency is formed as the intramural gas surrounds the gas-filled lumen of the bowel. Later, as frank necrosis develops, the mucosal folds tend to disappear and the internal surface becomes relatively smooth.

In association with the intramural gas, filling of the portal veins with gas produces linear branching translucencies in the peripheral parts of the liver (Fig. 13-34); these two findings form a highly significant roentgen complex for the diagnosis of intestinal necrosis.

ASCITES

When the patient is in the supine position ascitic fluid accumulates in the pelvis and ascends to either side of the bladder, causing a somewhat triangular density (dog ears) on either side of the bladder. It then extends into the paracolic gutters, more on the right than on the left, where it displaces the colon medially, usually more on the right than on the left. As more fluid accumulates, the inferior border of the liver is obscured; the liver is displaced medially when more than 2000 ml are present. There is enough difference in density between the liver and ascitic fluid to be detected on plain film study.[29] Therefore, the medial displacement can be observed. When present, it is a reliable sign of ascites.

When roentgenograms are obtained with the patient supine, free fluid in the peritoneal cavity causes a generalized increase in density of the abdomen. The margins of the liver, spleen, and kidneys become indistinct and the psoas muscle margins also become poorly visualized. Normally the lower lateral margin of the liver can be identified. If fluid is present in the area the liver edge becomes indistinct or disappears altogether. It should be noted that in emaciated individuals the margins of the abdominal viscera are seen very poorly because of a lack of fat around the viscera, which normally offers contrast because of its more radiolucent nature. If gas is present within loops of small bowel these loops are spread apart and the soft-tissue space between contiguous gas shadows is increased over the normal. Fluid in the flanks causes increase in the soft-tissue space between the radiolucent flank stripe (properitoneal fat line) and the adjacent gas-filled colon, as indicated in the foregoing. It also causes an outward bulging and increased definition of the properitoneal fat line. In roentgenograms obtained with the patient upright the fluid sinks to the most dependent part of the abdominal cavity and forms a homogeneous increase in density. This is limited to the pelvis if the amount of fluid is small or it may extend higher if a large effusion is present. The upper boundary of the fluid is not sharp, but the density gradually diminishes superiorly. It is limited inferiorly by a convex margin and frequently delineated from the urinary bladder by a narrow translucent zone. If gas is present in the small intestine, the loops float above the fluid and thus may not

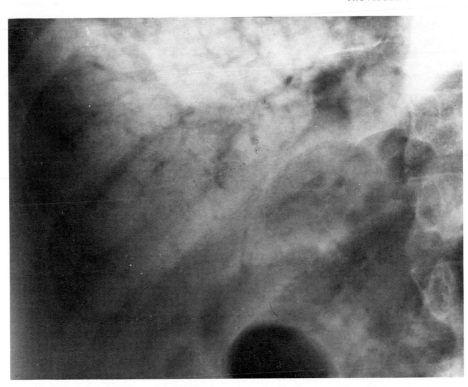

Fig. 13-34. Gas within the portal vein secondary to intestinal necrosis. The gas is seen as branching translucent shadows extending into the periphery of the liver.

be found within the pelvis as they normally would be. Similar findings are to be noted in roentgenograms obtained with the patient in the lateral decubitus position in which the fluid is seen to be sinking to the dependent side and the gas-filled loops of bowel are seen to be rising. If fluid for one reason or another should be loculated, it will not shift in position but remain in the same position regardless of the position of the patient. Such loculations may simulate the appearance caused by solid tumors or abscesses and usually the differentiation is not possible from roentgen observation. Small amounts of fluid may produce only increased pelvic density in films exposed with the patient upright as compared to those exposed with the patient supine; this is very difficult to assess, however, since there is normally an increase in pelvic density when an individual is upright. Fluid may occasionally accumulate between the gastric fundus and the left hemidiaphragm to simulate an infrapulmonary pleural effusion.

INTRA-ABDOMINAL ABSCESSES

The shadow of the abscess may be visualized as an area of increased density, particularly if it is surrounded by gas-filled loops of bowel. Frequently, however, it is too indistinct in outline to be recognized clearly except as a zone of ill-defined density. The signs of generalized peritonitis may be present, including separation of the gas-filled loops, because of exudate on the surface of the bowel wall or fluid in the peritoneal cavity. A paralytic ileus is likely to be found in association with the infection so that loops of the small intestine and the colon are very often distended. The shadow of an abscess may be confused with that of a tumor or even with a fluid-filled strangulated loop of bowel (the pseudotumor sign of Frimann-Dahl, *q.v.*) (see Fig. 13-13). Correlation of the roentgen observations with the clinical findings is essential in many of these cases in order more clearly to evaluate the roentgen findings.

If the abscess has developed as a result of perforation of the stomach or bowel, gas may enter it; or gas may form as a result of infection by gas-forming organisms (Fig. 13-35). When this happens, the interior of the abscess may have a mottled radiolucent appearance caused by gas bubbles intermixed with necrotic material or pus (Fig. 13-36). In upright or lateral decubitus roentgenograms a gas-fluid level may be demonstrated if the cavity contains pus. This may be confused with gas accumulations within the bowel. Distinguishing features include the constancy in position of the gas shadows regardless of the posi-

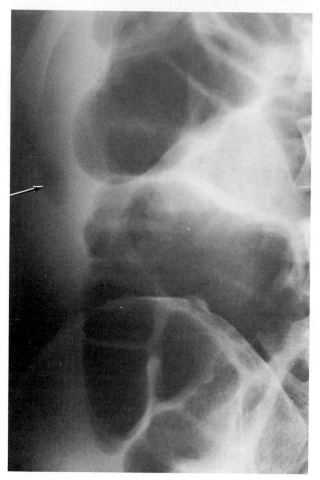

Fig. 13-35. Acute abscess of the appendix. The right colon is distended with gas, and there is also some gas in the distal ileum which is very slightly distended. **Arrow** indicates gas in an abscess resulting from a ruptured retroperitoneal appendix.

tion of the patient when multiple roentgenograms are obtained and constancy of the shadows in serial roentgenograms; at times the location of the shadows clearly indicates them to be outside the lumen of the bowel. Barium enema or barium-meal studies may show the lesion responsible and reveal the sinus tract leading from the lumen to the abscess (*e.g.*, a ruptured colonic diverticulum).

Ruptured aortic aneurysm with dissection of blood into the retroperitoneal fat may produce a mottled appearance that simulates the mottled gas sometimes observed in retroperitoneal abscess.[38] Because the differentiation may be very difficult in obese patients, the possibility of ruptured aneurysm must be consid-

ered, particularly if there are no clinical signs of infection.

SUBDIAPHRAGMATIC ABSCESS

Infection in the subphrenic space is more common on the right side than on the left. The earliest roentgen findings are those of elevation of the hemidiaphragm and restriction of its motion (Fig. 13-37). The limitation of motion may be local and of varying degrees of severity. These changes are not diagnostic of a subdiaphragmatic abscess, since other causes may be responsible for them. It is necessary at this stage, therefore, that the roentgen findings be considered in conjunction with the clinical signs and only when there is evidence to indicate the likelihood of a subphrenic abscess are these observations to be considered significant. During the immediate period

Fig. 13-36. Intra-abdominal abscess secondary to perforation of a carcinoma of the colon. The accumulation of mottled gas shadows **(arrows)** is extraluminal as shown by constancy in several other examinations and confirmed by surgical exploration.

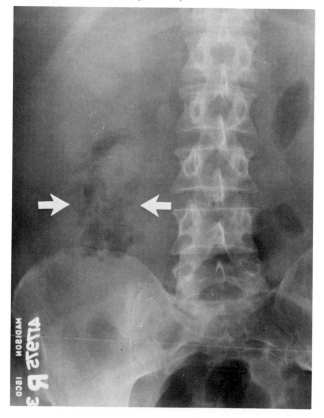

after upper abdominal surgery, it is not at all uncommon to find the diaphragm elevated, especially the right leaf, and its motion restricted because of abdominal distention or pain or a combination of both. This sign must be interpreted with particular caution during the postoperative period.

The next change to be observed is an inflammatory pleural reaction at the base of the lung and the development of pleural effusion. The fluid usually is not purulent and is sometimes referred to as a "sympathetic effusion." Once an appreciable amount of fluid has formed, the diaphragm becomes obscured and it may be difficult to determine its position. Examination of the chest with the patient recumbent and in right and left lateral decubitus positions may cause enough shifting of the fluid to allow at least a partial visualization of the diaphragm.

Gas formation within the abscess cavity is rather frequent and can be demonstrated in upright or lateral decubitus roentgenograms. These should always be obtained as a part of the study of a suspected or known subdiaphragmatic abscess. The gas surmounting the fluid leads to the formation of a fluid level and this gives one of the most significant roentgen findings for the diagnosis (Fig. 13-38).

The signs of a left-sided subphrenic abscess are similar to those just described. In addition, displacement of the stomach downward, medially, and often anteriorly may be seen. Sometimes the displacement can be recognized by the position of the gastric air bubble; at other times the introduction of a small amount of barium–water mixture may be needed to more clearly outline the entire stomach and demonstrate the evidence of the extragastric mass.

The roentgen findings in perirenal abscess are discussed in Chapter 20.

FOREIGN BODIES

A scout roentgenogram is useful for determining the presence or absence of opaque foreign bodies in the gastrointestinal tract or within the peritoneal cavity. In order to be sufficiently radiopaque to be visualized, metallic objects must be made of or contain one of the heavier metals such as iron, gold, or silver. Objects composed entirely of aluminum are of almost the same density as the soft tissues and therefore not readily visualized. During infancy and early childhood the swallowing of coins, pins, and nails is very common. Psychiatric patients in mental hospitals often swallow objects such as pins, paper clips, and the like. Roentgenograms are useful to confirm the

presence of the foreign body and to follow its course through the gastrointestinal tract.

Geophagia (dirt-eating) may result in the production of radiopacity in the gastrointestinal tract. The diagnosis is suggested by finding unusually radiopaque intestinal contents in a patient who has had no roentgenographic contrast studies and who is not taking medication containing radiopaque material.[10]

The presence of retained surgical sponges can be established if a radiopaque type of sponge has been used. There are several varieties of these sponges and they depend for radiopacity upon an insert of barium or metallic impregnated string or cloth. This type of sponge should be used routinely in surgical procedures within the body cavities. Because sponge counts occasionally indicate a missing sponge a roentgenogram of the abdomen obtained in the operating room before closing the incision will give the operating surgeon peace of mind if no radiopaque shadows are seen or will allow him to search for and remove the object before closure.

THE PANCREAS

ROENTGEN ANATOMY

The pancreas is situated along the posterior abdominal wall in the upper abdomen in intimate relationship to the stomach and duodenum. The head of the gland usually lies directly in front of the lumbar spine and is surrounded by the duodenal loop. The third portion of the duodenum crosses obliquely in front of the pancreas to its junction with the jejunum, where it forms the angle of Treitz. The central portion or body of the pancreas usually lies directly posterior to the body and antrum of the stomach, separated from it by the omental bursa, which in turn is bounded posteriorly by the pancreas and anteriorly by the posterior wall of the stomach. The tail of the pancreas is in contact with the medial surface of the spleen. The pancreas cannot be identified in roentgenograms of the abdomen. Its borders are indistinct and it blends with the soft tissues of the posterior wall of the abdomen. Arteriography of the celiac axis and superior mesenteric arteries in diseases of the pancreas, particularly carcinoma is discussed later in this chapter. Other than arteriography the roentgen diagnosis of pancreatic disease depends to a large extent upon observation of the changes produced in adjacent structures, particularly the stomach, duodenum, and transverse colon. Only when calcifications are found within the pancreas is there characteristic and direct roentgen evidence of disease. In spite of these draw-

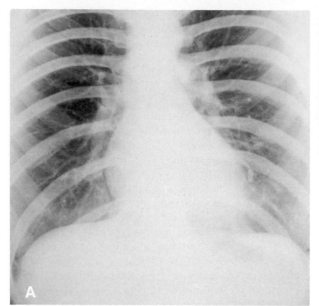

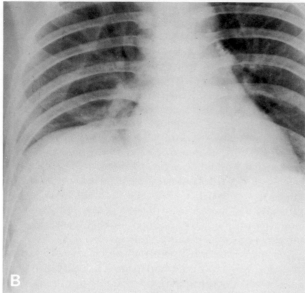

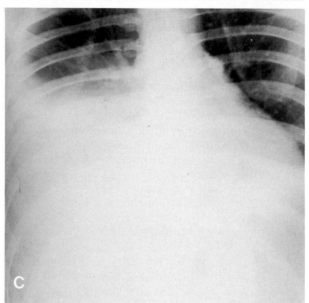

Fig. 13-37. Acute subphrenic abscess. **A.** Normal appearance of the lower chest before onset of the infection. **B.** Roentgenogram obtained several days after the onset of fever following a laparotomy shows elevation of the right hemidiaphragm. **C.** One week later, pleural effusion in addition to elevation of the hemidiaphragm is evident. The abscess was drained surgically. The pleural fluid was removed at thoracentesis; it was not purulent.

backs there are a number of roentgenographic findings in various diseases of the pancreas that offer considerable information, particularly when they are correlated with the clinical signs and symptoms. Scout roentgenograms of the abdomen as well as gastrointestinal studies with barium sulfate and angiography have a place in the study of the pancreas, as will be indicated in succeeding paragraphs.

Of the newer methods of examining the retroperi-

toneal structures, ultrasonography, which carries no radiation risk in addition to being noninvasive, should probably be performed first when pancreatic cancer or other disease is suspected. According to published reports, detection rates for separating patients with normal from abnormal pancreas are in the range of 85% to 90%. When ultrasound is negative or equivocal, computerized tomography may be very useful, particularly in patients who have a reasonable amount of retroperitoneal fat. In patients with reasonable possibility of pancreatic carcinoma, percutaneous needle biopsy guided by ultrasound is sometimes used.

ACUTE PANCREATITIS

In the presence of acute pancreatitis, roentgen examination may be of considerable value in helping to exclude the possibility of other causes of acute abdominal pain, such as calculi in the biliary or urinary tracts, ruptured peptic ulcer, and acute bowel obstruction. In addition, in many patients other findings will be present to direct attention to the pancreas as the site of disease. In general the roentgen findings must be interpreted in the light of clinical symptoms and signs since by themselves the changes may be too nonspecific to allow definitive diagnosis.

Preliminary or "scout" roentgenograms should include supine and upright projections as a routine with the addition of lateral decubitus views in patients with equivocal findings. Among the changes that may be observed are the following:

Regional or Localized Ileus ("Sentinel Loops"). Localized gas distention of one or more loops of bowel immediately adjacent to the pancreas may be found. The duodenum may be filled with gas or a loop of jejunum may be visualized in this manner (Fig. 13-39). In some cases a segment of the transverse colon is distended. The more localized the distention and the closer the relationship of the loops to the pancreas, the more significant is the observation. Fluid levels usually are present in the loops when upright or lateral decubitus views are obtained. When both the stomach and the transverse colon are distended with gas there may be an unusually wide soft-tissue space between them; normally they are in close relationship and separated by a thin space equivalent to the thickness of their walls. Because of its close relationship to the pancreas, gas distention of the duodenum is more suggestive of acute pancreatitis than is distention of a jejunal loop. The finding of localized gas distention of the midtransverse colon also is significant. All of the above findings are nonspecific and may be misleading, however.

Generalized Ileus. Not infrequently by the time the patient is examined roentgenologically the signs have become those of a more or less generalized adynamic distention. If there has been a spread of inflammation beyond the confines of the pancreas so that fairly extensive peritoneal inflammation is present, there may

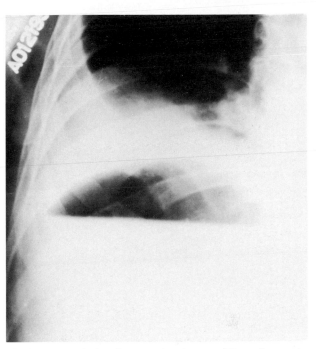

Fig. 13-38. Subdiaphragmatic abscess. There is an air-fluid level in the abscess cavity and a rather large pleural effusion.

be evidence of exudate separating the gas-filled loops. In the later or more advanced stages of the inflammation such generalized signs are frequent and by themselves are of little value in establishing the exact cause of the difficulty.

Pancreatic Pseudocyst. With extension of the inflammation beyond the confines of the pancreas, localized accumulations of fluid may form either in the immediate area of the pancreas or occasionally at some distance from it. These are known as pseudocysts. Such a mass may be visible as a soft-tissue shadow with ill-defined borders. When a collection of fluid forms adjacent to the pancreas or in the lesser peritoneal sac, displacement of the stomach, colon, and duodenum may indicate the presence of the lesion. The inflammation may spread to the subphrenic space and form a subphrenic abscess on either side although this complication is more frequent on the left. Spread to the subphrenic space results in elevation of the hemidiaphragm, restriction of its motion, and, within a short time, the development of pleural effusion. Rarely the infection may burrow through the diaphragm and cause an empyema or it may extend into the mediastinum with formation of a mediastinal ab-

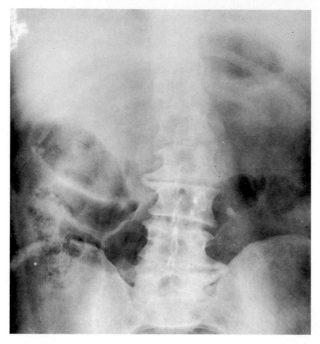

Fig. 13-39. Acute pancreatitis. There is some gas in distended loops of small bowel mainly in the right upper central portion of the abdomen. This localized adynamic ileus is not characteristic of acute pancreatitis but suggests the likelihood of acute inflammation in the area. When correlated with clinical findings, it may be highly suggestive in such cases.

scess. Many unusual presentations of pseudocysts with and without abscess formation have been described. Supraclavicular and retropharyngeal pseudocysts may occur in addition to mediastinal masses. They may also produce intrarenal, infrarenal, and presacral masses that may impinge on the ureter causing symptoms suggesting primary urinary tract disease. Rarely they may rupture spontaneously into the stomach or into the abdominal cavity.

Changes in the Lungs. As indicated in the preceding paragraph, extension of inflammation to the subphrenic space will cause elevation and fixation of the diaphragm. Linear streaks of density frequently can be visualized crossing the lung field in its basal portion in these patients. These linear shadows represent foci of platelike atelectasis and are the result of restriction of diaphragmatic motion. They are, of course, not specific for acute pancreatitis. Massive pleural effusion, usually on the left side, may also complicate pancreatitis. The fluid may have high

amylase levels and relatively high protein levels. Effusion is often chronic and tends to recur following thoracentesis.

Abdominal Fat Necrosis. Abdominal fat necrosis[5] may occur in the vicinity of the pancreas and of adjacent retroperitoneal fat and also in the omentum. Mottled areas of faintly visible radiolucency, most likely representing normal fat interspersed with the water density of hydrolyzed or saponified fat, may be present. The findings are subtle and require films of good technical quality (low contrast films with good detail) coned to the area of interest. Coned oblique films may be helpful. When present, this sign of fat necrosis is virtually pathognomonic of acute pancreatitis. Fat necrosis may be very extensive in these patients, since pancreatic lipase enters the blood stream by way of the lymphatics. It may cause osteolytic lesions of bone as well as occasional periosteal reaction and is the presumed cause of aseptic necrosis which is often observed in patients with pancreatitis.

Pancreatic Calculi. If the attack represents an acute exacerbation of a chronic pancreatitis, calculi may be visualized in some cases (Fig. 13-40) (see discussion of pancreatic lithiasis to follow).

Barium Meal Examination

Many patients with acute pancreatitis are too ill to be subjected to gastrointestinal examinations but important information can be obtained by barium meal examination. Some of the changes that may be observed in acute pancreatitis or during an acute exacerbation of chronic disease are the following:

Enlargement of the Papilla of Vater. The normal papilla is sometimes seen as a smoothly rounded, filling defect along the medial aspect of the descending duodenum approximately 1 cm in diameter and 0.5 cm in height. During the acute stage of pancreatitis the papillary defect enlarges. The mucosal folds of the duodenum adjacent to it become thickened. With a greater degree of swelling the pancreas may bulge into the duodenum and surround the ampulla, causing a defect that resembles a figure 3 in reverse. This sign is not specific for pancreatitis; it also occurs when the pancreas is enlarged as a result of neoplasm of the periampullary region.

Functional Disturbances of the Duodenum. The duodenal motility may be altered, often being increased over the normal. Peristalsis is hyperactive and re-

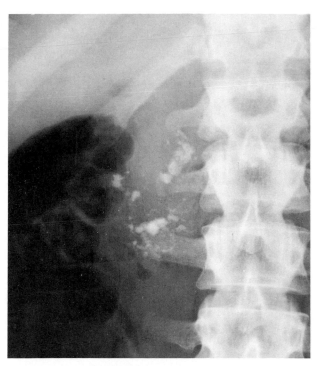

Fig. 13-40. Chronic pancreatitis. There is scattering of calculi in the region of the head of the pancreas which is enlarged.

verse peristalsis may be seen. The duodenum often is irritable as observed fluoroscopically. The mucosal folds may be altered, being coarsened or thickened.

Other Signs of Acute Pancreatitis. The left psoas muscle margin and the left renal outline may be blurred in the presence of acute pancreatitis. The left kidney at times is displaced slightly downward and outward. The stomach may be displaced forward if the pancreas is enlarged. Intravenous urography may reveal impairment of the left renal function if there has been sufficient pressure on the renal artery or vein to interfere with its circulation. Localized tenderness directly over the region of the pancreas may be elicited during fluoroscopic observation.

Enlargement of the Pancreas

Enlargement of the pancreas may be caused either by inflammation or neoplasm and in many cases it is impossible on the basis of roentgen examination to determine which condition exists. In some cases the invasive nature of a carcinoma may be apparent as it extends into the duodenum or the stomach. In others

the roentgen signs are minimal or completely absent. The chief roentgen findings that may be observed when the pancreas enlarges include the following:

Enlargement of the Duodenal Loop. Because the duodenum surrounds the head of the pancreas and is in intimate relationship to it, any appreciable enlargement of the pancreatic head causes widening of the duodenal loop. The duodenal curve becomes rounded (Fig. 13-41). This sign has long been described as one of the important roentgen features of pancreatic enlargement. It is of considerable diagnostic value when present but minor to moderate degrees of enlargement are difficult to recognize. The range of normal variation in the appearance of the duodenal curve is considerable and must be taken into account when considering the possibility of pancreatic enlargement. In obese individuals it is always more rounded and smooth than in persons of average habitus, and, in some of these, it may appear actually enlarged. This is caused by the high transverse position of the stomach and the accumulations of fat in the pancreatic area.

Forward Displacement of the Stomach. This is another sign difficult to evaluate unless the displacement is of considerable degree. The normal distance between the posterior surface of the stomach and the anterior border of the spine varies considerably in different persons and is much influenced by the habitus of the individual. A distended colon, the presence of ascites, or a large mass such as an ovarian cyst may elevate the stomach and cause the retrogastric space to appear unusually wide. The most accurate determination of the width of the retrogastric space is obtained by examining the patient in a supine position with a horizontally directed roentgen-ray beam passing transversely through the abdomen, the film cassette being placed along one side. This gives a lateral view of the abdomen with the stomach riding over the anterior surface of the pancreas. The stomach can be filled either with air introduced through a tube placed within it or with orally administered barium meal. The latter is generally preferred because of its simplicity. For standard examination the ordinary right lateral view of the stomach is adequate and is obtained as a routine procedure during examination of the upper gastrointestinal tract. A number of methods of measuring anterior displacement of the stomach and of the duodenojejunal junction have been described, but the variation in the normal is so great that the measurements are of questionable value.

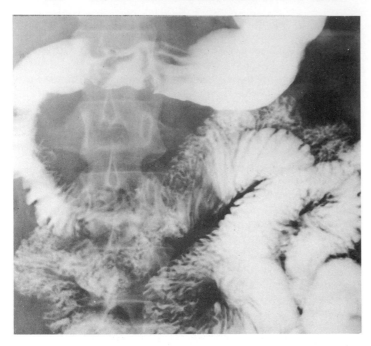

Fig. 13-41. Chronic pancreatitis. The duodenal loop has been widened by enlargement of the pancreatic head. There is also noted some flattening of mucosal folds along the inner side, particularly in the descending duodenum.

Changes in the Mucosal Pattern of the Duodenum. The effect of pancreatic enlargement upon the mucosal pattern of the duodenum often is a significant roentgen observation and is a more obvious sign of early enlargement than is rounding of the duodenal curve or forward displacement of the stomach. These folds may appear unusually thick and rigid. They may be flattened along the inner side of the duodenum and relatively normal on the outer (Figs. 13-42 and 13-43). When carcinoma of the head of the pancreas is present there may be invasion of the duodenal wall shown by a loss of mucosal pattern, with irregular nodular protrusions into the duodenal lumen; or constricted stenotic areas may be produced leading to duodenal obstruction. When the body of the pancreas is enlarged there may be evidence of compression of the transverse portion of the duodenum where it passes over the pancreas, the folds being flattened and the lumen of the duodenum narrowed in an anteroposterior direction.

Hypotonic Duodenography. This is a method for giving a more detailed study of the effects of pancreatic and other disease upon the mucosa of the duodenum. In brief, the technique consists in the intravenous or intramuscular administration of 1.0 to 2.0 mg glucagon (some prefer to use 30 to 60 mg of Pro-Banthine). The patient may be intubated and 100 to 200 ml of barium sulfate suspension instilled into the duodenum followed by the instillation of sufficient air to distend the duodenum.[12] Within about 5 to 10 minutes after injection of the drug, the duodenum becomes dilated and hypotonic with absence of peristalsis. When proper distention and barium coating of the duodenum are obtained, a number of spot films are obtained in projection which bring out the mucosal pattern of the duodenal loop. The finer detail of the duodenal mucosa is brought out to good advantage and the effects of pressure or invasion from a contiguous mass can be identified more easily than with a routine barium meal. The procedure is, in effect, an extension of the usual barium sulfate meal. The technique is also discussed in Chapter 17.

The Reverse Figure 3 Sign. Frostberg[21] originally called attention to a distinct alteration in the appearance of the inner wall of the descending duodenum in patients with pancreatic enlargement, which he described as a reverse figure 3. This is caused by swelling of the pancreas either from inflammation or neoplasm, with bulging of the gland into the duodenal lumen surrounding the papilla of Vater. It produces a smooth filling defect above and below the papilla that resembles a figure 3 in reverse (Fig. 13-44). It is a valuable sign of pancreatic disease but in itself does not distinguish between swelling caused by inflammation and that resulting from tumor.

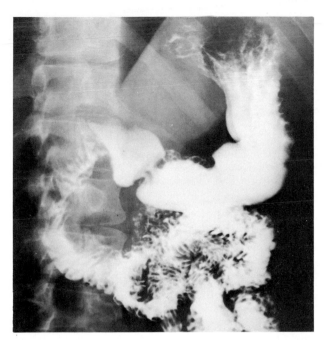

Fig. 13-42. Carcinoma of the head of the pancreas. There is a pressure defect on the inner side of the descending duodenum noted best inferiorly. The mucosal folds are somewhat flattened and distorted. The ampullary area projects slightly to the left producing a modified "E" sign.

Evidence of a Dilated Common Bile Duct. The common bile duct lies in close relationship to the duodenum, usually crossing just posterior to the junction of the first and second portions. Because of this close relationship, dilatation of the common duct may cause a pressure defect on the duodenum. This may be in the form of a bandlike compression or flattening of the duodenum, or a sharp angulation of the apex of the duodenal bulb and its continuation into the descending portion (see Fig. 13-42). The right lateral position is of value in showing this deformity but it also can be demonstrated frequently in the right anterior oblique position. This sign only indicates obstruction of the distal portion of the common duct but its significance in relation to pancreatic disease is obvious. Tumors of the periampullary region are prone to cause dilatation of the common duct and this may be the only roentgen abnormality that can be demonstrated.

The "Pad" Sign. The pad sign is a localized, smooth, pressure type of deformity, usually on the inferior surface of the gastric antrum or duodenal bulb, re-

sembling closely that which can be produced by applying pressure over the anterior abdominal wall by a pressure pad or by manual palpation (Fig. 13-45). Occasionally the pad defect is observed along the superior surface of the duodenal bulb or gastric antrum since the relationships of the stomach and pancreas need not be constant. This sign is best brought out by having the patient face the top of an upright fluoroscopic table and then tilting the table slowly toward the horizontal position under fluoroscopic observation. Pressure of the spine on the gastric antrum can simulate the pad sign when the patient is prone on the fluoroscopic table, but the effect of pressure from

Fig. 13-43. Carcinoma of the head of the pancreas. A mass **(arrow)** distorts the mucosa on the inner side of the descending duodenum. A little flattening of mucosal folds is noted above and below it.

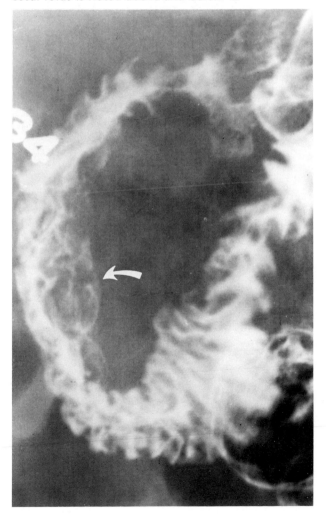

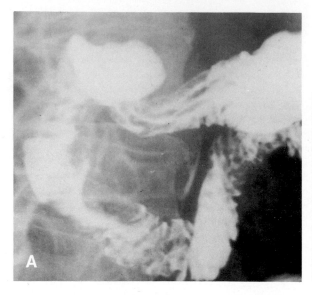

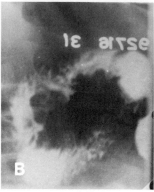

Fig. 13-44. Two patients with carcinoma of the head of the pancreas illustrating Frostberg's sign. The inner margin of the descending duodenum resembles a reversed figure 3. The mass appears more localized in **A** than in **B.**

an enlarged pancreas will appear before the table has reached a horizontal position. Careful palpation of the abdominal wall with the patient upright also may demonstrate this defect.

Visualization of the Common Bile Duct (Cholangiography). Using one of the cholecystographic media, such as iopanoic acid (Telepaque), it is sometimes possible to visualize the common duct when good gallbladder function is present. Even when the gallbladder is diseased, the common duct may be visualized if a double dose of iopanoic acid is administered. Demonstration of the duct occurs most frequently during the phase of gallbladder contraction following a fat meal. Therefore, a fat meal is usually necessary if demonstration of the common bile duct is desired. Another method for visualization of the common duct, intravenous cholangiography, is of value particularly when gallbladder disease interferes with its function or in patients in whom the gallbladder has been removed. This consists of the intravenous injection of iodipamide (Cholegrafin). We use a drip infusion technique. This material is excreted by the liver in a sufficiently high concentration so that the bile is radiopaque as it leaves the liver and thus the common duct may be outlined. These methods of examination are discussed in more detail in Chapter 14. If the common duct can be identified by rendering its bile content radiopaque, obstruction in the distal portion may be demonstrated because of the dilatation of the duct above the level of obstruction. These methods require reasonably good liver function and if

there has been very much liver damage results often are unsatisfactory. Then the method of direct puncture of a hepatic radicle through the abdominal wall and liver (percutaneous transhepatic cholangiography) may be used to demonstrate the presence of common duct obstruction and, often, the nature of the lesion responsible. This is discussed in Chapter 14.

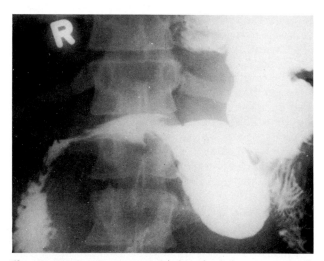

Fig. 13-45. Carcinoma of the head of the pancreas illustrating the "pad sign." A smooth pressure defect on the inferior surface of the duodenal bulb and distal gastric antrum indicates a mass in the region of the head of the pancreas.

Pancreatic Lithiasis

The formation of calculi within the ducts or possibly in the parenchyma of the pancreas gives one of the most striking and direct roentgen signs of pancreatic disease. In most cases the calcifications occur in association with chronic pancreatitis and the roentgen demonstration of them usually indicates the existence of this disease. Occasionally, however, pancreatic lithiasis is found in an individual who shows none of the clinical signs or symptoms of pancreatitis. Some investigators believe that all pancreatic calcifications form within the ducts; others consider that the concretions may form either in the ducts or in the gland parenchyma.

Pancreatic calculi are usually multiple and are seen in the roentgenogram as dense, small calcified areas throughout a portion or the entire gland. The effect is usually one of calcific stippling, since most of the stones are likely to be small (Fig. 13-46). The calculi are found most frequently in the head of the pancreas but it is not uncommon to have them widely distributed throughout the gland. When relatively few in number and limited to the region of the head, the stones may be overlooked in routine roentgenograms of the abdomen, obtained with patient in the supine or prone position, because the head of the pancreas usually lies directly over the upper lumbar vertebrae. They are seen to best advantage when the roentgenograms are obtained with the patient turned to a slightly oblique position that projects the pancreatic head to one side of the spine. If there is doubt concerning the nature of the shadows, a barium meal can be given and the relationship of the calcifications to the duodenal loop determined. In most cases the small dense and discrete calcifications clustered in the region of the pancreas make the diagnosis of pancreatic lithiasis not too difficult.

Although pancreatitis is by far the most common cause, there are other conditions in which pancreatic calculi may occur. These include hyperparathyroidism and advanced cystic fibrosis of the pancreas usually associated with diabetes mellitus. Rarely calcification is observed in ducts proximal to a pancreatic tumor or with a nonspecific ductal stenosis which has occluded them. Cystadenoma and cystadenocarcinoma of the pancreas may produce tumor calcification. Rarely there may be a radiating sunburst pattern of calcification in cystadenoma that is characteristic when it is observed.[47] Cavernous lymphangioma or hemangioma may be associated with phleboliths in and adjacent to the pancreas. A single case report of the "milk of calcium" type of density

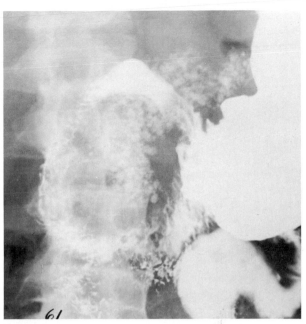

Fig. 13-46. Pancreatic lithiasis. Extensive calcifications in the head of the pancreas and extending throughout its body are noted on this barium study of the stomach and duodenum. Note also the enlargement of the duodenal loop, indicating enlargement of the pancreatic head. There is also some flattening of duodenal mucosa.

within the pseudocyst of the pancreas brings up another possible but rare cause of calcification in the pancreatic area.[52]

Renal and gallbladder calculi seldom cause difficulty in differential diagnosis because of the location and character of the shadows. Gallstones often are laminated while pancreatic calculi rarely are. In doubtful cases, cholecystography or intravenous urography may be used to localize the calculi in relation to these structures. Calcified lymph nodes cause the greatest difficulty. When the pancreatic calcifications are few in number they may resemble the appearance of calcified nodes rather closely. Roentgenograms of the barium-filled stomach and duodenum will help to localize the calculi and establish their position in relation to the pancreas. In most cases the small discrete calcifications distributed over a fairly wide area differ from the larger mulberry-type calcifications found in lymph nodes. Calcified plaques in the aorta or in branches of the celiac axis or other branches of the aorta also must be considered. Usually the linear nature of such plaques when they are viewed on edge or their curvilinear or circular shape when seen on end are sufficiently characteristic for proper identification.

Chronic Pancreatitis

The roentgen signs of chronic pancreatitis include the evidence of pancreatic enlargement, the presence of pancreatic calcifications, and changes secondary to pancreatic steatorrhea. The changes caused by enlargement of the pancreas have been enumerated and discussed in preceding sections of this chapter and, as indicated in the previous section, the roentgen demonstration of an enlarged pancreas frequently does not allow a differential diagnosis to be made between inflammation and tumor. The presence of pancreatic lithiasis is reasonably good evidence of the coexistence of chronic pancreatitis. Steatorrhea may be caused by disease of the pancreas, particularly by chronic pancreatitis. The clinical features of pancreatogenic steatorrhea resemble those of idiopathic sprue and the roentgen findings in the gastrointestinal tract may be similar (see Ch. 18). Some recent observations indicate that the small-intestinal changes are less severe in pancreatogenic steatorrhea than they are in the idiopathic form of the disease (nontropical sprue) and in some cases the small-bowel pattern may be normal or nearly so. Rather infrequently chronic pancreatitis may cause an osteomalacic picture in the skeletal system characterized by generalized demineralization of the skeleton and the occurrence of pseudofractures in some of the bones. These are highly characteristic of osteomalacia and are visualized as fissure-like defects or clefts extending transversely part way or completely through a bone. They represent fracture fissures filled with uncalcified osteoid. They are seen most frequently along the axillary borders of the scapulas, the inner margins of the femoral necks, and in the ribs. In patients with severe disease, however, they may be rather widely distributed in the skeleton.

Carcinoma of the Pancreas

The roentgen findings in carcinoma of the pancreas have been covered, to a large extent, in the section dealing with enlargement of the pancreas. Some observations concerning tumors of the periampullary region also have been made earlier in this chapter. As has been indicated, it often is impossible to distinguish between inflammatory and neoplastic enlargements of the gland. In some patients, direct invasion of the duodenum or the gastric antrum may have occurred and the infiltrative and destructive nature of the lesion may be readily apparent. For example, a carcinoma arising in the head of the pancreas may extend into the duodenum, causing an irregular nodular filling defect, loss of mucosal folds, abnormal fixation, stiffening of the duodenal wall, and ulceration. Partial or complete obstruction of the duodenum may be caused by carcinoma of the pancreas; this is an unusual complication of pancreatitis. The demonstration of pancreatic lithiasis in association with the signs of pancreatic enlargement is good evidence of the presence of chronic pancreatitis, although the possibility of coexisting carcinoma cannot be excluded entirely even in these cases.

The frequency of positive roentgen evidence in patients with pancreatic carcinoma depends upon the location of the tumor within the gland and to some extent upon its duration. Those lesions arising in the head of the pancreas, particularly in the periampullary region, will give positive roentgen findings more often and earlier than those that develop in the body or tail of the gland. In general, about 50% of all pancreatic carcinomas will show some evidence of their presence on roentgen examination if careful attention is paid to the early signs of pressure and invasion as has been noted. It is emphasized again that even when findings are present it may not be possible to state the nature of the lesion from roentgen examination alone and the diagnosis may have to be limited to that of a mass in or near the pancreas.

The detection of carcinoma of the pancreas early enough to permit surgical removal is a very difficult problem since the tumors may be asymptomatic until far advanced. There are a number of diagnostic methods in addition to hypotonic duodenography described previously. Selective superior mesenteric and celiac *arteriography,* sometimes followed by superselective catheterization of arteries supplying the pancreas, is used to demonstrate these neoplasms. The arteriographic findings include irregular encasement of arteries by the tumor, occlusion of arterial branches, compression of veins, and the presence of abnormal tumor vessels and tumor stain (Fig. 13-47).

Endoscopic retrograde cholangiopancreatography (ERCP) is also used. This permits retrograde opacification of the pancreatic duct. Many of the indications for this study have to do with the biliary tract disease, but it is used in patients with suspected pancreatic cancer and in patients with chronic pancreatitis when a surgical procedure on the pancreatic ducts is being considered. The findings in pancreatic cancer are those of duct obstruction and stenosis. Stenosis may be smooth or irregular with a rat-tail narrowing, while obstruction is abrupt. When there

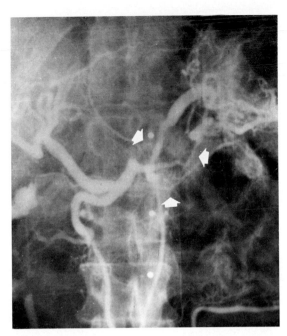

Fig. 13-47. Carcinoma of the pancreas. Celiac axis arteriogram shows obstruction, straightening, and narrowing of a group of vessels due to tumor encasement **(left and right arrows)**. There also is a small area of neovascularity **(lower arrow)**.

is stenosis of the common bile duct as well, there is a strong likelihood of pancreatic neoplasm. This method of examination is of limited value in tumors of the tail of the pancreas because of incomplete filling of the ducts in this region. Furthermore, it provides no information regarding resectability.

Ultrasonography is also used in the detection of pancreatic masses and is of special value in the diagnosis of pseudocysts. Solid pancreatic tumors may be detected, but there is no tissue specificity.

Computed tomography using body scanners provides for imaging of the pancreas, but differentiation between inflammatory and neoplastic masses is not possible with this method, and in thin patients the lack of retroperitoneal fat may make visualization difficult.

Percutaneous *fine-needle aspiration biopsy* is now being used to assess pancreatic disease as well as disease elsewhere in the abdomen and thorax.[23] For this procedure, a 23-gauge, 15-cm spinal type needle is employed. Localization of the mass to be biopsied may require angiography; this study is performed under fluoroscopic guidance or with ultrasonic control. The method has been in use for a relatively short time and has not been completely evaluated. How-

ever, results are promising, and it does permit histologic verification of tumor types.

Other Pancreatic Tumors

Cystadenoma. Cystadenoma is nine times more frequent in females than in males and tends to be large so that there is a palpable mass in about 80% of subjects.[43] In patients with this tumor the incidence of metabolic and endocrine abnormalities, including diabetes, obesity, sterility, infertility, thyroid dysfunction, and hypertension, is high. These abnormalities usually occur in the body or tail of the pancreas. Stromal and capsular calcification aids in roentgen diagnosis but occurs in less than 10% of these patients. The mass is also visible when the tumor is large. Localization as well as identification of a pancreatic mass is aided by barium studies of the gastrointestinal tract. Arteriography is virtually diagnostic when the tumor is hypervascular; displacement of major vessels, the presence of large feeding arteries, and pooling of contrast medium are the usual findings. Some are hypovascular or avascular and resemble pseudocyst angiographically. In these, differentiation is usually possible on clinical grounds since there is no history of pancreatitis or previous trauma in patients with this tumor.

Endocrine Tumors. Islet cell tumors may produce a number of hormones, including gastrin, secretin, insulin, and glucagon, normally secreted by the pancreas, as well as melanocyte-stimulating hormone, adrenocorticotrophic hormone, and serotonin which are not indigenous to the normal pancreas.[2] Clinical syndromes, such as the Zollinger–Ellison syndrome, the watery diarrhea hypokalemia, the achlorhydria syndrome, hyperinsulinism resulting in hypoglycemia, and hyperglycemia associated with hypersecretion of glucagon produced by the alpha-cell type tumor, may be present. The various clinical syndromes lead to the suspicion of the diagnosis. Rarely, islet cell tumors contain discrete nodular calcification which allows localization on plain films. Usually, selective pancreatic arteriography is necessary to detect and localize the tumor within the pancreas. The entire pancreatic blood supply must be selectively catheterized. The typical arteriographic findings in the arterial phase consist only of small, irregular arteries. In the capillary phase, the tumor is visualized as a round, well-marginated, dense stain. In some patients, large tumor vessels may be seen in the arterial phase producing an irregular mass with opacification persisting into the capillary phase. The tumors are small, and, if they are avascular or hypovascular, they cannot be demonstrated angiographically. A figure of 63% accuracy in identifying and localizing islet cell tumors by means of angiography has been reported.[24]

Pancreatic Cysts

True cysts of the pancreas are infrequent lesions from a roentgen point of view because they seldom become large enough to produce the signs of a pancreatic mass. They arise as a result of ductal obstruction, usually from a chronic pancreatitis. A more common lesion is the pancreatic pseudocyst. This represents an encapsulation of fluid caused by escape of pancreatic juice beyond the confines of the pancreas. It may follow an acute pancreatitis, a surgically produced injury to the gland, or trauma to the abdomen with rupture of the pancreas. The history often is that of a rapidly enlarging mass in the upper abdomen that follows one of the episodes just listed. When the stomach and duodenum are outlined with barium, the mass of the cyst causes a smooth, rounded, pressure enlargement of the duodenal curve. The stomach is pushed forward and it may be displaced upward or downward, often being freely movable over the mass so that the pressure defect varies upon the patient's change in position. The cyst may present itself at a distance from the pancreas although it usually is in close relationship. It may burrow in any direction.

Differentiation of a pancreatic cyst from other retroperitoneal masses may be difficult and often is impossible. To be considered in this connection are carcinoma of the pancreas, primary and metastatic neoplasms of the retroperitoneal lymph nodes, aneurysm of the abdominal aorta, and mesenteric cysts. Carcinoma of the pancreas usually does not reach the size that cysts commonly do and the invasive nature of the tumor may be evident. Fixation of the stomach to the tumor is frequent while this is less common with cysts, the stomach moving freely over the mass. Primary or metastatic tumors of the lymph nodes resemble carcinoma of the pancreas more than they do cysts. Mesenteric cysts usually are freely movable over a fairly wide area; pancreatic cysts are fixed.

THE LIVER

The homogeneous density of the liver in the right upper quadrant makes it rather easy to identify in roentgenograms of the abdomen. If not obscured by fluid or other pathologic changes within the thorax, the upper surface of the liver is outlined by the contour of the diaphragm. Part of the lower border of the right lobe usually is visible unless there is very little intra-abdominal fat to offer contrast or unless there is fluid in the peritoneal cavity. In these patients the liver blends imperceptibly with the general soft-tissue density of the abdomen. When the lower margin is not visualized, some information concerning the size of the liver can be obtained by noting the position of the gas-filled hepatic flexure of the colon. The lower margin of the left lobe of the liver cannot be identified.

The liver is transverse in position in persons of sthenic habitus; in the thin asthenic individual it assumes a much more vertical position and not infrequently the inferior edge of the right lobe extends to the plane of the posterior iliac crest. In certain of these individuals, notably in thin-waisted females, the medial surface of the vertically placed liver may

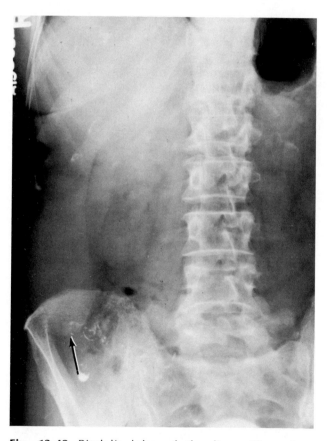

Fig. 13-48. Riedel's lobe of the liver. There is a tongue-like downward extension of the right lobe of liver **(arrow)**. This roentgenogram was obtained after evacuation of a barium enema.

present a V-shaped indentation so that the lower part of the lobe has a tonguelike downward extension. This is known as *Riedel's lobe* (Fig. 13-48). This formation causes the liver to project below the costal margin; it can be palpated and may lead to the erroneous impression of a mass.

LIVER SIZE

The determination of slight to moderate degrees of hepatomegaly by roentgen examination of the abdomen is difficult. The inferior costal margin is a good clinical landmark but it often is poorly localized in roentgenograms. When enlargement is present, several or all of the following signs are noted. Downward displacement of the hepatic flexure of the colon may be demonstrated (Fig. 13-49). The stomach is displaced toward the left and backward. Posterior displacement of the stomach occurs with enlargement of the left lobe of the liver. A localized mass projecting from the surface of the liver may result in a more localized pressure deformity upon the stomach. The right kidney often is displaced downward. The lower edge of the liver crosses the right psoas shadow (in the normal person it is above the psoas). There may be displacement of the duodenal bulb to the left of the midline or below the body of the second lumbar vertebra. There may also be elevation of the right hemidiaphragm. Gross determination of hepatic enlargement is possible by using these signs, but accurate determination of precise liver size cannot be made by examination of plain films.

TUMORS OF THE LIVER

In many cases it is impossible to determine the nature of a tumor involving the liver from plain abdominal roentgenograms alone. Primary and metastatic neoplasms often cause only the signs of local or general enlargement. Calcification within the tumor is occasionally present. Hepatoma, the most common primary tumor of the liver, will show areas of mottled calcification in about one-third of all patients having liver tumors. Otherwise hepatoma causes only general or local enlargement of the liver. In some patients the liver becomes very large. Cavernous hemangioma may calcify, and, characteristically, the calcifications are in the form of trabeculae radiating from a densely calcified center. Metastatic deposits from mucinous adenocarcinoma of the gastrointestinal tract may show areas of hazy calcification. Intrahepatic cysts may show calcification in the wall thus outlining the mass.

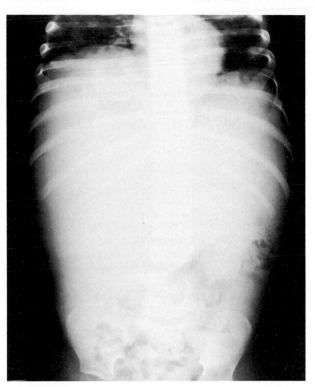

Fig. 13-49. Enlargement of the liver in a child with an undifferentiated carcinoma. The lower border of the greatly enlarged liver is outlined by gas in the displaced bowel.

Hepatic angiography is commonly used to evaluate liver masses.[36] In addition to determining the presence and nature of a mass, it defines the anatomic location, blood supply, and extent of the lesion. At times, arteriography should be supplemented by inferior vena cavography and portography or splenoportography. Isotope scanning may provide all of the information necessary regarding some hepatic masses, precluding the use of angiography; ultrasonography and computerized tomographic scanning are also employed. The ultimate place of these various modalities has not been determined as yet.

Opacification of the hepatic artery and its branches by a combination of catheterization of the celiac axis and its pertinent branches as well as the superior mesenteric artery is necessary. If the portal venous system requires study, selective catheterization of the splenic artery may be performed; this will permit visualization of the splenic and portal venous channels. Roentgen manifestations of intrahepatic neoplasms are varied. They include: (*1*) stretching or displacement of vessels; (2) evidence of neovascularity or tumor vascularity; (3) demonstration of one or more areas of avascularity; and (4) evidence of a tumor stain or blush in the hepatogram phase of the study. In the evaluation of liver metastases, the parenchymal or hepatogram phase is often more important than the status of the hepatic arteries. Parenchymal vascularity may be increased, decreased, or mixed, in which part of the tumor may be hypervascular and the remainder relatively avascular. Carcinoma arising from liver cells is usually a solitary hypervascular mass with enlarged feeding arteries, abnormal tumor vascularity, and increased parenchymal staining. Arteriovenous shunting is also frequent, particularly in the hepatomas; the latter may be multifocal. If surgical treatment is contemplated, examination should include visualization of the portal vein and its major branches to determine the presence or absence of venous invasion by the tumor. Since hepatomas tend to invade the inferior vena cava, this vein should be studied in the preoperative patient. Tumors arising in the ducts are usually relatively avascular, therefore the major finding tends to be encasement of branches of the hepatic artery by a tumor. Figs. 13-50 and 13-51 are examples of changes in a hepatic arteriogram produced by tumor vascularity in the arterial and capillary phases.

As indicated previously, a cavernous hemangioma may contain calcium which suggests the diagnosis. A hemangioma may be very large and involve most of the liver or there may be multiple hemangiomas. The arteriographic findings of normal arterial branches with ringlike clusters of small vascular spaces observed in the late arterial phase that remain opacified past the venous phase are quite characteristic. Early venous drainage does not occur.

Focal nodular hyperplasia, which is pathologically similar to hepatic adenoma, is usually associated with the use of oral contraceptives. It produces a well-circumscribed hypervascular lesion with prominent parenchymal staining and may be solitary or multiple. Blood supply may be from the periphery or from a central vessel with feeding arteries radiating outward. When multiple, the major diagnostic problem is concerned with metastatic disease.

LIVER ABSCESS

The roentgen signs of liver abscess usually are too indefinite to permit a diagnosis from plain roentgenograms. The size of the liver may be increased. Occasionally, gas within an abscess permits a definite diagnosis on plain film studies. If the abscess is near the superior surface there may be some restriction of motion of the right side of the diaphragm on fluoroscopic examination. Linear strandlike densities may be seen in the basal lung owing to atelectasis. If the abscess extends into the subphrenic space the roentgen signs become those of subphrenic infection. Infection may extend to the pleura or even to the lung with the development of a lung abscess. Amebic abscesses cause changes similar to those of abscess from other causes. Radioisotope scanning of the liver may demonstrate the abscess as a "filling defect." On hepatic arteriography the abscess is seen as an avascular area within the liver. Radioisotope scanning and hepatic arteriography are complementary procedures and, in conjunction with the clinical signs and symptoms, often allow a correct diagnosis to be made.

Abscess within the liver may also be detected by ultrasonography. Since this is a noninvasive procedure, it is often used as the initial study in patients with suspected hepatic abscess. Needle aspiration may be guided by ultrasonic localization.

CALCIFICATION WITHIN THE LIVER

Small, discrete, calcified areas, usually multiple, are occasionally seen within the liver. Often there are similar shadows within the spleen. These lesions probably are old, healed foci of tuberculosis or histoplasmosis. Current opinion leans toward the belief that widely disseminated calcified lesions of this nature are most often the result of a previous infection with *Histoplasma capsulatum*. Occasionally one or several larger areas of mottled calcification are visualized within the liver substance; these usually are the calcified residues of previous abscesses. *Echinococcus cysts* frequently involve the liver but are rarely seen in the United States. The cysts often are multiple and calcification in the wall is of common occurrence. Congenital cysts of the liver may be associated with polycystic disease of the kidneys. The calcified wall, if present, is usually thinner than is seen with hydatid disease and the cysts tend to be of uniform size (see Fig. 13-25). Primary hepatic tumors, including hemangioma, hemangioendothelioma, heptoblastoma, hepatoma, cholangiocarcinoma, and dermoid cyst, may also contain enough calcium to be visible on plain film radiographs. Hepatic metastases from mucinous carcinoma of the colon or breast and from cystadenocarcinoma of the ovary may also calcify. Rarely, metastases from other tumors may calcify.

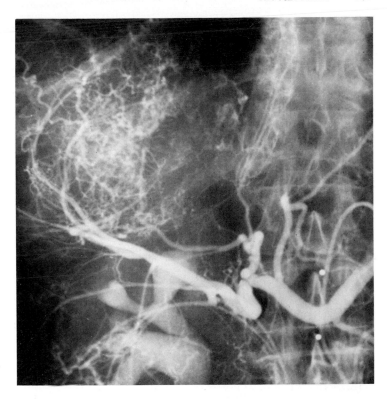

Fig. 13-50. Metastatic leiomyosarcoma of the liver. This arteriogram shows downward and lateral displacement of branches of the hepatic artery with extensive filling of tumor vessels in the right lobe of the liver.

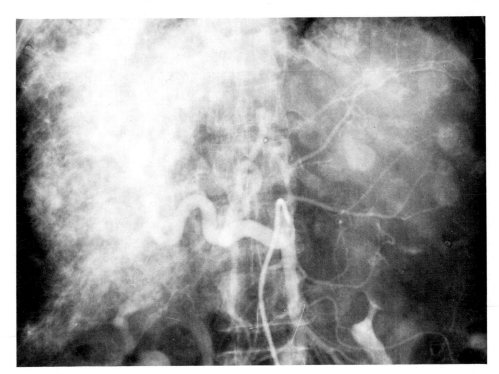

Fig. 13-51. Same patient as shown in Figure 13-50 during the capillary phase of the angiogram. Note the mottled blush throughout the right lobe of the liver and the more discrete, rounded areas of tumor blush on the left.

INCREASED DENSITY OF THE LIVER

A homogeneous increase in density of the liver is found in some patients with hemochromatosis (bronze diabetes), presumably because of the heavy deposition of iron that occurs in this disease. The spleen is affected in the same manner. When diffuse increase in density of these organs is seen in abdominal roentgenograms, particularly when the organs are found to be enlarged, the diagnosis of hemochromatosis should be given consideration.

Another cause of increased density of the liver and spleen is the presence of retained thorium dioxide. This substance may have been used as a contrast agent for cerebral arteriography at some previous time. Thorium dioxide (Thorotrast) is picked up by the cells of the reticuloendothelial system and retained by them almost indefinitely. It is a very radiopaque substance and even the amount ordinarily used for cerebral arteriography (15 to 30 cc) may be sufficient to cause a relatively permanent increase in density of the liver and spleen. Some years ago this substance had a rather wide usage for contrast visualization of these structures but it is not employed at the present time since there is evidence that it is carcinogenic. It possesses a low degree of radioactivity which probably accounts for the carcinogenesis.

GAS WITHIN THE PORTAL VEINS

Gas within the portal veins is a rare condition. It may develop as a complication of mesenteric thrombosis or other cause of intestinal gangrene. The gas is found in the form of linear and branching shadows (see Fig. 13-34). Characteristically it is found in the more peripheral parts of the liver. This aids in distinguishing portal vein gas from gas in the biliary tract. The condition carries a grave prognosis, since it usually indicates intestinal gangrene. In addition to mesenteric thrombosis, other forms of intestinal obstruction may be responsible.

HEPATIC TRAUMA

Because rupture of the liver may cause extensive hemorrhage and shock, immediate surgery is imperative. However, the rupture may be less extensive and cause lesser amounts of extrahepatic bleeding or intrahepatic hematoma or both. Plain films may then show progressive increase in hepatic size or hepatic displacement by a subcapsular or intraperitoneal hematoma.

Arteriography may show extravasation at the site of injury, displacement of arteries by hematoma, delayed filling of arteries in localized areas, arteriovenous fistula with shunting from hepatic arteries to portal veins, intrahepatic arterial aneurysms, and, rarely, an arterial–biliary fistula.

Since splenic and hepatic injury are often produced by the same traumatic event, angiography should include the study of both organs when there is doubt regarding the extent of injury.

THE SPLEEN

The spleen lies in the posterior part of the abdomen in the left upper quadrant directly below the left leaf of the diaphragm and lateral to the fundus of the stomach. Its medial surface is in relationship to the stomach and the tail of the pancreas. Visualization of the spleen in routine roentgenograms of the abdomen is variable. The lower pole often is outlined by gas in the splenic flexure of the colon and the medial surface by the gastric air bubble or by the colon, which may lie medial to the spleen. Rarely, a tongue-like extension of the spleen projects into the space between the fundus of the stomach and the diaphragm, causing a filling defect that resembles closely that of an intramural tumor of the fundus. Infrequently the spleen is located below its usual position or it may be movable and descend when the patient is examined in an upright position. Such an abnormal location may cause it to be mistaken for a tumor mass.

Congenital absence of the spleen is a rarity. It has been reported along with associated anomalies. These include partial situs inversus and multiple congenital cardiovascular anomalies. The liver may show symmetric lobulation, the left lobe being as large as the right. Symmetric lobulation of the lungs may also be present, with three lobes on the left, the same as the right.

Increased density of the spleen is found in hemochromatosis and after the intravenous injection of thorium dioxide (see preceding discussion "Increased Density of the Liver").

ENLARGEMENT OF THE SPLEEN

Splenomegaly usually is demonstrated more readily and with greater accuracy in roentgenograms than is a comparable enlargement of the liver. Even slight to moderate degrees of enlargement often make the splenic shadow easily visible as it presses against the stomach and colon and is outlined by the gas in these

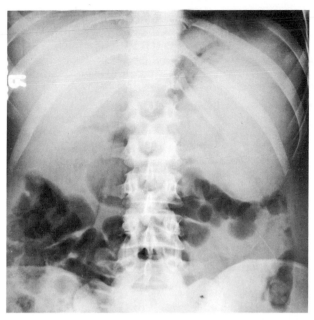

Fig. 13-52. Splenomegaly. The spleen displaces the stomach toward the midline, and the splenic flexure of the colon downward. It forms a well-defined mass in the left upper quadrant.

structures (Fig. 13-52). When the stomach is filled with barium, pressure of the enlarged spleen on the greater curvature usually is obvious. When very large, the spleen may displace the entire stomach toward or even beyond the midline. The splenic flexure of the colon is displaced downward. The left kidney also is pushed downward as the spleen increases in size. When significant enlargement occurs, the left side of the diaphragm may become elevated.

CALCIFICATION IN THE SPLEEN

It is very common to find multiple, small round or ovoid calcified foci distributed throughout the spleen (see Fig. 13-23). These may be phleboliths within the splenic veins or the healed lesions of some widely disseminated infection. In the past, tuberculosis has been thought to be responsible for these lesions but current opinion favors the belief that they represent the healed foci of histoplasmosis. There often are similar foci distributed extensively in the lungs and occasionally in the liver.

Chronic brucellosis may produce unique calcifications which measure 1 to 3 cm in diameter, are multiple, and consist of a flocculent calcified center

around which is a radiolucent area surrounded by a laminated calcified rim[1]

Calcified splenic cysts are infrequent. In the United States they are usually simple cysts, often of congenital origin. Occasionally a posttraumatic hematoma may become cystic with a calcified wall. A calcified cyst forms a rounded ringlike shadow, easily recognized because of the calcification outlining the wall of the cyst. Echinococcal disease is a frequent cause of calcified intraabdominal cysts in many foreign countries. It is a rare disease in persons who have spent their entire lives in the United States. The calcified wall of an echinococcal (hydatid) cyst often is thicker and coarser than a simple cyst. Multiple cysts are the rule.

Angiography can be used to determine the size and number of cysts as well as to localize them. When the cysts are active, there is usually a dense halolike vascular stain outlining their periphery; since inactive cysts show no such vascularity, angiographic findings reflect the biologic as well as the anatomic characteristics of the lesion. Similar findings have been observed in hepatic ecchinococcus cysts.

Splenic infarcts are infrequent causes of calcified areas within the spleen. The calcification may appear in the form of a wedge if the infarct is seen in profile or as a more rounded or oval-shaped area if seen *en face*. Unless calcified, splenic infarcts are not demonstrable in roentgenograms.

RUPTURE OF THE SPLEEN

In many individuals suffering a traumatic rupture of the spleen, the severity of the clinical symptoms and rapid loss of blood into the abdominal cavity lead to operative intervention without roentgen investigation. In those patients in whom bleeding ceases temporarily or in whom there is slow bleeding over a period of days, roentgen examination is helpful. Plain-film study is also used when clinical findings arouse suspicion of splenic injury, but are not diagnostic of it.[6] A number of signs have been described in rupture of the spleen including (1) prominent mucosal folds on the greater curvature of the stomach, (2) gastric dilatation, (3) displacement of the stomach to the right or downward, (4) separation of intestinal loops by intraperitoneal fluid, and (5) pleural reaction at the left base. They are not specific and are of limited value if present. A significant observation is that of a progressively increasing mass in the splenic area in serial roentgenograms covering a period of several hours or days after an episode of trauma. The escape of blood into the peritoneal cavity can be detected on supine plain-film study in most instances. The fluid (blood) is observed in the pelvis above and behind the bladder. Larger amounts extend into the flanks and displace the colon medially so that there is a band of water density between the extraperitoneal fat (flank stripe) and the colon on either side, usually more on the right than left. This is also a very significant observation.

Definite visualization of a normal splenic outline is good evidence that splenic rupture does not exist. The observation of one or more fractures in the lower left ribs should call attention to the possibility of splenic injury when the other signs are equivocal.

Splenic arteriography is a useful procedure when rupture of the spleen is suspected.[7, 30] Among the significant findings are (1) extravasation of the contrast material into the splenic parenchyma, and (2) simultaneous visualization of the splenic artery and vein indicating rapid shunting by way of the sinusoids. Other findings that have been described include (1) stretching of splenic arterial branches, (2) distortion and irregular opacification of the spleen with segments of avascularity indicating sites of rupture and hematoma, and (3) splenic enlargement. It is recommended that splenic arteriography be performed in all patients in whom doubt exists and other examinations have proved inconclusive. If splenic rupture is not recognized, a subcapsular hematoma may develop resulting in the production of a left upper quadrant mass. Symptoms may be vague and confusing. Splenic arteriogram demonstrates an avascular mass surrounding and compressing the spleen.

Cases of so-called spontaneous rupture of the spleen have been described in which rupture occurs without obvious trauma; a diseased spleen is probably a prerequisite. The initiating trauma in these cases may be so slight as to be considered insignificant. The roentgen findings are the same as those occurring after acute traumatic ruptures.

SPLENOPORTOGRAPHY

Splenoportography consists in the visualization of the splenoportal venous system, and the liver parenchyma to some extent, by the injection of a radiopaque contrast substance. This may be done in one of several ways. The first method introduced consisted in injection of the material into the splenic pulp by direct splenic puncture. The contrast substance passes rapidly into the splenic vein, then into the portal vein and the liver (Fig. 13-53). Normally tributaries to these veins do not fill by reflux. However, if there is obstruction anywhere from the sple-

nic to the hepatic veins there will be reflux into the mesenteric and gastric veins and if varices are present they will be opacified. Obstruction of the splenic or portal veins can be demonstrated, usually owing to thrombosis or to occlusion by pressure or invasion from a malignant tumor or inflammatory process in the vicinity. If the splenic and portal veins are patent but collaterals are demonstrated, portal hypertension is present usually owing to intrahepatic block, most commonly cirrhosis (Figs. 13-54 and 13-55). In cirrhosis the intrahepatic branches of the portal vein fill but are thin and attenuated, and during the phase of small vein and capillary filling (i.e., the hepatogram phase) the liver may show a mottled appearance. The procedure has its greatest usefulness in the study of portal hypertension particularly when surgical measures for relief are being considered. It is the best method for the radiographic demonstration of the presence and extent of varices. If the obstruction is in the hepatic veins, usually owing to thrombosis (the *Budd–Chiari syndrome*), the intrahepatic portal branches tend to be dilated.

Portography also may be done using the umbilical vein. The lumen of this vein does not become occluded after its function ceases. It is exposed and cannulated through a supraumbilical, extraperitoneal "cut-down." The method has the advantage of eliminating the possibility of hemorrhage which is present when direct splenic puncture is done.

Direct portography has been done using general anesthesia and a small, paraumbilical incision. A tributary of the portal vein, usually a branch of a mesenteric vein, is cannulated and the contrast material injected.

Adequate visualization of the splenoportal system usually can also be obtained during the venous phase of splenic or celiac axis angiography (Fig. 13-56). Direct splenic artery catheterization is preferred if the main reason for making the study is to visualize the venous system. This method is now used generally as a replacement for direct splenic puncture.

MISCELLANEOUS CONDITIONS

PSEUDOMYXOMA PERITONEI

This rare but interesting condition is caused in most patients by the rupture of a malignant mucocele of the appendix or of a pseudomucinous cystadenoma or cystadenocarcinoma of the ovary leading to the formation of masses of gelatinous material over the surface of the peritoneum. For practical purposes, in the male, the condition is caused only by rupture of a

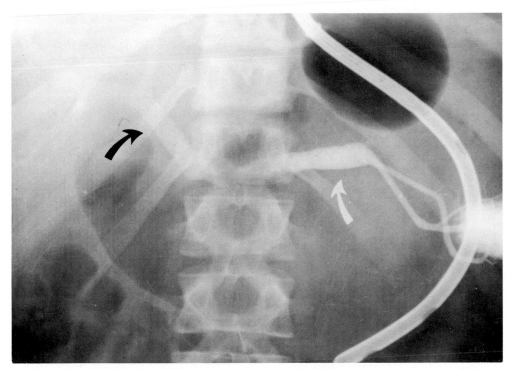

Fig. 13-53. Splenoportogram—normal findings. The contrast material was injected directly into the spleen. A small amount remains in the splenic pulp. There has been rapid passage of the material into the splenic **(white arrow)** and portal **(black arrow)** veins. There is no filling of collaterals and therefore there is no evidence of obstruction or of portal hypertension.

malignant mucocele of the appendix. The release of a large quantity of mucinous material causes a foreign-body type of peritonitis with thickening and fibrosis. The implantation of tumor cells on the surface of the peritoneum results in the formation of daughter tumors and cysts. These cysts also may rupture. The walls of the cysts may become calcified, giving numerous ringlike calcifications widely distributed throughout the peritoneal cavity. This is extremely rare. There are no other roentgen diagnostic signs of the disease and there is nothing characteristic about the appearance of the masses; usually individual mass shadows cannot be identified. In later stages, bowel obstruction may supervene and the roentgen findings then become those of obstruction.

MESENTERIC CYSTS

Mesenteric cysts are infrequent lesions but when present often have fairly characteristic roentgen findings. The cystic mass can be visualized as a sharply outlined, round shadow of soft-tissue density. Characteristically, the mass is freely movable and is displaced readily by altering the position of the patient or by palpation. Multiple-position roentgenograms are useful in demonstrating this mobility. When the intestinal tract is outlined with barium sulfate, particularly during a small intestinal study, the mass is sharply delineated as it is surrounded by the barium-filled loops of bowel. Unless very large, no obstructive signs are present and the bowel is displaced but not invaded or compressed. Calcification of the wall of the cyst is seen occasionally.

LIPOMAS

Lipomas or liposarcomas occasionally develop in the retroperitoneal tissues and they have been reported as occurring in the mesentery. It is sometimes difficult to determine if one is dealing with an actual fatty tumor or simply with a localized accumulation of fat ("depot fat"). Because fat is more translucent than

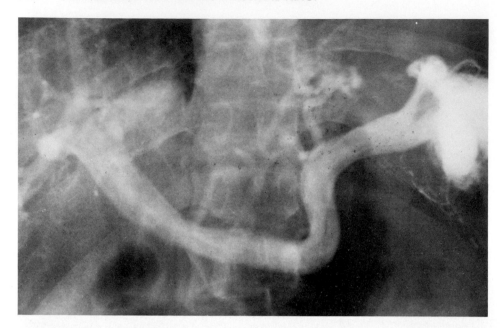

Fig. 13-54. Splenoportogram demonstrating varices in the gastric fundus and lower esophagus. The injection was made directly into the spleen.

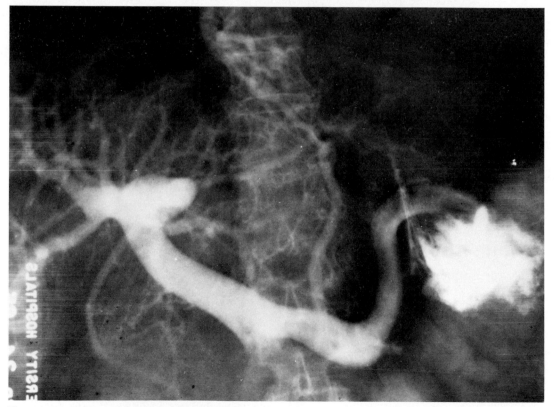

Fig. 13-55. Splenoportogram showing filling of varices of the osophagus after direct splenic injection, indicating portal obstruction.

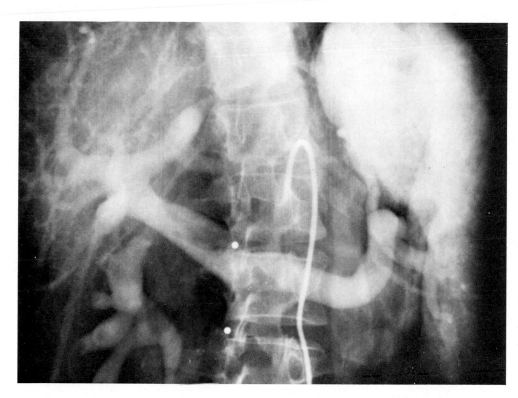

Fig. 13-56. Splenoportogram following celiac axis injection of contrast material. The tip of the catheter is in the celiac axis. Splenic and portal veins are patent, and there is no filling of other veins to indicate portal hypertension.

other soft tissues, a lipoma of any appreciable size may be visualized as an area of lessened density (Fig. 13-57). The translucency of fat is clearly shown when such a tumor develops in an extremity where it can be easily seen. In the abdomen, soft-tissue differentiation is not as good so that the lipoma must be fairly large for this sign to be obvious. Even when not clearly translucent, a disparity in the size of the mass and its radiographic density may be a lead to the correct diagnosis in some cases.

ANOMALIES OF THE ANTERIOR ABDOMINAL WALL

Omphalocele

In this condition there is a defect of the anterior abdominal wall at the umbilicus. Abdominal viscera are prolapsed into the anterior sac covered by a translucent membrane of amnion-peritoneum. The size of the sac and its contents are variable. Usually a portion of the small bowel is within the sac. Mesenteric attachment is usually abnormal, often fixed only by the superior mesenteric artery. This predisposes to volvulus of the midgut. Roentgen findings consist in the presence of mass that may contain loops of gas-

filled bowel, and, if partial volvulus has produced dilatation, it can be detected. The presence of liver in the sac may also be detected on roentgen examination.

Congenital Deficiency of the Abdominal Muscles (Prune-Belly Syndrome)[17, 53]

This syndrome occurs mainly in males (95%). It is characterized by the following triad: (1) deficient abdominal muscles of varying extent and degree; (2) undescended testes; and (3) urinary tract anomalies including renal dysplasia, ureteral and bladder dilatation secondary to a decrease or absence of muscle fibers, vesicoureteral reflux, patent urachus, urachal cyst, bladder diverticula, and dilatation of the posterior urethra. All of these anomalies are not present in all patients. Less commonly, cardiac defects, gastrointestinal anomalies such as malrotation, and skeletal anomalies may also occur. Plain-film findings include protuberant abdomen with bulging flanks, gaseous distention of the bowel, flared lower ribs, and wide interpubic distance. Urographic studies show ureteral, bladder, and posterior urethral dilatation and bladder diverticula. Rarely, some mottled calcification may be observed in the bladder wall or in an associated urachal cyst.[14]

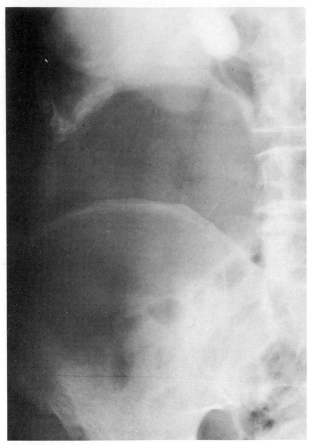

Fig. 13-57. Retroperitoneal lipoma. A large radiolucent mass below the right kidney contains fat which accounts for its lack of density. (Courtesy of Dr. Wayne Rounds)

REFERENCES AND SELECTED READINGS

1. ARCOMANO JP, PIZZOLATO NF, SINGER R et al: A unique type of calcification of chronic brucellosis. Am J Roentgenol 128: 135, 1977

2. AUERBACH RC, KOEHLER PR: The many faces of islet cell tumors. Am J Roentgenol 119: 133, 1973

3. BARON MG, WOLF BS: Splenoportography. JAMA 206: 629, 1968

4. BAUM S, NUSBAUM M: The control of gastrointestinal hemorrhage by selective mesenteric arterial infusion of vasopressin. Radiology 98: 497, 1971

5. BERENSON JE, SPITZ HB, FELSON B: The abdominal fat necrosis sign. Radiology 100: 567, 1971

6. BERK RN: Changing concepts in the plain film diag-

nosis of ruptured spleen. J Can Assoc Radiol 21: 67, 1970

7. BERK RN, WHOLEY MH: The application of splenic arteriography in the diagnosis of rupture of the spleen. Am J Roentgenol 104: 662, 1968

8. BOOKSTEIN JJ, REUTER SR, MARTEL W: Angiographic evaluation of pancreatic carcinoma. Radiology 93: 757, 1969

9. BRYK D: Functional evaluation of small bowel obstruction by successive abdominal roentgenograms. Am J Roentgenol 116: 262, 1972

10. BYRNE WJ, CIPEL L, BULER AR et al: Chronic idiopathic intestinal pseudo-obstruction syndrome in children. J Pediatr 90: 585, 1977

11. CALVY GL, DUNDON CC: Roentgen manifestations of acute intermittent porphyria. Radiology 58: 204, 1952

12. CARSEN GM, FINBY N: Hypotonic duodenography with glucagon. Radiology 118: 529, 1976

13. CLAYTON RS, GOODMAN PH: The roentgenographic diagnosis of geophagia (dirt eating). Am J Roentgenol 73: 203, 1955

14. CREMIN BJ: Urinary tract anomalies associated with agenesis of the abdominal walls. Br J Radiol 44: 767, 1971

15. DAVIS WS, ALLEN RP, FAVARA BE et al: Neonatal small left colon syndrome. Am J Roentgenol 120: 322, 1974

16. EATON SB, BENEDICT KT JR, FERRUCCI JT et al: Hypotonic duodenography. Radiol Clin North Am 8: 125, 1970

17. FRANKEN EA JR: Anomalies of the anterior abdominal wall. Classification in roentgenology. Am J Roentgenol 112: 58, 1971

18. FREY CF, REUTER SR, BOOKSTEIN JJ: Localization of gastrointestinal hemorrhage by selective angiography. Surgery 67: 548, 1970

19. FRIEDLAND GW, RUSH WA JR, HILL AJ: Smythe's "inspissated milk" syndrome. Radiology 103: 159, 1972

20. FRIMANN-DAHL J: Roentgen Examinations in Acute Abdominal Diseases, 3rd ed. Springfield, IL, CC Thomas, 1974

21. FROSTBERG N: Characteristic duodenal deformity in cases of different kinds of perivaterial enlargement of the pancreas. Acta Radiol [Diagn] (Stockh) 19: 164, 1938

22. GELFAND DW: The liver: plain film diagnosis. Semin Roentgenol 10: 175, 1975

23. GOLDSTEIN HM, ZORNOZA J, WALLACE S et al: Percutaneous fine needle aspiration biopsy of pancreatic and other abdominal masses. Radiology 123: 319, 1977

24. GRAY RK, RÖSCH J, GROLLMAN JH JR: Arteriography in the diagnosis of islet-cell tumors. Radiology 97: 39, 1970

25. KANTER IE, SCHWARTZ AJ, FLEMING RJ: Localization of bleeding point in chronic and acute gastrointestinal

hemorrhage by means of selective visceral arteriography. Am J Roentgenol 103: 386, 1968

26. KEEFE EJ, GAGLIARDI A, PFISTER RC: The roentgenographic evaluation of ascites. Am J Roentgenol 101: 388, 1967

27. LEONIDAS JC, BERGEN WE, BAKER DH et al: Meconium ileus and its complications. Am J Roentgenol 108: 598, 1970

28. LEVIN B: Mechanical small bowel obstruction. Semin Roentgenol 8: 281, 1973

29. LOVE L, DEMOS TC, REYNES CJ et al: Visualization of the lateral edge of the liver in ascites. Radiology 122: 619, 1977

30. LUNDSTRÖM B: Angiographic demonstration of rupture of the spleen. Acta Radiol [Diagn] (Stockh) 10: 1451, 1970

31. MILLER RE: The technical approach to the acute abdomen. Semin Roentgenol 13: 267, 1973

32. MILLER RE, NELSON SW: Roentgenologic demonstration of tiny amounts of free intraperitoneal gas: experimental and clinical studies. Am J Roentgenol 112: 574, 1971

33. MOSS AA, GOLDBERG HI, BROTMAN M: Idiopathic intestinal pseudo-obstruction. Am J Roentgenol 115: 312, 1972

34. NEBESAR RA, POLLARD JJ: Portal venography by selective arterial catheterization. Am J Roentgenol 97: 477, 1966

35. NEBESAR RA, POLLARD JJ: A critical evaluation of selective celiac and superior mesenteric angiography in the diagnosis of pancreatic diseases, particularly malignant tumors: facts and "artefacts". Radiology 89: 1017, 1967

36. NEIMAN, GOLDSTEIN HM: Angiography of benign and malignant hepatic masses. Semin Roentgenol 10: 197, 1975

37. NEUHAUSER EBD: The roentgen diagnosis of fetal meconium peritonitis. Am J Roentgenol 51: 421, 1944

38. NICHOLS GB, SCHILLING PJ: Pseudoretroperitoneal gas in rupture of aneurysm of abdominal aorta. Am J Roentgenol 125: 134, 1975

39. NIXON GW, CONDON VR, STEWART DR: Intestinal perforation as a complication of the neonatal small left colon syndrome. Am J Roentgenol 125: 75, 1975

40. POCHACZESKY R, CALEM WS, RICHTER RM: Umbilical vein portography. Radiology 89: 868, 1967

41. POLLARD JJ, FLEISCHLI DJ, NEBESAR RA: Angiography of hepatic neoplasms. Radiol Clin North Am 8: 31, 1970

42. POPPEL MH: The roentgen manifestations of relapsing pancreatitis. Radiology 62: 514, 1954

43. PRESSMAN BD, ASCH T, CASARELLA WJ: Cystadenoma of the pancreas. Am J Roentgenol 119: 115, 1973

44. QUELOZ JM, CAPITANIO MA, KIRKPATRICK JA: Wolman's disease. Radiology 104: 357, 1972

45. RIAN RL, EYLER WR: Aortic, iliac and visceral arterial lesions. Radiol Clin North Am 5: 409, 1967

46. RIGLER LG: Roentgen signs of intestinal necrosis. Am J Roentgenol 94: 402, 1965

47. RING EJ, EATON SB JR, FERRUCCI JT JR et al: Differential diagnosis of pancreatic calcification. Am J Roentgenol 117: 446, 1973

48. SANDS WW: Extraluminal localized gas vesicles. An aid in the diagnosis of abdominal abscesses from the plain roentgenograms. Am J Roentgenol 74: 195, 1955

49. SCHWARTZ SS: The differential diagnosis of intestinal obstruction. Semin Roentgenol 8: 323, 1973

50. SEAMAN WB: Motor dysfunction of the gastrointestinal tract. Am J Roentgenol 116: 235, 1972

51. TOMCHIK FS, WITTENBERG J, OTTINGER LW: The roentgenographic spectrum of bowel infarction. Radiology 96: 249, 1970

52. VAN NOSTRAND WR, RENERT WA, HILEMAN WT: Milk-of-calcium of the pancreas. Radiology 110: 323, 1974

53. WELCH KH, KEARNEY GP: Abdominal musculature deficiency syndrome: prune belly. J Urol 111: 693, 1974

54. WIOT JF, FELSON B: Gas in the portal venous system. Am J Roentgenol 86: 920, 1961

55. WOLFSON JJ, ENGEL RR: Anticipating meconium peritonitis from metaphyseal bands. Radiology 92: 1055, 1969

14

THE GALLBLADDER AND BILIARY TRACT

THE PLAIN ABDOMINAL OR SCOUT ROENTGENOGRAM

As the first step in the radiologic investigation of the gallbladder a preliminary or scout roentgenogram of the abdomen can be useful.[21] The position of the gall bladder may vary widely. It may be situated high in the right upper quadrant in the obese individual or overlie the lower lumbar spine or even the right ilium in those of asthenic habitus. Its relation to the inferior edge of the liver and the hepatic flexure of the colon remains fairly constant regardless of the habitus. The liver edge usually can be visualized in roentgenograms of the upper abdomen, and the hepatic flexure of the colon often is seen because of its gas and fecal content. Location of these structures aids in identifying the approximate site of the gallbladder. The descending duodenum and the gallbladder also are related closely in their anatomic locations and if the duodenum can be visualized, either because it contains air or because it has been rendered opaque as part of a barium meal examination, the position of the gallbladder becomes more certain. Rarely, the gallbladder will be found to the left of the midline.

The normal gallbladder is visualized rarely in scout roentgenograms. If it is enlarged, as in hydrops, it may be seen as a mass along the undersurface of the liver. An excess amount of gas in the hepatic flexure of the colon or gas distention of the small intestine aid in outlining the mass. Visualization of a normal-sized but pathologic gallbladder with thickened walls happens occasionally, but it always is difficult to be certain that the shadow in question actually represents the gallbladder and not some other structure such as the first portion of the duodenum filled with fluid, or another loop of fluid-filled bowel seen on end. In general, the diagnosis of a pathologic gallbladder is seldom justified on the basis of an apparent visualization in a scout roentgenogram unless it is enlarged or unless some of the other findings described in the following sections of this chapter are present.

As a reference, a series of papers, "Methodology and Diseases," dealing with most aspects of gallbladder and bile duct disease is recommended.*

* Gallbladder and Biliary Tract: Methodology and Diseases. Seminars in Roentgenology 11: Numbers 3 and 4, 1976.

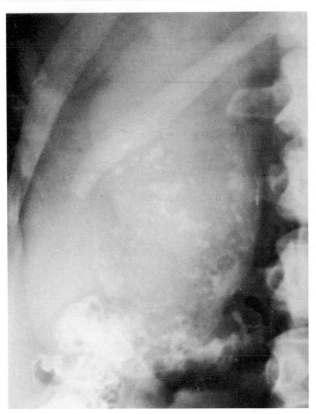

Fig. 14-1. Calcification in the wall of the gallbladder. There is an incomplete shell formed by irregular plaques of calcium in the gallbladder wall. The barium in the colon is a residual of an earlier study of the colon.

Calcification of the Gallbladder Wall

Extensive calcification of the gallbladder wall is an infrequent finding but is an obvious sign of a diseased organ. The calcified wall forms an oval-shaped density corresponding to the size and shape of the gallbladder (*porcelain gallbladder*) (Fig. 14-1). Because the incidence of carcinoma in porcelain gallbladder is relatively high, prophylactic cholecystectomy is probably warranted if the patient is a suitable surgical candidate.

A single large calculus may fill the gallbladder and if only its outer layer is calcified it may closely resemble calcification of the wall; at times it is impossible to distinguish between the two conditions. Much less common is the presence of mottled calcifications in gallbladder carcinoma which resembles that observed in mucous-producing adenocarcinoma of the colon.

Gallstones

A scout roentgenogram of the gallbladder area will demonstrate gallstones if they contain sufficient calcium to be radiopaque (only about 15% of gallstones fall within this category). The chief constituent of most gallstones is cholesterol. Other constituents include bile pigments and calcium salts, usually calcium bilirubinate, and, rarely, calcium carbonate. Most stones (approximately 90%) are mixed but do not have enough calcium to be visible roentgenographically. Stones composed of pure cholesterol or a mixture of cholesterol and bile pigments are nonopaque to roentgen rays. In fact, cholesterol has a density somewhat less than that of the soft tissues of the body and occasionally a large cholesterol stone may be demonstrated as a negative shadow because of the decreased radiopacity of the stone in comparison to the density of the liver and other abdominal structures immediately around it. In order for a stone to be radiopaque it must contain calcium. Opaque gallstones vary greatly in their roentgen appearances but in general they have a dense outer rim and a more transparent center (Fig. 14-2). The dense portion consists of calcium bilirubinate or carbonate while the transparent center is composed of cholesterol or bile pigment or both. Sometimes gallstones are laminated, consisting of alternating opaque and transparent rings. If multiple, gallstones usually are faceted. Occasionally a calculus is seen that has a dense opaque center surrounded by a transparent outer zone. Some of the larger stones, particularly those of cholesterol type, may show a stellate fissuring of the center with gas-filled fissures present (the *Mercedes-Benz* or crow's-foot sign). The fissures are even more transparent than the surrounding cholesterol and aid in visualization of the calculus as a negative density, which may be observed on a plain film, rather than an opaque one. Opaque stones must be differentiated from a variety of other causes of localized increased density in the right upper quadrant, including calcification of the costal cartilages, calcified foci in the liver, calcified lymph nodes, renal stones, warts and moles on the skin surface, film artifacts, and foreign material in the gastrointestinal tract. As a rule, the position of the shadow or shadows in relation to the liver edge and the hepatic flexure, the ringlike or laminated character, and the faceted contour make correct recognition possible. Differentiation from renal stones usually is made without difficulty if roentgenograms are obtained with the patient rotated to an oblique position. A gallstone that may overlie the renal shadow in the anteroposterior roentgenogram will be displaced away from the kidney in the

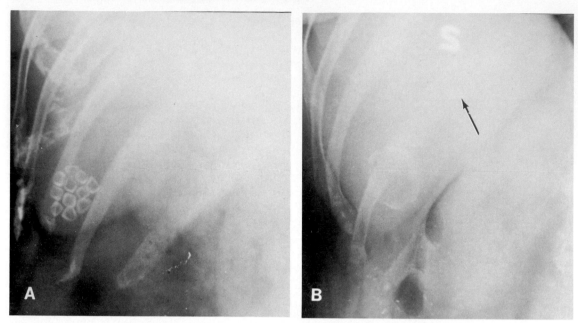

Fig. 14-2. Opaque gallstones. **A.** A number of faceted calculi with radiolucent centers are seen. **B.** A single, large, ring-contoured calculus with a transparent center is evident. The smaller calculus **(arrow)** is impacted in the cystic duct.

oblique projection. Multiple exposures aid in distinguishing gallstones from other calcareous shadows or similar densities for the same reason, *i.e.,* they either reveal the shadow remaining in the gallbladder area regardless of the relation of the patient to the roentgen film or they show displacement away from the gallbladder region, indicating clearly that the shadow cannot represent a gallstone.

Gas in the Gallbladder or Biliary Ducts

Gas within the gallbladder or the biliary ducts always is abnormal. Gas may enter the gallbladder from the intestinal tract because of a fistula between the two, as a result of a surgical anastomosis, or because of a patulous sphincter of Oddi. Spontaneous biliary fistulas usually develop between the gallbladder and the duodenum, less frequently between the transverse colon and the gallbladder. A common cause is ulceration of a large gallstone through the wall into the adherent duodenum. The stone, because of its size, may become impacted in the small intestine and cause a *gallstone ileus* (obstruction). Cholecystoduodenal fistula also may be caused by perforation of a duodenal ulcer. Any malignant tumor arising in the vicinity may cause a fistulous communication between the intestinal tract and some part of the biliary

duct system or the gallbladder. Gas in the biliary ducts is recognized without difficulty (Fig. 14-3). It forms a Y-shaped translucent shadow in the right upper quadrant corresponding in position to the common and right and left hepatic ducts. At times there is extensive filling of the smaller hepatic radicles. If the gallbladder is present and the cystic duct patent or if the fistula is between it and the intestine, it too becomes visible as a gas-filled structure.

Rarely, gas may enter the biliary tract because of a patulous sphincter of Oddi, a finding that may be confirmed by noting, during a gastrointestinal barium study, that the barium mixture refluxes into the common duct through the ampulla of Vater.

Infection with gas-forming organisms may be a cause of gas formation within the gallbladder, within its walls, or in both places. *Emphysematous cholecystitis* is a rare entity characterized by an acute infection of the gallbladder. It is found mainly in patients with poorly controlled diabetes but has been observed in others. The organisms involved are usually *Clostridium welchii* or *Escherichia coli.* Roentgenograms reveal gas within the gallbladder lumen, in the wall of the gallbladder, or in the pericholecystic tissues. It may be distributed throughout all these areas. It is probable that gas distention of the gallbladder lumen occurs first and that subsequently there is extension

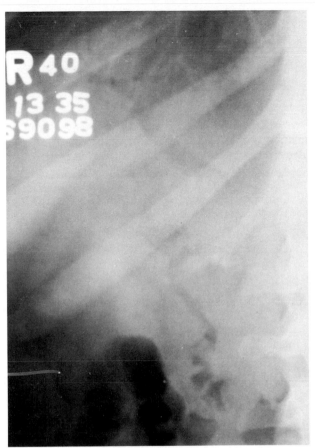

Fig. 14-3. Gas in the biliary ducts. The patient had a carcinoma of the head of the pancreas with a fistula between the common duct and the duodenum.

of the gas into the wall and later into the pericholecystic tissues. In the early stages a fluid level may be present if upright roentgenograms are obtained. In other instances the gallbladder contains only gas and is distended. In the early stages, gas is absent in the biliary ducts since there is almost universally obstruction of the cystic duct. Later the infection may spread into the ducts and gas then will be visualized within them. When gas is present in the wall of the gallbladder it forms a rim of translucent bubbles or streaks outside of the gallbladder lumen and roughly paralleling it. The roentgen appearance at this stage is diagnostic. When only the gallbladder lumen contains gas it may be mistaken for a normal gas accumulation in the stomach or intestine. It may also be necessary to exclude the possibility of an internal biliary fistula as a cause for the gas. The lack of gas in the biliary ducts is against the diagnosis of a fistula.

Barium studies may be required at times for differential diagnosis. Later, when gas bubbles form in the wall of the gallbladder, the diagnosis can be made from scout roentgenograms.

Gas in the Portal Veins

Accumulation of gas in the portal veins is an unusual finding sometimes seen in association with necrosis of the small bowel secondary to mesenteric thrombosis or other cause for devitalization of the bowel wall such as necrotizing enterocolitis. The gas appears roentgenologically in the form of fine linear translucent streaks, usually in the periphery of the liver (see Fig. 13-38). It resembles to some extent the changes seen in cholecystoduodenal or cholecystocolic fistual. However, in this latter condition the abnormal gas shadows are found in the common duct and central hepatic radicles and have a characteristic branching pattern. Gas in the portal veins is found in the peripheral parts of the liver. It carries a grave prognosis and most patients succumb to the primary disease, most frequently mesenteric thrombosis. In addition to the portal veins, gas may be found within the walls of the gangrenous segments of bowel in the form of linear streaks or bubbles (pneumatosis cystoides).

Changes in the Stomach and Duodenum

Alterations in the stomach or the duodenum may be caused by gallbladder disease, but the signs are difficult to interpret in many cases and are not too reliable. An enlarged gallbladder may cause a smooth, pressure defect on the superior surface of the duodenal bulb when the latter has been filled with barium mixture during a gastrointestinal examination. Adhesions between the gallbladder and the duodenum may cause irregularity in contour of the duodenal bulb that may at times be difficult to distinguish from duodenal ulcer. Adhesions also may cause a sharp angulation between the first and second portions of the duodenum or between the stomach and duodenum. They rarely cause obstruction of the pylorus or the duodenum.

CHOLECYSTOGRAPHY

Cholecystography is the roentgen method of choice for study of the gallbladder. It consists of making the bile sufficiently radiopaque to outline the gallbladder. Cholecystography is also a test of gallbladder function since it depends upon the ability of the gallbladder mucosa to concentrate the bile stored within it by removing water.

Technique of the Examination

There are several contrast agents available for oral cholecystography. They are: Telepaque (iopanoic acid), Bilopaque (sodium tyropanoate), Oragrafin (sodium and calcium ipodate), and Cholebrine (iocetamic acid). Oragrafin and Bilopaque are more water-soluble and are better absorbed than Telepaque, which is the most widely used agent in the United Stattes at the present time.

When Telepaque is used, fat should be included in the noon meal the day before the examination to avoid bile stasis and increase bile flow. Fat should probably be omitted in the evening meal since it delays gastric emptying. There is a wide variety of opinion regarding dietary preparation, however. Filming should be done no less than 14 hours or no more than 19 hours after ingestion of Telepaque. Using Oragrafin or Bilopaque, the type of evening meal seems to make little difference in absorption. Filming can be done in 10 to 12 hours, since peak radiographic opacification occurs sooner than with Telepaque. The agents are supplied in tablet or capsule form; the dose is 3 gm. It has been suggested that opacification is improved when Telepaque tablets are ingested over a 6-hour period rather than over the usual 10- to 20-minutes. Food is withheld after ingestion of the contrast agent until the roentgen examination is completed the following morning. Water and coffee or tea without cream may be taken. A series of roentgenograms of the gallbladder region is made on the morning after ingestion of the contrast agent. Although it is theoretically desirable, we do not routinely obtain a plain film of the abdomen prior to the examination. We routinely secure upright spot films using fluoroscopy with compression or decubitus views of the gallbladder in addition to a right anterior oblique prone and often a posteroanterior prone view; one film or a combination of films should include the entire abdomen. If obvious calculi are detected on the initial upright films, we usually do not obtain any more exposures, particularly in young patients. In the event that the gallbladder is not visualized or is poorly seen, we usually give a reinforcing dose of 3 gm of Oragrafin calcium granules.[6] Films are made 4 or 5 hours later. Tomography is used if there are questionable findings and when the gallbladder is not visible. We do not give a fatty meal routinely, but when opacification is poor or there is questionable irregularity of the gallbladder wall,

postfat-meal films are obtained. All films are monitored immediately and appropriate additional measures are taken, *e.g.,* tomograms, fat meal, or reinforcement dose of Oragrafin. We use the Oragrafin in lieu of the "double dose."

Numerous variations of the techniques just described have been reported, many of which can result in an adequate study of the gallbladder.

With large doses of present-day cholecystographic media it is possible to render the bile radiopaque as it is excreted by the liver and the gallbladder may be opacified even though its mucosa is diseased. Because of this, some investigators prefer not to use reinforcement techniques. The ability to render the gallbladder visible, however, does increase the chance for the detection of nonopaque calculi even though it does make the examination less sensitive as a test of function.

The drugs mentioned have few side reactions when given in the dosages specified. Occasionally, nausea or mild diarrhea will develop. Sensitivity to iodine is a definite contraindication to administration of any cholecystographic medium since all drugs now employed for this purpose depend upon iodine for their radiopacity. Other contraindications to the use of Telepaque or related compounds include obstructive jaundice, vomiting, diarrhea, and severe liver or renal disease.

Physiology of the Procedure

The drugs used for cholecystography contain a high percentage of iodine. Iopanic acid has an iodine concentration of 66.68% and the others have similar concentrations. The drug is absorbed from the gastrointestinal tract and secreted by the liver. The bile as it comes from the liver ordinarily does not contain enough of the drug to be radiopaque. The gallbladder receiving the bile concentrates it by removing water. The amount of iodine in the bile then becomes sufficient to make it radiopaque (0.25% to 1.0% iodine) and a dense shadow of the gallbladder, or more accurately, of its contents, results. In order for this to happen the mucosa of the gallbladder must be intact and functioning normally. If the gallbladder wall is diseased, usually as a result of chronic cholecystitis, the organic iodide is rapidly reabsorbed from the inflamed mucosa and failure of gallbladder visualization results. In some cases, failure of the gallbladder to reabsorb water is most likely a factor in nonvisualization. When the maximum capacity of the liver for excretion of the contrast agents is reached, further increase in plasma concentration results in renal excretion of the material. The following possibilities must be taken into account whenever nonvisualization occurs:

1. The patient did not take the drug or did not retain it.

2. Obstruction at the cardia or the pylorus may have prevented the material from entering the small intestine. Roentgenograms may show the medium remaining in the esophagus or stomach in these cases.

3. There may be faulty absorption in the small intestine. Severe diarrhea may influence the result.

4. The liver function may be impaired to the point where an insufficient amount of the material is secreted. The examination should not be performed if liver function is impaired seriously. Results are unsatisfactory in the presence of obstructive jaundice.

5. Obstruction of the cystic duct may prevent entrance of the bile into the gallbladder.

6. The gallbladder may have been removed at some previous time.

7. Disease of the gallbladder may have damaged the concentrating ability of the mucosa to the point where no shadow results.

8. The gallbladder may be in an unusual location and not be visualized on the film.

Ultrasonic "Cholecystography"

Although the role of ultrasonic cholecystography remains to be completely evaluated, there are definite indications for its use at the present time. It should be employed in pregnant patients and in those allergic to contrast media as well as in patients with suspected acute cholecystitis in whom early diagnosis is necessary. It is also useful in patients with jaundice in whom intravenous cholangiography and oral cholecystography are contraindicated. In addition, there are some patients in whom oral cholecystography shows reasonable function and no stones but whose symptoms suggest cholelithiasis. Since ultrasonography is capable of detecting calculi in some members of this group, this set of circumstances is another indication for the procedure.[3]

Results

The results of the oral cholecystography can be expressed in one of the following ways:

Normally Functioning Gallbladder without Stones. The normally functioning gallbladder without stones has become opaque so that its shadow is clearly visualized and the density of the shadow is uniform with no filling defects indicative of stones (Fig. 14-4A). Contraction of the gallbladder in response to a fatty meal is the result of the production of a hormone by the mucous membrane of the small intestine; this hormone is called cholecystokinin. There is considerable variation in the response of the gallbladder to a fatty meal (Fig. 14-4B) and evidence of contraction is not required for the results to be considered normal.

Cholecystokinin has been used in a number of studies to cause contraction of the gallbladder and possibly reproduce the patient's pain. Results have been equivocal and this is still considered an investigational drug.

Using contrast substances such as iopanoic acid (Telepaque) and sodium ipodate (Oragrafin), visualization of the cystic and common bile ducts is possible in many of the patients who have normally concentrating gallbladders. The best filling is obtained in the postfat-meal roentgenogram, particularly if this is a right lateral decubitus view. The cystic duct has a twisted corkscrew appearance caused by the valves of Heister. Its diameter varies between 0.2 and 0.3 cm. The diameter of the normal common bile duct varies from about 0.2 to 0.7 cm. It varies from time to time in the individual patient, the smaller measurement being most frequently obtained during the early phase of gallbladder contraction. The ability to visualize the ducts makes it possible to demonstrate partial obstruction, provided that gallbladder function remains reasonably good. Visualization of the bile ducts with Telepaque in the cholecystectomized patient is discussed later in the section on "Cholangiography."

Normally Functioning Gallbladder with Stones. The gallbladder has concentrated normally and a good shadow is present but stones are visualized as filling defects in the shadow (Figs. 14-5 and 14-6). Thus, nonopaque calculi can be demonstrated where otherwise they could not be seen. Because about 85% of all gallstones are of the nonopaque variety (chiefly cholesterol stones), the method is a very useful one providing the concentrating ability of the organ has not been lost. For the demonstration of very tiny calculi the postfat-meal roentgenogram often gives the best results, since the decreased size of the gallbladder makes it possible to see the small defects more clearly (Figs. 14-7 and 14-8). The "layering phenomenon" also is used to demonstrate small calculi. When the roentgenogram is obtained with the patient upright or in a lateral decubitus position the stones, being of similar composition and having the same specific gravity in each individual case, tend to form a transverse layer in the bile (Fig. 14-9). Some-

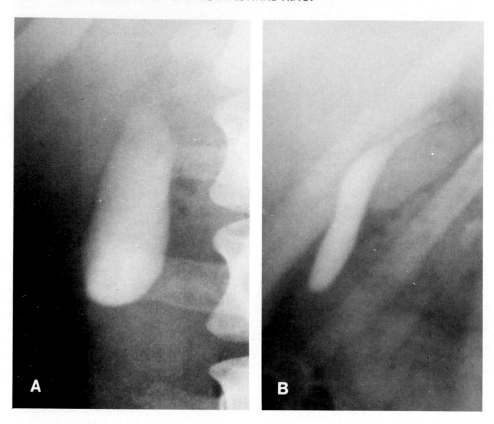

Fig. 14-4. Normally functioning gallbladder without stones **A.** Initial film. **B.** Film exposed 20 minutes after a fatty meal.

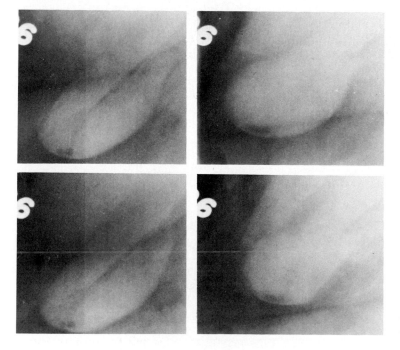

Fig. 14-5. A series of upright spot films. The patient had at least two small radiolucent calculi which, in these films, are noted to be dependent.

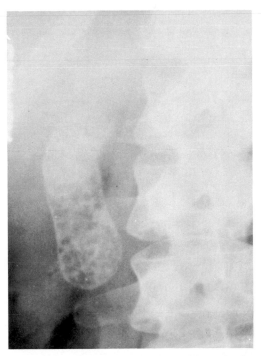

Fig. 14-6. Nonopaque calculi. The cholecystogram shows enough gallbladder function to outline clearly the numerous calculi within it.

times the stones gravitate to the dependent part of the gallbladder, particularly if they contain any calcium salts; at other times they float in the bile but invariably at the same level (Fig. 14-9). Thus it becomes possible, by bringing a number of small calculi into the same plane with reference to the beam of roentgen rays, to visualize them more easily than if they were spread out indiscriminately as they would be with the patient in the recumbent position. The explanation for floating of gallstones within the bile is based on the fact that bile tends to stratify in different layers with different specific gravities. The stones seek the level corresponding to the specific gravity of the calculi. The right lateral decubitus roentgenogram (Kirklin's position) also is useful in displacing the gallbladder away from gas shadows in the bowel and is a part of the routine series of roentgenograms made during cholecystography. The left lateral bending position may also be useful in moving the gallbladder away from confusing gas shadows. Gas bubbles in the duodenum may overlie the gallbladder in some positions and closely resemble stones. Larger accumulations of gas in the colon may interfere with clear visualization of the gallbladder. By the use of multiple positions and tube angulations it is possible, as a rule, to obtain one or more roentgenograms free of overlying gas shadows and thus allow correct interpretation. Gas in the duodenum does not remain

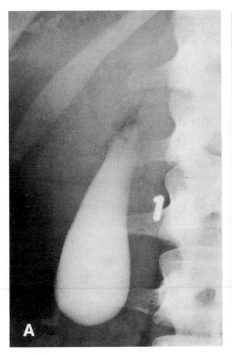

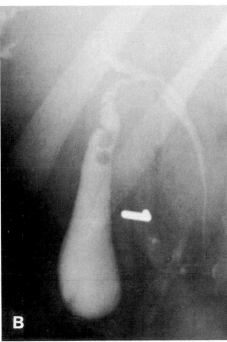

Fig. 14-7. Nonopaque calculi. **A.** Initial film before the fatty meal. **B.** Lateral decubitus film showing the two calculi near the cystic duct. The patient was in a decubitus position with the right side down; horizontal beam was used. The patient had had a fatty meal. Note the good filling of the cystic duct and partial filling of the common hepatic and common ducts.

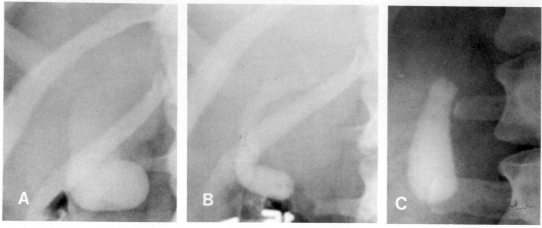

Fig. 14-8. Nonopaque calculi. **A.** The gallbladder has concentrated reasonably well. There is a little mottled appearance due to a large number of radiolucent stones. These faint, rounded lucencies, which measure 1 or 2 mm in diameter, are seen to better advantage in **B.** Roentgenogram secured after the patient had a fatty meal. **C.** Note the uniform density in a normal gallbladder of another patient in contrast to the mottled appearance of the calculi seen in **A** and **B**.

constant in position for very long and may have disappeared completely in some of the later roentgenograms.

Theoretically a calculus might contain enough calcium evenly distributed through it to make it of exactly the same density as the bile around it and thus be obscured during cholecystography. This chance for error is eliminated if a scout roentgenogram is obtained prior to the cholecystographic procedure, since the calculus will be radiopaque. Actually a calculus seldom is of homogeneous density and the chance for error is minimal. Compression upright spot films are very useful in this situation, and tomography is also helpful.

Cholelithiasis is very common, and stones are often observed in gallbladders which are well opacified. They are not uncommon in children, and there may be a higher percentage of calcified stones in children than in adults. An analysis of 367 cases[8] showed about 50% visible on plain films. In this group, 81% of the children had no evidence of hemolytic anemia.

Nonfunctioning Gallbladder with Stones. In the nonfunctioning gallbladder with stones a shadow of the gallbladder does not appear but opaque stones are present. Such calculi of course can be demonstrated in scout roentgenograms but the failure of

visualization during cholecystography gives the added information that the cystic duct is obstructed or that damage to the gallbladder wall has occurred; usually this indicates cholecystitis.

Nonfunctioning Gallbladder. In a nonfunctioning gallbladder the gallbladder is not visualized and no opaque calculi can be seen. Provided that the extraneous factors, as listed earlier, that may influence the examination can be eliminated, this finding indicates gallbladder disease in a very high percentage of patients. If there is doubt concerning the accuracy of the test, the examination can be repeated, using a double dose of the contrast material. However, we use the reinforcement technique with calcium ipodate. When no opacification is observed following this procedure, we consider the gallbladder to be abnormal. A third dose of contrast agent usually adds no information and carries some risk, particularly in the presence of hepatorenal disease. If there is a clinical doubt as to the presence of gallbladder disease, the examination may be repeated in 4 to 6 weeks. We have observed a number of patients in whom a normal study was obtained after that interval. The explanation for this is not clear, but acute or subacute gallbladder disease at the time of the first examination is possible.

The most common cause for a nonfunctioning gallbladder is chronic cholecystitis with stones. Salzman[21] and others have reported on the use of multiple doses of Telepaque for the opacification of gallstones that are otherwise nonopaque in a nonfunctioning gallbladder. The method consists in giving 3-gm doses of the drug each day for 3 or 4 days (1 gm after each meal), with subsequent roentgenography of the gallbladder. At times the margins of a stone may become opaque after this procedure, allowing its recognition. The method has been successful even in patients with jaundice who have one or more stones impacted in the common duct. We have abandoned the use of this method, however.

Subnormally Functioning Gallbladder. In a subnormally functioning gallbladder a shadow of the gallbladder is visible but it is faint and below the expected normal in density. The density may be so low that the presence or absence of stones cannot be determined. Usually it is advisable to repeat the examination, using a double dose of the contrast material or, preferably, the immediate administration of 3.0 gm of calcium ipodate as previously described with reexamination 5 hours later. Frequently, on reexamination much better visualization is obtained and a better idea of the function and the presence or absence of stones results. If the repeat examination again shows only a faint shadow a diagnosis of subnormal function can be made. Tomography may be useful in detecting calculi in these patients. With present-day contrast material it is unusual to find a faint gallbladder shadow and the diagnosis of subnormally functioning gallbladder is not made very often. As has been mentioned, lack of contraction alone, occurring after the fatty meal, is not sufficient to warrant a diagnosis of poor function or of gallbladder disease, but, if the gallbladder shows definite decrease in size, it is probably normal even though its density is less than is usually considered normal. Persisting faint shadows sufficient to indicate subnormal function and with failure of contraction after the fat meal are usually the result of chronic cholecystitis. The overall accuracy of cholecystography is very high (95% or more), and it is a very safe procedure. However, since 15% to 25% of patients require a second or reinforcement dose, there is room for improvement. New drugs and methodology hopefully may further improve the technique and results. Ultrasonography is recommended to establish a positive diagnosis of cholelithiasis after equivocal cholecys-

tography or in the nonvisualized gallbladder. It may be appropriate as a primary procedure in special situations such as iodine sensitivity.

TUMORS AND TUMORLIKE CONDITIONS OF THE GALLBLADDER

In addition to tumors, a number of conditions may produce tumorlike fixed defects in the gallbladder which may be visible on cholecystography. The following is a working classification:

> Polypoid (nontumorus)
>> Cholesterol polyp—cholesterolosis when multiple
> Inflammatory polyp
> Hyperplastic
>> Adenomyoma, adenomyomatosis
> Benign Epithelial Tumors
>> Papilloma
>> Adenoma
>> Fibroma
>> Hemangioma
>> Lipoma
>> Neuroma
>> Leiomyoma
>> Myxoma
> Cystlike
>> Epithelial cyst
>> Mucocele
> Heterotopic
>> Gastrointestinal mucosa
>> Pancreatic tissue
>> Hepatic tissue
> Congenital defects
> Malignant tumors
>> Carcinoma
>> Carcinoid
>> Sarcoma
>> Metastatic

Cholesterolosis

Not infrequently one encounters one or more small, round, translucent defects that are attached to the gallbladder wall. These vary in size from 1 to 2 mm to 6 to 8 mm. Their attachment to the wall is determined by lack of movement and failure to layer when

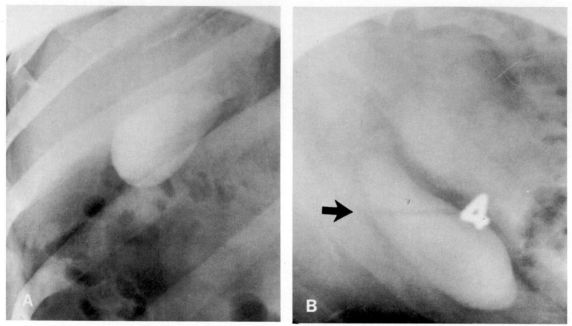

Fig. 14-9. Layering of gallstones. **A.** Film exposed with the patient in the supine, slight right posterior position. No definite calculi are observed in the gallbladder which concentrates satisfactorily. **B.** Film exposed with the patient in the right lateral decubitus position. The horizontal beam clearly defines a translucent line **(arrow)** parallel to the top of the examination table. The tiny calculi are too small to be visualized as individual defects.

roentgenograms are obtained with the patient in upright and lateral decubitus positions as well as in a recumbent position, and by noting that the defect, when viewed tangentially, is not separated from the gallbladder wall by a layer of contrast material. A large number of polypoid lesions have been reported showing these findings, the most frequent are cholesterol polyps (Fig. 14-10), adenomas, and adenomyomas. In one series of 17 proved cases, 11 lesions were found to be cholesterol polyps.

A *cholesterol polyp* is not a tumor but consists of a small collection of cholesterol crystals beneath or on the epithelial surface. It may form a sessile mass or be attached to the wall by a thin, delicate stalk. The lesion may be single or multiple, most frequently the latter. The designation of *cholesterolosis of the gallbladder* has been used for this entity (see Fig. 14-10). It also has been called lipid gallbladder and "strawberry gallbladder" because of the gross appearance of multiple tiny collections of cholesterol on the surface of reddened mucosa resembling strawberry seeds. The gallbladder with cholesterolosis tends to concentrate the contrast material unusually well and to show increased contraction after the fat meal.

According to Jutras and associates, cholesterolosis is one of the noninflammatory conditions. They have termed the condition *hyperplastic cholecystoses,* which also includes the entity known as adenomyomatosis.

Adenomyoma usually is found at the fundus of the gallbladder as a smoothly elevated or sessile mass, often with a central dimple, when viewed in tangent. Rokitansky–Aschoff sinuses are frequently associated findings. Jutras and Levesque[12] consider adenomyoma to be a localized form of *adenomyomatosis,* one of the hyperplastic cholecystoses; this is by far the most common of these lesions, all of which are characterized by the presence of Rokitansky–Aschoff sinuses or diverticula. A second form is generalized; in this the sinuses are present throughout the gallbladder wall. The third form is segmental; in this the involved area is usually narrowed, with sinuses visible in a circumferential distribution at the site of nar-

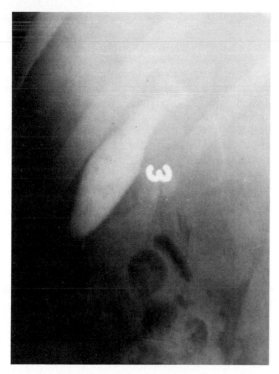

Fig. 14-10. Cholesterolosis of the gallbladder. There is good concentration in the gallbladder, and the common duct is faintly outlined. There are a number of very faint, irregular, translucent defects whch remained in comparable position in upright and decubitus projectons. These represent small accumulations of cholesterol, in and beneath the gallbladder mucosa, which project into the lumen. At times they may become pedunculated.

rowing. Some authors believe that the diagnosis should be suspected in any septated gallbladder. The diagnosis depends on careful technique; postfat-meal studies are helpful and often essential for its determination. The Rokitansky–Aschoff sinuses consist of tiny projections of the gallbladder mucosa into or through the muscularis, resulting in small diverticulumlike outpouchings when they become filled with the contrast medium. The appearance is one of multiple, tiny, beadlike densities paralleling the gallbladder lumen and separated from it by a thin translucent space. When these sinuses are particularly tiny and numerous, the appearance may be that of a fine, almost linear band of density paralleling the lumen. Some, if not all, of the patients with adenomyomatosis have symptoms of gallbladder disease, with relief of symptoms following cholecystectomy. The entities are characterized by a noninflammatory hyperplasia of one or more elements of the gallbladder wall. The cause is not known.

Adenoma

Adenoma is a true benign tumor resembling adenomas found in other parts of the gastrointestinal tract. It may be sessile or pedunculated. The term *papilloma* has been used when the surface has a papillary or villous appearance. Most adenomas are small, measuring a few millimeters in diameter and are often observed best on the postfat-meal or compresson study. As far as roentgen diagnosis is concerned it usually is impossible to distinguish one of these lesions from the others which appear as small, fixed defects; roentgenologists often report them as "polypoid lesions." On chance alone, cholesterol polyp is the most likely diagnosis in a given case.

The remaining lesions listed in the classification given in the introduction to this section are very rare and cannot be differentiated on cholecystography. The radiologic findings are as follows: small, round, radiolucent, fixed filling defect in the gallbladder wall, usually found in a normally functioning gallbladder and observed best on postfat-meal study. They may be multiple.

In general, many observers agree that, in the absence of significant symptoms, it is advisable to refrain from performing a cholecystectomy when single or multiple, small, fixed defects are found in a normally functioning gallbladder. Repeat cholecystograms can be obtained at intervals and if no change in size of the lesion or in function occurs, only interval reexaminations are necessary.

Occasionally, on repeat study, the defects will have disappeared. This happens because the thin pedicle attaching the lesion to the gallbladder wall may break allowing the polyp to float free. It may remain in the gallbladder simulating a small stone or pass through the ductal system into the duodenum.

Because they believe that the possibility of carcinoma cannot be excluded when a fixed defect is found, some investigators have recommended cholecystectomy in all patients showing this type of defect. We favor the more conservative approach, as has just been outlined, on the basis of available evidence.

Carcinoma of the Gallbladder

The diagnosis of carcinoma of the gallbladder is made very rarely on cholecystography. By the time of the initial examination, the tumor has become so large or has produced obstruction so that opacification of the gallbladder is impossible. There is often associated chronic inflammatory disease with or without stones which may also cause nonfunction. Because of the high incidence of carcinoma in patients with calcification of the gallbladder wall (porcelain gallbladder), the diagnosis of carcinoma should be entertained whenever calcification is observed. Rarely, mottled calcification may occur in the tumor similar to that noted in mucous-producing tumors of the colon.

Plain films may outline a mass in patients with very large tumors. Angiography has been used chiefly in evaluating the regional spread of gallbladder carcinoma. Usually the tumor is discovered late, however, so that the prognosis is very poor. Other primary malignant tumors are very rarely found in the gallbladder, and metastases to the gallbladder also are very rare. Among the lesions reported to metastasize to the gallbladder, melanoma seems to be somewhat more frequent than carcinoma.

Miscellaneous Conditions of the Gallbladder

Hydrops of the Gallbladder. Hydrops results in nonvisualization during cholecystography because the cystic duct is obstructed. The gallbladder is enlarged and this often is sufficient for it to be seen as a mass along the inferior edge of the liver (Fig. 14-11). Gray scale ultrasonography can readily identify gallbladder distention and confirm its enlargement.

Adhesions. Adhesions may distort the outline of the opacified gallbladder. However, considerable variation in the shape and position of the normal gallbladder exists and the diagnosis of pericholecystic adhesions should be made with considerable reservation in most patients.

Milk-of-Calcium Bile. Milk-of-calcium bile is a condition in which the gallbladder becomes filled with an accumulation of bile containing a high percentage of calcium carbonate. It follows obstruction of the cystic duct. Because the high concentration of calcium carbonate in the bile makes the entire gallbladder opaque the shadow resembles very closely that of a normally functioning gallbladder during cholecystography. Usually the obstruction of the cystic duct is caused by a calculus and this also is of the opaque calcium carbonate variety so that it is clearly visualized (Fig. 14-12). This is a good diagnostic sign. Layering may be observed on horizontal-beam films

to help confirm the diagnosis. Usually the gallbladder is small and does not change in size after a fat meal; if a scout roentgenogram was obtained prior to cholecystography the shadow, of course, would be present before the administration of the contrast material. A normal-sized gallbladder filled with milk-of-calcium bile may resemble a normally functioning gallbladder, however. In addition to the amorphous calcium carbonate material the gallbladder may contain calculi.

CONGENITAL ANOMALIES

Phrygian Cap Gallbladder

In this developmental anomaly an incomplete septum extends across the fundus separating it partially from the body. The fundus appears to be folded over the body, resulting in a caplike appearance (Phrygian cap, a conical cap represented in Greek art as that worn by orientals and identified in modern art with the so-called liberty cap). The deformity has no clinical significance but must be differentiated from localized adenomyomatosis (Fig. 14-13A).

Hourglass Gallbladder

In this anomaly the gallbladder is divided into two locules by a partial septum in its midportion. Occasionally a trilocular gallbladder is found (Fig. 14-13B).

Double Gallbladder

The gallbladder may be bifurcated with both sacs emptying into a common cystic duct or with individual cystic ducts. This is a rare anomaly. A rather common finding, possibly related to double gallbladder, is a diverticulumlike projection from the gallbladder; this usually involves the fundus.

Left-Sided Gallbladder

Rarely, the gallbladder is found to the left of the midline while the position of the liver is normal. If small-sized roentgenograms are used that include only the area usually occupied by the gallbladder, this condition may be missed and an erroneous diagnosis of a nonfunctioning gallbladder be made. In malpositions of the liver, the gallbladder is also in a similar anomalous position.

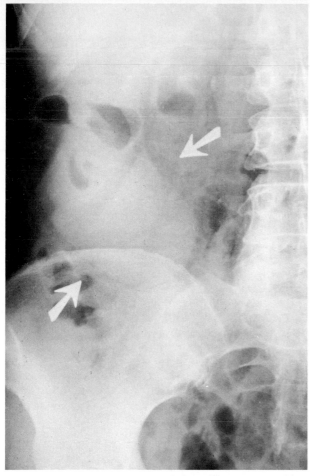

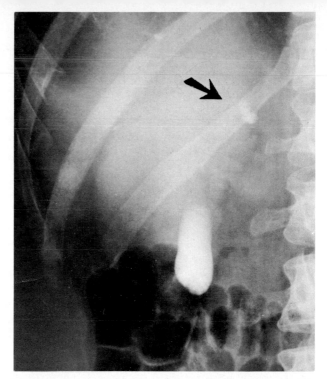

Fig. 14-12. Milk of calcium bile. The gallbladder is very dense. The **arrow** indicates a dense calculus that was impacted in the cystic duct. The patient had been given no iodinated contrast material.

Fig. 14-11. Hydrops of the gallbladder. The **arrows** point to the greatly enlarged gallbladder projecting downward from the lower hepatic border.

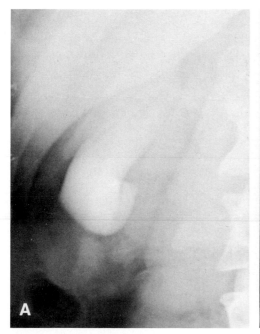

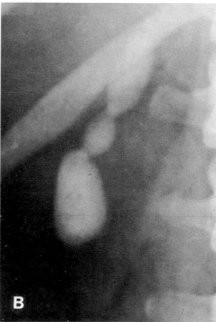

Fig. 14-13. Congenital anomalies of the gallbladder. **A.** Phrygian cap. The fundus appears to be folded over the body. **B.** Trilocular gallbladder. Partial septa divide the gallbladder into three locules. Several small calculi are noted in the most dependent one.

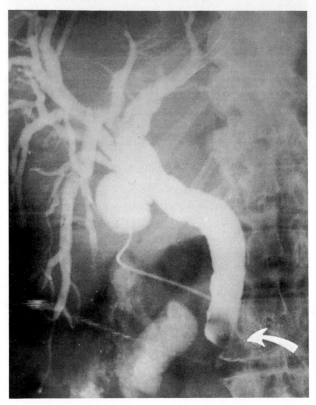

Fig. 14-14. Operative cholangiogram. The contrast material was injected into the gallbladder at the time of surgery. The **arrow** indicates a stone impacted in the distal end of the common duct.

Intrahepatic Gallbladder

In this anomaly a part or all of the gallbladder lies within liver substance. The condition can be recognized, or at least suspected, if the relationship of the gallbladder to the liver edge is studied carefully. Multiple roentgenograms with the patient in different positions and with different angulations of the roentgen-ray tube usually are necessary in order to make certain that the position of gallbladder shadow over the liver is not just an artifact of projection.

Absence of the Gallbladder

Congenital absence of the gallbladder has been reported but is a very rare anomaly. Usually the cystic duct is absent also. This must be differentiated from end-stage inflammatory disease and also from ectopia of the gallbladder.

Hypoplasia of the gallbladder occurs in about one-third of patients with mucoviscidosis.

THE BILIARY TRACT

METHODS OF EXAMINATION

Cholangiography

Cholangiography is a procedure whereby the biliary ducts are filled with an opaque material so that roentgen demonstration of the ductal system may be obtained.

Operative Cholangiography

This procedure consists in the injection of a contrast material, such as Renografin 60 or Renografin 76, directly into the ductal system or into the gallbladder at the time of surgical exploration. If the material is injected directly into the gallbladder the contents of the gallbladder are aspirated and from 40 to 50 cc of the contrast substance are injected. If injected directly into the common duct, from 10 to 15 cc are ample unless the duct is dilated. A portable roentgenray generator is brought into the operating room to obtain the roentgenograms. Usually the surgeon punctures the common duct with a 20-gauge needle and injects the solution directly into it. The roentgenograms are processed immediately for inspection in order to allow evaluation of the condition of the ducts before the abdomen is closed. The greatest problem with this examination is likely to be with the technique. In addition to careful injection to avoid the introduction of air bubbles into the ducts, careful radiographic technique is essential. Most errors of interpretation probably result from inadequate films and poor technique, although tiny stones may be missed on adequate films. Some surgeons recommend (and most radiologists concur) the routine use of operative cholangiography during cholecystectomy performed for treatment of nonmalignant disease, since the incidence of postcholecystectomy common duct stones is 10% to 20% in patients in whom the examination was not performed. The method is particularly useful to determine if any calculi are present within the common or hepatic ducts that cannot be palpated by the surgeon. Visualization of the ducts without filling defects and with evidence of free extension of contrast material into the duodenum enables the surgeon to be certain that no calculi remain and that there is no obstruction in the distal part of the duct. Calculi are visualized as negative filling defects within the denser shadow of the contrast material (Fig. 14-14). Air bubbles may be confused with calculi.

Postoperative Cholangiography

After T-tube drainage of the common duct the contrast material can be injected directly into the duct through the drainage tube to determine if the duct is patent and functioning satisfactorily before the tube is removed. The injection should be made under fluoroscopic control and films exposed as necessary during the procedure. Care should be taken that all air is removed from the system, and that all films are monitored while the patient is still on the table. Normally a free flow of contrast material into the duodenum is observed and the ducts can be seen to be free from defects indicative of residual stones. If calculi are present they are seen as negative defects within the contrast medium (Fig. 14-15). Obstruction due to strictures and neoplasm can be recognized by failure of entrance of material into the duodenum and the dilatation of the ductal system above the site of obstruction. In our institution, cholangiography is carried out in most cases of common duct drainage before the T-tube is removed.

Intravenous Cholangiography

Meglumine iodipamide (Cholegrafin) is used in this examination to outline the biliary duct system. It is the only agent available for use in the United States at present. Ioglycamide (Biligram) is used widely in Europe; iodoxamate (Cholevue) is a new agent now being studied. Indications for the use of intravenous cholangiography include: (*1*) nonopacification of the gallbladder on cholecystography; (*2*) biliary symptoms following cholecystectomy; (*3*) preoperative study of the biliary tree in patients with gallstones; (*4*) evaluation of ducts in patients with pancreatitis; and (*5*) suspected acute cholecystitis. Its use in this latter situation is controversial since nonvisualization is common, and a 24-hour film is required to make certain that the gallbladder does not fill. Contraindi-

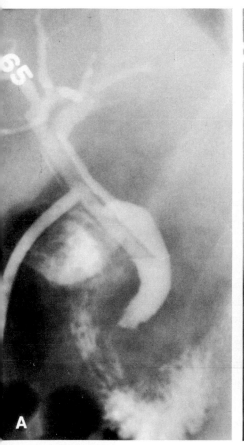
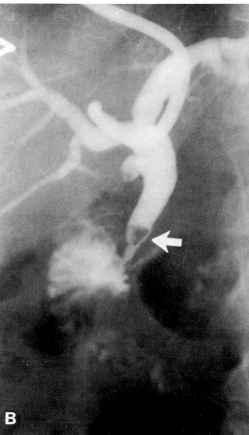

Fig. 14-15. Postoperative T-tube cholangiogram. **A.** An example of a normal study. The contrast material outlines the common duct and some of its hepatic tributaries. Some contrast material is noted in the duodenum. **B.** In this patient there is a residual stone in the lower end of the common duct. It is visualized as a triangular, translucent defect **(arrow).** Obstruction is not complete since there is some contrast material in the duodenum.

cations to the use of intravenous cholangiography include: (*1*) iodine hypersensitivity and (*2*) hepatorenal disease, which is a relative contraindication.

Cholografin depends on a high concentration of iodine for its radiopacity. It is administered intravenously in doses of 20 cc for the average adult patient with the injection being given slowly over a 10-minute period or it can be given by the slow, drip-infusion technique over a longer period of time. We use the drip infusion technique mainly because the patients appear to have less reactions to this than to the injection method of administration. Benadryl or other antihistamines may be given to minimize allergic reactions such as pruritus, erythema, and hives. The second type of reaction, *i.e.,* nausea and vomiting, appears to be related to injection rate. Hypersensitivity, resulting in hypotension, dyspnea, nausea, and vomiting are unusual in our experience, but may be treated by administration of (*1*) Adrenalin (0.3 ml of 1:1000 solution given subcutaneously); (*2*) Benadryl (50 mg injected intramuscularly or intravenously); (*3*) corticosteroids (100 mg of Solu-Cortef given intravenously) and; (*4*) oxygen. The material is secreted rapidly by the liver and appears in relatively high concentrations in the bile in from 10 to 15 minutes after injection. The concentration is sufficient to make the ducts opaque to roentgen rays (Fig. 14-16). Ordinarily a series of roentgenograms of the gallbladder region is obtained, beginning at 20 to 30 minutes after injection and spaced at intervals of 20 to 30 minutes. While the timing of the exposures will depend upon the results noted in the first roentgenogram, the usual spacing is 20, 30, 45, and 60 minutes. The technique is varied from patient to patient as the roentgenograms are processed immediately. Tomograms are obtained routinely when optimal opacification is noted. If the gallbladder is present and the cystic duct is patent the gallbladder may be visualized from 1 to 2 hours after injection. The examination is carried to 4 hours if opacification has not occurred earlier. Some believe that 24-hour radiographs should be obtained to insure optimal visualization of the gallbladder. Since preparation of the patient includes hydration, a fat-free liquid breakfast and lunch, if necessary, are given before the examination. There is no unanimity of opinion regarding the use of a fatty meal the day prior to the examination. If necessary, a cathartic is given the night before the examination.

In many patients a sufficient amount of the Cholografin is excreted by the kidneys so that a pyelogram is obtained. If liver function is diminished, renal excretion of the substance is increased and, in the pres-

ence of serious liver damage, roentgenograms reveal only opacification of the renal pelves and calyces and no visualization of the biliary ducts.

The caliber of the normal common bile duct postoperatively is on the order of 5 to 6 mm, the same as in normal ducts visualized by intravenous or oral cholangiography. In our experience the common duct may be somewhat larger than this and we have allowed an upper limit of normal to be 10 mm. When the greatest diameter of the duct exceeds this figure the finding should be considered as evidence of some type of obstruction.

Caution must be exercised in the interpretation of these observations, however, and correlation with the clinical history and the physical findings is needed in

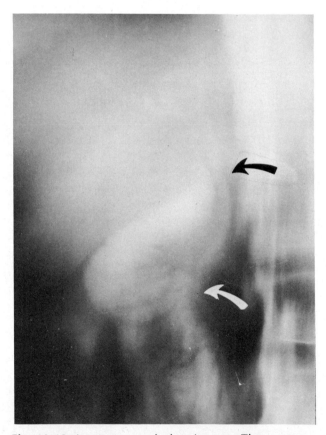

Fig. 14-16. Intravenous cholangiogram. The common duct is opacified, and there is some opaque material in the duodenum. Some of the hepatic ducts can be faintly visualized. All of the ducts appear normal in diameter. The **white arrow** points to the region of the ampulla. The **black arrow** indicates the common duct.

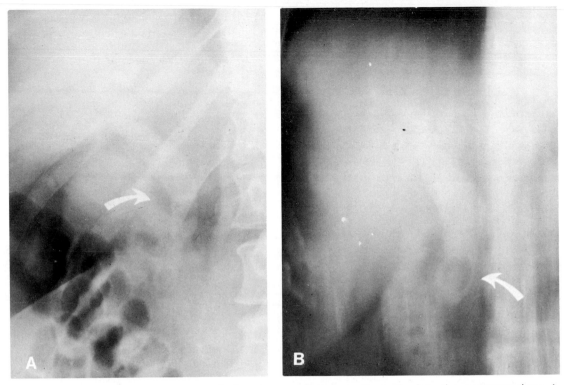

Fig. 14-17. Intravenous cholangiogram demonstrating calculi in the common duct. **A.** The **arrow** indicates the common duct in which there are two, faceted, radiolucent calculi. The duct is somewhat dilated. **B.** Tomogram of another patient. The **arrow** indicates the site of a large, common-duct stone that has caused some dilatation of the duct but is not completely obstructing it since there is some opacification of the duodenum.

borderline cases. The finding of an enlarged duct may indicate spasm of the sphincter of Oddi, stricture formation, tumor infiltration, or impaction of a calculus. Calculi may be demonstrated within ducts that are of normal caliber. They are recognized as negative or filling defects in the shadow (Fig. 14-17). Difficulty in interpretation caused by gas shadows in the intestinal tract is considerable despite the use of tomography. It is possible to have partial obstruction of a duct that is not found to be dilated on cholangiography. If the causative lesion cannot be identified (stone, stricture, etc.), Wise and O'Brien[25] use what they have called the time-density-retention concept. Briefly, their concept states that if the density of the common duct is greater at 120 minutes than at 60 minutes postinjection, partial obstruction is present. By using this criterion they found considerable improvement in the diagnostic accuracy of the procedure.

If the gallbladder has not been removed but is not visible after oral cholecystography, the intravenous injection of Cholografin may show it or may, by failure of visualization, suggest that the cystic duct is occluded and that the radiopaque bile cannot enter. Opacification of the gallbladder may not occur, however, even though the cystic duct is patent. If the cystic duct is patent the gallbladder may become opaque even though its wall is seriously diseased because concentration of the bile by the gallbladder mucosa is not required. Another sign of extrahepatic duct obstruction is opacification of intrahepatic ducts prior to visualization of the common bile duct. This is a reversal of the normal sequence of opacification which probably reflects biliary stasis in the presence of distal obstruction.

In the cholecystectomized patient the cystic duct may dilate to the point where it simulates a "reformed" gallbladder. The clinical significance of the so-called "reformed" gallbladder has been in dispute. In most cases in which a remnant of the cystic duct or even the neck of the gallbladder is visualized it is doubtful that clinical significance can be attached to the finding. The gallbladder, itself, does not reform.

In some patients it is possible to visualize the common duct after cholecystectomy by the oral administration of large doses of Telepaque. A dose of 6 gm, or twice the amount used for cholecystography, frequently will show the duct even though the gallbladder is severely diseased or has been removed. The material is secreted by the liver in a high enough concentration so that the concentrating ability of the gallbladder is not needed to make the bile radiopaque. This method has been supplanted by intravenous cholangiography; we do not use it.

Percutaneous Transhepatic Cholangiography

This procedure consists in direct needle puncture of the common duct or one of the hepatic ducts through the abdominal wall and liver. Evans and Mujahed[7] list the following indications for the procedure:

1. To differentiate between obstructive and non-obstructive jaundice
2. To help establish the precise site and cause of obstructive jaundice
3. To diagnose congenital anomalies of the bile ducts
4. To decompress the obstructed biliary system

The examination is carried out under fluoroscopic control. Many workers now use the Chiba University "skinny needle" because of improved ability to cannulate small (normal in size) bile ducts. An anterior subcostal approach appears to be favored by most over a lateral approach, but use of the Chiba needle may change this. Once a duct is entered, as determined by injection of a small amount of Hypaque 50 or other organic iodide, additional contrast medium is injected until a diagnostic cholangiogram is obtained. Bile may be withdrawn if ducts are dilated, but the major objective is to obtain good opacification of the ducts. Major complications are uncommon and are mainly those of bile peritonitis or hemorrhage. Cholangitis with liver abscesses is also a complication in patients with partially obstructing lesions. It is generally recommended that operation should follow the examination in jaundiced patients if there is obstruction of the common duct. In many hospitals, surgery is scheduled immediately after the procedure providing that a surgical lesion is present. In most patients the examination is performed to determine the nature and location of biliary ductal obstruction.

Examples of findings on transhepatic cholangiography are shown in Figures 14-18 (carcinoma of the papilla of Vater), 14-19 (impaction of stone in the common duct), and 14-20 (obstruction of the common hepatic duct).

Transjugular Cholangiography

The transjugular approach to ductal cannulization has been described by Weiner and Hanafee.[23] It is used to minimize the complications of the procedure. The original article written by these authors should be consulted for technical details. Although this method is not widely used, it has some advantages which include: (1) safety—it eliminates the need to traverse the peritoneal cavity and puncture the liver capsule; (2) a high success rate; (3) provision of the ability to perform concurrent hepatic studies;[19] and (4) obviation of a need for immediate surgery. Disadvantages include: (1) complexity of the procedure and (2) the need for special skill and equipment.

The procedure should not be employed in patients with acute cholangitis. The possibility of biliary–venous reflux warrants the routine use of antibiotics. Anatomic variations in the venous system, although rare, may prohibit employment of procedure.

Infusion Tomography of the Gallbladder

This examination, developed largely by Moncada and associates, has been used by them in the diagnosis of acute cholecystitis.[16] First a scout film is obtained to aid in determining the technical factors for tomography. Then, 300 ml of a 30% solution of methylglucamine diatrizoate is infused intravenously in a 15- to 20-minute period. Tomograms of the gallbladder area are obtained, beginning at a level of one-third the distance from the anterior abdominal wall to the table top and proceeding forward at 0.5-cm intervals. Acute cholecystitis is said to be present if a gallbladder wall thicker than 1 mm is demonstrated in one or more tomographic sections. Low KV technique is stressed (in the 76 kVp range). In Moncada and associates' initial group of 137 patients, 96% accuracy was documented. No false-positive finding was reported, but there was one false-negative in a patient with gangrenous cholecystitis. Hypervascularity of the acutely inflamed wall probably accounts for its good visualization. The examination shows promise for rapid diagnosis of acute cholecystitis but is evidently of little value in the diagnosis chronic biliary disease.

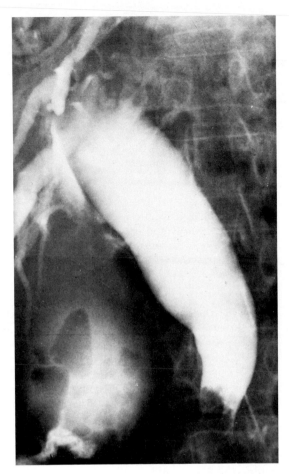

Fig. 14-18. Carcinoma of the papilla of Vater. This transhepatic cholangiogram shows an irregular obstruction near the distal end of the common duct. There is great dilatation of the common duct. A number of translucent calculi are noted within the partially opacified gallbladder.

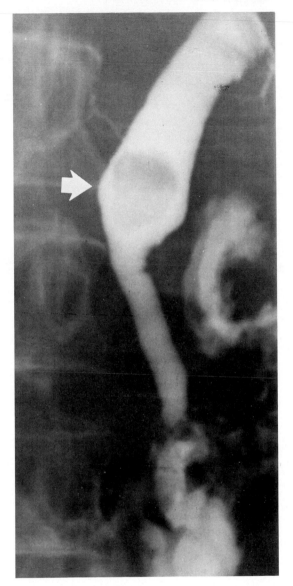

Fig. 14-19. Transhepatic cholangiogram showing a stone **(arrow)** impacted in the common duct which has caused only partial obstruction evidenced by the fact that there is contrast material distal to it in the duct and in the duodenum.

Computerized Tomography of the Gallbladder and Biliary Tract

The place of computed tomography in the examination of the gallbladder and biliary tract has not yet been determined. It is likely that this expensive procedure will not replace conventional cholecystography. It will probably be most useful in the study of patients whose gallbladder cannot be visualized, and in those in whom difficulty in differentiating obstructive from nonobstructive jaundice is experienced. The gallbladder and biliary tree are visible on CT scans and at times calculi may be detected when they are not evident on roentgenograms. Computerized tomography is a noninvasive method and therefore may replace transhepatic and endoscopic retrograde cholangiography in some patients. Ultrasonography, which is

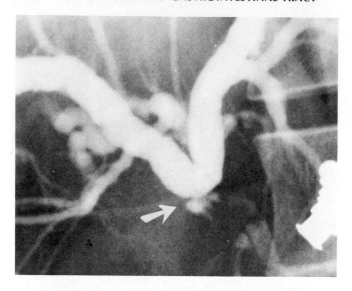

Fig. 14-20. Obstruction of the common hepatic duct just below the junction of the right and left hepatic ducts **(arrow).** This was an iatrogenic lesion demonstrated by means of transhepatic cholangiography.

less expensive and carries no radiation hazard, is also capable of detecting biliary duct dilatation and gallstones. The ultimate relationship of the two methods and their place in the diagnosis of biliary disease is yet to be determined.[13]

Endoscopic Retrograde Cholangiography

This method of examination of the biliary duct system also permits catheterization of the pancreatic duct. It entails the use of a fiberoptic duodenoscope. The procedure requires experienced endoscopists, radiologists, and an x-ray room equipped with image intensification and television. One major advantage is that it renders examination of the pancreatic duct possible. Indications are similar to those for transhepatic cholangiography except, with it, the pancreatic duct may be examined. Complications include acute pancreatitis, septic cholangitis, aspiration pneumonia, drug reactions, and instrumental injury. The success rate appears to be related to the skill of the endoscopist and is not related to biliary duct dilatation as in the case of transhepatic cholangiography. Its place in the examination of the biliary tree does not appear to be definitely established as yet, however.

Nonoperative Extraction of Biliary Duct Stones

The procedure of nonoperative extraction of stones retained in the biliary ducts under fluoroscopic control is now widely used. It has been popularized chiefly by Burhenne.[5] After waiting for approximately 5 weeks after cholecystectomy, another T-tube cholangiogram is obtained to locate the stones. Either a steerable catheter or guidewire is introduced into the sinus tract after the T-tube has been removed. The catheter is positioned with its tip beyond the location of a retained stone. A stone basket is introduced through the catheter positioned distal to the stone, opened, and then withdrawn in an attempt to snare the retained stone. Burhenne reports a success rate of 95% in a series of 217 patients. There were no fatalities in this series; the 5% morbidity rate was attributed to fever, subhepatic bile collection, extravasation, pancreatitis, sepsis, and vagotonic shock. All signs and symptoms disappeared within 24 hours. In order to facilitate nonoperative extraction, Burhenne recommends that surgeons use no less than a number 14 French T-tube brought out through a lateral stab wound to aid postoperative instrumentation should this become necessary.

DISEASES OF THE BILIARY DUCTS

CONGENITAL DUCT ANOMALIES

One of the most common of these anomalies is an accessory right hepatic duct which empties into the cystic or main hepatic duct. The major intrahepatic ducts may have other anomalous terminations and the same is true with the common hepatic and common bile ducts. Duplication of the latter two ducts has also been described. *Caroli's disease* is a form of ductal ectasia characterized by segmental saccular dilatation of the intrahepatic bile ducts usually recognized in adult life because of complications consisting of biliary calculi, cholangitis, and liver abscess.[18] This is a familial disease, probably inherited as a Mendelian recessive trait, frequently associated with other anomalies such as cystic disease of the kidney and pancreas as well as medullary sponge kidney. The diagnosis depends on visualization of dilated ducts and is most often made on operative or T-tube cholangiography, since intravenous cholangiography often shows insufficient opacification for diagnostic purposes.

Congenital strictures are very rare, the great majority of strictures being secondary to previous surgery. Opacification of the biliary tree is necessary for making the diagnosis. *Biliary atresia* may develop *in utero* but it probably is not congenital since chronic inflammatory disease involving the ducts and surrounding tissue is believed to cause obliteration of the lumen which may be segmental and irregular. This condition and neonatal hepatitis both cause persistent jaundice in the neonate and may actually represent the same disease, namely, hepatitis with a component of sclerosing cholangitis. On cholangiography, irregular areas of stenosis, dilatation, and poor arborization are noted.

Choledochal Cyst

Choledochal cyst is a rare malformation consisting of cystic dilatation of a segment of the extrahepatic bile ducts which usually involves the common bile duct. There are a number of theories regarding its etiologic background; probably the most compelling is that of Babbitt and associates[1] who postulate that anomalous insertion of the common duct into the pancreatic duct several centimeters from the ampulla of Vater results in reflux of pancreatic secretion into the common duct causing dilatation that eventually may become very marked. The pressure in the common duct is less than that in the pancreatic duct, resulting in the reflux. Recurrent cholangitis is common; this leads to fibrosis, resulting in obstruction of greater or lesser degree causing further dilatation. It is usually observed in childhood and is more common in girls than in boys. The clinical triad of abdominal pain, jaundice, and a palpable mass in the right upper quadrant of a child is not always present, but is significant when present and suggests the clinical diagnosis. The roentgen signs are essentially those of a mass in the gallbladder area. This mass may become very large and, as it does so, it displaces the duodenum anteriorly and to the left. Visualization of the gallbladder and the dilated common duct is usually not to be expected during cholecystography, but it

has been reported infrequently. Intravenous cholangiography may be useful in making the diagnosis if hepatic function is adequate. If hepatic function is not adequate, transhepatic cholangiography may be used to make the diagnosis. When biliary obstruction is incomplete, success has been reported with use of ^{131}I rose bengal. Ultrasound and CT scanning are also being used to make the presumptive diagnosis. Percutaneous transhepatic cholangiography has the advantage of outlining the duct system as well as the cyst.

Choledochocele

This is a rare anomaly consisting of dilatation of the intraduodenal portion of the common duct in the region of the ampulla of Vater. If the sac opacifies on intravenous cholangiography, the appearance is very similar to that of a uterocele with a saclike termination of the common duct.

Ductal Ectasia

In ductal ectasia, in addition to Caroli's disease, minimal segmental dilatation of the intrahepatic ducts is sometimes observed; this often causes no symptoms. *Diverticula* have also been observed involving the biliary tree. These anomalies are very rare.

Other Anomalies

Structural variations in the biliary tree, anomalous position, congenital diaphragm, and localized stenosis have also been reported but are extremely rare.

NEOPLASMS

Carcinoma

Biliary duct carcinoma is rare, and obstruction of the common duct by tumor is more commonly caused by carcinoma of the pancreas than by carcinoma of the common duct. Cholangiographic appearance is that of narrowing or occlusion of the common bile duct. The narrow segment is usually short and well demarcated but may be associated with an irregular polypoid intraluminal mass. If the mass is relatively smooth, it may resemble a calculus. Biliary duct carcinoma may also be very extensive and produce areas of stricturelike narrowing with proximal dilatation and an irregular appearance of the duct. This sclerosing type of bile duct carcinoma may closely resemble sclerosing cholangitis. Percutaneous or retrograde fiber-optic cholangiography is often necessary to outline biliary duct carcinoma. Other biliary duct neoplasms are exceedingly rare. Cholangiocarcinoma may occur anywhere within the biliary system but is most frequent in the common bile duct. The junction of the main hepatic and cystic ducts is the second most common site. As indicated earlier, the multicentric type tends to be very extensive and simulates sclerosing cholangitis.

Benign Tumors

Although exceedingly rare, benign tumors of the bile ducts such as papilloma and adenoma may occur, usually in the ampullary region. Roentgenographic findings consist of a filling defect or obstruction of the involved duct. Since the margins may be smoothly rounded, this type of tumor may closely resemble a calculus. Other benign lesions such as leiomyoma, fibroma, heterotopic pancreas, or gastric mucosal and inflammatory pseudopolyps may occur but are also rare.

Extrinsic Tumors

The porta hepatis may be involved by metastases from a variety of tumors resulting in more or less obstruction of the biliary duct system; and carcinoma of the pancreas may extend into the extrahepatic ducts or distort them. At times, it is impossible to differentiate primary biliary duct carcinoma from pancreatic carcinoma on the basis of cholangiography. Angiography is helpful in the differentiation. Angiographic findings consist of arterial encasement and fine neovascularity and there are usually angiographic signs of bile duct dilatation in primary duct carcinoma as well as evidence of arterio-arterial collaterals and venous obstruction. Lucencies observed in the hepatogram caused by dilated ducts tend to be cylindrical in contrast to the rounded or oval pattern of metastatic lesions.

OTHER LESIONS

Biliary Duct Calculi

These calculi are usually secondary to gallstones even in patients whose gallbladder has been removed since the source of common duct stones observed in these patients is usually retained intrahepatic or extrahepatic calculi. This is an important reason for using operative cholangiography. Primary common duct stones may occur, however, but usually are the result of a stricture in the common duct or sometimes in a large cystic duct remnant. Cholangio-

graphic findings are those of a smooth, well-defined filling defect producing a meniscus and more or less obstruction resulting in dilatation of the ducts proximal to the stone. This dilatation plus the smoothly rounded meniscus is quite characteristic.

Pseudocalculus Defect

A defect or obstruction of the distal end of the common duct usually indicates calculus, tumor, edema in the ampullary area, or spasm in this region. An uncommon defect,[17] it is most likely caused by prominence of muscle in the distal end of the common duct. On cholangiography, the upper border is outlined; it is convex upward, may be smooth or somewhat irregular, and usually involves the entire lumen without stretching or dilating the duct. It is not altered by antispasmodic agents. It does not cause obstruction and at fluoroscopy or cineradiography it can be observed to disappear during relaxation and reappear during the contraction phase at the distal end of the common duct. It produces no pain, is probably permanent rather than transient, and is most likely caused by prominence or an unusual arrangement of the muscle at the choledochoduodenal junction. The clinical and cholangiographic features described differentiate it from the lesions mentioned in the preceding paragraphs.

Stricture of the Common Duct

Over 90% of benign biliary strictures are secondary to surgical procedures. In addition to congenital stenosis, inflammatory disease, erosion by a gallstone, and external blunt trauma are the major nonsurgical causes of stricture of the common duct. Cholangiography demonstrates the obstruction. This finding, along with the history, usually provides the diagnosis.

Sclerosing Cholangitis

This rare inflammatory disease of the biliary duct system is characterized by fibrosis and stricture formation leading to biliary obstruction and cirrhosis. On cholangiography, strictures of varying lengths are seen in the intra- and extrahepatic ducts. The smaller radicles are obliterated resulting in a pruned-tree appearance. Other ducts have an irregular or beaded contour. Despite the strictures, dilatation is minimal. This lesion must be differentiated from diffuse sclerosing carcinoma of the bile ducts. There appears to be a little more duct dilatation in the latter as a general rule, but this finding is not very helpful in an individual patient. Patients with ulcerative colitis, regional enteritis, retroperitoneal fibrosis, and Riedel's thyroiditis have an increased incidence of sclerosing cholangitis for reasons that are not clear.

Cholangiolitic Hepatitis

This is a chronic intrahepatic disease of unknown cause. It results in diffuse and focal narrowing along with varying degrees of shortening and diminished branching of the intrahepatic biliary duct system, as observed on cholangiography. The disease must be differentiated from sclerosing cholangitis, but, in the latter, in addition to the intrahepatic disease, the extrahepatic bile ducts are involved. The diffuse scirrhous type of carcinoma causes similar changes, but there tends to be more proximal dilatation and the lesions are more sharply defined in carcinoma than in cholangiolitic hepatitis.[14]

Cholangitis

Ascending or acute obstructing cholangitis is usually secondary to common duct obstruction. Cholangiography outlines dilated ducts, but there are no specific radiographic findings to indicate cholangitis unless the acute suppurative process is severe and is complicated by small liver abscesses that communicate with bile ducts. When such abscesses are present, a specific diagnosis may be made when correlating the findings with the clinical condition of the patient.

Pyogenic Cholangitis. Chronic pyogenic cholangitis, which is common in the Far East, may be seen in Asian immigrants in the United States. Roentgen findings include: (*1*) decrease in arborization of intrahepatic radicles; (*2*) abnormal branching pattern with obtuse or right-angle branching; (*3*) areas of dilatation along with some areas of rapid peripheral tapering suggesting the appearance of an arrowhead; (*4*) radiolucent calculi; and (*5*) dilatation of the common duct up to 3 or 4 cm.[9]

Parasitic Diseases

Parasitic infestation of the bile ducts is rare. The roundworm, *Ascaris lumbricoides,* is an intestinal parasite that may migrate into the biliary tract. It may then cause partial obstruction. On cholangiography the worm is readily recognized because of its size and shape. This condition is occasionally encountered in the United States. *Liver flukes,* which are endemic in the Far East, may also involve the bile ducts where they appear as curved, crescentic defects or semilunar defects that may also cause duct dilatations.

Chronic Pancreatitis

Typical findings on cholangiography in patients with chronic pancreatic inflammation consist of a long stricture in the distal common duct with slightly dilated or normal proximal ducts. The transition of the stricturelike narrowing may be abrupt at the margin of the pancreas. There may be some tortuousity of the narrow area. Complete common-duct obstruction is rare.

REFERENCES AND SELECTED READINGS

1. BABBITT DP, STARSHAK RJ, CLEMETT AR: Choledochal cyst: a concept of etiology. Am J Roentgenol 119:57, 1973
2. BERK RN, CLEMETT AR: Radiology of the Gallbladder and Bile Ducts. Philadelphia, WB Saunders, 1977
3. BERK RN, LEOPOLD GR: The present status of imaging of the gallbladder. Invest Radiol 13:477, 1978
4. BORNHURST RA, HEITZMAN ER, MCAFEE JG: Double-dose drip infusion cholangiography: analysis of 107 consecutive cases. JAMA 206: 1489, 1968
5. BURHENNE HJ: Non-operative extraction of stones from the bile ducts. Semin Roentgenol 11:213, 1976
6. CRUMMY AB: Same day re-enforcement oral cholecystography. Wis Med J 65:84, 1966
7. EVANS JA, MUJAHED Z: Percutaneous transhepatic cholangiography. Semin Roentgenol 11:219, 1976
8. HARNED RK, BABBITT DP: Cholelithiasis in children. Radiology 117:391, 1975
9. HO CS, WESSON DE: Recurrent pyogenic cholangitis in Chinese immigrants. Am J Roentgenol 122: 368, 1974
10. JUHL JH, COOPERMAN LR, CRUMMY AB: Oragrafin, a new cholecystographic medium. Radiology 80:87, 1963
11. JUTRAS JA: Hyperplastic cholecystoses. Am J Roentgenol 83:795, 1960
12. JUTRAS JA, LEVESQUE HP: Adenomyoma and adenomyomatosis of the gallbladder: radiologic and pathologic correlations. Radiol Clin North Am 4:483, 1966
13. KRIEGER J, SEAMAN WB, PORTER MR: The roentgenologic appearance of sclerosing cholangitis. Radiology 94:369, 1970
14. LEGGE DA, CARLSON HC, DICKSON ER et al: Cholangiographic findings in cholangiolitic hepatitis. Am J Roentgenol 113:16, 1971

15. MENUCK L, AMBERG J: Bile ducts. Radiol Clin North Am 14:499, 1976

16. MONCADA R, CARDOSO M, DANLEY R et al: Acute cholecystitis: 137 patients studied by infusion tomography of the gallbladder. Am J Roentgenol 129:583, 1977

17. MUJAHED Z, EVANS JA: Pseudocalculus defect in cholangiography. Am J Roentgenol 116:337, 1972

18. MUJAHED Z, GLENN F, EVANS JA: Communicating cavernous ectasia of the intrahepatic ducts (Caroli's disease). Am J Roentgenol 113:21, 1971

19. RÖSCH J, ANTONOVIC R, DOTTER CT: Transjugular cholangiography. Semin Roentgenol 11:227, 1976

20. SACHS MD: Routine cholangiography, operative and postoperative. Radiol Clin North Am 4:547, 1966

21. SALZMAN E: Opacification of bile duct calculi. Radiol Clin North Am 4:525, 1966

22. TURNER FW, COSTOPOULOS LB: Percutaneous transhepatic cholangiography. A study of 115 cases. Can Med Assoc J 99:513, 1968

23. WEINER M, HANAFEE WN: A review of transjugular cholangiography. Radiol Clin North Am 8:53, 1970

24. WISE RE: Current concepts of intravenous cholangiography. Radiol Clin North Am 4:521, 1966

25. WISE RE, O'BRIEN RG: Interpretation of the intravenous cholangiogram. JAMA 160:819, 1956

15

THE ESOPHAGUS

In this and succeeding chapters, examination of the gastrointestinal tract by means of contrast material introduced into it, either orally or given as an enema, will be considered. The material most frequently used for contrast visualization of the intestinal tract is barium sulfate. Various companies manufacture barium sulfate expressly for roentgen diagnostic purposes and only material in containers bearing such a label should be used. Barium sulfate is completely inert in the gastrointestinal tract and it is very radiopaque. It is insoluble in water and is given, orally and rectally, as an aqueous suspension. Commercial preparations are available that contain suspending agents that help to keep the heavy powder from settling too rapidly. Such mixtures also serve to coat the mucosal surfaces somewhat better than plain barium–water mixtures.

Water-soluble iodinated compounds such as Hypaque and Gastrografin, may also be used as contrast agents. These compounds have a limited field of usefulness in roentgen studies of the gastrointestinal tract, including the esophagus.

Each part of the gastrointestinal tract will be dealt with separately in the discussions to follow and the techniques of examination will be found under the specific anatomic subdivisions. The colon is examined by means of a barium mixture given as an enema and this is commonly referred to as a *barium enema examination*. The esophagus, stomach, duodenum, and upper part of the jejunum are examined together by means of a barium mixture given orally; by common usage this is referred to as an *upper gastrointestinal series* (GI series). When the esophagus is studied specifically, the term *esophagram* (barium swallow) is applied. The mesenteric small intestine is not included routinely as a part of the upper gastrointestinal study. If it is to be examined this is done as a continuation of the gastrointestinal series by following the oral meal as it passes through the small bowel; this is referred to as a small-intestinal examination or as a *"small bowel study."*

Modern fluoroscopes are equipped with a device whereby a roentgen-film cassette can be brought in front of the patient being fluoroscoped and an exposure made using the fluoroscopic tube as the source of roentgen rays. Such a device enables the fluoroscopist to obtain a film image of something observed on the fluoroscopic screen within a second or two after it is seen. This makes it possible to record, on film, rapidly changing images and transient defects in the barium shadow which otherwise might be difficult to register. These roentgenograms are referred to as "spot films," since they usually cover only a small field and the examiner "aims" the exposure at a definite area. Spot films are very useful in gastrointestinal roentgenography because of the changing contours of the viscera brought about by peristalis and respiration and by palpation on the part of the examiner.

VIDEO AND CINERADIOGRAPHY

With modern image intensifiers it is possible to obtain motion studies of the gastrointestinal tract. This technique, *cineradiography,* has the advantage of recording on film the rapidly changing images seen fluoroscopically and allows a more leisurely viewing than does fluoroscopy as well as repeated viewings of the various parts of the gastrointestinal tract. The quality of reproduction is very good. It is possible to televise and videotape the image, also allowing more than one individual to view the procedure and to review the tape following the examination. Remote-control systems also are available; these allow the examiner to control the apparatus from an adjacent shielded control room. Television fluoroscopy and videotaping have become important adjuncts in the examination of the gastrointestinal tract.

The esophagus is examined routinely as a part of the study of the upper gastrointestinal tract. In addition it may be investigated because of specific complaints referable to it. The technique of examination will of necessity vary, depending on the presence or absence of a lesion, the amount of obstruction, and the like.

METHODS OF EXAMINATION

Preliminary Roentgenograms

The contracted esophagus may be visualized as a narrow stripelike shadow in the upper mediastinum in frontal roentgenograms of the chest. Also the external wall of the barium-filled esophagus may occasionally be visualized, particularly in the lower third in lateral and oblique roentgenograms, as it is outlined by the air-filled lungs adjacent to it. Roentgenograms of the neck and thorax without contrast material in the esophagus are useful for the detection of opaque foreign bodies. Such roentgenograms also may demonstrate the dilated fluid-filled esophagus of achalasia. In congenital esophageal atresia the dilated, air- or fluid-filled upper esophageal segment may be outlined. It may cause some forward displacement of the trachea. If perforation of the esophagus is suspected, plain-film roentgenograms may reveal air or fluid in the mediastinal tissues or in the pleural cavities. Occasionally a carcinoma of the esophagus may produce an abnormal shadow posterior to the trachea or widening of the mediastinum. However, in most lesions affecting the esophagus an adequate examination requires the use of contrast material to outline its lumen.

Contrast Visualization

Materials. A suspension of barium sulfate powder in water is the contrast material used for most esophageal examinations. The same mixture used for the examination of the stomach and small intestine is satisfactory for the preliminary study of the esophagus. For a more detailed study of the mucosa and to elicit small defects a thicker mixture may be needed. Only enough water is added to barium sulfate to form a creamy paste. This is given in tablespoonful amounts. There are a number of commercially prepared barium mixtures available for use in the study of the esophagus. Esophatrast, Barosperse, and HD 5000 were found to be equally satisfactory by Miller and associates.[28] Oily Dionosil sometimes is used in place of barium, usually because of the possibility of aspiration of the material into the tracheobronchial tree or because a fistula exists between the two. It is often used in examining the esophagus of the newborn when atresia is suspected. However, the danger from aspiration of barium sulfate is not great; in fact it has been recommended as a contrast agent for bronchography. When the possibility of aspiration exists the examiner should use caution regardless of the contrast agent used.

Having the patient swallow a small pledget of cotton soaked in the barium mixture is useful when examining for the presence of small or sharp foreign bodies such as fish bones. A small piece of bread soaked in the barium mixture is used occasionally to demonstrate the ability of the esophagus to transport solid food. Such a bolus may elicit spasm better than the liquid mixture. To determine the maximum diameter of a stricture, gelatin capsules of various sizes filled with barium powder or barium tablet can be given. By noting the largest size capsule or tablet that will pass through the stricture, an idea of its maximum diameter can be obtained.

Techniques of Examination. The pharynx is outlined by barium very briefly as the patient swallows. The bolus moves so rapidly that fluoroscopy is not very satisfactory, making cineradiography the best technique by means of which the swallowing mechanism can be studied along with the anatomy of the pharynx. Frontal and lateral views are obtained after the patient has been given a barium paste which coats the mucosa so that it can be outlined after the main bolus has passed into the esophagus. Because of the danger of aspiration, thick barium paste probably should not be used when the patient's history indicates considerable difficulty in initiating swallowing and when fluoroscopy with use of a small amount of thin barium, confirms this abnormality. Plain films, xeroradiograms, and tomograms are also used to demonstrate pharyngeal, laryngeal, and upper tracheal anatomy. Examination of the larynx is discussed in Chapter 22.

The technique of examination of the esophagus varies somewhat with the problem presented by the patient. We usually give the patient a liquid suspension of barium first, followed by barium paste. The patient is examined fluoroscopically in the upright and in the recumbent position. The visualization of esophageal varices and evaluation of esophageal strictures may be improved by the use of Pro-Banthine (propantheline bromide) given intramuscularly in 30-mg doses. This drug is contraindicated in patients with glaucoma or obstructive uropathy, however. Atropine in doses of 0.5 mg given intravenously may also be used. Abdominal compression along with the Trendelenburg position may be employed to keep the esophageal lumen dilated if this is necessary. Several methods of double-contrast examination have been described. These are used when it is necessary to obtain good detail of esophageal mucosa. A mouthful of barium followed by water is given by some.[76] The barium coats the mucosa and the water dilates the esophagus. Others administer a combination of Barosperse and a gas-forming substance, such as Seidlitz powders, giving the acid and base separately followed by a bolus of barium.[39] Spot films are obtained during fluoroscopic observation, and overhead films may be obtained as needed when fluoroscopy is completed. If the stomach is to be examined, this should be done before water or barium paste is given since either may interfere with the examination of the stomach.

Cinefluorography or fluoroscopy with videotaping are of particular value in the study of motility disorders of the esophagus.[9, 44] A change in motor activity of the esophagus often takes place with increasing age. In some patients, peristaltic waves may be slow, shallow, and at times traverse only the upper esophagus; in others, they are absent altogether. Tertiary contractions (curling) are common and often involve the lower one-half to one-third of the esophagus. The lower esophageal sphincter may not relax completely since the normal primary contraction may not be present. As a result, there may be some dilatation of the esophagus. Despite alteration in function, many of the patients are asymptomatic.

THE NORMAL ESOPHAGUS

ANATOMY

The esophagus begins at the level of the cricoid cartilage in the neck. It passes to the right of the transverse aortic arch, with which it is in close relationship. The arch causes a smooth indentation on the barium-filled esophagus; this becomes more prominent with advancing age (Fig. 15-1). The right branch of the pulmonary artery passes anterior to the esophagus; the left main bronchus crosses it directly below the level of the aortic arch and may cause a slight, smooth indentation in the barium shadow. The distal part of the esophagus lies to the right of and anterior to the descending thoracic aorta. In elderly persons in whom the aorta is elongated and tortuous, it may displace the lower part of the esophagus forward. The descending aorta in these patients usually executes a curve to the left and may project beyond the left cardiac margin in posteroanterior roentgenograms. The esophagus remains in close relationship to the right aortic border and will also curve to the left and then back to the midline as it descends through the diaphragm. Extrinsic compression of the distal esophagus by a dilated, tortuous, and rigid aorta in this area may cause partial esophageal obstruction, termed *dysphagia aortica,* particularly in elderly women. Smooth, eccentric esophageal narrowing adjacent to the dilated aorta is readily recognized fluoroscopically in this condition. Motor disturbances (presbyesophagus) plus the compression probably cause the condition.

The distal part of the esophagus lies directly behind the posterior surface of the heart and thus it is in close relationship with the left atrium. The abdominal portion of the esophagus is of variable length and the exact anatomy of this segment is in dispute. This is discussed more fully in the following section, "Normal Deglutition."

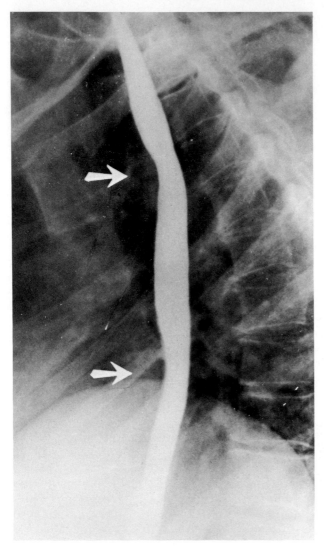

Fig. 15-1. Normal esophagus. The barium outlines the esophagus in this right posterior oblique view which is just off the lateral. The **upper arrow** indicates the indentation produced by the transverse aortic arch and the lower **arrow** indicates the slight impression at the level of the left atrium.

Normal Deglutition

The act of swallowing is a complicated process that has been under recent investigation by means of roentgen cinematography. As an extremely brief description of this complicated act it may be stated that the bolus to be swallowed is pushed backward by the tongue which is elevated toward the hard palate. The uvula and soft palate rise to close off the naso-

pharynx. The larynx rises, the glottis is closed, and the epiglottis tips backward over the laryngeal vestibule. The bolus passes rapidly through the pharynx, the hyoid bone is elevated and moves posteriorly, the pyriform sinuses momentarily fill, and the bolus is propelled into the esophagus by a powerful contraction of the pharyngeal muscles. The pharynx momentarily forms a funnel-like conduit for the bolus from the base of the tongue into the upper esophagus. Then the functional upper esophageal sphincter composed of the cricopharyngeus muscle and the uppermost 1 to 2 cm of intrinsic esophageal muscle contract, closing the upper esophagus, and the airway opens. The contraction wave continues down the esophagus as the primary persistaltic wave.

With the subject in the upright position, once a liquid bolus has reached the esophagus, it passes rapidly through the cervical portion, propelled by the stripping peristaltic wave that is a continuation of the propulsive contraction of the pharynx. Gravity is the major factor in further progress of the material through the remainder of the esophagus. Peristalsis ordinarily is not visible except as a contraction wave behind the advancing bolus, which serves to strip the residue into the stomach. With thick barium paste, and particularly if the swallowing act is performed with the patient in a horizontal position, the material is propelled by a broad contraction that passes rapidly down the esophagus. This is known as the primary wave or contraction. After the esophagus has been emptied of the major portion of the material there is a general relaxation and in the normal resting phase the esophagus remains in a slightly relaxed state. If the initial primary wave has not emptied the esophagus of most of the material a second wave ensues; other waves may follow until no more contrast material remains. These contractions, which are not initiated by swallowing, are called "secondary waves."

There is much variation in this process. Ordinarily movement is much slower in older than in younger individuals; often the first swallow is arrested at the level of the diaphragm and may remain there until more swallows have been taken. On deep inspiration the diaphragm seems to act as a pinchcock, closing the esophagus until exhalation is performed.

With rapid swallowing the entire esophagus remains filled except the cervical portion, which contracts rapidly after each swallow. The margins of the distended esophagus are smooth. The pressure indentation by the aortic arch is readily seen. The portion in contact with the left atrium of the heart will pulsate with the atrial pulsations. If, when the esophagus is in the contracted state, a thick barium paste has been given, sufficient paste will cling to the walls to outline the mucosal folds. These become visible as thin, vertical, stripelike shadows paralleling the long axis of the esophagus; the stripes represent barium caught in the valleys between the folds. Normally only three or four folds are present (Fig. 15-2). Frequently a smooth indentation is noted on the posterior wall of the upper end of the esophagus. This is called the "esophageal lip" and is believed to be caused by the transverse fibers of the cricopharyngeus muscles. It has no clinical significance.

Frequently, as the esophagus contracts behind a bolus of barium, the lower end becomes dilated, the primary wave stopping before it reaches the level of the diaphragm. A pouchlike dilatation of the esophagus results. After a few moments this segment usually contracts, pushing the retained barium mixture into the stomach, and it does not fill again until another swallow has been taken. This dilated segment is known as the *phrenic ampulla* or suprahiatal pouch (Figs. 15-3 and 15-4). It is of importance because of the necessity for distinguishing it from an esophageal hiatal hernia, which it closely resembles. The lower esophageal sphincter or vestibule extends from slightly above the level of the hiatus to the cardia; it straddles the hiatus, is difficult to localize anatomically, and is 2 to 4 cm in length.

The anatomic junction between the esophagus and stomach is termed the "cardiac orifice" or "cardia." A considerable amount of investigative work has been done, much of it in recent years, on the anatomy and physiology of the distal end of the esophagus and the mechanisms for closure of the cardia to prevent reflux of stomach contents into the esophagus. There have been differences of opinion regarding the presence of an abdominal portion of the esophagus, the exact site of esophageal closure, and the mechanism whereby competency of the cardia is maintained. It is no longer believed that the junction of esophageal and gastric mucosa represents the cardia or the site where closure occurs. The mucosal junction often is irregular with fingerlike projections of one type of mucosa into the other. Gastric mucosa also may continue a considerable distance above the level of the diaphragmatic hiatus. Also, it has been shown by Palmer and others, using metal clips attached to the mucosal junction at the time of esophagoscopy, that it is not fixed but that there is a certain amount of up and down migration of the mucosa on the muscularis with swallowing or even during the resting state. The nature of a given segment, *i.e.,* whether it is functionally esophagus or stomach, is determined not by the type of epithelial lining, but by

the character of its motor activity or peristalsis and the pressure gradient within it.

Roentgenologically, the junction between esophageal and gastric mucosa may not be obvious. The transition from three to four vertical parallel folds in the contracted esophagus to the larger, more tortuous, or crinkled folds of the stomach may be distinct, but in some individuals the esophageal folds appear to be directly continuous with the gastric folds and pass without interruption into the stomach. Also, when gastric mucosa extends some distance above the diaphragm, as in Barrett's esophagus, the fold appearance is that of esophagus rather than stomach. This becomes significant when the diagnosis of a small hiatal hernia is being considered.

According to Wolf and associates[42] the term "esophagogastric junction," refers to a segment about 5 cm in length between the body of the esophagus and the stomach. The upper part of this tract, about 3 cm in length, consists of the phrenic ampulla which extends to the diaphragmatic hiatus. Between the ampulla and body of the stomach is another tubular structure which is intra-abdominal in location and designated as the "submerged segment" or "abdominal gullet." This part is lined by squamous epithelium proximally and cylindric epithelium distally. Because the closing mechanism appers to lie at the level of the diaphragm, the opinion has been expressed that this represents the lower esophageal sphincter, at least from a functional viewpoint.

The mechanism whereby the lower end of the esophagus is closed, thus preventing reflux from the stomach, is not agreed upon. With but few exceptions, investigators have failed to find evidence of a true anatomic sphincter in the lower end of the esophagus, *i.e.,* a localized thickening of the circular muscle. Nevertheless, most observers agree that the muscle must exert a sphincterlike action and this is known as the physiologic sphincter. It is also generally agreed that this sphincteric action is relatively weak and that there must be some other mechanism to aid it. For a long time the pinchcock action of the diaphragm has been considered to be one of these factors. The right crus of the diaphragm surrounds the hiatus, encircling the esophagus in a slinglike manner. On deep inspiration, contraction of the diaphragm can be seen fluoroscopically, closing the esophagus and preventing swallowed material from passing through into the stomach. On expiration, as the diaphragm relaxes, the swallowed material passes readily into the stomach.

The obliquity of the insertion of the esophagus into the stomach also has been considered to be important. The direction of the esophagus in relation to the fundus results in a sharp angular sulcus or incisura between the two. This sulcus is deepened when the fundus is distended. Another possible mechanism is the presence of a valvelike action of a lip of mucosa along the left border of the cardia. The final answers to these problems remain unsettled but, roentgenologically, the point of closure, and therefore what may be termed the functional sphincter, appears to lie at the level of the diaphragm, extending 1 to 2 cm above and below it.

The normal distended esophagus has a smooth surface. When it is collapsed, longitudinal folds are seen in the lower one-half to two-thirds. They are thin and smooth. Occasionally, a pattern of transverse folds is séen in the distal third of the esophagus.[15] They are 1 to 2 mm thick, cross the width of the esophagus without interruption, and are transient so that they may be seen on only one or two of a number of spot films exposed during an examination. They are probably of no significance and may represent contraction of the muscularis mucosa alone without contraction of the muscularis propria.

The "Curling Phenomenon"

Curling is an alteration of motility seen rather frequently in elderly individuals and occasionally in younger persons. It is brought out to best advantage when the examination is performed with the patient recumbent. As the mass of barium descends into the lower part of the esophagus and distends it, multiple ringlike contractions rapidly appear and disappear, recurring at short intervals until finally a peristaltic wave moves the bolus into the stomach (Fig. 15-5). This condition also is known as *"corkscrew esophagus"* and *"beaded esophagus,"* and as *tertiary contractions* of the esophagus. In most instances it does not seem to be of clinical significance and does not cause symptoms. Occasionally the contractions are particularly deep and lasting and the contraction rings divide the esophagus into multiple dilated segments. Some patients with this more severe form of curling complain of dysphagia. This usually is intermittent and often is initiated by the swallowing of poorly chewed food. Also, in this severe form of curling, diverticulumlike outpouchings may be seen between two or more of the contractions. These may be only temporary and as the spastic contractions relax the outpouchings disappear. "Curling" is a major finding in presbyesophagus, as noted in the following paragraph.

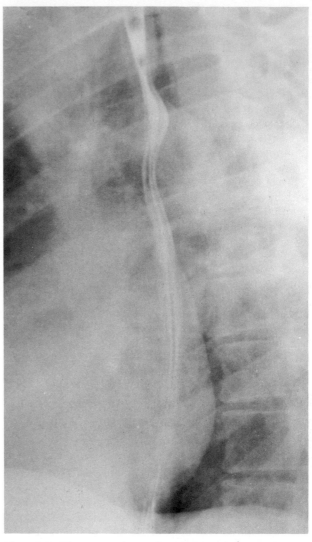

Fig. 15-2. The normal esophagus in a contracted state. Note the thin, longitudinal, mucosal folds.

DISORDERS OF MOTILITY

Presbyesophagus

The term "presbyesophagus" is used to describe an abnormality of esophageal motility associated with aging. However, the condition may be present in patients of middle age as well. Although most patients are asymptomatic, moderate dysphagia may be noted at times, particularly when they are eating solid foods. The primary perstaltic contraction is impaired, and there is an increase in nonpropulsive random contractions—tertiary contractions or curling. This

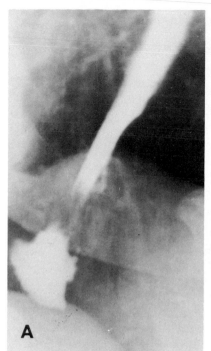 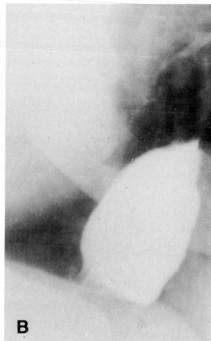

Fig. 15-3. The phrenic ampulla of the esophagus. **A.** The ampullary area is partially filled with barium, and a local dilatation is noted. **B.** The ampulla is filled. Dilatation, as compared with the portion of the esophagus above it, is noted.

phenomenon tends to involve the lower one-third to one-half of the esophagus, but may be more generalized. The lower esophageal sphincter may fail to relax occasionally and, in some patients, consistently. In the latter instance, usually some moderate dilatation of the esophagus is present.[9, 44]

Achalasia

Achalasia, often referred to as cardiospasm, is considered to be caused by a deficiency in esophageal innervation with a decrease or absence of the myenteric plexus—the ganglion cells of Auerbach.[38] The result is failure of relaxation of the lower esophageal sphincter or vestibule. There is also lack of normal persitalsis in the remainder of the esophagus although, at times, some shallow primary waves may be observed in the upper one-third to one-half. Random, nonpropulsive waves are common. A positive reaction to the Mecholyl test is considered to confirm the diagnosis. This consists in the production of a tetanic, nonperistaltic contraction of the distal one-half to two-thirds of the esophagus following subcutaneous administration of 10 mg or less of Mecholyl. It may cause severe pain in some patients. The condition usually occurs in adults ranging in age between 30 and 50 years, but rarely may occur in children.

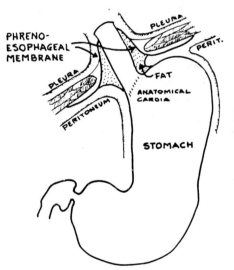

Fig. 15-4. Diagram illustrating the anatomy of the gastroesophageal junction. (Based on Harrington)

Roentgen Findings. The obstruction in achalasia is noted at or near the level of the diaphragm. Dilatation of the esophagus varies from moderate to severe. In the patients with marked dilatation the esophagus is often elongated and may be somewhat tortuous or angulated with the distal end curving to the right and

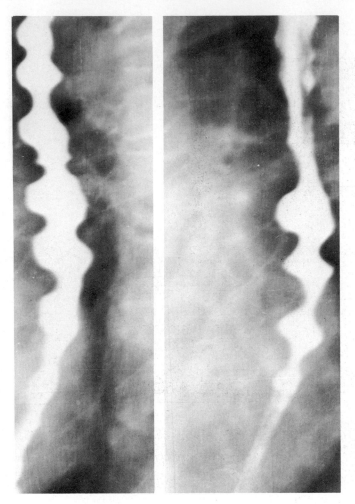

Fig. 15-5. Irregular or tertiary contraction noted on both films (exposed a short time apart) represents the so-called "curling phenomenon" which is observed in presbyesophagus.

back to the midline just above the diaphragm (Fig. 15-6).

Fluid and food in the dilated esophagus may cause mediastinal widening that may extend from the thoracic inlet to the diaphragm. An air–fluid level is commonly seen. At fluoroscopy the absence of normal persistaltic contractions may be observed along with some nonpropulsive random contractions. Small amounts of the barium mixture may pass intermittently into the stomach during the examination, but, in many instances, the greater portion of the meal is retained in the dilated esophagus. The distal end of the esophagus tapers smoothly to a point at about the level of the diaphragm.

Aspiration occurs commonly in patients with achalasia so that a recurrent bout of pneumonia or a chronic, low-grade pulmonary inflammatory process may be present. Pulmonary lesions are often asymptomatic but may lead to respiratory symptoms which overshadow the dysphagia resulting from achalasia.

Carcinoma of the esophagus may occur proximal to the area of achalasia, presumably the result of chronic esophagitis secondary to stasis. Because of the long-standing dysphagia and also because of the presence of much retained food and fluid in the esophagus, the diagnosis is made late in the course of the neoplasm. Some observers believe that the retention esophagitis of achalasia is premalignant and that all patients with this condition should have periodic esophagoscopy and esophagography with a careful search for a malignant lesion.

Diffuse Esophageal Spasm

Diffuse esophageal spasm is a clinical syndrome characterized by intermittent dysphagia and chest pain, repetitive contractions of the esophagus, and thickening of the esophageal wall. The symptoms are

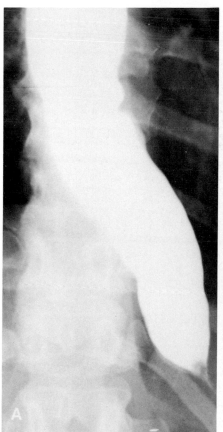
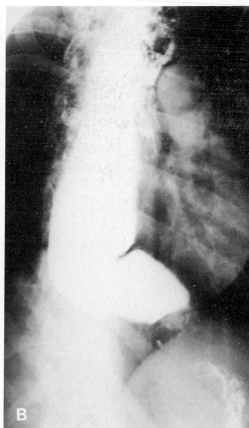

Fig. 15-6. Achalasia of the esophagus (cardiospasm). **A.** In this patient the characteristic dilatation and tapering of the lower end of the esophagus are seen. **B.** In this patient the esophagus is elongated as well as being dilated. This elongation is frequently observed in patients with a long history of the condition.

usually intermittent and are often elicited by swallowing a large bolus of food or fluid. Roentgen findings are variable since the spasm is intermittent (Fig. 15-7). Diffuse contraction of a long segment of esophagus may be observed, however, often during an attack of pain. In other patients the contractions will be intermittent and random, resembling tertiary contractions. The thickening of the esophageal wall can sometimes be demonstrated on films of good quality. The cause is uncertain; it is possible that there may be multiple causes. Some workers believe that diffuse spasm is due to an abnormality of the vagal sensory system.

Transient Postvagotomy Dysphagia

Dysphagia is common in the postvagotomy period. Usually it is transient and requires no treatment other than temporary exclusion of solid foods in the diet. The roentgen findings consist of a persistent tapered narrowing of the terminal 3 to 4 cm of the esophagus. The condition usually disappears spontaneously 2 to 6 weeks after the surgery.

Cricopharyngeal Achalasia

Cricopharyngeal achalasia is one of the causes of upper esophageal dysphagia. It may result from a number of neurologic diseases that interfere with normal relaxation of the cricopharyngeus muscle at the initiation of swallowing. Obstruction may be partial or complete. Because of danger of aspiration, Oily Dionosil is used for the examination of the upper esophagus when this condition is suspected. The amount of obstruction can be estimated and the possibility of other abnormalities excluded. Cricopharyngeus myotomy is the treatment of choice but is not always successful.

Chalasia

Chalasia, the reverse of achalasia of the lower esophageal sphincter, is found during the immediate postnatal period and is a cause of vomiting in infants. The esophagus is dilated, and there is diminished peristaltic activity. Free reflux of gastric content into the esophagus is observed (Fig. 15-8). The condition

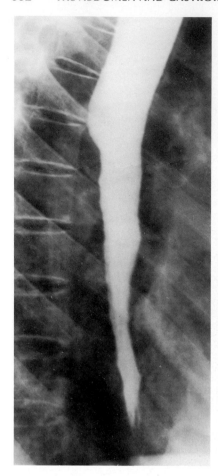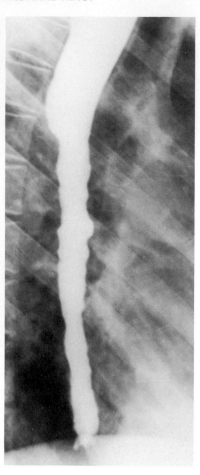

Fig. 15-7. Diffuse spasm of the lower half of the esophagus. These two films, exposed at short intervals apart, indicate the changing contour of the involved esophagus.

tends to disappear within a short time and is believed to be caused by incomplete development of neuromuscular control of the lower esophagus. If vomiting and reflux persist, the possibility of hiatus hernia must be considered in these infants.

Chalasia of the Cricopharyngeus

This is a condition involving the pharyngoesophageal sphincter in which sphincteric activity is diminished or absent. It is very rare and has been observed in one condition, myotonic dystrophy. Manometric studies show absence of the normal resting pressure in the cricopharyngeal region in some of these patients and a longer duration of the period of relaxation than is normal in others. The roentgen sign is the observation of a continuous column of barium extending from the hypopharynx into the cervical esophagus when the patient is not swallowing, indicating absence of the normal high-pressure zone. When the

condition is less marked, slow or delayed closure of the sphincter will be noted.[38]

SECONDARY MOTILITY DISORDERS

Progressive Systemic Sclerosis (Scleroderma)

Esophageal involvement is quite common in patients with scleroderma. The characteristic motility defect is failure of the primary propulsive wave to continue normally into the lower half of the esophagus. The patients must be studied in a horizontal position in order that this abnormality may be observed to best advantage. When they are in the horizontal position, the barium may remain in the esophagus for a considerable length of time. Other findings consist of dilatation, shortening, gastroesophageal reflux, and hiatus hernia (Fig. 15-9). Stricture secondary to reflux esophagitis may also be present. In the chest film the condition can often be suspected when a moderately dilated, gas-filled esophagus is observed.

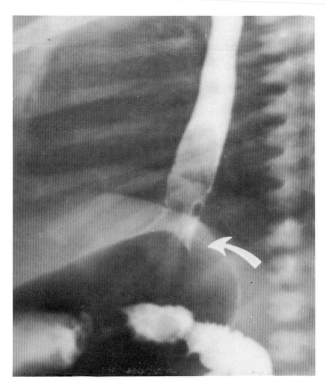

Fig. 15-8. Chalasia of the esophagus in a newborn infant. The **arrow** points to the patulous cardia. The barium in the esophagus has refluxed into it from the stomach.

Other connective-tissue disorders such as *lupus erythematosus* or Raynaud's disease may cause similar changes, but these are uncommon in our experience. Rarely, *amyloidosis* involving the esophagus may simulate the appearance of scleroderma there. *Dermatomyositis* causes abnormalities in the striated muscle and tends to begin in the pharnyx and extend to involve the upper third of the esophagus, but may also involve the smooth muscle of the lower two-thirds as well. Roentgen findings show the presence of air in the upper esophagus on plain film study. Barium studies show reflux into the nasopharnyx, persistence of barium filling in the valleculae (a positive vallecular sign), distended pyriform sinuses, aspiration, lack of constriction of the upper esophageal sphincter, and distention of the upper esophagus.

Other Causes of Motor Disorders

Diabetes mellitus, particularly in patients with neuropathy of long duration, may have dysphagia due to diminution of the normal progressive primary con-

tractions in the esophagus. There is some resultant dilatation, delay in emptying, and tertiary contractions. A number of neuromuscular disorders are also associated with esophageal motor dysfunction, but these may also be associated with pharyngeal dysfunction which is more disabling. *Chagas' disease,* caused by *Trypanosoma cruzi,* may produce changes in the esophagus that are indistinguishable on roentgen examinatin from those due to achalasia.

CONGENITAL ANOMALIES

ATRESIA OF THE ESOPHAGUS

Complete congenital occlusion of the esophagus is a relatively frequent anomaly, the site of obstruction usually being in the upper third just below the level of the sternal notch. The types of esophageal atresia, according to Vogt's classification, are as follows:

Type I. Complete absence of the esophagus
Type II. Atresia of the esophagus with both upper and lower segments ending in a blind pouch (no fistula)
Type III. Atresia of the esohagus with tracheoesophageal fistula
  a. Fistula between the upper segment and the trachea
  b. Fistula between the lower segment and the trachea, the upper ending blindly
  c. Fistula between the trachea and both esophageal segments

In type II the length of the atretic segment is variable but usually is fairly short. Occasionally extensive agenesis of the lower part of the esophagus has been found. The most frequent type is IIIb and this has been reported to constitute from 85% to 90% of all cases. The next most frequent lesion is type II.

Roentgen Observations. Preliminary roentgenograms of the chest and abdomen in anteroposterior and lateral directions are obtained. If the atresia is of either type IIIb or IIIc, air will be present in the gastrointestinal tract (Fig. 15-10). With the other types of atresia the abdomen will be completely free of air. The presence or absence of intestinal air, therefore, is important in distinguishing between the types of defect. Plain roentgenograms may show aspiration pneumonitis or atelectasis. The upper esophageal segment may be outlined by swallowed air and/or fluid secretions. Dilatation of the proximal segment

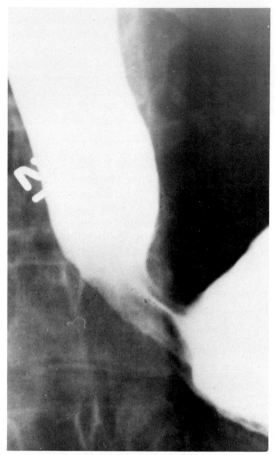

Fig. 15-9. Scleroderma involving the esophagus which is dilated and atonic. Free reflux from the stomach into the esophagus was noted at fluoroscopy.

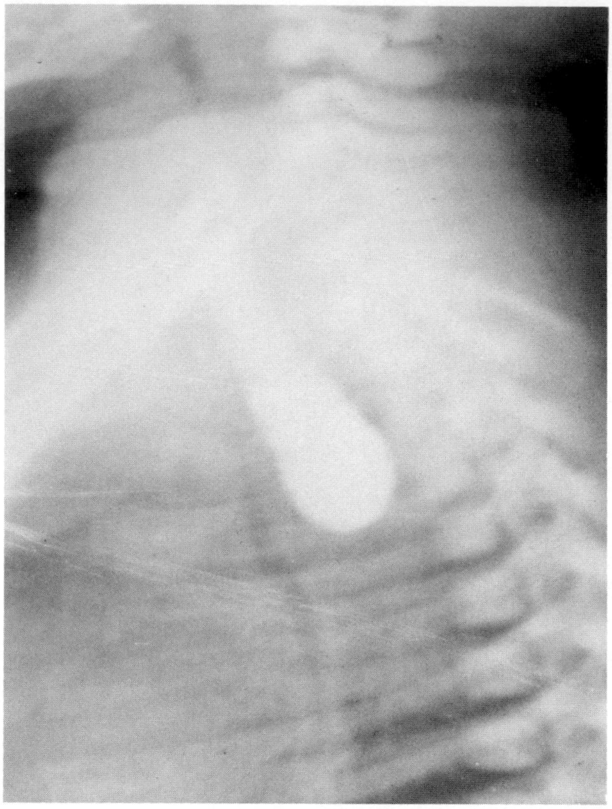

Fig. 15-10. Congenital esophageal atresia. This is a type III–b atresia in which the gas noted in the stomach indicated a connection between the lower end of the esophagus and the tracheobronchial tree. The short atretic segment of the esophagus above is outlined by contrast material.

may be sufficient to cause some forward displacement of the trachea.

The next step in the examination is to insert a soft-rubber catheter into the upper end of the esophagus (under fluoroscopic guidance) as far as it will go. A small amount of Oily Dionosil or barium sulfate, usually not more than 2.0 cc, is injected. This will outline the lower end of the segment and clearly demonstrate the presence of the atresia. If the anomaly is of either type IIIa or IIIc, the oil will flow into the trachea and be aspirated into the tracheobronchial tree. It is for this reason that Dionosil rather than a barium mixture has been recommended, because aspiration of any appreciable amount of the insoluble barium might cause severe respiratory embarrassment. A large amount of oil also is dangerous

because it can fill the small bronchi to the point where respiratory difficulty may develop. It is wise, therefore, regardless of what medium is used, to inject the material into the esophagus with caution, always under fluoroscopic guidance and with only enough of the contrast material to establish the presence and the type of the defect. The length of the distal segment may be determined by reflux of air or barium injected into the stomach in patients with gastrostomy.

In type IIIb, which is most frequent, there is usually an area of noncontraction above and below the anastomosis following repair. This may cause problems because the primary contraction doesn't continue through this segment downward to the inferior sphincter. The distal esophagus, including the sphincter, may be contracted when the bolus reaches its upper end (below the anastomosis). Also, relaxation in the absence of a bolus may result in gastroesophageal reflux.

As a rather rare variation of type IIIc, a small fistulous opening may be present between the esophagus and the trachea but with little or no narrowing of the esophageal lumen. This is the so-called H type of tracheoesophageal fistula. There may be slight esophageal narrowing at its site. The incidence of this anomaly is very low, comprising only 1.8% to 4% of all tracheoesophageal atresia–fistula complexes. The fistula is usually high, at or above the thoracic inlet. It extends obliquely downward from the posterior tracheal wall to the anterior esophageal wall. Aspiration of esophageal contents may cause intermittent pneumonia as well as choking and coughing during feeding. Chronic aspiration pneumonia may also be present. Oily Dionosil is the contrast agent of choice to use when the presence of this lesion is suspected. A nasal catheter is passed into the distal esophagus, and the Dionosil is injected in small increments under fluoroscopic control, employing cine recording or video taping for careful study later. The prone position or an oblique prone position is used to allow the tract to fill by gravitation. If the fistula is not found, a thin barium mixture may be used. Water-soluble media are contraindicated since they are very irritating to bronchial mucosa. Because the tract is usually small and may be plugged by mucous, it is a good idea to repeat the examination in a day or two if clinical symptoms suggest an H-type fistula. Esophageal air may be present in this condition and suggests the diagnosis in the presence of appropriate clinical symptoms and signs. Esophageal motility is usually normal in this condition.

Esophageal atresia and tracheoesophageal fistula are associated with congenital malformations involving other systems. The most common appear to be anomalies of the skeletal system, which may be rather minor, involving vertebrae and ribs. Cardiovascular anomalies are next in incidence and include atrial septal defect, ventricular septal defect, and tetralogy of Fallot as well as more complex cardiac anomalies. Other gastrointestinal anomalies such as duodenal and anal atresia have also been reported.

LARYNGOTRACHEOESOPHAGEAL CLEFT

Failure of normal separation of the foregut into trachea and esophagus may be represented by a cleft limited to the larynx, cricoid, and upper trachea. A large common cavity may be demonstrated by a combination of laryngogoscopy and fluoroscopic spot films. The H-type T-E fistula is another form of failure of normal separation of the foregut; the most severe form is the involvement of the entire trachea and adjacent esophagus, the persistent esophagotrachea.[10]

CONGENITAL STRICTURE OF THE ESOPHAGUS

Congenital stricture of the esophagus is an uncommon lesion and represents an incomplete occlusion. The lesion can be diagnosed without much difficulty on roentgen examination. It results in a smooth fusiform narrowing of the esophageal lumen, causing a variable degree of obstruction. About one-half occur in the middle third of the esophagus. There is usually dilatation above the stricture. In the newborn such a stricture is almost invariably of congenital origin. In the older infant or child it may be impossible to distinguish between a congenital stricture and one of acquired origin caused by the swallowing of caustic material, since the roentgen appearances may be similar. Usually acquired strictures are multiple and involve longer segments of the esophagus.

Esophageal Web

Esophageal web may also be congenital and occur as an isolated anomaly or in association with a congenital stricture. It is circumferential and causes obstruction, with proximal dilatation; the roentgenographic appearance is similar to that of a lower esophageal ring.[18, 32]

Cartilagenous Esophageal Ring

Tracheal cartilage and other tracheobronchial remnants may produce local esophageal narrowing, often distally, but may occur at any point in the esophagus. Radiographic findings of local narrowing associated with long, tiny intramural clefts representing ducts of tracheobronchial glands are characteristic. The appearance is similar to that of intramural pseudodiverticulosis, an acquired lesion of adults.

DUPLICATION OF THE ESOPHAGUS

Duplication of the esophagus is a rare congenital anomaly. A closed duplication results in a cystic mass lined with esophageal epithelium and filled with fluid. It is found, as a rule, in the central or posterior portion of the mediastinum. The cyst may enlarge rapidly during infancy causing symptoms of pressure upon the other mediastinal structures. Most esophageal cysts or duplications, therefore, are discovered during the first few years of life. The lesion is seen as a rounded or oval-shaped mass lying within or along a border of the mediastinum in close relationship to the esophagus. There are few features to distinguish this lesion from a variety of other tumors and mass lesions that may occur in the mediastinum; surgical exploration usually is necessary. Occasionally the cyst is lined with gastric or other type of epithelium.

Open duplication of the esophagus is another extremely rare developmental anomaly in which the lumen of the duplication is patent and communicates with the normal esophagus resulting in a double lumen.[12] Rarely it may be associated with gastric duplication or with partial pericardial defect.

DISEASES OF THE ESOPHAGUS

DIVERTICULA

Diverticula are common lesions in the esophagus as they are in most other portions of the gastrointestinal tract and they may be found in any part of the structure. Diverticula of the esophagus may be either of the pulsion or traction type but almost all are acquired lesions; congenital diverticula are exceedingly rare. The most significant from a clinical point of view is the one that develops along the posterior wall of the upper end of the esophagus at its junction with the pharynx (Zenker's diverticulum). This is an acquired pulsion type of diverticulum that forms at a site of anatomic weakness between the oblique and circular fibers of cricopharyngeus muscle in the pharyngoesophageal wall. The diverticulum may cause symptoms of difficulty in swallowing because of retention of food and consequent pressure upon the cervical portion of the esophagus at the level of the thoracic inlet.

Diverticula of the intrathoracic portion of the esophagus are found mainly in its middle third, in the region of the lung hila. Most of them probably are of traction type, caused by pull from fibrous adhesions following infection of mediastinal lymph nodes. Calcified nodes frequently can be demonstrated adjacent to the diverticulum, the nodes being the end result of previous infection, often primary tuberculosis.

Diverticula in the lower end of the esophagus (epiphrenic) are most often of pulsion type. They are seen frequently associated with the curling phenomenon, probably developing as a result of increased pressure in the areas between the contraction rings.

Most esophageal diverticula other than the Zenker's type are asymptomatic and are incidental findings during a gastrointestinal roentgenographic examination. Within the thorax a diverticulum has adequate space to enlarge without causing pressure upon vital structures; it usually does not retain material to any appreciable degree, and secondary complications are infrequent. A large diverticulum in the distal end of the esophagus just above the level of the diaphragm may be symptom-producing because of its large size and the retention of food within it (Fig. 15-11) (epiphrenic diverticulum).

Roentgen Observations. The diverticulum is visualized as an outpouching or sac protruding from the esophageal lumen and connected to it by a narrow neck (Figs. 15-12 and 15-13). The sac has a rounded contour in most cases; small traction diverticula may have a more pointed contour. The Zenker's type often reaches a large size (8 to 10 cm or more). This diverticulum as it enlarges extends downward and posteriorly, eventually reaching into the posterior mediastinum. The opening of the sac then is near the upper margin and retention of swallowed material is enhanced. The distended sac pushes the esophagus forward and, confined by the thoracic inlet, pressure obstruction will develop. This type of diverticulum may retain the barium mixture for many hours or even days. Diverticula in the remainder of the esophagus usually have their openings situated along one side of the pouch, retention of barium may be only for short periods, and some of the smaller ones may not be visualized at all unless the examination is conducted with the patient recumbent. Large epiphrenic diverticula may retain barium for some time, however.

Intramural Diverticulosis

This condition, sometimes termed *pseudodiverticulosis*, is characterized by the presence of multiple small outpouchings often associated with esophageal narrowing which may be tonic contraction in some instances and stricture in others. Its etiologic background is controversial. In some cases, autopsy has shown that the projections represent dilated ducts of esophageal glands associated with chronic esophagitis, often moniliasis. In others, the lesions appear to be mucosal herniations secondary to increased pressure in patients with obstruction of the esophagus. In either type the diverticula have been observed to decrease or disappear when the underlying condition is treated.[3, 30, 41]

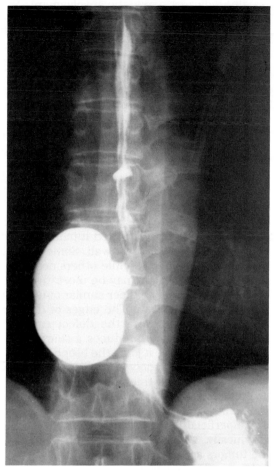

Fig. 15-11. Diverticulum of the lower end of the esophagus. This diverticulum is a little higher than the usual epiphrenic diverticulum.

Intraluminal Diverticulum

This rare condition is probably secondary to intraluminal herniation of a weblike stricture caused by adhesions. A pulsion-type diverticulum is formed which closely resembles the better-known intraluminal diverticulum of the duodenum on roentgen examination.[37]

TUMORS OF THE ESOPHAGUS

Benign Tumors

Polypoid Tumors. Polypoid tumors are uncommon and various types cannot be differentiated radiographically since they all appear as intraluminal

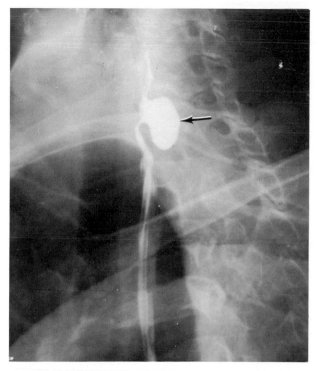

Fig. 15-12. Pharyngoesophageal diverticulum (Zenker's type). The **arrow** indicates the small diverticulum arising posteriorly at the pharyngoesophageal junction.

masses, often pedunculated, causing varying amounts of obstruction.

Leiomyoma. Leiomyoma is the most common benign tumor of the esophagus. The roentgenographic manifestations are those of an intramural tumor (rarely multiple) with a sharp angular junction between the mass, producing a filling defect and the esophageal wall. The extraluminal portion of the mass may be visible as it projects into the mediastinum and is outlined against adjacent lung. Despite the large size of some of these lesions, they usually cause no dysphagia. They cannot be differentiated from other extramucosal intramural tumors. Rarely, an intrathoracic thyroid glad may simulate an intramural esophageal tumor. Rarely, esophageal leiomyomas may contain enough calcium to be visible radiographically. The few studied angiographically were hypovascular.

Pseudotumor. Lower esophageal pseudotumor may be caused by varices, fundal plication used in treatment of reflux or hiatus hernia, or by retrograde pro-

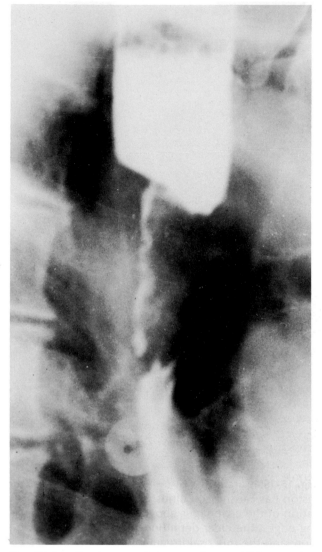

Fig. 15-16. Carcinoma of the esophagus. This annular lesion is clearly defined at the upper and lower ends. The lumen is narrow and irregular. There is some overhanging of edges and some obstruction manifested by the dilatation above the lesion.

tracheobronchial fistula and is present to some extent in all such cases.

In the lower end of the esophagus, carcinoma occasionally is of a fungating type, causing a bulky, lobulated, filling defect but with only moderate obstruction. Extension of a carcinoma of the distal esophagus to involve the cardiac end of the stomach may occur, but extension of a gastric lesion into the lower esophagus is more common, often producing a

bulky lesion as has been indicated. It may be impossible from roentgen examination to determine where such a tumor originated (Fig. 15-17B).

Infrequently a carcinoma of the esophagus causes a smooth, fusiform type of stricture, resembling closely the appearance of a benign fibrous stricture. The edges do not overhang but taper smoothly. Most benign strictures found in patients within the carcinoma age period occur in the lower end as a result of esophagitis or follow the ingestion of caustic materials and the resulting chemical esophagitis. Any stricture above the level of the distal few inches of the esophagus in a patient in the carcinoma age period with no history of ingestion of caustic material should be considered most likely caused by carcinoma. An exception occurs in Barrett's esophagus in which a stricture may form in the midesophagus. Esophagoscopy and biopsy should be performed if there is any doubt.

Superficial spreading esophageal carcinoma and leukoplakia may produce diffuse, fine nodular lesions that cannot be distinguished. Similar lesions have been described in *acanthosis nigricans* which may also cause a diffuse granular pattern similar to that of moniliasis.[22]

Rarely, carcinoma of the distal end of the esophagus causes an appearance closely simulating achalasia. The esophagus is greatly dilated and atonic. The lower end tapers gradually. The stricture caused by the tumor usually is at or close to the level of the diaphragmatic hiatus. Close observation may show a certain amount of irregularity of the stricture margins and absence of mucosal folds. A slight degree of overhang may be present at either end. These changes are in contrast to the smoothly narrowed segment in achalasia. If one finds an appearance similar to achalasia developing in an older individual without previous symptoms related to the esophagus, carcinoma should be suspected and esophagoscopy and biopsy should be performed.

Metastasis to regional nodes and lymphatics is common, and the lesion often extends up and down the esophagus in the submucosa. Hepatic metastasis may occur but this happens less frequently than in carcinoma of the stomach. Skeletal metastases, chiefly to the vertebrae and ribs, are often a result of direct extension by way of lymphatic or venous channels.

Lymphoma

The most common manifestation of lymphoma is extrinsic compression by masses of nodes. Direct involvement of the esophagus is uncommon. Diffuse

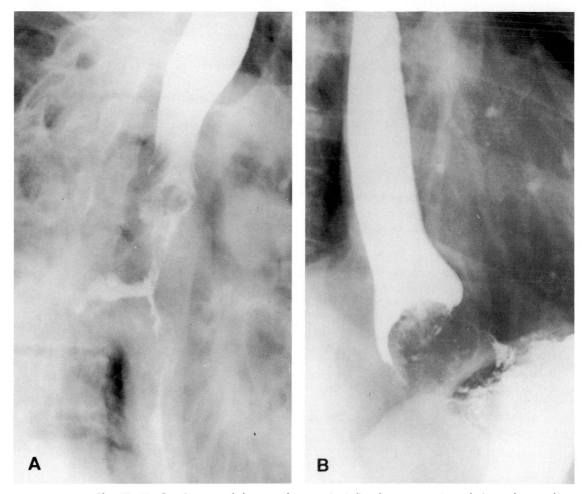

Fig. 15-17. Carcinoma of the esophagus. **A.** A fistulous tract extends into the mediastinum. The tumor has caused a long, irregular narrowing of the esophagus. **B.** This lesion is more localized than that shown in **A** and is a polypoid or fungating carcinoma which forms a bulky mass in the lower esophagus but is only partially obstructing. Many of these tumors represent primary adenocarcinoma of the stomach which has extended upward into the lower esophagus.

intramural submucosal involvement may occur, resulting in narrowing and a nodular appearance of the lumen.

ESOPHAGITIS AND ESOPHAGEAL ULCER

Esophagitis is said to be the most common disease affecting the esophagus. It is probable that mild forms of transient inflammation may occur very frequently but, because of the brief duration of the lesion and the lack of significant symptoms, roentgen and endoscopic examinations may not be requested.

The frequency of esophagitis in autopsy subjects is surprisingly high. Burke discovered 96 cases of acute and chronic inflammation in a series of 570 autopsies. This high incidence in patients coming to necropsy probably results from multiple factors including debilitation, the lowered resistance of the tissues to trauma and infection during the terminal state, relaxation of the cardia allowing regurgitation of gastric juice, frequent vomiting, and the use of a stomach tube or negative-suction apparatus.

Chemical Esophagitis

The swallowing of caustic materials, such as household lye, or an acid, such as sulfuric acid, will cause a severe erosive inflammation of the esophagus. Highly concentrated caustic material may cause necrosis and ulceration; the latter may be detected radiographically by intramural retention of the contrast agent, often associated with atony and distention with an air-filled esophagus. The ulcers manifested by intramural retention of barium may also extend into the stomach. Patients with atony initially, develop strictures later and those with deep ulcerations may develop gangrene with perforation.[25] In other patients the esophagus may appear rigid with persistent narrowing and absence of peristalsis; the mucosa is irregular owing to edema and mucosal changes. These patients also develop stricture later.[13] Others may experience irritability initially with lack of normal primary contractions. As the inflammation subsides, fibrosis and scar-tissue formation develop; the end result is usually one or more fibrous strictures. Roentgen examination may not be performed until after the acute inflammation has subsided and then it is undertaken to determine the location and extent of stricture formation. The strictures are most frequent at the sites of anatomic narrowing where the caustic material may have been held up momentarily. Thus they are seen at the level of the thoracic inlet, at the level of the aortic arch, and at or above the level of the diaphragmatic hiatus. The strictures are characterized by tapering edges and the fact that they are relatively long and also multiple (Fig. 15-18). If the injury has been very severe and if proper treatment has not been carried out, complete obstruction may develop.

Acute Ulcerative Esophagitis

In addition to ulcerative or erosive inflammation developing as a result of the ingestion of caustic materials as described in the preceding paragraph, acute ulcerative esophagitis is seen occasionally in patients with peptic ulcer, usually a duodenal ulcer, or following operation for relief of an ulcer. The cause of the disease is undetermined, but frequent vomiting, the use of a decompression tube in the esophagus, and the trauma and shock associated with upper abdominal operations seem to be of importance. The same lesion has been observed in patients with persistent vomiting from other causes (*e.g.,* pernicious vomiting of pregnancy). The regurgitation of highly acid gastric juice undoubtedly plays an important role although other factors may enter the picture.

Roentgen Observations. The roentgen findings (Figs. 15-19 and 15-20) in acute ulcerative esophagitis are as follows:

The involvement is limited to the lower third to half of the esophagus.

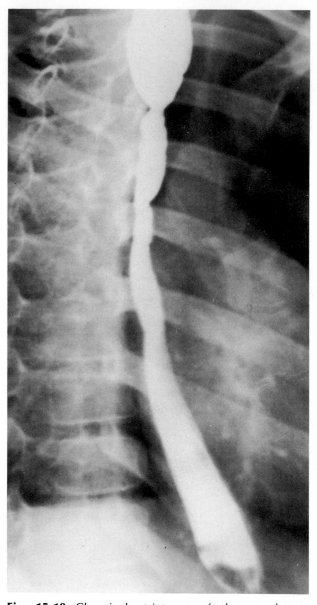

Fig. 15-18. Chemical strictures of the esophagus. Multiple areas of stricture formation are shown. They were caused by ingestion of caustic household cleaner containing lye.

The first evidence is that of esophageal spasm, which usually is intense. This causes a diffuse narrowing of the affected portion and results in varying degrees of obstruction. The spasm may relax intermittently to allow passage of the barium mixture into the stomach.

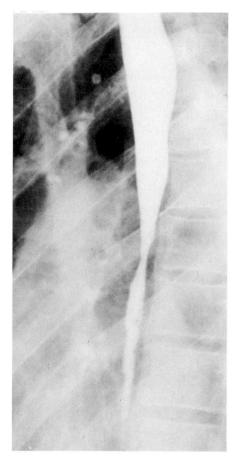

Fig. 15-19. Acute esophagitis. The patient developed signs and symptoms of esophageal obstruction following gastric resection. There was intense spasm which persisted throughout the examination and involved the lower half of the esophagus. It resolved in about 3 weeks.

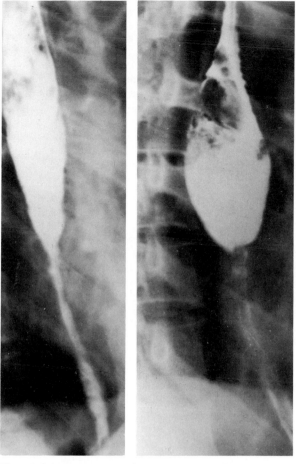

Fig. 15-20. Peptic esophagitis which developed in a patient suffering from pernicious vomiting of pregnancy. The esophagus remained contracted throughout the examination. Note the retained food causing irregular radiolucencies in the barium above the lesion.

After a short period, often only a matter of a few weeks, the deformity may become fixed because of fribrosis. The resultant obstruction may be severe and occasionally becomes complete. There is a complete absence of peristalsis in the involved segment.

The mucosal folds normally seen in the contracted esophagus are absent and the surface appears smooth or, occasionally, finely granular. In the early stages of the disease a fine roughening of the margin of the lumen may be noted, apparently representing the effects of the superficial ulceration that is present; in the late stages after the disease has sub-

sided to a fibrous stricture the margins become smooth.

Reflux Esophagitis

In some individuals, reflux from the stomach into the esophagus may occur frequently, and the acid gastric juice that then flows into the esophagus promotes the development of esophagitis. There may or may not be a hiatus hernia associated with the reflux. Diagnosis of the phenomenon is very difficult to make on radiographic study since the inflammation is often intermittent and may not be present at the time of the examination. In some instances, reflux may occur during the examination and may not occur in normal circumstances. The water siphonage or provocation test may be used,[7] but a number of false positive findings are produced and there may be false negatives as well. For this test the patient is placed in a right posterior-oblique supine position after barium has been administered. In this position the barium mixture will gravitate to the cardia. Several swallows of water are then given. As the lower esophageal sphincter relaxes to allow passage of the water, barium may reflux into the esophagus. This is considered a positive reaction. One of the symptoms of gastroesophageal reflux is heartburn. The acid–barium test is sometimes used in patients with this symptom. This consists in observing esophageal peristalsis during perfusion with barium sulfate containing 0.35% hydrochloric acid (pH 1.7). Delayed emptying and nonperistaltic contractions are the indicators of a positive reaction and in some patients the pain is reproduced. This most likely detects sensitivity of the esophagus to acid perfusion but does not necessarily indicate symptomatic reflux even though the reaction to the test is positive.

Roentgenographic Signs. In its early stages, reflux or peptic esophagitis produces slight limitation of distensability of the distal esophagus, slight irregularity of esophageal margins, and some irritability. These signs are minimal and although the diagnosis may be suggested in the presence of appropriate symptomatology, positive roentgen diagnosis cannot be made. Later on there is irregularity of the distal esophagus as a result of an abnormal mucosal pattern along with an area of stenosis. In some patients an actual ulcer crater can be observed in the distal esophagus, and hiatus hernia may be present (Fig. 15-21). In patients with peptic esophageal ulcer the incidence of duodenal ulcer is high. The stenosis may vary in severity but is seldom complete. In patients with the so-called short esophagus type of hiatus hernia, peptic esophagitis is virtually always present,

Peptic Ulcer of the Esophagus

The relation between ulcer of the esophagus, esophagitis, duodenal ulcer, and hiatus hernia is a close one.

Roentgen Observations. The roentgen evidence of esophageal ulcer is similar to that of ulcer in other parts of the gastrointestinal tract and depends upon the visualization of the ulcer crater as an outpouching or barium-filled pocket. The crater often is shal-

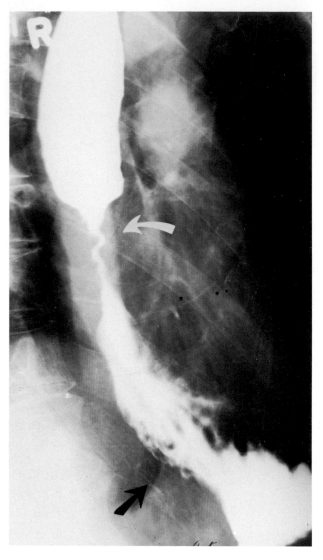

Fig. 15-21. Chronic peptic esophagitis. The **white arrow** outlines a small ulcer in the region of a stricture which is near the gastroesophageal junction. The **black arrow** indicates the level of the diaphragm. A considerable amount of stomach is noted above the diaphragm. This is the so-called "short-esophagus" type of hiatus hernia.

low and may be difficult to visualize unless seen tangentially.

Mucosal relief studies often show thickened mucosal folds radiating away from the edges of the crater, similar to the configuration seen in gastric or duodenal ulcers.

Spasm often is prominent and may cause a diffuse narrowing of the lumen around the ulcer. This nar-

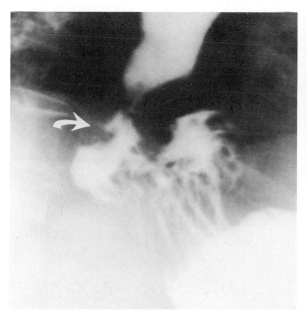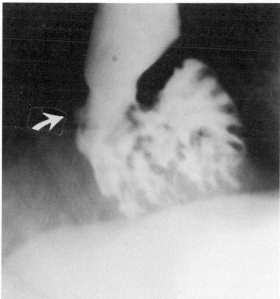

Fig. 15-22. Esophageal ulcer with an associated sliding or axial hiatus hernia. The lower esophagus was widely patent and free reflux from the stomach into the esophagus was noted at fluoroscopy. **Arrows** indicate the site of the ulcer.

rowing is characterized by its inconstancy during fluoroscopic observation.

A hiatal hernia is found in a high percentage of patients (see Figs. 15-22 and 15-23).

Usually the lumen of the esophagus is narrowed for a short distance above the ulcer and sufficient fibrosis may have developed to cause high-grade obstruction. The appearances then are those of a fibrosing esophagitis with the addition of the ulcer crater.

Less frequently the esophageal lumen is widely patent, the cardia relaxed, and free reflux from the stomach into the esophagus occurs (Fig. 15-22). This nonstenotic variety has been considered as a possible precursor to the stenotic lesion, representing the phase of the disease whereby the relaxed cardia allows free regurgitation of acid gastric juice into the esophagus. The ulcer crater must be searched for rather carefully in some of these patients because, in the absence of spasm and fibrosis, there is no narrowing or obstruction to draw attention to the lesion (Fig. 15-23).

Other Inflammatory Lesions

Candidiasis (Moniliasis). *Candida albicans,* usually a harmless fungus, may produce esophagitis of varying severity in patients with chronic debilitating disease, particularly those on steroid therapy, cancer chemo-

therapy, or antibiotics.[17, 19] Candida infection of the mouth may or may not be present along with the esophagitis. The most common radiologic finding is that of diffuse disease involving the esophagus producing a shaggy mucosal outline with numerous ulcerations accompanied by diminished peristalsis, and sometimes segmental narrowing. Clinical symptoms include dysphagia and retrosternal pain. Aperistalsis or atony may be the first sign of inflammation in candidiasis of the esophagus, but it may also be an early manifestation of other types of esophagitis. Rarely candidiasis appears to cause a chronic process with deep ulcerations simulating intramural pseudopolyposis. Another unusual manifestation is that of localized polypoid lesion without evidence of the infection elsewhere.

Herpes Simplex. Herpes esophagitis is usually observed in adults with a debilitating illness, such as that due to malignant disease, and sometimes it occurs in infants.[24, 27] Roentgenographic findings in some patients simulate those of candidiasis with small ulcerations, nodular filling defects, and mucosal edema producing thickening of the longitudinal esophageal folds. In two infants reported with the disease, the abnormality progressed to organic stricture simulating caustic ingestion, thus herpes simplex is a possible cause of organic stricture in

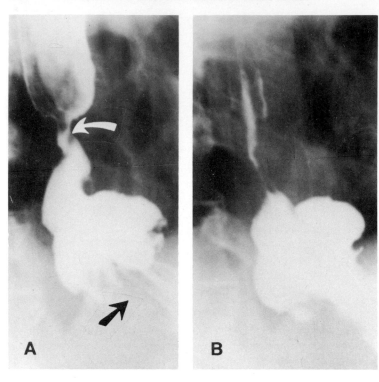

Fig. 15-23. Esophageal ulcer which is identified by the **white arrow** in **A** and is not clearly identified in **B**. The esophagus is short, there is a hiatus hernia, and the **black arrow** at the level of the hiatus indicates that it is wide.

the absence of a history of ingestion of a caustic substance.

Crohn's Disease (Regional Enteritis; Regional Ileitis). Regional enteritis rarely involves the esophagus, but when its presence is proved elsewhere in the body, esophageal abnormalities must be looked upon with suspicion.[8] Roentgen findings are variable. In some patients, flat, thickened mucosal folds progressing to typical cobblestone pattern with absence of peristalsis has been described. A stenosing form also occurs exhibiting conelike tapering, prestenotic dilatation, and stenosis that may be so complete as to require bypass or resection. Fistulous tracts are unusual but they do occur. Skip areas have not been described.

VARICES OF THE ESOPHAGUS

Dilatation of the veins of the lower part of the esophagus occurs chiefly as a result of cirrhosis of the liver but may result from splenic vein thrombosis, the esophageal veins serving as channels to bypass the obstructed portal system and splenic veins. Upper esophageal varices are caused by compression of the superior vena cava or azygos vein and are relatively rare.

The roentgen demonstration of esophageal varices by gastrointestinal examination is not always successful and the examination may yield negative results in patients who are later proved to have varices. These varices also may be difficult to demonstrate at autopsy after the veins have collapsed. When they are suspected, the roentgen examination of the esophagus must be carried out with particular care in these patients in order to elicit signs of their presence. The use of 30 mg of Pro-Banthine (propantheline bromide) is helpful in the demonstration of varices, as indicated earlier. Maximum enlargement occurs after about 10 minutes with the patient in the horizontal position. With the patient in expiration in the left posterior oblique (supine) position,[6] films are exposed 10 minutes after administration of a thick barium mixture and (if it is used) 5 minutes after administration of Pro-Banthine. Cinefluorography is also useful in some instances.

Roentgen Observations. The dilated veins project into the lumen of the esophagus and cause tortuous linear defects in the barium shadow (Figs. 15-24 and 15-25). These defects vary from time to time, being less prominent when the esophagus is distended and becoming more obvious when the patient is examined in the recumbent position or when the intra-ab-

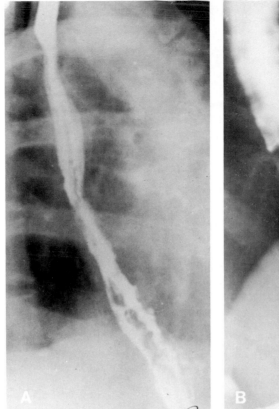

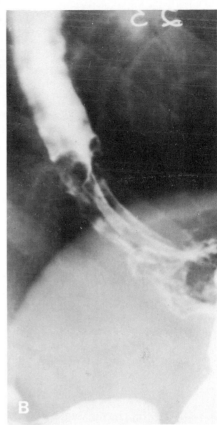

Fig. 15-24. Esophageal varices. **A.** The linear tortuous defects represent dilated veins. **B.** The varicosities are somewhat larger just above the level of the diaphragm than elsewhere.

dominal pressure is raised as during a Valsalva maneuver. The defects become obliterated temporarily by a primary contraction wave.

Small varices are best demonstrated by using a thick barium paste that clings to the mucosal surface. After most of the material has passed into the stomach, enough will remain on the surface to form a thin coating on the mucosa. Spot films are particularly valuable to obtain serial roentgenograms of the esophagus in various degrees of filling and contraction because the defects produced by the varices may be seen well in only one or perhaps several of the multiple exposures. When varices are extensive there may be some delay in passage of barium through the lower part of the esophagus. The varices frequently involve the gastric fundus, causing a tortuous thickening of the mucosal folds.

The best radiographic method for the detection of varices is the opacification of the dilated veins themselves and the demonstration of the collateral blood flow. This is accomplished by angiographic methods or splenoportography. However, endoscopy is often used as an initial study and, if varices are observed, no diagnostic radiographic examination may be necessary. If the patient is bleeding and the site is obscured by blood in the esophagus, splenoportography

Fig. 15-25. Esophageal varices. These films of the same patient were exposed at short intervals apart. They illustrate extensive varices of at least the lower half of the esophagus.

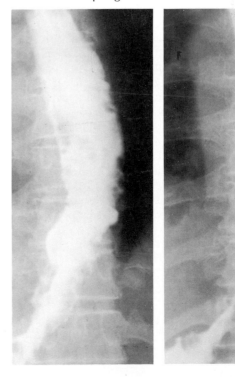

may be necessary. If the patient's spleen is not enlarged, celiac and mesenteric arteriography may be advisable to detect a possible arterial bleeding site. Venous embolization has been used successfully for bleeding esophageal and gastric varices as a temporary measure prior to performance of a definitive venous shunting procedure.

FOREIGN BODIES

Metallic Foreign Bodies

Metallic objects, such as pins, coins, and small toys, are swallowed frequently by infants and young children. Except for aluminum and some of the lighter alloys, the metals are very radiopaque and easily visualized during fluoroscopy and in roentgenograms. The latter must be obtained with short exposure times to eliminate motion; otherwise the shadow of even a fairly large object may be blurred to the extent that it cannot be seen. Objects made of aluminum may be impossible to detect during fluoroscopy or on roentgenograms because the density of this metal is so nearly equal to that of the soft tissues of the body. Because a "swallowed" foreign body will occasionally move upward into the posterior nares or nasopharynx and lodge there, this area must also be examined.

Nonopaque Foreign Bodies

Nonopaque foreign bodies can only be demonstrated after the ingestion of a barium mixture. If the foreign body has caused a complete or nearly complete obstruction, the diagnosis is made without difficulty. Occasionally the swallowing of a large solid bolus, such as a piece of poorly chewed meat, will result in the bolus becoming impacted, usually in the lower end of the esophagus just above the level of the diaphragm. The resulting defect when barium is given may resemble that of a completely obstructing carcinoma. The short duration of symptoms and absence of complaints prior to the onset of obstruction point to the benign nature of the lesion. Usually, after a few days, the bolus becomes sufficiently softened so that it will pass spontaneously into the stomach. Food impactions have been relieved quickly by the intravenous administration of glucagon, however. Impacted solid objects of wood or other nonopaque material are seen infrequently; the obstruction resulting from such foreign bodies may be complete or incomplete.

Impacted Bone

Pieces of chicken bone or other meat bones may be swallowed accidentally and, if large enough, will become impacted. The favorite site of impaction is in the cervical part of the esophagus at or just above the level of the thoracic inlet. Lateral roentgenograms of the neck will demonstrate most of these foreign bodies since the bones are radiopaque. Care must be taken not to confuse a normal ossification of the laryngeal cartilages for a bony foreign body. Such ossification is invariably present in these cartilages in adults. Small calcified or ossified areas may be seen to overlie the upper end of the esophagus in the lateral roentgenogram and are a possible source of error. Familiarity with the appearance of these cartilages is the best insurance against mistakes.

With very small foreign bodies such as fish bones or other small sharp objects that may have penetrated the mucosa and thus become lodged, the defect in barium filling caused by the foreign body may be so small that it cannot be seen readily and the shadow of the opaque bone may be too small to be detected. Diagnosis then depends upon the following:

1. A temporary delay in the passage of a solid or semisold barium-containing mass such as a gelatin capsule filled with barium sulfate powder or a lump of bread soaked in barium–water mixture. This is caused by localized spasm at the site of the foreign body.

2. Delay in the passage of a small wisp of cotton that has been soaked in the barium–water mixture. This is particularly useful in detecting the presence and location of objects such as fishbones.

Complications of Foreign Bodies

Penetration of the esophageal wall may result in a periesophageal abscess or a more diffuse mediastinitis. If the penetration occurs in the cervical area, air shadows may be visible in the soft tissues of the retroesophageal space. The soft-tissue space between the larynx, trachea, and the spine may be widened. Barium mixture may extend into a sinus tract. If the injury occurs within the thorax, mediastinitis may result. The mediastinal shadow becomes broadened at the level of the lesion and streaks of air may be visible in and along the mediastinal borders. Extension of infection can lead to pleural effusion. Stridor or recurrent pneumonia caused by an esophageal foreign body not known to have been ingested may occur in children.[40]

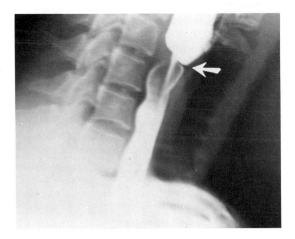

Fig. 15-26. Plummer–Vinson web in the upper end of the esophagus **(arrow).**

MISCELLANEOUS CONDITIONS

Esophageal and Hypopharyngeal Webs

Mucosal webs of the esophagus occur chiefly in the cervical area at the pharyngoesophageal junction or in the hypopharynx (Figs. 15-26 and 15-27). They arise from the anterior wall but may extend laterally on one or both sides. Occasionally they are circumferential. Most of the patients in whom they are observed have no evidence of the Plummer–Vinson syndrome, which consists of dysphagia and an iron-deficiency anemia. Most patients have no dysphagia or other symptoms related to the esophagus. Occasionally, multiple webs are observed. They are often difficult to see on films, since they are visible only when the esophagus is distended. Cine studies have been the most useful in making the diagnosis. Most of them appear to be of no clinical significance.[32]

Lower Esophageal Ring

Schatzki and Gary,[36] and Ingelfinger and Kramer[21] have reported the occurrence of a symmetric, thin, ringlike contraction in the lower end of the esophagus several centimeters above the diaphragm. The diameter of the lumen at the level of the ring varies from a few to as much as 38 mm (Fig. 15-28). The smaller rings of less than 10 to 12 mm are prone to cause symptoms of intermittent dysphagia, usually present over a period of years. The cause of the ring has been the subject of speculation but it now is recognized as representing the junction between

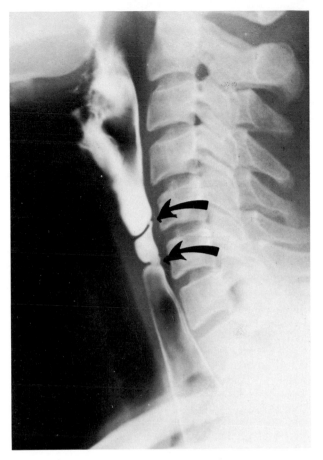

Fig. 15-27. Two esophageal webs are present **(arrows).**

esophageal and gastric epithelium. Because of this, some authors consider that the demonstration of a ring indicates some degree of upward displacement of the gastric mucosa, or a sliding hiatal hernia. As noted before, others consider the type of motor activity of the segment below the ring as determining whether it is, functionally, esophagus or stomach and that, in most cases, the segment will show an esophageal type of peristalsis.[5]

In addition to this mucosal junction ring, Wolf, Heitman, and Cohen[42] have described a functional ring 1 to 2 cm above it. It varies in length and caliber and usually disappears completely with maximum filling. They have called it the "A ring" or "contractile ring." When both rings are present, as in many patients with small, sliding hiatal hernias, the segment of esophagus between the rings shows a variety of configurations which distinguish it from the esophagus proximal to it.

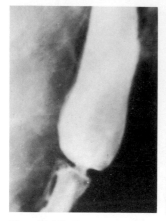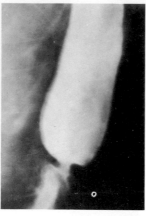

Fig. 15-28. Lower esophageal ring (Schatzki's ring). Observe the thin, circular constriction at the lower end of the esophagus which was noted to persist throughout the examination.

Spontaneous Rupture of the Esophagus

Spontaneous rupture of the esophagus is an infrequent lesion that usually follows forceful vomiting. The lesion occurs more frequently in males than in females. Other causes that have been noted include convulsive seizures, straining at stool, and childbirth. The rupture occurs in a normal esophagus. In most subjects the tear has been found in the lower end of the esophagus along the left lateral wall. Clinically the symptoms of vomiting followed by low thoracic pain and evidence of subcutaneous emphysema in the neck are considered highly significant for the diagnosis. Roentgenograms may reveal translucent streaks of air in the mediastinal tissues or in the cervical area. Pneumothorax, usually on the left side, is frequent. Escape of gastric contents through the rent causes a diffuse increase in density of the lower posterior mediastinum extending to both sides of the midline. Pleural effusion may be present. Infrequently these manifestations occur on the right side. In most of these patients the fistula may be demonstrated by the swallowing of Gastrografin. However, if this procedure reveals no abnormality, barium suspension should be used to obtain better visualization of mucosal detail. However, when the tear is superficial as in the Mallory–Weiss syndrome, it may not be detected radiographically. Bleeding may be the major complication in such patients. Selective arteriography is the radiographic method of choice in the actively bleeding patient. The diagnosis depends on the demonstration of extravasated contrast medium. Submucosal or intraluminal hematoma may cause partial esophageal obstruction in these patients, but

this is usually a very temporary phenomenon. Spontaneous submucosal hematoma may occur in patients with bleeding tendency or in those on anticoagulant therapy.

Barrett's Esophagus

Barrett's esophagus consists of extension of columnar epithelium for varying distances into the esophagus, often to the region of the middle third. An esophagus lined by this type of epithelium is more susceptible to ulceration and inflammation with stricture formation than is the normal esophagus. There is some difference of opinion as to the cause of this condition, but most now believe that it is an acquired lesion, probably secondary to reflux esophagitis. Roentgenographic findings are related to the secondary changes and include evidence of stricture in the midportion of the esophagus or higher, mucosal irregularity (most likely indicating inflammatory disease), and, sometimes, an ulcer crater. Many of these patients have an associated sliding esophageal hiatus hernia and most have a dilated esophagogastric junction. The presence of a mid-esophageal stricture alone should suggest the diagnosis in the absence of previous history of ingestion of a caustic substance.[4]

Difficulty in Swallowing Caused by Pharyngeal Paralysis

Among the less common causes of difficulty in swallowing are conditions that lead to weakness or paralysis of the muscles of deglutition, such as bulbar palsy and myasthenia gravis. The roentgen findings are rather similar in these diseases although they usually are more severe when the bulbar centers are involved. Plain roentgenograms of the neck reveal the dilated air-filled pharynx. When, during fluoroscopy, the patient is asked to swallow a mouthful of barium it will be noted that there is difficulty in pushing the material into the pharynx by the action of the tongue. Once in the pharynx the barium is held there for a variable time with only weak contractions or, in advanced cases, with complete absence of motor activity by the pharyngeal muscles. The pharynx is dilated and atonic and the barium collects in the pyriform sinuses and epiglottic vallecula, remaining there for a time before gradually passing into the esophagus (Fig. 15-29). This retention facilitates aspiration of the material into the trachea and this is almost invariably noted during the attempted swallowing of the barium. There may be sufficient aspiration to cause severe respiratory embarrassment and the ex-

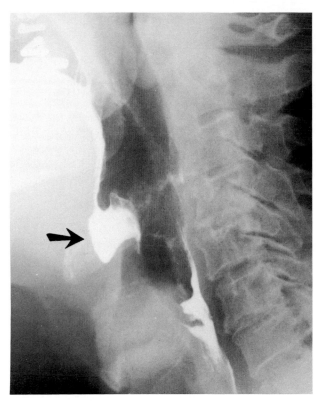

Fig. 15-29. Bulbar palsy. Barium has accumulated in the vallecula **(arrow)**. The pharynx is dilated and filled with air. This amount of air is not visualized in the normal pharynx during the resting phase.

amination is not without hazard. There also tends to be reflux of material into the nasal cavities. Except for a thin coating that remains on the mucosa the normal pharynx does not retain barium. In myasthenia gravis there is less atonicity of the pharynx and in general less difficulty in swallowing unless the muscular weakness is pronounced. There is difficulty in propelling the bolus into the pharynx and movements of the tongue are weak and ineffective. Also, rapid fatigue of deglutition is noted; it returns to near normal after a rest or after administration of an anticholinesterase drug.

REFERENCES AND SELECTED READINGS

1. ADLER RH: What is the cardia? JAMA 182: 1045, 1962
2. ALLISON PR: Reflux esophagitis, sliding hiatus hernia and the anatomy of repair. Surg Gynecol Obstet 92: 419, 1951
3. BOYD RM, BOGOCH A, GREIG JH et al: Esophageal intramural pseudodiverticulosis. Radiology 113: 267, 1974
4. BURGESS JN, PAYNE WS, ANDERSEN HA et al: Barrett esophagus. The columnar-epithelial-lined lower esophagus. Mayo Clin Proc 46: 728, 1971
5. CAUTHORNE RT, VANHOUTTE JJ, DONNER MW et al: Study of patients with lower esophageal ring by simultaneous cineradiography and manometry. Gastroenterology 49: 632, 1965
6. COCKERILL EM, MILLER RE, CHERNISH SM et al: Optimal visualization of esophageal varices. Am J Roentgenol 126: 512, 1976
7. CRUMMY AB: The water test in the evaluation of gastroesophageal reflux. Radiology 87: 501, 1966
8. CYNN WS, CHON HK, GUREJHIAN PA et al: Crohn's disease of the esophagus. Am J Roentgenol 125: 359, 1975
9. DODDS WJ: Current concepts of esophageal motor function: clinical implications for radiology. Am J Roentgenol 128: 549, 1977
9a. Editorial: Gastrin and the gastroesophageal sphincter. JAMA 217: 1098, 1971
10. FELMAN AH, TALBERT JL: Laryngotracheo-esophageal cleft. Radiology 103: 641, 1972
11. FLEISCHNER FG: Hiatal hernia complex. JAMA 162: 183, 1956
12. FRANK RC, PAUL LW: Congenital reduplication of the esophagus. Report of a case. Radiology 53: 417, 1949
13. FRANKEN EA JR: Caustic damage of the gastrointestinal tract: roentgen features. Am J Roentgenol 118: 77, 1973
14. FRANKEN EA JR: Gastrointestinal Radiology in Pediatrics. p. 23. Hagerstown, Harper & Row, 1975
15. GOHEL VK, EDELL SL, LAUFER I et al: Transverse folds in the human esophagus. Radiology 128: 303, 1978
16. GOLDSTEIN HM, DODD GD: Double contrast examination of the esophagus. Gastrointest Radiol 1: 3, 1976
17. GONZALEZ G: Esophageal moniliasis. Am J Roentgenol 113: 233, 1971
18. HAN SY, MIHAS AA: Circumferential web of the upper esophagus. Gastrointest Radiol 3: 7, 1978
19. HO CS, CULLEN JB, GRAY RR: An unusual manifestation of esophageal moniliasis. Radiology 123: 287, 1977
20. HUTTON CF: Plummer-Vinson syndrome. Br J Radiol 29: 81, 1956
21. INGELFINGER FG, KRAMER P: Dysphagia produced by contractile ring in lower esophagus. Gastroenterology 23: 419, 1953
22. ITAI Y, KOUGURE T, AKIYAMA Y et al: Radiological manifestations of esophageal involvement in acanthosis nigricans. Br J Radiol 49: 592, 1976
23. JOHNSTONE AS: Observations on the radiologic anatomy of the oesophagogastric junction. Radiology 73: 501, 1959
24. LALLEMAND D, HUAULT G, LABOUREAU JP et al: Lesions

of the larynx and esophagus in herpes simplex infection. Ann Radiol 17: 317, 1974

25. MARTEL W: Radiologic features of esophagogastritis secondary to extremely caustic agents. Radiology 103: 31, 1972

26. McNALLY EF, KATZ MI: The roentgen diagnosis of diffuse esophageal spasm. Am J Roentgenol 99: 218, 1967

27. MEYERS C, DURKIN MG, LOVE L: Radiographic findings in herpetic esophagitis. Radiology 119: 21, 1976

28. MILLER RE, CHERNISH SM, BRUNELLE RL: Comparative double blind study of esophageal barium pastes. Gastrointest Radiol 2: 163, 1977

29. MISSAKIAN MM, CARLSON HC, ANDERSEN HA: The roentgenologic features of the columnar epithelial lined lower esophagus. Am J Roentgenol 99: 212, 1967

30. MONTGOMERY RD, MENDL K, STEPHENSON SF: Intramural diverticulosis of the esophagus. Thorax 30: 278, 1975

31. NEUHAUSER EBD, BERENBERG W: Cardio-esophageal relaxation as a cause of vomiting in infants. Radiology 48: 480, 1947

32. NOSHER JL, CAMPBELL WL, SEAMAN WB: The clinical significance of cervical esophageal and hypopharyngeal webs. Radiology 117: 45, 1975

33. PALMER ED: An attempt to localize the normal esophagogastric junction. Radiology 60: 825, 1953

34. RAMSEY GH, WATSON JS, GRAMIAK R et al: Cinefluorographic analysis of the mechanism of swallowing. Radiology 64: 498, 1955

35. ROGERS LF: Transient post-vagotomy dysphagia: a distinct clinical and roentgen entity. Am J Roentgenol 125: 956, 1975

36. SCHATZKI R, GARY JE: The lower esophageal ring. Am J Roentgenol 75: 246, 1956

37. SCHREIBER MH, DAVIS M: Intraluminal diverticulum of the esophagus. Am J Roentgenol 129: 595, 1977

38. SEAMAN WB: Functional disorders of the pharyngoesophageal junction: achalasia and chalasia. Radiol Clin North Am 7: 113, 1969

39. SKUCAS J, SCHRANK WW: Routine air contrast examination of the esophagus. Radiology 115: 482, 1975

40. SMITH PC, SWISCHUK LE, FAGAN CJ: An elusive and often unsuspected cause of stridor or pneumonia (the esophageal foreign body). Am J Roentgenol 122: 80, 1974

41. WELLER MH, LUTZKER SA: Intramural diverticulosis of the esophagus associated with postoperative hiatal hernia, alkaline esophagus and esophageal stricture. Radiology 98: 373, 1971

42. WOLF BS, HEITMANN P, COHEN BR: The inferior esophageal sphincter, the manometric high pressure zone and hiatal incompetence. Am J Roentgenol 103: 251, 1968

43. WRIGHT JT: Allison's and Johnstone's anomaly. Am J Roentgenol 94: 308, 1965

44. ZBORALSKE FF, DODDS WJ: Roentgenographic diagnosis of primary disorders of esophageal motility. Radiol Clin North Am 7: 147, 1969

16

The Stomach

METHODS OF EXAMINATION

PRELIMINARY ROENTGENOGRAMS

The use of preliminary or scout roentgenograms in the diagnosis of perforation of the stomach is discussed in Chapter 13. Roentgenograms prior to the administration of contrast material are also useful to detect or exclude the possibility of the presence of metallic foreign bodies. Some swallowed air is almost always present in the normal stomach and when the patient is examined in an upright position an air–fluid level can be visualized in the fundus. Displacement of the gastric air bubble may indicate the existence of an extrinsic mass or the normal contour of it may be deformed by intrinsic tumor. If there is ample intra-abdominal fat the external surface of the stomach occasionally can be seen at least in part. Thickening of the gastric wall caused by scirrhus carcinoma sometimes can be identified in this way. These aspects are discussed more fully under the specific disease categories concerned.

CONTRAST VISUALIZATION

The esophagus, stomach, and duodenum are examined as a unit and what has been said about the conduct of the examination in the discussion dealing with the esophagus is equally true for the stomach and duodenum.

CONTRAST MATERIAL

The thin, barium–water mixture is the standard opaque meal for study of the stomach and duodenum. This consists of 125 gm of barium sulfate to 180 cc of water. This amount is adequate for fluoroscopic examination in most patients. If there is a delay between completion of the fluoroscopic examination and the making of roentgenograms or if gastric emptying is unusually rapid, an additional 40 to 60 cc of the mixture is given. If the small intestine is to be examined an additional 120 to 180 cc of the mixture should be given routinely after completion of the preliminary fluoroscopic study. A number of commercial preparations containing various suspending agents are available for this purpose. Several of them are quite satisfactory; the preparation used is a matter of the radiologist's personal preference. Water-soluble iodinated compounds are also used for the examination of the upper gastrointestinal tract, particularly when perforation is suspected. Gastrografin is the one most commonly employed. Some radiologists prefer these iodinated compounds to barium in the study of small bowel obstruction, but, in our experience, barium is far superior in assessment of this obstruction. When possible it is preferable to instill the iodinated compounds through a tube. They are hypertonic and act somewhat like a saline laxative. Also they become considerably diluted in the distal small bowel. They do not cling to the mucosa as does barium and they are not as satisfactory for mucosal relief studies. It has been shown experimentally that barium sulfate does not become impacted in the small intestine in the presence of obstruction, and clinical experience confirms this. Thus if the colon can be ruled out as the site of the obstruction, usually by means of a barium enema, it is safe to give barium orally.

Double-Contrast Method

The double-contrast method of examining the stomach was introduced in Japan to develop a more accurate means for detecting small gastric carcinoma.[22] Gas-producing (CO_2) granules or powders are administered with a relatively thick barium mixture and a silicone antifoaming agent such as simethicone. A number of variations of the method have been introduced in the United States including the use of Pro-Banthine in doses of 5 to 10 mg given intravenously, or glucagon administered in doses of 0.5 to 2 mg, to produce hypotonia and allow complete distention of the stomach. Glucagon is more satisfactory than Pro-Banthine because of less side effects, but it is expensive and at times difficult to obtain. We use it only in patients having an unusual amount of gastric contraction which interferes with the examination. Gelfand and Hachiya[15] tested several barium preparations and found HD 250% weight/volume (E–Z EM Corporation) to be superior to suspensions of greater viscosity and less density. We use this preparation and find it very satisfactory. A number of methods of administration of the barium and the gas-forming materials have been described.[17, 26, 27] The object is to coat the mucosa of the entire stomach and distend the stomach with gas in order to obtain a good double-contrast demonstration of all portions of the gastric mucosa. This usually requires rotating the patient on the horizontal table and sometimes elevating the head or foot of the table. Upright stud-

ies with forward bending are sometimes of value in patients with a high transverse or cascade stomach. (Studies are now under way in Japan in the use of proteinase to dissolve the mucous and promote better coating of the gastric wall.) It may also be necessary to repeat the turning maneuvers to recoat an area when there is poor coating or a question of a pathologic condition noted on the preliminary spot films. All films are checked before the patient leaves the department to ensure that a thorough study has been made.

Fluoroscopy

Fluoroscopy is an essential part of the examination of the stomach as it is for other parts of the gastrointestinal tract. It is more than a method for obtaining spot films. The ability to "see" and "feel" at the same time is a valuable part of the procedure. To the trained fluoroscopist, the look and feel of an area of stomach wall infiltrated by carcinoma is unmistakable. With fluoroscopy, peristalsis can be observed rapidly and the effect of a lesion on peristaltic activity easily determined. Spot films are obtained to record what is seen under the fluoroscope or to show finer detail that cannot be recognized by fluoroscopy. Unfortunately, palpation is more difficult when an image intensifier is used because of the bulkiness of the machine. The use of a television monitor by the examiner instead of the viewing mirror of the intensifier obviates most of this difficulty. Unless the patient is too ill to stand, the examination is begun with the fluoroscopic table in an upright position and the patient standing behind the fluoroscopic screen. Unless there are specific complaints referable to the esophagus, attention is first centered on the cardia and the first few swallows of the barium mixture are watched as they pass through the cardia and then "canalize" the stomach. Pressure by the fluoroscopist's lead-gloved hand is used to spread the material over the surface of the stomach and into the mucosal folds (see Fig. 16-4). In this way the undistended stomach is examined for filling defects, ulcer craters, pliability of walls, and integrity of mucosal pattern. Some authors have stressed that manual palpation should be avoided during fluoroscopy. They feel that even though the hand is protected with a leaded glove, some radiation may reach the examiner's skin. They prefer using specially constructed palpating spoons and other compression devices. However, we have found that satisfactory palpation can be done in most cases by keeping the protected fingers directly outside of the edge of the coned-down roentgen-ray beam. When palpating for deep masses the fluoroscope can be turned off momentarily. When this preliminary survey detects definite or questionable abnormalities, spot films can be obtained under fluoroscopic guidance with or without compression to bring out the maximum detail of the lesion or the area in question. The remainder of the barium mixture then is given and the esophagus is examined. Frequently the duodenum will begin to fill while the preliminary survey of the stomach is being made. If it does not, pressure applied over the antrum after the stomach is more completely distended usually will cause the duodenal bulb to fill and this is examined for contour deformities, ulcer craters, filling defects, and other abnormalities. After the duodenum has been studied thoroughly, and the spot films obtained, if desired, attention is returned to the stomach and search is again made for evidence of organic disease in the more distended organ. The examination usually is continued by lowering the table into a horizontal position and with the patient in various positions. In this manner the margins of the stomach can be brought into profile, peristaltic waves can be observed as they pass along the curvatures, filling and emptying of the duodenal bulb can be studied, and posturing can be used to bring out ulcer craters and filling defects to best advantage. For the demonstration of posterior-wall ulcers it is helpful to lower the table to about 45 degrees from the upright and turn the patient slightly toward the right. The ulcer crater then will fill with barium and the air overlying it makes a good "double contrast." The Trendelenburg position may also be used if necessary in the study of cardia or antrum.

Roentgenograms

After completion of the fluoroscopic study the patient is given another 60 to 90 cc of the barium mixture and overhead films are obtained with the patient prone in a right anterior oblique position. This is the most useful position to show both stomach and duodenum to advantage. As a rule we also obtain right lateral, prone, and supine roentgenograms, and any additional projections needed for optimal visualization of an area in question. A number of different routines are used in various departments, all aimed at a complete examination of the stomach.

Numerous studies have been undertaken to compare the accuracy of gastrointestinal radiology, using the single and double contrast, with endoscopy. Most of these show that endoscopy is superior in outlining mucosal erosions and small linear ulcers, particularly in the presence of enlarged mucosal folds. Also a study[30] comparing single and double contrast with endoscopy as a control has been made. The error rate for the standard examination was 20.5%, and for the double contrast, 19.5% (the average of two radiologists). The error rate declined by almost 50% when both methods were used, suggesting a complementary role of the two. The ultimate place of the double-contrast study of the stomach remains to be determined. If not used routinely, it will certainly be employed to delineate mucosal detail in patients with suspected tumors or other mucosal lesions.

With good technique the fine mosaic pattern of the areae gastricae can be clearly defined in the antrum. This area consists of a complex series of grooves present in the gastric mucosa usually in the antrum. The larger of the grooves define regular islands 3 to 5 mm in diameter. The barium collects in the grooves and may also outline a number of small pits which represent gastric glands. In cross section, the appearance is that of fine serrations of the mucosal surface. When the areas are particularly prominent with deeper grooves, the appearance is known as *état mammelonne;*[39] this is not believed to indicate any significant abnormality.

Cinefluorography

With the use of the image intensifier, good movies of the gastrointestinal tract can be obtained and this method is employed by some, particularly in the study of areas of questionable alteration in pliability. Also it is possible to store the image on television tape for play-back at any desired time.

Abdominal Arteriography in Gastrointestinal Bleeding

Arteriography of the abdominal vessels has been found useful in the study of acute and chronic gastrointestinal bleeding when other studies have failed to show a causative lesion. The vessels of the celiac axis and the superior and inferior mesenteric arteries can be catheterized by the percutaneous technique of Seldinger, usually by employing the femoral artery approach. Vascular lesions such as hemangiomas and arteriovenous malformations can be visualized readily. Other tumors may be identified at times owing either to their vascularity or because they displace or occlude normal vessels. The actual bleeding point can be visualized in many cases by the finding of local extravasation of contrast material into the gastrointestinal lumen (Fig. 16-1). Bleeding from gas-

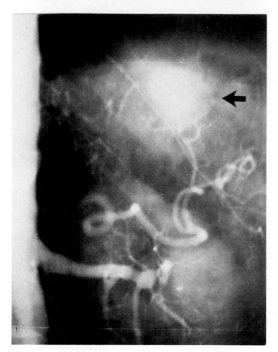

Fig. 16-1. Bleeding gastric ulcer demonstrated by abdominal aortography. There is a cloudy density in the gastric fundus **(arrow)** representing contrast material extravasated into the lumen from a bleeding ulcer.

tric or duodenal ulcers, various kinds of tumors, and from colonic diverticula has been diagnosed in this way. Most investigators agree that arteriography should be carried out in all patients in whom the source of bleeding cannot be found by other methods. The source of bleeding could not be determined until arteriography was employed in 22% in one reported series. In acute bleeding it has been recommended that arteriography be the initial radiographic procedure if endoscopy fails to find the source or if blood obscures the source. Bleeding must be brisk because it is generally agreed that active bleeding of 1.5 ml per minute is the least that can reasonably be expected to be detected by angiography. When bleeding is chronic, not brisk, and not detected endoscopically, barium studies of the upper gastrointestinal tract should be undertaken. If a bleeding site is found, the direct selective injection of vasopressor substances has controlled the hemorrhage in some patients, at least temporarily. Embolization is now used extensively for control of bleeding in a number of areas including the stomach. Various substances including autologous blood clots, gel-

foam, and synthetic substances such as iso-butyl cyano-acrylate have been used successfully in controlling arterial bleeding in the stomach. The bleeding vessel is selectively catheterized, and the material is introduced under fluoroscopic control. Autologous clots, gelfoam, balloon occlusion, iatrogenic paravenous hematoma, sclerosing agents, or combinations of these have been used to obliterate bleeding veins in the esophagus and stomach.[35]

In addition to its use in a problem case of gastric and duodenal bleeding, angiography is also employed to assist in confirming the presence of a questionable mass lesion in the stomach, showing its site of origin, size, and blood supply, but it is now used largely when other diagnostic studies have failed to solve a diagnostic problem involving the stomach.

Anticholinergic Drugs

The use of Pro-Banthine (propantheline bromide) to reduce muscle tone and peristalsis in the duodenum when searching for minor defects, particularly in pancreatic disease, has been widespread. Glucagon, because of the virtual absence of side effects, has replaced it to some extent. Anticholinergic drugs also can be used to reduce or eliminate spasm in the stomach, small intestine, and colon when spasm interferes with satisfactory filling or to rule out spasm as a cause for a defect that might indicate a serious organic lesion such as carcinoma. The usual dose of Pro-Banthine is 30 mg administered intramuscularly. This drug usually produces hypotonia in 5 to 10 minutes without significant side effects. Its effects usually wear off about 15 to 20 minutes after onset. The usual contraindications to the use of atropine and similar drugs should be noted; these include glaucoma, prostatism, and serious cardiovascular disease. Glucagon is a safer drug but is costly and sometimes difficult to obtain. The dose varies from 0.5 to 2.0 mg.

ANATOMY AND PHYSIOLOGY

ANATOMIC DIVISIONS AND TERMINOLOGY

1. Cardia: The junction of the esophagus and stomach.
2. Fundus: That part of the stomach above the level of the cardia.
3. Body of the stomach: The central two-thirds from the level of the cardia to the proximal part of the pyloric antrum.

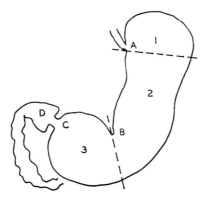

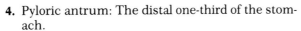

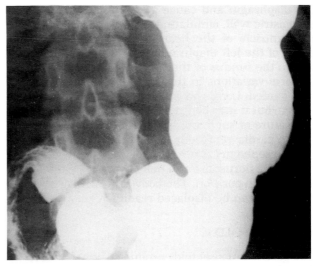

Fig. 16-2. Diagram of the normal stomach to show the major anatomic divisions. **(1)** Fundus; **(2)** body; **(3)** antrum; **(A)** anatomic cardia; **(B)** incisura angularis; **(C)** pyloric canal; **(D)** first portion of the duodenum or duodenal bulb.

Fig. 16-3. Roentgenogram of a normal stomach and duodenal bulb. Compare with the diagram in Figure 16-2. Note three peristaltic waves: a shallow one near the fundus, a deeper one near the incisura angularis, and a very deep one in the antrum.

4. Pyloric antrum: The distal one-third of the stomach.
5. Pylorus: The junction of the stomach and duodenum.
6. Pyloric canal: The channel through the pylorus. In the roentgenogram this measures about 7 to 8 mm in width and 5 mm in length.
7. Sulcus angularis: A relatively acute angle formed at or just below the middle of the stomach on the lesser curvature, becoming particularly pronounced when the stomach is of the J or fishhook form. It marks the boundary between the stomach and the pyloric antrum.

FORM AND POSITION OF THE STOMACH

The form and position of the stomach vary greatly in different individuals. In the person of asthenic habitus the stomach tends to lie in a vertical position having the form of a J or fishhook. In the sthenic individual it lies more transversely and in the very obese it assumes the shape of a "steer horn." In between these two extremes are many variations. The average shape of the normal stomach lies between the elongated fishhook contour and the more transverse and thus tends to assume the form of a shallow J or a reverse L (Figs. 16-2 and 16-3). An interesting variant is the type of stomach known as a *cascade* form. In this condition the fundus hangs downward and to the left, lying behind the body of the stomach, and with a

sharp angle formed between the two portions. The fundus usually is enlarged and when the meal is taken with the patient upright the major portion of it will accumulate in the dilated fundus before spilling over into the distal part of the stomach. The cause of this type of stomach is debatable but in many of these individuals the transverse colon is high in position, usually the result of obesity, and it is probable that this is responsible for the configuration in most cases.

THE FUNDUS AND CARDIA

The fundus of the stomach normally lies close to the left leaf of the diaphragm. The soft-tissue space between the fundic air bubble and the air-containing lung represents, therefore, the combined thickness of the gastric wall and the diaphragm. This measures on the average about 1 cm. Any appreciable increase in width of this soft-tissue space usually indicates a pathologic process involving the gastric wall, the subphrenic space, or the diaphragm. Exceptions occur when this space is unusually thick and yet nothing is found to account for it at the time of surgical exploration. The space is thicker in obese individuals and this must be allowed for in interpretation. Occasionally a tonguelike extension of the spleen may extend into the space between the fundus and

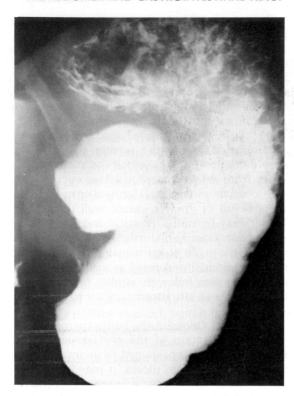

Fig. 16-7. Giant benign ulcer of the lesser curvature of the stomach illustrates the very large size that some ulcers may attain. This ulcer has penetrated the gastric wall and its base rests on the liver.

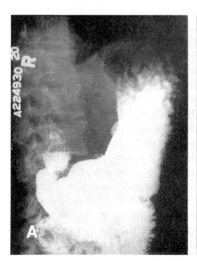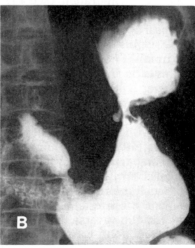

Fig. 16-8. Benign gastric ulcer. **A.** Shallow crater on the lesser curvature of the stomach. **B.** Benign ulcer on the lesser curvature of the stomach with a deep incisura on the greater curvature directly opposite the ulcer crater.

Spasm results in an inconstant and irregular narrowing of the involved area that can be effaced by palpation and that changes in contour as a result of peristalsis. Hypertrophy of the pyloric muscle results in a more or less fixed narrowing that may involve the immediate prepyloric segment of the stomach for a distance of several centimeters or more (see Fig. 16-28). Under fluoroscopic observation the narrowing usually changes slightly from time to time and is not fixed completely. Mucosal folds can be identified within the narrowed area and this, plus the slightly changing contour, helps to identify the lesion and distinguish it from an infiltrating annular carcinoma.

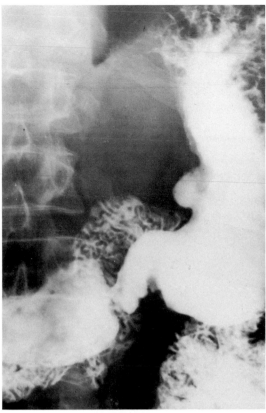

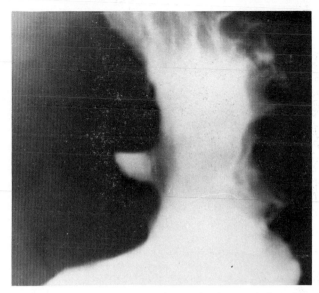

Fig. 16-9. Benign ulcer on the lesser curvature of the stomach. The base is smooth and there is a smooth halo of induration around the neck.

Fig. 16-10. Benign gastric ulcer. The base of the ulcer is pointed. This seems to occur during healing in many instances. There is a fairly wide collar of edematous tissue in the stomach around the crater's edge.

Fig. 16-11. Benign gastric ulcer. There is a translucent halo or collar **(arrow)** around the orifice. Scarring or spasm has resulted in shortening of the lesser curvature leading to some distortion of the gastric antrum.

Changes in the Mucosal Folds. The tendency for a spokelike radiation of folds away from the base of the ulcer crater has been noted. The folds often are thickened throughout the stomach when gastric or duodenal ulcer is present, probably a manifestation of increased gastric acid output. This relationship probably accounts for the observation that prominence of mucosal folds is more common in duodenal than in gastric ulcer.

Palpable Mass. If the ulcer has penetrated and become walled-off by inflammatory tissue a mass may be palpable, but in the usual case a palpable mass does not exist.

Gastric Retention. Retention of material in the stomach for abnormally long periods of time or frank evidence of pyloric obstruction is an extremely variable finding and depends to a large extent upon the location of the gastric ulcer. If the lesion is near the py-

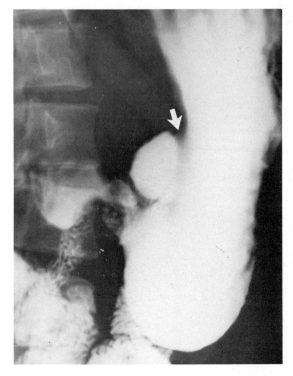

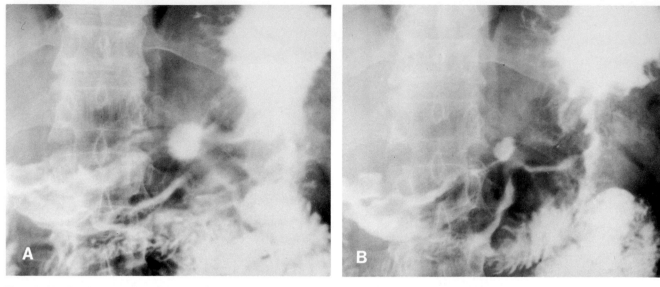

Fig. 16-12. Benign gastric ulcer on the posterior wall of the stomach near the lesser curvature. The films were exposed with the patient in the supine position in order that the crater be outlined best. **A.** Initial film. **B.** Roentgenogram obtained 1 month later. Some decrease in the size of the ulcer is apparent after a month of treatment.

Fig. 16-13. Benign gastric ulcer. **A.** Large crater observed on the initial study. **B.** Three weeks later, distinct decrease in the crater's size is evident. The patient had been on medical therapy in the interval. Note that the crater appears more pointed at this time than at the initial examination.

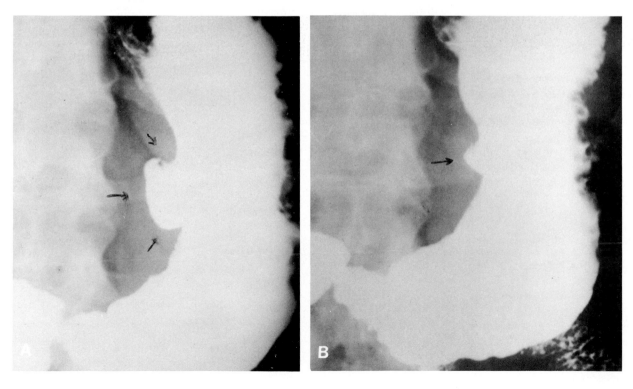

lorus there may be enough interference with emptying to cause a significant degree of obstruction. Even ulcers situated higher up on the lesser curvature often cause some retention because they interfere with normal peristaltic activity and because they cause pylorospasm. In other instances, even in the presence of a large gastric ulcer, the stomach empties promptly.

Pyloric or "Channel" Ulcer. A characteristic syndrome has been described in patients with pyloric ulcer. This consists of atypical epigastric pain, episodes of nausea and vomiting, and weight loss. Intermittent obstruction probably accounts for the symptoms. In our experience, this syndrome is not present in most patients with pyloric ulcer, however.

Double-Channel Pylorus. This is a form of gastroduodenal fistula in which an accessory channel connects the lesser curve of the distal antrum with the duodenal bulb. This channel is therefore above the pylorus. The cause in most, if not all, cases is peptic ulcer disease, and an ulcer lies in or immediately adjacent to the fistulous channel in most instances.

Differential Diagnosis of Benign and Malignant Ulcers

The term "carcinomatous or malignant ulcer" is used for a lesion that initially was a benign ulcer but that subsequently underwent carcinomatous change. There is not complete agreement as to whether a benign ulcer ever becomes malignant, but the pathologists with whom we are associated believe that this happens occasionally. The term "ulcerating carcinoma" is used for a lesion that was carcinomatous from the beginning but, with the development of central necrosis and ulceration, the gross features are essentially those of an ulcer. To avoid confusion in this discussion the term "ulcerating carcinoma" will be used for both. Ulcerating carcinomas of a type that might be confused with benign gastric ulcer are uncommon. It has been reported that only about 5% of all ulcers are malignant and therefore the chance for any ulcer being a carcinoma is small. Nevertheless, there are certain roentgen findings that are quite useful in differentiating the two lesions:

1. Benign ulcers usually are sharply marginated and round or slightly ovoid when viewed *en face*. Malignant ulcers often are of irregular shape and uneven in depth.

2. Benign ulcers project beyond the gastric lumen. An exception occurs when there is a mound of edem-

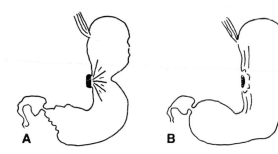

Fig. 16-14. Diagram illustrating benign **(A)** and malignant **(B)** ulcers on the lesser curvature of the stomach. The ulcer crater of the benign lesion projects outside of the normal lumen, the mucosal folds radiate away from its base in a spokelike fashion, and the edges of the crater tend to be undermined slightly. Irregular spasms narrow the antrum and incisura opposite the crater. The malignant ulcer **(B)** does not project beyond the gastric lumen. The halo surrounding it is irregular and nodular. The pattern of the mucosal fold is obliterated at the edges of the halo.

atous and inflamed tissue around the crater as described previously. The malignant lesion usually lies within the outline of the lumen because it develops in a mass of tumor tissue (Fig. 16-14).

3. The edematous halo surrounding a benign ulcer is relatively smooth and fades gradually at the periphery. In carcinomatous ulcers the halo is wider, often nodular, and usually more sharply demarcated from normal stomach wall at its periphery. The crater may be situated off center in relation to the halo.

4. When viewed in profile the combination of an intraluminal crater surrounded by a nodular halo resembles the *meniscus sign* or *complex* first defined by Carman and later elaborated by Kirklin. The surface of the barium-filled crater facing the gastric lumen was described originally as being concave, giving the appearance of a meniscus. However, more commonly the internal surface is convex. The floor of the crater tends to be flat (Fig. 16-14B), sometimes rounded (externally convex), or irregular and nodular.

5. Spokelike radiation of mucosal folds is characteristic of a benign ulcer. In carcinoma, radiating folds are unusual and, when present, they do not extend to the edge of the crater and tend to be more irregular than in benign ulcer.

6. The size and location of the ulcer no longer are considered to be important in differential diagnosis. Formerly it was believed that an ulcer crater larger in

diameter than 2.5 cm was, in all probability, malignant. The same was true of an ulcer on the greater curvature. It is now well established that benign ulcer can occur anywhere in the stomach although greater-curvature ulcers are infrequent. Some benign ulcers reach a very large size and some ulcerating carcinomas are small.

7. Under proper therapy, most benign ulcers decrease in size, the halo of edema regresses, and eventually the crater and the induration around it disappear. Some decrease in size should be noted at the first reexamination, usually performed within 3 weeks of the initial study (see Fig. 16-13B). Unfortunately, some benign ulcers heal very slowly or not at all in spite of proper medical management.

On the other hand, some ulcerating carcinomas may appear smaller on reexamination. There are several possible reasons for this. The inflammatory element may improve under therapy. Food particles or blood clots may fill the crater so that it cannot be completely outlined by the barium mixture. Also growth of neoplastic tissue may encroach on the crater decreasing its size. It is important, therefore, to determine whether the halo of induration is also decreasing as the ulcer crater appears to diminish in size. If it does not, one should view the lesion with considerable suspicion, and follow-up examinations should be obtained until the lesion has healed, even though endoscopic biopsy has revealed no carcinoma.

CARCINOMA OF THE STOMACH

A number of classifications of carcinoma of the stomach have been suggested, based upon pathologic characteristics. From a roentgen point of view it is sufficient to consider the following types: (1) polypoid or fungating, (2) infiltrating, (3) ulcerating, and (4) mixed types. Certain roentgen characteristics are common to all gastric carcinomas regardless of the pathologic type. The tumor stiffens the gastric wall where it is involved by the neoplasm; the soft, pliable appearance of the normal stomach, as brought out by palpation during fluoroscopy, is lost; peristalsis does not pass through the lesion; the normal mucosal pattern over the surface of the tumor either is destroyed completely or altered markedly in its appearance.

Fungating Carcinoma

In the fungating or polypoid type of gastric carcinoma (Figs. 16-15 to 16-17) the tumor forms a mass that projects into the gastric lumen and causes a filling defect in the barium shadow. The surface of the defect is irregular or nodular. Superficial or deep ulcer pockets may be present but the evidence of ulceration is less obvious than is the mass of the tumor. The mucosal folds are completely absent over the surface of the lesion. The defect is constant, rigid, and reproducible throughout the examination or at repeat examinations. The junction of the filling defect and the gastric wall usually is distinct and often forms an acute angle, giving an effect of overhanging edges (Figs. 16-5 and 16-6). With small lesions the defect is limited to one wall or one curvature; larger lesions completely encircle the stomach and cause an irregular, fixed narrowing of the gastric lumen.

Infiltrating Carcinoma

The infiltrating type of gastric carcinoma does not cause a distinct intraluminal mass but rather infiltrates the gastric wall, spreading in or beneath the mucosa.

Scirrhous Carcinoma. The scirrhous form of carcinoma is characterized by its infiltrating nature and by the fact that the tumor evokes a pronounced fibrous-tissue response in the gastric wall. The wall becomes thickened and rigid at the site of the tumor and peristalsis does not pass through it. The mucosal folds usually are obliterated; in their stead the surface has a fine granular or occasionally a rough, cobblestone appearance. Scirrhous carcinoma may be local or general. In the latter lesion the limits of the process are poorly defined as a rule and there is a gradual transition from normal to abnormal. Because of this and the absence of a distinct filling defect, the detection of early lesions is extremely difficult, particularly in the fundus or the upper third of the stomach where peristalsis normally is feeble or absent and palpation is difficult (Fig. 16-18). Eventually the infiltration of the tumor may involve practically the entire stomach and it is this extensive lesion that is sometimes called the *leather bottle stomach* or *linitis plastica* (Fig. 16-19). Characteristically this type of carcinoma does not obstruct the orifices until late; in fact the cardia and pylorus often are held open by the rigid gastric walls, so that the liquid barium mixture literally pours through the stomach into the duodenum and it is difficult to keep sufficient filling for adequate observation. The localized form of scirrhous carcinoma behaves somewhat differently. It tends to encircle the gastric lumen rather early in its development and cause a more or less localized narrowing of the lumen. This lesion is most frequent in the pyloric

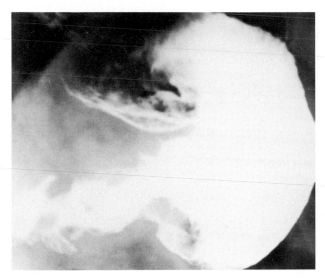

Fig. 16-15. Large fungating or polypoid carcinoma involving the distal one-third of the greater curvature and the distal two-thirds of the lesser curvature.

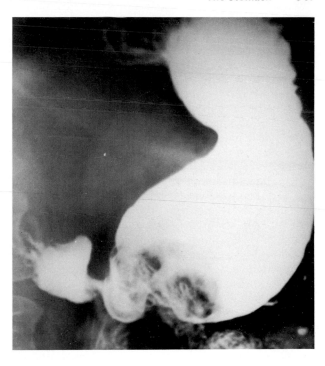

Fig. 16-16. Polypoid carcinoma arising on the greater curvature side of the gastric antrum. The masses project into the lumen and appear as radiolucencies, since they displace barium.

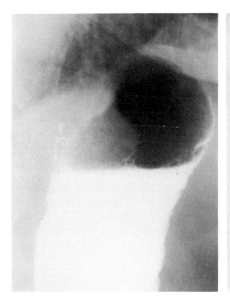
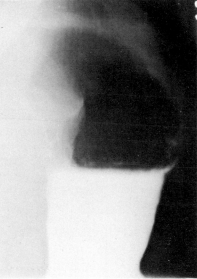

Fig. 16-17. Polypoid carcinoma of the gastric fundus. These films, exposed with the patient standing after having been given barium and gas-producing material, reveal a somewhat irregular polypoid mass in the region of the cardia. The soft-tissue mass is clearly outlined despite a lack of good mucosal coating.

antrum, where it results in an annular stricturelike narrowing. The limits of the lesion are more sharply defined than in the generalized or linitis plastica form of the disease and obstruction of the pylorus may develop relatively early. Occasionally, the outer wall of the stomach can be visualized and the great thickening caused by the tumor can be confirmed.

There are a number of benign lesions which may cause antral narrowing, wall thickening, and a decrease in peristalsis and which, therefore, may stimulate scirrhous carcinoma. Most of these are described elsewhere in this chapter. They include Crohn's disease, syphilis, sarcoidosis, tuberculosis, eosinophilic gastroenteritis, pseudolymphoma, ingestion of corrosive materials, irradiation, and amyloidosis.

Superficial Erosive Spreading Carcinoma. This type of tumor differs from the scirrhus by the absence of appreciable fibrosis and by the tendency for ulceration. An intraluminal mass is not a prominent feature. The involved area in the wall is stiffened and rigid. Ulceration occurs in a higher percentage of patients and the ulcer cavity may be the most obvious roentgen deformity. Because there is no intraluminal mass, the ulcer crater may project outside the gastric lumen when viewed in profile. Characteristically the wall around the ulcer is stiffened for some distance and fails to transmit peristalsis. The mucosal pattern is destroyed over the surface of the infiltrated area in most patients. Rarely the tumor has been observed to spread beneath the mucosa, leaving the folds intact, or else causing them to appear unusually thick. This appearance resembles closely that seen in some malignant lymphomas. If the lesion is limited to a moderate-sized area along one curvature, one or several incisuralike indrawings of the opposite curvature may be present. When ulceration develops, the ulcer pocket is more irregular than is seen in a benign ulcer, there is little tendency for the edges to overhang, the area of stiffness and induration around the crater is larger than in benign ulcer, and the mucosal pattern is obliterated in the vicinity or else is altered.

Mainzer, Amberg, and Margulis[28] have reported their experience with this lesion and note the controversy in the literature concerning the roentgen findings. The roentgen appearances in their patients fell into four main categories: (*1*) gastric ulcer, (2) polypoid filling defect, (3) contracted lesser curvature or antral rigidity, and (4) normal stomach. The ulcers were interpreted as benign. Those showing antral rigidity or contracted lesser curvature simulated a healed gastric-ulcer deformity. The polypoid lesions usually were small and often thought to be benign.

Their findings emphasize the need for early diagnosis of this lesion because of the high curability rate, *e.g.*, a 93% 5-year survival rate in one series.

Early in its development, this type of tumor is very difficult to detect because the roentgen signs are minimal. The local rigidity may not alter peristalsis very much, the mucosal irregularity may be minimal, and the ulcers or erosions may be very difficult to detect and, when visible, may be quite smooth and not rigid. It is in the detection of these early lesions that good double-contrast studies are of particular value.

Ulcerating Carcinoma

Ulceration may develop in any gastric carcinoma. As used here the term "ulcerating carcinoma" is meant to imply a lesion in which necrosis has led to deep ulceration with the ulcer cavity dominating the gross picture (Fig. 16-20). When a polypoid or fungating carcinoma develops extensive necrosis to the point where the lesion is predominantly an ulcer, the ulcer is of the meniscus type (described under the heading "Differential Diagnosis of Benign and Malignant Ulcers"). This is because the ulcer forms within a mass that projects into the lumen and thus the cavity of the ulcer will not extend beyond the luminal margin as a rule. When an infiltrating carcinoma ulcerates, the cavity of the ulcer does project outside the lumen when viewed tangentially and resembles a benign ulcer in this respect. Differences between the two are mentioned in the preceding section. The question as to the frequency with which a benign ulcer may undergo malignant transformation has not been settled, but it probably is an infrequent occurrence.

Mixed Types

It is to be expected that many gastric carcinomas will show roentgen features of more than one of the types described in the foregoing. A predominantly fungating tumor may undergo extensive ulceration, an infiltrating carcinoma may develop fungating characteristics, or different parts of a single tumor may resemble several of the types described. This is particularly true in advanced lesions, as many of these are when first examined.

Calcification in Gastric Neoplasms

Rarely, calcifications may be found in gastric carcinoma. In the reported cases this has been a mucinous type of adenocarcinoma, as is true when calci-

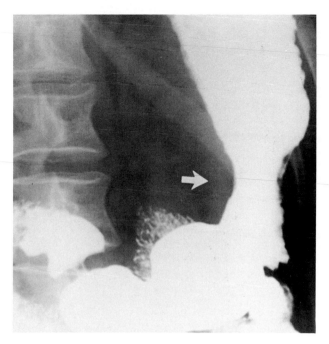

Fig. 16-18. Scirrhous carcinoma. There is moderate fusiform narrowing of the lumen **(arrow).** At fluoroscopy this was noted to be fixed with absence of peristalsis in the area. The margins of this lesion are not clearly defined.

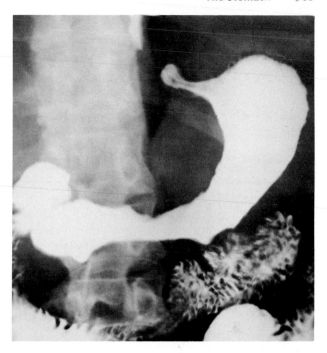

Fig. 16-19. Scirrhous carcinoma of the stomach (linitis plastica). All but the distal 1 or 2 cm of the stomach is involved by the lesion which has infiltrated and thickened the wall, producing a stiff, rigid structure.

fication occurs in carcinoma of the colon. Benign tumors may calcify and we have reported an example occurring in a leiomyoma of the gastric fundus.[10]

Gastric Remnant Carcinoma Following Gastric Resection

The incidence of recurrent carcinoma following gastric resection is decreasing with improved surgical techniques. There appears to be a higher incidence of gastric carcinoma in patients who have had resection for benign disease, the carcinoma having developed in the gastric remnant, than in the general population although there is some disagreement regarding this. Roentgen findings in the gastric remnant are similar to those in the intact stomach, but roentgen examination is more difficult because the area is not palpable, there is often some distortion secondary to the surgical procedure, and air contrast studies may be difficult because an open anastomosis does not permit adequate gastric distention or the retention of barium.

GASTRIC LYMPHOMA

Although malignant lymphoma may involve the stomach, it is rare that the gastric lesion is the only manifestation of the disease. Since the tumor may involve the stomach in a number of ways, the roentgen findings are variable. Some of these lymphomas resemble carcinoma of the fungating type so closely that roentgen differentiation is impossible. Others are ulcerating and may simulate either benign or malignant ulcers. Still others consist of multiple ulcerating lesions producing the so-called "target" or "bull's-eye" sign that has been described more frequently in gastric metastases. The infiltrating type may be very extensive, causing gross thickening of mucosal folds and of the gastric wall so that there is little peristalsis and the stomach is not distensable (Fig. 16-21). Multiple tumors (*i.e.,* tumor of the stomach and another in the colon or small bowel) should suggest the possibility of lymphoma. *Hodgkin's disease* may involve the stomach and, as in other lymphomas, the lesions are variable. Some gastric lymphomas simulate a benign or malignant ulcer. Others may resem-

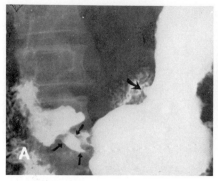
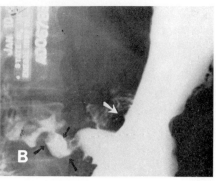

Fig. 16-20. Gastric ulcers, benign and malignant. **A.** The initial examination reveals a benign ulcer on the lesser curvature near the sulcus **(upper arrow).** The **lower arrows** point to another ulcerating lesion on the greater curvature side of the distal antrum. This lesion does not project beyond the lumen and is bounded by an irregular nodular halo. **B.** After several weeks of medical treatment the benign ulcer has decreased in size, leaving only a small, pointed projection **(white arrow).** The malignant ulcer has increased in size **(lower arrows).**

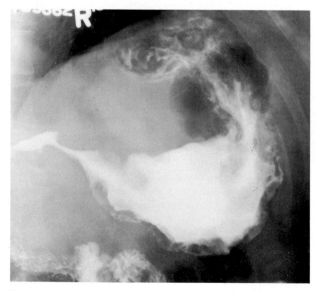

Fig. 16-21. Lymphosarcoma of the stomach. The tumor has infiltrated the gastric wall very extensively, resulting in gross thickening of the gastric rugal pattern, stiffening of the wall, and loss of the normal mucosal pattern. There is also a large extragastric component causing downward displacement of the duodenojejunal junction at the ligament of Treitz.

ble scirrhous carcinoma and some appear as a large intraluminal mass that cannot be differentiated roentgenographically from carcinoma.

GASTRIC SARCOMA

Primary sarcomas of the stomach are rare. Leiomyosarcoma is the most common. Neurogenic sarcomas, fibrosarcoma, and liposarcoma are extremely rare. These lesions arise in the gastric wall and form intramural masses of varying sizes that often are lobulated, frequently have a sizable extra-gastric component, and sometimes exhibit mucosal erosion and a central ulceration. The various types cannot be differentiated radiographically from each other or from their benign counterparts.

METASTASES TO THE STOMACH

Gastric metastases are unusual but certain tumors do tend to involve the stomach occasionally, breast carcinoma and melanoma being the most common. The patterns of involvement vary. The typical "target" or "bull's-eye" masses occurring in melanoma metastases are caused by ulcerations extending moderately deep into the tumor masses. Metastases from carcinoma of the breast and from bronchogenic cancer may also produce this type of lesion. A diffuse infiltrative metastatic tumor may be produced by breast carcinoma. Solitary polypoid or intramural masses also may be caused by hematogenous metastases.

BENIGN GASTRIC TUMORS

Gastric Polyps

Adenomatous polyps of the stomach are similar in all respects to polyps of the colon. Polyps develop less frequently in the stomach than they do in the colon. Because of the effects of active peristalsis in the stomach, a gastric polyp may develop a fairly long pedicle. When situated near the pylorus the pedunculated polyp is prone to prolapse through the pylorus into the duodenum and thus may be a cause of pyloric obstruction. Otherwise, bleeding is the only symptom to be expected. There may be one or several polyps present in the individual patient; rarely a diffuse polyposis of the gastric wall is encountered. Inflammatory or hyperplastic polyps also are found in the stomach and resemble in all respects the roentgen appearances of true adenomatous polyps. The diagnosis cannot be made purely from roentgen examination.

The incidence of gastric adenomatous polyps in patients with the Peutz-Jeghers syndrome is higher than that in the general population. Gastric polyposis also occurs in the *Cronkhite-Canada* syndrome associated with malabsorption, alopecia, hyperpigmentation, and atrophy of the nails.[29] There is a loss of albumin and electrolytes accompanied by steatorrhea. Familial polyposis of the colon is also associated with some increase in incidence of gastric polyps which may be adenomatous or hyperplastic. Syndromes in which gastrointestinal polyposis is a major feature are listed in Table 16-1.[23]

Villous adenoma is also a polypoid mass that is occasionally found in the stomach. The frondlike irregularities of the adenoma are very similar to those in the colon which are much more common.

Roentgen Observations. A polyp causes a smoothly rounded, translucent defect in the barium shadow. If the polyp has a pedicle, the defect caused by the polyp may move over a distance of several centimeters under the influence of peristalsis. The pedicle may be visualized as a narrow stalklike defect extending from the head of the polyp to the margin of the stomach. If the polyp is sessile, no motion of it in relation to the gastric wall is seen. A polyp of less than 0.5 cm in diameter is difficult to detect on roentgen examination unless situated directly on one of the curvatures where it can be visualized easily in profile (Fig. 16-22). The normal tortuosity of gastric mucosal folds offers difficulty in recognition of small lesions because of the similarity to polyps that may be produced when these folds are a little thickened. Occasionally a more or less generalized thickening and tortuosity of the gastric mucosal folds is found, the folds causing polyplike defects when they are seen on edge. It often is impossible to determine if one is dealing with a multiple polyposis of the stomach or a hypertrophied mucosa. Most frequently it is the latter condition that is, in fact, an inflammatory type of polyposis or polypoid hyperplasia.

A prolapsing polyp may cause the signs of pyloric obstruction with obvious gastric retention and delay in gastric emptying. Peristaltic waves are deep and vigorous and there is some degree of gastric dilatation. During fluoroscopy the defect caused by the polyp may change position, being seen in the pyloric antrum at times and then prolapsing into the duodenal bulb (Fig. 16-23). When situated within the bulb, the head of the polyp produces a circular and centrally placed filling defect. The stalk may be visible, extending through the pylorus and causing a puckering of the wall of the stomach at its point of origin. It may be possible to dislodge the polyp from the duodenal bulb by manual palpation during the fluoroscopic study.

Most gastric polyps are small, smooth, clearly demarcated, and benign. When lobulated and irregular they are more likely to be malignant. However, endoscopic examination with biopsy, if indicated, is usually performed.

Pseudopolypoid Masses

A number of conditions causing mucosal or submucosal masses may simulate polyps. These include gastric varices; small submucosal tumors such as lipoma, leiomyoma, fibroma, and neurolemmoma; inflammatory pseudopolyps; postoperative changes such as suture granulomas and small masses made up of redundant mucosa; prolapse of mucosa through the esophageal hiatus; and aberrant pancreatic and hepatic tissue. Lipomas near the pylorus may become pedunculated.

INTRAMURAL GASTRIC TUMORS

A variety of intramural nonmucosal tumors occur in the stomach but as a group these lesions are uncommon. Among these tumors of intramural origin one will find leiomyomas, neurofibromas, lipomas, and the like. Since it often is difficult to identify accurately the histologic nature of many of these tumors, some authors prefer to describe them simply as "spindle-cell tumors." The most common tumor in this group is the leiomyoma. Any of these lesions may occur as sarcomas.

Table 16-1. Polyposis Syndromes

	FAMILIAL COLONIC POLYPOSIS	GARDNER'S SYNDROME	JUVENILE POLYPOSIS	PEUTZ-JEGHERS SYNDROME	TURCOT SYNDROME	CRONKHITE-CANADA SYNDROME
Components	Multiple colonic polyps	Colonic polyposis; sebaceous cysts; osteomas; desmoid tumors; mesenteric fibromas	Gastrointestinal polyposis	Gastrointestinal polyposis; mucocutaneous pigmentation (melanin)	Colonic polyps; central nervous system tumors (usually glioblastomas)	Generalized polyposis; hyperpigmentation; alopecia; atrophy of the nails
Inheritance	Mendelian dominance	Mendelian dominance	Probably familial type	Mendelian dominance; variable penetrance	Few cases; questionable autosomal recessive	None
Onset of symptoms	Childhood and early adolescence	Average 30 yr.	Average 6 yr.	Childhood and adolescence	Childhood and young adult	42–75 yr.
Major symptoms	. . .	. . .	Bleeding; prolapse of polyps	Intussusception; bleeding	Central nervous system	Diarrhea
Anatomical involvement by polyps	Colon only; diffuse	Colon (diffuse); occasionally stomach and duodenum	Anywhere in the gastrointestinal tract, mainly in the colon; less numerous than in familial polyposis	Anywhere in the gastrointestinal tract; predominantly in the small intestine	Colon	Anywhere in the gastrointestinal tract, predominantly the stomach and colon
Pathology	Adenomas	Adenoma	Hamartoma	Hamartoma	?	? adenoma; predominantly cystic glandular dilatation
Malignant potential	Colorectal cancer in 2/3	High probability of colorectal cancer; likelihood of periampullary cancer	None	Low or none	Probably	Multiple carcinomata (2 of 15 patients)
Associated findings	. . .	Follicular odontomas; dentigerous cysts	Heart lesions; malrotation; hydrocephalus; congenital amyotoma; porphyria	Granulosa theca-cell tumors of the ovary may occur in 5% of female patients	. . .	. . .

(Koehler PR, Kyaw MM, Fenlon JW: Diffuse gastrointestinal polyposis with ectodermal changes. Radiology 103, 589, 1972.)

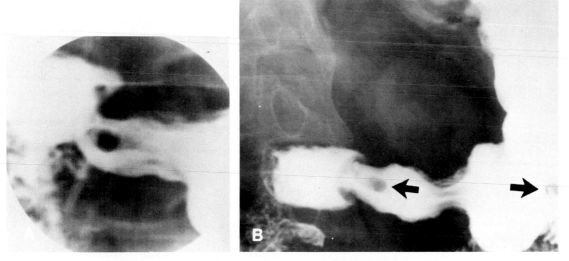

Fig. 16-22. Gastric antral polyp. **A.** Spot film. **B.** Film made after fluoroscopy. The distal antral defect **(left arrow)** points to a small polyp. The **right arrow** points to a polyp near the greater curvature.

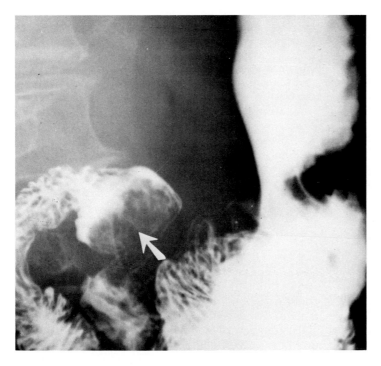

Fig. 16-23. Prolapsed pedunculated polyp of the gastric antrum. The head of the polyp is in the duodenal bulb **(arrow),** but other reontgenograms and fluoroscopy showed that it moved back into the stomach intermittently.

The following groups of rare submucosal tumors may be recognized as intramural roentgenographically, but may also simulate polypoid tumor. *Granular cell myoblastoma* is a rare benign intramural mass that may ulcerate.[1] This tumor also occurs in the skin, breast, mouth, and tongue. *Adenomyoma* or *myoepithelial hamartoma* may rarely produce a submucosal mass in the stomach, usually near the pylorus.[25] Many of these tumors contain pancreatic tissue. *Leiomyoblastoma* is another rare intramural tumor originating in smooth muscle, usually in the antrum.[13] *Carcinoid tumor* occasionally arises in the stomach, usually appearing as an intramural mass, but rarely it may be polypoid.

Grossly the intramural tumor is usually well circumscribed and encapsulated (Fig. 16-24). The tumor bulges into the gastric lumen but is covered by mucosa. An ulcer often develops on the summit of the mass and this may be a cause of gastric hemorrhage (Fig. 16-25). Otherwise, these lesions usually are asymptomatic.

With the larger lesions, and particularly those that are frankly malignant, the major portion of the tumor may grow to the outside, causing little intraluminal deformity but with a bulky exogastric mass.

Roentgen Observations. A small intramural tumor nodule resembles a sessile gastric polyp closely, causing a circumscribed, rounded, filling defect (Fig. 16-24) that is best brought out by pressure over the lesion. It may be impossible to distinguish between the two. If an ulcer has formed, it will be visualized as a pocketlike shadow of barium extending into the mass from its inner surface. Gastric peristalsis is not altered unless the lesion is large or unless it is malignant and has begun to invade the gastric wall. A lipoma, being relatively soft, may change shape under the influence of palpation or peristalsis. Most gastric lipomas are too small for the lucency of fat to stand out clearly from the adjacent gastric wall, a sign that is helpful in diagnosing lipomas of the peripheral soft tissues. Large lesions, as has been indicated, may show very little intragastric protrusion but the large exogastric mass may cause displacement of the stomach, suggesting that the lesion is entirely extrinsic. In some patients it is impossible to be certain if the lesion originated within or outside of the stomach.

ABERRANT PANCREATIC NODULES

Nodules of pancreatic tissue occasionally are found in the wall of the stomach but are somewhat more frequent in the first and second portions of the duodenum. Some of these nodules are almost microscopic in size and cause no roentgen signs. Others may measure up to 1 cm or more in diameter and be large enough to produce a filling defect. The defect of an aberrant pancreatic nodule is identical to that of a small intramural tumor, as described in the preceding section, and there frequently is no certain way to differentiate between them on roentgen examina-

tion. One sign that is helpful when present is the demonstration of a small central pit or niche on the surface of the nodule. Because pancreatic nodules are found in the proximal part of the duodenum while other intramural lesions are uncommon in this location, any such duodenal defect is more likely to be a pancreatic nodule than some other type of lesion. Ulceration may develop on the surface of a pancreatic nodule and bleeding may result; usually, however, the lesions are asymptomatic.

GASTRIC VARICES

In portal hypertension, varices of the gastric fundus are nearly as frequent as varices of the esophagus. They may also involve the body of the stomach. In the absence of esophageal varices, splenic vein occlusion between the left gastroepiploic vein and the coronary veins is likely when the gastric body is involved. The appearance on barium study is similar to that of varices in the esophagus. The varices may resemble giant folds, but tend to be serpentine and are readily compressible. Celiac arteriography can be used to confirm the diagnosis.

CHRONIC GASTRITIS

The problems concerning the significance of gastritis as a clinical entity and the roentgen patterns of the disease have not been completely settled. Gastritis as an accompaniment of other diseases of the stomach (*e.g.,* carcinoma, ulcer) is common. Gastritis of severe degree may result from the ingestion of acids and caustic substances. The major types of chronic gastritis are usually considered to be the atrophic and the hypertrophic.

Roentgen Observations. In *chronic atrophic gastritis* the mucosal folds are thinned and scanty. The normal serrations seen along the greater curvature are lacking. Many patients with these roentgen findings have atrophy without inflammation. In some the stomach is hypotonic giving it the semblance of scirrhous carcinoma. Morphine administered in a dose of 8 mg increases gastric tone and the amplitude of peristalsis temporarily, allowing pliability to be observed and thus aiding in differentiation of the gastritis from carcinoma.[40] Many patients showing histologic evidence of chronic gastritis have a normal roentgen mucosal pattern and the diagnosis of chronic atrophic gastritis often cannot be made on roentgen findings alone.

In the *chronic hypertrophic type,* similar diagnos-

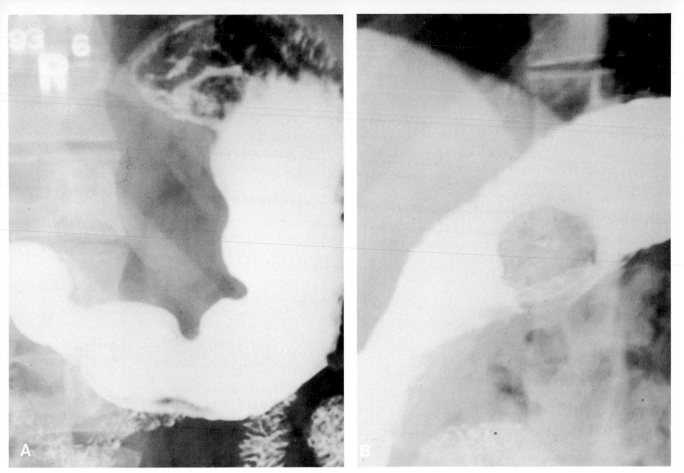

Fig. 16-24. Intramural gastric neurofibroma. **A.** The lesion is not outlined in this posteroanterior projection. **B.** The tumor defect is clearly visible along the greater curvature of the upper body of the stomach in this nearly lateral projection.

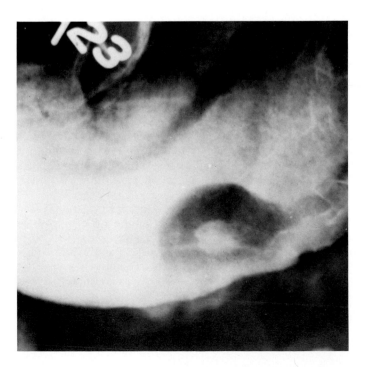

Fig. 16-25. Leiomyoma with a central ulcer crater near the greater curvature of the stomach. This is an example of a "target" or "bull's eye" lesion which may also occur in metastatic disease such as melanoma of the stomach.

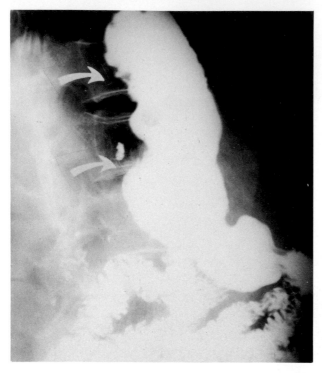

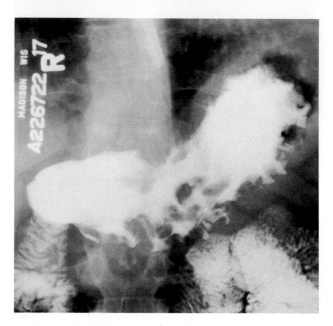

Fig. 16-27. Menetrier's disease. There is considerable thickening of the gastric mucosal folds, particularly in the gastric fundus and body.

Fig. 16-26. Giant gastric rugae in the area of the **arrows** suggest the possibility of carcinoma, but biopsy indicated that localized hypertrophic gastritis was responsible for the giant rugae.

tic difficulties may be encountered. The following changes may be found:

Thickening of the Mucosal Folds. Thickening and increased tortuosity of the mucosal folds as a sign of gastritis must be interpreted with considerable caution because of the wide variation in the normal size of these folds. There is no complete agreement as to what the maximum width of a mucosal fold in the stomach should be. As has been observed, a widened fold in the antrum is of more significance than one in the fundus because in the latter location the folds normally are thicker and more tortuous than in the distal part of the stomach. It has been suggested that a fold shadow measuring 0.5 cm in width in the antrum is probably abnormal, whereas a fold shadow of the same width in the upper part of the body or in the fundus is probably not abnormal. In general, localized thickening is more significant than a generalized prominence and may indicate a localized hypertrophic gastritis. Occasionally a rather marked thickening of mucous-membrane folds occurs in a lo-

calized area of the stomach sufficient to cause a filling defect that may resemble carcinoma rather closely. (Fig. 16-26). Surgical exploration and resection may be necessary to settle the problem. This condition is uncommon and is known as *giant hypertrophy of gastric rugae,* or *Menetrier's disease* (Fig. 16-27). In one form of the disease the involvement is predominantly in the middle third involving the greater curvature or both curvatures. However, the lesion may affect any part of the stomach with massive, localized thickening of rugae. At times the tortuous thickened folds resemble a mass of polyps. In another type of the lesion the mucosa is stretched over the mass and the surface may be quite smooth. The lesion is less common in the pyloric area. Some patients with Menetrier's disease have a considerable loss of protein, leading to hypoproteinemia and intestinal edema. Excess mucus secretion is common in this situation and may add to the mottled effect of the lesion. Eosinophilia and anemia are often present.

Stiffness of the Folds. Of equal and possibly greater importance than thickening of the folds is unusual stiffening of them. Normal gastric folds tend to be completely obliterated or nearly so as the stomach is distended with barium mixture. Folds also are flattened and decreased in width as peristaltic waves pass over them. In the antrum during antral systole, normal folds disappear except for the presence of fine hairline stripes representing thin valleys between the flattened folds as the antrum contracts over them. Normal folds can be obliterated if sufficient pressure is applied over the abdominal wall or the stomach is distended with gas. Stiffened folds also may be thrown into tortuous elevations that resemble polypoid defects and the differentiation from adenomatous polyps may be difficult if not impossible.

Antral Gastritis. Probably the most significant form of gastritis from the roentgen standpoint is that which involves the antrum of the stomach. This is a fairly common condition. There may be a localized thickening of the mucosal folds as noted in a preceding section. The prepyloric area of the stomach is likely to be uniformly narrowed for a distance of several centimeters or even more, proximal to the pylorus; the narrowing is concentric and usually not entirely constant during flurposcopic observation. Peristalsis through the area is deficient but seldom completely lacking. The antral wall is thickened and relatively stiff but lacks the complete rigidity of an annular carcinoma. These changes possibly are caused by associated pyloric muscle hypertrophy secondary to the chronic spasm and inflammation. Similar findings are noted in the adult form of hypertrophic pyloric stenosis. In some cases the mucosal folds are unusually thin and scanty suggesting an atrophic type of gastritis. Superficial ulcer craters may be present although frank ulceration is the exception. The lesion must be differentiated chiefly from an annular carcinoma of the antrum (Fig. 16-28). Significant roentgen differential points include:

1. The change from normal gastric wall to involved segment is a smooth one and there are no overhanging edges.

2. The narrowing is even and concentric in antral gastritis; in carcinoma the involvement may be greater on one curvature than on the other.

3. Mucosal folds are present through the contracted area in antral gastritis, they are absent in carcinoma.

4. There almost always is some flexibility of the wall in antral gastritis and, if fluoroscopic observation is carried out carefully or serial roentgenograms are obtained, slight relaxation and contraction may be determined. The wall, in annular carcinoma, is completely rigid.

Reflux Alkaline Gastritis. In patients who have had partial gastrectomy for peptic ulcer, an alkaline gastritis may result from reflux of intestinal content into the gastric stump. This is usually found late—2 or more years following surgery. Roentgen findings consist of enlarged mucosal folds, chiefly adjacent to the anastomosis, which may prolapse into the jejunum in Billroth II anastomoses. There may be an ulcer on the gastric side in contrast to the usual stomal ulcer which is on the jejunal side. This may be the cause for the relatively high incidence of gastric remnant cancer in the these patients who have had gastrectomy for treatment of ulcer disease.

Chemical (Corrosive) Gastritis. Inflammation of the stomach from the swallowing of caustic substances such as lye or strong acids may cause an extensive fibrosis of portions of the gastric wall. Early roentgen findings are varied; in many cases of alkali ingestion the gastric acidity tends to protect the stomach. In severe injury there is usually early gastric distention, sometimes with intramural gas secondary to mucosal destruction. Mucosal folds are edematous and coarse, and there may be large bullae of the mucosa. In injuries this extensive the stomach usually becomes small and fibrotic. Involvement of the prepyloric area is frequent and pyloric obstruction may result. In some patients the end result of an extensive chemical gastritis may be a deformity that resembles a scirrhus carcinoma in many respects. The lumen of the stomach is generally narrowed and the gastric walls show loss of pliability. The history is important in the evaluation of this lesion.

Ferrous Sulfate Ingestion. Children attracted by the bright color of ferrous sulfate tablets may ingest them. Soon thereafter the tablets or dissolved iron compound may be visible on plain films. Nausea, vomiting, acidosis, shock, coma, bloody diarrhea, and death may follow ingestion of as little as 1 gm. If the child survives, stricture of the gastric antrum may occur as a late complication. It may cause high-grade obstruction requiring surgical relief.

Emphysematous Gastritis. The term "emphysematous gastritis" refers to the presence of gas in the gastric wll usually caused by infection by a gas-forming organism. Generally it is not used to refer to the gas sometimes observed in the gastric wall following ingestion of corrosive material. Also, gastric infarction may produce a similar roentgenographic picture. Usually emphysematous gastritis is a complication of phlegmonous gastritis. When gas-forming organisms cause the inflammation or phlegmon of the gastric wall, emphysematous gastritis results. The patients

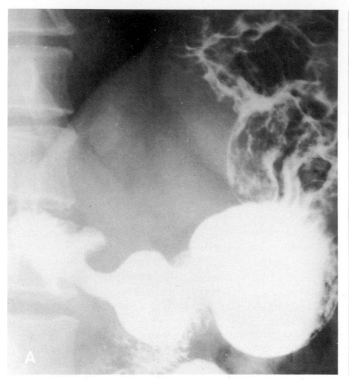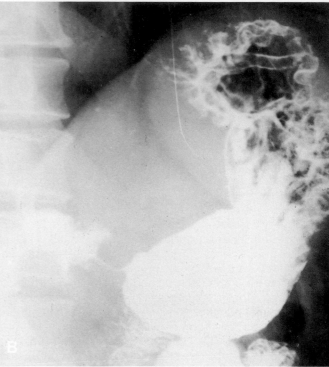

Fig. 16-28. Antral gastritis. There is narrowing of the gastric antrum in the immediate prepyloric area. By comparing the two roentgenograms (**A** and **B**) a contour change is noted. During fluoroscopy, the stomach in the prepyloric area did not expand any more than is depicted in **A.** The mucosal pattern in the upper portion of the stomach is very coarse.

are critically ill, and the mortality rate is high. Plain abdominal films show the presence of gas within the wall of the stomach. These, combined with the history, usually serve to make the diagnosis.

GRANULOMATOUS DISEASES

Crohn's Disease of the Stomach

A number of cases of this entity have been reported in the literature but the disease must be considered as distinctly infrequent. It corresponds, pathologically, to the same disease found in the small intestine (regional enteritis), granulomatous colitis in the colon, and the infrequent similar lesions found in the esophagus and duodenum. The roentgen findings include (1) involvement of the gastric antrum in most patients; (2) associated disease in the duodenum; (3) multiple, tiny or shallow ulcers; (4) thickened mucosal folds and cobblestone mucosal relief in some patients; (5 lack of antral distensibility; and (6) antral narrowing which may also involve a portion of the body. The appearance may resemble that of scirrhous carcinoma. The roentgen diagnosis is difficult to make unless there are associated changes, in the duodenum or elsewhere in the small intestine, characteristic of regional enteritis.

Gastric Tuberculosis

Involvement of the stomach by tuberculosis is extremely rare. In most of the cases, ulceration may be widespread. Extensive thickening of the gastric wall in which fistulous tracts may occur, and relative fixation and nondistensibility have been reported. Since the findings are not very specific, the diagnosis must be made by bacteriologic and histopathologic means.

Gastric Syphilis

Syphilitic involvement of the stomach is extremely rare. We have seen one patient in whom the roentgenographic findings resembled those of scirrhous carcinoma involving the body and antrum of the stomach. The mucosal folds are effaced and there is rigidity and lack of normal peristalsis in the area. Gumma of the gastric wall may produce a mass or masses indistinguishable from carcinoma.

Gastric Sarcoidosis

Rarely the stomach is involved in patients with sarcoidosis. Granulomas in the gastric wall may produce no roentgen signs but their predilection for the antrum may produce thickening of the antral wall, antral narrowing, and some nodularity of the mucosa.

Herpes Simplex

In immunosuppressed patients, herpes simplex may be generalized and involve the esophagus and stomach.[21] In a case reported recently, multiple, coarse nodules separated by interlacing crevices and shallow ulcers were demonstrated by radiography.

Eosinophilic Gastritis

Eosinophilic gastritis is a rare granulomatous disease that often involves the proximal small bowel as well as the distal stomach. In such an instance, the term *eosinophilic gastroenteritis* is preferred.[18] Usually eosinophilia is present; in most instances the gastric form is confined to the antrum in which there is an eosinophilic infiltration detectable microscopically. Roentgen findings are those of narrowing and rigidity of the antrum in which enlarged mucosal folds are often apparent. At times, mucosal irregularity produces a cobblestone effect that predominates over enlarged rugal folds. Pyloric obstruction, which may be present in some degree, is the cause of symptomatology in these patients. The condition is believed to be an allergy, but the specific antigen or antigens are not known. It is not to be confused with eosinophilic granuloma of the stomach which is an inflammatory lesion that takes the form of a polyp, usually present in the antrum. The granuloma is compromised largely of eosinophils. It is not related to eosinophilic granuloma of bone (histiocytosis X). *Polyarteritis nodosa* may cause gastroenteric changes that resemble those of eosinophilic gastroenteritis.

Allergic Granulomatosis

In allergic patients with Loeffler's syndrome, occasional massive gastric involvement is observed. Radiographic findings of thick, distorted mucosal folds and intramural masses are often transitory. Biopsy reveals multiple allergic granulomas throughout the gastric wall, *e.g.*, submucosa, muscularis, and subserosa.

MISCELLANEOUS ABNORMALITIES

Scleroderma

Gastric manifestations of scleroderma are uncommon but not rare. They consist of diffuse hypotonia with prolonged emptying time; mucosal folds may be effaced, resulting in a smooth gastric outline.

Gastric Pseudolymphoma

This benign proliferation of lymphoid tissue may resemble lymphoma when the stomach is involved.[7] Although the cause is unknown, this pseudolymphoma most likely represents a reaction to chronic peptic ulcer. Radiographic findings are varied. Some of these lesions appear as tumor masses while others are manifest as large gastric rugae. The most common finding, however, is that of a well-defined, benign-appearing gastric ulcer or ulcers with unusual thickening of mucosal folds resulting in some decrease in gastric volume and in peristaltic activity.

Benign Lymphoid Hyperplasia

Benign lymphoid hyperplasia of the gastrointestinal tract is characterized by an increase in size and number of lymphoid follicles. It's occurrence in the stomach is unusual; it is much more commonly found in the colon. It usually involves the gastric antrum and is manifested radiographically by multiple small defects producing a granular nodularity as well as an increase in gastric mucosal folds. Rarely, umbilicated polypoid lesions are observed. The diagnosis is made on biopsy since pseudolymphoma and lymphoma can produce a comparable appearance. At times the findings are minimal, there being only a slight increase in the serrated appearance of the areae gastricae. However, when this increase accelerates to a point where a fine nodularity causes multiple filling defects with a scalloped margin, the possibility of lymphoid hyperplasia must be considered, although the differentiation between normal and abnormal is difficult.

Radiation Injury

The stomach is relatively resistant to radiation; with large doses used in treatment of adjacent neoplasms, however, pre-pyloric or pyloric ulcers may be produced. The mucosa is thickened with prominent folds, and there may be edema 3 to 6 weeks after completion of therapy. Mucosal pattern may then become irregular, indicating the presence of multiple, superficial erosions. Finally, the involved gastric wall becomes rigid with little peristalsis resembling the changes of scirrhous carcinoma, particularly when the antrum and distal body are involved.

The Zollinger-Ellison Syndrome

This syndrome consists of:

1. Fulminating peptic ulceration. The majority of ulcers occur in the duodenal bulb but an atypical location of the ulcer, as in the distal duodenum or proximal jejunum, is found in about 40% of the patients.[8]

2. Marked hypersecretion of hydrochloric acid by the stomach.

3. Nonbeta islet cell tumors of the pancreas. Ectopic locations of the tumors (stomach, duodenum, etc.) occur in about 10% of patients.

4. If only partial gastric resection is performed, recurrence of an ulcer takes place in the majority of patients.

In some of these patients the pancreatic tumor is part of a syndrome with multiple tumors in other endocrine glands including the parathyroid, thyroid, pituitary, and adrenal. Severe diarrhea is among the clinical symptoms experienced by many patients. The basic abnormality is the secretion of large amounts of the hormone gastrin by the tumor. This causes the hyperchlorhydria and the resultant symptomatology.

Roentgen Observations. The roentgen findings include[8, 29]:

1. Increased gastric fluid content after overnight fasting.

2. Thickened, tortuous, gastric rugae resembling Menetrier's disease.

3. Peptic ulceration. An atypical location of the ulcer (other than the duodenal bulb or stomach) should alert the examiner to the possibility of this syndrome.

4. Dilatation of the duodenum, particularly the descending portion. The mucosal folds are thickened and coarse. In the early stage, spasm and irritability may cause apparent narrowing of the descending duodenum.

5. Changes in the small intestine resembling a malabsorption syndrome. Mucosal fold changes similar to those seen in the duodenum, increased fluid content, hypermotility, and segmentation are commonly encountered. Complete loss of folds may be seen in some segments similar to the "moulage sign" of sprue.

6. Failure of the ulcer to heal under medical therapy. After partial gastric resection, stomal and proximal jejunal ulcers develop in the majority of patients, sometimes within a few weeks after operation.

Foreign Bodies

A wide variety of indigestible foreign material may be swallowed and become lodged in the stomach and this is particularly frequent in children and among individuals who are psychotic. Most of the swallowed objects are metallic, including such objects as pins and coins. Even objects such as spoons and knives may be swallowed, particularly by the mentally deranged. Diagnosis is made without difficulty on plain-film examination because of the extreme density of the metallic foreign bodies.

Certain food substances may result in the formation of indigestible food balls (phytobezoars) in the stomach, the most common of these being persimmons. The continued ingestion of hair, usually by psychotic individuals, may result in the formation of a hair ball (trichobezoar).

Roentgen Observations

1. Metallic objects are readily visualized and the relationship to the stomach identified by the position of the object and its relation to the gastric air bubble. If necessary a small amount of barium–water mixture can be given to localize the object more certainly.

2. Nonmetallic objects can be visualized only after the ingestion of a barium–water meal. They will cause filling defects in the barium shadow. A foreign body is characterized by the fact that the defect can be displaced by manual palpation and by altering the position of the patient. The most common cause for such defects is retained food particles. Reexamination often will clarify the problem if doubt arises concerning the nature of the shadow or shadows.

3. *Bezoars* are visualized as masses within the gastric lumen, often of a sufficiently large size to

nearly fill the stomach. The barium mixture will be observed to flow around and completely surround the mass so that, no matter in what position the patient is placed, a layer of barium can be seen between the defect and the gastric wall. The barium mixture may penetrate into the interstices of the mass and remain after the rest of the stomach is empty; this results in a persistent mottled shadow that is characteristic of a bezoar. Phytobezoar formation is relatively frequent following surgery for ulcer disease in which vagotomy and partial gastric resection or vagotomy and pyloroplasty have been performed. Oranges appear to be the most common ingredients of these bezoars.

Gastric Diverticula

Diverticula of the stomach are uncommon, being found only about once in every 1500 to 2000 gastrointestinal examinations. Diverticula are usually located on the posterior wall of the gastric fundus close to the cardia. It is believed that such diverticula are in all likelihood acquired lesions rather than congenital ones. The fact that practically all gastric diverticula occur in a localized area of the fundus has been explained on the basis of this being a region of anatomic weakness so that diverticulum formation can occur more readily here than elsewhere. Diverticula in the prepyloric area are much less frequent. The sac may contain an island of pancreatic tissue. In the majority of patients it is doubtful if gastric diverticulum is the cause of clinical complaints. A rare case of a tumor, either carcinoma or sarcoma, developing in a gastric diverticulum has been reported. Bleeding from a diverticulum, usually the result of ulceration, also has been reported but is an uncommon occurrence.

Roentgen Observations. The diverticulum when filled with barium is visualized as a smoothly rounded outpouching connected to the stomach by a narrow neck (Fig. 16-29). While these pouches or sacs vary in size the majority are small, measuring several centimeters in diameter. Retention of the barium mixture in the pouch for hours after the rest of the stomach is empty is the rule. If follow-up roentgenograms of the abdomen are obtained, the small, round barium shadow will remain in the region of the gastric cardia long after the remainder of the stomach has emptied. A gastric diverticulum can be distinguished from a gastric ulcer without difficulty by its characteristic shape, the typical location, by the absence of spasm, and by the retention of contrast material for hours after the stomach is empty.

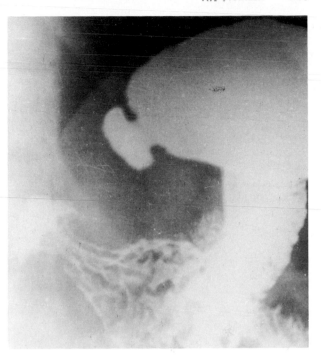

Fig. 16-29. Diverticulum of the gastric fundus. This is a typical location for gastric diverticula.

Hypertrophic Pyloric Stenosis

There are two major forms of hypertrophic pyloric stenosis, the infantile and the adult. In the infantile type the sex ratio is four boys to one girl and there seems to be a genetic factor involved. Onset of vomiting in an infant 3 to 5 weeks of age is the usual clinical presentation. There may or may not be a palpable pyloric tumor. The adult type probably is not related to the infantile although the cause is obscure in many patients. In some it appears to develop on the basis of a preexisting antral gastritis as a result of the chronic inflammation and the long-continued spasm. In others it is seen in association with a chronic ulcer and in these it may result from chronic pylorospasm. In still other patients an etiologic factor is not evident and perhaps some of these represent hypertrophy persisting into adult life, following an earlier infantile type of lesion.

In the patients reported by du Plessis,[11] atrophic gastritis was present in all those who had biopsy or surgical resection. du Plessis believes that the probable cause is a congenital deficiency in the longitudinal muscle over the pyloric canal with hypertrophy of the circular muscle and that the gastritis, gastric ulceration, and mucosal strictures are secondary.

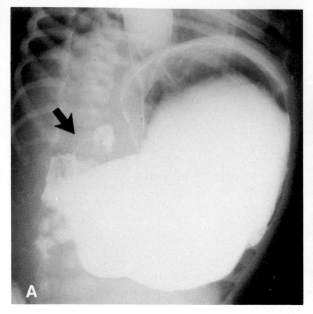

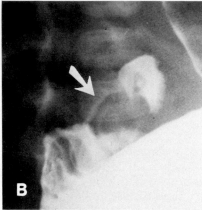

Fig. 16-30. A. Infantile hypertrophic pyloric stenosis. Note the thin, stringlike shadow of barium extending through the narrowed elongated pylorus **(arrow).** The stomach is dilated, but no deep obstructive type of peristaltic waves are noted on this film. **B.** Spot film showing the string sign **(arrow).**

Roentgen Observations

Infantile Type. The stomach usually is enlarged but pronounced gastric dilatation is not common. Deep peristaltic waves occur intermittently but these force only small quantities of the barium mixture through the pylorus with each wave and the gastric emptying time is delayed. As the barium is forced through the pylorus into the duodenum by peristalsis, the pyloric canal is visualized as a narrow elongated tract from 1 to 2 cm in length. The appearance is one of a thin "string" of barium (Fig. 16-30). The diameter of this segment may vary slightly from time to time but never becomes entirely normal. The double track sign is caused by a central mucosal fold in the pyloric area, so that barium forms a streak or track above and below it. This is a good but not infallible sign, since a contracted antrum can simulate it. As the duodenal bulb becomes visualized, its base often is seen to be concave because of the thickened pyloric muscle bulging into it. There is often a decreased amount of air in the small bowel in these infants.[37]

Adult Type. The roentgen signs are similar to the infantile form except that they are somewhat easier to demonstrate. The narrow elongated pyloric canal may measure 3 to 4 cm in length (Fig. 16-31). The caliber often changes slightly during fluoroscopic observation and mucosal folds can be demonstrated as thin, stripelike shadows paralleling the long axis of the antrum. A concave indentation in the base of the

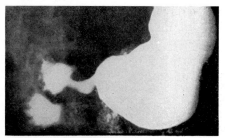

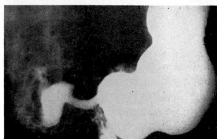

Fig. 16-31. Adult type of benign hypertrophy of the pylorus. There was persistent elongation of the pylorus in this patient. The mucosa appears smooth, but this lesion has to be differentiated from antral carcinoma, which may cause narrowing and elongation of the antrum in a manner quite similar to this.

duodenal bulb is often seen owing to the hypertrophied muscle. In the adult, gastric emptying often occurs at a normal rate and the stomach empties within an average length of time. Occasionally, gastric retention occurs and in rather uncommon instances a fairly high-grade obstruction may develop at the pylorus.

The lesion must be differentiated from an annular carcinoma of the gastric antrum. The chief differential points include: (1) The presence of mucosal folds in the constricted area. (2) Concavity of the base of the duodenal bulb. This may also occur in the presence of an annular carcinoma although it is more commonly seen in benign hypertrophy. (3) Slight changes in contour of the narrowed prepyloric area during fluoroscopic observation and as demonstrated in serial roentgenograms. (4) A smooth rather than an abrupt change from normal to abnormal gastric wall often demarcated by a transverse fold. (5) Incisura of the greater curvature of the elongated canal. (6) Regular and symmetrical shape and contour. (7) Deep peristalsis without much gastric dilatation. (8) The presence of a benign ulcer, usually near the incisura. (9) Absence of a palpable mass.

None of these signs is absolutely specific for a benign lesion but a combination of them is significant.

ESOPHAGEAL HIATAL HERNIA

Herniation of a part of the stomach through the esophageal hiatus is one of the common lesions of the upper gastrointestinal tract. The frequency of diagnosis of the lesion depends to some extent on whether the small, inconstant protrusions of gastric mucosa, so-called "hiatal insufficiency," are included. Also some have considered the esophagogastric junction to be at the site where squamous esophageal and columnar gastric epithelium meet. Since it is not infrequent to find the epithelial junction above the diaphragmatic hiatus, these cases would be considered as hiatal hernias. Others believe that the motor activity of the distal segment is the determining factor. If esophageal peristaltic waves pass without interruption through the distal segment, it would be considered, functionally, a part of the esophagus regardless of the type of epithelium present. We subscribe to this opnion which, of course, will lead to fewer diagnoses of small, asymptomatic lesions. Also the esophagogastric junction may move upward slightly above the hiatus when the normal individual is swallowing. Therefore, the term "hiatal insufficiency" is sometimes used in equivocal cases.

Demonstration of a hiatal hernia is best accomplished when the patient is examined while in a recumbent position. Some examiners use a bolster or some other compression device to increase intra-abdominal pressure. The barium mixture can be fed through a drinking tube and the cardia observed as the patient is rotated into various positions. Usually the hernia will fill readily when the patient is in either a supine or a right lateral position. The Valsalva maneuver is useful to show small hernias and to determine the competency of the cardia. Fixed hernias of any appreciable size often can be recognized in chest roentgenograms, the fundus of the stomach and the gas-fluid level within it forming a recognizable shadow in the lower part of the posterior mediastinum. A contracted prepyloric segment is found in about 15% of patients with hiatal hernia, which is termed by some "pseudohypertrophic stenosis." The cause is not clear. There also appears to be some correlation between patients with obscure pulmonary fibrosis and hiatal hernia with gastroesophageal reflux. Some authors believe that rumination in infants and children is caused by hiatal hernia or other esophageal pathologic process.

Types of Hiatal Hernia (Fig. 16-32)

Sliding (Axial) Hernia. The most common hiatal hernia is the sliding or axial type, the herniated portion consisting of the gastric fundus, with the cardia displaced above the level of the hiatus. The esophagus usually is somewhat kinked or buckled in its lower portion and the cardiac orifice lies along the posteromedial side of the fundus. The hiatus often is very wide, measuring 3 to 4 cm in diameter. In some cases the hernia is inconstant and reducible. In others it is fixed in the thorax. Reflux of material from the stomach into the lower esophagus is frequent in this type of hernia and is generally considered to be the important factor in the subsequent development of esophagitis and esophageal stricture (Figs. 16-33 and 16-34).

Paraesophageal Hernia. The paraesophageal type of hernia is much less frequent than the sliding. It is characterized by the fact that the cardia remains at or below the diaphragm, the fundus herniating through the hiatus to lie along the distal part of the esophagus. The esophagus remains of normal length and reflux through the cardia does not usually occur.

Short-Esophagus Type of Hernia. The short-esophagus type is also axial and resembles the sliding except that the esophagus is shortened and the cardia is sit-

Lesions of the body of the pancreas displace the stomach forward.

Transverse Colon. Upward displacement of the stomach may be due to a mass in the transverse colon if the mass is large. However, usually no deformity is present secondary to a mass in the transverse colon.

Other Masses. Any intra-abdominal mass, if large enough, may cause some displacement of the stomach. Thus, a very large ovarian cyst may elevate the stomach considerably. Mesenteric cysts may do likewise. Retroperitoneal sarcoma, metastatic enlargement of lymph nodes, and aneurysm of the abdominal aorta are examples of other mass lesions that may deform and displace the stomach.

REFERENCES AND SELECTED READINGS

1. ASTON SJ, TOMPKINS RK: Granular cell myoblastoma of the stomach. Ann Surg 177: 228, 1973
2. BAUM J, NAUSBAUM M, BLADEMORE WS et al: The preoperative radiographic demonstration of intra-abdominal bleeding from undetermined sites by percutaneous selective celiac and superior mesenteric arteriography. Surgery 58: 797, 1965
3. BERENS SV, MOSKOWITZ H, MELLINS H: Air within the wall of the stomach. Am J Roentgenol 103: 310, 1968
4. BLOCH C: Roentgen features of Hodgkin's disease of the stomach. Am J Roentgenol 99: 175, 1967
5. BOIJSEN E, WALLACE S, KANTER IE: Angiography in tumors of the stomach. Acta Radiol [Diagn] (Stockh) 4: 306, 1966
6. BURNS B, GAY BB JR: Menetrier's disease of the stomach in children. Am J Roentgenol 103: 300, 1968
7. CHILES JT, PLATZ CE: Radiographic manifestations of pseudolymphoma of the stomach. Radiology 116: 551, 1975
8. CHRISTOFORIDIS AJ, NELSON SW: Radiological manifestations of ulcerogenic tumors of the pancreas. The Zollinger-Ellison syndrome. JAMA 198: 511, 1966
9. CRONKHITE LW, CANADA WJ: Generalized gastrointestinal polyposis. An unusual syndrome of polyposis, pigmentation, alopecia and onychotrophia. N Engl J Med 252: 1011, 1955
10. CRUMMY AB, JUHL JH: Calcified gastric leiomyoma. Am J Roentgenol 87: 727, 1962
11. DU PLESSIS DJ: Primary hypertrophic stenosis in the adult. Br J Surg 53: 485, 1966
12. EVANS JA, WEINTRAUB S: Accessory pancreatic tissue in the stomach wall. Am J Roentgenol 69: 22, 1953
13. FAEGENBURG D, FARMAN J, DALLEMAND S et al: Leiomyoblastoma of the stomach. Radiology 117: 297, 1975
14. FERRUCCI JT JR, BENEDICT KT JR: Anticholinergic-aided study of the gastrointestinal tract. Radiol Clin North Am 9: 23, 1971
15. GELFAND DW, HACHIYA J: The double contrast examination of the stomach using gas-producing granules and tablets. Radiology 93: 1381, 1969
16. GHAHREMANI GG: Nonobstructive mucosal diaphragms or rings of the gastric antrum. Am J Roentgenol 121: 236, 1974
17. GOLD RP, SEAMAN WB: The primary double contrast examination of the postoperative stomach. Radiology 124: 297, 1977
18. GOLDBERG HI, O'KIEFFE D, JENIS EH et al: Diffuse eosinophilic gastroenteritis. Am J Roentgenol 119: 342, 1973
19. HARPER RAK, GREEN B: Malignant gastric ulcer. J Fac Radiol 12: 95, 1961
20. HOWARTH FH, COCKEL R, ROPER BW et al: The effect of metoclopramide upon gastric motility. Clin Radiol 20: 294, 1969
21. HOWILER W, GOLDBERG HI: Gastroesophageal involvement in herpes simplex. Gastroenterology 70: 775, 1976
22. ICHIKAWA H et al: Practical X-ray Diagnosis of the Stomach for the Detection of Early Gastric Cancer. Tokyo, Bunkodo, 1965
23. KOEHLER PR, KYAW MM, FENLON JW: Diffuse gastrointestinal polyposis with ectodermal changes. Radiology 103: 589, 1972
24. KOEHLER PR, SALMON RB: Angiographic localization of unknown acute gastrointestinal bleeding sites. Radiology 89: 244, 1967
25. LASSER A, KOUFMAN WB: Adenomyoma of the stomach. Am J Dig Dis 22: 965, 1977
26. LAUFER I: A simple method for routine double-contrast study of the upper gastrointestinal tract. Radiology 117: 513, 1975
27. LAUFER I: Assessment of the accuracy of double contrast gastroduodenal radiology. Gastroenterology 71: 874, 1976
28. MAINZER M, AMBERG JR, MARGULIS AR: Superficial carcinoma of the stomach. Radiology 93: 109, 1969
29. MARSHAK RH, LINDNER AE: Radiology of the Small Intestine. Philadelphia, WB Saunders, 1970
30. MONTAGNE JP, MOSS AA, MARGULIS AR: Double blind study of single and double contrast upper gastrointestinal examinations using endoscopy as a control. Am J Roentgenol 130: 1041, 1978
31. NELSON SW: The discovery of gastric ulcers and the differential diagnosis between benignancy and malignancy. Radiol Clin North Am 7: 5, 1969
32. OCHSNER S: Benign ulceration on the greater curvature of the stomach: report of seven proved cases. Am J Roentgenol 75: 312, 1956

33. PALMER PES: Giant hypertrophic gastritis. J Fac Radiol 9: 175, 1958

34. PAUL LW, BENKENDORF C: Retrograde jejunogastric intussusception. Radiology 73: 234, 1959

35. PEREIRAS R, VIAMONTE M JR, RUSSELL et al: New techniques for interruption of gastroesophageal venous blood flow. Radiology 124: 313, 1977

36. REESE DF, HODGSON JR, DOCKERTY MB: Giant hypertrophy of the gastric mucosa (Menetrier's disease). A correlation of the roentgenographic, pathologic, and clinical findings. Am J Roentgenol 88: 619, 1962

37. RIGGS W JR, LONG L: The value of the plain film roentgenogram in pyloric stenosis. Am J Roentgenol 112: 77, 1971

38. SAWYER KC, HAMMER RW, FENTON WC: Gastric volvulus as a cause of obstruction. Report of seven cases. Arch Surg 72: 764, 1956

39. SEAMAN WB: Editorial: The areae gastricae. Am J Roentgenol 131: 554, 1978

40. SILBIGER ML, DONNER MW: Morphine in the evaluation of gastrointestinal disease. Radiology 90: 1090, 1968

41. TEIXIDOR HS, EVANS JA: Roentgenographic appearance of the distal esophagus and stomach after hiatal hernia repair. Am J Roentgenol 119: 245, 1973

17

THE DUODENUM

METHODS OF EXAMINATION

The roentgenologic examination of the duodenum is carried out as an integral part of a gastrointestinal series during and after the study of the stomach. The same filming technique is used as for the stomach since the duodenum is shown along with the stomach in the routine roentgenograms and with spot films obtained as needed in the individual case.

In order to outline the distended duodenum completely and to visualize the mucosal pattern clearly, *hypotonic duodenography* may be used. This method of examination consists of the administration of 1.0 to 2.0 mg glucagon intravenously or intramuscularly to produce hypotonia of the duodenum.[15] The patient is intubated and 100 to 200 ml of barium suspension are instilled into the duodenum followed by the introduction of air through the tube in an amount sufficient to distend the duodenum. Then spot films and radiographs are obtained in several projections, making certain that good mucosal detail of the entire duodenum is obtained. Pro-Banthine (30 mg) is used by some but in comparison with glucagon, it has more side effects, which persist for 4 to 6 hours, and its use is contraindicated in patients with glaucoma, prostatism, cardiac arrhythmias, or myocardial infarctions. Massive gastric dilatation has also been reported following the administration of 30-mg doses of Pro-Banthine. In Europe, Buscopan (hyoscine-N-butyl-bromide) is widely used and appears to be effective in 20- to 40-mg doses. It is said to produce no significant side effects and to be superior to glucagon and Pro-Banthine.[2] *Tubeless hypotonic duodenography*[11] may also be employed to avoid the necessity of inserting a nasogastric tube. Gas-producing mixtures such as Seidlitz powders and sparklets may be used to distend the duodenum. In our experience, this method is satisfactory in most patients; when it is unsuccessful, a tube can be inserted as described above. Hypotonic duodenography is employed to provide a detailed study of the mucosal fold pattern and of the fine anatomic features in the ampullary area. It is useful in patients with carcinoma in the distal common duct, ampulla of Vater, or pancreas, but is not as helpful in the assessment of pancreatitis.

Arteriography of the duodenum can be accomplished by celiac axis catheterization or by selective catheterization of the hepatic artery. Metoclopramide (Maxeran, Nordick Pharmaceuticals, Laval, Quebec, a drug with cholinergic effects, has been used extensively in Europe since the 1960s in the examination of the duodenum and small bowel. Given intramuscularly or intravenously in a dose of 10 to 20 mg, it stimulates gastric peristalsis, relaxes the pylorus, and allows prompt filling of the duodenum (see section "Contrast Visualization" in Chapter 18). The effects of the drug are noted within minutes after administration. Small-intestinal transit also is increased, shortening the time needed for a complete upper gastrointestinal series and small-bowel study.

ROENTGEN ANATOMY AND PHYSIOLOGY

The superior or first portion of the duodenum has a distinct roentgen appearance that differs considerably from the remainder. As viewed in profile, it has a triangular shape with the base at the pylorus and the apex continuous with the descending duodenum. Because of its shape it is known as the duodenal bulb or cap (see Figs. 16-2 and 16-3). The mucosal folds in the bulb are relatively sparse and usually disappear completely when the bulb is distended. Peristaltic contractions resemble those of the stomach and tend to occur in rhythm with gastric peristalsis. A collection of barium, simulating an ulcer or a filling defect, resembling a small mass may occur at or near the inferior aspect of the duodenal bulb, at the junction of the bulb and the descending duodenum. Since the defect changes with peristalsis and compression and has a typical location, there should be no difficulty in distinguishing it from a pathologic lesion.

The second or descending portion of the duodenum is retroperitoneal in location and has no mesentery. The change in the roentgen appearance from the first to the second portions is striking (Fig. 17-1). The latter has a rich mucosal pattern, even when distended, with crisscrossing folds of mucosa (the valvulae conniventes or folds of Kerkring) causing a fine serration of the margins when the surface is coated with barium mixture. Peristalsis is relatively rapid with broad waves sweeping the contents forward into the jejunum. Peristaltic waves never empty the lumen completely of barium as long as gastric emptying is in progress and a thin layer will coat the mucosal surface even after passage of a wave. The papilla of Vater is located on the inner side of the descending portion and is visualized as a small

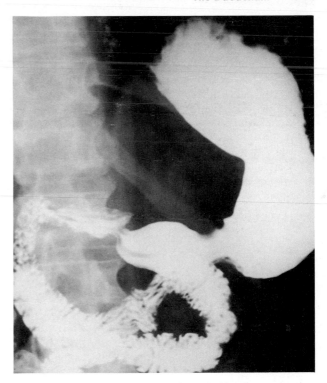

Fig. 17-1. The normal stomach and duodenum.

filling defect or localized mucosal irregularity. Other anatomic features observed in hypotonic duodenography in some patients[7] consist of a promontory or medial projection along the medial contour of the descending duodenum resulting in slight widening of the lumen. The lateral wall maintains a smooth continuity. When the promontory is present, usually there is a straight segment below it for 2 to 3 cm which is flat and devoid of valvulae.

The remainder of the duodenum resembles the descending portion. The duodenum surrounds the head of the pancreas and the ascending portion passes over the body of the pancreas to its junction with the jejunum at the angle of Treitz.

The superior mesenteric artery crosses the third portion of the duodenum just proximal to the angle of Treitz. In asthenic persons, pressure from this vessel may cause the appearance of mild duodenal obstruction with the duodenum somewhat dilated in its proximal portion and with reverse peristalsis occasionally seen (*the superior mesenteric artery syndrome*). This is a controversial syndrome; the diagnosis is made by exclusion, if at all. Most of the reports indicate that it occurs in asthenic patients with debilitating disease or trauma that leaves these patients emaciated and often immobilized. Duodenal dilatation is present, but obstruction is not complete and can be relieved by change to a prone or an oblique-prone position. Reverse peristaltic or churning movements occasionally are noted in otherwise normal-appearing individuals without there being any signs of obstruction. The visualization of churning movements in the duodenum, therefore, need not be of significance and it is probable that such movements can be initiated by deep palpation on the part of the examiner.

ANOMALIES OF THE DUODENUM

CONGENITAL OBSTRUCTION

Intrinsic

Duodenal Atresia. Congenital stenosis or atresia may be caused by delay or arrest in development at some stage in the formation of the duodenum. The duodenum is a frequent site of high gastrointestinal obstruction in the newborn. The increased incidence of duodenal obstruction in newborn mongoloids due to atresia and also to annular pancreas has been reported frequently. If the obstruction is complete, the stomach and the duodenum down to the level of the atresia will be distended with swallowed air; no gas will be visualized in the gastrointestinal tract below this level. Rarely an anomalous termination of a Y-shaped hepatopancreatic duct permits small amounts of gas to enter the duodenum below the atresia. One arm of the "Y" enters above and the other below the site of atresia. Gas can then enter the upper arm and gain access to the distal segment by way of the lower arm of the "Y." The atresia is distal to the ampulla of Vater in 75% of these patients. Incompetence of the sphincter of Oddi may be associated with neonatal duodenal obstruction, in which instance gas may be observed in the biliary ducts. Also gas has been reported in the portal venous system in neonates with duodenal obstruction and no evidence of infection.[18]

The diagnosis of duodenal atresia can be made from plain-film roentgenograms of the abdomen that will clearly show the gas distention of the stomach and the dilated proximal portion of the duodenum, with absence of gas elsewhere in the tract (the "double-bubble" sign). If a contrast substance is given it will stop at the level of the atresia (Fig. 17-2). If there is only a partial obstruction, gas will be visible below the duodenal level but distention of the stomach will

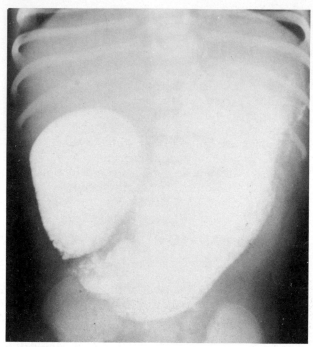

Fig. 17-2. Congenital atresia of the duodenum. Barium outlines the large stomach and a greatly dilated proximal duodenum to the stomach's right. Note that there is no gas beyond the proximal duodenum.

be present and the distended segment of duodenum may also be recognized by gas filling. The diagnosis can be confirmed by giving a small barium–water meal or one of the iodinated compounds such as Hypaque or Gastrografin, but this is seldom necessary. If a water-soluble, iodinated compound is used, it should be aspirated, since retention may cause gastritis with mucosal erosions and hemorrhage. We prefer the use of a small amount of barium for the roentgenographic study of these patients.

Partial obstruction may be caused by stenosis or incomplete atresia.

Duodenal Stenosis. Obstruction is incomplete in duodenal stenosis; otherwise, duodenal stenosis is similar to duodenal atresia. In duodenal stenosis, gastric and upper duodenal dilatation are present, but there is gas in the small bowel distal to the duodenum. After aspiration of fluid and gas, a small amount of barium is introduced which outlines the stenotic area and, hopefully, will fill the distal duodenum sufficiently to identify the position of the ligament of Treitz so that the possibility of the presence of malrotation can be excluded or confirmed.

Congenital Duodenal Diaphragm. This congenital anomaly is similar to the diaphragm or web sometimes observed in the gastric antrum. Usually a small orifice or aperture which may be eccentric is present. This anomaly is now believed to be the cause of *intraluminal duodenal diverticulum,* the latter being produced by peristalsis proximal to the partial obstruction which gradually pushes the diaphragm distally in the lumen of the duodenum until it resembles a wind sock. If this "sock" fills with barium, it appears as a dense, sausage-shaped intraluminal diverticulum, the thin wall of which may be outlined by barium in the duodenum distal to the opening. At times, an eccentric opening will allow barium to extend into the duodenum distal to it without filling the elongated diaphragm in which case the intraluminal diverticulum has the appearance of a radiolucent mass. Some authors believe that the intraluminal diverticulum is either a form of duplication or an intraluminal extension of an intramural diverticulum, but most now think that it is the result of a partially obstructing duodenal diaphragm. At times, both the common bile duct and pancreatic duct empty into the sac.

Extrinsic

Congenital Peritoneal Bands or "Veils." Cholecystoduodenocolic bands or membranes are of congenital origin and may cause obstruction of the duodenum in the infant. More often they do not, and are found with considerable frequency in the adult. They may cause a certain amount of deformity and distortion of the duodenal outline, particularly of the bulbar portion, and this deformity may be confused with that due to duodenal ulcer. Persistence of a mesoduodenum may allow the duodenum to twist upon itself, resulting in volvulus and consequent obstruction. Although these bands are of developmental origin, they may remain asymptomatic until adult life is reached, at which time obstructive phenomena may appear (Fig. 17-3). Symptomatic peritoneal bands in the adult, however, must be considered as relatively uncommon lesions.

Congenital peritoneal bands occurring in association with faulty rotation of the gut during its final stage of development may cause obstruction of the duodenum in the infant and occasionally in the adult. The site of obstruction is more frequent in the third portion of the duodenum than elsewhere. If the colon is examined by means of a barium enema, its abnormal position and the failure of complete rotation may be obvious. Otherwise the diagnosis of the type of du-

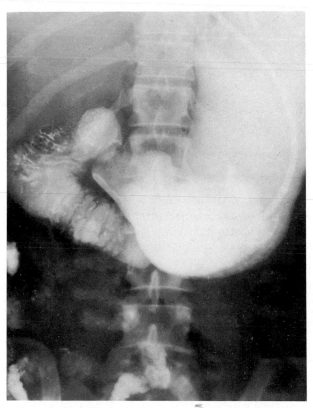

Fig. 17-3. Partial obstruction at the duodenojejunal junction caused by volvulus in this patient with a rotation anomaly of the gut. The stomach and duodenum are dilated. Because the obstruction is not complete some barium is present in loops of bowel distally. These loops are not enlarged. Note that they lie almost entirely on the right side. This patient's colon is on the left.

odenal obstruction cannot be made with certainty and the roentgen findings will resemble those described for duodenal atresia earlier in this chapter.

Isolated Incomplete Rotation of the Duodenum. This is a variant of malrotation in which the colon is in its normal position. Normally, the duodenum develops anterior to the superior mesenteric vessels, rotates 90 degrees to the right of the superior mesenteric artery, then backward and to the left 90 degrees, bringing it near the artery, and finally 90 degrees to the left into its natural position beneath and to the left of the artery as it enters the abdomen from the yolk sac. In isolated incomplete rotation, progress is arrested before the final 90-degree rotation and the duodenum is fixed and kinked in an abnormal position along the

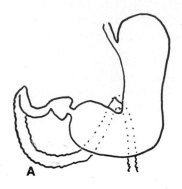
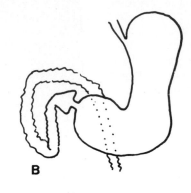

Fig. 17-4. Diagram illustrates two common anomalies involving the duodenum: **A.** Redundancy of the proximal duodenum. **B.** Duodenum inversum.

vessels. In approximately 10% of these patients some duodenal obstruction is present. If a barium enema study alone is done, the incomplete rotation cannot be detected; an upper gastrointestinal study is needed to determine the incomplete rotation with demonstration of the malposition of the duodenum and upper jejunum. Midgut volvulus does not usually occur in association with this anomaly.[8]

Annular Pancreas. Annular pancreas usually produces a partial duodenal obstruction and is usually found distal to the duodenal bulb. Associated anomalies such as malrotation, duodenal diaphragm, and peritoneal bands may be present. Findings are similar to those of duodenal stenosis and the roentgen diagnosis depends upon the demonstration of a smooth annular constriction, usually occurring in the upper part of the descending duodenum. In the adult, this lesion must be differentiated from a primary malignant tumor and from an ulcer of the second portion of the duodenum. In the former, the constriction is usually more irregular and involves a longer segment of the duodenum. The mucosal pattern is destroyed through the area of constriction. Ulcers of the post-bulbar portion of the duodenum depend on demonstration of an ulcer crater. In the very young infant, annular pancreas must be differentiated from congenital bands and veils. However, the defect of annular pancreas is usually longer than that of congenital bands or veils. The exact nature of the lesion is very difficult to determine prior to surgery, and the roentgen diagnosis is often limited to that of an obstructing lesion of the proximal duodenum.

Other Causes. In addition to the causes of duodenal obstruction described in the foregoing, there are other rare causes. These include duplication cysts, which may be large enough to cause obstruction, and other rare tumors. The majority of cases, however, are due to stenosis or atresia, congenital bands or volvulus, abnormal fixation, or annular pancreas.

REDUNDANCY OF THE SUPERIOR PORTION

The superior portion of the duodenum may be unusually long and hang downward as a loop between the bulb and the superior duodenal flexure (Fig. 17-4). Such elongation has no clinical significance but it may be mistaken for a deformed bulb caused by an ulcer.

DUODENUM INVERSUM

As a minor anomaly of rotation, the duodenum may loop to the right rather than to the left so that the descending and ascending portions tend to overlie one another; or, the ascending portion may actually lie to the right of the descending crossing to the left, at or above the level of the pylorus to its point of junction with the jejunum (see Fig. 17-4). The jejunum is in normal position and the rest of the small bowel is usually in normal situs.

RIGHT-SIDED DUODENUM

As part of a more extensive rotation anomaly, the duodenum together with the jejunum and the ileum may lie largely to the right of the midline with the colon on the left side of the abdomen (nonrotation of the bowel; see Ch. 18).

DUPLICATIONS

Congenital duplication of the duodenum is a rare anomaly but corresponds essentially to the same type of lesion that may be found in any other part of the gastrointestinal tract. It consists of a closed cystic mass of variable size that develops in the wall of the duodenum. The coats of the cyst reproduce the coats of the duodenum or some other part of the intestinal tract. Thus the lining of the cyst may be gastric or colonic mucosa instead of duodenal. The cystic mass may be submucosal intramural, or subserosal. When large it is impossible to determine the exact nature of such a mass from its roentgen features and it generally shows only the characteristics of an intramural tumor, with a smooth-surfaced mass bulging into the duodenal lumen but with mucosa intact over the surface. The lesion, if of any appreciable size, may cause obstruction. The small duplications are usually asymptomatic. Roentgen diagnosis, if at all possible, is usually limited to that of an intramural mass and an etiologic diagnosis is hardly possible. Duplications are apt to give rise to symptoms rather early in life because of the increasing size of the mass as fluid accumulates within it. This is also true of those involving other parts of the gastrointestinal tract. In small intramural duplications, alterations in shape on compression or during peristalis suggest its cystic nature, but lipoma may have similar characteristics.

DISEASES OF THE DUODENUM

DUODENAL ULCER

Duodenal ulcer is the most frequent organic lesion encountered in the upper gastrointestinal tract. The ratio of duodenal to gastric ulcers is on the order of 4 or 5 to 1. Most duodenal ulcers develop in the first portion of the duodenum, the duodenal bulb. A less common site is at the junction of the first and second portions or in the immedite proximal part of the descending portion; these are called postbulbar ulcers. Below this level ulcers in the duodenum are extremely rare. Ulcers in the duodenal bulb may form on any wall or surface, although they are somewhat more frequent on the posterior wall and along the lesser curvature than elsewhere.

Roentgen Observations

The Ulcer Crater. The demonstration of the ulcer crater is as important in the diagnosis of a duodenal ulcer as it is in the recognition of a gastric ulcer and represents the one positive roentgen sign of the lesion. When visualized on edge the ulcer crater projects as a niche, similar to the niche of a gastric ulcer except for its smaller size (Fig. 17-5). Frequently the crater is not seen directly on edge but rather is visualized *en face,* and is brought out to best advantage by applying compression over the bulb. As the barium content is expressed out of the more pliable portion of the bulb, the crater remains filled because of its rigid walls and appears as a dense round spot (Fig. 17-6). If a proper amount of compression is used so that a thin coating of barium remains on the mucosa, the folds can be seen to radiate outward from the crater as they do with gastric ulcers. The crater usually is small and less than 1 cm in diameter. Infrequently a very large crater, several centimeters in diameter, may be present (giant crater) (Fig. 17-7; see also Fig. 17-12). Such a crater may be so large as completely to replace the bulb and may actually be mistaken for a normal bulb. The constancy of its shape and persistent retention of barium with inability to express barium out of it on manual palpation are significant findings. The crater of a duodenal ulcer may be difficult to visualize when the general contour of the bulb is extremely irregular and deformed by scar tissue and it may be impossible to state at times whether an ulcer crater is present or whether the deformity is only the result of scar-tissue formation from a previous ulcer. With an acute duodenal ulcer the bulbar outline may be normal and only when compression is used will the lesion be identified. This is particularly true when the crater is directly on the anterior or the posterior wall, where it may be difficult to bring the lesion into relief so that the projecting niche becomes visible.

Marginal Deformity. Regardless of the site of the ulcer crater, the margins of the duodenal bulb usually show some irregularity in contour as a result of one or more incisurae. These are similar to the incisurae that may develop on the greater curvature opposite a gastric ulcer on the lesser curve, and in the early stages are spastic in nature; later on they may become fixed as a result of scar tissue. In the presence of an acute ulcer, marginal deformity may be slight or entirely absent and what deformity is present is caused by spasm. This may be inconstant and vary during the examination. With more chronic ulcers, deformity becomes fixed and as fibrosis and scarring develop the normal contours of the bulb become completely lost. Once this stage is reached, the deformity is permanent even though the ulcer heals (Fig. 17-8). One of the common deformities seen in chronic duodenal ulcer is that which resembles a collar button. The apex of the bulb is constricted, leaving rounded projections at the base adjacent to the pylorus. The appearance resembles that of a collar button very closely and this type of deformity is characteristic of a chronic ulcer involving the apex of the

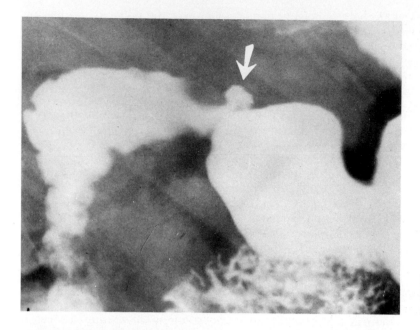

Fig. 17-5. Duodenal ulcer. The ulcer crater **(arrow)** projects from the superior surface near the base of the bulb.

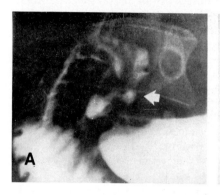
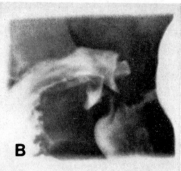

Fig. 17-6. Duodenal ulcer. **A.** The ulcer crater is easily seen in the central base of the duodenal bulb **(arrow). B.** Roentgenologic study of same patient shown in **A** after 6 weeks of treatment. The crater has disappeared, but the duodenum is distorted, indicating residual scarring.

bulb (Fig. 17-9). A wide variety of deformities of the duodenal bulb may occur as a result of chronic or recurring duodenal ulcer, however.

Postbulbar Ulcer. Duodenal ulcers occurring distal to the bulb usually develop on the inner side at the junction of the bulb and the descending duodenum. The crater projects as a niche and an incisura forms on the opposite side, causing a rather classic deformity (Fig. 17-10). The incisura represents an indrawing of the lateral wall of the duodenum that tends to become fixed and permanent as a result of scar tissue. Becasue of the location, an ulcer at this site may be obscured by the overlapping shadows of the bulb and the descending duodenum. There is considerable similarity in the appearance of all post-

bulbar duodenal ulcers. When chronic or recurring, they may result in an eccentric ringlike stricture of the upper descending duodenum.

Complications of Duodenal Ulcer
Bleeding. Although bleeding is not a contraindication to barium study of the upper gastrointestinal tract unless the patient is in shock, this examination is not usually undertaken as an initial study. Endoscopy is usually performed first and is most useful when the source of bleeding is in the proximal duodenum, but if bleeding is massive, its site of origin may not be determined. Since the accuracy of localization by angiography is improved when bleeding is massive, this study can be performed (Fig. 17-11). Selective catheterization of the bleeding vessel then per-

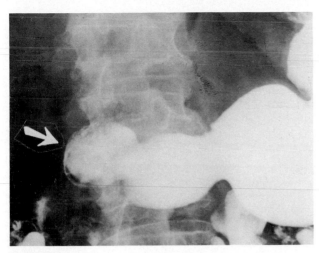

Fig. 17-7. Giant duodenal ulcer. The crater is the size of the normal duodenal bulb in this patient.

mits the use of vasoconstricting drugs or embolizing the bleeding artery to control bleeding. Therefore, angiography may be used as a therapeutic measure even though the bleeding site has been identified by other methods.

In chronic or intermittent bleeding manifested by hematemesis or melena, when endoscopy fails to locate the site, barium study of the upper gastrointestinal tract is indicated. When patients drink barium through a straw while in a supine position, they usually swallow enough air to provide a reasonable air contrast study of the proximal duodenum. The patients may be chronically ill and weak, but the examination can be performed with little compression and with the patient recumbent if necessary.

Obstruction. Duodenal ulcer is the most frequent cause of pyloric obstruction. When only a partial obstruction exists, the stomach may empty itself within a normal period of time or there may be a small amount of retention after overnight fasting. Fluoroscopically, peristaltic waves are vigorous, they are increased in depth, and one wave follows another at relatively close intervals. In this stage the antrum often appears somewhat enlarged during the period of antral diastole but contracts promptly as a result of peristalsis. The periods of peristaltic activity may last for a minute or two and alternate with periods of quiescence. With increase in the degree of obstruction the stomach is unable to empty itself within the usual time and gastric retention is found at the time of roentgen examination. Hyperactive peristalsis may

still occur, but the periods of activity are shortened and the stomach becomes more and more atonic. Eventually the obstruction may increase to the point where little emptying occurs through the pylorus and large amounts of fluid accumulate within the stomach. The stomach may become huge and, with the patient in the upright position, hang down into the lower abdomen or pelvis. At this stage the muscular activity has become greatly diminished and the stomach is, in fact, decompensated. Roentgenologic examination of such a stomach is hampered greatly by its size and by the retention of the fluid and food. Preliminary gatric aspiration and lavage may remove some of the material but seldom empties the stomach completely. Unless there is some passage of the barium mixture through the pylorus, it may not be possible to determine the cause of the obstruction. If the pylorus and duodenal bulb are visualized, the cause usually is apparent and it can be decided whether a duodenal ulcer is responsible or whether the lesion is on the gastric side of the pylorus (*e.g.,* a gastric ulcer or carcinoma). In difficult cases, reexamination after a period of several days, during which time repeated aspirations are undertaken or continuous gastric suction is carried out, may allow a more definitive examination to be made.

Perforation. Some of the roentgen findings in perforation of the gastrointestinal tract are described in Chapter 13, in the section entitled "Pneumoperitoneum" in which the escape of gas and its detection in roentgenograms of the abdomen are discussed. The most frequent cause of so-called "spontaneous pneumoperitoneum" is rupture of an ulcer. A posterior-wall duodenal ulcer may perforate into the lesser omental sac and the gas and fluid may accumulate and be loculated in this area. Air from a perforated posterior-wall ulcer may dissect along the retroperitoneal fascial planes and be visualized as linear streaks or bubbles along the psoas sheaths or as a more localized accumulation of gas bubbles in the posterior abdominal wall. Rarely, a perforated duodenal ulcer will cause pneumatosis of the jejunum and distal duodenum. Subserosal dissection of gas from the ulcer is the probable cause. There may also be penetration into the bile duct, resulting in a choledochoduodenal fistula.

In roentgenograms demonstrating a spontaneous pneumoperitoneum, Frimann–Dahl has called attention to the fact that at times gas within the duodenal bulb may clearly outline the deformity caused by an ulcer or even show the crater of the ulcer; in these instances the diagnosis of the cause of the perfora-

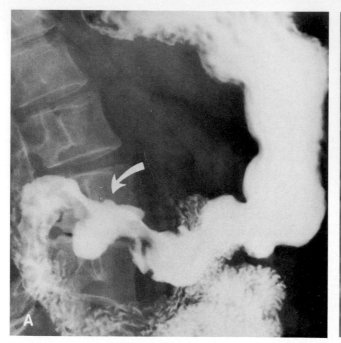 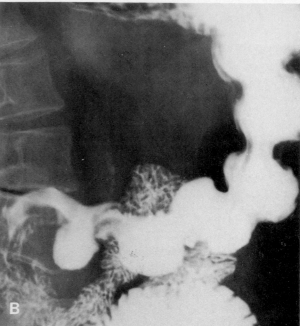

Fig. 17-8. Duodenal ulcer. **A.** The duodenal bulb is deformed, and there is a small crater projecting as an ulcer niche on the lesser curvature side **(arrow). B.** Six weeks later the crater has disappeared, but the contour of the duodenal bulb remains abnormal.

tion can be made without a barium-meal examination. In patients with suspected perforation and no pneumoperitoneum, a small amount (50 ml) of Gastrografin may be given by mouth 5 to 10 minutes before abdominal and chest films are obtained. Extravasation will occur by way of the perforation in a high percentage of patients.[9]

If the roentgen examination is not carried out for a period of 5 or 6 hours after the perforation has occurred, a certain amount of adynamic ileus is almost always present. Gas accumulates in loops of small intestine and in the colon, although the distention is seldom very severe. Evidence of free fluid may be suggested by blurring of the inferior edge of the right lobe of the liver which, normally, can be seen. These latter signs, of coure, are not specific for perforation.

A perforated ulcer may become walled-off and later, when the patient is examined by means of a barium meal, a sinus tract may be demonstrated as it fills with the barium. An example of this is shown in Figure 17-12.

Double Pyloric Canal. This condition, actually a gastroduodenal fistula, secondary to peptic ulcer, has been described in Chapter 16.

Concomitant Gastric Ulcer. Many believe that patients with duodenal ulcers may develop gastric ulcer

Fig. 17-9. Duodenal ulcer. This is an example of a "collar-button" type of deformity. **Arrow** indicates the ulcer crater, which is visible as a small, dense area along the inferior surface near the constriction.

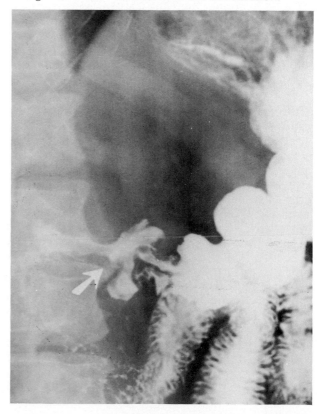

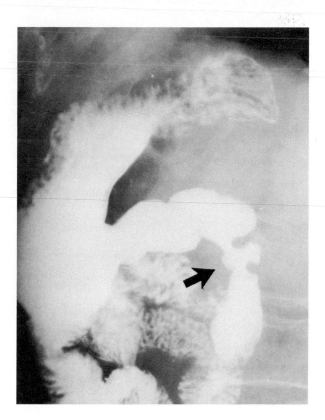

Fig. 17-10. Postbulbar duodenal ulcer. The **arrow** indicates the ulcer crater on the inner surface of the upper part of the descending or second portion of the duodenum. The crater with one or more incisurae opposite it is typical of an ulcer in this location.

Fig. 17-11. Bleeding duodenal ulcer demonstrated by arteriography. The gastroduodenal artery, arising as a branch of the hepatic artery, leads to a dense accumulation of extravasated contrast material in the duodenal bulb **(arrow).**

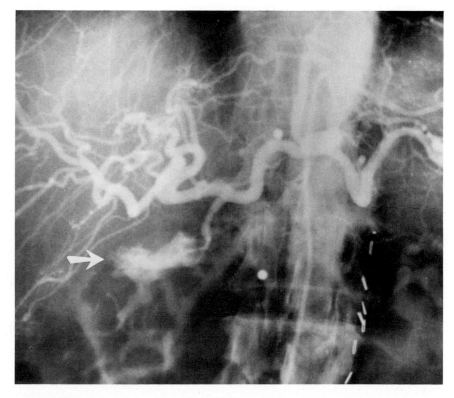

as a complication, caused either by excessive antral stimulation resulting in hypersecretion and gastric ulceration or by reflux of alkaline duodenal content into the antrum where alkali gastritis may develop leading to gastric ulcer. On the other hand, the presence of duodenal ulcer makes it unlikely that gastric carcinoma will develop. The nature of this relationship is uncertain but may have to do with gastric acidity.

Healing of Duodenal Ulcer. If an ulcer crater has been demonstrated at the initial examination, its progress can be followed by serial studies. Disappearance of the ulcer crater indicates healing of the ulcer. The general contour deformity of the bulb usually does not change since it is, in most instances, caused by scarring and fibrosis. The importance of crater demonstration therefore becomes obvious, because bulbar deformity alone may give no clue as to the presence of an active ulcer (see Figs. 17-6 and 17-8). In patients with acute duodenal ulcer and no previous history of ulcer disease, healing may leave no residual deformity, however.

DIVERTICULA OF THE DUODENUM

Duodenal diverticula are found very frequently during roentgen examination of the upper gastrointestinal tract. They are acquired lesions that may form in any part of the duodenum but the most common site is along the inner side of the descending duodenum close to the ampulla of Vater. Duodenal diverticula vary greatly in size from those that measure on the order of 1 cm in diameter to an occasional large one that measures from 8 to 10 cm in size. Giant diverticula measuring up to 20 cm in diameter have been described arising from the outer (right lateral) aspect of the duodenum. Although duodenal diverticula are usually considered to be asymptomatic lesions of no clinical significance, an occasional, very large diverticulum, by retention of food, may cause symptoms of partial upper gastrointestinal obstruction. In rare instances, ulceration within a diverticulum has been reported as a cause of upper gastrointestinal tract bleeding. Rarely the "blind loop" syndrome may apparently be caused by a duodenal diverticulum in which bacterial activity gives rise to vitamin B_{12} deficiency, hyperchromic anemia, and diarrhea.

A single diverticulum is the rule but occasionally two or more are found and, in an infrequent patient, multiple diverticula of the duodenum are present, associated with multiple diverticula of the jejunum.

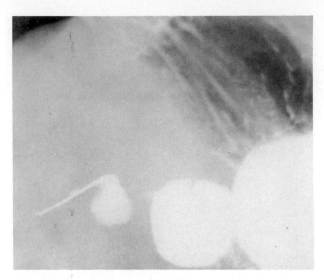

Fig. 17-12. Duodenal ulcer with a fistulous tract secondary to previous rupture. The rounded accumulation of barium represents a large ulcer crater that is almost as large as the normal duodenal bulb. The narrow tract extends beneath the right lobe of the liver for a distance of about 3 cm.

Roentgen Observations. Diverticula of the duodenum resemble those occurring elsewhere in the gastrointestinal tract. The diverticulum consists of a projecting sac which, when filled with barium mixture, appears as a pouchlike projection that is connected by a narrow neck to the duodenal lumen (Fig. 17-13). The diagnosis is made without difficulty. Diverticula in the distal part of the duodenum may be obscured by barium in the stomach; also, when the stomach is palpated or compressed over a diverticulum, a false impression of an ulcer crater in the gastric wall may be obtained. A diverticulum can be distinguished from a duodenal ulcer by the smooth, rounded, pouchlike appearance, the absence of spasm, and the lack of distortion of mucosal folds about the orifice. Also the mucosa of the orifice and of the diverticulum is smooth. At times an accumulation of gas or nonopaque food material may be found within the diverticulum, producing a filling defect. This is usually inconstant and may disappear or otherwise change in appearance during observation. At times it may be necessary to repeat the examination to make certain that one is not dealing with a neoplasm developing within the diverticulum. Rarely the common bile and pancreatic ducts enter a duodenal diverticulum. This can be suspected when an irregularity resembling the papilla is observed in a divertic-

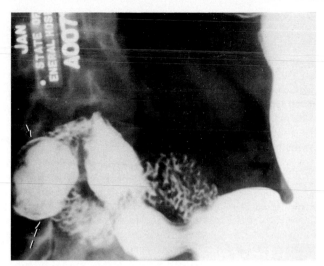

Fig. 17-13. Diverticulum of the second portion of the duodenum **(arrows).**

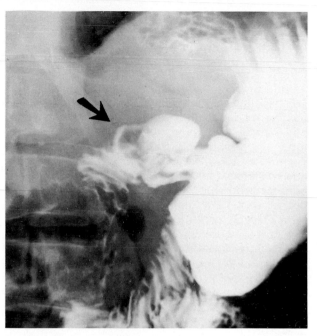

Fig. 17-14. Benign polyp of the duodenum **(arrow).**

ulum arising close to the usual entrance of these ducts. Endoscopic retrograde cholangiography (ERCP) or transhepatic cholangiography would be necessary to confirm the diagnosis, however. As a rare occurrence, a diverticulum of the duodenum may be entirely intraluminal. It is visualized as a pocketlike accumulation of barium projecting within the duodenal lumen. It occurs in the region of the ampulla of Vater and may be a cause of partial obstruction. It has been described more fully in the section on congenital duodenal diaphragm in this chapter. Rarely a large cholodochocele may appear as an intraluminal mass and resemble an intraluminal diverticulum.

TUMORS OF THE DUODENUM

Considered as a group, neoplasms of the duodenum are rare. Primary tumors are less frequent than is secondary invasion of the duodenum by carcinoma of the pancreas, the common bile duct, or other contiguous structures.

Benign Tumors

Benign polyps or adenomas originating in the duodenum are rare. The roentgen signs are similar to those of polyps elsewhere in the gastrointestinal tract. The polyp causes a sharply circumscribed, rounded filling defect in the barium shadow (Fig. 17-14). Air bubbles and food particles can be excluded by noting the

constancy of the defect. Occasionally a repeat examination is needed to be certain that one is dealing with an organic lesion. The polyp often has a pedicle and it may move over some distance under the effect of peristalis. The pedicle may be visualized as a stalklike shadow and at its point of attachment an inward tenting of the wall may be caused as the stalk is put under tension by a peristaltic wave. Adenoma of Brunner's glands may also present as polypoid intramural masses, whereas hypertrophy of Brunner's glands appears as multiple intramural masses projecting into the lumen of the duodenal bulb. Occasionally a pedunculated polyp of the gastric antrum will prolapse intermittently through the pylorus and the head of the polyp may be found in the duodenal bulb (see Fig. 16-23). Such a prolapsing polyp may lead to the signs and symptoms of intermittent pyloric obstruction.

A tumor that forms within the duodenal wall beneath the mucosa is called an intramural–extramucosal tumor. A variety of benign tumors occur in the duodenum but as a group they are uncommon. The most frequently encountered are leiomyomas, lipomas, adenomatous polyps, and Brunner's gland adenomas. Less common lesions include ectopic pancreas, neurofibromas, angiomas, hamartomas, fibromas, carcinoids, and duplication cysts. Of these lesions, lipomas may change shape under the influence of peristalsis because of the usual softness of the tumor. This may be a helpful differential sign but a few cases of duplication cysts also have been reported showing a similar finding so that it probably is not completely specific for lipoma. The defect caused by an intramural lesion is characterized by the fact that mucosal folds are visualized over its surface. The defect forms a smooth, convex bulge into the lumen, and usually a fairly sharp angle is formed by the junction of the defect and the normal duodenal wall. Ulceration may develop on the surface of the tumor and the ulcer crater may fill and be visualized as a dense, round shadow representing the barium-filled pocket, the "target sign." Occasionally the tumor develops largely beneath the serosa and the major portion of it may project outside of the duodenal lumen, so that little narrowing of the lumen or evidence of obstruction is present. The roentgen diagnosis of aberrant pancreatic nodules has been considered in the section dealing with these lesions in Chapter 16. Only the larger nodules that measure at least a centimeter in diameter are likely to cause sufficient deformity of the duodenal lumen to be visualized roentgenologically and it usually is impossible to determine the histologic nature of such a lesion from roentgen examination alone. The usual diagnosis is that of an intramural lesion, type undetermined. A sign that may be of value in differential diagnosis consists in the demonstration of a fine, hairline extension of barium from the duodenal lumen into the defect caused by the mass. This has been interpreted as evidence of a pancreatic duct opening from the nodule into the duodenal lumen. Closed duplications of the duodenum or so-called "enterogenous cysts" also may reveal roentgen signs indistinguishable from those of other intramural masses. Other duplication cysts may be large enough to cause obstruction of the duodenum. Extrinsic benign lesions such as pancreatic pseudocyst may also cause obstruction. Rarely, gallbladder disease with fistula into the duodenum and impaction of stones there may be responsible for duodenal obstruction.

Duodenal *varices* presenting as intramural masses projecting into the duodenal lumen may occur in patients with portal hypertension or with extrahepatic portal obstruction. Their appearance is similar to that of esophageal varices. They are observed with the patient in the prone position; they disappear on pressure and are not observed when the patient is in the upright position. They must be differentiated from hypertrophy of Brunner's glands and small tumors that produce intramural masses projecting into the duodenal lumen.

Carcinoma of the Duodenum

About 45% of small-bowel carcinomas arise in the duodenum; 35% are located in the first portion, 45% in the second portion, and 10% each in the third and fourth portions. The incidence is higher in patients with Gardner's syndrome than in the general population, even though antecedent polyps are not present. Adenocarcinoma of the duodenum is similar to carcinoma elsewhere in the gastrointestinal tract. There may be multinodular filling defects, ulceration with mucosal destruction, and/or rigidity and constriction of the lumen or obstruction, which is seen most frequently in infiltrating lesions. The mucosal pattern is absent over the surface of the lesion and the defect is constant, fixed, and rigid, resembling essentially the same type of defect encountered in carcinoma elsewhere in the gastrointestinal tract (Fig. 17-15). Some degree of obstruction is the rule and the duodenum above the lesion will be dilated. Gastric retention and moderate gastric dilatation often are noted. These carcinomas may be difficult to differentiate from primary pancreatic carcinoma, ampullary carcinoma, lymphoma, metastases, and sometimes, from inflammatory disease. Angiography may be very helpful in determining the site of origin of the lesion and CT scanning will probably play a role as well.

The findings in carcinoma arising in the biliary duct system have been described in previous chapters.

Villous Adenoma

Villous adenoma is a rare tumor in the duodenum. Roentgenologically, its cauliflower appearance with a lacy network of barium outlining the fronds is similar to that of villous adenoma in the colon.

Sarcoma

Leiomyosarcoma, although rare, is the most common sarcoma of the duodenum. It produces a lobulated intramural filling defect often with central ulceration or sinus-tract formation. The latter extends into the necrotic central portion of a mass which may be large and bulky. Similar changes are present in benign, smooth muscle tumors, but, when the lesion is greater than 5 cm in diameter, the chances are that it is sarcoma. Much of the mass may be extramural and its size will not be recognized on barium studies. On arteriography, neovascularity and venous stasis can be shown unless extensive necrosis is present. Other duodenal sarcomas are extremely rare.

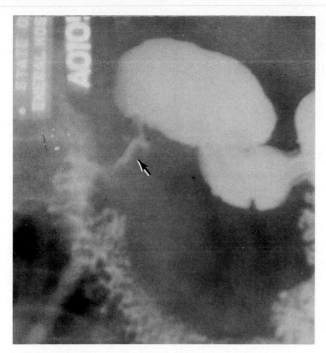

Fig. 17-15. Carcinoma of the second portion of the duodenum **(arrow).** The lesion is annular and causes an irregular constriction similar to that due to carcinoma elsewhere in the gastrointestinal tract. Although the obstruction is incomplete the duodenal bulb is distended.

Lymphoma of the Duodenum

Lymphoma is rare in the duodenum since its incidence increases from the pylorus to the ileocecal valve. Radiographic manifestations include multiple small nodules producing a cobblestone appearance, a form in which the wall may be diffusely infiltrated, a polypoid form, an invasive form with mesenteric lymph-node enlargement producing large extraluminal masses, and a form in which there is communication through multiple fistulas between intraluminal masses and adjacent bowel. Also, there may be spread of gastric antral lymphoma submucosally to involve the duodenal bulb and proximal descending duodenum causing contour deformities, filling defects, and ulcerations that are also observed in the stomach.

Duodenal Metastases

Rarely the duodenum may be invaded by adjacent gastric carcinoma. Also it may be invaded or distorted secondarily by carcinoma of the proximal transverse colon, occasionally with production of a duodenocolic fistula. Rarely, retroperitoneal node involvement from distal tumors may distort and/or invade the duodenum.

DUODENITIS

Duodenitis is a frequent accompaniment of duodenal ulcer. As a separate entity without associated ulceration it probably is infrequent and the diagnosis can not be made on roentgen examination. The clinical signs and symptoms are essentially those of ulcer.

The roentgen findings that have been described include (1) irritability of the duodenal bulb, (2) inconstant deformity of the bulbar outline, and (3) coarsening of the mucosal folds probably caused by excessive activity of the muscularis. However, these signs can occur in the normal person and they cannot be depended upon as evidence of duodenitis and therefore the diagnosis by radiographic methods is tenuous, at best.

REGIONAL ENTERITIS (CROHN'S DISEASE) OF DUODENUM

The duodenum is an infrequent site of regional enteritis. The stomach is often involved when the duodenum is involved in this disease. The findings vary considerably as in other portions of the bowel. In some of these patients there are spiculated ulcers, linear ulcers, and a cobblestone appearance, usually associated with some narrowing. In others there is stenosis of varying lengths and degrees with effacement of the normal mucosal pattern (Fig. 17-16). Also, there may be filling of the biliary and pancreatic ducts by way of fistulous communications or through a diseased ampulla of Vater. When the duodenum is involved, the disease is usually present elsewhere in the small bowel; this is often characteristic and helps to confirm the diagnosis.

DUODENAL TUBERCULOSIS

Isolated involvement of the duodenum by tuberculosis is extremely rare in the United States but is occasionally encountered in undeveloped countries.[3] The most common site of involvement of the gastrointestinal tract is the ileocecal region. Radiographic findings in the duodenum are those of small, superficial, multiple ulcerations usually observed in an area where the mucosa is thickened, resulting in narrowing of the lumen. Long, narrow ulcers, located be-

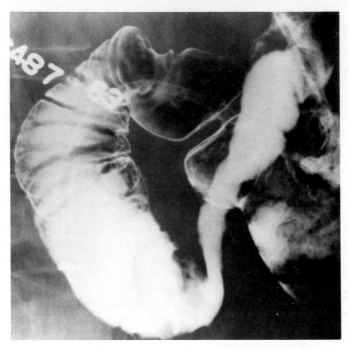

Fig. 17-16. Regional enteritis (Crohn's disease) involving the third and fourth portions of the duodenum. It is manifested by the long, relatively smooth stricturelike narrowing noted on this hypotonic duodenogram.

tween the thickened folds may resemble those of Crohn's disease. Caseation with abscess formation may lead to fistula and the development of sinus tracts; involvement of adjacent nodes may result in indentation of the duodenum, at times sufficient to cause obstruction. Fibrosis is common and strictures of the second portion result. Crohn's disease is the major consideration in the differential diagnosis, but the lesions also may resemble those of duodenal carcinoma.

OTHER CONDITIONS

Hypertrophy of Brunner's Glands

Infrequently the duodenal glands of Brunner may become enlarged sufficiently so that they cause nodular defects in the bulbar outline. Hypertrophy of these glands usually follows and is associated with gastric hyperacidity; it is thought to be a protective response against hyperacidity. Roentgenologically the enlarged glands cause multiple nodular defects in the bulbar shadow, giving it a mottled or cobblestone appearance. The walls of the bulb remain pliable and its motility is undisturbed. The process may be mistaken for a polyposis of the duodenum. Occasionally, a single gland will undergo hypertrophy causing a small, solitary, intramural mass which cannot be distinguished from other intramural tumors.

Periduodenal Adhesions

Inflammatory adhesions, particularly between the gallbladder and the duodenum, are frequent. These may cause a distortion in the outline of the bulb or a flattening of its superior surface. The duodenal bulb may form a sharp angle with the pyloric antrum or there may be an unusually sharp angulation between the bulb and the descending portion of the duodenum. At times the deformity caused by adhesions may resemble that of a duodenal ulcer rather closely and differentiation may be difficult. As noted in the section on "Duodenal Ulcer," the demonstration of the ulcer crater is a highly reliable sign and in its absence the diagnosis of duodenal ulcer often is presumptive.

Prolapse of Gastric Mucosa through the Pylorus

When the mucosa of the gastric antrum is redundant it may prolapse through the pylorus under the influence of active peristalsis. Slight degrees of mucosal prolapse are observed frequently during gastrointestinal examinations. There has been a difference of opinion concerning the significance of this finding. Some have believed it to be a frequent cause of symptoms related to the upper gastrointestinal tract and have considered it to be a cause for bleeding.

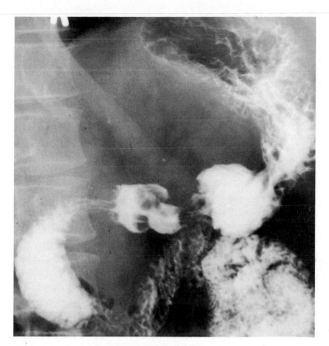

Fig. 17-17. Prolapse of gastric mucosa through the pylorus. The base of the duodenal bulb is indented by prominent gastric mucosal folds that have prolapsed into it.

Other observers have stated that, in the majority of patients, demonstrable prolapse of mucosa through the pylorus has little if any significance as far as symptoms are concerned. While the lesion may be a cause for gastrointestinal bleeding, this is probably an unusual complication. Evidence has been presented to show that the same type of defect can be demonstrated in individuals who are having no gastrointestinal symptoms and one should be cautious about attributing much significance to its presence.

Roentgen Observations. Typically, prolapse of the gastric mucosa results in a lobulated filling defect in the base of the duodenal bulb leading to an irregular concavity of the base of the bulb (Fig. 17-17). Mucosal folds in the prepyloric area of the stomach usually can be traced through the pylorus and can be seen to be continuous with the small nodular defects in the base of the bulb. The resulting defect has been likened to that of an open umbrella. When the prolapse is extensive, the folds may fill the major portion of the bulb as a gastric peristaltic wave passes through the antrum. As the wave relaxes the folds tend to return into the antrum and the defect in the base of the bulb will diminish or completely disap-

pear. The defect caused by mucosal prolapse resembles in some ways that resulting from hypertrophy of the pylorus. It is distinguished from the latter by the inconstancy of the defect and its intensification by peristalsis in the antrum, by the nodular type of filling defect, and by a lack of narrowing or elongation of the pyloric canal on the gastric side. Prolapsed mucosa can be differentiated from the defect caused by a prolapsing gastric polyp (Fig. 17-18) by the continuity of folds in the antrum with those in the bulb and by the multiplicity of nodulations in the defect (umbrella sign) rather than a single mass.

Intramural Hematoma of the Duodenum

Hematoma of the duodenum usually follows abdominal trauma, or it occurs in patients subject to bleeding tendencies such as in hemophiliacs or in those receiving anticoagulants. Roentgen examination reveals evidence of an intramural mass without sharply demarcated margins. The valvulae conniventes appear stretched, producing a "coiled-spring" appearance (Fig. 17-19). Also, the pointed projections of the valvulae have been likened to a picket fence. In other patients the hematoma forms a more circumscribed

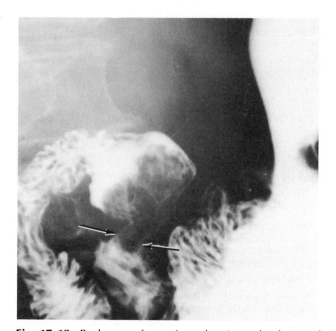

Fig. 17-18. Prolapse of gastric polyp into the base of the duodenal bulb. Note the large mass encroaching on the base of the duodenal bulb. **Arrows** outline the base of the pedicle in the prepyloric area of the stomach.

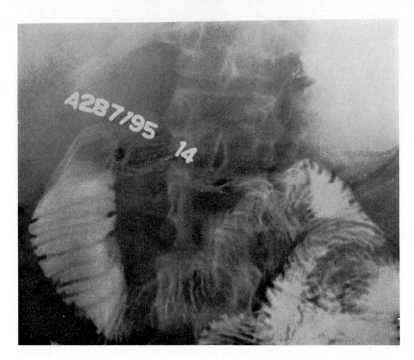

Fig. 17-19. Intramural hematoma of the duodenum in a patient with hemophilia. The lesion is largely confined to the third and fourth portions of the duodenum. Note the parallel or picket-fence arrangement of the folds and the lack of sharp definition of the margins of the duodenal abnormality.

intramural mass with well-defined margins. Obstruction of some degree is usually present and may be complete. The hematoma regresses spontaneously and reexamination in a few days to a week will show the improvement. Because of the hazards associated with surgery in hemophilia and other causes for spontaneous bleeding, accurate diagnosis is very important. In traumatic cases there is a predilection for hematomas to occur in the retroperitoneal or fixed portion of the duodenum. The right psoas margin may be obliterated owing to associated retroperitoneal bleeding. In hemophiliacs and others with bleeding tendencies the hematoma may occur elsewhere in the gastrointestinal tract.

Blunt Duodenal Trauma

In addition to intramural hematoma, secondary to blunt abdominal trauma as indicated in the previous paragraph, rupture of the duodenum may occur.[19] Roentgenographic findings may be subtle since the perforation in these patients is usually in the second and third portions of the duodenum, which are retroperitoneal. Gas dissecting into the perirenal and psoas area may produce a bubbly or mottled pattern of radiolucencies in the right flank. Psoas muscle may be obscured by the presence of associated retroperitoneal blood or fluid. Nonspecific conditions such

as scoliosis and segmental ileus may also be noted. These latter findings are only suggestive, at best. Early diagnosis is possible only by careful search of technically good roentgenograms of the abdomen in patients involved in accidents in which there is blunt upper abdominal trauma.

REFERENCES AND SELECTED READINGS

1. ABELL MR, LIMOND RV, BLAMEY WE et al: Allergic granulomatosis with massive gastric involvement. N Engl J Med 282:665, 1970
2. ARYE-SMITH G: Hyoscine-N-Butylbromide (Buscopan) as a duodenal relaxant in tubeless duodenography. Acta Radiol [Diagn] (Stockh) 17:701, 1976
3. BLACK GA, CARSKY EW: Duodenal tuberculosis. Am J Roentgenol 131:329, 1978
4. DODD GD, FISHLER JS, PARK OK: Hyperplasia of Brunner's glands. Report of two cases with review of the literature. Radiology 60:814, 1953
5. DODD GB, NAFIS WA: Annular pancreas in the adult. Am J Roentgenol 75:333, 1956
6. EATON SB, BENEDICT KT JR, FERRUCCI JT et al: Hypotonic duodenography. Radiol Clin North Am 8:125, 1970
7. FERRUCCI JT, JR, BENEDICT KT, PAGE DL et al: Radio-

graphic features of the normal hypotonic duodenogram. Radiology 96:401, 1970

8. FIROR HV, HARRIS VJ: Rotational abnormalities of the gut: re-emphasis of a neglected facet, isolated, incomplete rotation of the duodenum. Am J Roentgenol 120:315, 1974

9. FRASER GM, FRASER ID: Gastrografin in perforated duodenal ulcer and acute pancreatitis. Clin Radiol 25:397, 1974

10. FREE EA, GERALD B: Duodenal obstruction in the newborn due to annular pancreas. Am J Roentgenol 103:321, 1968

11. GOLDSTEIN F, ZBORALSKE FF: Tubeless hypotonic duodenography. JAMA 210:2086, 1969

12. GOLDSTEIN HM, ROGERS LF, FLETCHER GH et al: Radiological manifestations of radiation-induced injury in the normal gastrointestinal tract. Radiology 117:135, 1975

13. JONES CW JR: Regional enteritis with involvement of the duodenum. Gastroenterology 51:1018, 1966

14. MARTEL W: Hypotonic duodenography without intubation. Radiology 91:387, 1968

15. MILLER RE, CHERNISH SM, ROSENAK VD: Hypotonic duodenography with glucagon. Radiology 108:35, 1973

16. ROBERTS SW, HAMILTON WW: Regional enteritis of the duodenum. Radiology 86:881, 1966

17. SERRANO JF, McPEAK CJ: Primary neoplasms of the duodenum. Surgery 59:199, 1966

18. SHAW DG: Intrahepatic gas shadows in neonatal duodenal obstruction. Arch Dis Child 47:300, 1972

19. TOXOPEUS MD, LUCAS CE, KRABBENHOFT KL: Roentgenographic diagnosis in blunt retroperitoneal duodenal rupture. Am J Roentgenol 115:281, 1972

18

THE MESENTERIC SMALL INTESTINE

ANATOMY AND PHYSIOLOGY

The mesenteric small intestine begins at the duodenojejunal junction and ends at the ileocecal valve. When coated with a thin layer of barium the jejunum shows a prominent mucosal pattern. The folds stand out clearly as a network of crisscrossing lines and with finely serrated edges. This pattern is produced by the folds of Kerkring or valvulae conniventes and resembles that seen in the duodenum distal to the bulb. The mucosal surface of the ileum is much smoother and even mild distention tends to obliterate what folds are present. In the jejunum, on the other hand, the folds of Kerkring are not obliterated even when there is severe distention of the bowel.

The junction between the jejunum and ileum is not distinct, the folds gradually becoming fewer. The jejunum usually occupies the upper central, left side, and lower central portions of the abdomen; the ileum is found in the right lateral abdomen and within the pelvis. There is much variation, however, in the location of the different parts of the small intestine and there often seems to be a change in the same individual at different times. Because of its mesentery the loops of small intestine move freely and often change considerably in position in serial films (Fig. 18-1).

The junction of ileum and colon forms an anatomic landmark that can be recognized without difficulty by the roentgenologist. The lips of the ileocecal valve project into the lumen of the cecum for a short distance and the superior lip is more prominent than the inferior (see Fig. 19-3). Occasionally the valve stands out more clearly than usual and causes a circular filling defect along the cecal margin. At times the ileocecal valve is situated on the posterior wall of the cecum and, if the valve is a prominent structure, pressure over it causes it to appear as a round filling defect in the barium-filled cecum that may be mistaken for a polypoid tumor. Usually there will be a small amount of barium caught in the opening of the valve and this results in a dense shadow in the center of the translucent area. This is usually elliptical in shape and crevices between folds may radiate outward from the center in a spokelike manner. This configuration is typical of a thickened ileocecal valve when it is visualized *en face*.

Peristalsis in the jejunum is active and rapid. Pro-

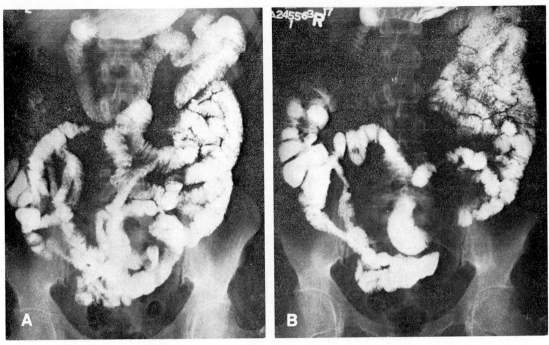

Fig. 18-1. Normal small intestine. Roentgenograms obtained ½ hour **(A)** and 1 hour **(B)** following administration of a barium meal. Note the change in distribution of the loops of small intestine and the change in mucosal pattern from jejunum to ileum. The meal is in the ascending colon on the 1-hour film.

pulsive movements begin in the duodenum and may progress into the jejunum for a considerable distance within a matter of seconds before they gradually cease. Such peristaltic rushes may transport a bolus of barium for a considerable distance along the small intestine and it is common to find barium in most of the jejunum in a matter of several minutes after the meal has begun to leave the stomach. In addition to peristaltic rushes, areas of segmental contraction occur that do not serve to propel the intestinal contents but rather seem to be a mechanism for mixing and bringing the fluid into intimate contact with the absorbing surfaces of the bowel.

Peristalsis in the ileum is much slower, the gradient, of course, being a gradual one. Propulsive waves are relatively infrequent, at least as compared to the jejunum, and they move at a slower rate. Thus the progress of a meal, after an initial rapid propulsion through the upper and midportions of the jejunum, slows considerably in the lower small intestine and it often requires from 1 to 1½ hours or even longer for a barium–water meal to reach the cecum. So much normal variation occurs, however, that it is difficult to set a limit for the transit time through the small in-

testine. To be noted also is the fact that the times given are for a barium–water mixture. Food leaves the stomach at a much slower rate and small-bowel progress also is much slower.

If food is given after the stomach is empty of the barium–water mixture, or nearly so, there usually is a prompt acceleration of small-bowel motility and a rapid propulsion of the mixture into the colon if it has not already reached the large bowel. The small-bowel transit time can be affected by many other factors. Drugs such as morphine may cause a pronounced delay in motility. Fear, excitement, nausea, and the like may affect motility adversely. Patients with severe or poorly controlled diabetes often show a considerable delay in gastric emptying and in small-bowel motility. One should use considerable caution before interpreting minor degrees of variation in the appearance of the small intestine on a single film as evidence of derangement of function or as a sign of organic disease.

The normal diameter of the jejunum is no more than 25 mm and that of the ileum no more than 20 mm. A diameter ranging from 25 to 30 mm is borderline, and any measurement over 30 mm definitely signifies abnormality. Narrowing is significant only if the area is consistently narrower than that of the adjacent intestinal lumen and/or there is persistent dilatation proximal to it. The jejunal folds (valvulae) do not usually exceed 2 mm in width; larger folds are almost invariably abnormal, particularly when they appear to be wavy.[38]

METHODS OF EXAMINATION

SCOUT FILMS OF THE ABDOMEN

As discussed in Chapter 13, preliminary or scout films of the abdomen are the method of choice for the initial study of small-bowel obstructions of acute nature and this aspect of small-intestine roentgenology will not be discussed further in this section. In the presence of a partial chronic obstruction of the small intestine there may be little or no accumulation of gas above the site of obstruction and the diagnosis then will depend upon contrast visualization. The lesions of nonobstructive character will ordinarily not be recognized until contrast study of the tract has been carried out unless they are large enough to be visible as a soft-tissue mass, contain calcium or gas, or displace gas-containing bowel.

CONTRAST VISUALIZATION

Contrast visualization of the small intestine is to a large extent a continuation of the roentgen study of the upper gastrointestinal tract as detailed in previous sections. The same barium–water mixture is used. It is essential that a nonflocculating barium sulfate containing a suspending agent be employed in order to bring out satisfactory mucosal detail. It usually is preferable to increase the amount of the mixture if small-intestine study is to be done and additional amounts of barium suspension to a total of 500 to 600 ml should be given after completion of the fluoroscopic study of the stomach and duodenum. Mixing of the barium sulfate with ice-cold normal saline solution instead of plain water has been recommended by some to hasten the transport of material through the small intestine and thus shorten the time needed for the examination.

Among the drugs that increase small-intestinal motility, *neostigmine* has been preferred by some. It is given intramuscularly in doses of from 0.5 to 0.75 mg for an average-sized adult after completion of fluoroscopy of the upper intestinal tract. Another drug, used extensively in Europe, which has been found useful in increasing gastric, duodenal, and jejunal peristalsis and relaxation of the pylorus is *metoclopramide*.[24] It is given intravenously in a dose of 10 to 20 mg. Within minutes, increase in gastric peristalsis is seen, the pylorus relaxes, and there is rapid filling of the small intestine. The mean small-intestinal transit time was found to be 55 minutes. The drug is of low toxicity.

The addition of 10 ml of Gastrografin to the routine barium mixture also has been advocated as a means of acclerating the small-bowel transit time. In our experience, Gastrografin's hypertonicity results in dilution of the barium to a degree that this method is not a very satisfactory one. We do not ordinarily use drugs to increase transit time.

The routine small-intestine study consists of a series of roentgenograms of the abdomen obtained at certain intervals after the ingestion of the barium mixture (Fig. 18-1). While this will vary among patients, depending upon the particular clinical problem at hand, and to some extent on the initial fluoroscopic observations of gastric and duodenal motility, the roentgenograms usually are obtained at the end of 30 minutes, 1 hour, and 1½ hours. If the barium–water meal has made normal progress and has reached the colon the examination is discontinued. If the head of the barium column remains in the small intestine, another film is exposed in 30 to 60 minutes. Additional films up to 24-hours or more may be necessary when partial obstruction is present, thus the examination is modified as necessary to fit the clinical situation. Usually the stimulation of peristalsis following eating will have caused a general advance of the barium mixture into the colon. Because of this we sometimes have the patient eat a small meal when transit is very slow. We routinely use fluoroscopy with compression to study the ileocecal area as well as areas where a lesion or a question of a pathologic process is observed, since all films are monitored during the examination. If more information is needed or if the routine roentgen study does not demonstrate a lesion when the clinical evidence suggests that one may be present, examination can be repeated with fluoroscopic observation carried out at frequent intervals. Palpation then can be used to separate overlying loops and occasionally a small lesion will be visualized that cannot be seen in the routine roentgenograms. The accuracy of the method is probably increased by the use of fluoroscopy routinely at frequent intervals, but routine roentgen study will serve a useful purpose if its limitations are kept in mind and there is recourse to fluoroscopy when indicated, as has been described, and to reexamine when necessary. In general, the accuracy of detection of disease in the mesenteric small intestine by roentgen methods is less than that in other parts of the gastrointestinal tract. This is due to the multiplicity of loops of bowel, the difficulty in separating them and visualizing individual segments clearly, and to the fact that, in many individuals, particularly those of an asthenic habitus, much of the small intestine lies deep in the pelvis and cannot be palpated nor can the loops be otherwise separated from one another. In spite of these drawbacks, roentgen examination of the small intestine is an extremely useful procedure and a great deal of information can be obtained from it.

Water-Soluble Contrast Agents

The use of water-soluble iodinated compounds has been recommended for the study of the small intestine when obstruction is present or suspected. However, investigative and clinical experience has shown that barium does not become inspissated above a small-bowel obstructive lesion and does not change a partial obstruction into a complete one. The water-soluble compounds are hypertonic and become considerably diluted in the lower small bowel. In children and in some adults, this can lead to enough fluid shift into the bowel to produce shock. Also, when water-soluble compounds are used the mucosal pattern is difficult to identify. A barium sulfate mixture, therefore, can be employed safely and allows better visualization even when obstruction is present. Only in patients with suspected perforation is the use of water-soluble iodinated compounds (usually Gastrografin) indicated. There may be occasional exceptions, such as in patients having acute high jejunal obstruction, but often no contrast studies are necessary because plain films and clinical findings are sufficient to make a strong presumptive diagnosis prior to surgery.

Intubation Methods

A double-lumen tube of the Miller-Abbott or Harris type can be passed into the small intestine and the opaque mixture injected directly into the bowel. At times this is done when the tube has been used to decompress the bowel above an obstruction. When the tip of the tube has progressed as far as it will go, the barium is injected under fluoroscopic control. In this way the exact site and the nature of the obstructing lesion sometimes can be identified.

Schatzki recommended the use of a small-intestinal enema for examining this part of the intestinal tract. The method consists in passing of a single-lumen tube into the upper jejunum and then allowing a barium–water mixture to flow slowly but steadily into the bowel. As a result the entire length of the small intestine can be filled at one time. A number of modifications of this method have been introduced. These include: (1) the use of a guidewire for rapid manipulation of the tube into the distal duodenum; (2) the injection of air when the entire small bowel is filled with barium, to produce a double-contrast study[13]; (3) the use of glucagon or Pro-Banthine to stop peristalsis in conjunction with the double-contrast study[31]; and (4) the use of an antifoam agent. A low-density barium suspension is necessary to outline lesions when loops are superimposed and cannot be displaced by compression or positional changes. Because good preparation is essential, low-residue diets and oral cathartics are used. The double-contrast method is not widely used routinely, but is valuable in certain instances in which small-bowel disease is strongly suspected but has not been confirmed by other means.[43]

Reflux Method

It is possible in some patients and with suitable technique to fill most or all of the small intestine by reflux of a barium enema through the ileocecal valve.[37] The filling is done under fluoroscopic control. We have had no personal experience with this method which has been ussed primarily for the detection of organic filling defects.

Arteriography

In some patients, selective superior mesenteric or celiac axis arteriography may give useful information if routine barium studies have revealed no abnormality. The method is particularly valuable if there has been acute or chronic bleeding from the gastrointestinal tract and a source of blood loss cannot be found. In some patients having acute hemorrhage the bleeding point may be identified because of leakage of contrast material into the lumen (see Fig. 17-11). In other patients the lesion responsible may be identified, such as an hemangioma or arteriovenous malformation. Other tumors, particularly if they show abnormal tumor vessels or a tumor stain or blush, can be visualized. In cases of acute hemorrhage, gastrointestinal arteriography is carried out as the initial procedure to be followed by barium studies if necessary. Selective injection of vasopressor substances may be used to control bleeding, at least on a temporary basis, after the bleeding point has been located. If this fails, embolization of autologous blood clot or Gelfoam or one of the newer synthetic materials may be used to control bleeding so that surgical treatment can be delayed until the patient's condition has improved.

ANOMALIES OF THE SMALL INTESTINE

DUPLICATIONS

In the chapters dealing with other parts of the gastrointestinal tract mention has been made of congenital duplications. This malformation is also found in the small intestine, somewhat more frequently in the ileum than elsewhere. The duplication may or may not communicate with the intestinal lumen. If it does it usually is of tubular shape, paralleling the normal gut and lying between the layers of the mesentery. A closed duplication is in the nature of a cyst. If small the cyst may lie within the wall of the gut; a larger lesion usually lies within the mesentery. The mucosal lining of the duplication may be that of any part of the gastrointestinal tract; gastric mucosa is present frequently. Associated anomalies such as spina bifida, hemivertebra, and meningocele are common.

If the duplication communicates with the intestinal lumen, a barium meal may cause its opacification but its recognition is often very difficult because of surrounding barium-filled intestinal loops and the tendency for these loops to overlie one another. The closed cystic type gives roentgen signs of a circumscribed soft-tissue mass displacing segments of bowel and perhaps compressing them. Those duplications that lie within the wall resemble other intramural tumors and may cause the roentgen signs of partial or high-grade obstruction. It is not possible to state the nature of such a lesion from the roentgen findings.

Duplication may be associated with atresia. Sometimes, calcification occurs in the duplicated segment. The finding of a small area of calcification associated with the signs of jejunal or ileal atresia may suggest the diagnosis. Otherwise, it can be made only at the time of operation or postmortem.

An unusual type of duplication of the small intestine, with a part of the duplicated segment lying within the thorax, has been reported infrequently. The duplicated segment forms a mass along the right posterior mediastinum. After a barium meal, the contrast material is found within the mass which communicates with the small intestine within the abdomen. This lesion is very rare.

ERRORS OF ROTATION

Embryologists divide the gut into three parts, the foregut (mouth to duodenojejunal junction), the midgut (duodenojejunal junction to the midtransverse colon), and the hindgut (midtransverse colon to the anus). The important segment concerned in errors of rotation is the midgut. This part of the tube grows very rapidly during the first weeks of life and, in order to have room, it herniates into the umbilical cord. Rotation of the midgut begins about the eighth week, during the period in which it lies outside the celomic cavity. The first stage is one of counterclockwise rotation with the superior mesenteric artery as the axis. The rotation is one of 180 degrees, which brings the postarterial segment anterior to the superior mesenteric artery. The second stage consists in a return of the gut to the abdomen and a further counterclockwise rotation of 90 degrees, making a total of 270 degrees. This occurs about the tenth week of life. The jejunum is the first part to return to the abdomen, followed by the ileum, cecum, and ascending and transverse colon. The small intestine collects in the left side of the abdomen and the cecum and ascending colon, the last parts to enter the abdomen, come to lie in the right hypochondrium. The third or final stage is completed at about the time of birth or shortly thereafter with completion of descent of the cecum into the right lower quadrant. Fixation of the cecum, ascending colon, and the duodenum takes place during the third stage. The anomalies of rotation that may occur depend upon the stage at which rotation was arrested. The return and rotation are sequential, therefore anomalies of rotation of the duodenum, mesenteric small bowel, or colon may occur independently.

First-Stage Arrest

First-stage arrest results in an omphalocele, a persisting herniation of the midgut into the umbilical cord. Occasionally other abdominal structures are present in the hernia such as the liver, spleen, or stomach. The diagnosis is a clinical one.

The vitelline duct, which connects with primitive midgut and yolk sac, may not obliterate following return of the gut to the peritoneal cavity. A *vitelline duct (omphalomesenteric cyst)* or a patent duct may result; more commonly a short segment connected to the gut persists, a *Meckel's diverticulum*. In the neonate the vitelline duct cyst may result in obstruction due to prolapse, intussusception, or volvulus. The cyst may contain gas and produce a characteristic appearance of a mass containing gas and fluid posterior to the umbilicus in an infant with obstruction.[19]

Second-Stage Arrest

Nonrotation. The gut may return into the abdomen without rotating. The small intestine is found in the right side of the abdomen and the colon in the left. This is an infrequent malformation and often is asymptomatic. On roentgen examination the distribution of the bowel is characteristic (Fig. 18-2). The entire colon lies to the left of the midline. The cecum is often near the midline but the ileocecal valve opens on the right side. A barium-meal examination will show the stomach and the first and second portions of the duodenum to be in normal position but the duodenojejunal flexure is absent; instead the entire jejunum is found to the right of the midline.

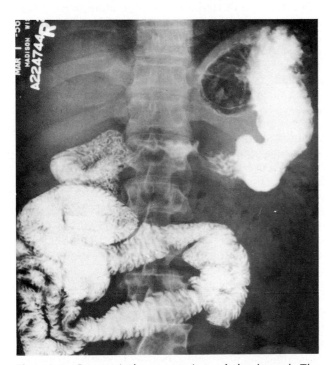

Fig. 18-2. Congenital nonrotation of the bowel. The stomach and first portion of the duodenum are in normal position, but the remainder of the duodenum and the jejunum lie almost entirely to the right of the midline. The colon was found to be on the left side of the midline in this patient.

Reversal of Rotation. This is a very rare anomaly in which rotation occurs in a clockwise manner. The duodenum comes to lie in front of the superior mesenteric artery and the transverse colon behind it. Obstruction from compression by peritoneal bands or from volvulus may occur.

Third-Stage Arrest

Anomalies of fixation occur as a part of third-stage arrest and these are much more frequent than complete failure of rotation (second-stage arrest). The attachment of the mesentery may be very short, while the length of the mesentery is abnormally long. This predisposes to volvulus of the entire midgut with or without compromise of its blood supply (see Fig. 17-3). There may be a failure of fixation of the cecum and the ascending colon; this predisposes to volvulus of the cecum (see Ch. 19). There also is a tendency to persistence of peritoneal bands or veils in these patients, with the possibility of compression or kinking of the bowel. Peritoneal bands may compromise the lumen of the duodenum and be a cause for high-intestinal obstruction in the newborn. One of the most frequent defects is a failure of complete descent of the cecum, which remains along the inferior surface of the liver. The appendix often remains in a retrocecal position with its tip pointing upward behind the cecum.

Volvulus of the Midgut

Volvulus of the midgut is a complication of malrotation that often occurs in the first weeks of life. It is the result of the anomalous long and/or narrow mesentery which contains the superior mesenteric artery in these infants. Signs of intermittent or persistent obstruction, usually in the duodenum, are manifest. Arterial and/or venous obstruction may be present. Upper gastrointestinal-series study is fast and direct, demonstrating the site and degree of obstruction and the position of the upper small bowel if obstruction is incomplete. Roentgen signs, in addition to evidence of obstruction, are the abnormal position of the ligament of Treitz, proximal jejunum in the right upper quadrant, and torsion of the duodenum. Since the examination may reveal a nearly normal state in the absence of obstruction (and volvulus), it should be performed when the infant is symptomatic.[3] Barium enema may be used to detect the position of the colon but is not necessary if the diagnosis of malrotation with volvulus and obstruction is made by the gastrointestinal examination. Angiography has also been

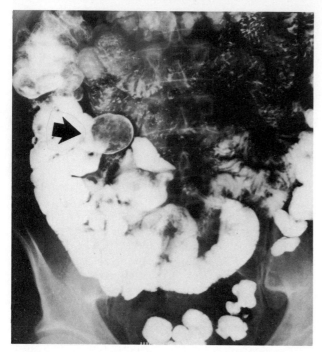

Fig. 18-3. Meckel's diverticulum. The **arrow** indicates the diverticulum which contains a little barium and some gas in the right central abdomen. The patient's chief complaint was intermittent gastrointestinal bleeding. When the patient was operated upon, heterotopic gastric mucosa was found in the diverticulum.

used as a diagnostic method; abnormal position of vessels indicates malrotation while torsion with narrowing or obstruction indicates volvulus.

MECKEL'S DIVERTICULUM

Meckel's diverticulum is reported to occur in from 1% to 4% of the population and is as frequent in males as in females. The cause is persistence of the omphalomesenteric duct at its junction with antimesenteric side of the ileum. Usually asymptomatic, Meckel's diverticulum may be a cause of hemorrhage, obstruction, intussusception, acute inflammation, or perforation. Heterotopic islands of gastric mucosa may be present; ulceration may result and be the source of the blood loss. Roentgen demonstration of a Meckel's diverticulum is difficult and often requires meticulous technique and careful observation. As a rule the diverticulum is located in the lower part of the ileum where overlapping of loops of small intestine make it difficult to visualize all segments clearly; those loops lying within the pelvis cannot be separated by palpation. Because of the usual shape of the diverticulum, elongated and tubular with a wide ostium, it does not retain the barium very well and even when completely filled can easily pass for a segment of bowel.

Occasionally a Meckel's diverticulum is demonstrated by retrograde filling of the ileum during a barium enema. More often the lesion is discovered during a small-bowel study (Fig. 18-3). Those that are visualized usually are saclike, rather than elongated and tubular, and have a narrow neck and ostium. The saclike character of the lesion causes it to retain barium after the rest of the meal has progressed into the colon. Upright roentgenograms may demonstrate a gas-fluid level within the sac.

Occasionally the diverticulum is very large and may contain air and fluid, producing an air–fluid level on horizontal-beam films. Calculi may be present and may aid in the identification of the diverticulum. Gastric mucosa in its wall may be detected by scintiscanning with 99mTc-Na pertechnetate. If there is brisk bleeding, angiography may be used to locate the site of hemorrhage and sometimes to determine its cause. Rarely, an ulcer within a Meckel's diverticulum has been demonstrated on small-bowel study. Infrequently, an internal hernia through the mesentery of a Meckel's diverticulum has been reported.[11]

ATRESIA AND STENOSIS

Congenital atresia may involve the small intestine as well as other parts of the gastrointestinal tract. There may be more than one site of atresia. The signs of bowel obstruction develop in the immediate postnatal period. Roentgen examination is useful in establishing the level of the lesion. The diagnostic findings are described in Chapter 19 in the section entitled "Atresia and Stenosis of the Colon." Figure 18-4 illustrates an example of atresia of the small intestine. A few cases of small-bowel atresia have been reported in which the ileum distal to the atresia opened directly into the peritoneal cavity, indicating possible danger from barium-enema studies if the obstruction is in the distal ileum. Atresia may be a complication of meconium ileus and evidently is caused by volvulus which may occur *in utero* in these patients. Atresia in the jejunum or ileum is not as commonly associated with other anomalies as is duodenal atresia. Agenesis of the dorsal mesentery, high jejunal atresia, and prepnatal occlusion of the superior mesenteric artery associated with the distal small bowel coiled around a vascular stalk, without a true mesentery, and supplied by collateral branches from the ileocolic and the

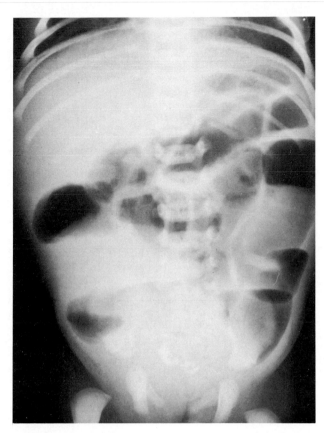

Fig. 18-4. Congenital jejunal atresia. There are numerous loops of dilated, gas-filled bowel, all of which were found to be jejunum. It is not possible to differentiate small and large bowel in such a patient, and barium enema is needed to exclude the possibility of a colonic obstruction. Note a small amount of residual barium in the recto-sigmoid.

middle and right colic arteries is termed the "apple-peel" small bowel. Mortality rate is high because of the vascular insufficiency of the small bowel.[28]

Stenosis is less common than atresia and is usually severe, producing high-grade obstruction. Symptoms in both conditions occur in the first 24 hours of life.

DISEASES OF THE SMALL INTESTINE

NEOPLASMS

A variety of neoplasms may develop in the small intestine, including carcinomas, carcinoids, leiomyomas, leiomyosarcomas, lymphosarcomas, and the like. In the Mayo Clinic series,[18] leiomyoma was the most frequent type. Other tumors included adenomas, lipomas, fibromas, myxomas, neurofibromas, hemangiomas, and their malignant counterparts. Many of these lesions appear as localized, polypoid filling defects and resemble one another in their roentgen appearances and in their tendency to cause intussusception. Some of them may be multiple; these include leiomyoma, neurofibroma, adenoma, and lymphoma. Hemangioma is sometimes recognized because of the presence of calcified phleboliths—calcified thrombi in the dilated vascular spaces. As a group, neoplasms of the small intestine are uncommon. The clinical manifestations usually result from the development of obstruction or are caused by bleeding or a combination of the two.

Roentgen Observations

Signs of Obstruction. Obstruction may result in the accumulation of abnormal amounts of gas and gas distention of loops of small bowel with gas–fluid levels present when roentgenograms are obtained with the patient upright or in a lateral decubitus position. These signs have been described in Chapter 13. As a rule the obstruction must be fairly severe in order to produce these changes. Because obstruction caused by small-bowel tumors often is intermittent in character with asymptomatic periods, roentgen examination performed during the time when symptoms are present may give valuable information. The temporary nature of the obstructive signs is probably the result of episodes of intussusception. If roentgen examination is carried out during a period when there is complete absence of obstructive symptoms it may be difficult to detect the lesion. When a barium meal is given, obstruction is demonstrated by the obvious dilatation of the barium-filled loops of bowel above the level of the lesion. When obstruction is minimal or early this may be the first clue to the presence of the tumor (Fig. 18-5). The gastric emptying rate may be delayed and the progress of the meal through the small bowel slowed. The wide range of normal should be kept in mind and unless there is dilatation of the bowel as well as a delay in progress, the diagnosis of an obstructive lesion is hardly justified. If the examination is performed during a period of intussusception, the diagnosis may be made during contrast filling. The intussusception causes a local dilatation of the bowel. The barium mixture caught in the crevices of the dilated intussusceptum produces a "coiled-spring" appearance. This is always highly suggestive of intussusception when it occurs in any part of the gastrointestinal tract. Frequently, there is complete obstruction associated with the intussusception and the nature of the lesion responsible may not be obvious.

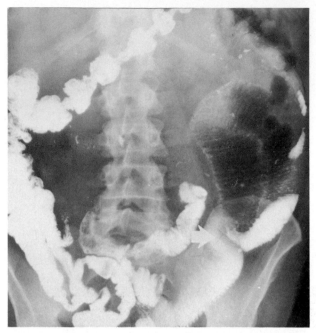

Fig. 18-5. Partial obstruction of the jejunum. The **arrow** indicates the site of obstruction caused by a malignant lesion. Note that the obstruction is incomplete and that loops distal to it are normal in caliber.

Filling Defect. If the lesion has caused a complete obstruction or a nearly complete one so that the barium mixture does not extend through the area of the lesion and outline its lumen, the roentgen diagnosis may be limited to that of an obstructing process. If obstruction is incomplete the filling defect of the tumor may be visualized (Fig. 18-6). In general, such defects resemble those caused by similar tumors in the esophagus, stomach, and colon. Thus, carcinomas are likely to encircle the lumen, producing an annular constriction with irregular narrowing of a short segment and with the margins of the lesion sharply demarcated from the normal and with overhanging edges. An intramural mass, such as a *leiomyoma,* causes a smooth-surfaced filling defect with intact mucosa over the surface except where ulceration may possibly have developed (Fig. 18-7). The ulcer may be very deep and resemble a sinus tract, particularly in leiomyosarcoma, in which necrosis may be so extensive that a large, irregular cavity may be demonstrated. A leiomyoma may also become very large and bulky and result in a sausage-shaped mass projecting into the intestinal lumen. Because the bowel wall is not completely fixed or infiltrated by the tumor, obstruction may be relatively moderate even when the tumor is large. Occasionally a leiomyoma or

Fig. 18-6. Small intestinal neoplasms. **A.** Primary adenocarcinoma **(arrow)** causing an irregular filling defect which is partially obstructing. **B.** Lymphoma **(arrow)** involving the lower jejunum. The lesion is large and bulky, with a large, irregular ulcer, but causes relatively little obstruction.

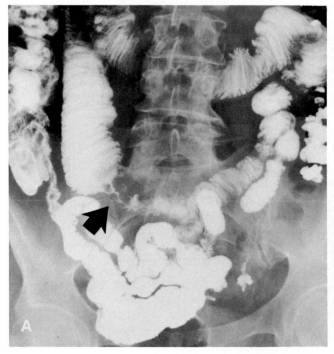
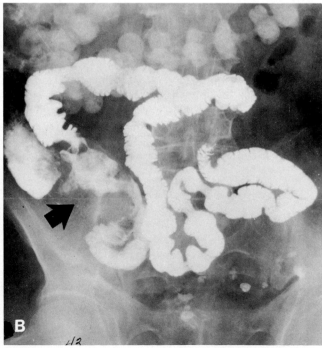

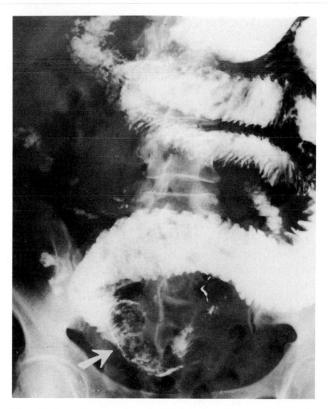

Fig. 18-7. Leiomyoma of the lower jejunum **(arrow).** The large, smooth, oval filling defect produced by the tumor causes partial obstruction. Note dilatation of the bowel above the tumor.

its malignant counterpart may grow almost completely extrinsic to the bowel lumen and thus cause little or no deformity in the barium outline. Such a tumor may not be identified as arising from the bowel wall unless it does develop to the point where it causes obstruction. Small tumors may not cause any signs of obstruction and the only clinical symptom may be that of bleeding. Very careful investigation with multiple roentgenograms, fluoroscopy, and spot films may be required to locate such a lesion. It is in some of these patients that selective superior mesenteric arteriography can often provide diagnostic information by demonstrating the bleeding site.

Plexiform neurofibromas, in which multiple adjacent nerve trunks are involved, occurring on the mesenteric side of the small bowel, produce multiple nodular masses. They appear to occur only in association with neurofibromatosis. A palpable abdominal mass is usually present in this condition.[16]

Lymphosarcoma involving the small intestine may appear in several forms. In one, the lesion presents as a discrete, polypoid, intramural mass. In another, it is more infiltrating, causing a ragged, irregular defect. Ulceration and excavation may occur so that the lumen through the lesion is actually larger than the normal. Fistulous communication with adjacent loops of bowel is not uncommon. In still another type the disease occurs in the form of multiple, small, nodular defects, causing a coarse scalloping of the bowel wall. The disease is most frequent in the ileum where the greatest amount of lymphoid tissue is present. Gastric and colonic lesions may accompany the small intestinal disease. In some patients, lymphosarcoma presents as a predominantly mesenteric invasive form in which single or multiple extraluminal masses exert extrinsic pressure on the adjacent bowel, producing a spruelike pattern.[22] Segmentation and flocculation similar to that seen in sprue occur in some patients. The lesion may be very difficult to distinguish from some other conditions that cause the malabsorption syndrome but there often are nodules projecting into the lumen suggesting the neoplastic nature of the process.

Hodgkin's disease involving the small intestine resembles lymphosarcoma except that narrowing and stricture formation secondary to the fibrotic reaction associated with Hodgkin's disease tend to be more severe than in lymphosarcoma. Extensive necrosis excavation and apparent dilatation in the region of the lesion are less common in Hodgkin's disease. Multiple lesions are frequent and the stomach and colon may be involved.

Carcinoid tumors are relatively uncommon in the small intestine but in some series they have been reported as being the most frequent tumor. If small the tumor may produce only a localized filling defect; larger lesions may cause intussusception or obstruction. The tendency for carcinoid to invade the contiguous mesentery and to cause fibrosis is to be noted. This may result in angulation and kinking of the bowel, aggravating the obstruction. A segment of the bowel may become encased by extension of the desmoplastic reaction from the mesentery, resulting in diffuse narrowing of the lumen in the area involved. There may also be thickening of mucosal folds. Calcifications within the tumor appear to be common in the form of one or two small, smooth, ringlike spherical densities. Arteriographic study reveals: (1) a stellate or radiating pattern of distal ileal branches; (2) arterial narrowing, smooth or irregular, ranging from minimal stenosis to complete occlusion; (3) venous occlusions with no filling of draining veins; and (4) a tumor stain that in many of these tumors seems to be reasonably characteristic, but may be noted in mesenteric fibrosis.[5] In contrast to carcinoids of the appendix, those in the small intestine are often malignant. In some cases there results a so-called *carcinoid syndrome* consisting of chronic diarrhea, flushing and cyanosis of the skin, respiratory distress, and right-sided cardiac disease. These clinical signs in association with roentgen evidence of a small-intestinal tumor are highly suggestive of the diagnosis.

Adenomas, lipomas, and *fibromas* resemble one another. The lesions may be single or multiple and cause a sharply outlined, polypoid-type filling defect of variable size. They often cause intussusception.

The Peutz–Jeghers Syndrome. This entity, transmitted as an autosomal dominant trait, consists of multiple, polypoid lesions in the gastrointestinal tract associated with a peculiar oral pigmentation. The pigment is melanin and appears in round, irregular spots at the mucocutaneous junction of the lips and in the mouth. The intestinal lesions are most commonly found in the small bowel but also occur in the colon and stomach. They represent hamartomas rather than true polyps. Often they are very small and difficult to identify in roentgenograms particularly in the jejunum where there is a rich fold pattern. They resemble other polypoid lesions and may be sessile or pedunculated. Their multiplicity and small size are suggestive signs; the diagnosis is confirmed by the presence of oral pigmentation.

Carcinoma, metastatic to the bowel, is usually multiple. A wide variety of roentgen appearances have been described depending on whether the lesion involves the wall of the intestine or the mesentery or both, the presence or absence of obstruction and of ulceration, and the size of the individual mass. As a rule, hematogenous metastases are multiple and are located chiefly on the antimesenteric border of the small bowel, while metastatic seeding tends to occur in the mesentery and on the mesenteric borders of the small bowel, usually the distal ileum. Stretching and fixation of mucosal folds results from mesenteric and peritoneal implants, while the hematogenous metastases are the ones that may ulcerate. The seeded metastases tend to follow the flow of ascitic fluid and most of them occur in the right lower quadrant.[35] *Metastatic malignant melanoma* is likely to cause multiple, nodular or polypoid filling defects. Central necrosis and ulceration may occur causing a "target deformity," a dense, barium-filled central crater surrounded by the sharply marginated nodular mass.[33] The tendency for this tumor to metastasize to the intestinal tract has been noted frequently.

Direct Invasion. Direct extension of invasive tumors to the small bowel is less common than is their extension to the colon. A right renal neoplasm may invade the duodenum, however, as will adjacent neoplasm of the pancreas or common bile duct. Extension by way of lymphatics may also occur, chiefly from the colon to the duodenum, but such extension to jejunum and ileum is much less common.[44]

REGIONAL ENTERITIS; CROHN'S DISEASE

Regional enteritis is an inflammatory disease of the small intestine, the cause of which is unknown. It develops most frequently in the distal ileum. The disease can involve the proximal part of the ileum, the jejunum, the duodenum, the stomach, and, rarely, the esophagus. The term "regional enteritis" is preferred since it recognizes the wide distribution of the disease throughout the small intestine. In the colon the disease has been called *granulomatous colitis* or *Crohn's disease* (see section "Granulomatous Colitis" in Ch. 19). An acute form of ileitis is seen, particularly in children. The patients often are operated upon because of an erroneous diagnosis of acute appendicitis. Based on study of resected specimens, some authors believe that this is an acute exacerbation of chronic disease which may have been relatively asymptomatic previous to the acute episode. In many patients, however, there is spontaneous improvement with disappearance of symptoms, and the disease does not recur. The roentgen changes resemble the early findings in regional enteritis. It should be noted that in children, particularly during adolescence, *hyperplasia* of *lymphoid follicles*, may be normally present in the distal ileum causing numerous tiny projections on the mucosal surface or a fine, cobblestone mucosal relief. This should not be misinterpreted as evidence of early regional enteritis.

Roentgen examination of a patient suspected of having regional enteritis should be initiated with a barium-enema study. If the lesion involves the terminal ileum, this segment may fill by reflux through the ileocecal valve and it can be studied to good advantage during fluoroscopy. If the terminal ileum does not fill, barium is given orally and a small-bowel study made as described previously. This procedure also is essential for the detection of lesions in the more proximal part of the small intestine and for determination of the presence or absence of obstruction.

Roentgen Observations

Nonstenotic Phase. When filled by reflux during a barium enema the ileum is seen to be normal in caliber or irregular and slightly narrowed. The mucosal folds may be blunted or thickened. They may be distorted and rigid. As they become thicker, irregular, and indistinct, they may appear to be partially fused. When ulceration develops, the normal fold pattern is lost, and the mucosal surface develops a rough cobblestone appearance. Linear ulcers, if present, are seen as longitudinal crevices filled with barium. When transverse ulcers are also present, the cobblestone appearance is produced. Multiple, smooth defects are caused by islands of inflamed mucosa. The involved area may become increasingly narrow, leading to the stenotic phase. Spastic contractions, an indication of irritability, may be noted fluoroscopically. If filling occurs proximal to the area of involvement, the change from an abnormal to a normal ileal pattern is abrupt.

Following an oral barium meal, there often is an initial delay in progress through the lower ileum. The head of the barium column will not move into the colon until food is given; then it moves rapidly through the involved segment. This is probably caused by fixation and rigidity which prevents normal peristalsis. The involved segments become somewhat straightened. Thickening of the walls results in separation of loops.

Stenotic Phase. As the disease becomes more chronic it is characterized by marked inflammatory induration of the wall of the bowel and of the mesentery (Fig. 18-8). The segment has a fixed, rigid appearance as shown in serial roentgenograms. The internal surface becomes smoother or finely irregular with complete absence of a mucosal fold pattern. The diameter of the lumen is narrowed, sometimes uniformly, at other times in a more irregular manner. Apparently owing to irregular fibrosis and contraction, diverticulumlike outpouchings called pseudodiverticula may form, usually in the antimesenteric side. With increasing fibrosis the lumen may be narrowed to a diameter of only a few millimeters. When the segment is filled with barium the appearance resembles that of a string and is known as "the string sign" (Fig. 18-9). This now is the stenotic phase of the disease. The length of the involved segment is variable but may extend for a foot or more. Skip areas also are common, that is, two or more involved segments separated by normal bowel.

Fistula formation is common in regional enteritis. The fistulas may be between adjacent segments of small intestine of between small bowel and colon, vagina, urinary bladder, or skin surface. Perianal fistulas are frequent. The tracts often can be identified in roentgenograms. Abscess formation owing to extension of the disease beyond the confines of the bowel also occurs with some frequency. The thickened bowel wall and mesentery, enlargement of regional lymph nodes, and the formation of abscesses results in an inflammatory mass that displaces loops of bowel away from the area of disease (Fig. 18-10). A soft-tissue space, therefore, will surround the involved bowel where normally there would be other segments of small intestine. The medial wall of the cecum often shows a concave indentation caused by the inflammatory mass surrounding the terminal ileum. Because of its rigidity the terminal ileum often develops a goosenecked shape as it curves downward into the pelvis from the ileocecal valve. The lips of the valve become thickened and cause characteristic biconcave filling defects in the medial wall of the cecum.

Although the bowel may be markedly stenotic, obstructive signs may be minimal. When stenosis does occur the bowel above the lesion becomes dilated with excess fluid and gas present.

Jejunal Disease. Regional enteritis may affect a segment of bowel above the terminal ileum; the roentgen findings may be similar for lesions above the terminal ileum as for those in it. Sometimes the disease occurs as a skip lesion above a diseased terminal ileum. At other times the jejunum is the primary site of the disease. The early mucosal changes are similar to those noted in the ileum. During the stenotic phase there often are multiple constricted areas with dilated segments in between. Fistula formation is less frequent with jejunal than with ileal disease. A long, stringlike area of narrowing is also less frequent in jejunal lesions; rather, areas of constriction alternate with areas of dilatation. The strictures usually have a smooth lumen with tapering ends. Occasionally ulceration may cause irregularity of the margins. We have observed a few patients with jejunal involvement proved by biopsy in whom the only finding was diffuse thickening of the valvulae and perhaps a little rigidity and slight dilatation. The appearance was very similar to that of edema of the jejunal wall. In some, the process regressed to the point where no roentgenographic alteration could be detected. In others, the appearance was unchanged for months. Duodenal involvement is uncommon. It has been described in Chapter 17 in the section entitled "Regional Enteritis (Crohn's Disease) of the Duodenum." Gastric and esophageal involvement has been described in the chapters dealing with those areas.

There is an increased incidence of ankylosing spondylitis, usually confined to the sacroiliac joints, in patients with regional enteritis. There also appears to be a slight increase in incidence of small bowel carcinoma in these patients. The inflammatory changes

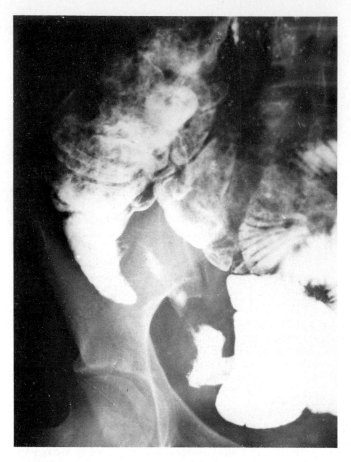

Fig. 18-8. Regional enteritis (Crohn's disease). The distal ileum is narrowed, and there is loss of the normal mucosal pattern. A surrounding inflammatory mass has displaced adjacent loops of bowel and produced a concave indentation on the medial wall of the cecum.

Fig. 18-9. Regional enteritis involving the terminal ileum. The **arrow** indicates the abnormal ileum which is narrowed and produces the "string" sign.

tend to obscure the neoplasm, so it is often discovered late.

After surgical resection and anastomosis there is a great tendency for Crohn's disease to recur in the bowel adjacent to the anastomosis.

NODULAR LYMPHOID HYPERPLASIA

Hyperplasia of the lymphoid follicles may affect the small intestine, the colon, or both. In the preceding section of this chapter, mention is made of hyperplastic follicles in the terminal ileum in older children as a normal finding. When it occurs in other parts of the intestinal tract or during age periods other than adolescence it is called *nodular lymphoid hyperplasia*. It may be associated with dysgammaglobulinemia;[21] these patients are susceptible to infections and *giardiasis* involving the bowel is said to be common. Nodular lymphoid hyperplasia has been reported in patients with sarcoidosis also. It appears to be an essentially benign condition, the result of a variety of stimuli. The increased incidence during childhood and adolescence has been noted. The roentgen find-

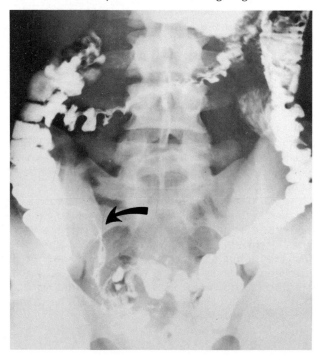

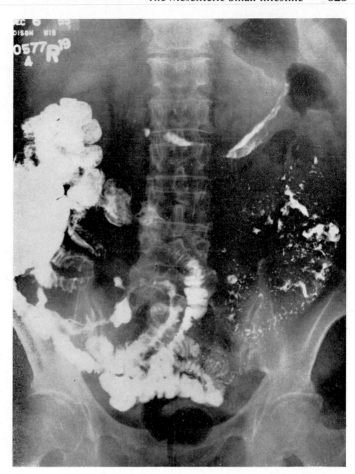

Fig. 18-10. Regional enteritis involving a long segment of the ileum which is narrowed irregularly. Several small extensions of barium represent fistulas. The inflammatory mass associated with the disease has displaced adjacent loops. Despite the extensive disease in this patient, there is very little obstruction.

ings consist of numerous tiny nodular projections on the mucosal surface (Fig. 18-11). The individual lesions usually measure from 1 to 3 mm in diameter and are so small that they are difficult to identify in the jejunum where mucosal folds are most prominent. The lesions may be widespread or limited to a shorter segment of bowel. A localized area of inflammatory disease resembling regional enteritis but due to giardiasis, may be found in the duodenum or jejunum. Sometimes, *systemic mastocytosis* may cause a fine nodulation in the small intestine closely resembling lymphoid hyperplasia. The most prominent feature of lymphoid hyperplasia, however, is thickening of the wall and coarsening of the mucosal folds in the duodenum and proximal jejunum. These patients are very intolerant to alcohol and, following its ingestion, mucosal folds become progressively thicker, secretions in stomach and small bowel increase, and there may be pylorospasm. In lymphoid hyperplasia of the colon the nodules resemble the lesions of *familial*

polyposis and biopsy is necessary to distinguish the two conditions. In the nodular form of lymphosarcoma the lesions usually are larger. The same is true of *metastatic melanosarcoma* and other metastatic tumors. Other diseases to be considered in differential diagnosis include the *Peutz–Jeghers syndrome* and *Gardner's syndrome.*

TUBERCULOSIS

The incidence of tuberculous ileocolitis has decreased considerably in recent years and it has become a rare disease in general hospital radiologic practice. Tuberculosis of the intestinal tract is usually localized to the distal part of the ileum, the cecum, and the proximal part of the ascending colon. While the lesions may be limited either to the ileum or to the colon, most often both are involved. Since intestinal tuberculosis may be secondary to pulmonary disease, evidence of lung involvement is important in

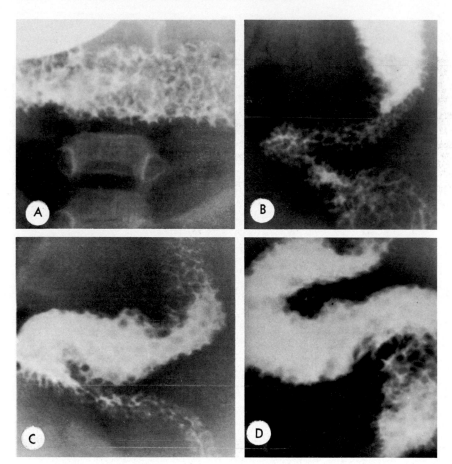

Fig. 18-11. Nodular lymphoid hyperplasia. **A.** Segment of transverse colon. **B–D.** Portions of sigmoid colon in various degrees of filling and contraction. The multiple, tiny, nodular projections on the mucosal surface are similar to those found in nodular lymphoid hyperplasia of the small intestine. (Wolfson JJ, Goldstein G, Krivit W, Hong R: Am J Roentgenol 108: 610, 1970.)

establishing the diagnosis and in distinguishing tuberculosis from other diseases, particularly regional enteritis.

Roentgen Observations. After the oral administration of barium there may be an initial delay in progress through the lower part of the small intestine but, after several hours, occasionally only following the taking of food, there will be noted a rapid propulsion of the barium through the ileocecal area. Serial roentgenograms or fluoroscopy may demonstrate temporary filling but the tendency is for the inflamed segments to remain empty. One finds, as a result, barium filling of proximal ileal loops, filling of the colon distal to the ascending portion, but a very incomplete filling of the terminal ileum and cecum. A similar phenomenon may be seen in regional ileitis, particularly the acute form of the disease, and it is not specific for tuberculosis (*Stierlin's sign*).

When examination is by means of a barium enema, the cecum and often the entire ascending colon are found to be very irritable. Only in very chronic disease is such irritability absent. The bowel fills momentarily, only to undergo a mass contraction with propulsion of the mixture from the ascending into the distal colon, and the patient may be unable to retain the enema. The terminal ileum is difficult to fill and once filled does not tolerate the barium very well.

In the later stages of the disease, irritability is less pronounced. Deep and large ulcers may form. These, combined with scarring and fibrosis, cause the lumen to become very irregular (Fig. 18-12). If limited to a small area, the lesion may have a superficial resemblance to carcinoma. The margins of the defect, however, are not as sharply demarcated from the normal bowel as in carcinoma; there are no overhanging edges or sharp angular junctions between the filling defect and the bowel wall. It is unusual to have cecal disease without involvement of the terminal ileum. More often the disease is so extensive and predominantly ulcerative that its resemblance to car-

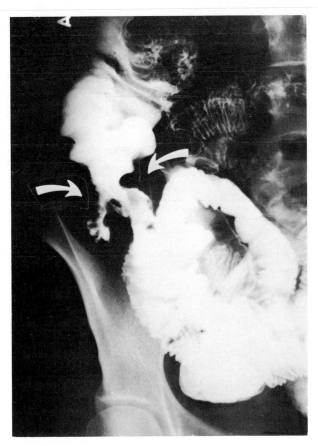

Fig. 18-12. Ileocecal tuberculosis. Note the irregular contraction of the cecum and the irregularity of the margin of the ileum adjacent to the ileocecal valve **(arrows).**

cinoma is remote. There is a tendency for it to skip areas, leaving normal bowel in between sites of disease. The smooth, uniform, stringlike constriction often seen in regional ileitis does not develop; instead, irregularity in width of the ileal lumen is the rule. In difficult cases the presence or absence of pulmonary tuberculosis may be a very important factor in diagnosis. Without evidence of tuberculosis elsewhere, it is virtually impossible to distinguish tuberculous ileocolitis from Crohn's disease radiographically.

MALABSORPTION AND RELATED SYNDROMES

Abnormal changes in the small intestine first described in sprue were later found in a number of other entities. These are now generally grouped under the designation of the *malabsorption syn-* *drome.* The main fault in this syndrome is defective absorption of carbohydrate, protein, and fat from the small bowel. The result is steatorrhea with passage of bulky, foul-smelling, high-fat content stools. Various deficiency states may thus be induced, including osteomalacia and rickets, with loss of weight and anemia among the clinical signs. Marshak and Lindner[33] have listed more than 25 conditions which may cause the malabsorption syndrome.

Some investigators[23] have not been able to find any specific signs which would allow differentiation between one of these entities and the others on roentgen study. Other writers, however, believe that differentiation can be made in many cases based upon the alterations in the small-bowel patterns.[33] The changes seen in sprue form a classic pattern for this syndrome (Fig. 18-13). In addition, a few of the more important diseases that enter into the differential diagnosis of sprue will be considered, including Whipple's disease, amyloidosis, and scleroderma. Other diseases such as regional enteritis and lymphosarcoma are discussed elsewhere in the appropriate sections.

Sprue

Celiac disease in children and nontropical sprue in adults are generally considered to be the same disease. Tropical sprue may be a different entity but the roentgen findings in the gastrointestinal tract are similar to those of the other two diseases. The changes described in the following are related to one another and are usually all present in any individual patient although varying in degree.

Dilatation. This is present in practically all patients and tends to be most severe in the lower half of the jejunum. However, the extent and severity of dilatation varies among patients. In severe disease the dilatation may be marked, resembling that in mechanical obstruction. However, in these patients, there is ineffective and disordered peristalsis, which tends to prolong transit through the area, rather than hyperperistalsis as observed in obstruction. The cause of dilatation is unknown.

Segmentation. This is another important finding in sprue and refers to the accumulation of barium mixture in segments of variable length and separated by empty segments containing no barium mixture. Segmentation may involve much of the small intestine but tends to be more severe in the distal jejunum and ileum than elsewhere. It may be delayed or immediate; as noted on a small bowel study the delayed form

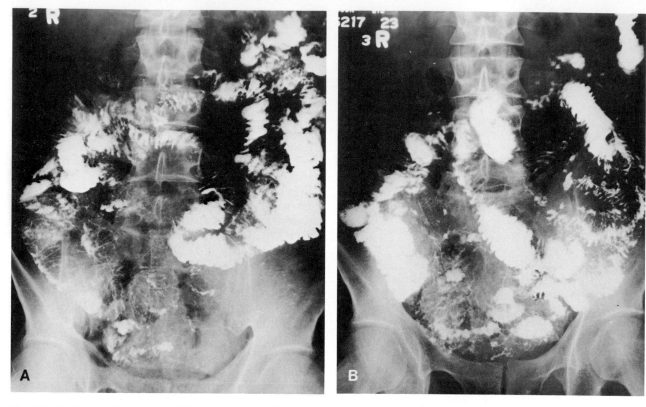

Fig. 18-13. Sprue. Two-hour **(A)** and 3-hour **(B)** studies made after the patient was given a barium meal. These demonstrate extensive segmentation, a coarse mucosal pattern, and some dilatation as well as flocculation of barium. The flocculation is most marked in the distal jejunum and ileum.

is more common. It is accompanied by an excessive amount of fluid and probably caused by it.

Changes in Mucosal Folds. The folds tend to be thinned and often are decreased in height. In some patients, however, the folds appear thickened and the valleys between the folds are widened. The fine, crinkled appearance of the normal valvulae conniventes is lost. Some segments of jejunum may show a complete absence of folds, the margins being quite smooth and tubular. This appearance has been termed the "moulage sign" and is one of the significant findings in sprue. It is associated with segmentation and dilatation. Simple distention will not completely obliterate the folds, even though it is severe.

Hypersecretion. Increased fluid content in the bowel lumen is shown by a tendency for the barium to be scattered in flecks and blotches (flocculation) and by the presence of air–fluid levels in upright roentgeno-

grams. Because there are physical differences in barium suspensions, some of which appear to flocculate more readily than others, the observer must become accustomed to the barium used in the department for the study of the small bowel.

Alterations in Motility. The transit time of barium mixture through the small intstine may be normal, decreased, or accelerated. Because of the wide range of transit times in normal individuals, this finding often is difficult to interpret unless the motility—increased or decreased—is clearly abnormal. It is somewhat dependent on the volume of barium employed.

Transient Intussusception. It is not uncommon in sprue to find the characteristic appearance of intussusception in one or several segments. The intussusception is nonobstructive and transient and the cause is not known. The diagnosis is based on the findings of a localized filling defect with stretched and thinned valvulae conniventes overlying it (*i.e.*, the coiled-spring appearance).

Rare Observations in Sprue and Celiac Disease. These are: (*1*) At times there is duodenal involvement, with thick mucosal folds that may be decreased in number and asymmetrical in distribution, associated with varying degrees of duodenal dilatation. (*2*) Multiple small-bowel ulcerations occasionally occur, presumably as a complication of sprue. (*3*) Colonic ulcers have been reported, but are extremely rare. (*4*) Intramural small-bowel hemorrhage may also complicate sprue. (*5*) There appears to be an increased incidence of lymphosarcoma and carcinoma of the small bowel in patients with sprue and celiac disease.

Differential Diagnosis. In addition to other causes for the malabsorption syndrome, differential diagnosis includes mechanical small-intestinal obstruction. Irregular dilatation, segmentation, flocculation, and the moulage sign are characteristic of sprue. In obstruction, the bowel is dilated uniformly above the obstructing lesion and the barium column tends to be continuous; also the loops of bowel appear to be under tension forming arched curves across the abdomen. In sprue the intestinal loops are flaccid and atonic. If the obstruction is partial the bowel distal to the block is normal in caliber or collapsed and the transition from dilated to collapsed bowel is abrupt.

Among the miscellaneous causes of the malabsorption syndrome are: (*1*) diverticula, blind loops and strictures in which overgrowth of intestinal bacteria may led to macrocytic anemia as well as malabsorption syndrome; (*2*) a number of surgical procedures, particularly those in which there has been resection or bypass of the principal areas of absorption in the duodenum and jejunum; (*3*) pancreatic and hepatic diseases; (*4*) severe diabetes; (*5*) intestinal lactase deficiency; and (*6*) a number of dermatologic conditions such as dermatitis herpetiformis, psoriasis, and exfoliative erythroderma.[34]

Whipple's Disease

Patients with Whipple's disease have steatorrhea, diarrhea, abdominal pain, weight loss, and arthralgia. Lymphadenopathy and polyserositis are noted on physical examination. The basic and characteristic histologic feature is the presence, in the lamina propria and in lymph nodes, of macrophages which are Sudan-negative and periodic acid-Schiff (PAS) positive. The wall of the intestine, along with the mesentery, is thickened and edematous. The roentgen findings in the gastrointestinal tract are similar to those of sprue and some authors have noted difficulty in making the differentiation between sprue and Whipple's disease. Marshak and Lindner[33] stress the findings of thickened mucosal folds, more in Whipple's disease than in sprue, and a lesser degree of dilatation, segmentation, and flocculation in Whipple's disease than in sprue. In fact, dilatation, segmentation, and flocculation may be absent altogether in Whipple's disease. In Whipple's disease the thickened folds are more prominent in the jejunum than elsewhere. Also, the folds may be slightly nodular and have a "wild" and redundant appearance (Fig. 18-14). The lumen may be normal or slightly dilated. Seven of eight patients with Whipple's disease reported by Phillips and Carlson[41] had coarse folds and slight dilatation of the small bowel (lumen over 25 mm in diameter and folds over 2 mm in thickness). Five patients had minimal to moderate flocculation of barium, but there was no segmentation. Similarity of Whipple's disease to intestinal lymphangiectasia and amyloidosis has been noted. Correlation with clinical findings and biopsy is essential in most cases.

Scleroderma
(Progressive Systemic Sclerosis)

Involvement of the esophagus is common in scleroderma but other parts of the gastrointestinal tract also may be affected. The major histologic alteration is atrophy of the muscularis and replacement by fibrous tissue. In the small intestine the changes of a malabsorption syndrome may be seen. As in the esophagus, atony and hypomotility occur with varying degrees of dilatation (Fig. 18-15). The delayed transit time plus the dilatation may be severe enough to strongly suggest a small-bowel obstruction. Usually the mucosal folds are not widened or blunted, but a narrowed distance between them, most marked in the jejunum and proximal ileum, associated with a sharp spiculation of the valvulae has been reported. Narrowed distance between the mucosal folds was noted in about two-thirds of 18 cases reported. Intussusception was observed in three patients. In more advanced disease the formation of saccules or pseudodiverticula is characteristic. This also is seen in the colon. The other findings reported in sprue, such as segmentation, flocculation, and hypersecretion, are uncommon. The occurrence of *pneumatosis intestinalis* (intramural gas) in scleroderma has been documented. Small-bowel changes in *dermatomyositis* are similar to those of sclero-

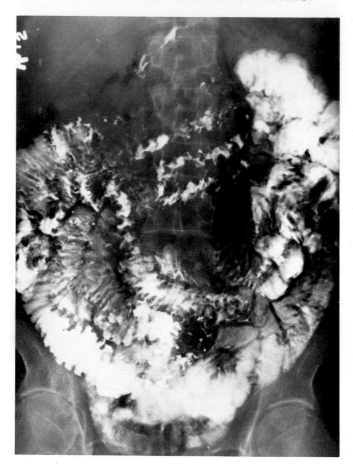

Fig. 18-14.   Whipple's disease. The mucosal folds of the small intestine are thickened and irregular. Some segments are moderately dilated. The barium mixture is diluted in some areas by increased fluid, and there is some segmentation.

derma except that dilatation of the bowel often is more severe.

Amyloidosis

Amyloid infiltration of the gastrointestinal tract is frequent in amyloidosis. The most significant roentgen finding in the small intestine is a thickening of the mucous membrane folds which may involve the entire small bowel. If there is an associated malabsorption syndrome there may be a mild degree of segmentation, flocculation, and dilatation, but changes in the folds remain the most obvious abnormality. The folds may become sufficiently thickened to efface the valvulae in some areas. Occasionally the dilatation may become more severe and clinical manifestations of mechanical obstruction may occur, along with prolonged transit time, representing a form of intestinal pseudo-obstruction.[27] The differentiation between Whipple's disease and amy-

loidosis is difficult and often impossible on roentgen study.

Intestinal Lymphangiectasia

Intestinal lymphangiectasia, first described about 18 years ago, is one of the diseases that causes loss of protein from the gastrointestinal tract with resulting hypoproteinemia. Some patients develop malabsorption. Study of microscopic sections reveals edema and dilatation of lymphatics throughout the mucosa and submucosa. The disease may be present in infants and is thought to be congenital in such patients. When it develops later in life it apparently is acquired, but the pathogenesis is uncertain. Chylous ascites is often present, particularly in infants. The most characteristic roentgen change is that of a diffuse, symmetric thickening of the mucosal folds due to edema. Hypersecretion also is noted, but the other changes seen in the "sprue pattern," such as seg-

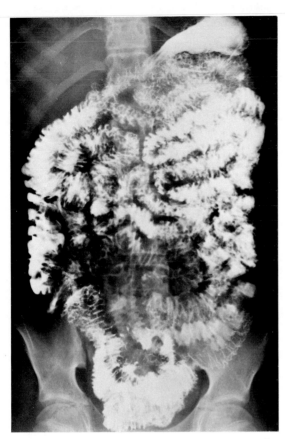

Fig. 18-15. Scleroderma of the small intestine. The mucosal folds are thickened, particularly in the lower abdomen. There is also some thickening in the wall causing slight separation of loops.

mentation and dilatation, are usually minimal or absent. The differentiation from Whipple's disease and amyloidosis may be difficult to make on roentgen study. The same is true of the other entities that may cause intestinal edema.

Hypoproteinemia; Intestinal Edema

There are a number of diseases that can cause excessive loss of protein from the gastrointestinal tract with resulting hypoproteinemia. These include such entities as Menetrier's disese, intestinal lymphangiectasia, regional enteritis, ulcerative colitis, lymphosarcoma, and Whipple's disease. These diseases have frequently been listed under the term *protein-losing enteropathies*. Rarely, multiple inflammatory polyps of the small bowel and cystic lymphangioma of the mesentery are associated with protein-losing en-

teropathy. The etiologic basis of these conditions has not been definitely established. The hypoproteinemia causes noninflammatory intestinal edema. The roentgen findings in patients with intestinal edema consist of generalized and uniform thickening of the mucosal folds (Fig. 18-16), interference with normal motor activity of the bowel, thickening of the wall of the intestine, and, in some, ascites. Some dilatation of the intestinal lumen often is seen, but segmentation and flocculation are absent. Because the intestinal walls are thickened, some widening of the soft-tissue spaces between adjacent loops may be seen. The uniformly thickened folds with a continuous column of barium in the lumen has been likened to a stack of coins. The changes often are seen to best advantage in the jejunum.

Hypoproteinemia also occurs as a result of kidney or liver disease (cirrhosis) and the roentgen signs of edema of the bowel become apparent. It also has been found in a variety of other conditions such as congestive heart failure, burns, allergy, the Zollinger–Ellison syndrome, sprue, neoplasms, histoplasmosis of the small intestine with giant villi and secondary protein-losing enteropathy, the Cronkite–Canada syndrome, and constrictive pericarditis,

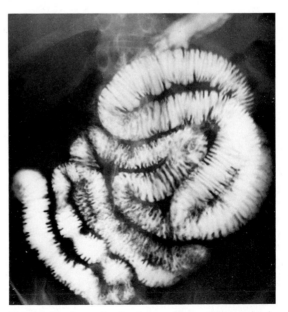

Fig. 18-16. Intestinal edema. The uniform thickening of mucosal folds is characteristic and was shown at autopsy to represent submucosal edema in this patient who had carcinoma of the pancreas.

among others. A correlation with the clinical findings is helpful in evaluating the roentgen findings of intestinal edema. The symptoms are those of the primary disease and not of the intestinal edema. The primary disease (*e.g.*, regional enteritis, Menetrier's disease, lymphosarcoma) often can be identified with considerable assurance from the roentgen appearances, but, in other instances, the signs are only those of edema. Many of the diseases that cause intestinal edema also cause a malabsorption syndrome and it has been speculated that some of the changes seen in malabsorption are the result of edema.

Immunoglobulin Disorders[31]

Marshak and Lindner[33] have classified immoglobulin disorders into primary and secondary groups. The primary disorders include a group of variable immunoglobulin deficiencies: hypogammaglobulinemic sprue, hypogammaglobulinemia with pernicious anemia and atrophic gastritis, nodular lymphoid hyperplasia of the small bowel, and giardiasis. The second group is that of selective IgA (immunoglobulin class A) deficiency including IgA deficient sprue and nodular lymphoid hyperplasia of the small bowel. The secondary disorders may be divided into the following: (*1*) decreased immunoglobulin synthesis or increased synthesis of abnormal immunoglobulins which include plasma-cell dyscrasias, Waldenstrom's macroglobulinemia and alpha chain disease, lymphosarcoma, and chronic lymphatic leukemia; (*2*) increased immunoglobulin breakdown and loss which include the exudative gastroenteropathies and intestinal lymphangectasia; and (*3*) amyloidosis. Also, Marshak and Lindner have organized the roentgen findings into: (*1*) sprue or malabsorption pattern in hypogammaglobulinemic sprue and IgA deficient sprue; (*2*) multiple nodular defects in lymphoma and variable immunoglobulin deficiency; (*3*) inflammatory changes secondary to giardiasis; and (*4*) thickening of small intestinal folds as in amyloidosis, lymphoma, macroglobulinemia, lymphangectasia, and plasma-cell dyscrasias. Several of these conditions are described in more detail in this chapter.

DIVERTICULOSIS

Diverticulosis of the jejunum is an uncommon but not rare entity characterized by a few or many diverticular outpouchings. The outpouchings, or sacs, vary in size from tiny ones up to some measuring 2 cm or more. They arise on the mesenteric side of the bowel wall. Occasionally they are very numerous and often are associated with diverticula of the duodenum. Diverticula in the jejunum show the roentgen characteristics of diverticula elsewhere in the gastrointestinal tract, consisting of smooth-walled sacs communicating with the lumen through narrow necks. In some patients there is an associated *malabsorption syndrome*. Isolated diverticula also occur in the terminal ileum. Acute infection of a diverticulum may cause symptoms and signs simulating those of acute appendicitis. Other complications include recurrent spontaneous pneumoperitoneum, obstruction secondary to ileal or jejunal diverticulitis, and perforation which may be detected radiographically by observation of a tract leading from a diverticulum into an adjacent abscess or by the presence of pneumoperitoneum. These complications are rare, however.

INTUSSUSCEPTION

Ileoileal intussusception is much less common than ileocolic intussusception, which is discussed in Chapter 19. In ileoileal intussusception the absence of pain and later appearance of bleeding often result in a delay in diagnosis. For roentgenographic study, barium may be given orally because the obstruction is in the small bowel. Slight dilatation of the bowel proximally may be noted. If only the central channel of the intussusception fills, a narrow central ribbon of barium may be the only other sign of the prolapse. If the channel is occluded, only a small nipplelike projection into the channel from the dilated small bowel may be observed. If there is less obstruction, some barium may pass through, then extend in a retrograde manner to outline the leading mass and form a typical coil-spring pattern. Hydrostatic reduction is usually unsuccessful in ileoileal intussusception. In children, ileoileal intussusception may arise spontaneously, but in the adult it most often develops as a result of an intraluminal tumor or sometimes of an intramural mass. Usually the actual tumor cannot be identified even though the diagnosis of intussusception is made.

MESENTERIC VASCULAR OCCLUSION

Acute Mesenteric Occlusion

The occurrence of acute obstruction of the superior or inferior mesenteric arteries or veins due to embolus or thrombosis results in an acute, severe illness with infarction of the bowel, necrosis, peritonitis, and, usually, death. Most patients are too ill for barium studies to be performed. The plain-film findings in acute mesenteric occlusion have been discussed in Chapter 13.

Segmental Ischemia

If the vascular occlusion occurs gradually and there is an adequate collateral blood flow, infarction may not develop and there are no positive roentgen changes. Also if the occlusion involves a small branch vessel and perforation does not occur, the patient may survive and later show roentgen findings that become fairly characteristic. This has been called segmental ischemia or, depending on the location, ischemic jejunitis, ileitis, or colitis.

Abdominal roentgenograms may reveal positive signs of the disease in some patients. One or several segments of small intestine will be outlined by gas in the lumen. Thickening of the bowel wall can be identified if two segments lie adjacent to one another. The luminal surface may become smooth with effacement of the normal fold pattern (or haustral sacculations in the colon). The segments appear rigid and the appearance does not change significantly in serial films exposed over a period of several days. If necrosis of the intestinal wall develops, intramural gas sometimes is seen as thin, radiolucent, gas stripes paralleling the bowel lumen (*i.e., pneumatosis intestinalis*). Gas in the portal vein branches within the liver is found infrequently but carries a grave prognosis; most patients succumb to the disease. The combination of intramural gas and portal vein gas form a significant roentgen diagnostic complex for intestinal necrosis. If a small-bowel barium study is performed the involved segment shows thickening of mucosal folds and nodular indentations along the margins (called "thumbprinting" or "scalloping") due to submucosal hemorrhage or edema. As the edema increases the folds become greatly thickened and the lumen may be narrowed. If diffuse ulceration develops the folds become effaced and the lumen becomes smooth. This is more obvious in the jejunum because of the greater number of folds present normally. With healing and fibrosis one wall may become flattened and shortened and multiple sacculations or pseudo-diverticula form on the opposite border. Further fibrosis leads to a rigid tubular appearance followed shortly by stricture formation and dilatation of the bowel above the stricture. The strictured area is usually several inches long and is characterized by smooth tapering ends and a concentric lumen. The entire gamut of these changes occurs rapidly, often only a matter of several weeks from onset to stricture formation. Similar changes occur in the colon when it is involved by segmental ischemia. In the earlier stages the appearance may resemble that of intramural hemorrhage. When stricture formation develops, regional enteritis must be considered in differential diagnosis. Clinical symptoms may be helpful but are sometimes misleading.

Once the tentative diagnosis of ischemia is made, angiography with selective catheterization of the superior mesenteric artery and of the celiac and inferior mesenteric arteries, if necessary, may be used to confirm the diagnosis. The site of obstruction may be identified and the major collateral vesels defined. This information is invaluable when surgery is to be performed. Small-vessel occlusion may be extremely difficult to identify, and the same is true of small-vessel disease, which may alter the blood supply to one or more segments of the bowel.[25]

When mesenteric infarction is present but no site of obstruction can be identified the condition is called *nonocclusive mesenteric ischemia.*

INTESTINAL PARASITES

The demonstration of roundworms (*Ascaris lumbricoides*) in the intestinal tract is possible when a small-intestine study is carried out. The worm may be visualized as an elongated, tubular filling defect in the barium-filled loop of bowel (Fig. 18-17). Because the worm may ingest some of the barium, it is not uncommon to find a thin, dense, stringlike shadow centrally situated within the filling defect produced by the body of the worm. This stringlike shadow represents the barium-filled gastrointestinal tract of the worm. Follow-up roentgenograms after the bowel has emptied itself of the barium mixture (3 to 5 hours after ingestion) may then show the persisting string of barium, which may remain for some hours. The usual location for these defects is in the distal jejunum and proximal portion of the ileum. Only occasionally are worms recognized in the colon.

Tapeworms also can occasionally be demonstrated in the small intestine as long, linear translucencies. A tapeworm is differentiated from a roundworm because of its greater length and by the absence of the stringlike barium shadow outlining the intestinal tract of the worm as the tapeworm does not have an alimentary canal.

Giardiasis

Infection with *Giardia lamblia* does not produce any significant inflammatory disease in most individuals, but, in patients with dysgammaglobulinemia who are infected with this organism, symptoms of the infection are relatively frequent. This organism can also

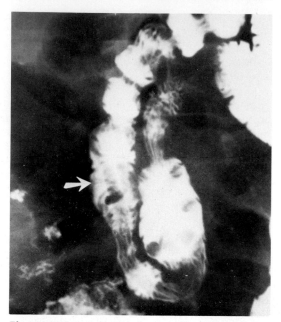

Fig. 18-17. Ascaris in the small intestine. The worms are shown as elongated **(arrow)** and round translucencies in this loop of small intestine.

cause symptoms of disease when it is a heavy contaminant of water supplies. In infection with *Giardia lamblia,* radiographic findings are those of increase in size of the distal duodenal and upper jejunal mucosal fold pattern as well as irritability. There also may be flocculation and segmentation as well as slight narrowing of the lumen with distortion as well as enlargement of the folds. Transit through the jejunum may be very rapid.

Strongyloidiasis

Strongyloides stercoralis is a helminthic parasite that enters the body through the skin, passes through the lung, and is later ingested to produce inflammation in the duodenum and jejunum. Edema and thickening of the mucosal folds, sometimes with nodular intramural filling defects, are found in the duodenum and jejunum caused by invasion of the bowel wall by the parasites who deposit their ova there. At times, the infestation is very severe and may cause paralytic ileus; ulceration may also occur. The changes may closely resemble those of Crohn's disease from which it must be differentiated. The parasite is common in the tropics but is endemic in the southern United States as well. Other parasitic infestations are rare in this country.

DISACCHARIDASE DEFICIENCY

Because they are necessary for the digestion of sugars, deficiency of lactase, sucrase, or fructase may give rise to symptoms of abdominal discomfort and distention, flatulence, and diarrhea. Lactase deficiency is said to be the most common abnormality of the small intestine. Normally, it is present in the epithelial cells of the small bowel. Suitable roentgen study may demonstrate significant changes. The patient is given a nonflocculating barium mixture to which has been added 25 to 50 gm of lactose. Interval films of the small intestine will show a dilution of the barium in the small bowel, dilatation of loops, and a decreased transit time so that the head of the barium column will be in the colon at the end of 1 hour or sooner. These signs are accompanied by abdominal cramps and diarrhea. It has been recommended that lactose be added to the barium mixture for all small-bowel examinations since it does not alter the quality of the study if there is no lactase deficiency.

INTRA-ABDOMINAL HERNIAS

Hernias affecting the intestinal tract may be either external or internal. The diagnosis of external hernia is essentially a clinical problem and roentgen examination is used chiefly to determine the contents of the hernial sac and to demonstrate how much, if any, obstruction is present. A description of the roentgen aspects of external hernia is given in Chapter 19 and will not be repeated here.

In internal hernias the intestinal protrusions are entirely within the peritoneal cavity. The abnormal sac or pouch may have been caused by trauma. More frequently the rent in the mesentery or peritoneum follows a surgical procedure. Also, some internal hernias develop on the basis of congenital defects with the formation of abnormal pouches or fossae. The incidence of intra-abdominal hernias in clinical practice is low. The congenital hernias, in particular, may exist without producing symptoms. When symptoms are caused by an internal hernia they are usually those of bowel obstruction.

Of the congenital types of internal hernia, those involving the paraduodenal fossae are generally considered to be the most important; left paraduodenal hernia is about four times as frequent as the right-sided type. When complete obstruction of the intestine is caused by an internal hernia, the roentgen findings are those of bowel obstruction (*q.v.*), and the nature of the causative lesion seldom can be stated. In those lesions causing only partial obstruction the diagnosis is possible in some cases. The same

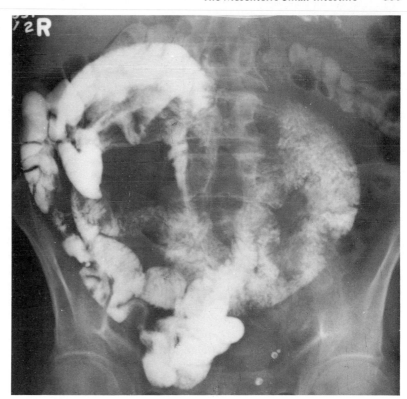

Fig. 18-18. Internal abdominal hernia into the left paraduodenal fossa. A large portion of the jejunum lies within the hernial sac, the margins of which are outlined by the barium-filled small bowel within it.

is true of the asymptomatic hernias. The roentgen findings depend upon the site of the hernia and the amount of bowel involved, but, in general, consist in the visualization of an abnormal accumulation of the barium-filled loops of small intestine into a sac-like configuration (Fig. 18-18). The afferent and efferent loops may be identified as they enter and leave the sac. There may be an abnormal retention of barium within the herniated loops and, if partial obstruction is present, the bowel above the level of the hernia will be dilated. The colon often is found in an abnormal position and the relationships of the colon and small intestine may be distinctly abnormal.

MISCELLANEOUS CONDITIONS

Radiation Injury

The small bowel is the most radiosensitive part of the gastrointestinal tract. At 4500 rads, there is some risk of ulceration, perforation, fibrosis, and obstruction. With larger doses, there may be severe pain, nausea, vomiting, bloody diarrhea, and abdominal distention. Later changes are those of thickening of the wall causing separation of loops. Chronic changes include narrowing with formation of stricture which may involve lengthy segments. The intestinal loops may be fixed, matted together with some kinking and twisting. These late changes may result in some obstruction. Mesenteric fibrosis may create traction and augment the angulation and kinking sometimes observed.

Eosinophilic Gastroenteritis

The gastric manifestations in this syndrome have been described earlier. The inflammation usually involves the stomach and proximal small bowel. The jejunal wall is thickened. The valvulae conniventes are widened and thickened. They may be distorted in severe involvement, resulting in irregular angulation and a saw-tooth contour. When involvement becomes very severe, the valvulae may be effaced. There are usually some regular nodular defects associated with the other changes that can produce a cobblestone appearance in some instances. The thickening of the bowel wall may produce narrowing in some patients. If these findings of the small bowel are associated with involvement of the distal gastric antrum in a patient with eosinophilia and a history of allergy, the diagnosis can be strongly suspected.

Bezoars

Bezoars of the small intestine are found most commonly in patients who have had gastric resection. They are usually phytobezoars, with oranges being their most common cause. In patients with small-bowel strictures, solid material may fail to pass through the stricture, remain in the intestine, and later on appear as an enterolith when calcium is added. As indicated previously, stones are sometimes observed in patients with Meckel's diverticulum.

Cystic Fibrosis

In cystic fibrosis the duodenum is involved somewhat more frequently than the remainder of the small bowel. The findings are those of nodular mucosal changes with a coarse, smudged appearance of mucosal folds particularly in the duodenum. In the jejunum, the changes are relatively mild and consist of thickened folds along with slight dilatation and sometimes the malabsorption pattern. Meconium ileus equivalent in older children or adults may result in small-bowel distention proximal to fecal masses in the ileum. Changes in the colon are striking; these are described in Chapter 19.

Henöch–Schoenlein Purpura

Henöch–Schoenlein purpura is a disease found primarily in children. It is manifest by nonthrombocytopenic purpura, joint pain, and gastrointestinal symptoms. There are no radiologic findings unless submucosal hemorrhage and edema involving the bowel, either locally or in a somewhat diffuse pattern, are present. These produce mural defects or "thumbprinting," on the roentgenogram. In some instances, large, local intramural hemorrhage may result in intussusception. Edema may cause enlargement of valvulae as well as thickening of the bowel wall. Increased secretions may cause blurring of mucosal folds that may become effaced if the edema is severe. Marked increase in secretions causes dilution and flocculation of the barium. Obstruction may be produced by a large hematoma in some instances. The disease is self-limited and healing of the bowel is complete without residual effects.[30]

Abetalipoproteinemia

This autosomal recessive disease is characterized by malabsorption of fat, atypical retinitis pigmentosa, and progressive neurologic deterioration. There is absence of plasma betalipoproteins and reduced serum cholesterol, phospholipids, and vitamin A. The patients have steatorrhea which may be erroneously diagnosed as due to sprue. Roentgen findings consist of some dilatation and some thickening of mucosal folds throughout the entire small bowel. There may also be some thickening of haustra and abnormally prominent folds in the colon. Mild dilatation is present as well as some dilution by increased secretions. Segmentation and flocculation are sometimes observed. The diagnosis depends upon laboratory findings.

Potassium Depletion States

Potassium deficiencies are frequently associated with ileus and are most commonly encountered in the postoperative patient, particularly when the operation has required intestinal manipulation. Hypokalemia may also occur in association with acute conditions such as gastric or small bowel obstruction, ulcerative colitis, dysentery, and infantile diarrhea. Chronic conditions causing hypokalemia include ileostomy diarrhea, biliary fistula, chronic obstruction of the gastrointestinal tract, chronic renal salt loss, prolonged overuse of cathartics, and use of diuretics. The ileus which may occur in any of these conditions may be caused by a number of factors, but intestinal distention is often reduced significantly following potassium replacement. Therefore, hypokalemia must be considered in patients with ileus (distention), particularly in those having postoperative distention.[29]

REFERENCES AND SELECTED READINGS

1. BAKER HL, GOOD CA: Smooth-muscle tumors of the alimentary tract: their roentgen manifestations. Am J Roentgenol 74: 246, 1955

2. BALIKIAN JP, NASSAR NT, SHAMMA'A MH et al: Primary lymphomas of the small intestine including the duodenum. Am J Roentgenol 107: 131, 1969

3. BERDON WE, BAKER DH, BULL S et al: Midgut rotation and volvulus. Radiology 96: 375, 1970

4. BISCHOFF ME, STAMPFLI WP: Meckel's diverticulum: with emphasis on the roentgen diagnosis. Radiology 65: 572, 1955

5. BOIJSEN E, KAUDE J, TYLEN U: Radiologic diagnosis of ileal carcinoid tumors. Acta Radiologica [Diagn] (Stockh) 15: 65, 1974

6. CLEMETT AR, FISHBONE G, LEVINE RJ et al: gastrointestinal lesions in mastocytosis. Am J Roentgenol 103: 405, 1968

7. CLEMETT AR, MARSHAK RH: Whipple's disease. Roent-

gen features and differential diagnosis. Radiol Clin North Am 7: 105, 1969

8. COHEN WN: Gastric involvement in Crohn's disease. Am J Roentgenol 101: 425, 1967

9. COHEN WN: Intestinal lymphangiectasis. Radiology 89: 1080, 1967

10. CROHN BB, JANOWITZ HD: Reflections on regional ileitis, twenty years later. JAMA 156: 1221, 1954

11. DALINKA MK, WUNDER JF: Meckel's diverticulum and its complications with emphasis on roentgenologic demonstration. Radiology 106: 295, 1973

12. DEEB PH, STILSON WL: Roentgen manifestations of lymphosarcoma of the small bowel. Radiology 63: 235, 1954

13. EKBERG O. Double contrast examination of the small bowel. Gastrointest Radiol 1: 349, 1977

14. FERRUCCI JT, BENEDICT KT, PAGE DL et al: Radiographic features of the normal hypotonic duodenogram. Radiology 96: 401, 1970

15. GELFAND DW: High density, low viscosity barium for fine mucosal detail on double-contrast, upper gastrointestinal examinations. Am J Roentgenol 130: 831, 1978

16. GINSBURG LD: Eccentric polyposis of the small bowel. A possible radiologic sign of plexiform neurofibromatosis of the small bowel and its mesentery. Radiology 116: 561, 1975

17. GOLDSTEIN HM, POOLE GJ, ROSENQUIST CJ et al: Comparison of methods for acceleration of small intestinal radiographic examination. Radiology 98: 519, 1971

18. GOOD CA: Tumors of the small intestine. Caldwell Lecture, 1962. Am J Roentgenol 89: 685, 1963

19. GROSFELD JL, FRANKEN EA JR: Intestinal obstruction in the neonate due to vitelline duct cysts. Surg Gynecol Obstet 138: 527, 1974

20. HERBST J, FRIEDLAND GW, ZBORALSKE FF: Hiatal hernia in "rumination" in infants and children. J Pediatr 78: 261, 1971

21. HODGSON JR, HOFFMAN HN II, HUIZENGA KA: Roentgenologic features of lymphoid hyperplasia of the small intestine associated with dysgammaglobulinemia. Radiology 88: 883, 1967

22. HOROWITZ AL, MEYERS MA: The "hidebound" small bowel pattern in scleroderma: characteristic mucosal fold pattern. Am J Roentgenol 119: 332, 1973

23. ISBELL RG, CARLSON HC, HOFFMAN HN II: Roentgenologic-pathologic correlation in malabsorption syndromes. Am J Roentgenol 107: 158, 1969

24. JAMES WB, MELROSE AG: Metoclopramide in gastrointestinal radiology. Clin Radiol 20: 57, 1969

25. JOFFE N, GOLDMAN H, ANTONIOLI DA: Barium studies in small bowel infarction. Radiology 123: 303, 1977

26. LAWS JW, SPENCER J, NEALE G: Radiology in the diagnosis of disaccharidase deficiency. Br J Radiol 40: 594, 1967

27. LEGGE DA, WOLLAEGER EE, CARLSON HC: Intestinal pseudo-obstruction in systemic amyloidosis. GUT 11: 764, 1970

28. LEONIDAS JC, AMOURY RA, ASHCRAFT KW et al: Duodenojejunal atresia with "apple peel" small bowel. Radiology 118: 661, 1976

29. LOWMAN RM (Editorial): The potassium depletion states and postoperative ileus. The role of the potassium ion. Radiology 98: 691, 1971

30. MACPHERSON RI: The radiologic manifestations of Henoch-Schoenlein purpura. J Can Assoc Radiol 25: 275, 1974

31. MARSHAK RH, HAZZI C, LINDNER AE et al: Small bowel in immunoglobulin deficiency syndromes. Radiol Clin North Am 14: 477, 1976

32. MARSHAK RH, KHILNANI M, ELIASOPH M et al: Intestinal edema. Am J Roentgenol 101: 379, 1967

33. MARSHAK RH, LINDNER AE: Radiology of the Small Intestine. Philadelphia, WB Saunders, 1970

34. MARSHAK RH, LINDNER AE, MAKLANSKY D: Ischemia of the small intestine. Am J Gastroenterol 66: 390, 1976

35. MEYERS MA: Clinical involvement of mesenteric and antimesenteric borders of the small bowel loops. Gastrointest Radiol 1: 49, 1976

36. MIERCORT RD, MERRIL FG: Pneumatosis and pseudoobstruction in scleroderma. Radiology 92: 359, 1969

37. MILLER RE, LEHMAN G: Localization of small bowel hemorrhage. Complete reflux small bowel examination. Am J Dig Dis 17: 1019, 1972

38. OSBORN AG, FRIEDLAND GW: A radiological approach to the diagnosis of small bowel disease. Clin Radiol 24: 281, 1973

39. OU TL, BANK S, MARKS IN et al: Benign lymphoid hyperplasia of the gastric antrum. Another cause of "etat mammelonne". Br J Radiol 50: 29, 1977

40. PAUL LW, WINSTON MC: Focal constricting inflammatory lesions of the small intestine. Am J Roentgenol 81: 616, 1959

41. PHILIPS RL, CARLSON HC: The roentgenographic and clinical findings in Whipple's disease. Am J Roentgenol 123: 268, 1975

42. POCK-STEEN O CH: Roentgenologic changes in protein-losing enteropathies. Acta Radiol [Diagn] (Stockh) 4: 681, 1966

43. SELLINK JL: Radiologic examination of the small intestine by duodenal intubation. Acta Radiol [Diagn] (Stockh) 15: 318, 1974

44. SMITH SJ, CARLSON HC, GISVOLD JJ: Secondary neoplasms of the small bowel. Radiology 125: 29, 1977

45. SOS T, MEYERS MA, BALTAXE HA: Non-fundic gastric varices. Radiology 105: 579, 1972

46. TOD PA: Radiological facets of malabsorption. Australas Radiol 12: 121, 1968

47. WERBELOFF L, BANK S, MARKS IN: Radiological findings in protein-losing gastroenteropathy. Br J Radiol 42: 605, 1969

48. ZBORALSKI FF, AMBERG JR: Detection of the Zollinger-Ellison syndrome: the radiologist's responsibility. Am J Roentgenol 104: 529, 1968

19

THE COLON

METHODS OF EXAMINATION

PRELIMINARY ROENTGENOGRAMS

It is good practice to obtain a scout roentgenogram of the abdomen prior to the introduction of contrast material into any part of the gastrointestinal tract. In the examination of the colon the conditions in which plain roentgenograms are of value include (1) obstructing lesions; (2) perforations manifested by free intraperitoneal gas; (3) foreign bodies; (4) calcifications; (5) retained opaque media; (6) bony abnormalities; (7) organ enlargements or displacements; and (8) soft-tissue masses. These and other abnormalities have been discussed in Chapter 13.

CONTRAST VISUALIZATION

The Oral Meal

Barium given orally and followed through the gastrointestinal tract by means of serial roentgenograms is of limited value for the detection of organic lesions of the colon and is rarely used; however, it may give some information in functional abnormalities of the bowel and it is useful in the investigation of errors of rotation. If obstruction of the colon is known to be present or is suspected, barium sulfate should not be given by mouth because of the likelihood of its becoming impacted above the obstruction. In general the roentgen study of the colon for the detection of organic disease depends upon a barium-enema examination.

Barium-Enema Examination

Preparation of the Colon. For satisfactory examination it is necessary that the colon be cleansed thoroughly of fecal matter. This is essential in obtaining an adequate examination of the colon. The accurate identification of small polyps is possible only when there are no confusing shadows caused by retained fecal lumps. Also, it is imperative that the mucosa be clean and well coated with barium in order that early mucosal lesions of inflammatory bowel disease may be detected. Therefore, the preparation of the patient for the examination is of vital importance. Various combinations of diets, laxatives, and preparatory enemas are used in the United States and elsewhere; this is probably an indication that none of them is entirely satisfactory. If possible, we like to have our patients on a clear liquid diet for 24 to 48 hours prior to the examination. Two ounces of castor oil are given the evening before the examination. We have tried other laxatives such as Dulcolax (bisacodyl) and X-Prep (anthraquinoidal glycosides) but, in our opinion, they have not been as effective as castor oil. On the morning of the examination the patient is given a 2000-ml tap-water enema in the x-ray department approximately 1 hour before the procedure is to be started. We have not resumed the use of tannic acid since it has been re-released by the Federal Food and Drug Administration. Our experience before its use was prohibited was that it did promote good to excellent evacuation of the bowel which greatly enhanced the value of the post-evacuation film. When the upper gastrointestinal tract and the colon are to be examined, we prefer to do the upper gastrointestinal examination first since it gives us an added day for dietary preparation; residual barium on the day of the colon examination indicates inadequate preparation. The absence of barium suggests, but does not ensure, that preparation is adequate.

The preparation of the infant colon is generally similar to that for the adult patient, particularly if the examination is being done for the detection of polyps. Less drastic procedures are adequate for most other conditions, such as the identification of errors of rotation, partial or complete obstruction, and megacolon. *The introduction of a large quantity of water into the colon should be avoided in a patient with megacolon because of the danger of causing water intoxication.* For those patients in whom castor oil is not used, one or two cleansing enemas of warm tap water will suffice. Because fluid and electrolyte balance are of vital importance to a critically ill infant or child, an isotonic solution can be used for the cleansing enema.

When ulcerative colitis is known to be present or when diarrhea is a significant symptom, castor oil or other cathartics should be omitted. In these cases we have found it advantageous to use warm, normal saline solution for the cleansing enema. This should be given slowly to avoid overdistention of the colon and the quantity of the enema should be reduced. Frequently 200 to 300 cc of solution are sufficient to remove fecal residues and accumulations of mucus and allow good visualization of the mucosal surface.

Barium Mixtures. A number of barium mixtures are available for use in the study of the colon. For a standard barium enema, we use the pre-packaged Baracoat enema bag which contains 16 ounces of micronized barium sulfate by weight (MacBick). For air-contrast barium enemas, we use HD 85, which contains 85% weight/volume barium sulfate (Lafayette Pharmacal). We use up to 500 ml of this preparation, undiluted, per examination.

In the past we added "fluffy" tannic acid powder to the barium mixture to promote evacuation of the barium enema and give a better mucosal pattern in the post-evacuation study. However, because of some evidence that tannic acid might be toxic, particularly to the liver, its use was banned by the Federal Food and Drug Administration. Recently the use of Clysodrast and tannic acid (no more than 0.25% tannic acid) has received approval. It promotes colonic peristalsis and precipitates mucus that might otherwise cling to the mucosa. The result is an improved post-evacuation study. Present contraindications include: (1) patients under 10 years of age, (2) pregnancy, and (3) known or suspected ulcerative disease. We have not resumed its use, but believe that it definitely promotes evacuation of the colon.

Many authors have advocated the use of high kilovoltage technique in roentgenography of the filled colon in order to visualize small polyps more easily. Roentgenograms obtained with kilovoltages above 100 often allow one to "see through" the dense barium shadow and small filling defects are not likely to be obscured by the layer of barium overlying them.

Technique of Examination: The Conventional Barium Enema. The barium mixture is introduced into the colon by gravity, using a disposable barium-enema unit. The container is placed from 2 to 3 feet above the top of the fluoroscopic table. The mixture is allowed to flow into the colon slowly in order to avoid overdistention of the rectum which may precipitate defecation. If difficulty is encountered or expected a small balloon catheter can be used in place of the rectal tip, the balloon being inflated under fluoroscopic control, preferably by the examiner. If ulcerative colitis is present or if there is a rectal stricture a balloon should not be used because of the danger of rupture of the rectum. When there is doubt about the presence of a rectal pathologic condition, the radiologist should perform the rectal examination himself before inserting a balloon catheter.

The flow of mixture is observed by fluoroscopy from the moment it enters the rectum until satisfactory filling of the colon has been obtained or the examination is discontinued for other reasons. The patient is rotated into various positions to bring the flexures and the loops of sigmoid into profile. Manual palpation with the lead-glove protected hand or, preferably, a palpating device such as a palpating spoon, is used to separate overlying loops, to determine the pliability of the walls, and to bring out small intraluminal defects. When the barium column reaches the cecum the flow is discontinued. Ordinarily there will be reflux into the terminal ileum either when the cecum fills or later during evacuation of the enema. When the ileum fills, this segment of the small intestine can be examined; also it locates the ileocecal valve and this is an anatomic landmark that assures that the entire colon has been filled. At times, ileal filling is a disadvantage because the barium-filled loops may obscure some part of the colon that is under suspicion or in which a lesion has been found. The sigmoid often is hidden in this way, therefore, we prefer to take all necessary spot films of the rectosigmoid early in the examination, before there is filling of the right colon. Filling of the ileum should be avoided if a double-contrast examination is to be done, as described in a later paragraph. Sometimes, ileal filling can be prevented by stopping the flow of mixture when the head of the column has reached the hepatic flexure. The pressure that has been built up in the distal colon, combined with manual palpation, may cause the ascending colon and cecum to fill. A slow administration of the enema and avoidance of too much distention of any part of the colon also may prevent reflux, at least until after the patient has been allowed to evacuate the enema.

During filling, spot roentgenograms of suspicious areas or of any region that is difficult to visualize in standard roentgenograms, such as the flexures and the sigmoid loops, are obtained. We have no fixed pattern for spot-filming other than to spot-film the flexures, sigmoid, rectum, and ileocecal area, but vary our procedure from patient to patient, depending upon the nature of the problem.

After completion of fluoroscopy, roentgenograms of the abdomen are obtained with the patient in (*1*) a prone position, (*2*) left lateral position, and (*3*) the prone, 35-degree caudad angled position for the rectosigmoid (or preferably in the prone, 45-degree right anterior oblique position with 35-degree caudad angulation). Other projections also may be indicated. Then evacuation of the mixture is allowed and a postevacuation roentgenogram is obtained. Variations from this more or less routine procedure may be necessary. We rarely use the Chassard–Lapiné view because it is so difficult and uncomfortable for our patients, many of whom are elderly. Fluoroscopy after the patient has evacuated the mixture may be useful.

The Double Contrast Enema. There is a considerable difference of opinion among radiologists and clinicians as to whether the double contrast enema should be used in special situations following a conventional enema or whether it should be used routinely without preliminary barium studies. We prefer to use the double contrast enema (*1*) in patients in whom the conventional enema has shown polyps or a suspicion of polyps, (*2*) when there is a single polyp demonstrated on the conventional examination, (*3*) in the follow-up of small polyps, (*4*) in patients in whom conventional enema has failed to find the source of chronic blood loss, and (*5*) in patients in whom a suspicious lesion of any type is not definitely diagnosed on the initial study. Whenever the conventional study has not provided all of the information desired or has not answered a clinical problem, the double contrast study may be of value.

The double contrast enema examination should not be performed for at least 24 hours after sigmoidoscopy if at all possible; after a rectal or sigmoid biopsy we prefer to wait a week or more before undertaking it. Although a number of authors use the double contrast study in the examination of patients with ulcerative colitis and granulomatous colitis, we have been hesitant to do this; also barium studies of any kind are contraindicated in patients with toxic megacolon. Perforation of the colon is another contraindication to both types of barium studies.

Technique. Many variations in the method of carrying out the examination have been described by Welin, Miller, Laufer, and others.[27] Some prefer a method used by Laufer. The examination is started with the patient in the prone position, and barium is allowed to flow to the splenic flexure during the insufflation of air which follows immediately; the patient is then rotated with his left side elevated. Appropriate spot films of the sigmoid colon are obtained during this maneuver to avoid overlapping if the terminal ileum should fill later. By the time the patient is rotated 90 degrees the barium should be in the right colon and additional air is introduced under fluoroscopic control. Then the table is moved to the upright position and the barium is drained from the rectum. Additional air is introduced and double contrast views of the rectum and flexures are obtained. Then the table is returned to the horizontal position for double contrast views of the sigmoid and cecum. Additional spot films may be obtained when there is any redundancy or when a lesion is observed in any part of the colon (Fig. 19-1). The overhead films are then obtained consisting of a posteroanterior, anteroposterior, and right and left lateral decubitus views,

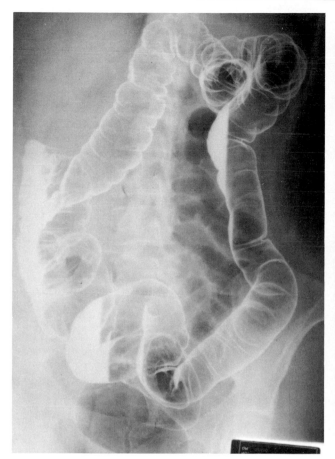 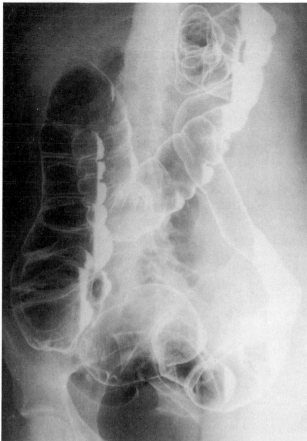

Fig. 19-1. Double contrast examination of the colon. These lateral decubitus projections, obtained during double contrast examination, show such good coating of the mucosa that any mucosal lesion present could be detected during the examination. Several additional films are obtained, including spot films of any questionable area.

and a prone angled view of the rectosigmoid. The latter view may be obtained with the patient in the right anterior oblique prone position when the sigmoid is redundant. The position can be monitored fluoroscopically if necessary for proper angulation. All films are viewed before the patient leaves. A simple method used by many is to fill the colon to the cecum or nearly so, let the patient evacuate, and then introduce the air.

A drug with an anticholinergic effect, such as propanthaline bromide (Pro-Banthine) in 30- to 60-mg doses given intramuscularly, atropine in 0.25- to 1.0-mg doses given orally, or glucagon in 1- to 2-mg doses given intramuscularly or intravenously, is used routinely by some, and, if needed, by others, to lessen spasm and discomfort during the examination. Some use Valium (diazepam) in 5- to 10-mg doses, given orally, to relax the patient during the examination. We use glucagon only when spasm of the colon is a problem during the examination.

Other Methods. *Water Enema.* This is used to show the increased radiolucency of a lipoma, once the lesion has been identified as a mass on regular barium-enema study. We have tried this method several times but do not find it very helpful.

Water-Soluble Media. A water-soluble medium such as Gastrografin, Hypaque 50, and Renografin 76 is occasionally used in special situations. These media have no place in the routine examination of the colon since they are hypertonic, irritating, do not coat the mucosa, and are very expensive. There are several special situations in which they are used, however.

These include suspected perforation when the demonstration of its exact site is important and, possibly, in patients with the meconium plug syndrome. Injudicious use can be disastrous, however. When Gastrografin is used in patients with obstruction, if some of this medium flows into the colon proximal to the obstruction and cannot be evacuated, cecal perforation may result from increased pressure caused by fluid accumulating as a result of hypertonicity of the material. Also, Gastrografin appears to have contributed to bowel necrosis in newborns when retained in the colon and may substantially alter fluid balance in these neonates. Tween 80 (polysorbate) is a stool emulsifier and surface-active substance; it is an oily, yellow fat that is not broken down or absorbed in the distal bowel.[43] An enema solution of 1% to 2% Tween 80 and isotonic sodium diatrizoate has recently been used by Wood and Katzberg[75] for the relief of meconium or fecal mass obstruction in infants and children. These authors believe that it provides a safe and simple technique for relief of intraluminal bowel obstruction in infants and children. It avoids the hazards of using a very hypertonic solution in patients with problems of fluid balance and of obstruction. However, there is some evidence in experimental animals that Tween 80 may play a major role in mucosal damage produced by Gastrografin when these substances are used together.

The Colostomy Patient. Examination of the colon in the colostomy patient poses problems, since castor oil usually cannot be used in this situation. Therefore, a liquid diet and irrigation are often employed in preparation of the patient for the examination. A number of devices are available to enable the patient to hold an enema tip in place while occluding the colostomy stoma. It is not wise to use a balloon-type catheter inflated inside the bowel in these patients since perforation is a definite possibility. The conventional enema study is not very difficult, but we have had problems with air contrast in these patients, particularly when they cannot cooperate very well. Giving an enema through an ileostomy stoma is performed in a manner similar to that of giving an enema through a colostomy stoma.

Arteriography. Arteriography of the mesenteric arteries, preferably by selective catheterization of the vessels, has been used to locate bleeding sites in the colon that cannot be detected by more conventional means. If bleeding is active and the rate exceeds 0.5 ml per minute, the bleeding site in the bowel may be demonstrated by selective arteriography. Some tumors can be identified by arteriography, particularly if they are highly vascular. However, many tumors are not highly vascular and routine barium enema study may be more reliable than arteriography in these situations.

THE NORMAL COLON

ANATOMY AND PHYSIOLOGY

The discussion to follow deals mainly with the appearance of the colon (*1*) when fully distended by means of a barium enema, and (*2*) when contracted after the barium enema has been expelled. These are the conditions under which most roentgenograms of the colon are obtained (Fig. 19-2). Only those aspects of anatomy and physiology of particular interest from a roentgen point of view will be included and the reader is referrred to standard texts dealing with these subjects for more basic information.

The Divisions of the Colon

The usual anatomic divisions of the colon can be recognized in most patients and ordinary anatomic usage is followed in the description of roentgenograms.

Ileocecal Valve, Cecum, and Appendix. The junction of the ileum and cecum is a most important roentgen landmark. While considerable variation exists in the structure of the normal valve, the studies of Fleischner and Bernstein[20] and of Lasser and Rigler indicate the following roentgen features to be of significance.

Of the two lips forming the valve the superior is the longer. As they project into the filled cecum from the medial side and are viewed in profile, these lips cause filling defects, one above the other and separated by a small extension of barium that may, if ileal reflux has occurred, be continuous with the barium-filled lumen of the ileum. The lips seen in this manner measure from 2 to 5 mm in width (Fig. 19-3).

If the ileocecal valve is on the posterior surface and compression is applied over the cecum the valve appears as a transverse, spindle-shaped filling defect with a small pocket of barium in the center representing the opening (see Fig. 19-3B).

Thickening of the valve lips is not infrequent. In some patients this is caused by an accumulation of fatty tissue; in others hypertrophy of the muscle coats is responsible; in still other patients it is caused by a protrusion of ileal mucosa beyond the valve lips. This

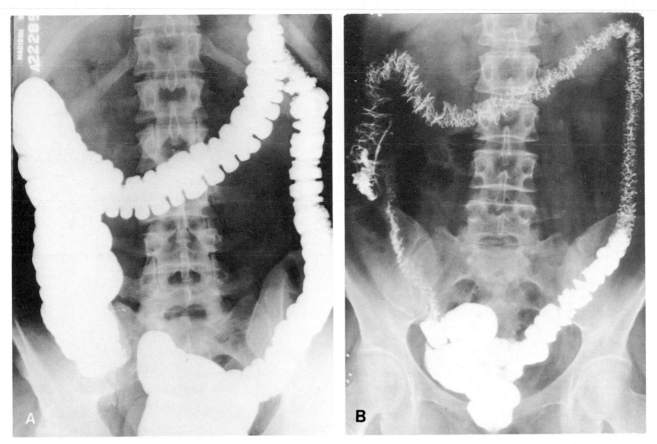

Fig. 19-2. Normal colon. **A.** The barium-filled colon with the patient in the prone position. **B.** Post-evacuation film showing much of the colon to be contracted with the mucosa in fine, crinkled folds. There has also been some reflux of barium into the terminal ileum and into the appendix, which is in a retrocecal position.

latter condition resembles closely the protrusion of gastric mucosa through the pylorus. The significance of these conditions is doubtful but the defect in barium filling caused by a prominent valve may resemble a polypoid or an intramural tumor. The correct interpretation depends upon establishing its relationship to the filled ileum, the smoothly rounded contour of the mass with a small accumulation of barium in the center indicating the valve opening, the occasional stellate radiation of mucosal folds from the center of the defect, and by changes in shape of the defect during examination when it is caused by mucosal prolapse.

The appendix arises from the base of the cecum on the side of the ileocecal valve. When the valve is on the posterior surface of the cecum the appendix almost always is in a retrocecal position. The ileocecal valve therefore serves as a fairly good indicator of appendiceal location. Following appendectomy and inversion of the appendiceal stump, a small polypoid defect in the base of the cecum may be visualized. This is caused by the invaginated stump and may resemble the defect of a true polyp. A history of previous appendectomy and the location of the defect aid in identifying it correctly (see Fig. 19-42).

The cecum is surrounded completely by peritoneum and thus has a fair degree of mobility. A portion of the ascending colon also may be surrounded by peritoneum and, in some individuals, there may be a distinct mesentery. In these the cecum and ascending colon are unusually mobile and the position of the cecum may vary widely from time to time. It is in these patients that volvulus of the cecum can develop.

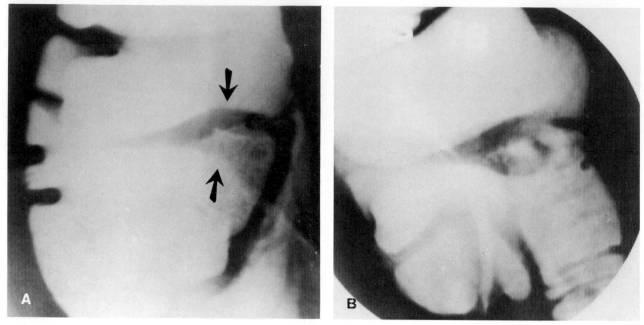

Fig. 19-3. The ileocecal valve. **A.** Compression film exposed during fluoroscopy, showing the terminal ileum projecting downward from the medial side of the cecum. The lips of the valve form a spindle-shaped lucency **(arrows). B.** Roentgenogram of another patient in whom the valve is more posterior and is seen *en face.* Note filling of the appendix and of the terminal ileum.

The Ascending Colon. Except for that portion immediately adjacent to the cecum, the ascending colon ordinarily is retroperitoneal in location and is covered by peritoneum only on the anterior surfce. At the hepatic flexure the colon turns toward the midline and forward to form the beginning of the transverse portion, and it acquires a mesentery. The length of the ascending colon is variable. In some persons it is very long and the cecum is situated within the pelvis.

The Transverse Colon. This part of the colon has a mesentery and is freely movable. It is displaced easily by manual palpation and by masses within the abdomen. It varies in length from one individual to another. In persons of asthenic habitus it may extend into the pelvis and overlie the sigmoid. The flexures also may be unusually low in such individuals. The position of the colon has little to do with its function in most cases and the diagnosis of visceroptosis should carry no implication that functional derangement must be associated. The transverse colon and the hepatic flexure occasionally are found interposed between the liver and the diaphragm (*Chilaiditi's syndrome*). This type of interposition is common, especially in mentally retarded or psychotic patients with chronic colonic enlargement, and sometimes it occurs in association with chronic lung disese, postnecrotic cirrhosis, or pregnancy. As a rule this displacement is a transient one and usually has no clinical significance.

The Descending Colon. The splenic flexure is one of the most fixed parts of the gastrointestinal tract, being held to the diaphragm by the phrenicocolic ligament. The flexure and the entire descending colon are retroperitoneal in position so there usually is no mesentery. Infrequently this is not true and a mesentery is present allowing a certain amount of medial and lateral movement. The junction of the descending colon and the sigmoid is indicated anatomically by the emergence of the colon from the retroperitoneal space and the development of a mesentery for the sigmoid portion. This occurs just below the iliac crest within the left fossa. This junction is usually not very distinct in roentgenograms and can be located only approximately.

The Sigmoid Colon. Having a long mesentery, the sigmoid colon is freely movable. The length is variable but usually the sigmoid executes one or two loops within the pelvis. It may be very long and extend upward on the left side as high as the splenic flexure. In other patients it curves to the right side as far as the cecum before turning back toward the midline and then to the left to its junction with the descending portion. Extreme elongation and mobility of the sigmoid predispose to volvulus.

The Rectum. The junction of the rectum and the sigmoid is not an abrupt one in roentgenograms, although anatomically it represents a change from the colon, which has a mesentery, to the rectum, which has none and lies in the retroperitoneal space. Proctoscopy is the method of choice for examination of the rectum; routine roentgen methods used in examining the colon should not be relied upon for diagnosis. Many rectal lesions, such as fungating carcinomas and ulcerative colitis, can be demonstrated clearly by roentgen examination, but other significant lesions usually are not identified. Inability to identify lesions by roentgen study is due chiefly to the great distensibility of the rectum. During the administration of the enema the rectum is filled with a large amount of barium and small lesions may be covered completely. Being situated within the pelvis it cannot be palpated during fluoroscopy and therefore palpation as an aid to roentgen diagnosis cannot be utilized. Double-contrast studies allow good visualization of the rectal mucosa, however.

Colon Anatomy

The colon is characterized by the presence of haustral sacculations and by the taeniae coli; these give it an appearance distinct from the remainder of the gastrointestinal tract. The taeniae are three longitudinal muscle bands that extend from the tip of the cecum to the lower part of the sigmoid and constitute the majority of the longitudinal musculature of this portion of the tract. The haustra are saclike pouches separated by crescentic folds made up of all the layers of bowel wall. The sacculations vary from 1 to 5 cm in length and are most constant in the right half of the colon. Haustra are variably present in the lower part of the descending colon and sigmoid, although usually demonstrable in these areas. The haustra are not completely fixed and serial roentgen studies carried out over a period of minutes show a constant change in the depth of the crescentic folds and in the width of the sacculations. This constant change leads to a certain amount of forward and backward movement, known as haustral churning. The diameter of the colon decreases from the cecum to the rectosigmoid junction.

The length of the colon varies greatly in the newborn and during infancy. Elongation of the sigmoid is the rule but the rest of the colon may be unusually redundant. The elongation tends to diminish as the child grows older but even in the adult one must allow a wide range of variation for the normal before considering that abnormal elongation is present.

After evacuation of the barium mixture, a thin coating usually remains on the mucosal surface. When contracted the mucous membrane is thrown into a network of folds, giving it a fine, crinkled relief (see Fig. 19-2). Occasionally, in the lower part of the descending and sigmoid areas, the folds are more or less parallel and run in the direction of the long axis of the bowel. Otherwise parallel folds of this type usually are seen only momentarily and in short lengths of the bowel; they are caused by the presence of a mass peristaltic contraction.

During the process of evacuation the colon contracts in length as well as in breadth; if redundant loops are present in the filled colon they often are reduced in length or disappear completely in the contracted state.

Mucosal Anatomy. The normal colonic mucosa is relatively smooth but there are small, linear indentations that are largely circumferential but sometimes longitudinal; these are called "innominate grooves."[21, 72] They are deep enough to retain barium and therefore may be visible on radiographs. Observed *en face*, they appear as a linear network pattern with the majority of the lines circumferential but enough of them are oblique and longitudinal to form the network. Where two of these lines cross, a small pit is formed that appears as a spiculation when silhouetted and as punctate densities when seen *en face*. The innominate grooves may not be apparent in the filled colon, but are visible on the postevacuation film and on air contrast studies of good quality. They are often observed in only one portion of the colon on a single examination. Some believe that the marginal spiculations and punctate collections are caused by filling of the crypts of Lieberkühn, but, because they are very small (0.8 to 1.0 mm), the pattern is probably created by the innominate lines and their junctions. The grooves must be differentiated from the small ulcers noted in early ulcerative colitis and also the network pattern must be differentiated from the minimal cobblestone pattern of early ulcerative colitis. The uniformity and clear definition tend to make the differentiation from ulcers. In ulcerative colitis the ulcers are irregular in size, shape, and distribution; they persist on repeated examination, may be somewhat blurred, and are associated with an abnormal mucosal pattern.

Movements of the Colon

The forward movement of contents in the cecum and ascending colon often seems to be the result only of the constant addition of material from the small intestine. Serial studies often show only a gradual forward movement of the head of the barium column, which may continue until it is well along in the transverse colon. The chief means of movement of fecal material into the distal part of the colon is by mass peristaltic contractions. In the normal individual these probably occur only a few times a day. During a barium enema examination when the colon has been made irritable by catharsis and by the distention from the enema, mass contractions are seen occasionally. Usually in these instances the contraction wave begins in the ascending colon, moving with moderate speed and pushing the colonic content before it. Within a few seconds the wave will have reached the descending colon or, occasionally, the sigmoid. Sometimes it may stop before reaching the splenic flexure. Once forward progress of the contraction has been halted the colon relaxes and usually refills. In some patients, while the contraction is in progress the desire to defecate is strong and the enema may be expelled.

Reference has been made to haustral churning movements in a previous paragraph. These are very slow movements and can be visualized only by exposing serial roentgenograms at intervals of from 15 to 30 seconds over a period of several minutes. They are studied to best advantage when the colon has been filled by means of a barium meal. The haustral movements are not believed to play any part in the forward propulsion of colonic content; rather the type of motion suggests that they are a means of constantly changing the material that is in contact with the colonic mucosa.

CONGENITAL MALFORMATIONS

ERRORS OF ROTATION

During its development the intestinal tract is described as consisting of the foregut, the midgut, and the hindgut. During early fetal life the midgut grows so rapidly that it cannot be contained within the abdominal cavity and it herniates into the umbilical cord. In time it returns into the abdominal cavity. During this process of herniation and return the gut undergoes a rotation of 270 degrees counterclockwise on the axis of the mesenteric artery. The process of rotation may be arrested at any stage. Faulty rotation of the gut during its development involves not only the colon but the small intestine as well. This condition is also discussed in Chapter 18.

Reversal of Rotation

Rotation in a clockwise direction is extremely rare and results because the postarterial rather than the prearterial segment enters the abdominal cavity first, passing behind the superior mesenteric artery from left to right. The transverse colon then lies behind the duodenum.

Complete Failure of Rotation

Complete failure of rotation is relatively infrequent. When this happens the jejunum and ileum are found in the right side of the abdomen and the colon in the left. The cecum may overlie the sacrum or may be to the left of the midline; the ileocecal valve is situated on the right side of the cecum. The diagnosis is made without difficulty on barium-enema examination if the colon is filled completely and the ileocecal valve identified. Serial roentgenograms after a barium meal will show the absence of a normal duodenal loop, the third portion of the duodenum turning downward and the jejunum being entirely on the right side of the abdomen. The condition usually is not a cause of symptoms.

Incomplete Rotation (Malrotation)

Incomplete rotation is common and is always associated with a defect in peritoneal attachment that is of greater clinical significance than the faulty rotation. The cecum is unusually mobile; the ascending colon is surrounded by peritoneum and may have a mesentery. The attachment of the mesentery can be very short. These conditions predispose to volvulus. On barium-enema examination the cecum is found in an abnormal position or, if normally situated, it is found to be abnormally mobile. If volvulus develops, the diagnosis often can be made by plain roentgenograms of the abdomen without the use of contrast material. Roentgen findings in volvulus of the sigmoid and cecum are described in Chapter 13 and volvulus of the midgut in Chapter 16.

Volvulus of the Transverse Colon

This is much less common than volvulus of the cecum and has less characteristic findings. Plain-film findings are those of a distended proximal colon, sometimes with a larger upper central loop. Two air–fluid levels are usually observed on horizontal-beam films. The distal colon is usually contracted and empty. Unless signs of perforation or peritoneal irritation or signs suggesting gangrene are present, barium-enema study should be performed. A "beak" sign is virtually pathognomonic if present but may not be demonstrable. At times, the site of obstruction may be rather smoothly rounded, and unless plain-film findings are strongly suggestive the diagnosis must be that of obstruction of unknown cause.

DUPLICATION OF THE COLON

Duplication of the colon is a rare anomaly. It may be limited to the colon or rectum, and it is usually partial. When duplication involves the entire colon, it may be associated with duplications of the lower urinary or genital tract or both. This type is often associated with other congenital anomalies.[38] Roentgen findings depend on the site and extent of the duplication. At times a soft-tissue density may compress the lumen and even cause obstruction of adjacent bowel. When the duplications communicate, they may be identified as gas-filled structures paralleling the colon. On barium examination, displacement or compression by the mass which cannot be observed on plain films may be evident; the mass may be elongated and is usually located along the mesenteric border when in the sigmoid colon. When it extends into the rectal area, the rectum is displaced forward. Urography or cystography may demonstrate a double bladder or urethra. Often the diagnosis cannot be made definitely on roentgenographic examination unless there is a communication. Rarely, calcification is present within the lumen of the duplicated segment.

IMPERFORATE ANUS

Imperforate anus is responsible for about 5% of cases of intestinal obstruction in the neonatal period. Roentgen examination is useful in determining if the lesion is "high" (above the pelvic floor) or "low" and the presence and nature of the frequently associated anomalies.

For many years the *inverted view* has been used to determine the length of the atretic segment (Fig. 19-4). This consisted of a lateral view of the inverted infant with a radiopaque marker placed on the perineum. The distance from the end of the rectal gas column to the marker was supposed to indicate the length of the atresia. There are, however, several possible sources of error: (1) since it may require 8 hours or more for swallowed air to reach the rectum the infant should be examined a number of hours after birth (24 hours or so). If the examination is undertaken too soon after birth an erroneous result may be obtained. (2) An accumulation of meconium in the rectum may prevent gas from entering it. (3) Another area of atresia higher up in the gastrointestinal tract may make the examination of no value as far as the rectum is concerned. For these and other reasons the inverted view is no longer recommended as a means for determining the length of the atresia.[13] It can be used, however, to show: (1) air in the bladder in male patients with rectourethral and rectovesical fistulas; (2) the mass of a dilated vagina (filled with fluid, air, or both) in the rare female cloacal anomaly; and (3) lumbosacral spinal anomalies that correlate well with urologic malformations that are found in two-thirds of male and female "high" lesions and one-third of male "low" atresias.

Berdon and associates[3] divide imperforate anus into four major groups, according to sex and whether there is a "high" or a "low" lesion. If there is a detectable perineal fistula, the atresia is classified as "low." If there is no detectable perineal fistula, it is considered a "high" lesion. More than 50% of males with a high atresia will show air in the bladder from a fistula to the urethra or bladder. If air cannot be demonstrated, voiding cystourethrography can be carried out to outline the fistula.

The spinal anomalies are mostly errors of segmentation. Kurlander[39] found that more than 70% of imperforate anus patients with anomalies of the sacrum had urologic anomalies. Because many of these anomalies are of a serious nature, diagnosis should be made as soon as possible, *i.e.,* within the first week of life. The urologic anomalies, in addition to those mentioned, include crossed ectopy, crossed fused ectopy, renal agenesis or nonfunction, hydronephrosis, and vesicoureteral reflux.

ATRESIA AND STENOSIS OF THE COLON

Atresia of the colon above the level of the rectum is infrequent. The atresia may be a complete discontinuity or, more rarely, an internal veil or diaphragm that occludes the lumen completely. In the first type the segments may be connected by a fibrous band or

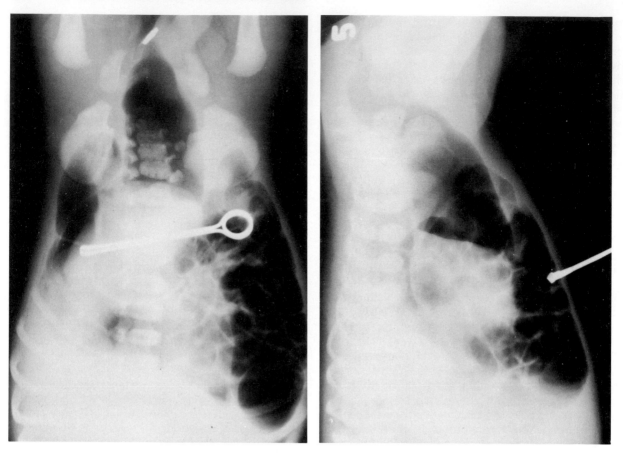

Fig. 19-4. Imperforate anus. The patient was inverted at the time that the films were exposed. There is a lead marker over the anal dimple. Gas extending into the rectum demonstrates a short atretic segment.

have no connection. There may be multiple areas of atresia with isolated blind segments joined by fibrous strands. The passage of meconium does not exclude the possibility of atresia but when cornified epithelial cells are absent in the meconium it is fairly good evidence that atresia exists.

Roentgen Findings. Plain-film roentgenograms of the abdomen may reveal the site of obstruction because of gas distention above it. It requires 6 to 8 hours after birth for swallowed air to reach the lower part of the colon. When atresia exists, the bowel gradually becomes distended with gas and fluid. It often is difficult to distinguish gas-distended loops of colon from small intestine in the infant because both become smooth-walled and tubular when distended. The persistence of haustra in the colon and of the valvulae conniventes in the jejunum, which is a dis-

tinguishing anatomic feature in the adult, even when the bowel becomes greatly distended, is not a distinguishing anatomic feature in infants. The position of the segments becomes important—the colon situated along the circumference of the abdomen and the small intestine within the central part. The colon is dilated up to the site of obstruction and there is only minimal to moderate distention of the small bowel. If there is doubt about the location of the obstruction a barium enema can be given. The colon below the atresia invariably has a small lumen. This has been referred to as "microcolon." If a membrane or diaphragm obstructs the colon, the membrane or diaphragm may be ballooned into the dilated colon proximal to it by the pressure of the barium, producing the "wind-sock" sign. If this sign is present, it suggests the presence of a membrane or diaphragm as the cause of obstruction.

If the atresia is in the small intestine and located in the duodenum or proximal jejunum the caliber of the colon may be normal. In distal jejunal or ileal obstructions the entire colon has a very small caliber. Microcolon occurs only when the colon has not been used, *i.e.,* when no meconium has passed through it. This should not be construed as the cause of the patient's difficulty; it is merely the normal appearance of bowel below the level of a congenital obstruction.

According to Berdon and associates,[4] atresia of the small intestine can occur if there has been volvulus of a segment of small bowel *in utero.* The volvulated segment undergoes infarction and necrosis and may eventually be absorbed, leading to atresia at the site of the obstruction. Meconium ileus is a frequent cause of the volvulus.

Incomplete obstruction or stenosis of the colon also is a rare condition. Symptoms depend upon the severity of the stenosis and are related to the degree of obstruction. Cornified epithelial cells usually can be found in the meconium, since swallowed amniotic fluid can pass through the gastrointestinal tract. Plain-film roentgenograms will show gas distention above the level of stenosis if the stenosis is at all severe. If these are not diagnostic, a barium enema can be given to outline the site and degree of stenosis.

Agenesis

Agenesis of the colon is extremely rare, except for the type in which a short segment of the right colon, usually the cecum, is present. There is often an associated fistula to the bladder or vagina. In neonates with this anomaly the cecum dilates enormously a few hours following birth.

MEGACOLON

Megacolon usually is considered as being of three types, organic, functional, and congenital (Hirschsprung's disease).

Organic Megacolon

Any lesion that causes a chronic partial obstruction of the colon may lead to a gradual enlargement of the bowel above the level of obstruction to a size where it may properly be called a megacolon. Because it requires a period of time for development, the lesions that cause it usually are benign. They include adhesive bands, chronic volvulus, congenital and acquired strictures, and the like. In our experience, adhesions and chronic or recurrent volvulus have been the

most frequent causes. The diagnosis of organic megacolon and its differentiation from the congenital type depend upon the history and the demonstration of the causative lesion. In congenital megacolon the onset of symptoms usually dates from birth; in organic megacolon the onset is later in life. The characteristic findings in congenital megacolon will be described subsequently and the diagnosis can be made without difficulty when they are present. The dilatation of the colon usually is less in organic megacolon than in congenital megacolon and the site of obstruction may be higher than the rectosigmoid. Megacolon caused by volvulus usually is recognized because of the demonstration of the volvulus or by the unusually redundant and mobile sigmoid if examined during a nonobstructive period.

Functional Megacolon

Functional megacolon results from faulty bowel habits in children and not infrequently in psychotic adult patients. The onset of symptoms may be early in life, but usually they do not date from birth. On digital examination the rectum is found filled with feces, in contrast to congenital megacolon in which the rectum usually is empty. Barium enema demonstrates dilatation of the entire colon, including the rectum. Enlargement of the rectum may be especially great and when distended with the barium enema it may fill the entire pelvis. The dilatation of the rest of the colon usually is not as pronounced as it is in congenital megacolon, the amount of impacted feces is less, and relief often is obtained at least temporarily by repeated enemas. A lateral view of the pelvis is often helpful in determining the diagnosis since large masses of fecal material in a dilated rectum differentiate the functional from the aganglionic megacolon.

Congenital Megacolon (Aganglionosis) (Hirschsprung's Disease)

Aganglionosis of the rectosigmoid results in a pronounced dilatation of the colon or a portion of it with hypertrophy of the walls of the dilated portion and with a normal-sized or narrowed segment in the rectum or the rectosigmoid region. Within the narrowed portion there is a marked diminution or a complete absence of the ganglion cells in the myenteric plexuses. The dilated colon is filled with a large amount of feces at all times.

According to current concepts the difficulty arises from a failure of development of the ganglion cells in the myenteric plexuses in the rectum and sigmoid. In turn this causes an interruption of peristalsis. There is an absence of the defecation reflex and a retention of feces above the aganglionic segment results. The proximal colon undergoes a gradual enlargement. The aganglionic segment usually is in the lower sigmoid and rectum but a long segment of bowel may be involved at times, including the entire colon. Rarely there is more than one aganglionic segment—zonal aganglionosis. This type of the disease should be considered in patients who fail to respond to resection of a low (rectosigmoid) aganglionic segment. Hypotonia of the urinary bladder frequently is present, indicating abnormality of parasympathetic innervation to the bladder as well as to the distal colon.

Aganglionosis is much more common in males than females, approximately 80% of patients being males. The symptoms begin at birth or shortly thereafter with constipation, abdominal distention, and vomiting. At first the distention may be relieved by enemas but eventually these become ineffective. The distention may vary from time to time. In some patients the development of symptoms is insidious but eventually the more or less typical pattern characteristic of the condition develops. In the older child it is usual to find the colon filled with masses of feces that can be palpated through the thin abdominal wall. Peristaltic waves may be observed. The patients often are malnourished and anemic.

Roentgen Observations. *Plain-Film Roentgenograms.* The diagnosis of megacolon often can be made from a simple roentgenogram of the abdomen. The widely dilated colon filled with fecal matter and gas results in a mottled shadow that is diagnostic of fecal impaction. The abdomen is distended and the diaphragm is elevated. The rectum and/or rectosigmoid is not distended and contains little or no gas or feces as observed on the lateral roentgenogram. In order to outline the aganglionic segment a barium enema may be necessary.

Barium-Enema Examination. A number of cases of sudden death following tap-water enemas have been reported in infants with Hirschsprung's disease. The cause of death is uncertain although some believe it is the result of water intoxication. Megacolon has a much larger absorptive surface than the normal and the superficial ulcerations frequently present contribute to rapid absorption of hypotonic solutions. The high pressure sometimes used to fill a dilated colon also may contribute to rapid absorption of water. Because there is a known hazard, certain precautions should be observed[65]: (*1*) Normal saline solution should be used for the barium enema and for preparation enemas. (*2*) As much of the fluid should be recovered as possible by siphoning or suction. (*3*) Use of high pressure should be avoided, an elevation of the enema container 2 to 3 feet above the table top being sufficient. (*4*) As soon as the aganglionic segment has been outlined, the procedure should be discontinued and there should be no attempt to fill the dilated segment.

As the barium is introduced the rectum is found to be of essentially normal caliber. At some place in the upper part of the rectum or the distal sigmoid the lumen may decrease slightly in caliber for a short distance or it may remain fairly normal. The transition from the normal or narrowed area to grossly dilated bowel is abrupt and the barium column passes into it without difficulty. (Fig. 19-5). No attempt should be made to fill the dilated colon; once the transition zone is adequately identified, the procedure should be discontinued as has been indicated.

In patients with a long aganglionic segment, difficulty in diagnosis may be experienced because of some variation in caliber of this segment. In some patients it may be larger than normal but comparison with the greatly dilated proximal colon will indicate that, although the aganglionic segment is long and dilated, the dilatation above it is greater and the transition between the two is abrupt. The difference in caliber and the sudden change are the important criteria in these cases. In some patients, only the upper sigmoid colon is dilated and elongated with the rest of the bowel relatively normal in caliber. In others the entire colon above the aganglionic area is greatly dilated. It can be seen, therefore, that appearances will vary somewhat among patients.

It is essential that the barium filling of the colon be done under fluoroscopic guidance. The transition between normal or narrowed bowel to dilated colon is seen to best advantage with the patient rotated to the left into a left posterior oblique or left lateral position. Otherwise the dilated colon often overlies the rectum and in routine roentgenograms may completely hide the significant lesion. Spot roentgenograms are useful to record the condition on film and they can be made with the patient in whatever position is found best to delineate the area.

In the newborn and the very young infant the classic signs of the disease may not be evident on roentgen examination even though normal bowel movements do not occur and there is abdominal distention and vomiting. When delay in colonic emptying occurs, follow-up films are obtained, including a lat-

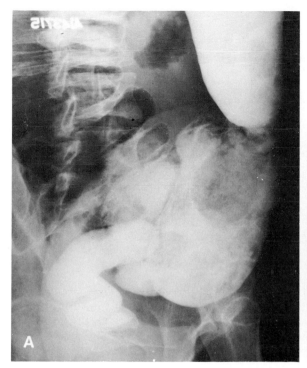
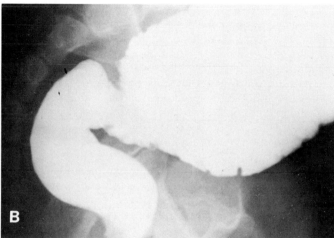

Fig. 19-5. Congenital megacolon. **A.** The barium-filled rectum and distal sigmoid of this patient are normal. There is an abrupt transition into a greatly dilated sigmoid colon which contains a considerable amount of fecal material. **B.** In this patient the findings of an abrupt transition from normal distal to grossly enlarged proximal colon are similar to those in patient **A.**

eral view of the rectosigmoid. Roentgenograms obtained 24 to 72 hours after barium enema will show residual barium in the colon above the rectal level, the rectum often being empty. At times, however, there may be 12-hour (or more) retention of barium in infants with the small left colon syndrome (immature left colon).[11] This finding is less significant in the older infant or the child because simple constipation may also cause colonic stasis. However, in constipation the barium tends to collect in multiple masses or boli rather than being more uniformly distributed as seen in Hirschsprung's disease. Also, the rectum may be empty in the latter condition and is usually full of barium in constipation.

Hope and associates[32] have described the occurrence of irregular, disorganized, spastic contractions in the aganglionic area which they consider to be significant in diagnosis in the neonatal period. However, the most important sign at this age period, if a transition zone cannot be demonstrated, is colonic stasis. Twenty-four-and 48-hour roentgenograms should be obtained if Hirschsprung's disease is a consideration

and they may simplify an otherwise difficult diagnostic problem. The diagnosis may be confirmed by rectal biopsy if roentgen findings are equivocal.

Aganglionosis of the Entire Colon

In this form of Hirschsprung's disease, radiographic findings may not be diagnostic since the colon may appear normal on barium enema.[10] The mortality rate is very high, probably because the condition is not recognized early. There are certain findings that suggest the diagnosis, however. These include: (*1*) The colon fills easily. (2) There may be a shaggy, irregular contour or areas of abnormal colonic contraction. (3) Free and rapid reflux into the terminal ileum may be observed. (4) If the terminal ileum is involved, there may be a transition zone with proximal dilatation in the terminal ileum. (5) There is a disparity in size of the colon and ileum, the dilated ileum contrasting with the narrow colon. (6) Barium is retained in the entire colon. (7) There is loss of redundancy of the flexures resulting in a short colon.

DISEASES OF THE COLON

CARCINOMA

Published statistics indicate that the majority of carcinomas of the large intestine can be visualized during proctosigmoidoscopic examination. Approximately 60% are found in the rectum and in the rectosigmoid region, another 10% in the remainder of the sigmoid, and the final 30% in the rest of the colon. The diagnosis of lesions in the rectum and distal part of the sigmoid should be made by proctosigmoidoscopy rather than by roentgen examination and a barium enema that fails to demonstrate abnormality is not considered adequate to exclude the possibility of a lesion in this area unless special procedures are used. Above the level of proctoscopic vision, roentgen examination is the method of choice.

From the roentgen point of view carcinoma of the colon occurs in three major types: (1) polypoid or fungating, (2) infiltrative or annular, and (3) completely obstructive. In general, carcinoma of the colon has roentgen features similar to those of cancer elsewhere in the gastrointestinal tract. These features have been discussed in appropriate sections. Carcinoma stiffens the bowel wall and causes a fixed defect, it destroys the mucosal pattern or alters it markedly, and it is prone to narrow the lumen and cause obstruction. Rarely, a fourth type involves a long segment of colon; this lesion is often a scirrhous type of carcinoma.

Polypoid or Fungating Carcinoma

When the colon has been filled with barium mixture a polypoid carcinoma is seen as an intraluminal mass or filling defect of variable size attached to the colonic wall by a broad base (Figs. 19-6 and 19-7). Characteristically the surface of the defect is somewhat irregular or lobulated; the edges of the lesion form an acute angle with the normal colonic wall; the mucosal pattern is lost completely over the surface of the defect. The larger bulky lesions often are described as fungating, a term that indicates a more advanced stage of growth. Areas of necrosis develop frequently in these large tumors and result in pocketlike accumulations of barium within the necrotic cavities. Small polypoid carcinomas resemble sessile benign polyps and often it is impossible to state from roentgen evidence whether such a lesion is benign or malignant. Polypoid carcinomas occur in all parts of the large intestine but they are the predominant type in

the cecum and ascending colon. In this location the tumor often reaches a large size before it causes enough symptoms to lead to the diagnosis; not infrequently the patient is examined only because of a refractory anemia or an unexplained fever or loss of weight. Polypoid carcinomas are not as likely to cause obstruction as the annular type, but bleeding is a common and often an early symptom.

Infiltrating or Annular Carcinoma

This type of carcinoma is characterized by infiltration of the wall rather than by a bulky intraluminal mass. It narrows the bowel lumen and when it has reached the stage of an annular growth, constriction is invariably present. The length of colon involved by an annular carcinoma seldom exceeds 4 to 6 cm. The edges of the lesion tend to overhang and form acute angles with the bowel wall. This is one of the features of carcinoma in all parts of the gastrointestinal tract. The constriction caused by the tumor usually is concentric and in some cases only a few centimeters long, which gives an appearance that has led to the designation of "napkin-ring carcinoma" (Figs. 19-8 through 19-10). The folds of mucosa are completely absent within the area of the lesion. The defect is constant and rigid and a mass often is palpable.

Obstructive Carcinoma

Either polypoid or annular types of carcinoma may cause complete obstruction although the annular type is more prone to do so. When obstruction to the retrograde flow of barium is complete, the information obtained by outlining the channel through the tumor is no longer available. Often the abrupt termination of the barium column and the evidence of overhanging edges at the distal border of the lesion can be identified. In other instances a partial outlining of the channel is obtained. In many, however, the appearance of the end of the barium column is not distinctive and the roentgen diagnosis must be limited to that of an obstructive lesion.

It is rather common to find complete or nearly complete obstruction to the retrograde flow of the barium mixture and yet to have few of the clinical signs and symptoms of bowel obstruction. In these patients, peristalsis apparently is able to keep semisolid material passing through the narrowed area but, when an enema is given, the retrograde flow and the hydrostatic pressure used close the narrow orifice. Even though these patients may be unob-

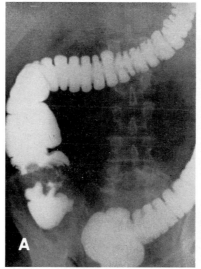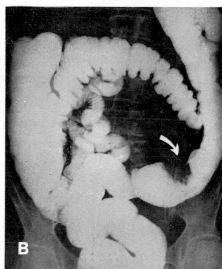

Fig. 19-6. Polypoid or fungating carcinoma of the colon. **A.** The large intraluminal lesion has not caused obstruction in this patient. The overhanging edges are characteristic. **B.** This patient has a small intraluminal lesion in the sigmoid. Note irregularity of the surface of the mass.

structed clinically it is very unwise to give barium by mouth because the chance for causing impaction is considerable. As the water is absorbed by the colon there is left the insoluble barium sulfate to form a hard, rocklike mass. An acute obstruction may be precipitated in such a case; at the least the impacted barium may be impossible to remove and adds to the surgical difficulties when resection is attempted or it may complicate the postoperative period.

Long-Segment Carcinoma

Occasionally an infiltrative carcinoma may involve a long segment of bowel.[26] The wall is invaded and the colon is narrowed in a stenotic or stricturelike fashion that resembles the narrowing sometimes observed in the stomach of patients with linitis plastica.

The roentgenographic findings in this type of neoplasm tend to resemble those of a long area of stenosis with tapered margins and partial preservation of the mucosal pattern. Because of the relative preservation of mucosa and the length of the lesion, long-segment carcinoma tends to resemble inflammatory disease. Histologically these lesions are usually scirrhous in type. Occasionally metastases to the colon may produce a similar lesion, and rarely lymphoma may have this appearance. The latter two lesions are virtually impossible to differentiate from primary carcinoma except that they are multiple somewhat more frequently. The primary long-colon type may metastasize to another area in the colon, however. The majority of long metastatic lesions arise in the stomach and involve the transverse colon by way of the gastrocolic ligament.

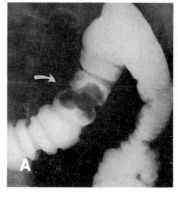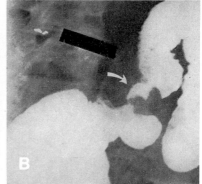

Fig. 19-7. A. Small polypoid carcinoma in the distal transverse colon **(arrow). B.** Annular carcinoma which also has some features of an intraluminal irregular polypoid mass. **(arrow).**

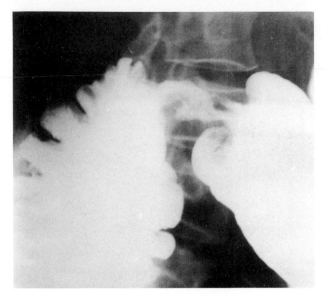

Fig. 19-8. Annular carcinoma of the hepatic flexure, displaying the so-called "napkin-ring" defect.

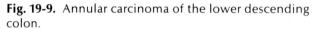

Fig. 19-9. Annular carcinoma of the lower descending colon.

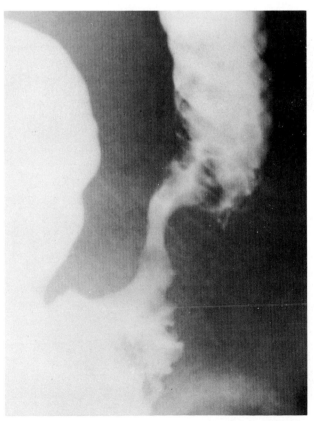

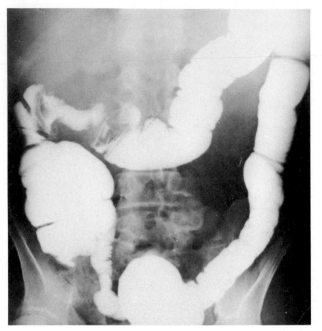

Fig. 19-10. Large carcinoma of the hepatic flexure. The lesion is extensive and shows polypoid and annular or infiltrating characteristics. It has not produced obstruction to retrograde flow of the barium.

Further Observations

Sinus Tracts and Fistulas. Sinus tracts extending into contiguous tissues or fistulous communications with other abdominal viscera are rather frequent complications of advanced carcinoma of the colon. During filling of the colon with barium mixture there may be noted extension of contrast material into a loop of small intestine through a direct fistulous communication. Similar fistulas may form between the colon and the urinary bladder, the gallbladder, or the stomach. It may be impossible in some of these cases to determine from which structure the tumor arose.

Other Inflammatory Changes. The development of inflammatory changes other than sinus tracts or fistulas is relatively common and at times the inflammatory aspect may overshadow the neoplastic. Inflammatory thickening or abscess formation adds to the mass characteristics of the cancer but also changes the roentgen features. The defect is increased in length and one or both ends of it may taper gradually rather than have an abrupt demarcation from the normal bowel. Thus, one of the characteristic signs of gastrointestinal carcinoma is lost. Fortunately, this usually affects only one end of the lesion and at the other the typical overhanging edges of a carcinoma defect remain. When an annular defect of more than 6 cm in length is found it is probable that there is an intramural or pericolic inflammatory mass associated with the carcinoma.

An ulcerating colitis may develop proximal to an obstructing lesion of any kind and may occur in patients with carcinoma. It is probably caused by ischemia secondary to elevated intraluminal pressure. Severe involvement may complicate resectional surgery undertaken for removal of the neoplasm.

Intussusception. Intussusception in the adult usually is caused by a tumor of sessile or pedunculated nature. Some are the result of lipomas or leiomyomas. Intussusception as a complication of colonic carcinoma occurs chiefly with the polypoid type involving the right side of the colon. The signs of intussusception predominate in the roentgen picture. As the barium column reaches the obstruction it widens out and the end of the column develops a concave or cup-shaped appearance as it surrounds the intussusceptum. The tumor responsible for the obstruction ordinarily forms the leading edge of the intussusceptum. In many cases, however, it cannot be clearly identified. Characteristically, ringlike shadows of barium mark the termination of the column, representing barium caught in the haustra of the intussuscipiens (Fig. 19-11). As the hydrostatic pressure of the enema becomes effective, the head of the barium column will move proximally for some distance but the concavity of its end is maintained. The intussusception may be reduced completely by this method and the defect of the tumor then becomes clearly apparent. At other times, reduction is incomplete and filling of the colon proximal to the obstruction is not attained.

Calcification. Mucin-producing carcinoma of the colon may occasionally contain enough calcium to be recognized radiographically. This is quite rare, however, and more commonly calcium deposits of the psammomatous type are observed in metastases from these lesions—mainly in the liver. A stippled or granular calcification, which may vary from minimal, poorly defined to dense, clearly defined areas, may be observed.

Multiple Tumors. The simultaneous presence of more than one colon carcinoma is not unusual, occurring in an estimated 2% to 4% of patients having carcinoma of the colon. There is also a high incidence

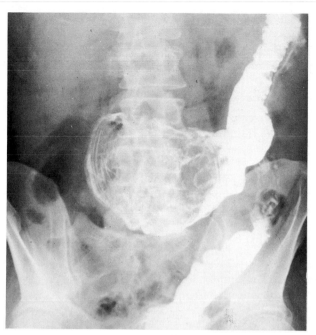

Fig. 19-11. Intussusception of the transverse colon caused by a polypoid carcinoma of the cecum. Note the coiled-spring appearance of mucosal folds in the proximal and distal portions of the large masslike filling defect.

of benign tumors, mainly adenomatous polyps, in patients with more than one malignant lesion in the colon. Also, there are certain conditions such as familial polyposis and chronic ulcerative colitis in which the incidence of both single and multiple colon cancer is high. In multiple lesions, if the distal tumor is partially obstructing, inability of the radiologist to prepare and to fill the proximal colon makes it virtually impossible to detect a proximal lesion.

Ureterosigmoidostomy and Colon Tumor. There is a definite increase in the incidence of adenocarcinoma of the sigmoid colon adjacent to an ureterosigmoidostomy stoma.[55] Also, since the urine-diverting procedure is often done to correct congenital anomalies, the patients are younger than the average patients with cancer of the colon, even though there may be a long span of time between the procedure and the appearance of a neoplasm. The cause is uncertain, but there are several theories: (1) Urine contains a carcinogen affecting colonic mucosa. (2) Chronic fecal irritation causes ureteral metaplasia and neoplasia. (3) A pseudopolypoid mucosal mass develops and becomes malignant. Whatever the cause, the high incidence should alert the radiologist to the possibility of malignancy if late ureterocolonic obstruction develops in patients who have had a ureterosigmoidostomy.

Differential Diagnosis

Inflammatory Masses. The most important lesion from the standpoint of differential diagnosis is a localized inflammatory mass and this usually is the result of diverticulitis with or without a frank abscess in the colonic wall or pericolic tissues. The inflammatory changes cause a narrowing of the lumen and this may be severe enough to result in complete obstruction. As the lesion encroaches upon the lumen a filling defect is produced when the colon is filled with barium. The differential signs are discussed later in this chapter under the heading "Diverticula."

Other inflammatory lesions that may be confused with carcinoma are infrequent. Hyperplastic tuberculosis in the cecum and ascending colon has been reported as causing a defect somewhat similar to carcinoma but this lesion is rare in general radiologic practice. An area of granulomatous colitis may resemble to some degree the defect of an annular carcinoma. However, this lesion usually involves a longer segment of bowel, the lumen may not be narrowed too greatly, the mucosal surface has a granular appearance, and the ends of the defect taper gradually, a characteristic of all inflammatory lesions. Infrequently, a nonspecific inflammatory granuloma is found in the colon and it may produce roentgenologic findings very similar to those of carcinoma. Because they are rare these lesions seldom enter into the differential diagnostic picture.

Amebic disease of the colon may present as a localized mass known as *ameboma*. In areas where this disease is endemic it has been suggested that most patients with a localized filling defect in the colon have a course of emetine therapy prior to any surgical procedure. This is because the lesion may mimic carcinoma very closely. If due to amebiasis, the lesion will improve promptly under adequate therapy.

Benign Polyps. With larger polyps it may be difficult to determine if the lesion is benign or not from its roentgen features. Small polyps, those less than 1 cm in diameter, usually can be kept under observation with reexamination at intervals of 3 to 6 months unless the lesion is a source of bleeding. The same is true of a polyp with a pedicle. The presence of a pedicle indicates that the lesion is not invading the bowel wall. The demonstration of a pedicle, therefore, is of considerable importance from the standpoint of treatment as well as diagnosis. The tip of a pedunculated polyp may show malignant changes, but polyps do not ordinarily invade the adjacent colon.

Extrinsic Masses. A variety of masses within the abdomen may cause pressure defects on the colon. As a rule the defect is a smooth one and often changes during the examination or can be made to disappear by altering the position of the patient or by the effect of manual palpation. The mucosa is intact, an important point in differential diagnosis because mucosal folds are not seen over the surface of a carcinoma defect. A malignant tumor from a neighboring structure may invade the colon and often it is difficult if not impossible to determine whether such a lesion is primary in the colon or not. If only the external wall is involved and the mucosa is intact, the demonstration of mucosal folds through the area of defect is significant.

Intramural Tumors. Tumors arising from elements of the bowel wall other than the mucosa are relatively infrequent. They include such lesions as lipomas, leiomyomas, and leiomyosarcomas. The roentgen features of a small, extramucosal, intramural tumor resemble those of a sessile polyp. The larger tumors of this nature often suggest polypoid carcinoma. The visualization of mucosal folds over the surface of the mass is of importance in establishing the intramural nature of the mass, but it may be difficult to be certain about this finding. Lipomas of the cecum are said to be a common cause of intussusception in the adult and in some instances a lipoma may actually develop a pedicle because of peristaltic pressure. If large enough, a lipoma may appear unusually translucent because of its fat content. In our experience, polyps and polypoid carcinomas have been more frequent causes of intussusception in the adult than have lipomas.

POLYPS

The term "polyp" often is used to include inflammatory as well as neoplastic lesions. Roentgenologists frequently use the term "polypoid lesion" because of inability to determine the histologic nature of many of the small masses that have similar gross features. Polyps of the colon are slightly more common in males than in females; multiple tumors are frequent. Their distribution in the various parts of the colon and the age incidence are similar to carcinoma. From 60% to 75% occur in the rectum or lower part of the sigmoid and are accessible to proctoscopic examination. The incidence of colonic polyps in routine autopsy series ranges from 7% to 12.5% and is much higher in some reports.[14]

The majority of colonic polyps are adenomas. The lesion may be sessile and attached to the colonic wall by a broad base, but the larger ones often have a pedicle caused by peristaltic pressure. The pedicle may be as much as 4 or 5 cm in length. Polyps vary greatly in size from tiny wartlike excrescences on the mucosal surface to lesions that measure several centimeters in diameter. The relation of polyps to carcinoma is an interesting one and opinions have been expressed repeatedly in the literature that a high percentage of carcinomas of the colon and rectum originate in preexisting polyps. Others, however, have disputed this and evidence has been presented to indicate that most polyps of the colon do not become malignant. As noted previously, the demonstration of a stalk, roentgenologically, is an important finding, since it indicates a lack of invasiveness on the part of the lesion.

Roentgen Observations. If the head of the advancing barium column is watched closely during fluoroscopy the defect of a polyp often is seen momentarily as the barium flows around it. If the polyp is small it soon becomes obscured as the segment fills more completely. Palpation with compression paddle or spoon helps to bring out the defect more clearly; compression cones and similar devices found on most modern fluoroscopes can be used to approximate the colonic walls. Sufficient pressure is used to squeeze most of the barium from the area, leaving a thin layer within which the small defect of the polyp will be visible.

A polyp causes a rounded, negative (translucent) filling defect in the barium shadow (Fig. 19-12). The edges are smooth and the margins sharply defined. If sessile, the defect does not move at any time during the examination. If it has a pedicle, the head of the polyp may move during filling and evacuation of the enema or be displaced by palpation. Occasionally a pedicle of considerable length is present and the polyp can move a distance twice the length of the pedicle. The pedicle may be visualized as a stalklike defect and its point of attachment is indicated by a slight indrawing of the colonic wall (Fig. 19-13).

The postevacuation roentgenogram is an impor-

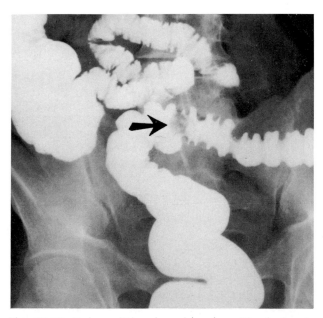

Fig. 19-12. Polyp of the sigmoid colon. The lesion is seen as a smooth, round, filling defect in the lumen **(arrow).**

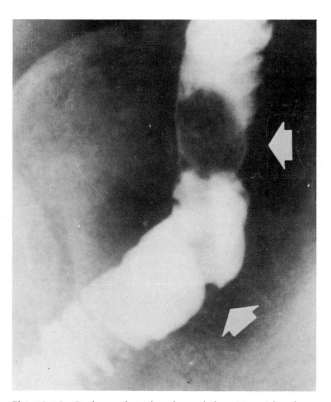

Fig. 19-13. Pedunculated polyp of the sigmoid colon. The **upper arrow** indicates the polyp and the **lower arrow** the point of attachment of its pedicle.

tant part of the roentgen examination for the detection of polyps. In the contracted state a thin layer of barium usually coats the mucosal surface, which then is seen as a network of fine folds. The polyp also is coated with barium and appears as a rounded mass displacing or replacing the normal mucosal relief (Fig. 19-14). The minimum size of a polyp that can be detected regularly on roentgen examination is variable, but is usually considered to be on the order of 0.7 to 1 cm. Practically all polyps of this size should be demonstrated, provided that proper cleansing of the colon has been obtained. Polyps smaller than this are often visualized if preparation has been good and if other factors, including location in an area accessible to visualization, are favorable. The identification of tiny polyps is accomplished most often when multiple lesions are present.

Double-contrast studies (see section on "Techniques of Examination" in the early portion of this chapter) are considered to be indispensable by many for the detection of polyps. It is of vital importance to have the colon free from fecal material in order to obtain a satisfactory and diagnostic double-contrast study of the colon. The ideal method of preparation has not been achieved, as indicated in the earlier discussion of colon preparation. When surrounded by air a polyp forms a positive shadow as it projects into the colonic lumen because it is of greater radiographic density than air. The surface usually is coated with a thin layer of barium, which is continuous with that coating the contiguous intestinal wall.

The question of the relationship of adenomatous polyps to cancer of the colon has not yet been settled. There are some radiographic findings that suggest malignancy in polypoid masses, however. They include the following: (1) Size—over 1 cm (or possibly over 1.5 cm). (2) Contour—irregularity of the surface. (3) Base—persistent indentation or irregularity of the mucosa at the base. (4) Pedicle—a short, thick pedicle doesn't exclude the possibility of malignancy, but a long (2 cm or more) pedicle makes cancer unlikely. Areas of malignancy have been observed histologically in such polyps, but it is doubtful that they represent invasive tumor. (5) Growth rate—malignant polyps grow at a more rapid rate than do adenomatous polyps; any increase in size observed on follow-up double-contrast studies must be considered as an absolute indication for surgical exploration.[70]

Differential Diagnosis.

Fecal Lumps. Small lumps of nonopaque fecal matter offer the greatest difficulty in differential diagnosis. A

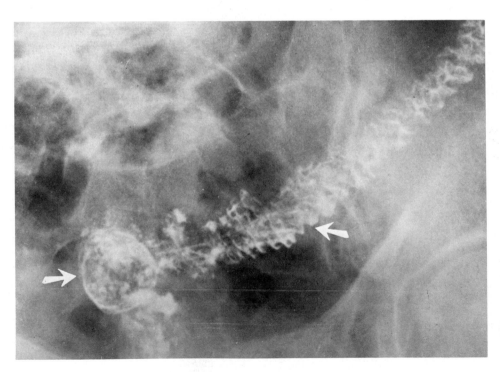

Fig. 19-14. Pendunculated polyp of the sigmoid colon. The **left arrow** points to the head of the polyp, which is coated with barium. The **right arrow** indicates the point of attachment of the polyp's long pedicle to the colonic wall.

lump of feces may move extensively as the mixture flows through the colon; it may disappear completely in postevacuation roentgenograms; or it may disintegrate while being palpated. The constancy of a polyp defect is one of its characteristic features. When there is doubt, re-examination is required and this should be done without hesitation whenever any question exists. Visualization of a pedicle, when one is present, is an extremely important finding and allows a diagnosis of polyp to be made with assurance (see Fig. 19-13).

Diverticula. A diverticulum may resemble a polyp to some extent in double-contrast roentgenograms if seen *en face* rather than in profile. If the diverticulum contains a nonopaque fecalith or air and has only a coating of barium on its surface, it will appear as a ringlike shadow. Also a diverticulum when seen *en face* may appear as a double ring, the inner one formed by the barium coating of the neck and the outer ring by the sac of the diverticulum. The air-filled sac of the diverticulum stands out with a greater translucence than does the adjacent bowel, while a polyp causes a shadow denser than the surrounding air (Fig. 19-15). Also, the polyp has a sharp inner border contrasted to the sharp outer border of a diverticulum when viewed *en face*.

Intramural Tumors. A sessile polyp may resemble an extramucosal intramural tumor very closely and the differentiation often is impossible on roentgen examination, particularly when the lesions are small. Actually, some intramural tumors become polypoid in their gross features and may develop a pedicle.

Pseudopolyps. In some patients with chronic ulcerative colitis, the coalescence of small ulcers into larger and deeper ulcerations with undermined edges may leave islands or tags of inflamed but otherwise intact mucosa. These tags cause small, round, translucent defects in the barium shadow that resemble true polyps very closely. In most cases it is impossible to distinguish a pseudopolyp from a true one and both may be present in the same patient (see Fig. 19-29). However, most of the polyps are inflammatory in these patients.

Polyposis Syndromes (Table 19-1)

Familial (Multiple) Polyposis. Familial polyposis or adenomatosis of the colon is a rare disease of hereditary or familial nature. In most patients the onset is during the second decade of life, but cases have been reported in which the disease has been found during early childhood. The familial aspects of the disease have been thoroughly studied by Dukes and by others. Apparently it represents a gene mutation which, if carried as a Mendelian dominant trait, appears in succeeding generations; if as a recessive

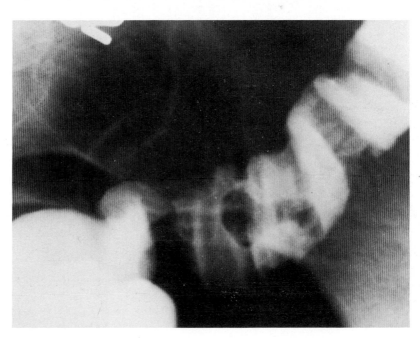

Fig. 19-15. Pedunculated polyp in the lower sigmoid. The small polyp and its pedicle are readily outlined.

Table 19-1. Clinical Features of Polyposis Syndromes

	FAMILIAL COLONIC POLYPOSIS	GARDNER'S SYNDROME	JUVENILE POLYPOSIS	PEUTZ-JEGHERS SYNDROME	TURCOT SYNDROME	CRONKHITE-CANADA SYNDROME
Components	Multiple colonic polyps	Colonic polyposis; sebaceous cysts; osteomas; desmoid tumors; mesenteric fibromas	Gastrointestinal polyposis	Gastrointestinal polyposis; muccocutaneous pigmentation (melanin)	Colonic polyps; central nervous system tumors (usually glioblastomas)	Generalized polyposis; hyperpigmentation; alopecia; atrophy of the nails
Inheritance	Mendelian dominance	Mendelian dominance	Probably familial type	Mendelian dominance; variable penetrance	Few cases; questionable autosomal recessive	None
Onset of symptoms	Childhood and early adolescence	Average 30 yr.	Average 6 yr.	Childhood and adolescence	Childhood and young adult	42–75 yr.
Major symptoms	...	...	Bleeding; prolapse of polyps	Intussusception; bleeding	Central nervous system	Diarrhea
Anatomical involvement by polyps	Colon only; diffuse	Colon (diffuse); occasionally stomach and duodenum	Anywhere in the gastrointestinal tract, mainly in the colon; less numerous than in familial polyposis	Anywhere in the gastrointestinal tract; predominantly in the small intestine	Colon	Anywhere in the gastrointestinal tract, predominantly the stomach and colon
Pathology	Adenomas	Adenoma	Hamartoma	Hamartoma	?	? adenoma; predominantly cystic glandular dilatation
Malignant potential	Colorectal cancer in 2/3	High probability of colorectal cancer; likelihood of periampullary cancer	None	Low or none	Probably	Multiple carcinomata (2 of 15 patients)
Associated findings	...	Follicular odontomas; dentigerous cysts	Heart lesions; malrotation; hydrocephalus; congenital amyotoma; porphyria	Granulosa theca-cell tumors of the ovary may occur in 5% of female patients	...	...

(Koehler PR, Kyaw MM, Fenlon JW: Diffuse gastrointestinal polyposis with ectodermal changes. Radiology 103: 593, 1972)

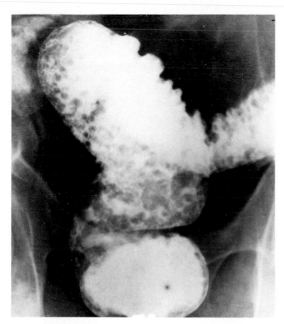

Fig. 19-16. Multiple familial polyposis of the colon. The polyps appear as numerous, round translucent defects involving the sigmoid and rectum.

trait, it may skip a generation unless both parents carry the gene. The only possibility of cure lies in a total colectomy; otherwise the usual course is the development of carcinoma of the colon unless death from other causes supervenes. During barium-enema examination, routine fluoroscopy may fail to reveal evidence of the disease because the polyps often are very small. Even in roentgenograms of the filled and contracted colon it may be difficult to visualize the lesions. The margins of the filled colon usually show a fine roughening, representing the defects of small polyps seen in profile (Fig. 19-16). Post-evacuation roentgenograms may show the larger polyps but the small ones may be lost in the crinkling of mucosal folds when the bowel contracts. The ideal method for roentgen demonstration is by means of double-contrast studies. Perfectly done, double-contrast roentgenograms reveal the innumerable tiny polyps as small nodules along the mucosal surface of the colon. Some of the tumors may be larger than others and easily seen by routine methods. Carcinomatous degeneration is often present in some of these even at the time the patient is first examined. The differentiation of familial polyposis of the colon from pseudopolyposis or polyposis developing during ulcerative colitis is not difficult since in the former the bowel is otherwise normal while in the latter condition the extensive changes of ulcerative disease are apparent. When ulcerative colitis has "healed," leaving only pseudopolyps, the differentiation may be more difficult. In the diffuse form of lymphosarcoma involving the colon, the thickened folds may suggest multiple polyps.

Peutz–Jeghers Syndrome. This entity consists of multiple polyposis of the small bowel, stomach, and colon associated with mucocutaneous pigmentation on the lips and sometimes in the mouth. Melanin is the pigment involved. The lesions are most frequent in the small bowel and are benign hamartomas rather than adenomatous polyps. The same is true of the gastric lesions. In the colon the lesions are relatively few in number and are often pedunculated. They appear to be mainly adenomatous polyps in contrast to the small-bowel lesions. In patients with the Peutz–Jeghers syndrome the incidence of gastric and colonic carcinoma is somewhat higher than in the general population, but the incidence of small-bowel cancer probably does not differ. There appears to be an increased incidence of ovarian tumors in the females with this syndrome. The small-bowel polyps may cause intussusception that is often transient. The other complication is bleeding that is usually not severe. The presence of the distinctive pigmentation is an important clinical finding which aids in the diagnosis. (See also section "The Peutz–Jeghers Syndrome" in Ch. 18.)

Gardner's Syndrome. This syndrome consists of colonic polyposis associated with osteomas of the skeletal system and various soft-tissue tumors.[34] The osteomas may occur in any bone but are most frequent in the calvarium, mandible, and other facial bones. They vary considerably in size from small areas of cortical thickening to larger, distinct masses having the density of cortical bone. The intestinal polyps occur mainly in the colon but may occasionally (in 5% or less) occur also in the stomach and duodenum. The colonic polyps are similar to the adenomatous polyps in patients with familial multiple polyposis, and there is a similar, extremely high incidence of colonic carcinoma as well as a relatively high incidence of periampullary carcinoma. As in familial multiple polyposis, colectomy is recommended because of the virtual certainty of malignant disease in the colon.

Lymphoid Hyperplasia. The condition known as benign or nodular lymphoid hyperplasia of the colon is similar to but less common than lymphoid hyperplasia in the ileum. It is often associated with dysgammaglobulinemia but may occur in otherwise normal children.[40] Roentgen findings may be very similar to those in familial polyposis. The manifestations are best seen in double-contrast studies of the colon and if the appearance of the nodules is slightly umbilicated, this is diagnostic. A tiny fleck of barium is noted in the center of the small, round, filling defect in the colon. Lymphoid hyperplasia most likely represents response of lymphoid tissue to a variety of stimuli in children. Tiny nodular filling defects up to 2 mm in diameter are very common in children under 5 years of age and probably represent a normal lymphoid follicular pattern, therefore the term "lymphoid hyperplasia" is reserved to designate nodules larger than 2 mm in diameter.

Cronkhite–Canada Syndrome. This rare syndrome consists of nonfamilial diffuse gastrointestinal polyposis predominantly in the stomach and colon, but also in the small intestine, with ectodermal changes consisting of alopecia and atrophy of the nails and pigmentation. Usually there is severe protein loss and it is generally considered to be one of the protein-losing enteropathies which is often fatal in females, but is not as severe in males. The polyps are inflammatory with cystic glandular dilatation and no tendency to undergo malignant change.

Juvenile Polyps. Polyps of the colon occurring in children have a different histologic appearance than the usual adenomatous polyp found in adults. They are benign inflammatory or retention polyps with numerous cystic spaces. There has been no reported instance of malignant degeneration. The polyps are usually few in number and may be solitary; occasionally they may also be present in the stomach and small bowel. The presenting complaint usually is that of bleeding from the rectum or an anemia from chronic blood loss. Occasionally the lesion may cause obstruction because of intussusception. The roentgen findings are similar to those of polyps of the colon in adults but their occurrence in children and the fact that they apparently do not become malignant are significant factors. Excisional biopsy is reported to be curative; however, the clinical manifestations should be sufficiently severe to warrant a surgical procedure.

Other Tumors and Tumorlike Lesions

As is true in other parts of the gastrointestinal tract, a variety of tumors of extramucosal, intramural nature are found in the colon, but as a group these tumors are not common lesions. They include lipomas, leiomyomas, leiomyosarcomas, and, rarely, such tumors

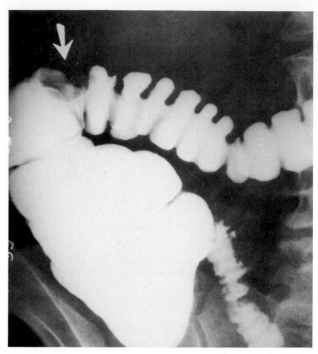

Fig. 19-17. Intramural tumor (lipoma) at the hepatic flexure of the colon **(arrow).**

as fibromas, hemangiomas, and extramedullary plasmacytomas (myelomas). Lipomas are found most frequently in the right side of the colon (Fig. 19-17). With the larger lipomas the tumor may appear unusually translucent.[46] Extensive segmental and diffuse generalized colonic lipomatosis has been reported in which the appearance is similar to that of extensive polyposis. This is extremely rare. Theoretically the demonstration of an intact mucosa over the surface of a mass should be good evidence of its nonmucosal origin. Actually, whether or not the mucosa is intact is difficult to determine in tumors of the colon for the mucosa over an intramural mass may be stretched and flattened so that folds cannot be identifed. Roentgen findings usually limit the diagnosis to that of a polypoid mass or lesion. Some intramural tumors even develop a pedicle because of the effects of peristalsis.

Lymphosarcoma of the colon may occur as a discrete, often bulky, intraluminal tumor simulating carcinoma, or as a diffuse involvement of a considerable length of colon, or it may have multiple nodules. The diffuse form is characterized by extensive submucosal infiltration, leading to thickening of the mucosal folds somewhat similar to that seen when this disease involves the stomach. The thickened tortuous folds give the appearance of multiple polypoid protrusions. Occasionally a local "dilatation" or "aneurysm" may occur similar to lymphosarcoma observed more commonly in the ileum. The terminal ileum is often involved in association with the colonic disease and gastric involvement also is common.

Endometriosis. The occurrence of implants on the peritoneal surface consisting of islands of tissue having the characteristics of normal endometrium is termed *endometriosis*. This condition is relatively common in women during active menstrual life. Endometrial implants in the wall of the rectum or sigmoid may lead to an inflammatory reaction since each implant functions as a miniature uterus during menstrual periods. This causes a fibrotic reaction and leads to the development of a constricting process that may produce the symptoms and signs of bowel obstruction. The important clinical features of endometriosis include: (*1*) occurrence in women of age range usually between 25 and 45 years; (*2*) high incidence of menstrual irregularities; (*3*) absolute or relative sterility; (*4*) long history of symptoms suggesting bowel obstruction with frequent exacerbations at the time of menstruation; (*5*) absence of cachexia of weight loss; (*6*) infrequent evidence of bleeding from the bowel; (*7*) high incidence of benign uterine tumors. The roentgen findings include: (*1*) a filling defect of varying size; (*2*) a sharp demarcation from normal to narrowed bowel similar to carcinoma; (*3*) an essentially intact mucous membrane; and (*4*) fixation and tenderness to palpation, especially at the time of menstruation (Fig. 19-18). While these features are characteristic, we have seen small defects that were difficult if not impossible to distinguish from those due to carcinoma. Correlation of roentgen and clinical observations is extremely important in these cases. Surgery may be required for diagnosis as well as treatment, particularly if the lesion simulates a malignant tumor.

Villous Adenoma. This unusual tumor is found chiefly in the rectum and rectosigmoid in patients of middle age or older. It is characterized pathologically by a soft, velvety mass made up of a large number of villi or frondlike projections from the base of the tumor. It is usually benign, but some observers believe that malignant degeneration occurs rather frequently. Clinically, there is an excess of mucus leading to frequent watery or mucuslike stools, sometimes resulting in hypoproteinemia and in fluid and electrolyte imbalance (particularly hypocalcemia).

On barium-enema examination the lesion may be seen to be of variable size from a few centimeters to that of a large and bulky mass encircling the lumen and causing an extensive filling defect. The appearance of the tumor may vary considerably in the filled and evacuated state of the colon as seen in barium-enema study. Characteristically, the margin is rough and serrated. There may be many streaks of barium

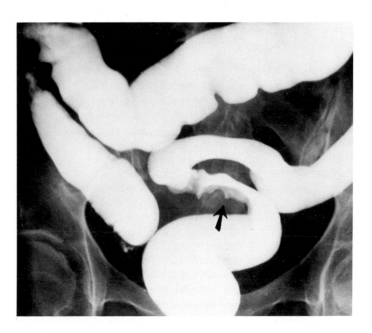

Fig. 19-18. Endometriosis. **Arrow** points to a mass caused by an endometrial implant.

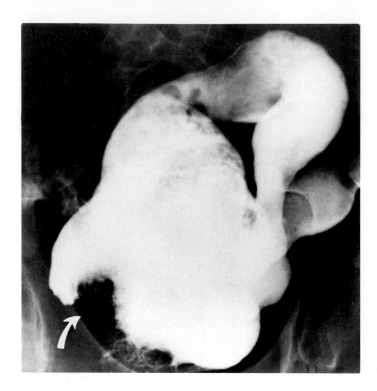

Fig. 19-19. Villous adenoma of the rectum. The lesion presents as a filling defect **(arrow)** with a ragged surface and with thin, linear extensions of barium into the tumor mass near the anal canal.

extending between the numerous villi (Fig. 19-19). In other cases the tumor's surface has a cobblestone appearance. These findings, taken in association with the clinical signs and symptoms, may allow a preoperative diagnosis.

DIVERTICULA

Diverticula are very common lesions in the adult colon. Their incidence increases in persons above the age of 40; most elderly persons have at least a few. Diverticula of the colon are acquired and form at points of anatomic weakness, usually at the sites where blood vessels perforate the muscular coat. Rarely, traction diverticula develop secondary to inflammatory disease of the mesenteric nodes. The sigmoid colon is most frequently involved but, in some individuals, diverticula are found throughout the length of the large intestine. An isolated diverticulum has been described as occurring in the cecum or elsewhere. As a rule, however, multiple diverticula are present and very large numbers are often seen. For reasons that are not clear, diverticula of the right colon cause significant bleeding more often than do those on the left. The lesions vary in size from tiny ones no more than 1 or 2 mm in diameter to some

that measure several centimeters; the majority are not more than a centimeter in diameter. Because minimal diverticulitis is very difficult to detect radiographically, some authors prefer the term "diverticular disease," which includes diverticulosis and diverticulitis. In patients with diverticula who develop granulomatous colitis, the diverticula decrease in size or disappear as the colitis develops, but tend to appear if the colitis improves.

Roentgen Observations. The presence of diverticula without the signs of inflammation is designated as *diverticulosis;* when inflammation is present the condition is termed *diverticulitis.* Some diverticula may be filled with fecal matter and not be visualized at all during a barium-enema examination. In others the sac may contain a fecalith but enough barium will enter to coat the wall; the diverticulum then appears as a ring shadow (Fig. 19-20). When the entire diverticulum fills with barium and is seen along the margin of the colon it forms a budlike shadow projecting beyond the confines of the barium-filled colonic lumen. If seen *en face* it appears as a dense round spot. Diverticula once filled with barium often retain the contrast material for days. Such retention does not appear to be harmful. Many times they be-

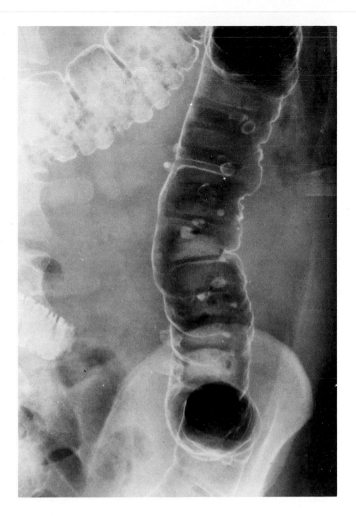

Fig. 19-20. Diverticula of the descending colon in a double-contrast study. Some of the diverticula appear as small, round densities when they contain barium. The others appear as rings when coated with barium and filled with air.

come visible only after the barium has been given orally; the barium meal often demonstrates the extent of a diverticulosis of the colon more clearly than does the barium enema.

Diverticulitis

Inflammatory reaction in a diverticulum may be limited to the sac and the pericolic tissues, while the wall of the colon may not be affected to any appreciable degree. The roentgen signs of inflammation often are meager in these cases. However, the initial inflammatory disease in a diverticulum may progress to perforation. This may be a microperforation with the associated inflammation correspondingly mild. Even larger perforations may be sealed over rapidly, leading to a localized abscess in the pericolic tissues of variable size. Multiple perforations may occur and the accompanying abscesses may communicate with each other. A fistulous tract usually can be seen extending into the abscess and the abscess cavity may partially fill with barium (Fig. 19-21).

On barium-enema study a small perforation may be visualized as a small, cloudy area of barium density around the site of the diverticulum. Local swelling from inflammation of the pericolic tissues as well as of the wall of the colon leads to formation of a mass. This causes a localized filling defect in the barium column. Larger abscesses cause correspondingly larger defects; the inflammatory reaction may be sufficient to result in partial or complete obstruction to retrograde filling. The inflammatory mass may surround the lumen causing narrowing of a short segment (Fig. 19-22) or appear as a unilateral filling defect encroaching upon the bowel lumen. Particularly

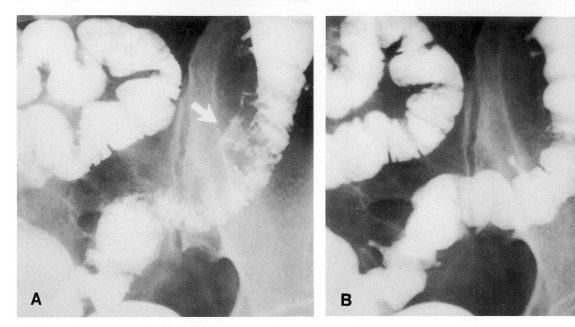

Fig. 19-21. Diverticulitis of the sigmoid colon with perforation and fistula formation. **A. Arrow** indicates the area of extension of contrast material beyond the lumen. Note thin, linear extensions above and below this triangular extravasation. **B.** Same patient shown in **A** several months later. The acute inflammatory reaction has subsided. The site of the previous fistula appears to be marked by a single, long diverticulum-like projection.

in the early stages, spasm is usually present and the area is irritable as seen under the fluoroscope. The appearance is that of narrowing of a relatively long (as compared to carcinoma) segment of bowel, usually in the sigmoid, with multiple diverticula that may or may not have local extravasation indicating perforation. The area may be spikelike in appearance owing to compression of haustra and possibly of diverticula. The mucosa is intact and the ends of the involved segment are tapered, not abrupt. Since much of the narrowing may be due to spasm, glucagon (1–2 mg by intravenous or intramuscular injection) or Pro-Banthine (30 mg) may be given. This often provides a much better study of the involved colon, since it may permit filling in areas not previously visible. In acute diverticulitis, the involved area is tender to palpation. However, such tenderness also may be found in carcinoma, particularly if there is much of an inflammatory element associated. At times a linear band or track of barium parallels the lumen and lies adjacent to it. This may also occur in granulomatous colitis and carcinoma, but appears to be most common in diverticulitis.[17]

If there is complete perforation which does not be-

come sealed off, pneumoperitoneum often can be demonstrated and, later, the signs of local or general peritonitis including adynamic ileus and exudate separating loops of bowel are evident. Diverticular perforation also may cause fistulous communications between the colon and urinary bladder or colon and vagina in females.

The differentiation from carcinoma may be difficult. The presence of overhanging edges at the margins of the filling defect, and the irregular eccentric lumen seen in carcinoma are significant (Fig. 19-23). The signs of walled-off perforation including the defect due to inflammatory mass, the demonstration of one or more fistulous tracts, the presence of diverticula in or adjacent to the filling defect, and spasm and irritability of the involved area are findings pointing to inflammatory disease. In many patients the diagnosis can be confirmed by progress examinations, carried out over a period of a few weeks, which will show a gradual subsidence and eventual disappearance of the signs of inflammation. If barium has extravasated into the abscess, a small amount may be trapped and continue to be visible for some time as a small fleck or patch of barium.

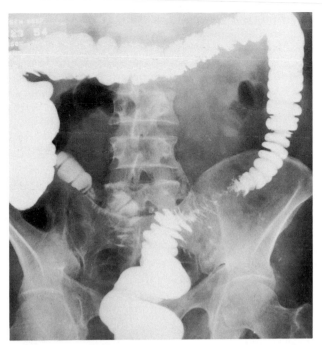

Fig. 19-22. Diverticulitis of the sigmoid colon. There is narrowing of the lumen over a relatively long segment. The ends of the lesion are tapered. A few diverticula are visible. There was tenderness to palpation over this lesion.

INFLAMMATORY DISEASE OF THE COLON

Chronic Idiopathic Ulcerative Colitis

In the majority of cases, chronic idiopathic ulcerative colitis begins in the rectum or lower part of the sigmoid and the diagnosis can be made by proctoscopy. In these patients, roentgen examination is useful to determine the extent and the severity of the disease above the level of proctoscopic vision. Less often the disease begins in the left side of the colon above the rectosigmoid and infrequently it has its origin in the right side of the colon. Ulcerative colitis sparing the rectum is infrequent.

Most cases of chronic ulcerative colitis have a subacute onset, subsiding gradually into a chronic course, but occasionally the onset is abrupt and the course is that of an acute, severe, fulminating infection. In still other cases the onset is so insidious that the nature of the disease is not recognized for some time. Pathologically it begins as a mucosal inflammation that in time spreads to involve all coats of the bowel wall. However, the inflammation remains most intense in the mucosa and submucosa. Small and su-

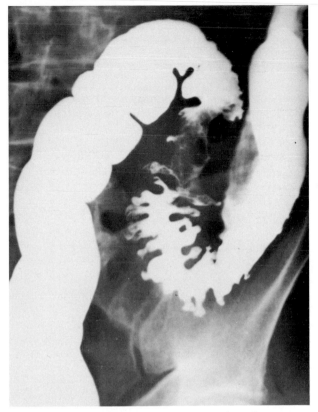

Fig. 19-23. Carcinoma in a patient with rather extensive diverticulosis of the upper sigmoid. In addition to the numerous diverticula, there is a well-circumscribed annular lesion with overhanging edges representing the tumor. It causes a pressure deformity on the adjacent segment of descending colon. In addition to the annular lesion, there is evidence of intraluminal exophytic masses.

perficial ulcers are a feature of this stage. In chronic disease the entire or the major part of the colonic wall may be denuded or there may be left islands of inflamed and hypertrophied mucosa. The wall becomes stiffened by fibrosis. When the disease is active, the wall may be very friable, therefore no type of balloon catheter should be used when barium-enema study is done in these patients.

Roentgen Observations

Early Changes. During the early changes of the disease, roentgen findings may be meager and the diagnosis can be established more readily by proctoscopy, unless the disease has begun above the rectosigmoid level. Usually the involved segment of colon is more irritable than normal as observed under the fluoroscopic screen. It may be difficult to keep it filled with barium and the patient suffers more distress from the enema than is usual. Otherwise fluoroscopy may show little in the way of abnormality. Roentgenograms of the filled colon demonstrate a persistence of haustral sacculations but the haustra are irregular in width and the septa separating them are thickened. The postevacuation roentgenogram often gives important information. Instead of the mucosa forming a crisscrossing network of fine folds, the folds are thickened and tend to course in a longitudinal direction (Fig. 19-24). The thin coating of barium on the surface appears finely stippled because of the innumerable tiny ulcers. When seen along the edges,

the ulcers cause numerous, tiny, spikelike projections. Rather similar tiny projections are seen occasionally in the normal colon. These are thought to result from barium filling of the innominate lines.[21] Edema may cause a fine granularity of the mucosa, which becomes coarser and more granular in appearance if the disease progresses to the phase of ingrowth of granulation tissue. If only part of the colon is involved, the demarcation between the diseased and normal bowel is not distinct. In the normal individual, longitudinal folds are sometimes seen in the lower descending portion of the colon during the postevacuation phase. However, the folds are finer than those seen in patients with ulcerative colitis

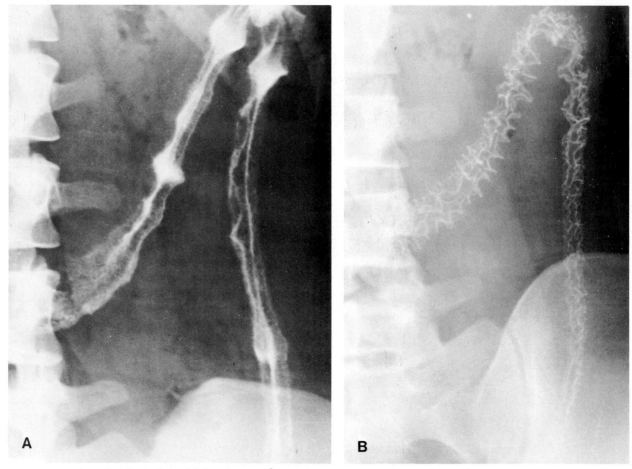

A   **B**

Fig. 19-24. Chronic ulcerative colitis. **A.** Postevacuation roentgenogram of a patient with chronic ulcerative colitis showing the appearance of the contracted colon. The mucosal folds are coarsened and thrown into a longitudinal pattern. **B.** Postevacuation roentgenogram of a normal colon showing the finely crinkled pattern of colonic mucosal folds in the same region as that shown in **A.**

and there is no stippling of the barium coating caused by the tiny ulcers. Normally, there are few if any haustra in the lower descending colon when it is distended and this should be taken into account when early ulcerative colitis is a possibility. The appearance of the mucosa is the significant feature in differentiation along with the presence or absence of the other signs of inflammation.

In the acute fulminating cases, roentgen findings during the early stages are even more difficult to evaluate. Some patients are critically ill and yet show a minimal amount of ulceration and inflammation on direct inspection; the severity of clinical signs and symptoms, therefore, does not always bear a direct relationship to the severity of pathologic changes. As a rule it is unwise to attempt a barium-enema study on a patient with acute fulminating disease because of the danger of perforation and the toxicity and prostration caused by the disease. If this study is undertaken, usually within a short time after onset of the acute disease, the margins of the barium-filled colon begin to appear rough and shaggy because of the presence of ulcers, edema, and inflammation of the mucosa. Excess secretions are present. Haustra may persist but the septa are thickened and vary in depth. In other cases an acute fulminating disease develops during the course of chronic ulcerative colitis. The disease is often accompanied by a *toxic dilatation of the colon* (toxic megacolon). A striking feature in abdominal roentgenograms in these patients is the marked colonic dilatation. The most severe involvement tends to be localized to the transverse colon (Fig. 19-25). Even when the entire colon is involved, the maximum dilatation is likely to be in the transverse segment. The diagnosis often can be made from plain roentgenograms. The mucosal surface, as outlined by the gas, is roughened with a shaggy or cobblestone appearance. Haustral markings are either absent or irregular in width and depth and the wall of the colon is thickened. Polyps or pseudopolyps cause rounded projections on the luminal surface of the affected bowel (Fig. 19-26), adding to the generally roughened appearance of the mucosal surface. Barium enema is contraindicated because of the danger of perforation of the colon, which is one of the major complications and may be recognized roentgenographically by the demonstration of free gas within the abdominal cavity. Perforation is an indication for immediate surgery.

The retrorectal soft-tissue space is increased to 1 cm or more in more than one-half of the patients who have ulcerative colitis.[13] This is measured from the posterior surface of the barium in the distended rec-

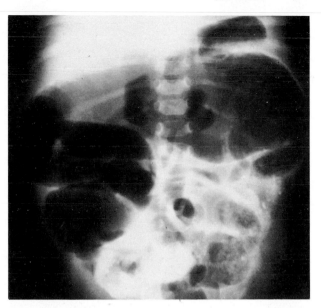

Fig. 19-25. Toxic megacolon associated with ulcerative colitis in a child. The ascending and transverse portions of the colon are greatly distended with gas.

tum to the sacrum at the S3–S5 level. However, this space may also be increased in patients with granulomatous colitis of the rectum and in those having other rectal inflammatory diseases, therefore the increase is of little help in making a differential diagnosis.

Later Changes. As the disease becomes more advanced and more chronic the roentgen pattern becomes characteristic. Haustra diminish in depth and eventually disappear. The lumen of the colon becomes uniformly narrowed and the bowel is shortened (Fig. 19-27). When the disease is of segmental distribution, as in right-sided colitis, the ends of the area of involvement taper gradually and the transition to normal bowel is not abrupt. The margins of the barium-filled lumen are finely roughened as a result of the miliary ulcerations. In the post-evacuation roentgenogram, when the colon is contracted, mucosal folds are absent; instead, the surface coated with barium residue has a granular appearance.

In still later stages the colon develops the characteristic "lead-pipe" appearance (Fig. 19-28). It fills very rapidly with only a few ounces of the mixture. The lumen is diffusely narrowed and the colon is greatly shortened. Occasionally one or more areas of smooth stricture formation are present.

Occasionally, ulcerative colitis begins in the right

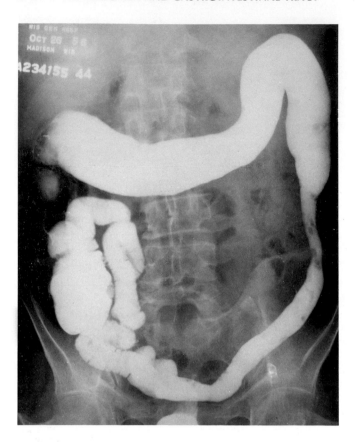

Fig. 19-26. Chronic ulcerative colitis. The entire colon is involved including the rectum. There is narrowing, shortening, and loss of haustrations. A few pseudopolyps are seen in the midportion of the descending colon.

side of the colon. When it does the appearance is similar to that seen in patients in whom the disease originates in the distal part of the colon.

When the cecum is involved by chronic ulcerative colitis, the ileocecal valve usually is widely patent and rapid filling of the terminal ileum results. The ileum may be dilated but otherwise normal. Involvement of the terminal ileum, the so-called "backwash ileitis," occurs in about 10% of cases of generalized ulcerative colitis. The appearance resembles regional enteritis except that the changes are less severe. Thickening of mucosal folds, due to edema, and spasm and irritability of the segment are the main findings. Narrowing usually is not pronounced and a string sign is not seen. If changes in the terminal ileum are the same as those seen in regional enteritis, the colonic disease is most likely granulomatous colitis rather than ulcerative disease.

Pseudopolyposis. During the later, ocasionally earlier, stages of chronic ulcerative colitis, polypoid or pseudopolypoid changes become frequent. The co-

alescence of small ulcers into larger and deeper ones with undermined edges may denude large areas of mucosa but leave islands or tags of inflamed or hypertrophied mucosa. These cause small, rounded translucent defects in the barium shadow that resemble those caused by true adenomatous polyps (Fig. 19-29). In fact, during proctoscopic examination such tags may be misinterpreted as true polyps.

Pseudopolyposis secondary to ulcerative colitis presents a typical roentgen appearance. In addition to the usual changes of narrowing, shortening, and loss of haustrations characteristic of ulcerative disease, numerous translucent defects will be seen. Those situated along the margin of the colon cause it to appear roughened (Fig. 19-29).

Rarely, localized giant pseudopolypoid masses may be observed in ulcerative colitis. They are manifested by a local intraluminal mass, single or multiple, that may be circumferential and closely resemble carcinoma. This type of lesion has also been observed in granulomatous colitis and in both diseases must be differentiated from carcinoma.

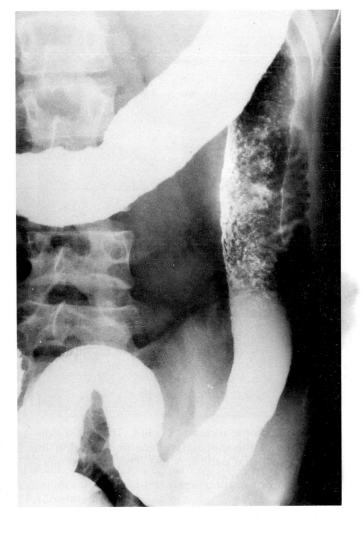

Fig. 19-27. Chronic ulcerative colitis. The left side of the colon is shown. Haustra are absent, and the mucosal pattern is grossly abnormal. Note the coarse granular appearance best observed in the air-containing upper descending colon.

Reversibility. It has been stated that complete reversal to normal may occur in chronic ulcerative colitis. Close observation, however, usually reveals that there is some persistent abnormality in the form of decreased distensability, some haustral abnormality, and often some persistent shortening of the colon. The disease in these patients may reactivate at any time.

Carcinoma. Carcinoma of the colon is one of the complications of chronic ulcerative colitis. The roentgen appearance in some of these patients is similar to that of carcinoma arising in an otherwise normal colon. In others, the tumor produces a stricturelike narrowing, usually relatively short, which may be central with smoothly tapering ends. Often, however, the lesion is an eccentric stricture with some mucosal irregularity. Any stricture of the colon encountered under these circumstances should be viewed with suspicion and warrants the consideration of surgical exploration.

Granulomatous Colitis

This form of colitis is also known as Crohn's disease of the colon because it is recognized as being the same disease as regional enteritis involving the small intestine. In contrast to ulcerative colitis, granulomatous disease tends to be right-sided and segmental and usually spares the rectum. Associated involvement of the terminal ileum is frequent and is virtually always present when the cecum is involved;

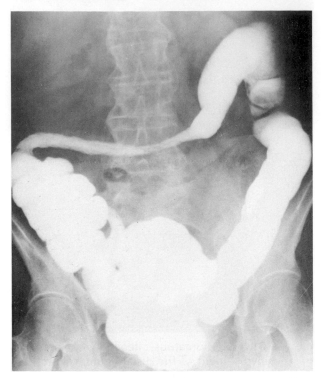

Fig. 19-33. Granulomatous colitis. This patient illustrates the segmental nature of the disease. The involvement is confined largely to the transverse colon where there is narrowing and gross abnormality of mucosal pattern as well as loss of normal haustrations.

litis in whom there is some question as to whether or not the incidence is actually increased.

There are a number of patients in whom there appear to be a few findings characteristic of each disease so that roentgen differentiation cannot be made. There may also be a problem in histopathologic diagnosis in some of these patients.[45]

The Double-Contrast Enema in Ulcerative Colitis and Crohn's Colitis. Numerous reports indicate that double-contrast enema study is a safe and very useful procedure in patients with ulcerative colitis and in those with Crohn's colitis and that it localizes the extent of the disease more accurately than do other studies.[41] Furthermore, the subtle, early changes are more readily recognized than in the conventional examination, so that the procedure aids in the differential diagnosis. There is some risk of exacerbating the disease, however. Other diseases that may enter the differential diagnosis include diverticulitis, segmental infarction, and, at times, some of the specific and nonspecific inflammatory diseases that may resemble

granulomatous colitis, particularly when there are skip areas.

Angiography has been used in an attempt to differentiate granulomatous from ulcerative colitis, but, although there is some difference of opinion, it appears that the angiographic features are nonspecific, therefore angiography is not an accurate method of differential diagnosis.[6]

Colitis in Behcet's Disease. Behcet's disease is an uncommon entity of unknown cause in which multiple systems are involved, including the skin, the mucous membranes with oral and genital ulcers, ocular inflammation, arthritis, central nervous system involvement, thrombophlebitis, and colitis. When the colon is involved, deep ulcerations with skip areas, mucosal nodularity, or polypoid thickening which resembles granulomatous more closely than ulcerative colitis are present.[25]

Tuberculosis

Tuberculosis of the colon usually is associated with disease of the terminal ileum. This site, namely the ileocecal region, is involved in 85% to 90% of patients who have gastrointestinal tuberculosis. No recognizable pulmonary tuberculosis is present in the majority of these patients. The disease may be segmental and may occur elsewhere in the colon, chiefly in the sigmoid. In the ileocecal area, the roentgen manifestations are those of narrowing, loss of haustrations in the colon, and ulceration of the mucosa in the area involved. Full thickness of the wall is involved so that the ulcers may be deep. Ileocecal tuberculosis can simulate Crohn's disease to the point where differentiation radiographically is not possible. Occasionally, it may produce a stricturelike lesion in some areas or an intraluminal mass with irregular polypoid filling defects simulating carcinoma in others. In this segmental form of the disease, there may be multiple lesions; their presence helps in the differentiation from carcinoma.

Amebiasis

The diagnosis of acute intestinal amebiasis depends almost entirely upon the demonstration of *Entamoeba histolytica* in the stool. In chronic, localized disease (ameboma) those lesions in the rectosigmoid area can be biopsied. Serologic tests for amebiasis also have been found helpful by some investigators. Roentgen examination may reveal changes in the colon, but in the majority of patients with amebiasis the findings essentially reveal no abnormality and the patient is treated successfully before chronic changes of roentgenographic significance develop. Pathologically the cecum, appendix, and ascending colon are involved initially in most of these patients. The next most frequent site is the rectosigmoid region. It is unusual to have the colon between these areas affected unless there is an overwhelming infection. The earliest mucosal change is superficial ulceration, which may produce a fine serrated appearance. Characteristically the ulcers are pinhead in size and separated from one another by normal mucosa. As the disease progresses the ulcers become deeper, larger, and confluent with undermining of their edges, simulating ulcers sometimes observed in granulomatous colitis. Spasm and loss of haustrations in the involved area(s) accompanies the ulcerations.

In some patients with amebiasis, barium-enema examination will demonstrate a deformity of the cecum. It has been reported that cecal deformity occurs in approximately one-third of patients whose stools are positive for *Entamoeba histolytica* and it is much more frequent when the disease is symptomatic; thus carriers who are asymptomatic are not very likely to show changes on roentgen examination. The cecal deformity is one of concentric narrowing and shortening with loss of haustral indentations (Fig. 19-34). The cecum often assumes a cone-shaped appearance. It usually is tender to palpation. The deformity of the cecum is believed to be caused by fibrosis from secondary infection and long-continued spasm. The ileocecal valve may be thickened, fixed, open, and incompetent, but roentgen evidence of disease of the adjacent terminal ileum is rarely present.

Lesions in the rectosigmoid portion of the colon are even more difficult to evaluate unless they occur in association with the rather typical cecal deformity. Stenotic narrowing is the rule but there is little to distinguish it from other lesions, particularly carcinoma. A localized, granulomatous, inflammatory mass, called an ameboma, is an occasional manifestation of the disease. It may develop in either the cecum or the rectosigmoid area and closely resemble carcinoma in its gross features. The roentgen differentiation may be difficult if not impossible. Usually there is less fixation than in tumor, and one end of the mass may have a tapered appearance rather than the abrupt shoulderlike change typical of carcinoma. An ameboma will decrease in size, as a rule, within 5 days under antiamebic drug treatment.

The combination of a cone-shaped cecal deformity and a local inflammatory (skip) lesion elsewhere in

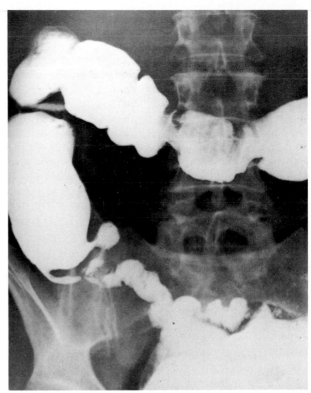

Fig. 19-34. Amebiasis of the cecum. There is much shortening of the cecum. Note that the ileocecal valve appears to be in the most proximal colon. The deformity is believed to be the result of fibrosis in patients with this disease.

the colon is very suggestive of amebiasis. Toxic megacolon is occasionally observed, which is similar in appearance to that in ulcerative colitis and is frequently complicated by perforation.

Tuberculosis can be distinguished from amebiasis without difficulty in most patients by the almost universal involvement of the terminal ileum as well as the cecum. The cecal deformity of amebiasis bears little resemblance to right-sided idiopathic ulcerative colitis that usually affects a much longer segment of the bowel.

A short segment of granulomatous colitis may offer some difficulty in diagnosis but usually the changes of granulomatous disease are sufficiently characteristic to allow differentiation.

Histoplasmosis

Although histoplasmosis may involve any portion of the gastrointestinal tract, the colon and distal ileum are the most common sites. Small nodules or ulcerations may result from the granulomatous process. The nodular lesions may become large enough to resemble pseudopolyps. There is often some constriction in the area of involvement, and there may be several lesions scattered in the colon. Large nodes may cause extrinsic pressure. In the distal ileum, thickening of the wall producing separation of loops similar to that in Crohn's disease along with some mucosal irregularity is observed. When ileocecal involvement is present, histoplasmosis may resemble Crohn's disease and, in the colon, lesions resembling those of tuberculosis and sometimes those of carcinoma are observed; these diseases, therefore, must be differentiated from histoplasmosis.[28]

Schistosomiasis

Rarely the rectosigmoid area is involved by schistosomiasis, usually in patients with disease of the bladder. Mucosal ulceration with edema, spasm, and a pericolic mass are present. Calcification has been observed in the wall of the colon in these patients similar to that noted in the bladder when it is involved.[59]

Chagas' Disease (Trypanosomiasis)

Although Chagas' disease is rare, it has been observed in the southern portion of the United States and is endemic in South and Central America. The organism responsible destroys autonomic ganglia in the gastrointestinal tract, mainly in the esophagus and colon. The chief manifestation in the colon is dilatation and elongation, which may involve segments of the colon but can involve the entire colon.

Salmonellosis and Shigellosis

Colitis caused by salmonellae or shigellae is manifested by ulceration, spasm, and edema; a loss of haustral pattern and a rather smooth appearance of the colon except for the superficial ulcerations may be observed. Another pattern is that of edema resulting in thumbprinting. Involvement may be diffuse or segmental. Shigellae involve the colon primarily while salmonellae are more prominent in the terminal ileum, although colon changes are also seen. The lesions respond to therapy leaving no residuals.

Necrotizing Enterocolitis

Necrotizing enterocolitis is largely a disease occurring in the first 5 days of life in infants with low birth-weight who have undergone stress, particularly hypoxia. Also there seems to be a causal relationship between indwelling umbilical arterial and venous catheters and the development of necrotizing enterocolitis. The disease is potentially lethal. It is characterized by bowel involvement varying from simple mucosal ulcerations to transmural necrosis of the bowel wall over long segments. Radiographic findings are: (1) intestinal distention; (2) gas in the wall of the involved bowel; (3) free air in the peritoneum, usually indicating perforation; and (4) gas in the portal venous system (Fig. 19-35). Ascites may also be present and is probably a sign of imminent perforation. The ascending colon and ileum are the areas most frequently involved, but any portion of the colon or small bowel may be affected. Surgery is indicated when perforation occurs; medical management has proved successful in patients without perforation. Formerly the mortality rate was extremely high, but with early recognition and prompt therapy the rate has decreased.

In the survivors, strictures may occur as a complication. Many times this narrowing apparently is reversible, however, so that surgical resection may not be necessary.[68]

Fig. 19-35. Necrotizing enterocolitis. Fine streaks of intramural gas are noted throughout most of the bowel. There is also a considerable amount of gas within the bowel loops. On the original film a suggestion of gas was also noted in the portal veins in this infant.

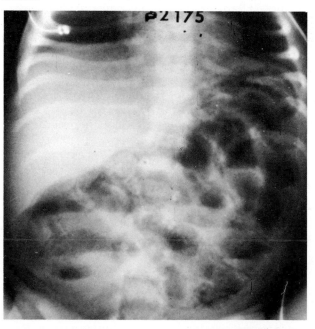

A relatively benign form of necrotizing enterocolitis has been recognized recently in which the radiographic findings consist of distention, pneumatosis, and portal venous gas, pneumoperitoneum, however, is not observed. If the distention is minimal, the prognosis is particularly good.[61]

Rarely, necrotizing enterocolitis occurs in adults in whom the radiographic manifestations are similar to those observed in infants having the disease. Barium studies are contraindicated in this disease because of the danger of perforation. Therefore, it is extremely important that good plain film studies be obtained and that these be examined carefully for evidence of pneumatosis of the involved bowel wall.

Pseudomembranous Enterocolitis

The pathogenesis of this disease is uncertain but an increasing number of cases have been described as occurring in debilitated patients on treatment with certain antibiotics. Clindamycin (Cleocin) seems to be the principal cause, but other drugs including tetracycline, penicillin, ampicillin, and lincomycin (Lincocin) also have been implicated. The plain-film findings consist of (*1*) unusual wide transverse bands replacing the normal haustral markings; (2) giant thumbprinting along the margins of the colon; (3) a finer pattern of scalloping within the more gross thumbprinting; (4) minimal distention. If the patient's clinical condition permits, a low-pressure barium-enema study can be performed with caution. This study is contraindicated, however, if the patient is toxic or has peritonitis or sepsis. Barium studies reveal a shaggy appearance of the colon caused by the pseudomembrane, and there may be some ulcerations in areas where there is no pseudomembrane. Prompt recognition of the condition is helpful so that use of the offending antibiotic can be discontinued and supportive measures instituted. Endoscopy is the diagnostic method of choice since the pseudomembranes are readily visible. The findings in the colon may be identical to those of ischemic colitis, and toxic dilatation may occur in some instances.

Recent evidence indicates that toxin-producing clostridia may actually be the cause of pseudomembranous colitis in patients on antibiotics.[1] These organisms are resistant to the antibiotic used for therapy, so they proliferate and reach high concentrations in the colon during the antibiotic treatment. It appears to be likely that pseudomembranous colitis associated with antibiotics is actually caused by a cytotoxin produced by colonic flora.

Lymphogranuloma Venereum

This venereal disease is caused by a virus and is especially common in black females living in the tropics. Rectosigmoid involvement leads to the formation of strictures of the rectum and lower colon almost exclusively in females. The mucosal surface may be ulcerated, and rectal fissures, rectovaginal fistula, and perianal abscess may complicate the disease. The diagnosis is usually made on rectal biopsy and confirmed by a complement fixation test or an intradermal (Frei) test. Roentgen findings consist of narrowing of the rectum with irregularity and ulceration occurring early in the course of the disease. Fistulous tracts may be demonstrated. Later on, fibrosis resulting in stricture causes varying degrees of narrowing, sometimes for as long a distance as 25 cm. The contour of the narrow colon is often irregular as a result of mucosal ulceration.

POSTRADIATION FIBROSIS

Following heavy doses of radiation to the pelvis, usually given for the treatment of cervical carcinoma, an intense inflammatory reaction may develop in the rectum and sigmoid. The acute reaction, if severe, includes ulceration which is usually superficial, but if damage is more extensive, deep, penetrating ulcers with perforation and abscess formation may occur. This is not ordinarily observed as a result of radiotherapy, however. The initial phase is followed by fibrosis and scarring and occasionally this becomes sufficiently severe to cause a stenosis of the bowel. The lesion is seen as a relatively long and smooth stricture affecting the upper rectum or sigmoid. The bowel may appear stiffened and fixed. The defect differs from that caused by an annular carcinoma by being of greater length and by the gradual tapering of its edges. Resection or colostomy may be required if stenosis is severe. The history of previous radiation to the pelvis of sufficient degree to cause damage to the bowel is important in determining the diagnosis.

SEGMENTAL ISCHEMIA OF THE COLON

Segmental ischemia may involve the colon as it does the small intestine.[12] Ischemic involvement of the colon is represented by a spectrum that varies from mild and chronic to acute with rapid progression to necrosis and perforation.[52] Angiography may be useful in making the diagnosis, but often no site of vascular obstruction is observed. Symptoms include crampy abdominal pain, distention, and bloody diarrhea. The distribution of the left colic artery is usually involved in the chronic or subacute occlusive type of the disease. Edema and submucosal hemorrhage produce a narrowing of the lumen and irregularity with scalloped indentations termed "thumbprinting"—rather characteristic findings. Superficial ulceration may be present but this is not a prominent factor on barium examination in these patients. Rarely, the barium will extend into an ulcer and become trapped in the colonic wall, but pneumatosis of the wall does not usually occur. In the majority of patients, there is gradual improvement, but there may be stricture formation as a late complication. On plain film study there may be enough gas in the involved colon to allow visualization of the characteristic thumbprinting so that the diagnosis can be made or at least strongly suspected, particularly in those patients with a typical history. As has been indicated, barium studies will show the characteristic appearance and follow-up shows rather rapid improvement.

In contrast to this relatively mild disease just described, the left colon may occasionally be involved in the acute extensive, nonocclusive bowel ischemia associated with congestive heart failure, digitalis intoxication, or peripheral occlusive arterial disease. Symptoms are those of sudden onset of severe abdominal pain, vomiting, diarrhea, gastrointestinal bleeding, abdominal distention, peritonitis, and shock. Prognosis is very poor in these patients. In either type of ischemia, early operative intervention is recommended when peritoneal irritation is evident or conservative therapy fails.

INTRAMURAL HEMORRHAGE

Intramural hemorrhage may occur in ischemia as indicated in the foregoing, in the colon following trauma to the abdomen, in patients taking anticoagulants, or in those suffering from a hematologic disorder such as hemophilia. The early roentgen changes depend upon the amount and distribution of intramural bleeding. Characteristically, on barium filling, multiple, concave indentations or filling defects along one or both walls of the involved area, called "thumbprinting" or "scalloping," are noted. Based solely on roentgen findings it may be impossible at this stage to determine whether ischemia or intramural hemorrhage caused by other conditions is present except that thumbprinting tends to be more severe in intramural hemorrhage than in ischemia. However, progressive examinations usually show a prompt regression of these findings in uncomplicated hemorrhage and an eventual return to normal. Also, intra-

mural hemorrhage usually involves a shorter segment of colon than does ischemia, may be more massive locally, and may occur at multiple sites. Regression is usually not as rapid in hemorrhage secondary to ischemia, and a permanent stricture, not caused by hemorrhage, may occur as a result of ischemia.

COLONIC BLEEDING

In the middle-aged or elderly person, intermittent bleeding from the colon may be caused by a number of conditions, the most common of which is *diverticulosis*.[8] A very high percentage of bleeding diverticula are in the right colon proximal to the hepatic flexure and nearly all bleeding diverticula are proximal to the splenic flexure. Carcinoma is a rare cause of acute rectal bleeding. *Arteriovenous malformations or vascular dysplasias* often present with intermittent colonic hemorrhage or chronic occult bleeding and are more common in the ascending colon than elsewhere.[2, 64] There is an apparent association of aortic stenosis with these vascular malformations. Often the lesions cannot be located on endoscopic and barium studies, and they are extremely difficult to find at surgery; therefore angiography is the diagnostic method of choice. When bleeding is active (0.5 ml or more/minute) its site may be manifested by extravasation of the opaque medium. The vascular lesion itself may be identified. There are slowly emptying dilated, tortuous, intramural veins. There may also be a vascular tuft representing dilated venules in the mucosa as well as early filling of one or more veins, indicating arteriovenous communication. Angiography also has the potential for selective infusion of vasoconstrictor drugs or embolization. These vascular dysplasias or ectasias are probably acquired degenerative lesions secondary to intermittent venous obstruction during muscular contraction or distention of the colon.

INFLAMMATION OF APPENDICES EPIPLOICAE

The appendices epiploicae are small, pedunculated, fat pads along the surface of the colon, covered by the visceral peritoneum of the colon. Cases of inflammation of one or more appendices have been reported. There may be torsion with gangrene, acute inflammation with suppuration, chronic inflammation, or (rarely) intussusception. In cases reported in the past the inflammatory process resembled a carcinoma in one patient; in another the appearance suggested an extrinsic mass; in a third patient there was spasm and edema of folds in the involved areas; and in a fourth patient there was only evidence of a reflex ileus. Calcification in the appendices has also been reported; it is a rare cause of intraabdominal calcification.

HERNIAS INVOLVING THE COLON

Herniation of a loop of colon into an inguinal or femoral hernial sac is very frequent. In left-sided lesions the sigmoid colon is the portion usually involved. The hernia can be demonstrated by barium enema and its reducibility determined during fluoroscopic examination. Occasionally a large scrotal hernia will contain a long segment of the bowel. On the right side, hernial sacs usually contain small intestine; infrequently the cecum will be present in the hernia. It is often impossible to distinguish an inguinal from a femoral hernia by roentgen examination; inguinal hernias are apt to be larger than femoral hernias. At times a volvulated loop of colon incarcerated within a hernia may be visualized because of the gas accumulation within the segment. At other times the loop will contain only fluid and the roentgen signs will be those of bowel obstruction.

Herniation of colon into an anterior abdominal wall sac is another common condition. The diagnosis of abdominal hernia is essentially a clinical one and roentgen examination only serves to determine the nature of the hernial contents and to demonstrate the signs of obstruction if such exist. Lateral roentgenograms of the abdomen are useful to show the presence of gas-filled loops of bowel within the hernia when incarceration of bowel is suspected.

Lumbar hernia is an infrequent lesion that usually follows trauma but occasionally occurs spontaneously. The hernia projects posterolaterally and the diagnosis is readily made on barium-enema study. Plain roentgenograms of the abdomen may show a gas-filled loop of colon within the hernia. Oblique projections to bring the area into profile show the lesion to best advantage.

Spigelian Hernia

A spigelian hernia is the result of a defect in the linea semilunaris lateral to the outer border of the rectus muscle, usually below the umbilical level at the point where the posterior sheath of the transverse abdominal muscle ends—the line of Douglas. Colon and/or small bowel may extend into the hernia which often enlarges laterally to appear near the anterosuperior spine of the ilium. Roentgen findings depend on the amount of bowel outside the peritoneal cavity and the amount of lateral dissection.

The colon is affected indirectly in many internal hernias but the major alteration most frequently is in the small intestine as discussed in Chapter 18.

FUNCTIONAL DISTURBANCES

Examination of the colon by means of a barium enema is of little value in the study of most functional disturbances. The use of castor oil catharsis and cleansing enemas for preparation often makes the bowel very irritable and spasm may be fairly intense. This method of examination has for its prime purpose the detection of organic disease rather than functional disturbances. An oral barium meal followed through the intestinal tract by means of serial roentgenograms may give some information concerning colonic stasis but the findings must be interpreted with considerable caution. Barium sulfate is not a food, it is insoluble in the gastrointestinal tract, and because of absorption of water from the colon the barium tends to become hardened. Because of this a colon that may function normally under ordinary circumstances may show evidence of barium stasis after an oral meal. As a general rule, therefore, the appearance of the colon after a barium meal cannot be relied upon for the diagnosis of disturbed colonic function. Clinically, the terms "irritable colon," "mucous colitis," "spastic constipation," and similar designations are employed rather frequently. These clinical states do not have associated gross pathologic findings and roentgen examination does not lend itself to the clarification of these problems.

The "Cathartic" Colon

Roentgen examination occasionally demonstrates rather pronounced changes in the appearance of the colon and terminal ileum in patients who have been habitual users of irritant cathartics. In patients with milder cases there is shortening of the cecum, which develops a conical shape resembling somewhat the deformity seen in some patients with amebiasis. The ileocecal valve lips are shortened and the valve is gaping. In those having the more severe cases the colon distal to the cecum shows diminution in haustral sacculations and becomes quite smooth; the lumen may be narrowed or enlarged, and, in the contracted state the mucosal folds assume a linear arrangement rather than a crisscross pattern. On the whole the appearance resembles in many ways idiopathic ulcerative colitis. The bowel, however, is not as stiffened, as it is in long-standing chronic ulcerative colitis, there is no history of diarrhea or bloody stools; instead, there is a history of ingestion of irritant cathartics over a period of many years (Fig. 19-36).

In patients who have developed the enema habit, using a daily or almost daily enema of soapsuds in order to obtain a bowel movement, a rather similar alteration in the appearance of the bowel has been observed by us. It is well to keep in mind these conditions when changes of this nature are found during barium-enema examination because they may be misinterpreted as evidence of chronic ulcerative colitis. As noted in the preceding paragraphs, correlation with the clinical history and findings is important.

INTUSSUSCEPTION

Ileocolic intussusception is very common in children less than 1 year of age (Fig. 19-37). The vast majority are invaginations of ileum into colon (ileocolic) with about 5% colocolic and the remainder ileoileal. Intussusception is an invagination of proximal into distal gut resulting in some angulation and compression of the mesentery and its vessels often causing impairment of venous drainage and then impairment of arterial flow. In young children, since no definite intraluminal mass is usually present, the cause is not clear. In older children and in adults, usually an organic lesion, such as Meckel's diverticulum or an intramural or intraluminal tumor, or hemorrhage is manifest. The onset is usually acute in a previously healthy child who has abdominal pain, is vomiting, and, later, has bloody mucoid stools. Clinical diagnosis may be made with reasonable certainty in the

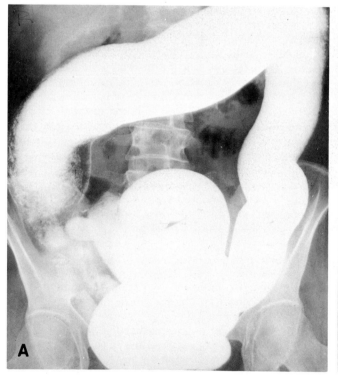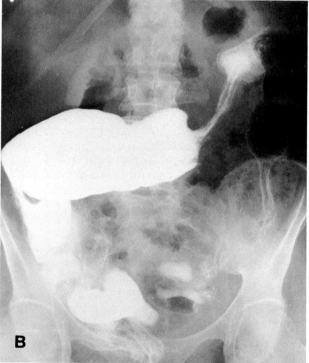

Fig. 19-36. The colon after prolonged ingestion of irritant cathartics. **A.** Roentgenogram of the barium-filled colon. **B.** Postevacuation film. The appearance of the filled colon resembles that of ulcerative colitis except that the colon is somewhat dilated. In the postevacuation film the mucosal folds appear grossly abnormal, suggesting those observed in chronic ulcerative colitis in some areas. It is important to correlate the roentgenographic findings with the history in such patients.

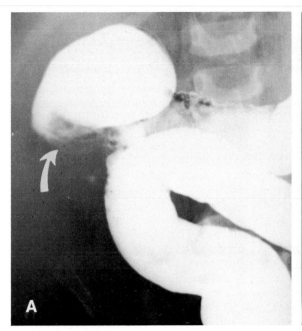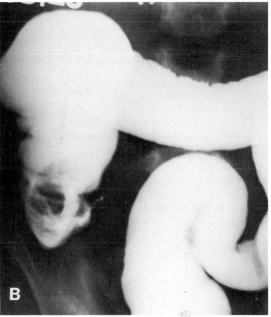

Fig. 19-37. Ileocolic intussusception in a young child. **A.** During barium-enema study the obstruction was encountered in the distal transverse colon but was gradually reduced to the point shown in this roentgenogram. The concavity of the barium column **(arrow)** marks the intussusceptum. **B.** This film shows further reduction. However, because reduction was not complete, surgical treatment was required.

majority of these patients who have an abdominal mass in addition to the symptoms. Plain films usually show some distention of the small bowel and may show a soft-tissue mass projecting into the colon. Barium enema is usually employed to confirm the diagnosis, and, in most radiology departments, is used to reduce the intussusception unless signs of peritonitis are present, in which case it is contraindicated. Sedation is often employed in an attempt to relax the child, and, some radiology departments, glucagon has been used to decrease colonic spasm as an aid to the reduction.[18] Radiologists must make certain that there is no residual ileoileal intussusception remaining after the ileocolic portion is reduced. When reduction fails or is incomplete, surgery is indicated.

THE POSTOPERATIVE COLON

Preparation of the postoperative colon for barium-enema examination depends to a large extent upon the nature of the operative procedure. If this has consisted of local excision of a polyp or resection with end-to-end anastomosis, the same preparation is used as for the standard examination, including castor oil catharsis and cleansing tap-water enemas. When a colostomy is present it usually is sufficient to irrigate the bowel through the colostomy opening, using a balloon catheter. If the rectum has not been removed as part of the operative procedure, the distal part of the colon is cleansed by means of tap-water enemas given in the usual manner.

If the rectum has not been removed, the lower part of the bowel can be examined by giving a barium enema rectally, and if obstruction is not present, the entire segment from the anus to the colostomy is examined by this means. If the bowel above and below the colostomy is to be examined at one sitting it is preferable to fill the distal part first. When this portion of the examination is completed, including obtaining postevacuation films, the proximal loop can be examined by using one of the stoma-occluding devices mentioned in the section on technique in the early portion of this chapter.

There may be clinical indications to reverse the procedure and examine the proximal loop first; some radiologists prefer this as a routine measure in patients who have had a colostomy.

End-to-End Anastomosis

For lesions in the lower part of the descending colon and in the sigmoid area, local resection with end-to-end anastomosis often is performed. The roentgen appearance of such an anastomosis varies somewhat with the time interval after surgery. Usually, after a period of several months, there will have been subsidence of the postoperative edema and after this period the appearance of the anastomosis does not change significantly. In many cases the site of the anastomosis is difficult to detect. When the segment is completely distended, a thin ringlike constriction may be visualized, but in some cases there is no change in the width of the lumen. Frequently a distinct and abrupt change in the mucosal pattern and the haustral indentations will indicate the site of the resection. Occasionally the postevacuation roentgenogram demonstrates these changes to better advantage than when the colon is completely distended. Because the normal findings may vary somewhat, many writers have recommended that a postoperative barium-enema examination be carried out on every patient who has had resection and end-to-end anastomosis for treatment of carcinoma within several months after the operation. This preliminary examination will serve as a reference for later studies and will be of aid in detecting early recurrences. It is pointed out that any irregularity or nodular defect along the suture line, no matter how small, should be viewed with suspicion unless a similar irregularity was seen in the immediate postoperative period. Only by careful observation and serial examinations is it possible to detect recurrent carcinoma at the site of resection when the lesion still is in an early stage. After it becomes more advanced the roentgen findings are no different than those seen in primary carcinoma of the colon. It is also important to remember that multiple tumors of the colon are not infrequent and that follow-up examinations are very useful in detecting early polyp formation and carcinomatous degeneration in polyps in other parts of the colon.

Resection of the Colon

Resection of the proximal colon with ileotransverse colostomy is another common operative procedure performed because of disease involving the right side of the colon. The roentgenologist should be informed of the presence of an anastomosis between the ileum and colon before the barium-enema examination is begun. Otherwise there may be rapid extension of the barium mixture through the anastomosis with rapid flooding of loops of small bowel so that the site becomes obscured. This may happen while the examiner's attention is centered elsewhere and by the time he becomes aware of the presence of an anastomosis the field may be hidden completely and the examination will be unsatisfactory. Recurrence of carcinoma is the stump of the resected colon is relatively uncommon. In these patients, recurrences are more likely to develop in the tissues at the site of the original lesion, in the draining lymph nodes, or as a metastatic spread to the liver. Barium-enema examination of the postoperative colon in these patients, therefore, is of value chiefly in demonstrating the patency of the ileotransverse colostomy and in the detection of possible new tumors in the colon that remains. These patients should have thorough preparation so that fecal matter is eliminated from the colon insofar as possible. Clear liquid diet is important in the preparation of these patients.

THE APPENDIX

Filling of the appendix occurs frequently during barium-enema examinations of the colon and it also can be demonstrated when delayed roentgenograms (*i.e.*, at 6, 24, and 48 hours) are obtained after the oral administration of barium. Failure of visualization of the appendix by either method is no indication that it is diseased, but the great majority of normal appendices will fill with barium on barium-enema examination. If the appendix does fill, some idea of its size, position, and mobility can be obtained. It is not uncommon to find the appendix remaining visible because of barium filling for days after the examination and it is doubtful if the demonstration of such stasis has any clinical significance. The diagnosis of chronic appendicitis cannot be made from roentgen findings. The retrocecal position of the appendix often can be established if the structure fills with barium; even if it does not, the posterior position of the ileocecal valve usually indicates a posterior location of the appendix as well.

ACUTE APPENDICITIS

Roentgen examination in acute appendicitis is usually limited to scout roentgenograms of the abdomen. Within a few hours after the onset of acute appendicitis, scout roentgenograms often will show the presence of one or several short loops of gas-filled ileum in the right lower quadrant. As a rule the distention is slight and fluid levels, in upright roentgen-

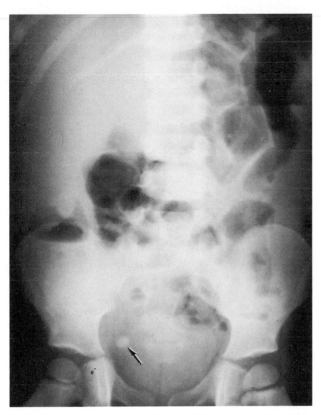

Fig. 19-38. Acute appendicitis with perforation. This film, exposed with the patient in the upright position, shows gas in the colon and small bowel, probably representing adynamic ileus. There is a calcified fecalith of the appendix **(arrow)** in the pelvis.

ograms, are either absent or short and inconspicuous. A fluid level may be demonstrated in the cecum in upright or left lateral decubitus views (Fig. 19-38). This is an important sign when taken in conjunction with other findings, provided an enema has not been given prior to the examination and there is no obstruction in the distal colon. In the presence of the latter, the entire colon will be distended rather than distention being limited to the cecum and ascending colon. In the presence of a spreading inflammation the signs of a more generalized ileus may develop. In later stages the soft-tissue spaces between the loops may be thickened as a result of spread of the inflammation and the presence of exudate on the serosal surfaces of the bowel. In some cases, blurring of the properitoneal fat line along the right lower abdominal wall is observed. This finding is difficult to interpret because visibility of the line varies considerably in normal individuals and as an isolated observa-

tion its value in the diagnosis of acute appendicitis is limited. Fluid density interposed between the colon and the flank stripe in the right lower quadrant, when present, is a suggestive sign in a patient with right lower quadrant pain. Indistinctness in the outline of the lower part of the psoas shadow and a scoliosis, concavity to the right, may be seen in some patients, but these signs alone are also difficult to evaluate.

In gangrenous appendicitis, local pneumatosis has been observed in the adjacent cecum, a reasonably reliable sign when correlated with clinical observations. In patients with fixed high retrocecal appendicitis, the inflammatory disease may produce indentations on the posterolateral aspect of the adjacent colon. Local spasm or irritability of the colon may be manifest as well. Skeletal-muscle splinting may produce a lumbar scoliosis, convexity to the left.[49]

Whenever the diagnosis of acute appendicitis is being considered, careful observation of the right lower quadrant of the abdomen for evidence of a calcified fecalith in the appendix should be made. The fecalith is seen as a round or ovoid shadow of calcium density and may be laminated (see Fig. 19-38). The size varies but usually is on the order of 0.5 to 1 cm. The fecalith frequently overlies the ilium and may be difficult to visualize because of the density of the bone. In some patients the fecalith is extruded from the appendix as a result of rupture and comes to lie within an abscess cavity. The fecalith may be visualized low in the right side of the pelvis when the ascending colon is long and the cecum abnormally low in position. It may resemble an ordinary phlebolith in the pelvic veins. Appendiceal fecaliths (coproliths) will be found in approximately one-fourth of children having acute appendicitis and in about one-half of these patients plain films of the abdomen will suggest an inflammatory process in the abdomen.

Contrary to popular belief that enemas are hazardous in patients with acute appendicitis, many now believe that the procedure is harmless and some think that it is useful in determining the diagnosis. Nonfilling of the appendix plus a mass that may distort the cecum or small bowel is suggestive but not diagnostic. A patent lumen virtually excludes the diagnosis of acute appendicitis, particularly when filling is complete including filling of the rounded appendiceal tip. Partial filling of the appendix does not exclude the possibility of inflammation, however.

If the appendix ruptures and a more extensive peritonitis develops, the roentgen signs become those of an adynamic ileus with evidence of peritoneal exudate separating the gas-filled loops of bowel. Rupture of the appendix rarely leads to pneumoperitoneum and the demonstration of free gas in the peritoneal cavity in upright or lateral decubitus roentgenograms is not to be expected.

APPENDICEAL ABSCESS

During the acute stage of the appendiceal abscess roentgen findings are usually limited to those of (*1*) adynamic ileus (see Fig. 13-32), (*2*) evidence of an ill-defined mass of soft-tissue density in the lower right quadrant with an absence of gas shadows in the area, (*3*) occasional identification of a calcified concretion or fecalith in the area, and (*4*) in some instances, formation of gas within the abscess visualized as small flocculent translucencies within the mass of the abscess (see Fig. 13-35). After subsidence of the acute phase, some patients are examined by means of a barium enema because the clinical signs have been atypical and the diagnosis remains in doubt. In these cases a barium enema often will show evidence of a mass adjacent to the tip of the cecum deforming it and causing a filling defect in the cecum (Figs. 19-39 and 19-40). There is local tenderness, the cecum is fixed in position, and careful study of roentgenograms will show mucosal folds and deformed but intact haustra. If the ileum fills by reflux through the ileocecal valve it may be displaced by the mass; its lumen may be narrowed irregularly and its mucosal folds thickened. In some of these patients the demonstration of a calcified fecalith within the mass is the most convincing diagnostic sign. The history of a recent episode of acute nature, the tender mass, and the location immediately adjacent to and fixed to the cecum are helpful corroborative signs.

TUMORS OF THE APPENDIX

Mucocele

Mucocele of the appendix is an uncommon lesion, its frequency in routine autopsies being reported as from 0.2 % to 0.5%. It is generally considered to arise as a result of a gradual occlusion of the appendiceal lumen with the development of a cystlike mass filled with a mucinous material. In addition to this benign type of lesion, there is a malignant form that is in fact a mucoid papillary adenocarcinoma of a low degree of malignancy. This tumor resembles a benign mucocele in its gross features but differs in behavior. Should rupture of a malignant mucocele occur, there may be implantation of epithelial cells on the surface of the peritoneum. These cells continue

to produce mucus and give rise to the condition known as pseudomyxoma peritonaei, which is described in Chapter 13 under the heading "Pseudomyxoma Peritonaei."

The roentgen diagnostic features of appendiceal mucocele are:

1. A sharply outlined round or ovoid soft-tissue mass in the right lower quadrant, usually having a fair degree of mobility. On barium-enema examination the mass is found to be attached to the cecum and to move with it (Fig. 19-41).

2. The cecum is displaced to some extent by the mass. It may be displaced laterally or medially, depending upon the position of the appendix.

3. Calcium deposits are common in the wall of the mucocele.

4. The appendix does not fill.

5. The mass may cause no cecal deformity if small; if larger, a smooth, pressure type of defect is seen with intact but distorted mucosal folds.

Intussusception of a mucocele into the cecum is a rare complication. When this happens the defect resembles that of a polypoid cecal tumor and the diagnosis of a mucocele cannot be made unless there is calcification in its wall.

Myxoglobulosis

Myxoglobulosis is a variant of mucocele in which the content consists of round or oval globules (3 to 10 mm) resembling tapioca or fish eggs, often with a calcified rim. The roentgen appearance is that of a mass similar to mucocele except that it contains multiple oval or round calcifications, usually circumferential but occasionally solid.[16]

Adenocarcinoma

Mention has been made in a previous paragraph of the mucoid papillary type of adenocarcinoma or malignant mucocele. There also is a solid so-called "colonic" type of adenocarcinoma arising in the appendix but it is a very rare lesion. This tumor soon invades the cecum and then it resembles a primary carcinoma of the cecum in its clinical and roentgen features. Earlier it may resemble an inverted appendiceal stump, a polyp, a small mucocele, or intussusception of the appendix.

Carcinoid Tumors

Carcinoid tumors are not limited to the appendix although they occur most frequently in this location. It

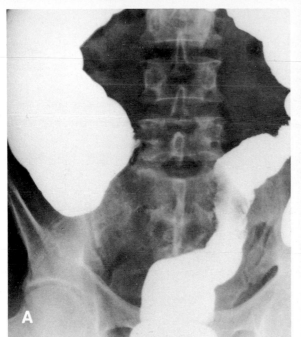 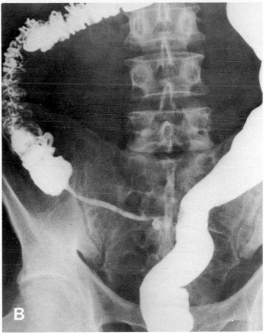

Fig. 19-39. Appendiceal abscess. **A.** Roentgenogram obtained 1 week after the onset of clinical symptoms. There is a mass between the cecal tip and the sigmoid, indenting both of these structures somewhat. **B.** Roentgenogram of the same patient shown in **A** obtained several months later. The appendix is now filled with barium, and there is a fecalith in its tip. The inflammatory mass has decreased considerably in size. Subsequent surgical exploration confirmed the diagnosis.

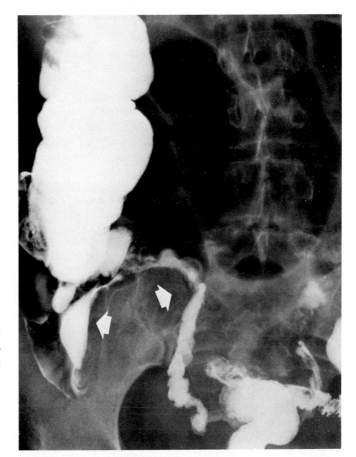

Fig. 19-40. Appendiceal abscess. Residual barium in the colon and distal ileum demonstrates a mass displacing the cecum and terminal ileum **(arrows).**

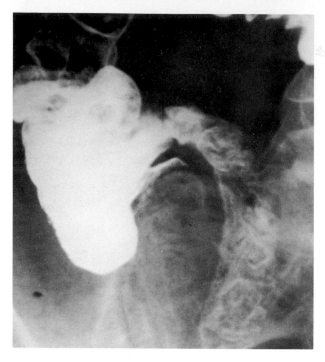

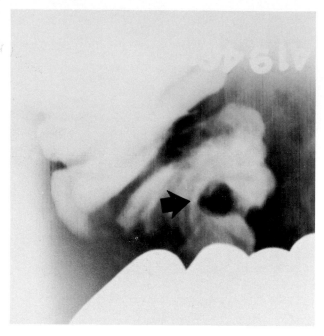

Fig. 19-41. Mucocele of the appendix. There is a thin shell of calcification partially outlining the mass which displaces the ileum medially and causes an indentation on the cecum medially.

Fig. 19-42. Appendiceal stump defect. The **arrow** indicates the site of an inverted appendiceal stump projecting into the base of the cecum.

is known that this tumor may develop in any part of the gastrointestinal tract. It is generally accepted that carcinoids arise from the silver-staining cells known as Kultschitzky's cells that are found in the crypts of Lieberkühn. Because of silver-staining properties the tumor also is known as an *argentaffin tumor* or *argentaffinoma*. Carcinoids, particularly those arising other than in the appendix, in addtion to being locally invasive, may metastasize. Carcinoids of the appendix are more likely to be single lesions and they show less tendency to metastasize than do carcinoids arising elsewhere in the gastrointestinal tract. In the small intestine, invasion of the wall and infiltration of the tumor into the mesentery leads to fibrosis, angulation of the loop, and an adherence of peritoneal surfaces. The combination of sharp angulation and a filling defect is an important roentgen sign of carcinoid of the small intestine. In the appendix, the roentgen diagnosis is hardly possible. The tumors often are small and situated in the tip of the appendix. Only in the event that the lesion invades contiguous structures, particularly the mesentery and ileum or cecal tip, is it likely to produce any roentgen signs. (Also see Ch. 18.)

Appendiceal Stump Defect

After appendectomy, invagination of the appendiceal stump may produce a filling defect in a tip of the cecum, which may resemble a polyp very closely (Fig. 19-42). The history of previous appendectomy and the location of the defect are important aids in establishing its nature.

OTHER CONDITIONS

Rarely *Crohn's disease* may be limited to the appendix when first observed. Roentgen findings in the few reported cases are those of a cecal deformity and a mass resembling and erroneously thought to be an appendiceal abscess.[67]

Intussusception of the appendix may be small and incomplete, involving only the appendix. At times, the entire appendix is intussuscepted (inverted) and appears as an elongated cecal mass. This is the most common type. In other patients, the inverted or intussuscepted appendix acts as the leading mass for a colonic intussusception. Appearance is similar to that of colonic intussusception due to other lesions.

REFERENCES AND SELECTED READINGS

1. BARTLETT JG, CHANG TW, GURWITH M: Antibiotic-associated pseudomembranous colitis due to toxin-producing clostridia. N Engl J Med 298: 531, 1978

2. BAUM S, ATHANASOULIS CA, WALTMAN AC: Angiodysplasia of the right colon: a cause of gastrointestinal bleeding. Am J Roentgenol 129: 789, 1977

3. BERDON WE, BAKER DH, SANTULLI TV, et al: The radiologic evaluation of imperforate anus. Radiology 90: 466, 1968

4. BERDON WE, BAKER DH, SANTULLI TV, et al: Microcolon in newborn infants with intestinal obstruction. Radiology 90: 878, 1968

5. BRAHME F: Granulomatous colitis. Roentgenologic appearance and course of the lesions. Am J Roentgenol 99: 35, 1967

6. BRAHME F, HILDELL J: Angiography in Crohn's disease revisited. Am J Roentgenol 126: 941, 1976

7. CAPITANIO MA, KIRKPATRICK JA: Lymphoid hyperplasia of the colon in children: roentgen observations. Radiology 94: 323, 1970

8. CASARELLA WJ, KANTER IE, SEAMAN WB: Right-sided colonic divertiula as a cause of acute rectal hemorrhage. N Engl J Med 286: 450, 1972

9. CASTLEMAN B, KRICHSTEIN HI: Do adenomatous polyps of colon become malignant? N Engl J Med 267: 469, 1962

10. CREMIN BJ, GOLDING RL: Congenital aganglionosis of the entire colon in neonates. Br J Radol 49: 27, 1976

11. DAVIS WS, ALLEN RP, FAVARA BE et al: Neonatal small left colon syndrome. Am J Roentgenol 120: 322, 1974

12. DUNBAR JD, NELSON SW: Nonangiographic manifestations of intestinal vascular disease. Am J Roentgenol 99: 127, 1967

13. EDLING NPG, EKLOF O: The retro-rectal soft-tissue space in ulcerative colitis. Radiology 80: 949, 1963

14. EKELUND G: On cancer and polyps of colon and rectum. Acta Pathol Microbiol Scand [A] 59: 165, 1963

15. FARMAN J: Vascular lesions of the colon. Br J Radiol 39: 575, 1966

16. FELSON B, WIOT JF: Some interesting right lower quadrant entities. Radiol Clin North Am 7: 83, 1969

17. FERRUCCI JT JR, RAGSDALE BD, BARRETT PJ et al: Double tracking in the sigmoid colon. Radiology 120: 307, 1976

18. FISHER JK, GERMANN DR: Glucagon-aided reduction of intussusception. Radiology 122: 197, 1977

19. FLEISCHNER FG, BERENBERG AL: Recurrent carcinoma of the colon at the site of the anastomosis. Roentgen observations. Radiology 66: 540, 1956

20. FLEISCHNER FG, BERNSTEIN C: Roentgen-anatomical studies of the normal ileocecal valve. Radiology 54: 43, 1950

21. FRANK DF, BERK RN, GOLDSTEIN HM: Pseudo-ulcerations of the colon on barium enema examinations. Gastrointest Radiol 2: 129, 1977

22. FRANKEN EA JR: Lymphoid hyperplasia of the colon. Radiology 94: 329, 1970

23. FRYE TA: Villous adenomas of the sigmoid colon. Radiology 73: 71, 1959

24. GIRDANY BR, BASS LR, SIEBER WK: Roentgenologic aspects of hydrostatic reduction of ileocolic intussusception. Am J Roentgenol 82: 455,1959

25. GOLDSTEIN SJ, CROOKS DJM: Colitis in Behcet's syndrome. Radiology 128: 321, 1978

26. GREENBAUM EI, FREEDMAN S: Neoplasia of the colon over a long segment. Clin Radiol 24: 416, 1973

27. HAMELIN L, HURTUBISE M: Remote control technique in double contrast study of the colon. Am J Roentgenol 119: 382, 1973

28. HAWS CC, LONG RF, CAPLAN GE: Histoplasma capsulatum as a cause of ileocolitis. Am J Roentgenol 128: 692, 1977

29. HEILBRUN N, BERNSTEIN C: Roentgen abnormalities of the large and small intestine associated with prolonged cathartic ingestion. Radiology 65: 549, 1955

30. HILL MC, GOLDBERG HI: Roentgen diagnosis of intestinal amebiasis. Am J Roentgenol 99: 77, 1967

31. HODGSON JR, SAUER WG: The roentgenologic features of carcinoma in chronic ulcerative colitis. Am J Roentgenol 86: 91, 1961

32. HOPE JW, BORNS PF, BERG PK: Roentgenologic manifestations of Hirschsprung's disease in infancy. Am J Roentgenol 95: 217, 1965

33. JOHNS ER, HARTLEY MG: Giant gas-filled cysts of the sigmoid colon: a report of 2 cases. Br J Radiol 49: 930, 1976

34. JONES EL, CORNELL WP: Gardner's syndrome. Review of the literature and report on a family. Arch Surg 92: 287, 1966

35. KAYE JJ, BRAGG DE: Unusual roentgenologic and clinicopathologic features of villous adenomas of the colon. Radiology 91: 799, 1968

36. KERRY RL, RANSOM HK: Volvulus of the colon. Etiology, diagnosis and treatment. Arch Surg 99: 215, 1969

37. KIRSH D, DROSD RE: Roentgen changes in diseases of the appendices epiploicae. Am J Roentgenol 81: 640 1959

38. KOTTRA JJ, DODDS WJ: Duplication of the large bowel. Am J Roentgenol 113: 310, 1971

39. KURLANDER GJ: Roentgenology of imperforate anus. Am J Roentgenol 100: 190, 1967

40. LAUFER I, DeSA D: Lymphoid follicular pattern: a normal feature of the pediatric colon. Am J Roentgenol 130: 51, 1978

41. LAUFER I, MULLENS JE, HAMILTON J: Correlation of endoscopy and double-contrast radiography in the early

stages of ulcerative and granulomatous colitis. Radiology 118: 1, 1976

42. LILJA B, PROBST F: Intestinal endometriosis. Acta Radiol [Diagn] (Stockh); 4: 545, 1966

43. LUTZGER LG, FACTOR SM: Effects of some water-soluble contrast media on the colonic mucosa. Radiology 118: 545, 1976

44. MARGULIS AR: Examination of the colon. In Margulis AR, Burhenne HJ (eds): Alimentary Tract Roentgenology. St. Louis, CV Mosby, 1973

45. MARGULIS AR, GOLDBERG HI, LAWSON TL et al: The overlapping spectrum of ulcerative and granulomatous colitis: a roentgenographic-pathologic study. Am J Roentgenol 113: 325, 1971

46. MARGULIS AR, JOVANOVICH A: Roentgen diagnosis of submucous lipomas of colon. Am J Roentgenol 84: 1114, 1960

47. MARSHAK RH, LINDNER AE: Ulcerative and granulomatous colitis. In Margulis AR, Burhenne HJ (eds): Alimentary Tract Roentgenology, p 742, St. Louis, CV Mosby, 1973

48. MARSHAK RH, MOSELEY JE, WOLF BS: The roentgen findings in familial polyposis with special emphasis on differential diagnosis. Radiology 80: 374, 1963

49. MEYERS MA, OLIPHANT M: Ascending retrocecal appendicitis. Radiology 110: 295, 1974

50. MIKITY VG, HODGMAN JE, PACINILLI J: Meconium blockage syndrome. Radiology 88: 740, 1967

51. MOERTEL CG, DOCKERTY MB, JUDD ES: Carcinoid tumors of the vermiform appendix. Cancer 21: 270, 1968

52. O'CONNELL TX, KADELL D, TOMPKINS RK: Ischemia of the colon. Surg Gynecol Obstet 142: 337, 1976

53. OESTREICH AE: Colon agenesis. Semin Roentgenol 9: 167, 1974

54. PARKS TG, CONNELL AM, GOUGH AD, et al: Limitations of radiology in the differentiation of diverticulitis and diverticulosis. Br Med J 2: 136, 1970

55. PARSONS CD, THOMAS MH, GARRETT RA: Colonic adenocarcinoma: a delayed complication of ureterosigmoidostomy. J Urol 118: 31, 1977

56. POCHACZEVSKY R, LEONIDAS JC: The meconium plug syndrome. Am J Roentgenol 120: 342, 1974

57. POCHACZEVSKY R, SHERMAN RS: Diffuse lymphomatous disease of the colon: its roentgen appearance. Am J Roentgenol 87: 670, 1962

58. POTTER RM: Dilute contrast media in diagnosis of lesions of the colon. Radiology 60: 500, 1953

59. REEDER MM, HAMILTON LC: Tropical diseases of the colon. Semin Roentgenol 3: 62, 1968

60. REEVES BF, CARLSON HC, DOCKERTY MB: Segmental ulcerative colitus versus segmental Crohn's disease. Am J Roentgenol 99: 24, 1967

61. RICHMOND JA, MIKITY V: Benign form of necrotizing enterocolitis. Am J Roentgenol 123: 301, 1975

62. SAMUEL E: Gastrointestinal manifestations of vascular disease. Proc R Soc Med 60: 839, 1967

63. SEAMAN WB: Unusual roentgen manifestations of large bowel cancer. Semin Roentgenol 11: 89, 1976

64. SPRAYREGEN S, BOLEY SJ: Vascular ectasias of the right colon. JAMA 239: 962, 1978

65. STEINBACH HL, ROSENBERG RH, GROSSMAN M, et al: The potential hazard of enemas in patients with Hirschsprung's disease. Radiology 64: 45, 1955

66. SWISCHUK LE: Meconium plug syndrome: a cause of neonatal obstruction. Am J Roentgenol 103: 339, 1968

67. THREATT B, APPELMAN H: Crohn's disease of the appendix presenting as acute appendicitis. Radiology 110: 313, 1974

68. TONKIN ILD, BJELLAND JC, HUNTER TB et al: Spontaneous resolution of colonic strictures caused by necrotizing enterocolitis: therapeutic implications. Am J Roentgenol 130: 1077, 1978

69. WEBER H, DIXON CF: Duplication of the entire large intestine (colon duplex). Am J Roentgenol 55: 319, 1946

70. WELIN S, YOUKER J, SPRATT JS: The rates and patterns of growth of 375 tumors of the large intestine and rectum observed serially by double contrast enema study (Malmö technique). Am J Roentgenol 90: 673, 1963

71. WICHULIS AR, BEAHRS OH, WOOLNER LB: Malignant lymphoma of the colon. A study of 69 cases. Arch Surg 93: 215, 1966

72. WILLIAMS I: Innominate grooves in the surface of mucosa. Radiology 84: 877, 1965

73. WOLF BS, MARSHAK RH: "Toxic" segmental dilatation of the colon during the course of fulminating ulcerative colitis: roentgen findings. Am J Roentgenol 82: 985, 1959

74. WOLFSON JJ, GOLDSTEIN G, KRIVIT W, et al: Lymphoid hyperplasia of the large intestine associated with dysgammaglobulinemia. Am J Roentgenol 108: 610, 1970

75. WOOD BP, KATZBERG RW: Tween 80 diatrizoate enemas in bowel obstruction. Am J Roentgenol 130: 747, 1978

76. WRIGHT LT, FREEMAN WA, BOLDEN JV: Lymphogranulomatous strictures of the rectum: a résumé of four hundred and seventy-six cases. Arch Surg 53: 499, 1946

77. YOUNG BR, SCANLAN RL: Roentgen demonstration and significance of the pedicle in polypoid tumors of the alimentary tract. Am J Roentgenol 68: 894, 1952

SECTION IV

THE URINARY AND FEMALE GENITAL TRACTS

20

THE URINARY TRACT

METHODS OF EXAMINATION

THE PLAIN-FILM ROENTGENOGRAM

Roentgen examination of the urinary tract should begin with a plain film of the abdomen exposed with the patient in a supine position. This roentgenogram includes the kidneys and the ureteral and bladder areas, and is commonly termed a KUB or scout film. If the patient is tall, an extra roentgenogram of the bladder is necessary. It is essential that the plain film be obtained before contrast medium is given for the excretory urogram. In this plain-film examination the renal shadows can be seen and their size, shape, and position noted. The presence of calcium in cysts, tumors, or stones can be detected along with vascular or lymph-node calcification in the area. Psoas muscle shadows are usually well outlined and asymmetry or other abnormalities can be noted. The ureters cannot be defined but radiopaque calculi may be detected along the course of the ureter. The shadow cast by the urinary bladder can often be identified. Vesical calculi can be outlined. Vascular calcifications, including phleboliths and arterial plaques, are frequently seen in the pelvis and must be differentiated from urinary calculi. This often requires special examinations. These conditions are discussed more fully in Chapter 13.

EXCRETORY UROGRAPHY

Preparation of the Patient

Excretory or intravenous urography is a relatively simple method of outlining the excretory system and is used widely for detection of disease involving it. Preparation for the examination consists of castor oil catharsis the evening before the study. Other cathartics used commonly are a senna preparation (X-Prep: Gray Pharmaceutical) and bisacodyl (Dulcolax: Boehringer–Ingelheim, Ltd.). Catharsis is usually necessary in bedridden patients who are hospitalized, to remove gas and fecal matter from the colon, since these tend to obscure the renal areas. In ambulatory patients, gas and feces are not as much of a problem. Mild dehydration is obtained by omitting fluids for the last 2 or 3 hours before the examination, and the meal before the examination also is omitted. Many variations of the method just described are in use and satisfactory urography often can be obtained with no preparation, particularly in ambulatory out-patients. Dehydration is not necessary for this examination, but it is well to omit fluids for the last hour or two before the study in order to prevent overhydration. Because there are situations in which dehydration is clearly contraindicated such as in patients having multiple myeloma or renal failure, those critically ill including neonates, the preparation is altered to fit the needs of each patient.

In infants and small children a carbonated beverage can be given to distend the stomach with gas. This displaces the bowel enough to allow visualization of the renal shadows through the gas-filled stomach. However, this method is not often used since we have found that it may make visualization worse rather than better.

Contrast Media

The contrast media are organic iodides which depend on their iodine content for radiopacity.[79] Those generally used in intravenous urography include the following:

1. Conray 60 (meglumine iothalamate) provides 28.2% iodine
2. Conray 400 (sodium iothalamate) 66.8%, 40% iodine
3. Hypaque 50 (sodium diatrizoate) 30% iodine
4. Hypaque M60 (meglumine diatrizoate) 28.2% iodine
5. Hypaque M90 (meglumine 60%, sodium 30% diatrizoate) 46.2% iodine
6. Hypaque 25 (sodium diatrizoate) 15% iodine (300 ml for infusion urography)
7. Renografin 60 (meglumine 52% sodium 8% diatrizoate) 28.8% iodine
8. Reno-M-60 (meglumine diatrizoate) 28.2% iodine
9. Reno-M-DIP (meglumine diatrizoate) 14.1% iodine (300 ml for infusion urography)
10. Renovist II (sodium and meglumine diatrizoate) 31% iodine
11. Isopaque 280 (meglumine and calcium metrizoate) 28% iodine
    The iodine is not free in these compounds and is excreted still bound to the molecule of contrast agent.

Because new contrast media are introduced at frequent intervals, the foregoing list very likely will be altered within the next few years. At the present time we are using Renovist II in "high" doses, 0.5 ml per pound body weight and find it a very satisfactory medium. Some institutions use somewhat higher doses than this. Our method delivers 0.34 mg of iodine per kilogram of body weight. In our hands, it is a satisfactory dose for patients with reasonably good renal function. These contrast media are excreted almost entirely by glomerular filtration with very little or no tubular resorption. When there is mild dehydration, there is more tubular resorption of fluid and therefore greater concentration of iodide in the urine producing better visualization of the collecting system. In children, high-dose urography is also used commonly. The dose ranges are as follows:[6] premature infants—no more than 4 ml/kg body weight; newborn full-term—10 ml; 1–6 months—12–15 ml; 6–24 months—15–25 ml; 2–5 years—25–30 ml; 5–10 years—30–45 ml.

Contraindications to intravenous urography are: (1) hypersensitivity to the contrast agent, (2) the presence of combined renal and hepatic disease, (3) oliguria, (4) a serum creatinine level over 7 mg/100 ml, and (5) multiple myeloma (unless the patient can be kept well hydrated during and after the study). All of these contraindications are relative and the value of potential information to be obtained must be weighed against the risk in each patient.

The contrast media are injected intravenously and are all organic iodides, which are filtered rapidly by the glomeruli. They may all produce reactions of varying severity so that certain precautions should be taken before their use. Sensitivity tests are not reliable and are not in general use since they have no predictive value regarding reactions to the contrast media. The most common symptoms are flushing, arm pain, nausea, vomiting, urticaria, asthma, allergic rhinitis, and other allergic manifestations. More severe reactions with such cardiovascular manifestations as pulmonary edema, hypotension, and cardiac arrest are life-threatening and must be treated promptly. Respiratory arrest or obstruction and central nervous system reactions, such as toxic convulsions and coma, may also occur. The radiologist should have a plan for response to a serious reaction and the equipment and medication to manage severe reactions should be immediately available whenever contrast media are injected. If a major reaction appears to be developing, treatment should begin at once, and a call for skilled help should be placed. Maintenance of an adequate airway is essential; oxygen should be given in all major reactions. Tables 20-1 and 20-2 indicate the various types of reaction and the method of treatment as well as list the representative drugs and their dosages.

In a nationwide survey[43] covering 3.8 million urograms, a death rate of 19 per million was found. This figure may be low, however.

The prophylactic use of drugs has been studied and discussed for many years. Some authors advise the prophylactic use of antihistamines in patients with a history of allergy, although there is no solid evidence to indicate that it has a definite value. Hypotension and bradycardia following the use of intravenous contrast agents appears to be a vasovagal reaction[3] that can be reversed promptly by administration of atropine intravenously, starting with 0.6 to 0.8 mg and increasing the dose until the desired therapeutic effect is observed. This has led to the suggestion by some that atropine might be used prophylactically in a dose of 0.5 mg given intravenously immediately before the contrast agent is injected.[116] There is also evidence to show that diazepam (Valium) is helpful in reducing the incidence of reactions by inhibiting reflex vagal bradycardia. In patients with asthma or hay fever, prednisone in 30- to 50-mg doses for 3 days before the examination may be useful. The presence of a nephrogram on a 10-minute film without opacification of collecting structures or ureters suggests systemic hypotension and may be an early sign of a vasovagal type of reaction to a contrast medium.[106]

Advanced Renal Failure. If factors such as cardiac failure and other causes of hypoperfusion such as hypovolemia from a variety of causes can be excluded, excretory urography is of value in the study of renal failure. Most authors advocate very high-dosage urography—doses approximating 600 mg I/kg body weight, which is twice the dose that we use in patients without failure. Dehydration should be avoided, and catharsis is usually contraindicated. The methylglucamine salts may be used on patients in whom sodium is restricted. When serum creatinine levels are up to 6 or 7 mg/100 ml, information of diagnostic importance can usually be obtained. At times, there is enough opacification to evaluate renal size and cortical thickness in patients with serum creatinine levels above 6 to 7 mg/100 ml. If necessary, the contrast medium can be removed by dialysis. The consensus seems to be that there is no particular advantage in *drip infusion urography* in these patients, but some prefer to use it. In this method, the contrast material is relatively dilute and is supplied in 300-ml bottles for drip infusion. It is a convenient method of delivering a large volume of contrast medium. In patients with renal failure, it is often necessary to obtain urograms over a period of time up to 24 hours. Tomography is used routinely in this group of patients. Ultrasound may provide similar information and should be considered before urography in patients with severe renal failure.

High-dosage urography makes total body opacification possible in infants. In premature and newborn infants, relatively larger doses of contrast medium are required; up to 4 ml (300 mg I/ml) per kilogram of body weight causes opacification of all vascular structures in these infants. It is therefore used in differential diagnosis of abdominal masses, both intra- and extrarenal.

Technique of Examination

Following intravenous injection of the contrast substance it is desirable to use some method to compress the ureters and thereby hold the material in the kidneys in order to outline the pelvis and calyces. A number of devices are available for this purpose. We have found that a compression band, under which a blood pressure cuff has been placed, is a useful device. When a pressure of 90 to 100 mm Hg is used the ureters are obstructed sufficiently to produce satisfactory filling. The band is placed just above the symphysis pubis so that the ureters are partially compressed as they pass over the pelvic brim. This method is simple and effective but there are other methods of compression that may be used and a variety of special divided compression devices are available. The Trendelenburg position is of some use when the patient cannot tolerate a compression device. Compression is not necessary in patients with obstruction and is inadvisable when the examination is being made because of a suspected ureteral calculus. When the examination is performed as a functional study it is also inadvisable to use compression. In patients with hypertension of suspected renal origin the early films are exposed without compression. Then compression may be applied, after a 5- to 10-minute film has been obtained, to produce complete filling for anatomic study. In patients with suspected aortic aneurysms or similar masses the use of compression is unwise.

The first roentgenogram is obtained approximately 5 minutes after injection and a second is obtained at 15 minutes. The compression band then is released and a third roentgenogram is secured. The voltage range (between 70 to 75 kVp) is important. We use tomography on most patients, usually between 1 and 5 minutes after injection of a bolus of contrast medium. A minimum of three tomographic cuts are obtained at one-centimeter intervals. Then additional

Table 20-1. Specific Treatment for Major Reactions to Contrast Media*

TYPE	DRUG	AVG. ADULT DOSE	COMMENTS
Cardiac and pulmonary arrest	See table of drug dosages		
Hypotension	Neosynephrine I.V. drip	10 mg in 500-cc I.V. solution	Oxygen
	Aramine I.V. drip	5 cc in 500-cc saline (50 mg)	Titrate to pt.'s usual BP with I.V. drip
	Levophed I.D.	Ampule in 500 cc normal saline or 5% dextrose in water	Trendelenberg position
Hypotension—vasovagal	Atropine I.V. if indicated	0.5–1 mg I.V. Repeat if indicated	Often transient and does not require drug. Vasopressors not recommended
Bronchospasm	Adrenaline S.C.	0.1–2 0.3 cc 1:1000 aqueous	
	Adrenaline I.V.	0.1–0.3 cc 1:1000 aqueous	Oxygen
	Aminophylline I.V.	10 cc in 10 min (250 mg)	Give I.V. slowly
	Solu-Cortef I.V.	2.0 cc (100 mg)	Give aminophylline slowly
Toxic convulsions	Nembutal I.V.	0.5 cc q. 2 min (25 mg)	Oxygen
	Valium I.V.	5 mg	May require Solu-Cortef 2.0 cc (200 mg) IV
	Solu-Cortef I.V.	100 mg	
Pulmonary edema	Oxygen		
	Morphine I.V. or	10 mg	Elevate upper torso
	Demerol I.V.	1.0 cc (50 mg)	Venous compression of extremities by rotation tourniquet
	Solu-Cortef I.V.	2.0 cc (100 mg)	
Laryngeal edema	Adrenaline I.V.	0.3	Oxygen
		0.1 cc 1:1000 aqueous	Endotracheal intubation
	Solu-Cortef I.V.	2.0 cc (100 mg)	May require tracheostomy
Hypertensive crisis due to pheochromocytoma	Regitine I.V.	1.0 cc (5 mg)	May require additional doses

* This table outlines treatment for major reactions to contrast media. Modified after Weigen and Thomas. (William B. Seaman, Chairman, Committee on Drugs, and American College of Radiology. Committee Report: Prevention and Management of Adverse Reaction to Intravascular Contrast Media, July, 1977)

tomograms are obtained as needed. Each film is monitored as the examination progresses. Then alterations in the procedure are made when indicated. Additional exposures of the bladder area may be necessary in some instances. We obtain a post-voiding film of the bladder in patients over 40 years of age, and in all those with incontinence. Oblique films are of value in patients with suspected ureteral calculi and in those in whom questionable calyceal abnormalities are observed on the anteroposterior films. When it is important to visualize the ureters, a film with the patient in the prone position is useful, since the ureters fill better in the prone than in the supine position. In some institutions, one roentgenogram in the prone position is obtained routinely; others obtain an upright film routinely. It is important to inspect each film to determine what additional films are needed. Fluoroscopy is sometimes useful to determine renal motion and study ureteral function. If excretion of contrast material is delayed it may be necessary to obtain roentgenograms for periods up to

several hours after injection. In patients with acute ureteral obstruction, such as is frequently present when a ureteral calculus is being passed, there is often a delay in excretion on the involved side. Delayed roentgenograms may show opacification of the renal pelvis and ureter down to the level of obstruction when the immediate roentgenograms will reveal only increased density of the renal parenchyma. Delayed roentgenograms are of value whenever there is delay in excretion. In patients with renal failure, preliminary tomograms are necessary as a baseline with which to compare the faint opacification of renal parenchyma and/or calyces and pelves, which appears after the contrast medium is injected. A number of variations of this technique are used. Most important is close monitoring of all films so that adequate visualization of the urinary tract is obtained in each patient. Special methods are used in patients with hypertension of possible renovascular origin. These are described in the section "Renovascular Hypertension" in this chapter.

Table 20-2. Adult Drug Dosages Used in Treating Severe Reactions

DRUG	ROUTE	USUAL DOSE	INDICATION	COMMENTS
Adrenaline 1:1000	S.C.	0.1–0.3 cc	Allergic reactions, asthma, etc.	Acts rapidly. Give stat
Adrenaline 1:1000	I.V.	0.2–0.5 cc q.s. 10 cc	Asystole in cardiac arrest	Improves cardiac tone. May induce vent.
	I.C.	physiol. saline		fib. or change "fine" fib. to "coarse" fibrillation
Aminophylline 3¾ gr	I.V.	250 mg in 10 cc	Bronchospasm, cardiac asthma, pul. edema	Inject 10 cc in 10 min slowly! Vasodilation. May cause hypotension
Aramine 1%	I.M.	0.2–1.0 cc	Hypotension	Rapid but brief action.
	I.V.	0.1–0.5 cc	Profound collapse	Titrate pt. to usual BP
Atropine SO$_4$ 0.6 mg/cc	I.V.	1.0 cc	Bradycardia, hypotension	Decreases vagal inhibition
Benadryl 1% (10 mg/cc)	I.V.	3.0–5.0 cc	Allergic reactions	I.V. antihistamines might cause drowsiness
Calcium chloride 10%	I.C.	5.0 cc	Asystole in cardiac arrest	Cardiotonic action similar to that of adrenalin
Demerol 5% (50 mg/cc)	I.V.	2.0 cc	Pulmonary edema, cardiac asthma	Good analgesic and sedative
Lasix	I.V. I.M.	20 mg in 2.0 cc	Pulmonary edema, cerebral edema	Slow injection. Separate syringe. Rapid diuresis
Nembutal 5% (50 mg/cc)	I.V.	2.0 cc	Toxic convulsions	Inject slowly. May cause respiratory depression
Regitine	I.V.	5.0 mg	Hypertensive crisis due to pheochromocytoma	Control by BP
Sodium bicarbonate 3.75 gm/50 cc	I.V.	50–150 cc	Acidosis in cardiac arrest	Give by slow injection as early as possible. Use freely
Solu-Cortef	I.V.	100–200 mg	Allergic reactions, status asthmaticus, profound collapse	Dose can be repeated
Papaverine	I.A.	40 mg in 1.0 cc	Arterial spasm	Dilute to 20 cc with physiol. saline
Xylocaine 1% (10 mg/cc)	I.V.	5.0–10 cc	Most cardiac arrhythmias, vent. fib.	Makes heart more responsive to defibrillation

(Courtesy William B. Seaman, Chairman, Committee on Drugs, American College of Radiology. Committee Report: Prevention and Management of Adverse Reaction to Intravascular Contrast Media, July, 1977)

RETROGRADE UROGRAPHY

Retrograde urography is another method used in the examination of the upper urinary tract. It is generally used to confirm findings suspected on intravenous urography and can also be used when the excretory urogram has been unsatisfactory or inconclusive. Cystoscopy and catheterization of the ureters is necessary for this examination. Roentgenograms are obtained following direct instillation of contrast mate-

rial into the pelves via the catheters. Media available for intravenous use diluted to 20% or 30% are satisfactory for retrograde pyelography. Occasionally air is used as a contrast substance, particularly when a radiolucent calculus is suspected and is not visible on excretory urography or on retrograde study using an opaque medium. Roentgenograms are obtained after 3 to 5 ml of a contrast medium are slowly introduced through ureteral catheter into the renal pelvis. The catheters are withdrawn and another roentgenogram is secured. Oblique views and delayed frontal views may also be necessary in some patients. The contrast medium may be injected by syringe or may be introduced by gravity with a vessel containing the medium no higher than 45 cm above renal level. Care should be taken to avoid overdistending the collecting system since the high pressure may produce backflow into tubules, interstitium, lymphatics, or (?) veins. The chief advantage of retrograde pyelography is that a dense contrast substance can be injected directly under controlled pressure so that visualization is good. The extent of impairment of renal function that may be present does not influence the degree of visualization. Excretory urography is a simpler and easier procedure because cystoscopy is not necessary. This is particularly important in children and it also has advantages in patients with renal injury or with anomalies such as duplication of the ureters. The excretory method also serves as a test of renal function, particularly of comparative function of the two kidneys. Its chief disadvantage is that visualization may be incomplete owing to failure of filling of portions of the excretory system. With the newer

contrast media and compression, excretory films of a quality comparable to retrograde studies can be obtained in many patients, eliminating the need for ureteral catheterization.

RENAL ANGIOGRAPHY

There are several methods for the radiographic study of the renal arteries. The use of a catheter, introduced percutaneously into the femoral artery by the Seldinger technique or by direct arterial cut-down of the femoral or ulnar artery, permits more variability in techniques than does the translumbar method. A midstream aortic injection is made first using 40 to 60 ml of one of the organic iodides mentioned earlier. This survey examination indicates location and number of renal arteries and may define abnormal lumbar vessels in patients with metastatic tumor (Fig. 20-1A). Then selective renal arteriograms are obtained by manipulation of the catheter tip under fluoroscopic control into the desired renal artery followed by injection of small amounts (10 to 15 ml of the opaque medium) into the artery. This has the advantage of

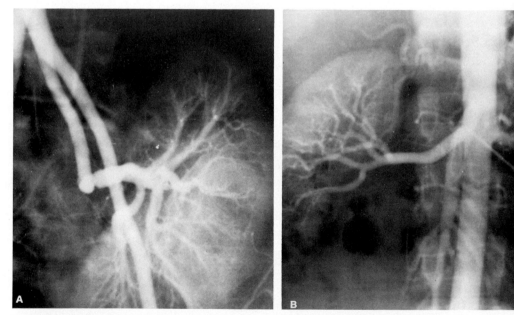

Fig. 20-1. A. Angiogram in the study of renal transplant. The percutaneous catheter technique was used to demonstrate the renal artery which is anastomosed to the internal iliac artery. **B.** Translumbar aortogram of a normal person. The needle tip is near the orifice of the right renal artery which is well filled and clearly defined. There is some filling of the left renal, the splenic, hepatic, and the superior mesenteric arteries as well as the aorta.

dense opacification of the renal artery and its branches that is needed in a detailed study of the vessels. The main disadvantages are that a small accessory vessel may be missed and multiple injections are required when multiple vessels are present. Simultaneous study of both renal arteries can be performed by placing the catheter equipped with multiple side holes at the proper level in the aorta (midstream aortic injection). Injection of 30 to 40 cc of 90% Hypaque or a similar medium usually results in satisfactory filling of both renal arteries. This method has the advantage of filling accessory arteries that may be present, as well as affording simultaneous visualization allowing comparison of the renal vessels on the normal and abnormal sides. Rapid film changers are used, programmed to radiograph arterial, nephrographic, and venous phases of the examination. Magnification techniques may be used to study vascular detail in one or both kidneys. Subtraction is also used on occasion for better visualization of vessels in renal disease. Epinephrine may be employed to improve accuracy in the diagnosis of renal masses.[15] As a rule, normal vessels constrict while tumor vessels do not, making their identification easier. "Inflammatory neovascularity" tends to constrict slightly.

TRANSLUMBAR AORTOGRAPHY

This examination has been largely supplanted by the Seldinger technique of percutaneous transfemoral catheterization which permits aortography and selective renal arteriography at the same time. The translumbar approach is used only in patients with advanced arteriosclerotic disease when catheterization is hazardous or impossible. A long needle is inserted directly into the abdominal aorta from a point just below the twelfth rib on the left. After making certain that the needle is in the aorta, the contrast medium is injected and roentgenograms are obtained using automatic changers (Fig. 20-1B).

RENAL VENOGRAPHY

Retrograde renal venography is performed by introducing a catheter into the femoral vein with the Seldinger technique, advancing the catheter through the vena cava into the main renal vein to the region of the point of division of segmental veins. The retrograde injection of contrast medium is not very effective because of the strong pressure of venous flow; because of this, epinephrine has been used in doses of 14 to 16 µg injected into the renal artery over a period of 40 seconds followed immediately by injection of an organic iodide, such as Renografin 76, into the vein. Amounts in the neighborhood of 30 ml are given over 2 to 3 seconds. This results in considerable improvement over simple retrograde venography. Others have tried balloon occlusion of the renal artery to temporarily halt the arterial flow to the kidney during the few seconds it takes to obtain the venogram. Filming sequence varies with individuals, but is approximately two films per second for 3 seconds following injection of the bolus. The examination is performed after a renal arteriogram has been secured so that the patency of the renal vein can be predetermined. Although they occur infrequently, renal vein valves may cause technical difficulty. The technique is used in assessment of inflammatory disease, in differentiation between congenital absence of a kidney and a small contracted, nonfunctioning kidney, in suspected renal-vein thrombosis, and in detection of avascular tumors. In other words, it is used in an attempt to make a definitive diagnosis when angiography has failed to do so.

NEPHROTOMOGRAPHY

The term "nephrotomography" was introduced in 1954 by John A. Evans and his colleagues to define a method of radiographic examination that has since been used extensively in the study of the kidneys. The basic technique consists of intravenous injection of a large amount of one of the iodinated contrast agents (50 ml or more) given in a bolus. Tomograms are then obtained at suitable intervals to secure visualization of the arterial supply of the kidneys (arterial phase). This is followed by a nephrogram phase during which tomograms are obtained at predetermined levels. The nephrogram phase is relatively easy to obtain; timing is more critical for the arterial phase. We no longer study the arterial phase in nephrotomography, preferring to use selective renal arteriography for this purpose. Excretory tomograms can then be secured in projections and levels needed to solve the problem at hand.

For an intravenous drip method described by Bosniak,[14] 150 ml Hypaque M 90% mixed with 50 ml glucose and water (125 ml contrast agent if the patient weighs less than 100 pounds) are used. Other media such as Hypaque M 75% (180 ml) and Renografin 76 (190 ml) have been employed with equally good results. The first 100 ml are given as fast as possible (in about 5 minutes), then the flow is slowed to about one-half and the tomograms are obtained. Scout tomograms are secured before the study starts to obtain optimum technique and levels. A range of 70 to 75 kVp and a tomographic arc of 25 to 30 degrees are used. At least five cuts at 1-cm intervals are obtained in both anteroposterior and oblique projections during the infusion of the last half of the contrast substance. Additional films may be exposed if necessary. Nephrotomography is used extensively as an adjunct to intravenous urography whenever a questionable defect or shadow is observed. Nephrotomography as an adjunct to excretory urography, or as part of the study, is being used by increasing numbers of radiologists since this method aids in determining the presence of renal masses, particularly in the detection of small masses that may represent early curable malignant disease. It also aids in the definition of the renal outline which may not be clearly visible on static films. Examples of the use of this technique are cited in the section of this chapter entitled "Simple Cysts."

PERCUTANEOUS ANTEGRADE PYELOGRAPHY (PERCUTANEOUS TRANSLUMBAR NEPHROSTOMY OR PYELOGRAPHY)

This examination consists of the placement of a needle or catheter (percutaneous nephrostomy) in the renal pelvis.[114] A posterolateral approach is used and the needle is inserted under fluoroscopic observation; in some institutions, ultrasound guidance is used alone or in combination with fluoroscopy. In addition to using percutaneous nephrostomy for diagnosis, a catheter may be placed for temporary drainage and, in some instances in which all surgical procedures are contraindicated, increasingly larger tubes may be positioned for longer-term drainage. The indications for such procedures include (1) short-term palliation in terminal disease; (2) as a temporizing measure prior to definitive diversion; and (3) to relieve obstruction when immediate surgery is contraindicated. In addition to the possibility of outlining the collecting system and defining the cause for obstruction, material can be obtained for cytologic and bacteriologic studies, and medication can be introduced through the tube if it is left in place.

VOIDING CYSTOGRAPHY OR CYSTOURETHROGRAPHY

The examination is used largely in the study of patients suspected of having lower urinary tract obstruction or vesicoureteral reflux, and in children with persistent or recurrent urinary tract infection in whom vesicoureteral reflux is a possibility. In essence, the examination consists of filling the bladder with radiopaque material (sodium or meglumine diatrizoate or iothalamate), usually to the point of producing discomfort.

The patient is examined before, during, and after urination. The examination should be performed on unanesthetized patients who have not had recent instrumentation. Bladder filling is checked during this part of the procedure. Fluoroscopy using image intensification is necessary to obtain an adequate examination. In addition, spot films (70- or 90-mm or conventional spot films) are used to record the findings. The fluoroscopy can also be recorded on video tape if desired, since no additional radiation is used. Films are exposed with the patient in the lateral or an extreme posterior oblique position for best visualization of the bladder neck and urethra. If there is vesicoureteral reflux, films are obtained to show the amount of reflux and also the size of the ureters and renal collecting system.

Some radiologists prefer a suprapubic needle puncture of the bladder for voiding cystourethrography in infants and children, believing that it is more physiologic and possibly safer since there is no urethral trauma and there appears to be less chance of infection of the lower urinary tract. This examination is performed with the patient under local anesthesia. A long 21-gauge needle is inserted into a full bladder through a low suprapubic site.[21, 44] Regardless of the method used, urinary vaginal reflux is the rule in girls 3 to 8 years of age, so suprapubic needle aspiration of urine for culture is another advantage of this method. Cinefluorography is not needed and its use entails unnecessarily high radiation exposures. The bladder, ureters, and sometimes renal pelves and calyces (when reflux is present), and urethra are examined during micturition.

CYSTOGRAPHY

Retrograde cystography is another method of studying the bladder. Following voiding, a catheter is inserted and the bladder is filled with opaque material, usually an organic iodide. During routine cystography, a small amount of contrast medium is absorbed from the bladder. If the agent remains in the bladder for a long period of time, there may be enough absorption to produce some opacification of the renal collecting system, so that an excretory urogram may be obtained. Among the indications for this technique are the study of patients with bladder tumors, diverticula, or calculi. Air is sometimes used in amounts of 100 to 200 cc to study the bladder wall.

Double contrast may also be used for the study of the bladder mucosa. One such method is the instillation of Aqueous Dionosil in amounts of 7 to 10 cc followed by air, carbon dioxide, or nitrous oxide, but we prefer to use one of the diatrizoates or iothalamate. Films are exposed with the patient in prone, supine, oblique, and decubitus positions. Filling can be monitored by fluoroscopy using image intensification; additional films may be obtained, depending upon the situation. Ultrasound has largely supplanted this technique.

EXTRAPERITONEAL PNEUMOGRAPHY

Extraperitoneal (retroperitoneal) pneumography can be employed to outline any retroperitoneal tumor or organ, but is used most frequently in the examination of the kidneys and adrenal glands. The presacral area is preferred as the injection site since single puncture can be used for examination of both sides and the risk of embolism is much less than when the lumbar injection site is used. The method is largely of historical interest.

Technique

The patient lies on his right side with knees drawn up. The skin surrounding the tip of the coccyx is prepared and a local anesthetic agent is injected into the skin at a point 1 to 2 cm below the coccyx. Then a spinal needle is inserted and, with the aid of a finger in the rectum, is directed upward along the anterior sacral wall for 3 or 4 cm. A vinyl catheter then may be inserted through the needle and anchored in place. This will allow additional gas to be injected as indicated during the procedure. Oxygen or carbon dioxide may be used as the contrast substance. Carbon dioxide is preferred because of its solubility which avoids the possibility of gas embolism. After checking to see that the needle is not in a vein, 2 or 3 cc of the gas are injected. The gas should flow easily. If not, the needle should be moved slightly. If perineal emphysema appears, the needle should be inserted at least 2 cm farther. Then a total of 500 to 800 cc of oxygen or 750 to 1500 cc of carbon dioxide can be injected at a pressure of 15 to 20 cm H_2O. The side to be examined should be elevated and if both sides are to be examined half of the gas is injected with the patient in the right lateral decubitus position and the other half with the patient in the left lateral decubitus position. Roentgenograms are obtained on completion of injection. Then additional films can be exposed as indicated. Two hours is the optimum time

for visualization of the retroperitoneal abdominal viscera when oxygen is used, but carbon dioxide is absorbed rapidly, so filming must be accomplished quickly after injection. The examination is relatively simple and safe since there are no large vessels in the retrorectal space. It is not an easy examination, however, and should be undertaken only when other methods have failed to determine the cause for the patient's symptoms or signs. With the advent of adrenal venography and CT scanning, there seems to be very little indication for this examination.

ROENTGEN ANATOMY

THE KIDNEY

The normal kidney is a bean-shaped structure that lies on either side of the lower thoracic and upper lumbar spine, usually between the upper border of the eleventh thoracic and the lower border of the third lumbar vertebrae. In the upright position, the kidney descends 2 or 3 cm. The right kidney lies approximately 2 cm lower than the left and both move slightly with respiration and with change in position. Usually the right kidney moves cephalad when the patient rotates from the supine to the prone position, while there is little, if any, change in position of the left kidney. The long axis is directed downward and outward, parallel to the lateral border of the psoas muscle on either side. In the lateral view the axis is directed downward and anteriorly, so that the lower pole is 2 to 3 cm anterior to the upper pole. When the patient is supine, the renal pelvis and proximal ureters lie well posterior to the anterior edge of the vertebral bodies. At L3, the average ureter is three-fourths of a vertebral width from the posterior vertebral margin. It then curves anteriorly to the level of the anterior vertebral border at L4; at L5 it is anterior to the vertebral body about one-fourth of the anteroposterior diameter of this vertebral body.[23] Renal size varies; the average length of the right kidney is from 12 to 12.7 cm while the left is 3 to 5 mm longer with an upper limit of a 1.5 cm variation in length. There is a relation between body height and renal length; as a general rule the kidney length in adults is 3.7 ± 0.37 times the height of the second lumbar vertebra measured on the same film using the posterior margins of the vertebral body. According to Batson and Keats,[8] 97% of normal kidneys are within the range between the height of L1 through L3 and the height of L1 through L4. In children between 1½ and 14 years of age the renal length is equal to the length of the first four lumbar bodies including the three intervening discs + 1 cm. In infants the renal size is relatively greater. In children the normal difference in renal length on the two sides may be up to 1 cm.

There is some variation in renal shape, particularly on the left side. Fetal lobulations may persist on one or both sides, producing rather clearly defined indentations or notches along the lateral aspect of the kidney. The left kidney may be generally triangular in shape with a local bulge or convexity along the left midborder sometimes termed a "dromedary hump." This may be related to the position of the spleen or may be a form of fetal lobulation or both. The kidney is visualized in roentgenograms mainly because of the presence of perirenal fat. The increased radiotransparency of fat gives soft-tissue contrast so that the outline of the kidney stands out from the surrounding soft tissues. The renal outline is better visualized in obese individuals than in thin persons and if there has been much wasting caused by chronic illness or malnutrition, the renal outlines may be very indistinct or completely invisible in roentgenograms of the abdomen. The kidneys lie in a retroperitoneal position. They are contained within the renal capsule and surrounded by perirenal fat which is enclosed within Gerota's (perirenal) fascia. Perirenal hemorrhage, pus, or urine tend to be contained within this fascia and can be recognized as a perirenal soft-tissue mass on plain films.

THE URETERS

The ureters normally course straight downward from the most dependent portion of the pelves to the midsacral region, then turn posterolaterally and course in an arc downward and then inward and anteriorly to enter the trigone of the bladder on either side of the midline. A slight amount of redundancy is common and alteration in size is frequently noted. Therefore, it is necessary to exercise care in making the diagnosis of ureteral stricture, displacement, or dilatation. There are three areas where normal narrowing of the ureter can be observed when it is filled with radiopaque material: the ureteropelvic junction, the ureterovesical junction, and at the bifurcation of the iliac vessels.

THE BLADDER

The normal urinary bladder is transversely oval or round; the inferior aspect normally projects 5 to 10 mm above the symphysis pubis. Its floor parallels the superior aspect of the pubic rami, while its dome is rounded in the male and flat or slightly concave in the female owing to the presence of the uterus above it. The size and shape of the normal bladder vary considerably. The wall of the bladder is smooth as outlined by opaque material used in urography or cystography. The bladder is in a higher position in children than in adults and is slightly higher in males than in females. The bladder is relatively larger in children than in adults. It should not be considered pathologically significant in children when the enlargement is symmetrical and the longitudinal diameter is greater than the transverse.

THE NORMAL UROGRAM

The renal pelvis varies considerably in size and shape but is usually roughly triangular with the base parallel to the long axis of the kidney. It may be conical with the apex contiguous to the upper ureter. The range of normal is wide; some pelves are long narrow tubes while others are large and globular. There is also a considerable variation in position of the pelvis in relation to the kidney. It may be almost completely within the renal outline (intrarenal) or almost completely extrarenal. The former is usually small while the latter is large. The average normal pelvis is partially intra- and partially extrarenal. Bifurcation or duplication of the pelvis is very common and is considered an anatomic variant rather than a congenital anomaly.

The calyceal system consists of major calyces that begin at the pelvis and extend into the kidney to the junction with the minor calyces. Each major calyx may be divided into a base adjacent to the pelvis, and an infundibulum that is more or less tubular and extends from the base to the apex, or distal portion, from which one or more minor calyces project. The minor calyx consists of a body or a calyx proper, beginning at the junction with the major calyx, and the fornix that surrounds the conical renal papilla and into which the latter appears to project. The anatomic shape of the minor calyx is fairly constant, but since this structure is projected in various planes in the urogram there is considerable apparent variation. When viewed *en face*, it resembles a circular life preserver with a dense periphery and a relatively radiolucent center. In profile the appearance is somewhat triangular with the apex of the triangle pointing toward the major calyx; the base points away from it and is sharply concave or cupped. In contrast there is marked variation in the shape of the major calyces, which can be long and narrow or short and broad (Figs. 20-2 through 20-5). There are usually two

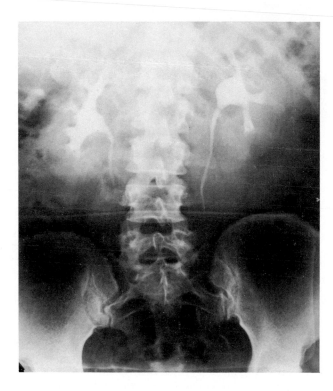

Fig. 20-2. Intravenous urogram of a normal person showing good filling of the pelves, calyces, and ureters down to about the level of the compression device, the superior portion of which overlies the lower fourth lumbar vertebra.

Fig. 20-3. Intravenous urograms of two normal persons. Compression is used in both of these subjects. This has resulted in a little blunting of the calyceal fornices. Renal outlines are better defined in **B** than in **A.** Note that there is some asymmetry on the two sides, particularly in **A.**

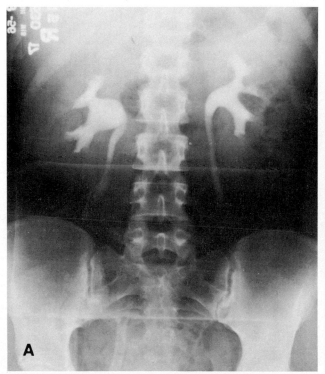

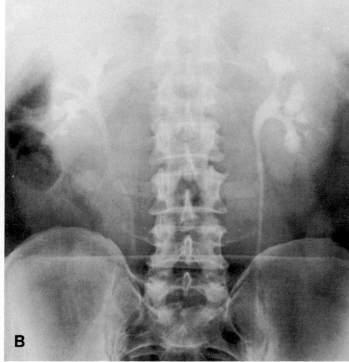

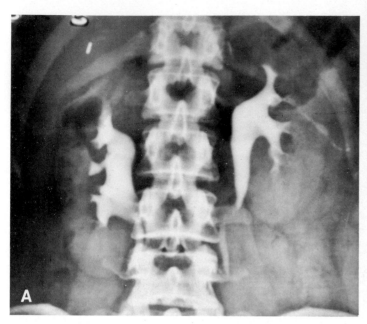

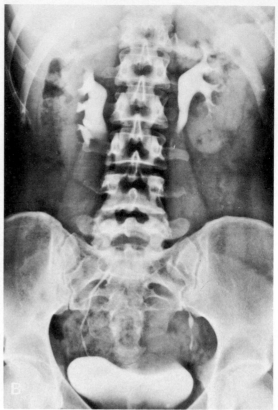

Fig. 20-4. A and B. Intravenous urograms of a normal person. The pelves and calyces are well filled. There is considerable asymmetry in this subject. The lower poles of the kidneys are particularly well outlined in A.

Fig. 20-5. Normal Intravenous urograms. A. Note the sharp and clearly defined calyces, particularly on the left. There is some asymmetry of major calyces, and there is a dromedary lump on the left. B. This patient has situs inversus. Note the gastric air bubble on the right. There is a little asymmetry, but this study demonstrates no abnormality.

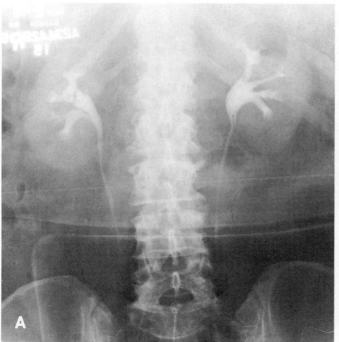

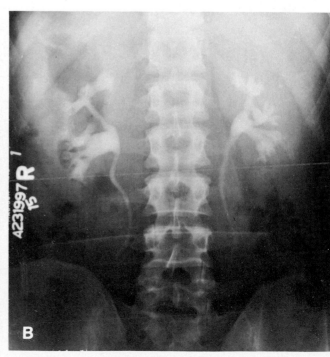

major calyces and six to fourteen minor calyces, but the number can vary widely. The calyceal system is not always bilaterally symmetric, which makes interpretation difficult in some instances. In the lateral projection the calyces are viewed obliquely and normally do not project anterior to the anterior aspect of the lumbar vertebral bodies. Cross-table lateral supine projections may be necessary to determine renal position in relation to the sagittal plane if the kidneys are unusually mobile.

There is a coordinated peristalsis that begins in the calyceal system of the kidneys. The kidneys alternately fill and contract and it is this activity that accounts for the variable appearance of the collecting system during intravenous urography. When the lower ureters are compressed, as described in the section entitled "Technique of Examination," peristaltic contractions are not as obvious. The discharge of urine from the pelvis into the ureter is accompanied by ureteral peristalsis. This occurs as broad waves at variable intervals (from four to twelve per minute). Ureteral peristalsis causes the ureter to have a variable caliber in different portions at the same time and a variation in contour in serial roentgenograms. The waves are visible as smooth areas of constriction or complete absence of filling that may separate one or more areas of slight dilatation. The effects of calyceal and ureteral peristalsis must be taken into account in the interpretation of intravenous urograms. Serial roentgenograms and fluoroscopy are of value in showing the rather wide variation in appearances of these structures from moment to moment.

Renal Backflow

The term "backflow" was initially applied to the escape of contrast material from the renal pelvis and calyces during retrograde pyelography as a result of an increase in intrapelvic pressure. The pressure is increased in intravenous urography by the use of compression devices. Acute ureteral obstruction also results in an increase of intrapelvic pressure. Since similar phenomena occur in these instances the term "backflow" has been carried over to describe changes observed in excretory urography. Backflow occurs in the normal kidney and its recognition and differentiation from that due to diseases of the kidney are therefore important.

There are two major types, pyelotubular and pyelosinus or pyelointerstitial. Pyelolymphatic and pyelovenous backflow are merely stages of the pyelointerstitial form. Pyelotubular backflow is the most frequent type; when it occurs during intravenous urography it probably represents stasis in the tubules in the papilla rather than actual backflow. Roentgen findings consist of a brushlike tuft of opacity radiating into the papilla from the minor calyx (Fig. 20-6). Pyelointerstitial (pyelosinus) backflow begins with minute rupture (painless) of the fornix of a calyx permitting the escape of contrast material or urine into the renal sinus, which is the loose adipose and connective tissue surrounding the pelvis and calyces and supporting a venous plexus. When the amount of extravasation increases it extends medially into the peripelvic area, into the perirenal fat within Gerota's fascia, and downward along the ureter. The extravasated material may enter the lymphatics to produce pyelolymphatic backflow. A much less common occurrence is pyelovenous backflow in which, presumably, the material enters the arcuate and other veins. There is some controversy as to whether or not this is ever demonstrated. Some investigators believe that the arcuate shadows observed in this condition are produced by perivascular extension of pyelosinus extravasation, not by filling of the veins, thus the term "pyelovenous backflow" is not accurate. All of the forms of backflow may be observed at one time (Fig. 20-6).

The roentgen findings in the early extravasation of the pyelointerstitial backflow consist of a hornlike projection of opaque medium extending from the fornix away from the papilla into the renal substance. As more material is extravasated it extends medially to the hilum and along the upper ureter, producing poorly defined densities in these areas. Pyelolymphatic backflow is manifested by opacification of lymphatic channels that extend from the hilum of the kidney medially toward the periaortic nodes. These channels tend to be redundant, somewhat tortuous, and branched (Fig. 20-7).

Extravasation of medium into the renal parenchyma also results when the catheter penetrates a calyx in retrograde pyelography. The roentgen appearance is variable, depending upon the amount and distribution of the extravasated material.

Arterial and Venous Impressions

Arterial impressions or indentations on the renal pelvis and infundibula were found in 18% of 150 patients studied by Nebesar, Pollard, and Fraley.[88] They occur three times more often on the right than on the left. The most common site is the superior infundibulum on the right. The impressions consist of smooth transverse or oblique indentations on the infundibu-

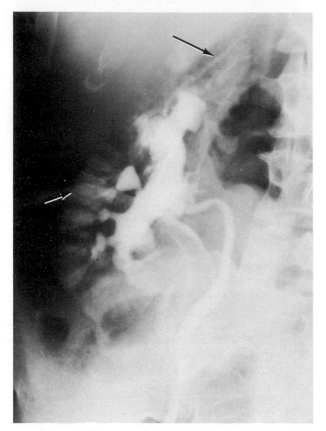

Fig. 20-6. Backflow. This retrograde pyelogram shows a marked amount of pyelolymphatic backflow **(upper arrow).** Pyelotubular backflow is outlined by the **lower arrow.** There is also some extravasation in the vicinity of the ureteropelvic junction representing interstitial backflow.

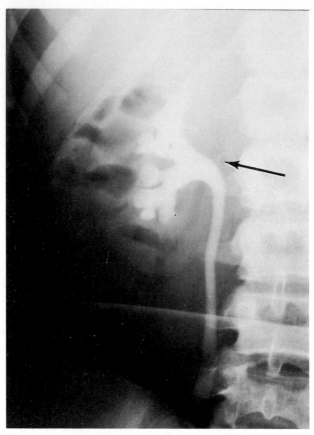

Fig. 20-7. Pyelolymphatic backflow. The **arrow** indicates the thin, tortuous opacified lymphatic channel just above the renal pelvis. The increased pressure resulting from a compression band evidently caused the backflow.

lum or pelvis. A slight delay in emptying of the upper pole calyces may be manifested by an apparent early opacification on the excretory urogram. Most of the involved vessels are ventral to the collecting system. They usually cause no symptoms and are significant only in that they must be differentiated from pathologic processes (Figs. 20-8 and 20-9). Occasionally, some infundibular obstruction is produced, leading to dilatation of calyces, pain, and occasionally to infection. Oblique as well as frontal projections are needed to make the diagnosis. Confirmation by angiography may be necessary when other causes are suspected. Occasionally a slightly tortuous renal artery, renal artery, renal artery aneurysm, or bulbous renal vein simulating a renal sinus mass (pseudotumor) is observed, particularly on a tomogram. The appearance is that of a round or oval mass in the renal sinus that is usually recognized as vascular, but angiography may be needed for differentiation in some instances.

Venous impressions on the superior infundibulum are not as common as those produced by arteries. Urographic findings are quite characteristic[78] and include a wide, smooth filling defect of the proximal part of the superior infundibulum that is usually best shown on the prone film. Venography can be used to confirm the diagnosis.

THE NORMAL CYSTOGRAM

The normal cystogram outlines the smooth-walled, rounded or oval bladder. The urinary bladder is usually filled to some extent durng excretory urography and this examination is often sufficient to out-

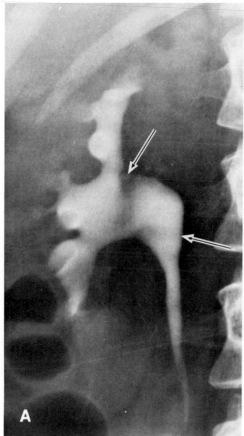 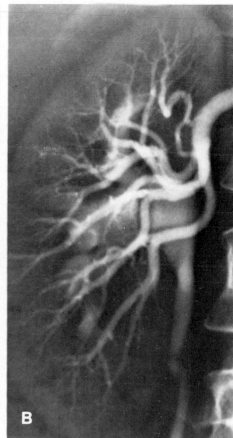

Fig. 20-8. A. Urogram showing arterial indentations producing a vertical lucency on the lateral aspect of the pelvis **(upper arrow)** and horizontal pelvic indentation **(lower arrow). B.** Selective renal arteriogram, on the same patient shown in **A,** demonstrating the relationship of arteries to the indentations noted in **A.**

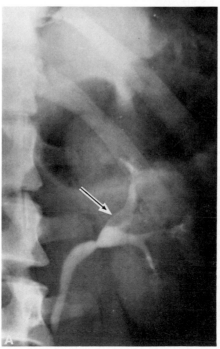 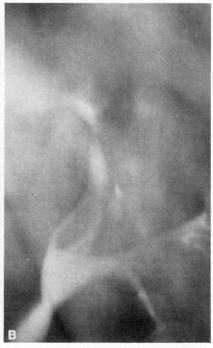

Fig. 20-9. A. Unusual vascular indentation causing a persistent elongated defect in the upper pole infundibulum on the left **(arrow). B.** Close-up of the defect which was persistent. Subsequent selective arteriogram showed a renal arterial branch causing the defect.

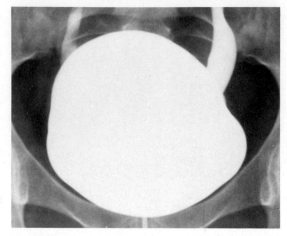

Fig. 20-10. Cystogram showing bilateral vesicoureteral reflux. The bladder outline appears normal.

line gross lesions. When additional study to the bladder is indicated by roentgen means, cystography is used (Fig. 20-10). Films are exposed in frontal, lateral, and oblique projections and, if necessary, upright and postvoiding roentgenograms may be obtained as indicated earlier.

ANOMALIES

Anomalies of the kidney and ureter result from errors in development.[67] The kidneys arise from a mass of renal mesenchyme at the upper end of the ureteral buds, which in turn arise from the lower end of the mesonephric (wolffian) ducts. The mesonephron is the excretory organ lower in the phylogenetic scale and, in the human, it functions for a short time in early embryologic development before becoming a part of the male genital system. The ureteral buds grow dorsally, lying close together as the renal mesenchyme differentiates. Each bud bifurcates into an upper and lower sprout to form the major calyces. The ureter is anterior to the kidney as the latter ascends from the upper sacral area to its position in the lower thoracic–upper lumbar region. As it ascends the kidney rotates to bring it lateral to the ureter in the midlumbar region. The renal blood supply is attained after the kidney reaches its normal adult position. The lower end of the ureter loses its relation to the wolffian duct and opens into the bladder in a higher and more lateral position. The wolffian duct migrates distally and its orifices eventually are situated in the distal portion of the floor of the prostatic urethra to become the ejaculatory ducts in the male.

The orifices of the wolffian duct become vestigal structures in the female.

ANOMALIES IN NUMBER

Renal Agenesis (Single Kidney)

The occurrence of a single kidney is a rare anomaly and great care must be taken when making a radiographic diagnosis of unilateral renal agenesis since a nonfunctioning kidney may not be readily visible. The single kidney tends to be larger in patients with agenesis of one kidney than in patients with secondary compensatory renal hyperplasia. Radiographic signs are an absence of a renal shadow on one side with an unusually large kidney on the other. The trigone is usually deformed with the ureteral orifice missing on the involved side, so that cystoscopy may confirm the diagnosis. At times, a portion of the lower ureter may be present in renal agenesis, however; therefore there may be no deformity of the trigone. Angiography confirms the absence of the renal artery but renal venography is said to be more reliable than arteriography in making the diagnosis of renal agenesis. Renal agenesis may be associated with other anomalies such as congenital heart disease and a neuromuscular deficit accompanied by a small pelvic outlet, sacral agenesis, and bladder hypoplasia (caudal regression). Surgical exploration is necessary at times to make certain of this anomaly.

Supernumerary Kidney

Supernumerary kidney is also a rare anomaly. The usual finding is that the third kidney is small and rudimentary, and the other kidney on the same side is often smaller than the normal kidney on the opposite side. Demonstration of the presence of a separate pelvis, ureter, and blood supply is necessary to make this diagnosis. Intravenous urography can be used to outline the excretory system of the supernumerary kidney if it is functioning and an abdominal aortogram will show the blood supply if that is necessary to confirm the diagnosis.

ANOMALIES IN SIZE AND FORM

Hypoplasia

Anomalies of renal size and form are much more common than anomalies in number. Hypoplasia on one side is usually associated with hyperplasia on the other. The hypoplastic or infantile kidney functions normally so that it can be seen on excretory urograms. It must be differentiated from the acquired

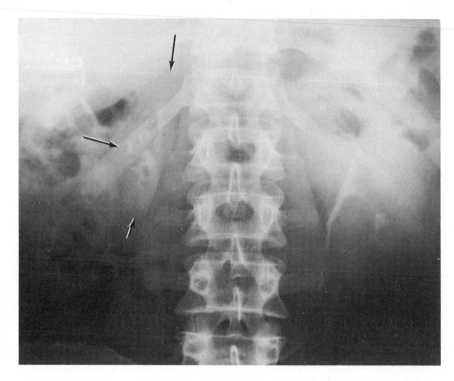

Fig. 20-11. Hypoplasia of the right kidney. Note the marked difference in size of the two kidneys. Function is present on the right kidney despite its small size. The limits are outlined by **arrows.**

atrophic kidney which is small and contracted secondary to vascular or inflammatory disease that has resulted in a decrease of renal parenchyma. In congenital hypoplasia the calyceal system and pelvis are small, and there is a normal relationship between the amount of parenchyma and the size of the collecting system (Fig. 20-11). In the secondarily contracted kidney, the pelvis and calyces tend to be normal in size so that the decrease in renal size is due to a parenchymal deficit. Furthermore, the function of the latter tends to be impaired. Despite these differences, it is often very difficult to distinguish between these two conditions without the use of renal arteriography. The size of the orifice of the renal artery is important; in hypoplasia it is small; in an atrophic kidney it is normal, but may taper to a very small size near the orifice.

Hyperplasia

The other anomaly in size, hyperplasia, is associated with agenesis or hypoplasia on the opposite side. Enlargement of the kidney is usually caused by conditions other than agenesis or hypoplasia, however, and is then more properly termed "compensatory hypertrophy." A number of disorders may cause renal enlargement; these include obstructive hydronephrosis, polycystic disease, other cystic or dysplastic disorders, neoplasm, renal vein thrombosis, acute infection, Waldenstrom's macroglobulinemia, hemophilia, acute arterial infarction, and duplication of the renal pelvis.[30] Often the enlargement is bilateral however, and there are clinical and laboratory findings and urographic findings which help to make the differentiation. Renal biopsy may be necessary in some instances. A number of conditions characteristically cause bilateral renal enlargement. They include: (1) acute glomerulonephritis; (2) lymphoma; (3) leukemia; (4) systemic lupus erythematosus; (5) polycystic disease; (6) bilateral renal vein thrombosis; (7) amyloidosis; (8) sarcoidosis; (9) sickle cell disease; (10) lipoid nephrosis; (11) lobular glomerulonephritis; (12) glycogen storage disease; (13) hereditary tyrosinemia and (14) total lipodystrophy.

FUSION ANOMALIES

Fusion anomalies represent an alteration in form of the kidneys and can often be recognized or at least suspected on plain roentgenograms of the abdomen (KUB films).

Horseshoe Kidney

The horseshoe kidney is the most common type of fusion anomaly. In this condition the lower poles of the kidney are joined by a band of soft tissues, the isthmus, which varies from a thick parenchymatous mass as wide as the kidneys themselves to a thin stringlike band of fibrous tissue. Rarely the upper poles are involved, the long axis of the kidney is reversed in this anomaly so that the lower pole is nearer the midline than the upper. There is also an associated rotation anomaly on one or both sides that varies in degree, usually more on the left. The calyces are directed backward or posteromedially rather than laterally. As a result they are seen on end or obliquely, which alters their appearance considerably (Fig. 20-12). The ureters tend to be somewhat stretched over the isthmus and partial obstruction on one or both sides is common (nearly 50%). This leads to dilatation of the pelvis (pyelectasis) and calyces (caliectasis) and may also lead to chronic inflammatory disease and the formation of calculi. The roentgen diagnostic features on the plain film are: (1) alteration in the axis of the kidneys; (2) mass observed connecting the lower poles; (3) renal enlargement if present; and (4) calculi if present. Urographic findings confirm these findings and in addition there are: (1) malrotation; with the pelves anterior or anterolateral in position; (2) nephrographic demonstration of the parenchymal isthmus connecting the lower poles (if present); (3) often varying degrees of dilatation of the collecting system on one or both sides; (4) possible nonfunction of one kidney because of massive obstructive hydronephrosis; (5) possible partial obstruction of both kidneys, usually at or near the ureteropelvic junction; (6) upper ureteral displacement which varies with the amount of malrotation.

Horseshoe kidneys are frequently supplied by multiple arteries and the isthmus is often supplied by anomalous branches of the common iliac on one or both sides.

Crossed Ectopy

Crossed ectopy with fusion, the unilateral fused kidney, is an anomaly of form that is much less common than the horseshoe kidney. It consists of fusion of the kidneys on the same side; the lower one is ectopic and its ureter crosses the midline to enter the bladder normally on the opposite side. Both kidneys are often lower in position than normal and various rotation anomalies as well as a wide variation in shape and type of fusion are noted. This anomaly is also frequently associated with partial obstruction, which results in inflammation and often in calculus formation. The "caked" kidney is a variation in which there is fusion of both upper and lower poles; with failure of rotation the calyces are directed posteriorly. The renal mass lies in or near the midline and is low in position, often overlying the sacrum. The ureters enter the bladder normally. A number of descriptive terms have been applied to other rare forms of fusion; all of these forms tend to result in obstruction, which

Fig. 20-12. Horseshoe kidney. **A.** Note the reversal of the long axis of the kidneys. There is very little rotation anomaly. The fusion inferiorly is faintly visualized on this reproduction. **B.** Marked rotation anomaly with inferior fusion. Also the right kidney has a somewhat ectopic position.

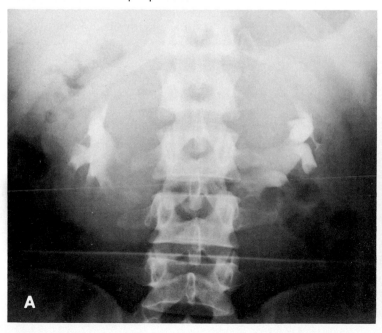
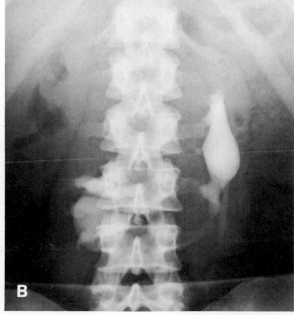

in turn causes hydronephrosis, infection, and calculus formation. These ectopic kidneys usually have an aberrant blood supply, often with multiple arteries. Extrarenal calyces occur rarely if the portion of the ureteric bud fails to invaginate the ectopic nephrogenic mass. The extrarenal calyx is large, probably because there is no supporting parenchyma, and mimics the blunt calyx due to obstruction or infection.

ANOMALIES IN POSITION

Anomalies of renal position are common. Malrotation has been described in the foregoing as being almost constantly present in fusion anomalies, but it also occurs as a single anomaly. (Fig. 20-13). It results from incomplete or excessive rotation and urographic study will indicate the degree of anomaly. Rotation anomalies are usually of little clinical significance unless associated with obstruction, but it is important to recognize them as anatomic variations that do not produce symptoms and are innocuous lesions. Retroperitoneal tumor masses may displace the kidneys and produce an alteration in rotation that must be differentiated from congenital rotation anomalies. Crossed ectopy may occur without fusion and the

findings are similar to those described in the preceding section except for the lack of fusion. The ectopic kidney is lower than the normal one in position and is usually described as a sacral or pelvic kidney, depending upon its position. Failure to visualize the kidney in its normal position should lead one to suspect ectopy and to look for it, since agenesis of a kidney is very rare. In many instances the kidney can be visualized only when contrast material outlines it, so that intravenous urography, radionuclide scanning, or retrograde pyelography may be necessary to indicate its position. If it is nonfunctioning, aortography may be used to identify the aberrant artery (arteries) to a pelvic kidney which may or may not appear as a pelvic mass on plain film. The pelvic mass representing an ectopic kidney may be discovered on study of the small bowel or colon as an extrinsic mass displacing bowel. Characteristically the ureter of an ectopic kidney is only long enough to reach from the renal pelvis to the bladder and this aids in distinguishing displacement of a normal kidney downward from one that developed in an abnormally low position. Superior ectopia of the kidney or thoracic kidney is probably more common than reports in the literature would indicate. The possibility of intrathoracic kidney should be considered in the differen-

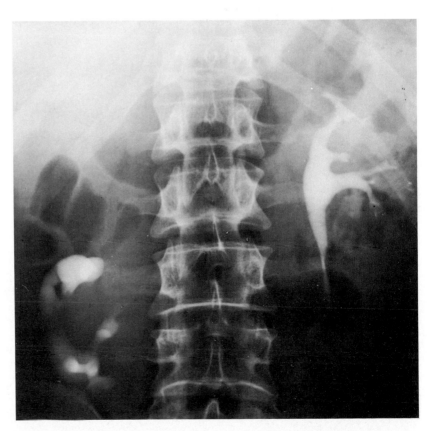

Fig. 20-13. Ectopic and malrotated right kidney. The calyces are dilated as compared to those in the normal left kidney.

tial diagnosis of masses of appropriate size projecting into the posterior thorax from below the diaphragm. An intrathoracic kidney is usually unilateral. It may be associated with herniation through the foramen of Bochdalek or a congenital eventration of the diaphragm posteriorly. Intravenous urography will readily identify the position of the kidney in these cases.

"Nephroptosis" is the term applied to abnormal downward displacement of the kidney. Roentgenograms obtained with the patient in the upright position normally show downward displacement of the kidney equal to the width of a lumbar vertebra. When the kidney is displaced more than this, ptosis is said to be present. The condition is more common on the right side than on the left; it is frequent in females but rare in males. It is of doubtful clinical significance since obstruction ordinarily is not produced and surgical intervention is rarely, if ever, indicated. Roentgen demonstration of this condition can be accomplished by obtaining an additional exposure during urography with the patient in an upright position. In the low position the kidney often rotates on its horizontal axis; the lower pole then lies more anterior than normal. Oblique views are necessary to measure true renal length when this occurs. Rarely there is enough mobility so that the kidney (usually the right) will move across the midline when a patient is in the appropriate lateral decubitus position. Also, one kidney may be displaced across the midline by an extrarenal mass, an acquired abnormality.

OTHER RENAL ANOMALIES

Aberrant papilla occurs occasionally. The papilla projects directly into the lumen of the infundibulum as a smooth, conical mass that appears round or oval when viewed *en face*. It bears no resemblance to a minor calyx in which a normal papilla projects. Other anomalies include multiple papillae entering a single calyx which may simulate blood clot or nonopaque stone.[69]

Megacalyces

The term "megacalyces" describes an anomaly consisting of enlargement of calyces in one or both kidneys associated wth underdeveloped renal pyramids. There is no evidence of obstruction. Function is normal. Because of calyceal size, there may be stasis with a tendency for stone formation. This may result in infection which may alter the urographic findings.[117]

Enlarged Column of Bertin

"Enlarged column of Bertin" is sometimes termed "pseudotumor" and it often congenital but may be acquired in patients with renal infections or other abnormalities that result in local hyperplasia.[52] The column of Bertin is normal cortical tissue that extends centrally between the papillae of the medullary pyramids. This may become large enough to simulate a mass and usually appears at the junction of the upper and middle thirds of the kidney, particularly in patients with incomplete renal duplication. The calyces and infundibula are displaced in patients with incomplete renal duplication. The calyces and infundibula are displaced but usually not distorted. This abnormality is best observed by nephrotomography which demonstrates: (*1*) partial or complete renal duplication; (*2*) a mass of homogeneous density contiguous with the renal cortex between the upper and middle pole infundibula; (*3*) a mass that opacifies as densely and often somewhat more densely than the surrounding parenchyma. When large-dose nephrotomography is used, the mass-like column of Bertin is often denser than the adjacent parenchyma. The same is often true in the nephrographic phase of renal arteriography.

Solitary Renal Calyx

A solitary renal calyx is an extremely rare anomaly in which one or both kidneys have a single calyx that drains the entire kidney into a somewhat bulbous tube that represents the pelvis. A number of other mammalian kidneys have a solitary calyx. This anomaly does not necessarily indicate renal disease, but other congenital anomalies may be associated with it.

ANOMALIES OF THE RENAL PELVIS AND URETER

Ureteropelvic Junction Anomalies

Ureteropelvic dysfunction or obstruction is the most common congenital anomaly of the urinary tract. It is usually bilateral but not always symmetrical. The left side is often more severely involved than the right. The amount of hydronephrosis depends on the severity of obstruction. In the neonate, when obstruction is marked it may be the cause of massive unilateral or bilateral renal enlargement. There is some controversy as to the cause of this anomaly, but the majority appear to be the result of an intrinsic abnormality that may be associated with such extrinsic abnormality as an aberrant vessel or band of fibrous tissue, either of which may angulate the ureter and tend to hold it in place while the pelvis dilates and may extend below the ureteropelvic junction. Whether these extrinsic lesions alone can produce obstruction is not certain. Rarely, an intrinsic mucosal fold or web may be present.[1] More often there appears to be abnormality in a muscle layer resulting in the dysfunction. If infection, often accompanied by reflux, occurs, fibrosis secondary to it may aggravate the condition.

Urographic findings vary with the severity of the condition. The caliectasis and pyelectasis are observed along with a somewhat rectangular extrarenal type of pelvis that is rather characteristic. Often the ureteropelvic junction is not dependent as in the normal individual, so the insertion of the ureter is high and posterior.

Duplication of the Pelvis and Ureter

Incomplete double ureter is formed when the renal bud divides too early or the division extends into the ureter.[56] The division varies from an exaggeration of the length of major upper and lower pole calyces to duplication of the ureter for most of its length. Complete duplication of the ureter may also occur. Each ureter has its own vesical orifice and the upper ureter usually drains the upper third of the kidney, while the ureter that drains the lower pelvis drains the lower two-thirds of the kidney (Fig. 20-14). The ureter that drains the upper pole is ventral to the lower one but crosses over and empties into the bladder in a lower and more medial position, and when one of the ureters empties in an extravesical location it is the one that drains the upper pelvis. Urographic recognition of duplication is simple when both pelves and ureters are opacified and should be suspected if only one of them fills since there will then be a segment of kidney without drainage. These anomalies of the pelvis and ureter may be unilateral or bilateral, with a tendency to be asymmetric. Occasionally multiple budding will result in multiple short upper pelves and ureters that are extrarenal in type. In this anomaly, each of several major calyces will have its own pelvis and upper ureter, which usually joins with the others to form a common lower ureter. It is not infrequent for one-half of a double ureter to be obstructed. Triple ureter has also been reported. There are several abnormalities related to duplication of the kidney and ureters, the most common being vesicoureteral reflux, ureterocele, and ectopic ureteral orifice. All may be associated with infection, and obstruction may complicate ureterocele and ectopic ureteral ori-

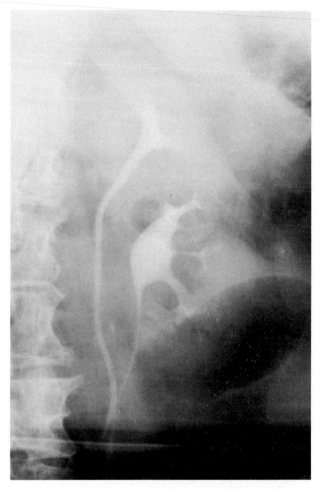

Fig. 20-14. Duplication of the pelvis and ureter. The upper pelvis drains the upper pole of the kidney while the lower pelvis drains the central portion of the kidney as well as the lower pole.

fice. When obstruction and/or infection result in nonfunctioning of the upper pole, the roentgenographic findings are varied. If there is a nonobstructive inflammatory lesion resulting in nonfunction, the findings are those of a calyceal system that drains only the central and lower pole of the kidney so the calyces are fewer than normal in number and the most superior calyx does not extend into the upper pole of the kidney. In order to make this determination, it is imperative that clear visualization of the outline of the upper pole be obtained. If there is a hydronephrotic mass, the upper pole will be enlarged, and the lower calyces that are filled may be displaced by the large upper pole mass, and there may also be some rotation of the kidney, the amount depending upon the size of the mass. If the mass is very large the entire kidney may be displaced laterally along with the upper ureter. There may or may not be calculi in the obstructed or infected upper pole.

Anomalies in Position of Ureteral Orifice

There are several possible anomalies in position of the ureteral orifice and this variation is usually better studied by cystoscopy than by radiographic means. In the male, the ureter may open into the seminal vesicles, the vas deferens, the ejaculatory duct, or the posterior urethra. In the female, the abnormal ureter may open into the urethra, beneath the urethral orifice near the hymen, or into the lateral vulvar wall, the uterus, the vagina, or, rarely, into the rectum. Although ectopic ureteral insertion is present in all patients with ureteral duplication, it also occurs in patients with a single ureter. The sites, symptoms, and radiographic findings are similar except that there is no duplication.

Ureteral Jet Phenomenon

The ureteral jet phenomenon is caused by a jet of opaque medium propelled by ureteral peristalsis, which may occasionally extend across the base of the bladder to the opposite side. The jet maintains the caliber of the ureter and simulates an anomalous ureter that opens on the opposite side of the trigone (Fig. 20-15). When present, it excludes the possibility of significant vesicoureteral reflux. When there is any question as to the cause of the apparent anomaly, another film will reveal a normal lower ureter in these patients.

Retrocaval Ureter

Postcaval or retrocaval ureter is limited to the right side except in situs inversus. It is caused by failure of the right subcardinal vein to atrophy; it persists as the adult vena cava. Normally, the right supracardinal vein persists as the vena cava. The abnormal relationship may cause partial obstruction, leading to hydronephrosis, infection, and calculus formation. The ureter passes to the left behind the inferior vena cava, then turns toward the right and courses downward in its normal position. In some cases there is redundancy of the ureter proximally, so that an S type, or fishhook or inverted J type, of deformity is produced. The site of narrowing or obstruction, if present, is proximal to the vena cava and is probably at the lateral edge of the psoas, and is caused by the pressure of the retroperitoneal fascia over the muscle. In other cases of retrocaval ureter with no redundancy, obstruction is less common and when present coincides with the lateral margin of the inferior vena cava.

The diagnosis can usually be made on urography. In addition to the abnormal course of the right ureter in the frontal projection, its posterior position in the lateral view can be observed. The diagnosis can be confirmed by inferior vena cavography with an opaque catheter in the ureter. The medial swing is usually maximum at L4-5 and occasionally as high as L3. There may be partial obstruction at the level of the lateral wall of the vena cava. Medial deviation of the ureter (medial to the vertebral pedicles) may also be caused by psoas muscle hypertrophy in muscular males and may occur as an anatomic variant usually at the L5 and S1 levels. Retroperitoneal fibrosis and abdominal aortic aneurysm may also cause medial deviation. The deviations in the retroperitoneal fibrosis are bilateral and there is no S- or J-shaped redundancy. Retroperitoneal masses with ureteral displacement must also be differentiated.

Ureterocele

There are two types of ureterocele, simple and ectopic. The simple ureterocele consists of an intravesical dilatation of the ureter immediately proximal to its orifice in the bladder. It usually results from a combination of ureteral orifice stenosis and a deficiency in the connective tissue attachment of the ureter to the bladder. It varies in size from a scarcely perceptible dilatation to one that is moderately large and resembles a cobra head in shape. There may be partial obstruction resulting in hydroureter. In general this type is smaller than the ectopic ureterocele. It occurs with equal frequency in males and females and is usually discovered in adults. A calculus in the intramural portion of the ureter may produce dilatation simulating ureterocele, but the calculus produces pain, and it is usually visible on the plain film. A tumor of the bladder, either primary or secondary, may also cause dilatation simulating simple ureterocele.

The ectopic type of ureterocele is four or five times more frequent than the simple type. It is usually discovered in childhood, and is much more common in females (6 or 7 to 1) than in males. It is more likely to be associated wth severe hydronephrosis, hydroureter, or infection than is the simple type.[35] Both types tend to occur in the presence of duplication of

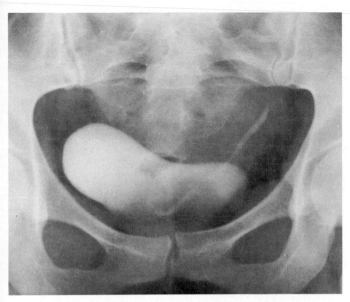

Fig. 20-15. Ureteral jet phenomenon. Note the apparent extension of the ureter across the midline. Cystoscopy revealed a normal position of the ureteral orifice on the left.

the ureter; the ectopic type is almost always associated with this anomaly. The ectopic ureterocele consists of the submucosal passage of the distal portion of the involved ureter within the vesical wall to terminate in the urethra rather than in the bladder as in the simple type. The submucosal portion of the ureter dilates and bulges anteriorly into the bladder to form the ureterocele. It may prolapse through the urethra to form a vulval cyst and usually extends posterior to the vesical neck and proximal urethra. It invariably involves the ureter from the upper pole of the kidney (Fig. 20-16).

The roentgen appearance of the simple type depends on whether the opaque medium fills the ureterocele. If it is filled the lesion is outlined by a radiolucent wall that stands out in contrast to the filled bladder as well as to the filled, dilated, distal ureter. When the ureterocele is not filled with opaque material it appears as a radiolucent mass within the opacified bladder in the region of the ureteral orifice. The shape may be somewhat fusiform with a narrow lower end resembling a cobra's head, but the larger ones tend to be more rounded in shape. When a calculus is present in the ureterocele, it is noted to lie on one side of the midline and remains there despite changes in the patient's position.

Ectopic ureteroceles are larger than the simple

ones and often extend to the anterior bladder wall when viewed in the lateral projection. The contact with the floor of the bladder is broad and extends to the internal urethral orifice. Obstruction of the other ureter is frequent and the extravesical portion may distort the bladder. Several conditions may simulate ectopic ureterocele; these include hydrometrocolpos and "cyst" of the seminal vesicle produced when the ectopic ureter inserts into the seminal vesicle. The condition is less frequent in males than in females, but in males the incidence of infection is higher, the malformation is more complex, and the frequency of a single collecting system is greater than in females. Eversion is also more common in males, and the tendency to prolapse into the posterior urethra causing bladder outlet obstruction is greater.

Intravenous urography is the roentgen method of choice in diagnosis of ureterocele. An eccentric mass encroaching on the bladder floor in a patient with duplication of the ureter is virtually pathognomonic.

Ureteral Diverticula

A single ureteral diverticulum is probably a congenital anomaly and may represent a dilated rudimentary branched ureter. When the diverticulum is filled with contrast medium, the diagnosis is easily made because the appearance is similar to that of a diverticulum elsewhere. Some of these diverticula have the appearance of a blind-end duplication without much dilatation and almost certainly are rudimentary or partially duplicated ureters. They are best demonstrated by retrograde pyelography, but may be apparent on an excretory urogram. Many diverticula are acquired and most authorities believe that multiple diverticula are almost always acquired, and are indicative of previous infection. They appear as ureteral outpouchings of various sizes and numbers, best seen on a retrograde pyelogram, but with good ureteral filling they may also be clearly defined on an excretory urogram.

Other Ureteral Anomalies

Transverse Ureteral Folds. In infants, a corkscrew appearance may be demonstrated in the upper ureters on an excretory urogram. This appearance is caused by thin, transverse folds that represent inward projections of the full thickness of the ureteral wall. They appear as horizontal folds measuring about 1 mm in thickness on the urogram, probably represent persistence of fetal tortuosity of the ureter, are of no clini-

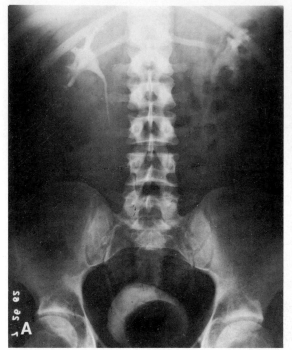

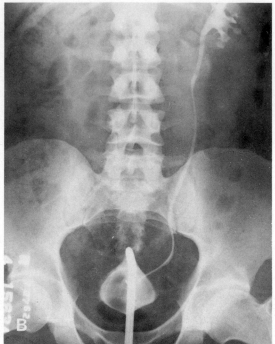

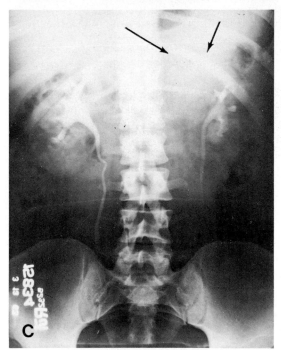

Fig. 20-16. Ectopic ureterocele. Note the large, rounded mass encroaching on the bladder, chiefly on the left side. The collecting system on the left drains the lower left kidney. **A.** Retrograde pyelogram **B,** in which a ureteral orifice in the normal position was catheterized, shows drainage of the lower kidney. The ectopic ureter draining into the ureterocele could not be catheterized. It drained the upper pole of the left kidney and was obstructed so that no function was present at the time of the urogram **C. Arrows** outline the upper pole of the kidney on the left.

cal significance, and represent a minor anatomic variant that occasionally persists into adolescence.

Vertical Ureteropelvic Striations. The vertical striations occasionally observed in the pelvis and upper ureter usually are associated with reflux and are probably secondary to infection, edema, and dilatation. However, in rare instances, they appear to be an isolated finding and in these they may represent a minor anatomic variant. They may be observed on excretory urograms or retrograde pyelograms.

Ureteral Valves. A ureteral valve is a very unusual anomaly that is manifested by the following: (1) anatomically demonstrable transverse folds of ureteral mucosa containing bundles of smooth muscle fibers; (2) obstruction above the valve and a normal ureter below it; and (3) no other evidence of mechanical or functional obstruction. It is usually unilateral and may be annular with a pinpoint opening or cusplike in appearance. It may occur anywhere in the ureter, although it is slightly more common in the lower ureter than elsewhere. The cause of this anomaly is uncertain.[1]

Patent Urachus and Urachal Cyst

The urachus represents the intra-abdominal remnant of the allantoic duct or caudal extension of it, which is continuous with the vesical portion of the urogenital sinus in embryologic development. Normally it constitutes the middle umbilical ligament. The allantois extends from the primitive urinary bladder through the umbilicus to the placenta. Four types of anomalies are possible: (1) complete patency; (2) patency at umbilical end or blind external type; (3) patency at vesical end or blind internal type; and (4) patency between bladder and umbilicus, which gives rise to urachal cyst. Urachal prominence or urachal remnant is observed fairly often in patients with high intravesicle pressure dating from birth or before birth. Examples are patients with myelomeningocele or posterior urethral valves. The blind external type and complete patency are usually recognized on inspection when the umbilical cord sloughs off but may be suspected earlier. Roentgen visualization can be obtained by using any of the organic iodides mentioned earlier in this chapter as contrast materials that can be injected into the umbilical end of the urachus. Cystography is needed to demonstrate the internal type. The findings are those of a smooth-walled tubal structure lying in the anterior midline that extends into the plane of a line between umbilicus and the bladder. The bladder may be distorted and elevated. The cyst may extend from the bladder to the umbilicus or end blindly when it begins at either end. When a cyst of the urachus is present without internal or external communication of the roentgen findings depend upon its size. If large, it may be noted as a midline, soft-tissue mass lying between the bladder and the umbilicus in the anterior abdominal wall. Gas-filled small intestine may be displaced and study of the small bowel by means of barium meal will show comparable displacement. Rarely calculi may form in a patent urachus or urachal cyst.

HYDRONEPHROSIS (OBSTRUCTIVE UROPATHY); (URINARY STASIS)

Regardless of its cause, chronic obstruction of the urinary tract leads to hydronephrosis, which indicates dilatation of the pelvis and calyces with progressive destruction of renal parenchyma. The terms "pyelectasis," "caliectasis," "ureterectasis," or "hydroureter" are more accurate in designating the location of the dilatation. The obstruction that produces hydronephrosis may be unilateral or bilateral, depending on the site of the lesion producing it. Unilateral obstruction is caused by a lesion at or above the ureterovesical junction, while bilateral obstruction may be caused by a lesion distal to that point. Bilateral obstruction above the ureterovesical junction is not uncommon, however, particularly in patients with congenital anomalies, and in these the hydronephrosis is usually asymmetric. Enlargement of the urinary collecting system including pelves, calyces, ureters, and bladder may result from causes other than obstruction, however.

NONOBSTRUCTIVE HYDRONEPHROSIS (URINARY STASIS)

There are several nonobstructive conditions that may cause dilatation of the renal pelvis and calyces and also of the ureters. Diabetes insipidus may be associated with relatively moderate hydronephrosis. Nephrogenic diabetes insipidus tends to cause a more severe degree of dilatation, often with tortuosity of the ureters in addition to the dilatation. In this condition there is a tubular abnormality with insufficient absorption of water, leading to a large volume of hypotonic urine.[83] Urinary tract infection tends to cause segmental or generalized dilatation (ileus) of the ureter with poor or reversed peristalsis leading to pyelectasis and caliectasis. This may be augmented by vesicoureteral reflux which is commonly found in association with urinary infections. The changes may decrease or disappear when the infection is successfully treated. Dilatation with stasis in the absence of urinary tract abnormality may also be caused by intra-abdominal inflammatory disease such as appendicitis or peritonitis—a finding similar to that of adynamic ileus involving the gut in patients with peritonitis. Excessive fluid intake (overhydration) may cause some dilatation. A variety of neurologic disorders are also associated with dilatation without obstruction. Minimal or moderate degrees of pyelectasis, caliectasis, and ureterectasis are observed in patients with vesicoureteral reflux and in those with urinary tract infection without reflux. An adynamic, short segment of upper ureter may also cause some dilatation of the pelves and calyces; this appears on a urogram as a short, narrow ureteral segment with dilatation above it.

CONGENITAL HYDRONEPHROSIS
(URINARY STASIS)

Congenital hydronephrosis is caused by a variety of lesions. In anomalies of position it is usually due to the abnormal relationship of the upper ureter to the kidney. Congenital strictures, bands, aberrant vessels, and valves may also produce hydronephrosis. In addition, there are instances of congenital hydronephrosis in which the cause is obscure; many of these are "neurogenic" in that they are associated with lesions of the spinal cord and with congenital megacolon. The dilatation is usually bilaterally symmetrical in patients with congenital megacolon. Congenital abnormalities then may result in either obstructive or nonobstructive uropathy. In neonates, ascites at birth may indicate obstructive uropathy, often secondary to posterior urethral valves, but a variety of lesions may cause the obstruction. Obstruction of the bladder outlet, ureteral atresia, presacral neuroblastoma, complex caudal anomalies including urethral and anorectal atresia, ureterocele, vesicle neck valve, and myelomeningocele have also been reported as rare causes of neonatal ascites secondary to obstructive uropathy. Pneumothorax and/or pneumomediastinum have been reported in a number of neonates with ascites secondary to urologic malformations.

Rarely, ureteropelvic junction obstruction may produce intermittent symptoms related to overhydration in patients who may have an aberrant vessel that produces some narrowing at the junction. In patients with these symptoms, urography with oral overhydration, Lasix given intravenously, or large-volume drip infusion may demonstrate the pyelectasis and caliectasis. As indicated earlier, duplication with ectopic ureteral insertion into urethra, and the like, often results in hydronephrosis of the upper collecting system; this is a congenital anomaly but acquired disease such as infection may be the major cause when obstruction is observed in the adult. Rarely, there is lower pole hydronephrosis in a duplicated kidney.

ACQUIRED HYDRONEPHROSIS
(OBSTRUCTIVE UROPATHY)

Acquired hydronephrosis is caused by a variety of lesions also; among them are tumors, calculi, strictures, operative procedures, and prostatic enlargement. Ureteropelvic junction obstruction is the most common type of bilateral obstruction above the bladder. It may be asymmetric, however. Congenital valves appear to be the most common cause of the obstruction, but an aberrant artery may contribute to obstruction or may cause it in some instances. Pregnancy is often associated with hydronephrosis that tends to be more severe on the right than on the left. Ureters are dilated to the pelvic brim. This may be caused by mechanical pressure but because there is little or no association with fetal position, the cause is not certain. The ureters are occasionally displaced laterally. Hydrocolpos and hydrometrocolpos tend to cause ureteral obstruction. Abdominal aortic aneurysm may compress the ureter or retroperitoneal bleeding, associated with aneurysm, may cause fibrosis leading to ureteral stricture and hydronephrosis. Granulomatous disease of the small intestine or colon (Crohn's disease) or both occasionally cause ureteral obstruction. There are all degrees of dilatation, and progression of the changes can be noted on serial examinations if the obstruction is not relieved.

Urographic Findings

The earliest urographic change in hydronephrosis is a flattening of the normal concavity of the calyx and blunting of the sharp peripheral angle produced by the papilla as it juts into the calyx. This change is reversible and is readily produced by a small increase in pressure. It is noted in normal individuals when a compression band is in place during urography. The pelvis enlarges gradually with increasing or prolonged obstruction, but pelvic and calyceal dilatation are not necessarily parallel. The next calyceal change is that of "clubbing," in which the concavity pro-

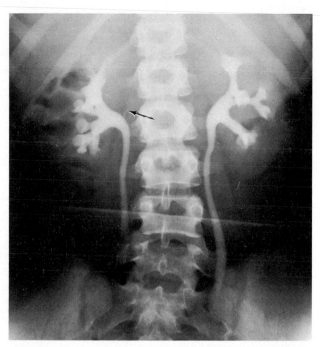

Fig. 20-17. Minimal bilateral hydronephrosis. The pelves are not enlarged, but there is a little blunting of the calyces. Note the minimal pyelolymphatic backflow on the right **(arrow).**

duced by the papilla is reversed (Figs. 20-17 through 20-19). Calyces then gradually enlarge with progressive destruction of parenchyma and enlargement of the collecting system of the kidney until the kidney becomes a nonfunctioning hydronephrotic sac in whch the normal anatomy is obliterated (Fig. 20-20). Renal function may be greatly diminished in severe hydronephrosis and there is accumulation of opaque material in the parenchyma adjacent to the grossly dilated calyces. This forms crescentic areas of faint opacification termed the "crescent" sign of hydronephrosis (Fig. 20-21). Later there may be faint opacification of the calyces themselves. Infection may be a complicating factor, tending to accelerate parenchymal destruction. When present, it produces more irregularity in the dilated calyces than is seen in uncomplicated hydronephrosis. Also there may be bleedng with clots in the dilated collecting system which may resemble intrapelvic tumor. When hydronephrosis is suspected as the cause for nonfunction and no signs of opacification are observed, a horizontal-beam radiograph obtaincd wth the patient in the upright or decubitus position may be helpful, since the contrast medium is heavier than urine and will layer in dependent portions of calyces. Erect films

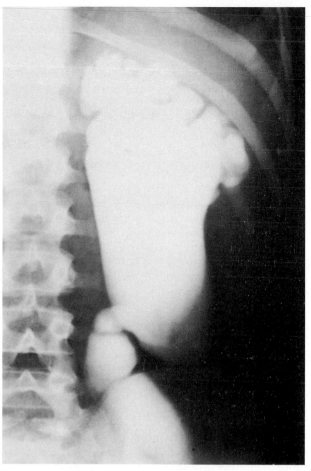

Fig. 20-18. Hydronephrosis and hydroureter in a patient with chronic pyelonephritis. A very thin rim of parenchyma is present. This is a retrograde pyelogram in a patient who had virtually no function in this kidney.

may also be helpful when equivocal shadows are observed that may represent contrast in dilated calyces. In the evaluation of patients with dilatation of the pelvis and calyces, particularly in children, it is important that the bladder be emptied before the urogram is obtained. A distended bladder may result in a false hydronephrosis, the cause for which is uncertain. When the bladder is empty, the "hydronephrosis" disappears. Vesicoureteral reflux may accentuate the dilatation of the upper urinary tract in these patients but does not appear to be the major cause.[19]

When complete obstruction persists, there is usually increasing hydronephrosis with so-called hydronephrotic atrophy resulting in loss of renal parenchyma of varying degrees. In some instances, func-

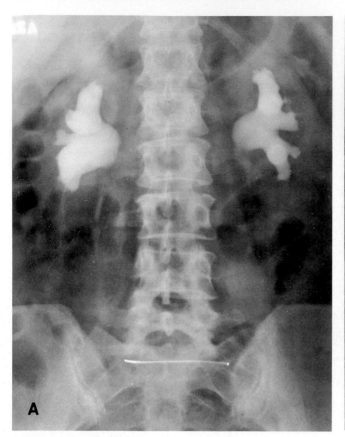 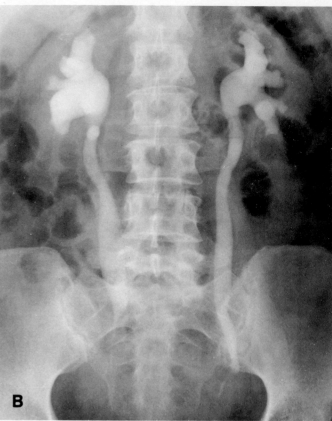

Fig. 20-19. Bilateral hydronephrosis showing the value of delayed films. **A.** Intravenous urogram, obtained 15 minutes after injection of a contrast medium, shows dilatation of pelves and calyces with no definite ureteral opacification. **B.** This film, exposed 90 minutes after injection of the medium, shows dilatation of ureters extending down to stricturelike narrowing which is a little higher on the right than on the left.

tion will return following relatively long periods of obstruction providing that some good renal cortex remains. Occasionally a combination of obstruction and ischemia may result in decreased renal size when the obstruction is relieved.

RENAL AND URETERAL CALCULI

Urinary tract calculi are formed in the pelvis, often in the region of the papillae, and calyces. The calculi may remain within the pelvis and gradually increase in size to form a cast of the pelvis and calyces. This represents what is known as the staghorn calculus

(Fig. 20-22). In other patients, multiple calculis may form within the calyceal system and they may be similar, or may vary considerably, in size. Calculi tend to be asymptomatic until they cause obstruction. Then the typical renal or ureteral colic is produced. Most renal calculi contain enough calcium to be visualized on roentgenograms. Calcium phosphate, calcium oxalate, and magnesium ammonium phosphate stones are the most common; the stones usually are composed of a mixture of chemical compounds since pure stones are relatively rare. Diamonium calcium phosphate and magnesium phosphate stones are uncommon. Cystine, urate, and xanthine stones are rare. Urinary stasis and infection are important fac-

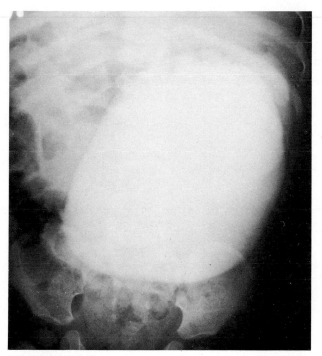

Fig. 20-20. Massive hydronephrosis in a child. The greatly dilated pelvis is opacified. It nearly fills the entire left abdominal cavity. Physical findings were those of a large, somewhat fluctuant abdominal mass on the left.

tors in promoting the formation of calculi, but the exact cause is not certain in many instances. Matrix calculi are a combination of about two-thirds muco-protein and one-third mucopolysaccharide; they are radiolucent and usually form in the presence of *Proteus* infection. This amorphous mucoprotein is present in stone formers but, since it is not present in normal urine, it probably plays a role in the formation of renal calculi. Hyperparathyroidism and other conditions with hypercalcemia, including some which cause dissolution of bone, may also be associated with calculi. They include osteolytic metastases, leukemia, multiple myeloma, and sarcoidosis. Gout and other conditions associated with high serum uric acid and hyperuricosuria increase the incidence of uric acid stones. Hyperoxaluria, whatever the cause, tends to promote formation of renal calculi. There is some evidence to indicate that calculi may also result from renal artery stenosis; the vascular insufficiency may cause parenchymal injury leading to calculus formation.

ROENTGEN FINDINGS

The roentgen findings are those of an opacity of varying size and shape overlying the urinary tract. Often the plain-film diagnosis is easily made, particularly when the calculus forms a cast of the pelvis or calyces or both. Excretory urography is often indi-

Fig. 20-21. Hydronephrosis, the crescent sign. **A.** Selective left renal arteriogram shows grossly stretched, narrow vessels with very few branches. Note the vessels stretched over the large renal pelvis medially. **B.** Later film shows the crescent sign caused by opacification in the thin rim of remaining renal tissue. Surgical removal confirmed the diagnosis of severe hydronephrosis. (Courtesy of Dr. Thomas L. Carter and Dr. Richard Logan)

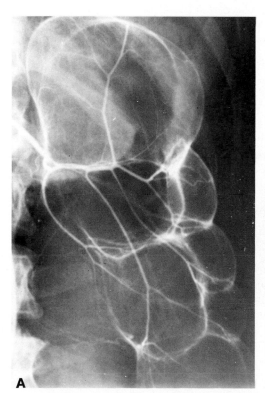

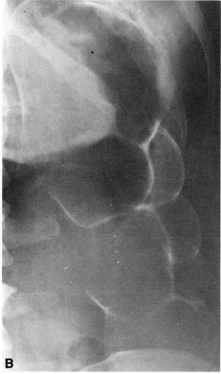

A

B

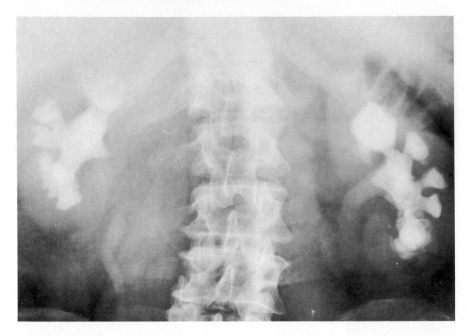

Fig. 20-22. Staghorn calculi. Note the calcification forming a cast of the pelvis and calyces on each side. Renal function was so poor that very little additional density was observed on these urograms. The ureters are faintly opacified however.

cated to ascertain the localization and to determine the condition of the calyceal system. Oblique and lateral views may be necessary in addition to frontal projections in order definitely to localize a calculus. Urography is also necessary to find radiolucent calculi. These calculi appear as negative shadows displacing the opaque medium. In patients with renal or ureteral colic there is usually delayed excretion by the involved kidney. The diatrizoates and other triiodinated media in the large doses used in urography are excreted almost entirely by glomerular filtration. With the acute obstruction produced by the passage of a ureteral stone, the intrapelvic pressure increases to the point where there is little or no glomerular filtration. Increasing density of the kidney (demonstrated by nephrogram) indicates accumulation of iodide, probably a result of accumulation of contrast material in the lumina of nephrons and collecting ducts, and eventually there is usually some opacification of the calyces, pelvis, and ureter. It is therefore important to obtain films until opacification is adequate to make the diagnosis. If the routine nephrograms show a prolonged density on the involved side, it is likely that films exposed at 30-minute or progressively longer intervals will show enough opacification to localize the site of the obstructing ureteral calculus and confirm its presence within the ureter (Fig. 20-23). If this method fails, an opaque catheter can be passed and the calculus localized in relation to it by means of frontal, oblique, and lateral roentgeno-

grams. The most common sight for ureteral calculi to lodge is at or above the ureterovesical junction in the pelvic portion of the ureter. Occasionally a calculus will have passed before the examination is completed and no obstruction is then visible. When the calculus has lodged at the ureterovesical junction for any length of time, it is not uncommon to note a localized radiolucent indentation on the bladder owing to edema above the ureteral orifice, even though the calculus may have been passed. Ureteral calculi are small in size (1 to 3 mm in diameter). In general these small stones pass quickly down the ureter to lodge at or near the ureterovesical junction. They tend to be parallel to the course of the ureter when they are oval or elongated. Most of them lie above a line drawn through the ischial spines. However, it should be recognized that angulation of the roentgen-ray tube or alteration of position of the pelvis may project these calculi lower in position. Larger calculi are not so likely to leave the renal pelvis and to become lodged in the ureter. Ureteral calculi tend to be round or oval in shape. If the calculus remains within the ureter for any length of time it may become elongated and increased in size; large stones found within the ureter usually mean that they have been present for a considerable period of time (Fig. 20-24). In patients with acute renal colic caused by an obstructing ureteral calculus, urography may demonstrate pyelointerstitial backflow, and it is likely that many small interstitial extravasations occur that are not seen.

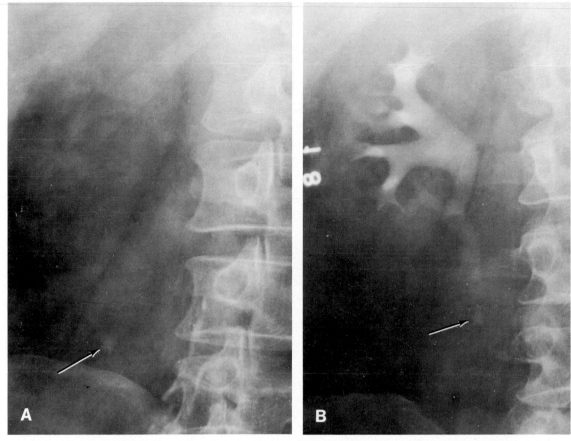

Fig. 20-23. Right ureteral calculus. **A.** Note the density **(arrow)** just above the right iliac crest in this right posterior oblique projection. **B.** Urogram shows slight dilatation of the ureter extending down to the site of the calculus. This roentgenogram was obtained at 90 minutes following the intravenous injection of contrast material. Earlier films showed no excretion on the right side, demonstrating that delayed films were essential to confirm the diagnosis of ureteral calculus in this patient.

Occasionally there may be a rather large amount of extravasation which usually migrates to the renal sinus in a peripelvic location; rarely the extravasation may extend laterally to a subcapsular position.

It is not uncommon to observe a single loop of gas-filled small bowel, usually in the left upper quadrant, in patients with acute renal colic. The site of the loop is not necessarily related to the position of the stone. Occasionally, extensive adynamic ileus may occur.

DIFFERENTIAL DIAGNOSIS

Suspected renal or ureteral calculus must be differentiated from all other calcifications that may occur in the renal areas and along the course of the ureters. Gallstones are usually multiple, tend to be faceted, and often exhibit typical concentric rings of calcium. Oblique roentgenograms will show their anterior position. Common duct and cystic duct stones may be opaque but they also lie anterior to the kidney and ureter. Calcification of costal cartilages is common and usually readily identified. Oblique projections will show the relationship of such shadows to the anterior lower thoracic wall if there is any doubt about the nature of the densities. Calcified mesenteric nodes and calcifications in the appendices epiploica usually move enough from one time to another to be differentiated from urinary calculi. The same is true of opaque material in the gastrointestinal tract, but it is frequently necessary to obtain more than one

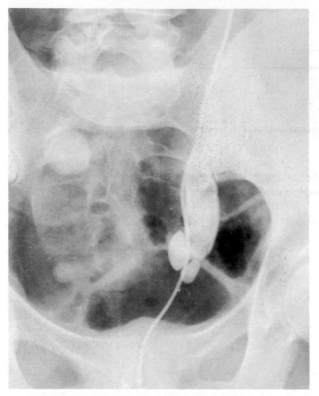

Fig. 20-24. Multiple large ureteral calculi on the left. The ureteral catheter indicates the relationship of the calculi to the ureter. The bladder is outlined by air.

roentgenogram to make the differentiation. Pancreatic calculi usually conform to the shape of the portion of pancreas and can be identified readily, but occasionally it is necessary to examine the stomach and duodenum by means of a barium meal to make certain of the position of the calculi. Calcification in cysts and tumors of the kidney and elsewhere in the abdomen must also be differentiated. The contour of the cyst wall can usually be identified and when calcified tumor is present, it is usually large enough to be visualized as a soft-tissue mass. Occasionally the lateral tip of a transverse process of one of the lumbar vertebrae may be easily visible in comparison to the remainder of the process and resemble a ureteral calculus; close inspection will suffice to make the differentiation. Vascular calcification, either in pelvic arteries or in veins (phleboliths) are generally the most difficult problems. Arterial calcification is usually along the course of a large artery and tends to be elongated as well as to outline the arterial walls, forming a ringlike density when seen in cross section and parallel lines when seen in longitudinal section.

Phleboliths often have a fairly typical appearance with a radiolucent central area and tend to be more rounded in contour than calculi. Phleboliths may have a central calcific nidus surrounded by a zone of lesser density, which in turn is surrounded by a denser periphery. Roentgenograms obtained in anteroposterior and oblique projections are often sufficient to exclude the possibility of urinary calculus as the cause for the density or densities present. If not, excretory urography with oblique and special views as needed, including delayed roentgenograms, usually will provide the diagnosis. If there still is doubt, cystoscopy with introduction of a radiopaque catheter into the ureter usually solves the problem. The ureteral stone stays in relation to the contrast medium in all projections. In any patient having symptoms suggestive of ureteral colic, importance should be attached to any calculus density, no matter how small, occurring along the course of the ureter, particularly if it is found in the region of the distal part of the ureter. Conversely, in a patient with no symptoms at all suggestive of ureteral colic, small rounded calcifications in the lateral aspect of the pelvis can usually be disregarded since they undoubtedly represent phleboliths. Occasionally a ureteral calculus may cause no pain, so that catheter studies may be indicated if the density closely resembles a ureteral stone in a patient without pain.

RENAL "MILK OF CALCIUM"

The term "milk of calcium" refers to a suspension of fine sediment containing calcium that is observed most commonly in a calyceal diverticulum or hydrocalyx with little or no drainage or in a so-called pyelogenic or calyceal cyst.[87] Films exposed with the patient erect show a horizontal level indicating that the calcium is in suspension. The appearance is quite similar to that observed in the "milk-of-calcium" gallbladder. Similar suspension of liquid or semisolid calcium has been observed in association with renal cysts and rarely it has been seen associated with hydronephrosis; on upright films, several levels of calcium are noted in calyces.

There are certain findings in plain films that suggest the diagnosis. These include: *1*) a somewhat peripheral location as compared to the central location of stones in the collecting system; (2) an unusually large area; (3) circular, or nearly circular, configuration; (4) faint calcification, particularly in relation to size; (5) diminishing density gradually toward the periphery; (6) indistinct margins. When these findings suggest the possibility, an upright or decubitus film can be obtained to confirm the diagnosis.

NEPHROCALCINOSIS

"Nephrocalcinosis" is the term used to describe calcium deposits within the renal parenchyma. Calcium is usually concentrated in the medullary pyramids but may be scattered rather diffusely throughout the entire renal parenchyma; the amount of calcification may vary considerably. This lesion is found in association with several diseases characterized by abnormally high concentrations of calcium or phosphorus resulting in precipitation of calcium phosphate in healthy renal tissue. Primary hyperparathyroidism is the best example of this group and nephrocalcinosis occurs in approximately 25% of patients with the disease, but renal lithiasis is more common than calcinosis. When the latter occurs, tiny calcifications confined to the medulla are usually present, with occasional larger calcifications occurring in the renal pyramids. Hypercalciuria of undetermned cause, hyperchloremic acidosis, hypervitaminosis D, milk-alkali syndrome, sarcoidosis, renal tubular acidosis, hyperoxaluria, carcinoma metastatic to bone, regional enteritis with secondary enteric hyperoxaluria, and idiopathic hypercalcemia are other conditions producing nephrocalcinosis. Another group is represented by patients with renal disease in which calcium is precipitated in damaged tissue. Normal blood calcium levels are usually present in this group, which includes patients with such renal diseases as chronic pyelonephritis, chronic glomerulonephritis, lower nephron nephrosis, and injury of distal convoluted tubules due to various causes. In chronic pyelonephritis, unequal distribution of relatively large deposits occurs. Calcinosis is rare in chronic glomerulonephritis; when present the findings of tiny granular calcifications scattered throughout the cortices of small kidneys are very suggestive of the diagnosis. Medullary deposits are found in "sponge kidney."

Roentgen findings depend on the extent of calcification. This varies from faintly visible, milky, granular densities to stippled calcification in the renal papilla and cortex (Fig. 20-25). The finding is relatively rare and it has been shown that there are many instances of histopathologically proved renal calcification in which the calcium cannot be visualized radiographically in the living subject.

Films of good quality in the low-kilovoltage range (70 to 76 kVp) exposed before contrast media are given are necessary to demonstrate small amounts of

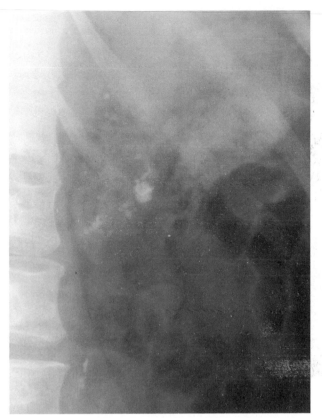

Fig. 20-25. Nephrocalcinosis. Note the stippled calcific densities overlying a rather small left kidney.

calcium. Coned views to include only the renal area as well as oblique views are often necessary, the latter to localize the calcium within the kidney. Tomography is also very helpful in demonstrating and localizing calcifications in the kidney. At times, calcification is seen on tomograms when it is not visible on the plain film.

Renal Tubular Acidosis

Nephrocalcinosis and nephrolithiasis are the radiographic findings in patients with renal tubular acidosis.[26] The nephrocalcinosis is manifest by dense calcium deposits in the medullary portion of the kidney. Those patients who lose calcium also have osteomalacia. The findings are chiefly in patients with distal tubular acidosis and not in those with the proximal form in whom there is only slight hypercalciuria. Radiographically, the dense medullary calcifications are somewhat similar to those observed in medullary sponge kidney, but the individual calcifications are larger in renal tubular acidosis and have less tendency to be oval or elongated than in medullary sponge kidney. Also, the calcification is somewhat more widespread in some patients.

INFECTIONS AND RELATED CONDITIONS

ACUTE PYELONEPHRITIS

There are few specific roentgenologic findings in the presence of acute pyelonephritis. Intravenous urography may be contraindicated during the acute phase, but a plain film may reveal some enlargement of the kidneys, particularly in severe acute infection. If excretory urography is carried out, findings in addition to those of renal enlargement suggest the disease. If the disease is unilateral, delayed appearance of contrast medium in the calyces and decreased excretion of contrast medium are easy to detect in the involved side when compared to the opposite, uninvolved side. There may be some dilatation and distortion of calyces, and papillary involvement indicated by irregularity is sometimes observed. The renal outline may be obscured in a local area, indicating spread of infection into or beyond the renal capsule. Ureteral enlargement may also be present, particularly in infants who also have more hydronephrosis than adults with acute infection. The dilatation (ileus) usually involves the proximal ureter. There may be longitudinal ureteral striations, parallel lines in the upper ureter, and similar involvement may be observed in the pelvis.[61]

Emphysematous pyelonephritis is a special form of acute pyelonephritis affecting diabetics or patients with urinary tract obstruction. The finding of gas in and around the kidney in an acutely ill patient suggests the diagnosis. The affected kidney usually does not function well. Gas-forming organisms recovered include *Escherichia coli* and *Proteus vulgaris*. Emphysematous pyelonephritis should be regarded as a complication of a severe necrotising infection, usually indicating extensive destruction of renal parenchyma, and having a poor prognosis.

RENAL ABSCESS

Acute suppurative infection of the renal parenchyma is usually hematogenous in origin and begins in the cortex. It is rare and unless recognized and treated early, there is often extensive destruction of renal parenchyma. The most frequent causative organsm

is the staphylococcus. When one or more small cortical abscesses develop in the parenchyma, no roentgen manifestation are present. If these small abscesses coalesce to form a large abscess, a plain-film roentgenogram often shows local enlargement of the kidney. The perirenal fat is blurred in the area of involvement so that the renal outlne tends to be indistinct. The involved kidney may be fixed during inspiration and expiration. The psoas muscle is often indistinct. There may be scoliosis with the concavity toward the involved side; this suggests the complication of perirenal abscess. Excretory urography is of value if there is enough function to outline the calyceal system. The findings are those of compression and displacement or obliteration of the calyces owing to the tumorlike mass produced by the abscess. The involvement may be local so that only one calyx is displaced, compressed, or obliterated. The other signs such as haziness of the renal outline and evidence of local enlargement are more clearly defined on the urogram than on a preliminary roentgenogram. Often the findings may indicate a mass that cannot be differentiated from other renal masses. The cortical abscess may break through into the collecting system, to appear as a cavity communicating with a calyx and simulating tuberculosis. A peripheral abscess may also break through the renal capsule and produce a perirenal abscess.

Clinical signs of infection may not be present in some patients, particularly when the course is prolonged and the infection is chronic. Therefore, the differentiation from tumor may be difficult; renal angiography is useful in making the distinction. Angiographic findings include late increased vascularity at the margin of the lesion, local stretching of the vessels over the mass, enlarged stretched capsular vessels if perirenal extension is present, absence of tumor vessels (no arteriovenous shunting indicated by early venous filling), presence of "inflammatory neovascularity," a nephrogram that is sometimes delayed and often mottled and loss of cortical definition. The term "inflammatory neovascularity" refers to an increased number of regular, often parallel, small vessels at the periphery of the abscess. The epinephrine response appears to be varied, according to some reports, but the inflammatory vessels contract in some patients to aid in differentiation from tumor vessels, which do not contract. A lucent defect at site of lesion, noted in the nephrogram, and a blush in the late capillary–early venous phase caused by the inflammatory neovascularity are also observed. Angiography permits differentiation in the majority of patients, but occasionally findings are equivocal;

gallium scanning and renal venography may be useful. The findings may simulate those of a necrotic, renal-cell carcinoma, however; therefore clinical findings are of great importance in the differential diagnosis.

RENAL CARBUNCLE

Renal carbuncle is distinguished from an abscess which is a local collection of pus in the renal parenchyma that may be fairly well encapsulated.[59] The carbuncle is a large conglomeration of many confluent abscesses. In the acute phase, plain films may show blurring of the renal outline and renal enlargement which may be local or general. On excretory urography and nephrotomography, the mass may be more clearly defined, with poor to complete nonvisualization of the collecting system. Calyces may be obliterated, stretched, or draped, and the nephrogram may show loss of the cortical–medullary junction in the area of involvement. Renal arteriography may show displacement of vessels with diminution in opacification and slow perfusion; at times the arterial branches will appear denuded. In the more chronic phase, the local mass is more clearly defined. Renal outline is more definite. There may be calcification within the mass. Renal function is usually better than in the acute phase, and there is displacement of the collecting system. On the nephrographic phase, an area of radiolucency is observed. Renal arteriography, at this time, may show an avascular mass or one with "inflammatory neovascularity." Differentiation from tumor may be difficult. Other studies such as renal venography and gallium scanning may be of value in these patients.

The clinical presentation of renal carbuncle may vary widely from an acute onset accompanied by sepsis to an insidious onset with vague symptoms. It must be differentiated from hypernephroma and from other inflammatory lesions, but at times the differentiation cannot be made except at operation.

PERIRENAL ABSCESS

Hematogenous infection may also result in perirenal inflammatory disease and abscess formation. The infection may actually arise in the perirenal area in addition to extending there as a complication of cortical abscess. Plain-film roentgenograms of perirenal abscess will show an absence of the perirenal fat shadow causing an indistinctness of the renal margin. When the abscess is confined within the perirenal (Gerota) fascia, the large space posterior and inferior to the kidney may fill with pus; this may be outlined as a mass that is confined chiefly to the infrarenal area, since the space is larger there than elsewhere. The lower pole of the kidney is obscured. Excretory urography may show upward, anterior, and either medial or lateral renal displacement depending on the site of the abscess. There may be some compression of the collecting system if the abscess is large. Fixation of the kidney by the infection is demonstrated on roentgenograms, exposed with the patient in the upright position, that show a failure of the normal descent. The psoas muscle shadow is enlarged and its margin blurred adjacent to the area of infection. Lumbar scoliosis with convexity away from the side of the lesion results from muscle splinting and is usually present. The diaphragm is often slightly elevated with areas of linear atelectasis in the basal lung manifested by small horizontal densities in the basal lung parenchyma.

Psoas abscess may displace the kidney and ureter, but does not ordinarily spread to involve the kidney (Fig. 20-26).

CHRONIC PYELONEPHRITIS (ATROPHIC PYELONEPHRITIS)

There has been much confusion in the literature regarding chronic pyelonephritis since the histopathologic findings do not distinguish this infection from a number of other diseases that cause similar histopathologic change. Furthermore, many patients with bacterial infection of the urinary tract do not develop morphologic changes in the kidney. The following criteria for the diagnosis of chronic, atrophic pyelonephritis were suggested by Hodson[60]: (*1*) The disease is centered in the medulla with scar eventually affecting the whole thickness of renal substance. (*2*) There is an irregular surface depression over the involved area. (*3*) The involved papilla is retracted with secondary dilatation of its calyx. (*4*) The dilated calyx has a smooth margin but variable shape. (*5*) Renal tissue adjacent to the involved area is normal or hypertrophied with a sharp definition between normal and abnormal. (*6*) Distribution is unifocal or multifocal, involving one or both kidneys. (*7*) There is decrease in size of the involved kidney.

Chronic bacterial infection of the kidneys usually starts as a focal process in the medulla, causing a localized area of fibrosis or scarring. As it progresses, the infection causes further scarring, resulting in loss of renal parenchyma, irregularity of the renal surface, and distortion of the calyx in the involved area. The calyces involved become clubbed. Renal

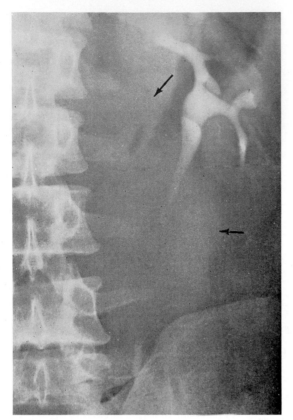

Fig. 20-26. Psoas abscess. Note the large psoas mass **(arrows)** which displaces the left kidney and upper ureter. It also compresses the ureter. This is a chronic abscess which is so well localized that the psoas shadow is clearly defined.

tissue between involved areas is normal or hypertrophied. Parenchymal loss may progress to the point where there are only a few millimeters of scar tissue between the capsule and the calyx. Unless there is obstruction or significant reflux the distribution of the lesions is uneven (Fig. 20-27).

According to Hodson[60] the disease usually begins in childhood, but it may not be recognized until early adult life. The earliest roentgen sign is a decrease in the amount of renal parenchyma, often in one pole of the kidney. Later the adjacent calyx or calyces exhibit clubbing. As the disease progresses, the findings become more generalized and are often bilateral but usually not symmetric. *Acute bacterial nephritis* in adults may produce a pattern of calyceal deformity that suggests papillary necrosis. Also it may produce focal calyceal clubbing and generalized renal atrophy that suggest the small, smooth kidney with papillary

necrosis usually associated with the more severe forms of analgesic uropathy. The roentgen appearance may be similar to that in chronic atrophic pyelonephritis except that the scarring does not extend to the renal capsule and, because of this, no irregularity of the renal surface develops. In other patients with adult-onset infection, focal scarring similar to that of chronic atrophic pyelonephritis, whch is presumably a childhood-onset disease, has been described.

As indicated, reflux as well as infection probably plays a part in the development of changes in the kidney, but it has also been shown that the scarring and atrophy are most marked in the areas in which there is intrarenal reflux in addition to the reflux into the collecting system. It is likely that infection plays a role in these patients also.

Hydronephrotic atrophy or obstructive atrophy of the kidney also causes progressive blunting of the calyces and narrowing of the renal parenchyma. However, this tends to be very symmetric in contrast to the irregular distribution of the scars of pyelonephritis. A similar appearance may be observed in patients with vesicoureteral reflux. Infection may be present in both of these conditions and it also can cause the focal parenchymal scarring which is found in pyelonephritis. When the disease begins in adult life, there is less scarring of the parenchyma, but the calyceal blunting is similar.

Renal angiography is frequently employed to assess the blood supply and is helpful in differential diagnosis. In pyelonephritis there is bilateral asymmetry of blood supply with decrease in caliber corresponding to the extent of the renal disease. The nephrogram phase outlines the irregularity of the cortical margin of the kidney. The intrarenal arteries are obliterated at the sites of severe disease and tend to be tortuous in areas of lesser involvement (Fig. 20-28).

XANTHOGRANULOMATOUS PYELONEPHRITIS

This form of severe chronic inflammation of the kidney is found predominantly in adult females. The clinical findings consist of a history of easy fatiguability and low-grade fever that may antedate urinary symptoms of dysuria, frequency, and a dull, aching flank pain sometimes associated with palpable flank mass. Recurrent attacks may occur. Calculi are common, and there may be parenchymal calcification. The disease is usually unilateral, but the opposite kidney is often involved by pyelonephritis. The pathologic process consists of granulomatous involvement

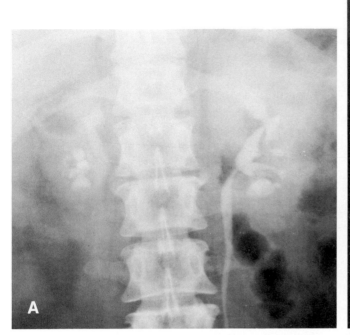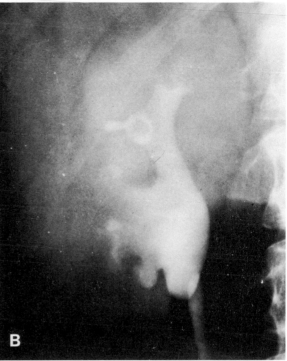

Fig. 20-27. Bilateral pyelonephritis. **A.** In the patient with chronic pyelonephritis, most of the calyces are blunted, some more than others. The right kidney is small, and the lower pole of the left kidney is also small due to parenchymal loss. **B.** In another patient with chronic pyelonephritis the upper pole calyces appear reasonably normal. Central and lower pole calyces are clubbed, and, on the initial film, marked decrease in lower pole parenchyma could be observed.

in the renal parenchyma, associated with foam cells, cholesterol slits, extensive fibrotic changes, and atrophic glomeruli. The process may be localized or involve the entire kidney; at times it may extend to produce a periureteric mass in the upper ureteral region. It may also extend to involve perirenal fat leading to the production of a fixed renal mass. Ureteropelvic junction obstruction may be a significant etiologic factor with secondary infection. *Proteus vulgaris* is commonly found in the urine but may not be the etiologic agent. Urographic findings consist of calyceal dilatation and blunting with irregularity of papillae, decreased cortical thickness, and ureteral deformity and stricture which may resemble changes due to extensive tuberculosis. In many, no function may be present. The kidney and psoas outlines may be indistinct. When obstructed, retrograde studies reveal dilatation and gross distortion of pelvis and calyces. In some patients a local mass resembling carcinoma is present; in others there is a poorly demar-

cated, diffuse mass, often associated wth greatly diminished or no renal function. The calculi are often staghorn in type, but small calculi may be present including obstructing ureteral stones. Angiography reveals displacement and stretching of intrarenal arteries with absence of small peripheral branches. Capsular and ureteric branches may be prominent. The nephrogram phase resembles that of hydronephrosis. In many instances the granulomatous mass cannot be differentiated from renal cell carcinoma by angiographic methods. CT scanning may be helpful if there is much xanthomatous material in the mass. Some authors suggest the use of renal venography in the differential diagnosis.

"PYELITIS" OF PREGNANCY

The term "pyelitis" is applied to renal infecton that sometimes accompanies pregnancy. Most pregnancies are associated with some degree of hydronephro-

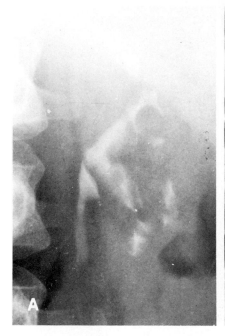

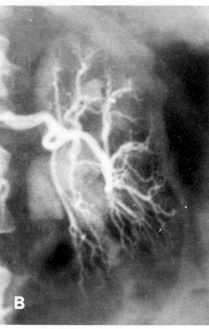

Fig. 20-28. Chronic pyelonephritis. **A.** Urogram shows poor filling and some distortion of the pelvis and calyces. **B.** Selective arteriogram shows tortuosity of arteries which appear pruned because the small branches are obliterated.

sis, usually more marked on the right than on the left. This is believed to be the result of mechanical obstruction caused by increased uterine size; it usually clears promptly following delivery. When infection occurs, however, urinary symptoms result from the combination of obstruction and infection. Urograms will outline the dilated calyces and there usually is associated dilatation of the ureter down to the brim of the pelvis (Fig. 20-29). Infection, when present, is usually of recent origin, so that there are no anatomic changes directly related to it unless the patient has had repeated infections in the past or has a chronic pyelonephritis.

RENAL PAPILLARY NECROSIS

Renal papillary necrosis, or necrotizing renal papillitis, is characterized by infarction of renal papillae, resulting in necrosis wth demarcation and sloughing of the involved tissue. The necrotic material may be passed in fragments or as a single mass or it may remain in the calyx. When it remains it may calcify peripherally to form a rather typical concretion. The cause of the necrosis is not clear but it is most likely that medullary ischemia can result from a number of insults. The condition is usually bilateral and may involve few or many papillae. It is more frequent in females than in males. Infection is not a prominent feature in necrosis associated with sickle-cell disease

or with phenacetin abuse. As has been indicated, the abuse of analgesics such as phenacetin over prolonged periods of time is associated with a chronic form of the disease and probably causes it. The large majority of cases of papillary necrosis of the chronic type probably are due to abuse of analgesics. A chronic form also may be associated with sickle cell disease (homozygous-S); with heterozygous S-hemoglobulinopathy, minimal papillary necrosis develops without signs or symptoms. Occasionally, chronic papillary necrosis may occur in patients having renal vein thrombosis and in those with obstructive uropathy in the absence of infection. An acute fulminating form associated with infection occurs in patients with diabetes mellitus and in patients with obstructive uropathy, particularly when infected. In the acute fulminatng form the diminished renal function may make excretory urography useless, but in most instances the diagnosis can be made with this examination. Therefore, retrograde pyelography is seldom necessary to make the diagnosis. Renal size is normal in the analgesic-abuse group of patients, but in those with the fulminant form the kidneys may be enlarged and kidney function decreased. Eventually there is enough destruction or atrophy to decrease renal size so that kidneys become small and smooth. Early papillary swelling may be very difficult to assess by excretory urography; the earliest manifestations suggesting the diagnosis are those of necrosis with

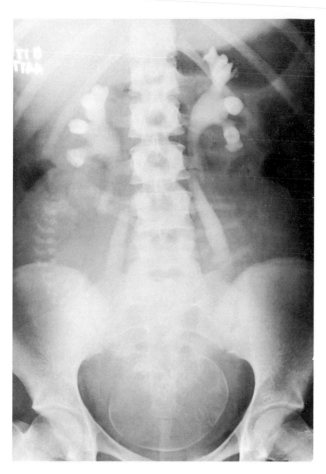

Fig. 20-29. Hydronephrosis in pregnancy. The patient had upper urinary tract infection. Combined with pregnancy, this condition is sometimes termed "pyelitis of pregnancy." A urogram obtained 2 months after delivery showed normal urinary tract. Hydronephrosis is present in the latter period of pregnancy in most gravid patients, but infection is relatively uncommon.

formation of tracts extending from the fornix into the parenchyma paralleling the long axis of the papilla. These manifestations may be difficult to evaluate since pyelointerstitial backflow may present the same appearance. If the necrosis with tract formation is evidenced in more than one film in the absence of calyceal dilatation, it is a suggestive early sign.

There are three forms of papillary sloughing. One is the central or partial type in which there is a tract extending from the tip of the papilla into it for varying distances. The shape of this cavity varies considerably from one calyx to another. In the second form, the necrosis occurs at the base of the papilla; this results in sloughing of the papilla. The papilla may remain in the kidney or be excreted. The third form of papillary sloughing is necrosis *in situ* in which the papilla remains attached, decreases in size, and eventually may calcify; it usually cannot be recognized until calcification occurs. A triangular radiolucent shadow ringed with a dense opaque shadow, the "ring shadow," may be observed when the necrotic papilla remains in the calyx. Eventually, a typical concretion may develop; it consists of a dense, calcified shell surrounding a radiolucent center. Late in the disease, scarring may result in some distortion. Ureteral involvement varying from slight irregularity to stricture formation is found occasionally. The diagnosis can be histopathologically confirmed if some of the sloughed material is passed and recovered from the urine. The increased incidence of the disease in recent years is attributed to its recognition as a chronic condition and possibly to increasing abuse of phenacetin.

BILATERAL ACUTE RENAL CORTICAL NECROSIS

This disease is characterized by bilateral, symmetric, ischemic necrosis of the renal cortex, with sparing of the medullary portion of the kidney and a thin rim of subcapsular cortex. It is a cause of acute renal failure which has terminated fatally in most instances. It may be associated with a number of antecedent conditions such as severe burns, multiple fractures, internal hemorrhage, severe infections, transfusions of incompatible blood, peritonitis, and others. It occurs frequently in pregnancy, often associated with abruptio placentae. With the advent of modern treatment, including hemodialysis, a number of patients have recovered partially from the disease and certain roentgen findings have been observed which suggest the diagnosis.

Initially the kidneys are usually enlarged. This is followed by a decrease in size of varying degrees. Faint cortical calcification in the form of a thin shell-like rim around the periphery of the kidney appears in 50 to 60 days following the onset. This is so faint that tomograms may be necessary for adequate visualization in patients suspected of having the disease. Tram-line or double-line calcification has also been reported. The calcification may extend into the interlobular septa, appearing as diffuse and punctate densities in the remaining cortical tissue.[92] The renal contour may be irregular and the calcification interrupted, depending upon the distribution of the disease. The renal pelvis and calyceal system appear normal but function is usually so decreased following recovery from the acute phase of the disease that retrograde pyelography is necessary to outline it.

PYELOURETERITIS CYSTICA, PYELITIS CYSTICA, AND URETERITIS CYSTICA

Pyeloureteritis cystica and ureteritis cystica are manifested by small suburothelial cysts which elevate the epithelium of the ureteral wall and sometimes the wall of the renal pelvis. These cysts appear as small radiolucent defects along the course of the ureter when it has been opacified by contrast substance. The appearance of multiple, small, mucosal filling defects is pathognomonic. The defects are usually more numerous in the upper ureter than elsewhere. They may become large enough to produce partial ureteral obstruction and range from microscopic size to 2 cm in diameter. Signs of active infection at urography are often present in these patients; or there may be a history of previous urinary-tract infection. Stones in the urinary tract are also common. The pathogenesis is unknown, however. The lesions may be unilateral (70%) or bilateral. The condition is relatively rare in the ureters and renal pelvis, and is extremely rare in the infundibula and calyces.

TUBERCULOSIS

Pathology

The kidney is involved by tuberculosis in a manner comparable to involvement of other organs. The infection is hematogenous. The organisms are filtered out by the glomerular capillary bed where they may produce small tubercles, most of which heal. Necrosis may occur and organisms migrate from the cortex to the region of the renal papilla where new tubercles are formed in the loop of Henle, leading to destruction of medullary tissue and ulceration. These early lesions are often multiple, but do not involve all the papillae. As the disease progresses, involvement of adjacent infundibula often leads to obstruction. Similar stricture formation leading to obstruction is found when there is ureteral involvement. The disease does not heal spontaneously and the destruction continues, producing irregular cavities adjacent to the calyces. Eventually this leads to virtual destruction of the entire kidney. If ureteral obstruction is not a factor, the kidney may gradually decrease in size or remain normal in size and gradually fill with caseous

material along with some calcium to form the so-called "putty kidney." If ureteral obstruction occurs before the kidney is destroyed and functionless, a large hydronephrotic kidney results, in which there are irregular cavities adjacent to the calyces. These anatomic changes are visible on urograms and form the basis for the roentgen diagnosis of renal tuberculosis. This diagnosis should always be confirmed, as in pulmonary tuberculosis, by demonstration of the organisms in the urine from the involved kidney. Even though the disease is hematogenous, the initial source, usually lung or bone, may not be detected. Calcifications in mediastinal and mesenteric nodes and in the liver and spleen may be present, however. Clinical evidence of renal involvement is unilateral in about 75% of patients even though the organisms have presumably been disseminated to both kidneys.

Roentgen Findings

The roentgen findings on plain-film examination are those of alteration in size of the kidney and calcification within it. These are nonspecific findings but may be suggestive, particularly if cloudy flocculent calcification outlines most of the renal shadow, indicative of extensive destruction of parenchyma—autonephrectomy. The calcification may be dense and irregular and lie within the renal outline, often in the cortical area. In the early stages of cortical involvement, no urographic findings are present and it is possible to have considerable parenchymal involvement without urographic change. The earliest finding is that of a slight irregularity of the involved calyx caused by ulcerative papillary lesions (Fig. 20-30). Further destruction is manifested by loss of the normal papilla and irregular ragged cavity formation (Fig. 20-31). Often this is associated wth a narrowing of the infundibulum to the affected calyx. The infundibulum may later become completely obstructed, so that the diseased area is not visible on retrograde pyelography. In this event there may or may not be enough function for visualization of the cavity on intravenous urography. Therefore, a careful evaluation of calyceal distribution in relation to the renal outline is necessary in all patients with suspected renal tuberculosis. Parenchymal destruction may result in cortical scarring with irregular narrowing of the parenchyma and irregularity of the renal outline. When the renal pelvis is involved, the mucosa is irregular owing to ulceration. Local constriction caused by fibrosis is also common and dilatation results when there is obstruction at or below the ureteropelvic junction. Ureteral involvement may result in stricture formation, which is often multiple; and mucosal infection can also produce small local nodules that appear as filling defects along the ureteral wall. The appearance is quite variable, ranging from that of a beaded to a corkscrew pattern to that of single or multiple strictures in some instances. In advanced involvement of the ureter it is common to find the ureter unusually straight, extending in a direct line downward from the renal pelvis to the pelvic brim without the usual slight curves seen in the normal ureter. The bladder, seminal vesicles, and vas deferens may also be involved in patients with renal tuberculosis. The bladder wall may be thickened and the bladder's capacity diminished. Tuberculous granulation tissue projecting into the bladder may resemble carcinoma in some instances. Irregular mottled calcification in these structures is a roentgen finding which suggests the diagnosis.

Urography is used in renal tuberculosis as a method of making an anatomic diagnosis, to be confirmed by bacteriologic study. It is also of value in following the renal lesion during treatment, in detecting complications, such as ureteral obstruction or infundibular obstruction, and in outlining the opposite kidney.

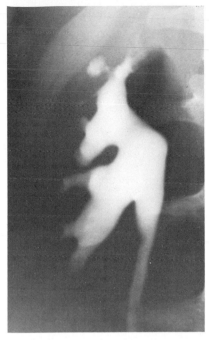

Fig. 20-30. Renal tuberculosis. The calyces of the upper pole are involved and are irregular as a result of adjacent parenchymal destruction.

Fig. 20-31. Renal tuberculosis. **A.** In this patient, extensive involvement with cavity formation is noted superiorly and centrally. There is also irregular narrowing of one of the upper central infundibula. **B.** This patient has a relatively normal right kidney, but the small, dense, irregular kidney on the left didn't change during urography. This left kidney represents the so-called "putty" kidney.

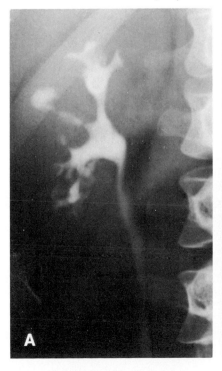

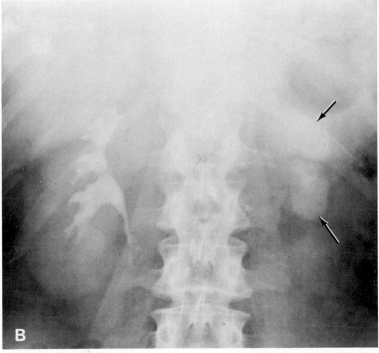

Differential Diagnosis

Differential diagnosis of calcium deposits must include consideration of renal calculi and nephrocalcinosis as well as cyst and tumor calcification. Calculi are usually more discrete and rounded than the calcification seen in tuberculosis. Tumor calcification often extends beyond the border of the kidney and tends to be less hazy and flocculent in appearance than in tuberculosis. Calcification in cysts occurs in the wall and tends to outline it in an arcuate form of varying size. This calcification also tends to extend beyond the shadow of the normal kidney. Urographic changes in chronic pyelonephritis consist of calyceal abnormality that may resemble early tuberculous involvement, but the change is usually more general than in tuberculosis. The same is true in renal papillary necrosis, which is usually bilateral and tends to be more extensive than renal tuberculosis. In some patients, granulomatous changes predominate to the extent that a renal mass is formed which must be differentiated from other renal masses. Usually other signs are present that aid in the diagnosis of these cases. *Brucellosis* may produce findings in the kidney identical to those due to tuberculosis, but it is very rare.

RENAL CANDIDIASIS

Because renal candidiasis usually occurs in patients who have a chronic illness or whose immune system has been altered, the following are important in its development: antibiotic therapy, prolonged use of indwelling intravenous catheters, treatment with adrenocortical steroids, chemotherapy, therapy with immunosuppressive agents, blood dyscrasias, diabetes mellitus, intravenous drug abuse, and chronic disease such as malignant neoplasm.[20] In systemic candidiasis, involvement of the kidney is common. Renal candidiasis may assume three forms that may be different stages of the same disease: (*1*) acute pyelonephritis in which the fungi proliferate in the renal tubules to form cortical and medullary abscesses with interstitial edema and renal failure; (*2*) a more chronic process with hydronephrosis and chronic pyelonephritis; and (*3*) disseminated candidiasis that involves several organs including the kidneys.[20] Excretory urography may demonstrate the multiple fungus balls in the renal pelvis and upper ureter in patients with pyelonephritis, but renal function may be so poor that retrograde studies are needed to reveal their presence. The appearance is one of shaggy, irregular filling defects in the renal pelvis, often extending into the infundibula and upper ureter. Acute papillary necrosis resulting from candidiasis is similar to that caused by other acute fulminating infections, except that, in candidiasis, more debris may be present in the calyces and pelvis representing the sloughed necrotic papilla plus the fungus balls (mycelia masses).

TRAUMA

The kidney lies in a well-protected area and is not frequently injured. In patients with chronic renal disease, however, relatively minor trauma may cause considerable damage. Direct force over the renal area is the usual cause of injury. Trauma to the kidney is manifested by hematuria, which may be gross or microscopic. When found after injury, blood in the urine indicates some type of renal damage or injury to the lower urinary tract. Intravenous urography, which is carried out as soon as possible after injury, using tomography and a high-dose technique is the primary radiographic diagnostic measure. It is a safe procedure and may lead to a definitive diagnosis of the extent of renal injury relatively soon after the trauma. Obviously, treatment for shock and other emergency measures may be necessary before urography is performed. The excretory nephrogram (1-to 2-minute film) is a good indicator of renal function. It is possible to check the presence and condition of the contralateral kidney if surgical removal of the injured kidney is contemplated. However, there are instances in which extravasation is not shown on the intravenous study because function is greatly reduced. Retrograde pyelography is indicated when excretion is poor or absent. The use of renal angiography in the posttraumatic period is indicated if there is diminution of renal function, since renal artery involvement with resultant thrombosis is not uncommon following renal trauma. It is the only method that will yield accurate information regarding damage to the blood supply. Renal arteriography is indicated whenever significant renal damage is present or suspected. Immediate surgical correction of the vascular lesion may prevent permanent renal damage in some instances. The anatomic and physiologic alterations produced by trauma may be caused by occlusive renal arterial change much more often than is now realized.

Selective renal arteriography is also used when (*1*) no function is demonstrated on the urogram, (2) preexisting renal disease is suspected, and (3) it is needed to confirm the integrity of the opposite kidney. This study is usually not necessary in patients with suspected renal trauma when the excretory urogram reveals no abnormality. Traumatic renal artery occlusion is the most serious injury and must be identified early by arteriography; thrombosis or avulsion may cause it.

The severity of parenchymal injury may vary from rupture of a calyx with extravasation into the parenchyma to more extensive fracture of parenchyma with subcapsular and parenchymal extravasation. When the injury is more severe the capsule may rupture with perirenal extravasation of urine as well as perirenal hemorrhage. These nonpenetrating injuries may be classified into: (1) contusion, (2) cortical laceration often with intrarenal hematoma, (3) calyceal laceration, and (4) fracture with laceration of capsule (a) with laceration of the collecting system and (b) without calyceal or infundibular laceration. Nonparenchymal injury, such as rupture of the renal pelvis and rupture of an anomalous extrarenal calyx, may also occur. Immediate surgical extirpation of the kidney may be needed in some instances when there is extensive fracture with retroperitoneal and intraperitoneal hemorrhage. The opposite kidney should always be studied by means of excretory urography before nephrectomy.

Roentgen findings depend upon the extent of injury. If perirenal hemorrhage is present the renal shadow, and sometimes the psoas shadow, is obliterated or enlarged. At times the hemorrhage remains localized in the perirenal area and produces a localized or generalized enlargement of the kidney that may simulate tumor. Rarely, calcification of a hematoma in or around the kidney may be seen as a late finding in renal trauma. Hemorrhage within the renal capsule may also produce local or generalized enlargement of the kidney. Accessory signs on plain-film roentgenograms are scoliosis, convexity to the opposite side indicating muscle spasm, gas in the small bowel in the vicinity of the injury caused by localized adynamic ileus, and fracture of an adjacent rib, vertebral body, or vertebral process. Urography demonstrates the amount of extravasation and may show calyceal compression and distortion caused by parenchymal and subcapsular accumulations of blood, urine, or both (Fig. 20-32). The amount of extravasation is not necessarily proportional to the parenchymal or vascular damage, however. Because posttraumatic distortion and stricture are important, urographic studies should also be carried out during

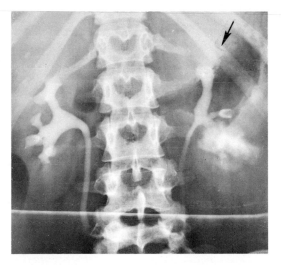

Fig. 20-32. Interstitial extravasation of opaque medium in the lower pole of the left kidney caused by trauma. The **arrow** indicates the site of a fracture of eleventh rib on the left.

or following convalescence to outline any residual deformity.

COMPLICATIONS OF RENAL TRAUMA

Persistent extravasation of urine through a calyceal or pelvic rent may result in a collection of urine in the perirenal space; this is termed a "urinoma" or "uriniferous perirenal pseudocyst." When the urinoma is large, the entire perirenal space bounded by Gerota's fascia may be filled. Sometimes the urinoma may be localized. When urine collects within the renal fascia, it causes elevation and lateral displacement of the lower pole of the kidney and medial displacement of the ureter. Since Gerota's fascia confines it, the urinoma appears as an elliptical mass oriented inferomedial to the lower pole of the displaced kidney.

An *arteriovenous fistula* may result from blunt trauma or from penetrating trauma. In many instances these fistulas close spontaneously while in others they persist and occasionally cause hematuria. A number have been reported to occur following renal biopsy. Angiography is required for determining the diagnosis. Hypertension, either transient or permanent, may result from occlusion or stenosis of the renal artery or one of its segmental branches. Subcapsular or perirenal hematoma followed by fibrosis with compression (Page kidney) may also cause hypertension. These abnormalities are usually diagnosed by renal arteriography, but the appearance secondary to hematomas may make differentiation from tumor very difficult. Calcification may develop in hematomas in and around the kidney as a late sequela of trauma. Strictures with resultant obstruction may also develop as a result of trauma to the urinary tract. Rarely, massive hemorrhage may occur late in patients with posttraumatic arteriovenous fistula or aneurysm. Selective arterial occlusion has been used successfully in some of these patients, obviating the necessity for surgery.

RENAL CYSTIC DISEASES

The classification of renal cystic diseases is difficult and there is much confusion in the literature because of many disagreements among pathologists. For our purposes the classification of Bernstein and Meyer[10] as modified by Elkin and Bernstein[37] is most useful (Table 20-3).

RENAL DYSPLASIA

Multicystic Kidney

Congenital multicystic disease of the kidney, Potter type II, is an uncommon disorder usually considered to be a severe form of renal dysplasia.[91] The bilateral form results in renal nonfunction, while the unilateral form, which is more common, carries a good prognosis if uncomplicated by other anomalies. There is absence of normal renal parenchyma, the pelvis is small or absent, and the ureter is hypoplastic, stenotic, or atretic. The nephrons which are present are hypoplastic with arrested development. The blood supply is variable. The kidney consists of a mass of cysts of varying size and is usually very large. Multicystic kidney is the most common cause of abdominal mass in infants. The opposite, uninvolved kidney is usually hypertrophied. At times the involved kidney is small and is distinguishable from aplastic kidney only by the presence of cysts. The disease usually presents as a unilateral flank mass in a healthy-appearing infant. The mass may be visible on the plain film. Excretory urography shows no function of the affected kidney and a normal appearance of the contralateral kidney. When the affected kidney is small it may be undetected until the patient reaches adult life.

When high-dose urography is used in infants, on the involved side the pattern of a large mass with opacification of vascularized strands of dysplastic tissue and cyst walls surrounding radiolucent cysts, no

Table 20-3. Classification of Renal Cysts*

I. *Renal Dysplasia*
  A. Multicystic kidney
  B. Focal and segmental cystic dysplasia
  C. Multiple cysts associated with lower urinary tract obstruction
II. *Polycystic Disease*
  A. Infantile polycystic disease
    1. Polycystic disease of the newborn
    2. Polycystic disease of childhood
      a. Congenital hepatic fibrosis
      b. Medullary tubular ectasia
  B. Adult polycystic disease
III. *Cortical Cysts*
  A. Trisomy syndromes
  B. Tuberous sclerosis complex
  C. Simple cysts
    1. Solitary
    2. Multiple
  D. Multilocular cysts
IV. *Medullary Cysts*
  A. Medullary sponge kidney
  B. Medullary cystic disease
  C. Medullary necrosis
  D. Pyelogenic cyst
V. *Miscellaneous Intrarenal Cyst*
  A. Inflammatory
    1. Tuberculosis
    2. Calculous disease
    3. Echinococcus disease
  B. Neoplastic-cystic degeneration of carcinoma
  C. Traumatic intrarenal hematoma
VI. *Extraparenchymal Renal Cysts*
  A. Parapelvic cyst
  B. Perinephric cyst

* Based on classification of Bernstein J. and Meyer R.[9] and Elkin M. and Bernstein J.[24]

nephrogram and no renal function are diagnostic, especially if cystoscopy and retrograde pyelography has demonstrated absence of one half of the trigone or atretic ureter on the involved side. Shell-like calcification may outline some of the cysts. Occasionally there will be delayed opacification of some of the irregular cystic spaces; there may be a small amount of functioning renal tissue scattered in the dysplastic kidney to account for this. Therefore, delayed films up to 24 hours should be obtained.[24] Arteriography reveals absence or hypoplasia of the renal artery, no nephrogram and no collateral vessels on the involved side. This is a benign lesion and need not be removed, once the diagnosis is made. Segmental multicystic renal dysplasia may also occur; in the cases reported by Daughtridge,[32] peripheral and central calcification was present which resembled that sometimes observed in renal-cell carcinoma. Arteriography revealed a sharply demarcated, avascular mass with no neovascularity. Differentiation from avascular tumor is difficult in this segmental form of the disease.

Multiple Cysts Associated with Lower Urinary Tract Obstruction

A number of conditions causing urinary obstruction in fetal life may lead to renal dysplasia. The most common occurrence is in infant males with posterior urethral valves. On excretory urography the dilated bladder, hydroureter, and hydronephrosis are observed if renal function is satisfactory. The cysts are not demonstrated, but their presence may distort the calyces and pelvis. They evidently develop *in utero,* and represent dilated cystic areas in the renal cortex resulting from increased pressure in the developing kidney caused by obstruction. Diagnosis usually is made on histologic study and rarely on urography.

POLYCYSTIC DISEASE

Infantile Polycystic Kidney

Infantile sponge kidney (polycystic disease of the newborn; congenital polycystic renal disease, Potter type I) is a rare condition, is genetically autosomal recessive, involves both kidneys and usually the liver. Most patients die in infancy with only an occasional one living into childhood, usually afflicted with hypertension and increasing renal insufficiency. The cortex and medulla are filled with radially oriented cysts.

There is bilateral renal enlargement which is easily detected on palpation of the abdomen in the newborn infant. Roentgen findings include massive renal enlargement which can be seen on the plain film. The nephrographic phase of the urogram is usually delayed and when it appears, tends to present a peculiar fuzzy, streaky, or striated appearance. Concentration is usually poor, so that the collecting system is faintly visualized at best. The kidneys retain the contrast medium for some time. Renal outlines are smooth and there is very little calyceal distortion.

Polycystic disease of childhood is a less severe form of polycystic kidney than that occurring in infants, and it allows a somewhat longer life span. The cystic lesions are not quite as extensive and the function is somewhat better than in the infantile form, but the streaky or striated appearance of the renal parenchyma is similar to that in the infantile disease.

Adult Polycystic Disease

The pathogenesis of renal polycystic disease is not completely understood, but the disease is transmitted as an autosomal dominant trait and is associated with cystic disease of the liver and occasionally of the pancreas and with berry aneurysms of the cerebral vessels. This anomaly, Potter type III,[91] results from an abnormal rate of division of tubules, irregular hyperplasia of portions of tubules left as the ureteral bud advances, and cystic dilatation of terminal portions of tubules. There is a reduced number of nephrons, which often are attached to collecting tubules at abnormal locations. The cysts maintain continuity with the nephron. They are numerous and often vary in size up to several centimeters. This sometimes results in marked renal enlargement and a lobulation or irregularity of renal outline is often present. Involvement is bilateral in 90% of these patients, but is not necessarily symmetric, so that renal enlargement is often unequal. The disease tends to be progressive, often leading to renal failure and death. When the diagnosis is made in an infant, it usually means that the condition is severe and the prognosis is poor. In adults the prognosis is generally fair unless there is marked renal failure. Urographic findings are usually characteristic enough to be diagnostic (Fig. 20-33). The nephrogram reveals numerous rounded, cystlike rarefactions and an irregular renal contour. In addition to the general renal enlargement there is extensive elongation of infundibula and calyces and irregular enlargement of calyces, but no calyceal clubbing is present. The infundibula often appear to partially surround the cysts of varying size and the calyces also are noted to stretch around the smaller cysts. This results in multiple, crescentic contours of the filled calyces and their infundibula and in elongation and thinning of infundibula. The minor calyces are often separated, but no irregularities are noted such as are found in infiltrating tumors. On plain-film roentgenograms the renal outlines are often indistinct despite the enlargement, owing to a decrease in perirenal fat. The bilaterality of the findings is of considerable aid in differential diagnosis. Rarely there may be curvilinear and central, amorphous calcifications in the renal cysts and also in the cysts of liver and spleen which may be present in this disease. There is a rough correlation between increasing renal size and the severity of the disease; an increase indicates increasing severity. Angiographic findings consist of stretching of vessels around the cysts and a decrease in density of the areas of involvement during the nephrographic phase of the examination. The

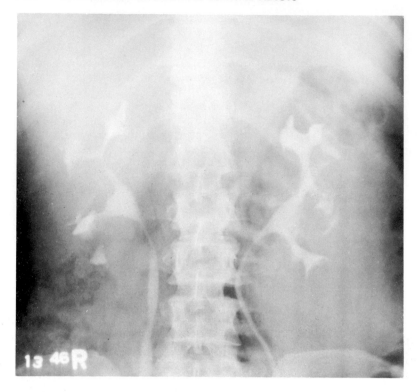

Fig. 20-33. Polycystic kidneys. Note the large, poorly defined kidneys and the stretching of infundibula and evidence of pressure on the calyces on both sides. The ureter on the left is displaced by a large cyst.

latter finding is quite characteristic and can be seen on nephrotomography.

CORTICAL CYSTS

Tuberous Sclerosis

Renal cysts are usually small and of tubular origin. Rarely, cortical cysts large enough to produce distortion have been reported. Angiomyolipoma of the kidney is found frequently in association with tuberous sclerosis. This tumor or hamartoma is described in the section on "Benign Tumors."

Simple Cysts

The simple renal cyst is often a silent lesion of little or no clinical importance but it is the most common unifocal renal mass. Cysts sometimes bleed and may become large enough to be noted as masses that can be palpated through the abdominal wall. In the latter instance they may cause renal damage by reason of their size, particularly if situated in a region where obstruction of the excretory system can occur. These lesions are usually unilateral and they may be solitary but often there are two or more and they may be so numerous that differentiation from adult polycystic

disease may be difficult. The roentgen findings depend on the location. The chief importance of the simple cyst is that it may simulate a tumor in its appearance. Plain-film roentgenograms may outline a smooth, local enlargement of the kidney. Occasionally (in 2% to 3%) there is a thin shell of calcium outlining the cyst wall or a portion of it (Fig. 20-34). It is much more common to see curvilinear calcifications in tumors of the kidney than in cysts. The cysts may reach massive size and actually dwarf the kidney (Fig. 20-35). Differentiation between a cyst and a tumor ordinarily cannot be made by plain-film study. Urographic findings consist of crescentic defects and stretching of the infundibula and calyces when the lesion arises close to the calyces. When the cyst arises further away, there is less calyceal change and when the cyst is in a subcapsular position there is little or no pressure deformity on the pelvis or calyces. The changes caused by a cyst are usually less marked than those produced by a tumor of similar size and location. There is often less distortion of calyces with cysts than with tumor.

The "claw" sign is thought by many to be very valuable in the identification of renal cysts. It consists of a triangular clawlike projection of renal parenchyma observed on the nephrographic phase of the renal angiogram or on nephrotomography (Fig. 20-36). The

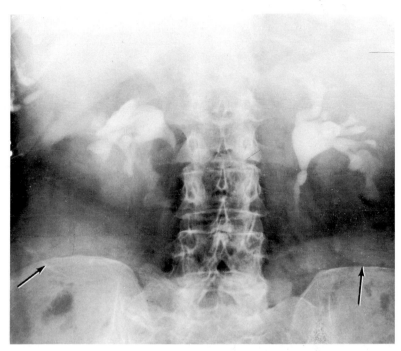

Fig. 20-34. Bilateral renal cysts. Note the relatively large size of the cysts with a faint rim of calcification on the right. **Arrows** outline the inferior aspects of the cysts.

following signs, when all are present, are quite reliable: (*1*) The lesion is peripheral so that at least one-fourth of its wall is visible. (2) The wall is very thin and smooth. (3) The claw sign is present. (4) The mass is lucent compared to the adjacent parenchyma and sharply demarcated from the renal parenchyma. (5) The entire wall is well visualized. If no exceptions to these signs are made, the lesion most likely is a cyst. Even if all of them are present, many physicians would do a cyst puncture or use ultrasound for confirmation. Following urography or arteriography, a small amount of iodine may enter a cyst and may cause a decrease in contrast between cyst and parenchyma, leading to more difficulty in differentiating the cyst from a tumor. Angiographic findings include displacement of vessels around a clearly defined, smoothly rounded, thin-walled mass, nonopacification of the mass during the nephrogram phase, and absence of abnormal ("tumor") vessels. For further discussion on the differentiation of cysts and tumors see the listing entitled "Renal Cyst" in the section entitled "Adenocarcinoma."

Multilocular Cysts

This condition is very rare. It consists of unilateral solitary cysts which contain numerous loculi that do not intercommunicate or connect with the renal pelvis. This abnormality is usually found in childhood.

Fig. 20-35. Moderate-sized cyst in the lower pole of the left kidney outlined by **arrows.** It produces some distortion of the lower pole calyces and infundibula. On the initial film the cyst showed less density than did the upper pole of the kidney where there was a good dense nephrogram.

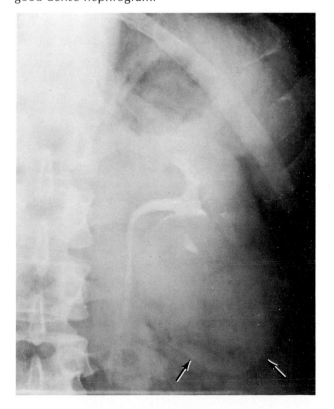

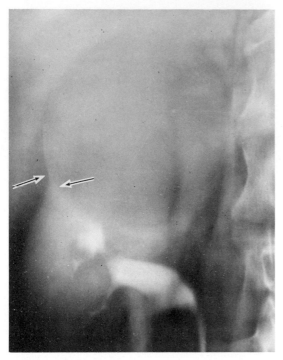

Fig. 20-36. The claw sign of a renal cyst **(arrows).** Nephrotomogram clearly outlines the smooth wall of the radiolucent cyst adjacent to the density of the opacified parenchyma.

The remainder of the kidney is normal. Potter classifies this lesion as a localized form of type II cystic disease (multicystic renal dysplasia). Others believe it to be a benign neoplasm, a multilocular cystic nephroma. Rarely, diffuse calcification is present, resembling that in renal-cell carcinoma, which makes differentiation prior to surgery virtually impossible. Abdominal mass is the major presenting complaint. Roentgen findings resemble those of simple cyst and include visible mass on the plain film. Distortion of the pelvis and calyces, depending on the size and location of the cystic mass, is noted on the urogram. Arteriography shows the mass to be avascular and vessels around it may be stretched, but no neovascularity or "tumor stain" is demonstrated.

MEDULLARY CYSTS

Medullary Sponge Kidney

Medullary sponge kidney is a form of cystic disease involving the medulla of the kidney. It has also been called precalyceal canalicular ectasia, renal tubular ectasia, cystic disease of the renal pyramids, cystic dilatation of the collecting tubules, and multiple cysts of the renal medulla. It is more frequent in males (about 2:1) than females; it has been reported in siblings but does not appear to be hereditary. The changes are confined to the renal medulla and consist of dilatation and cyst formation involving the collecting tubules in the renal pyramids. Calculi are frequently found in the cysts. The condition may be limited to a single pyramid, but is usually more extensive and is usually bilateral, but not necessarily symmetrical. Renal enlargement may be present when the lesions are general. The defect apears to be a developmental one involving the formation of the collecting tubules, but some authors believe that it is an unusual form of polycystic disease or related to it. Function is usually preserved and the disease does not appear to progress. However, there may be morbidity caused by infection and colic or both when calculi are passed. In the advanced disease, the extensive cyst formation in the medulla resembles a sponge. Microscopically the rounded, elongated, or irregular cysts present a varied appearance. The epithelium varies from transitional to squamous or columnar, normal tubules are reduced or absent, and some degree of inflammatory change is usually present. The cysts may contain calculi or masses of calcified debris.

The disease is usually discovered in persons of middle age, but has been found in children. Clinical symptoms may be absent, but recurrent infection results in pyuria and fever. Hematuria is common and renal colic may be the presenting symptom. Medullary sponge kidney has been associated with hyperparathyroidism in several instances. The mechanism is not certain, but the parathyroid adenoma in this condition may be secondary to a disorder of excretion of calcium by the abnormal kidneys and not a primary disease.

The roentgen findings are quite characteristic, even though the extent of the disease varies considerably. The plain film demonstrates the calculi when present. Their position and appearance is often diagnostic. The calculi are usually multiple, small, smoothly rounded or oval and occur in clusters or in a fanlike arrangement in the renal pyramids (Fig. 20-37). Intravenous urography is a better method of examination than retrograde pyelography, since the dilated tubules may not fill in a retrograde manner. In the urogram the dilated tubules are seen to be opacified unless infection has impaired renal function. Minimal dilatation produces a fine striated appearance; with increasing dilatation the appearance becomes more cystlike, with rounded or elongated cavities enlarging and often distorting the papilla and minor calyx (Fig. 20-37 and 20-38). Adjacent calyces may show a considerable difference in the degree of involvement. There is usually no difficulty in the roentgen diagnosis of typical sponge kidney, but in some instances pyelotubular backflow, renal tuberculosis, renal papillary necrosis, and nephrocalcinosis must be considered in the differential diagnosis.

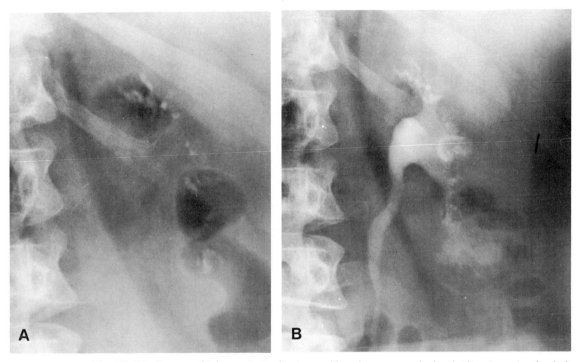

Fig. 20-37. Sponge kidney. **A.** Preliminary film shows mottled calcifications in the left kidney. **B.** Urogram of the patient shown in **A** demonstrates the relationship of the calcifications to several of the calyces. These calcifications are in dilated tubules in the renal papillae.

Fig. 20-38. Sponge kidney. **A.** Note calculi in typical medullary location. **B.** In addition to the calcifications, some dilated tubules are noted on this excretory urogram.

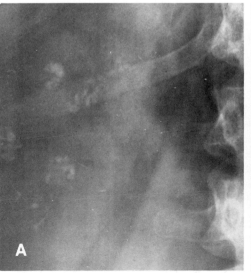

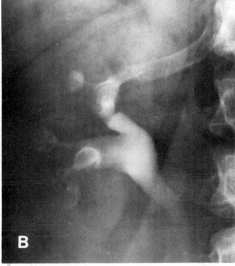

Medullary Cystic Disease (Nephronophthisis)

Nephronophthisis (familial juvenile nephronophthisis, medullary cystic disease of the kidney) is a rare disorder of unknown origin usually found in children and young adults. Anemia, polydipsia, polyuria, salt-wasting, and progressive uremia develop insidiously. Growth retardation, bone deformities, and hypocalcemic tetany occur in young patients. Urine has a low, fixed specific gravity with absence of protein or formed elements. Histopathologic findings consist of alternating areas of cystic dilatation and atrophy in the proximal and distal tubules with marked thickening of the basement membrane. Interstitial fibrosis with round-cell infiltration is prominent. Glomeruli show minor focal thickening early, progressing to sclerosis and periglomerular fibrosis.

Urographic study has been of limited value because of poor function, but, with high-dose urography and nephrotomography, minor calyceal blunting and uniform contraction of the kidneys are visible. In some patients, cystlike areas of lucency may be observed on nephrotomography. If these changes are correlated with the clinical and laboratory findings, the diagnosis should be suggested.

Renal angiography shows marked cortical-thinning, multiple cysts that spare the thin outer cortex, which is undulating because of the numerous cysts that also displace vessels. The cortex is best seen in the nephrogram phase of angiography.[80]

Renal Medullary (Papillary) Necrosis

See section on "Infections and Related Conditions" in this chapter.

Pyelogenic or Calycine Cysts

The term "pyelogenic" or "calycine" cyst (calyceal diverticulum) refers to the small cystlike spaces that often communicate with a calyx, but that occasionally are observed on urography to opacify despite no apparent connection with the adjacent calyx. This lesion may be a true congenital cyst, but cystlike structures of similar appearance may result from inflammatory destruction of parenchyma adjacent to a calyx or from inflammatory obstruction of a calyx. The diagnosis is made on intravenous urography when a small, rounded space fills with opaque medium (Fig. 20-39). The cysts are filled by their own tubules and so are visible despite lack of apparent communication with the calyceal system. In contrast

to the cysts in the renal pyramids as found in sponge kidney, the calycine cysts apparently arise from the fornix of the calyx and occur laterally rather than centrally in relation to the papilla. Although there is a difference of opinion as to the nature of the cysts that do not appear to communicate with the collecting system, these cysts are of little clinical significance unless infected and usually represent an incidental finding on urography. Surgical intervention is rarely necessary. Calculi are frequently formed in the cysts and are visible on plain roentgenograms. Rarely, milk of calcium is observed, with a fluid level evident on an upright film (Fig. 20-40).

EXTRAPARENCHYMAL RENAL CYSTS

Parapelvic Cysts

Parapelvic cysts are relatively rare and, unlike the simple renal cysts, they do not lie within the renal parenchyma. They are located and probably originate in the hilus of the kidney in close proximity to the pelvis and major calyces. Their origin is obscure. Some authors believe them to be of lymphatic origin; others believe that they are congenital cysts which arise from embryonic rests or from remnants of the wolffian body or from mesonephric remnants.

Roentgen findings are those of a mass in the renal hilus which causes compression and displacement of the pelvis and distortion and displacement of the major calyces and infundibula. Mild local caliectasis may result from partial obstruction resulting from compression. They do not contain calcium. The renal vascular pedicle may be displaced and distorted by the mass. They resemble lipoma of the renal hilus or lipomatosis when the latter results in a hilus mass.

Since there is no renal parenchymal interface with this type of cyst, the nephrographic phase of arteriography or nephrotomography is somewhat different than that seen in the simple cyst. The parapelvic cyst appears as a spherical mass of lesser density than the opacified renal parenchyma adjacent to it surrounded by a halo of fat that is more radiolucent than the cyst. When this halo of fat can be clearly seen to outline a smooth, round mass, the diagnosis can be made with a high degree of certainty (Fig. 20-41).

Perinephric Cyst (Pararenal Pseudocyst; Urinoma)

Pararenal pseudocyst is a term used to describe a complication of renal or ureteral injury. Pararenal pseudohydronephrosis, hydrocele renalis, hygroma

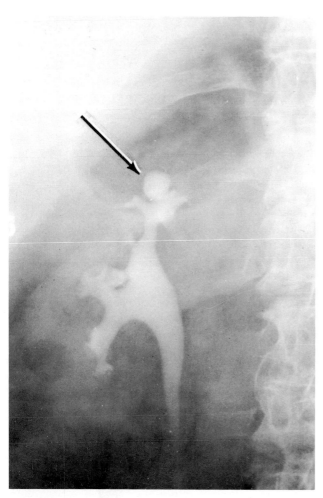

Fig. 20-39. Calycine cyst **(arrow).** The cyst communicates with one of the calyces of the upper pole.

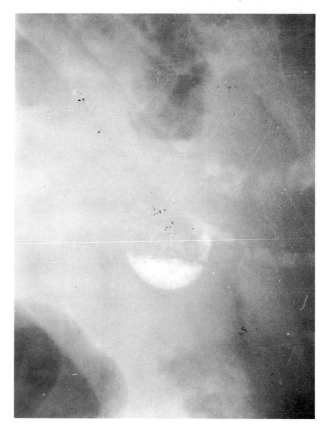

Fig. 20-40. Milk of calcium in a renal cyst. This film, exposed with the patient in the upright position, shows calcium, that is somewhat granular in appearance, in a cyst located in the central portion of the left kidney. There is also evidence of calcium in the cyst's wall.

perirenalis, perirenal cyst, and perinephric cyst are synonyms. Persistent extravasation of urine or blood or both following accidental trauma or surgery may produce a vicious cycle of extravasation, compression of the pelvis or upper ureter, and resultant hydronephrosis which may lead to eventual loss of renal function. Roentgen findings consist of a mass adjacent to the kidney, usually below it. The mass often displaces the kidney upward and rotates it laterally. Usually a definite line of separation between the mass and the kidney is observed. Intravenous urography may opacify the mass (if contrast extravasates into it) and will reveal the displacement of the ureter and kidney or both. Retrograde study may be necessary to confirm the diagnosis. This complication is

rare, but is one reason why follow-up urography is necessary in patients with renal trauma.

ECHINOCOCCAL (HYDATID) CYSTS

The kidney may be involved in patients with echinococcal infestation with formation of cysts similar to those noted in the liver and other parenchymatous organs. The cysts may have a calcified wall visible on plain-film study. Calcification occurs in 50% to 80% of these patients. The calcification may be similar to that found in tumors or cysts or may resemble renal calculi. Cysts are pear-shaped or round and may be closed, although most of them eventually open into a calyx and can be outlined by opaque medium upon urography and pyelography. Often the large cyst contains daugher cysts that are smaller and resemble a

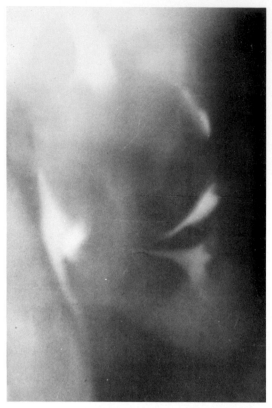

Fig. 20-41. Halo sign of a parapelvic cyst. Nephrotomogram shows ill-defined radiolucency caused by compressed renal sinus fat surrounding the smoothly rounded cyst in the renal hilus.

grapelike cluster of masses extending into the larger cyst or adjacent to it. The cysts deform the renal outline and calyceal system in a manner similar to the deformity produced by simple cyst. They do tend to obliterate the minor calyces and deform the major calyces to a somewhat great extent, however. They may reach very large proportions, and result in considerable compression of renal parenchyma and distortion of calyces. The discharge of daughter cells into the renal pelvis can produce colic. This discharge can be retroperitoneal and intraperitoneal also. The findings are those of renal mass and are not pathognomonic. When the cyst communicates with the collecting system, it may be seen to fill on excretory urography, so that the grapelike clusters of daughter cysts within it are visible—a highly suggestive sign.

Angiography may not be very helpful; it does demonstrate a thick wall and an avascular center, exclud-

ing the possibility of a benign cyst and suggesting the possibility of a tumor.

The cystlike lesions found in tuberculosis, neoplasms, and the like, are described in the appropriate sections.

RENAL VASCULAR ABNORMALITIES

RENAL ARTERY ANEURYSM

Aneurysms of the renal artery are not common, but are well known to radiologists because they have been observed to contain calcium in a high percentage of reported cases. In recent series in which angiography has been used to study the renal artery, the figure has changed. It is likely that no more than 25% to 30% of these aneurysms contain enough calcium to be roentgenographically visible. The diagnosis can usually be made on plain-film studies in the calcified group. The rounded, ring-contoured, calcified aneurysm maintains a constant relationship to the renal pelvis in various projections. About two-thirds are located at the bifurcation of the renal artery and one-third in the segmental branches. About one-half of those involving segmental arteries are intraparenchymal. They may be congenital, caused by atherosclerosis, or posttraumatic (often false aneurysms). Systemic hypertension is present in about 15% of patients with aneurysm of the renal artery. Angiography can be used for confirmation and is the only means of diagnosis when the aneurysm is not calcified. Bilateral renal aneurysms are relatively common (about 20%) so arteriography is indicated on the opposite side when an aneurysm, either calcified or noncalcified, is found on one side. In general the calcified aneurysms do not tend to rupture, but the incidence of rupture of uncalcified aneurysms is in the range of 25%. Because of the threat of rupture, renovascular hypertension, arterial thrombosis, or renal infarction, surgical repair should be considered for patients with noncalcified renal artery aneurysms.

POLYARTERITIS NODOSA

Multiple, small, intraparenchymal renal aneurysms are observed in polyarteritis nodosa. Renal involvement occurs in 80% to 100% of these patients. Similar microaneurysms are present in other viscera involved by this disease. In the kidney the multiple, small aneurysms involving the interlobar and accurate arteries are associated with scarring which results from thromboses and infarctions. The aneurysms may rupture to produce renal hemorrhage.

The infarcts produce pain and hematuria. Renal angiography outlines the aneurysms and its use is essential for making diagnosis. At times the small aneurysms found in this disease may regress spontaneously.

RENAL ARTERIOVENOUS FISTULA

Renal arteriovenous fistulas may be congenital or acquired and there are some in which the etiologic background is undetermined; these may be termed "idiopathic." The congenital malformations may be very large, and result in high-output cardiac failure, while others are very small and are of little, if any, clinical significance. Most arteriovenous fistulas in the kidney are acquired, especially following percutaneous biopsy, but others follow blunt or penetrating renal trauma or surgical procedures in the renal area, and some are secondary to renal neoplasms. Renal arterial disease occasionally may result in an arteriovenous fistula. Many of those formed following trauma, including that due to percutaneous renal biopsy, heal spontaneously. When these fistulas persist, hematuria and hypertension may occur as complications. Urograms and plain films are usually not very helpful in determining the diagnosis, but plain films may reveal calcification and, in the case of a large arteriovenous fistula, the collecting system may be displaced by the mass produced by the fistula. Arteriography reveals the fistula along with early venous filling and often it demonstrates venous dilatation and tortuosity secondary to the arteriovenous shunt. Renal function may be diminished on the side of involvement, depending on the severity of the shunt.

RENAL ARTERY OCCLUSION

Renal arterial occlusion is most commonly caused by embolism in patients with cardiac disease. Thrombosis also occurs, most often secondary to atherosclerosis, but sometimes it is caused by trauma. Regardless of cause, when a renal artery is occluded function is lost. Partial function may occasionally return in a year or more. The roentgen findings in acute renal arterial occlusion consist of urographic evidence of a nonfunctioning kidney of normal size in which retrograde pyelography shows no abnormality. A peripheral rim of opacified cortex may be observed during the nephrographic phase. Presumably this cortex is supplied by the collateral circulation of the renal capsule. Acute segmental infarction may be responsible for either complete nonvisualization on in-

travenous urography or a local failure of calyceal filling. The cause for the complete loss of function in these patients is not certain. It may be that a shower of small emboli accompany the segmental embolic block.[36] Following total renal infarction without infection the kidney decreases in size and usually remains nonfunctioning. Retrograde study reveals decrease in size of the calyceal system consistent with renal size. The late findings in segmental infarction are those of local decrease in size which may distort the kidney locally and cause an irregular contour. Renal arteriography is used to confirm the diagnosis in all types of arterial occlusion. Both left and right sides should be studied because involvement is frequently bilateral.

RENAL VEIN ANOMALIES

Valves are occasionally found in renal veins as has been indicated previously. There are a few reports of an anomaly of the left renal vein which consists of the formation of a venous ring around the aorta. Radiographically it is recognized as a bifurcation of the renal vein as it courses from the kidney to the vena cava.

RENAL VEIN THROMBOSIS

Thrombosis of the renal vein occurs more frequently in children than in adults. In adults, direct invasion, or extrinsic pressure by tumor, and thrombosis of the inferior vena cava are among the more frequent causes. Ileocolitis is considered the chief cause in children, but any condition which produces dehydration, acidosis, and hemoconcentration may be the inciting factor. In infants who have had intrauterine renal vein thrombosis, a faint lacelike calcification corresponding to intrarenal vascular structures may be observed at birth on plain-film study. Because diagnosis is difficult from a clinical standpoint, radiographic methods are of prime importance. The roentgen findings depend on the rapidity of the occlusion and its relation to the development of venous collaterals. In the acute, complete thrombosis with infarction and perirenal hemorrhage, the kidney is enlarged and intravenous urography shows no function. The renal arteriogram shows delayed flow through narrow, stretched, interlobar arteries. Opacification of the parenchyma is poor and the nephrogram phase is prolonged. Venous drainage cannot be identified. When the acute occlusion is partial, the kidney also becomes enlarged. Function as demonstrated by excretory urography is gradually regained in about 2

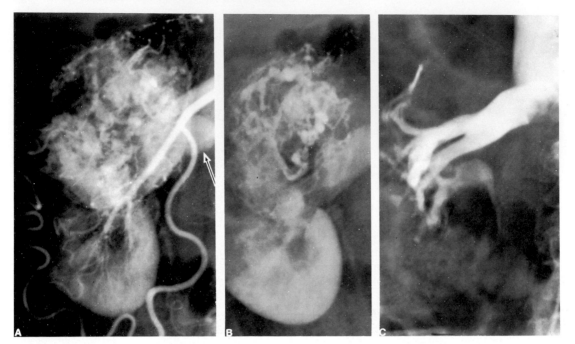

Fig. 20-42. Renal vein thrombosis. **A.** Renal arteriogram at 2 seconds shows a large vascular mass in the upper pole of the right kidney. Note the renal vein below the artery **(arrow). B.** Five-second film shows a continued opacification of the tumor and clear definition of the renal vein. **C.** Renal venogram. The tumor thrombus is clearly defined in the inferior aspect of the renal vein at its junction with the vena cava which is now outlined above the renal vein. Although there is partial obstruction of the renal vein, no collaterals are visible.

weeks as venous collaterals develop. In gradual occlusion, collateral circulation has time to develop and the roentgen examination may show no abnormality whatsoever. When renal arteriography is carried out, the venous phase may show extensive venous collaterals.

When renal vein thrombosis is suspected, excretory urography should be performed. If the diagnosis is supported by absence or decrease of function and increase in renal size, renal arteriography should be the next step in the radiographic study of the patient. Evaluation of the renal arterial supply, intrarenal pathologic state, venous collaterals, or absence of renal vein filling and possibly demonstration of the actual obstructive site can all be accomplished with proper timing of the examination (Fig. 20-42).

RENOVASCULAR HYPERTENSION

Renal arterial disease resulting in decreased arterial blood supply to the kidney long has been recognized as a cause of hypertension. Advances in vascular surgery have focused attention on this cause of hypertension, since surgical correction may relieve or diminish the severity of the disease. It is estimated that there are correctable renal lesions in 3% to 5% of hypertensive patients. Although numerous studies have been made, exact figures on the incidence are not available.

Certain clinical features have been used to indicate that renal artery stenosis is the cause of hypertension. They include (1) unexplained hypertension in a child or young adult or in a patient over age 50, especially if there is no family history of hypertension; (2) sudden onset of malignant hypertension in a patient known to have been mildly hypertensive in the past; (3) hypertension in a patient with known atheromatous disease; (4) the presence of an upper abdominal bruit; and (5) history of unexplained flank pain or renal trauma that suggests the possibility of renal vascular accident. However, the only finding which appears consistently in patients with renovascular hypertension is an upper abdominal high-pitched continuous bruit. Roentgen methods are essential in the study of patients with suspected renovascular hypertension. The excretory urogram and the isotope renogram are used as screening tests. There is some difference of opinion as to their relative value but most investigators use the urogram. The radioisotopic renogram may be used to detect decreased or delayed renal vascular flow and decreased functioning renal mass, therefore it is useful as a qualitative test of the amount of function in the two kidneys and also in following individual renal function. Combined with excretory urography in a patient with an upper abdominal bruit, it will detect nearly all patients who will benefit from correction of renovascular lesions.

The excretory urogram is modified in order to make it a more useful test in unilateral renal artery stenosis. The most common modification is the rapid-sequence method, with films exposed every minute for 3 to 5 minutes after rapid injection. The injection of the contrast substance should be rapid and no compression device is used. After the 5-minute film a compression band may be used for a 10- and 15-minute study, then removed if later films are indicated. Recently, the use of urography plus a diuretic given intravenously has been tried as a basis for screening. Reportedly, the diuretic causes normal kidneys to enlarge more than 10% in area, while it causes kidneys with renal artery stenosis to enlarge less than 5%. With furosemide as the diuretic, a high incidence of false positives and indeterminate results in patients without renal artery stenosis renders this screening method relatively valueless.[118]

The following urographic findings are significant in the diagnosis of renovascular hypertension and the presence of any one or a combination of them constitutes a positive study: (*1*) Since the right kidney is normally shorter than the left, a difference in renal size of 1.5 cm if the right is larger than the left or of 2 cm if the left is larger than the right kidney. (2) Appearance time: delay in appearance or a distinct decrease in volume of medium excreted; this was found to be the single most valuable sign in the Cooperative Study.[12] (3) The presence of vascular indentations on the upper ureter or pelvis or both which indicates development of collateral circulation. (4) Hyperconcentration observed on the later films manifested by a decrease in volume seen as lack of distention of pelvis and calyces and a simultaneous increase in density on the involved side. In evaluating density, equal volumes should be compared, since a large volume of low concentration of iodine may appear as dense as a small volume of high concentration. (5) Local atrophy (caused by segmental infarct), often best visual-

ized on a tomogram as areas of decreased concentration in the parenchyma. Even in patients with bilateral renal artery disease the findings just enumerated are pertinent, since the stenosis is usually more severe on one side than on the other and screening tests give positive results in about the same percentage. Urography is a safe, simple and inexpensive screening procedure, but an incidence of 10% false negatives was found in the Cooperative Study.[12] The incidence of false positives is not excessive, but the method does not permit discrimination between favorable and unfavorable responses to surgical procedures.

In a cooperative study of bilateral renovascular disease,[13] 60.7% of 250 patients had abnormal findings on urographic examination. When renovascular disease is nearly equivalent bilaterally, urograms are relatively insensitive, but the urogram was often helpful in making the decision between unilateral or bilateral operation.

Since only 3% of patients with hypertension have renovascular disease as a cause, many observers believe that screening should be abandoned or possibly used only in young patients (under 35 years), particularly if they have a bruit.

When the screening tests are positive or suggestive, anatomic localization of the renal-artery lesion by means of arteriography is indicated. This permits the study of the arteries on the "normal" side as well. Actually, the obstructed kidney is protected by the low pressure resulting from the stenotic lesion and is often more normal than the contralateral one.

Arteries may be studied by:

1. Translumbar aortography—direct aortic puncture. This method is rarely used in our department and does not permit selective studies.

2. Catheter techniques in which the percutaneous transfemoral method of Seldinger or direct arterial cut-down may be used. The opaque medium is injected into the aorta near the renal artery orifices. This is the best method for detecting multiple renal arteries. This is followed by selective renal arteriography in which the renal artery is catheterized and a small amount of medium is injected directly into it.

Arteriosclerotic disease is the most common cause of renal artery obstruction. Atheromatous plaques in the aorta may encroach on the orifice of the renal artery. When the renal artery is involved, single or multiple defects may be visible. Usually the lesion occurs in the proximal portion of the renal artery, very near its origin. It may cause a concentric or eccentric constriction of the artery. Poststenotic dilatation is common and aneurysm may be present. Diffuse involvement results in multiple irregularities in the lumen. The lesions are more common in males (60%) than in females (Fig. 20-43). The left renal artery is more often involved in a ratio of 3 to 2 when unilateral. Approximately one-third of patients have bilateral artery disease.

The other major cause of stenosis leading to renovascular hypertension is fibromuscular dysplasia (hyperplasia).[55] This disease may be seen in persons of any age, but is most common in young adult women (55% of the focal form and 85% of the multifocal disease is found in females). The lesions are bilateral in nearly 50% of patients. When unilateral, the right renal artery is involved in approximately 75% of patients. The process tends to involve the main renal artery and extend into its branches. The characteristic sites are in the middle and distal portions of the renal artery in contrast to the atherosclerotic involvement which is at or very near the origin of the artery (Fig. 20-44). Fibrous stenosis involves either intima or adventitia and perivascular tissues, while fibromuscular stenosis involves the media.

Kincaid and associates[65] classify fibromuscular dysplasia into the following gross morphologic forms:

1. Multifocal (62.4% of 125 patients); "string-of-beads" appearance caused by alternate areas of narrowing and mural aneurysms
2. Focal (7%); solitary stenosis less than 1 cm in length
3. Tubular (13.6%); elongated, smooth concentric stenosis
4. Mixed (16.8%); two or more of the above forms

All multifocal and most tubular lesions in their study were all of the medial type. A few of the tubular and focal lesions were intimal and two of the tubular were periarterial. In the multifocal form, there were rings of extreme hyperplasia of the fibrous components and rarely of the muscular elements of the media. They alternated with zones of extensive medial degeneration resulting in mural aneurysms. In the tubular form, mural aneurysms were not observed. The mural aneurysms may become very thin-walled, and enlarge beyond the perimuscular wall to become true aneurysms. Renal artery dissection may occur; there is a tendency to extend into primary or secondary branches of the renal artery and produce focal infarction. Occasionally renal artery aneurysm may cause partial obstruction leading to renovascular hypertension.

The presence of a renal vascular lesion does not

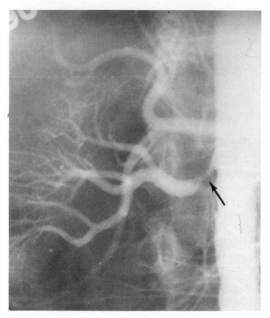

Fig. 20-43. Translumbar aortogram with good visualization of the renal artery. **Arrow** indicates the site of a stenotic lesion secondary to arteriosclerosis in this 63-year-old man with hypertension. Note the poststenotic dilatation of the renal artery.

mean that it is the cause of hypertension, since there are a number of factors involved in the production of this disease. Furthermore, there are many normotensive patients with severe renal artery disease. One likely hypothesis is that normotension is present when there is a balance between the available blood supply and the amount of functioning renal parenchyma. If the blood supply is reduced more than the functioning parenchyma, the resultant ischemia may cause hypertension. When major renal artery disease is present, there may be associated arteriolosclerosis of smaller renal vessels and other factors decreasing the amount of functioning renal parenchyma; this also reduces demand for blood, so that no ischemia is present and hypertension is not produced. It is therefore very difficult to assess hemodynamically significant stenosis. It is generally agreed that the presence of collateral vessels indicates significant stenosis. The principal value of pressure measurements across a stenotic area lies in exclusion of a gradient; this saves the patient from unnecessary exploratory surgery. Demonstration of a gradient indicates a significant stenosis, but it does not follow that the hypertension is curable by removal of the lesion causing the gradi-

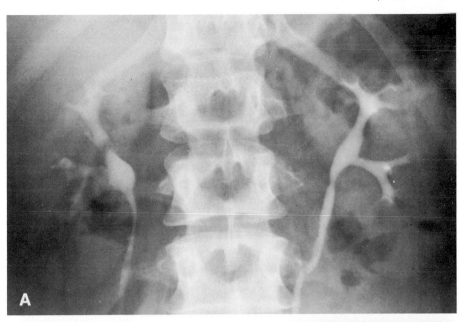

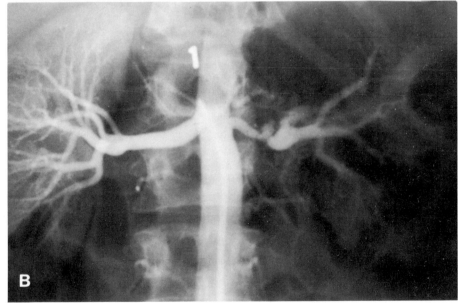

Fig. 20-44. Fibromuscular dysplasia in an 18-year-old woman with hypertension. **A.** This urogram shows very slight hyperconcentration on the left. There are a few minor indentations on the upper left ureter suggesting the possibility of collateral vessels. **B.** This arteriogram shows a normal right renal artery. On the left there are multiple constrictions with poststenotic dilatation. There is great delay in perfusion of the left kidney as compared with the right. Note the collateral arteries in and below the renal hilus.

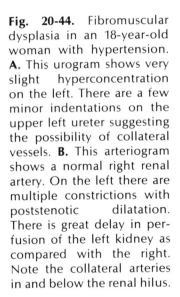

ent. As a general rule a stenosis of 70% with a lumen of 2 mm or below indicates a significant vascular lesion. Renal vein renin determinations and split-function studies are used in conjunction with renal arteriography in the assessment of patients with possible renovascular hypertension as candidates for surgery.

A number of renal lesions other than renal artery stenosis may cause hypertension. These include chronic pyelonephritis, hydronephrosis, Page kidney (constriction from any cause), arterial thrombosis, renal tumor, adult polycystic disease, polyarteritis nodosa, neurofibromatosis causing renal artery stenosis, and arteriovenous malformations or shunts. Other conditions causing hypertension that may be treated surgically include primary aldosteronism, pheochromocytoma, and, rarely, Cushing's syndrome.

TUMORS OF THE KIDNEY

BENIGN TUMORS

Benign renal tumors are rare and usually asymptomatic. Histologic types include adenoma, fibroma, lipoma, leiomyoma, hemangioma, and hamartoma; the renin-secreting juxtaglomerular cell tumor is very rare, and is usually small, but it may be seen on arteriography as an avascular mass surrounded by a denser rim of compressed parenchyma. There may be a few dilated, tortuous arteries present and, of crucial importance in the diagnosis, elevation of venous renin from the affected kidney. When the benign renal tumors are small, no roentgen signs are produced. If they attain sufficient size, a plain-film roentgenogram will reveal enlargement of the renal shadow at the site of the tumor. Urography may then show enough distortion of the calyceal system to make the diagnosis of renal tumor. It is also possible for one of these benign lesions to project sufficiently far into the pelvis locally to be recognized as a space-occupying mass. The chief importance of these benign renal tumors lies in differentiation between them and malignant disease of the kidney. This usually cannot be made with certainty on excretory urography. Rarely, a leiomyoma arising in the renal capsule will contain calcium resembling that observed in leiomyoma elsewhere. With the exception of hemangioma, the benign renal tumors are noted to be avascular on angiography. Some benign tumors may exhibit abnormal vascularity and malignant lesions may be completely avascular. Despite these pitfalls, angiography remains the best method of preoperative study of renal masses. Retroperitoneal masses arising near the kidney may be difficult to differentiate from renal tumors since they may distort the kidney and/or displace the upper ureter (Fig. 20-45).

Renal Angiomyolipoma

Renal angiomyolipoma (hamartoma) often can be differentiated from other benign tumors and from malignant renal tumors. It usually occurs in patients with tuberous sclerosis. It is a mixed mesodermal tumor composed of adipose, smooth muscle, and blood vessels in varying proportions. The tumors may be single or multiple, unilateral or bilateral. They occur without other lesions of tuberous sclerosis, but then may be a *"forme fruste"* of the condition. Clinical manifestations include signs of infection, pain, hematuria, or an asymptomatic abdominal mass.

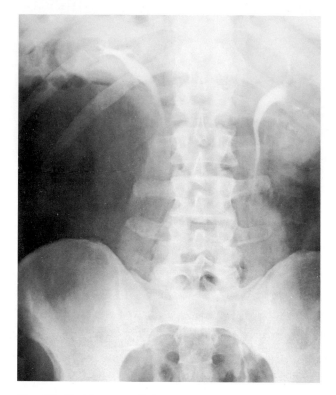

Fig. 20-45. Huge radiolucent tumor distorting the right kidney and ureter. This is a large retroperitoneal lipoma.

Urographic findings are those of a mass that enlarges the kidney, and distorts and displaces the pelvis and calyces. If there is much fat present, the radiolucent areas within the mass suggest the diagnosis. If multiple and bilateral, they may simulate polycystic disease. Renal angiography is the method used to differentiate this tumor from polycystic disease. The most striking finding is the presence of many, peculiar, small, regular outpouchings of the interlobar and interlobular arteries resembling berry aneurysms. In some patients the interlobular arteries terminate in the "aneurysms" resembling a cluster of grapes, in contrast to the irregular size and contour of the tumor vessels of hypernephroma. This appearance is present in the arterial phase and is obscured by the nephrographic phase. Later there is irregular puddling indistinguishable from that due to malignant tumor. The venous phase is normal, not early as in hypernephroma. Differentiation from renal-cell carcinoma may be very difficult or impossible, however. Polycystic disease is readily differentiated by means of angiography.

Lipomatosis of the Renal Sinus

This condition is also called fibrolipomatosis, fatty replacement, fatty transformation, lipomatous paranephritis, and lipoma diffusum renis. Since it may resemble tumor on urographic study, it is considered here. It consists of an excessive amount of fat in the renal sinus which distorts the renal pelvis, infundibula, and calyces to varying degrees. It is usually found as a replacement process in renal atrophy whatever the cause, but may occur in simple obesity. It is found in older age groups, usually in those over 50. The roentgen appearance may simulate renal tumor, peripelvic cyst, or polycystic disease. It is therefore important that differentiation be made since lipomatosis is not a surgical problem.

Roentgen Observations. The condition can usually be suspected on intravenous urography but nephrotomography is the examination that best outlines the changes and permits a positive diagnosis. The pelvis is flattened or irregularly indented on its lateral aspect; the infundibula are elongated, narrow, and often appear stretched. The calyces may be relatively normal but may be blunted and dilated in patients with pyelonephritis. At times the deposition of fat is localized so that tumor or cyst may be simulated, while the more diffuse type may resemble polycystic disease. The process may be unilateral or bilateral. When bilateral it is not necessarily symmetric. Involvement on the left is often somewhat greater than on the right. The infusion method of urography in conjunction with nephrotomography is usually diagnostic when this condition is suspected. This method of examination combines a good nephrographic phase with filling of calyces to bring out in sharp relief the relationship of the radiolucent fat to the opacified pelvis, calyces, and renal parenchyma (Fig. 20-46).

Renal Pseudotumor

The kidney is capable of hypertrophy and hyperplasia. When local, a mass (pseudotumor) may result which is difficult to differentiate from tumor. There may be compression of the pelvis and calyces, splaying of the calyces, and local enlargement with protrusion from renal surface. The calyces do not regenerate, so the masses do not contain these structures. In addition to the demonstration of a mass, excretory urography may reveal the signs of the renal disease which results in the regeneration of renal parenchyma including nonobstructive caliectasis and irregular thinning of cortex. The pseudotumor formed at the junction of the middle and upper third of the kidney in duplication, an enlarged column of Bertin, is an example of normal parenchyma resembling a tumor mass. Angiography reveals spreading of the arteries, but no tumor vessels or arteriovenous shunts are present, so there is no early venous filling. The capillary blush equals or exceeds that of the remaining renal parenchyma and there is no evidence of a wall or capsule.

A number of other conditions may resemble renal hilar or parenchymal masses. These include aneurysm of the renal artery, dilated vein(s), renal abscess, hematoma, xanthogranulomatous pyelonephritis, renal tuberculosis, and, most important and frequent, renal cyst.

MALIGNANT TUMORS

Malignant tumors of the kidney are of five general types: (1) adenocarcinoma (hypernephroma); (2) embryoma (embryonal adenosarcoma, Wilms' tumor); (3) carcinoma of the renal pelvis; (4) sarcoma; and (5) lymphoma, including leukemia. The adenocarcinoma or hypernephroma is the most common renal malignant neoplasm. This tumor usually arises in the upper or lower pole of the kidney and may attain great size before causing symptoms.

Adenocarcinoma (Hypernephroma) (Renal-Cell Tumor)

Plain-film roentgen findings consist of local or general enlargement of the kidney which varies with the size of the tumor. The renal outline tends to be preserved even though it may be lobulated, distorted, and irregular. This is because the lesions are limited by the renal capsule until far advanced. It is not unusual to note calcification within the tumor. The calcification may be irregularly scattered or curvilinear within the tumor. It may also be curvilinear or rimlike, outlining the periphery of the tumor. Renal displacement or tilting of the axis may result when there is a large medial mass in the upper pole or lower pole, or the entire kidney may be displaced if the tumor is large. Displacement of neighboring organs occurs when the tumor attains sufficient size. This may be apparent on a plain-film roentgenogram but it is often necessary to outline the colon and small intestine by means of a barium enema and small-bowel study to determine the amount and direction of displacement.

Urographic changes are due to the distortion produced by the tumor mass. Calyces are elongated, dis-

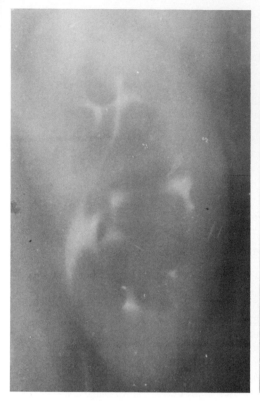
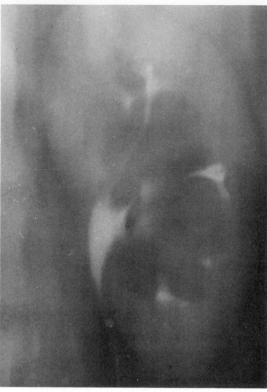

Fig. 20-46. Lipomatosis of the renal sinus. These tomograms show radiolucent fat in the renal sinus with elongation and narrowing of infundibula.

torted, narrowed, or obliterated. The renal pelvis may be altered in a similar manner. As a rule, hypernephroma produces more disruption of the normal pattern than does a cyst of similar size. Distortion of the calyces is particularly significant because cysts can elongate and compress them and cause a stretching of the infundibula. Filling defects in the pelvis can simulate epithelial tumors arising there, but the latter do not usually produce calyceal deformity. Large tumors may cause considerable displacement of the upper ureter and may also partially obstruct the pelvis or upper ureter (Fig. 20-47). There is usually enough function to visualize the pelvis and calyces on excretory urography, in contrast to the

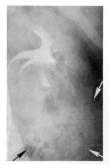
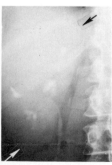
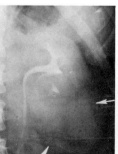
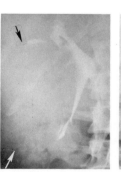
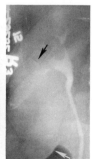

Fig. 20-47. These excretory urograms indicate various findings produced by renal carcinoma. Note the considerable distortion of the calyces sometimes associated with the tumor mass. **Arrows** indicate the tumor site in each case.

loss of function often noted in hydronephrosis, which may also produce renal enlargement. At times, renal infiltrative tumor involvement may be so extensive that no function remains. Also, function may be diminished by invasion and thrombosis of a renal vein. Occasionally infiltrating hypernephroma can cause renal enlargement without much distortion of the calyces, and subcapsular tumors can also reach considerable size without much distortion.

The malignant renal tumor must be differentiated from renal cyst. This differentiation may be impossible on excretory urography because tumor may simulate cyst. Excretory urographic findings[104] show the following characteristics:

Renal Cyst:

1. Kidney is normal in size.
2. Mass is attached to periphery of the kidney in many cases; sharp outlines, permitting measurement of diameter of mass; may be less dense than kidney tissue and produce a "double shadow."
3. Calcification may be curvilinear, but very rare.
4. Renal pelvis may be displaced or compressed.
5. Calyceal elongation is sometimes found usually in combination with calyceal displacement or compression.
6. Calyceal displacement often takes the form of "crowding" together of calyces.
7. Calyceal compression is common, particularly with centrally located cysts.
8. Calyceal amputation is rare.
9. Simple types of calyceal deformity are noted.
10. No calyceal deformity may be seen, particularly if cyst is subcapsular.
11. "Claw-sign" is present in nephrographic phase.

Renal Tumor:

1. Kidney is enlarged.
2. Mass is contiguous with body of kidney; indistinct outlines; mass often is denser than kidney and may obliterate psoas shadow.
3. Calcification is central, eccentric, or peripheral in location—curvilinear or amorphous.
4. Renal pelvis may be displaced, compressed, or invaded.
5. Calyceal elongation is sometimes found, often in combination with calyceal amputation.
6. Calyceal displacement often takes the form of separation of calyces.
7. Calyceal compression is common, particularly with centrally located tumors.
8. Calyceal amputation is very common.
9. Complex or bizarre types of calyceal deformity are seen.
10. No calyceal deformity may be seen if tumor is peripheral in location.
11. Pyelotumor backflow: an ill-defined pool of contrast medium infiltrating or outlining a necrotic tumor in which there may be an irregular cavitation.

It is generally agreed that renal angiography is an essential part of the roentgen study of patients with renal masses. Nephrotomography in conjunction with infusion urography is useful, but does not replace angiography (Figs. 20-48 and 20-49). In addition to its value in differentiating cysts and benign neoplasms from malignant lesions, angiography yields valuable information regarding the extent of the tumor, its blood supply, and the venous drainage in many instances. Some investigators advise cavography and direct catheterization of renal veins to obtain precise evidence of major renal vein invasion and also to aid in the differentiation of malignant and benign masses. Selective catheterization of the small retroperitoneal arteries (*e.g.,* inferior phrenic, middle adrenal, lumbar, and gonadal) to aid in the demonstration of extracapsular extension is sometimes use-ful. Epinephrine injected into the renal artery a few seconds preceding the injection of contrast medium may be a useful adjunct, especially in small tumors. The normal arteries contract and the tumor vessels that do not respond are more clearly outlined. This differential constriction may sometimes be observed in renal abscess or carbuncle, which makes the differential diagnosis difficult in these cases. Also, there may not be a differential effect in metastases to the kidney.

Another examination which is in wide use in the differentation of renal masses is percutaneous cyst puncture. When there is a reasonable certainty on ultrasound that a mass is cystic, it can be punctured directly under fluoroscopic control. Fluid is aspirated and checked for cells. Then an opaque material is injected and the cyst walls outlined. In the benign cyst,

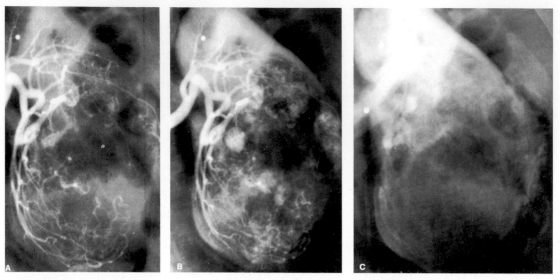

Fig. 20-48. Hypernephroma as seen on the selective renal arteriogram. **A.** At 1.5 seconds there are abnormal vessels within the lower pole mass while arteries surrounding it are stretched. **B.** At 3 seconds, more puddling and arteriovenous shunting is visible with many abnormal "tumor" vessels. **C.** At 16 seconds the renal vein is opacified. Note also the abnormal veins lateral to the mass, outside of the kidney.

Fig. 20-49. Renal cyst. Selective renal arteriogram shows normal vessels stretched around a radiolucent mass which is not as clearly defined as are many cysts; therefore cyst puncture is warranted.

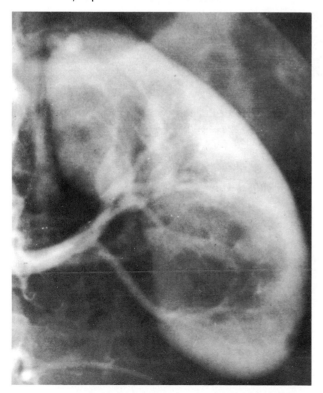

the aspirate is clear, the wall is smooth, and the Papanicolaou smear is negative. The wall is outlined by placing a contrast medium (Pantopaque, Hypaque, etc.) or air or both within the cyst. Methylene blue can be used to outline the needle tract if a tumor is suspected and surgery contemplated. Pantopaque seems to aid in regression or disappearance of the cyst, but there is a difference of opinion regarding its use in a cyst that is benign and causes little or no morbidity; we do not use it.

The evaluation of solitary renal masses should include the following procedures in the order given: (1) Intravenous urogram with tomography. (2) If a typical cyst—ultrasonography and cyst puncture including a study of the aspirate and a contrast study of the cyst. (3) If atypical cyst or solid mass—arteriography.[47] In some circumstances, abdominal CT scanning might be used before arteriography, and in others it might be used after arteriography.

When angiography suggests tumor, surgery is usually indicated. The ultimate use of CT scanning of patients wth renal masses is yet to be determined. Angiography is equivocal in approximately 5% of cases so that benign lesions may be mistaken for tumor and vice versa. Angiography with cyst puncture in questionable cases approaches 100% in accuracy. Contrast injection is necessary in these "cyst" punctures.

The angiographic findings in cyst consist of a thin wall, sharp margination, avascularity, stretched and displaced vessels, and no abnormal vascularity, pooling, or abnormality of venous filling. In renal-cell carcinoma there may be (1) relative avascularity of the entire tumor or a portion of it, (2) increased vascularity with irregular pooling, arteriovenous communcations with early venous fill, (3) abnormal circulation by way of capsular or extrarenal vessels, (4) lack of constrictor response to epinephrine in tumor vessels, and (5) venous collaterals and abnormal peripheral venous channels around the mass. Transcatheter embolization of renal-cell carcinoma has been carried out by several investigators.[51] Preoperatively it is done to aid in surgical removal since the embolization causes tumor vessels to collapse resulting in a decrease in operating time and blood loss. In patients with inoperable tumors, it is undertaken to relieve symptoms and reduce tumor size. A number of materials have been used for embolization, including autologous clot, gelfoam, isobutyl 2-cyanoacrylate, Ivalon (a polyvinyl alcohol), faromagnetic silicone, microspheres, muscle tissue, steel coils, and radioactive gold seeds. Balloon catheter occlusion has also been employed.[77]

Wilms' Tumor

The nephroblastoma, or Wilms' tumor, is the most common abdominal neoplasm of infancy and childhood. The majority arise in the first 5 years of life, but this tumor is rarely present at birth in contrast to fibromyomatous hamartoma of the kidney or to neuroblastoma. Wilms' tumor arises from embryonic renal tissue and tends to become very large. Visible enlargement of the abdomen is often the presenting complaint. Scout roentgenograms show the outline of the mass with displacement of neighboring structures and elevation of the diaphragm on the side of the lesion. These tumors occasionally contain calcium, in contrast to neuroblastoma (about 50% contain calcium) which also causes a large tumor mass in infants and children. Urographic findings are those of a large intrarenal tumor that distorts the pelvis and calyces and often displaces and partially obstructs the ureter. The distortion of the calyces tends to be less than with hypernephroma of similar size but is greater than in neuroblastoma, which often arises adjacent to the kidney and produces pressure upon it. Renal function may be impaired but there is usually enough to outline some of the calyces on urography and to differentiate this tumor from hydronephrosis causing massive renal enlargement (Fig. 20-50). Wilms' tumor tends to metastasize to the lungs

and periaortic nodes and may also extend locally by direct invasion. Calcification in metastases has been reported but is extremely rare. Angiography has been done in a few reported cases. Tumor stain is not common and no arteriovenous shunts are present to produce pooling or puddling. The tumor vessels are long and tortuous, resembling a creeping vine; they tend to be discrete, of large caliber, and an irregular diameter. Inferior venacavography is used to detect displacement, obstruction, and invasion of the vena cava.

Tumors of the Renal Pelvis

Tumors of the renal pelvis are of epithelial origin and present a different roentgen picture from adenocarcinoma of the renal parenchyma. There are two major types of malignant lesions, the transitional cell and the squamous cell epithelioma. Transitional cell tumors comprise nearly 90% of malignant tumors of the renal pelvis. They tend to be somewhat less invasive than the squamous cell type. The latter is very commonly associated with chronic infection, leukoplakia, or calculi. These tumors produce symptoms of hematuria, pain (obstructive type), and sometimes a palpable mass caused by obstructive hydronephrosis or large tumor with perirenal extension. On the plain film, there may be no sign of tumor. Because hematuria is an early sign, the patients are usually examined when the lesion is small and therefore difficult to detect. The tumor causes a filling defect in the pelvis or calyx that may be smooth or irregular and may be large or small. These defects are outlined on urograms as radiolucent areas projecting into the opacified pelvis or calyx (Fig. 20-51). Malignant tumors are generally more irregular than benign papillomas of the pelvis, but roentgen differentiation of the various cell types of renal pelvis tumors is not possible. The roentgen evidence of an infiltrating type of tumor may be minimal, but it may become very large and produce major alterations in the renal pelvis (Fig. 20-52). Blood clots and radiolucent calculi can produce similar defects. For this reason it is common practice to follow intravenous urography by retrograde pyelography when a filling defect is noted. If a blood clot or calculus has caused the defect, the second examination will show disappearance or alteration in size or position of it. Calcification may occur within this type of tumor but is uncommon. Ureteral and bladder implants occur frequently and they produce small defects similar to those caused by primary tumor in the kidney. Occasionally a tumor may invade and infiltrate the adjacent parenchyma to simulate renal-cell carcinoma. There are angiographic dif-

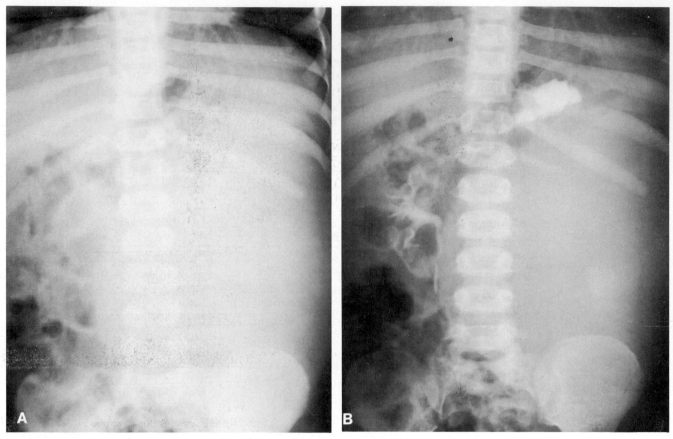

Fig. 20-50. Wilm's tumor. **A.** In the preliminary film a huge mass is noted in the left side of the abdomen. **B.** The excretory urogram shows function on the left side with several dilated calyces above the major mass. The right kidney appears normal, but the ureter is displaced slightly to the right by the tumor which extends across the midline.

ferences that may be helpful. The tumor is relatively hypovascular, there is no pooling or arteriovenous shunting or neovascularity. The residual parenchymal vessels are occluded or encased by tumor and narrowed. Because these angiographic findings may also be present in metastatic tumors of the kidney, angiography may not be very helpful in differentiation.

Squamous Metaplasia of the Renal Pelvis

Leukoplakia or squamous metaplasia of the renal pelvis is probably caused by infection or chronic irritation of other source. It is included here because it may resemble carcinoma of the pelvis and often pre-cedes squamous cell carcinoma of the renal pelvis. Infection is found in 80% of patients and 40% have had renal calculi. The patient may describe passing tissue or gritty material and the diagnosis is established by finding keratinized squamous epithelium in the urine. The condition is usually unilateral.

Radiographic findings are varied. Irregular areas in the renal pelvis partially surrounded by contrast material, large laminated masses presenting an onion-skin appearance, irregular plaques or bands producing linear striations, and roughening or wrinkling of the renal pelvis may be found. Any of these findings should suggest the diagnosis, but lucent calculi, hematoma, and, particularly, carcinoma of the renal pelvis must be considered in the differential diagnosis.

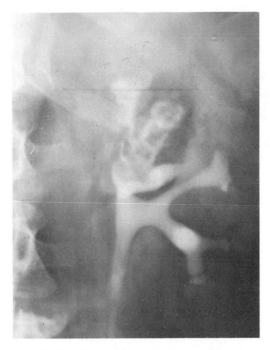

Fig. 20-51. Carcinoma of the renal pelvis. Note the irregular filling defects of the upper pole calyces and infundibula. The lesion was a transitional cell carcinoma.

Sarcoma

Sarcoma arising from the connective-tissue elements of the kidney is rare. Often retroperitoneal sarcoma arising in or near the kidney becomes so extensive that it is not possible to determine the site of origin even at autopsy. Fibrosarcoma, liposarcoma, leomyosarcoma, rhabdoymyosarcoma, and even osteosarcoma of the kidney have been reported. All are rare. Roentgen findings are those of a mass in the renal area that is often difficult to outline clearly and may obliterate the psoas shadow in its superior aspect. Urograms tend to show somewhat less distortion of the pelvis and calyces than is noted in a hypernephroma of similar size.

Lymphoma and Leukemia

Involvement of the kidneys in patients with chronic leukemia may occur late in the disease. In children with acute leukemia, renal involvement is more common than in the chronic form. The leukemic infiltrate tends to be largely cortical in location. The plain-film finding is that of renal enlargement,

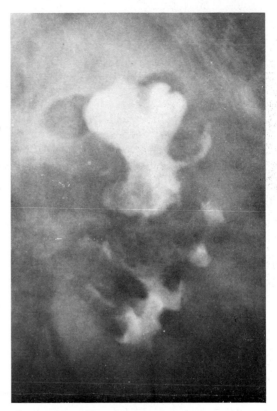

Fig. 20-52. Infiltrating carcinoma (transitional cell) of the renal pelvis. Note gross distortion of infundibula and calyces. The pelvis does not opacify because it is full of tumor.

usually bilateral. Urographic signs in addition to bilateral enlargement consist of enlargement of the renal pelvis without dilatation or evidence of obstruction, calyceal and infundibular elongation, and irregularity of renal outline. The findings may be caused either by leukemic infiltration or by edema and hemorrhage secondary to the disease.

The distribution of disease is somewhat more varied in the lymphomas. Diffuse infiltration causing renal enlargement, with distortion, elongation, and compression of the calyces, is the most common form of involvement. The disease may also be manifested by single or multiple tumor nodules or by perirenal masses resulting in displacement or distortion of the kidney. The solitary tumor nodules resemble masses produced by primary renal tumors and cannot be differentiated on the basis of roentgen findings alone. Multiplicity of tumor nodules should suggest the possibility of lymphoma. Some lymphomas with multiple renal masses may resemble polycystic disease on angiography. CT scans or ultrasonography demonstrate the solid nature of the masses. The kidney is involved by lymphosarcoma and reticulum cell sarcoma more frequently than by Hodgkin's disease. There are a few reports of angiography in these conditions. Some resemble renal cell carcinoma; others contain tumor vessels with a straight palisadelike appearance and others are hypovascular. Since most, if not all of these tumors, secondarily invade the kidney, signs of the disease elsewhere are very helpful in making the diagnosis.

The nephrotic syndrome has been reported in association with lymphatic leukemia and Hodgkin's disease with renal involvement. Another complication is hypertension caused by obstruction of a renal artery by the tumor.

MISCELLANEOUS RENAL CONDITIONS

Amyloidosis. Renal amyloidosis may be primary or secondary to chronic inflammatory disease. Plain-film findings include bilateral, symmetrical renal enlargement with normal collecting system. Late in the disease the kidneys may become small and have diminshed function. Angiographic findings recorded in a few reports include a slight decrease in renal artery size, pruning, tortuosity and irregularity of the distal interlobar arteries, a relatively homogeneous nephrogram, nonvisualization of the interlobar arteries, prominent extrarenal arteries, and uneven involvement of the kidneys. Renal vein thrombosis is common. When the disease is restricted to the renal pelvis, linear submucosal calcification outlining the pelvis may be noted.

Scleroderma. Renal scleroderma may show changes similar to those found in the kidneys of patients with advanced malignant hypertension. In patients with scleroderma the nephrogram phase of the roentgenographic examination is quite characteristic. Spotty lucencies are seen scattered throughout the kidney with a delay in arterial flow manifested by persistent filling of arteries during the nephrogram phase.[125]

Chronic Glomerulonephritis. Renal cortical calcification somewhat similar to that in patients who survive acute renal cortical necrosis is sometimes observed in patients with chronic glomerulonephritis. The kidneys of patients with chronic glomerulonephritis are small, and fine cortical calcifications are observed.

Multiple Myeloma. In multiple myeloma, renal involvement is the result of precipitation of abnormal proteins in the tubules. Roentgen findings are those of bilateral, smooth renal enlargement with a normal collecting system. Parenchymal thickness is increased. Later in the disease, renal failure with oliguria may result in small kidneys. In this disease, it is essential that the patient be well hydrated during excretory urography to avoid the risk of precipitation of abnormal urinary protein in the tubules.

Agnogenic Myeloid Metaplasia. When extramedullary hematopoiesis occurs in the renal hilus, it may simulate a parapelvic cyst or neoplasm.[102]

Hemophilia. Nonobstructive renal enlargement has been noted in patients with hemophilia. Its cause has not been established.

S-Hemoglobinopathy. Sickle cell hemoglobinopathy may be a cause of renal papillary necrosis. It may occur in SS, SC, and SA disease. Papillary necrosis in these patients is similar to that in analgesic-abuse patients. Bilateral renal enlargement has also been reported in patients wth S-hemoglobinopathies and in thalassemia, but it is not found in many of these patients.

Sarcoidosis. The hypercalcemia frequently observed in patients with sarcoidosis may result in nephrocalcinosis and/or nephrolithiasis. In addition, the granulomas of sarcoidosis may involve the kidney. The granulomatous disease is usually not severe enough to cause any recognizable alteration, but the nephrocalcinosis as well as renal calculi can be observed in this disease. Usually there is no deformity of the collecting system. There may be some irregularity of the renal outline secondary to scarring related to tubular atrophy in patients with long-standing hyperuricemia.

Radiation Nephritis. Acute radiation nephritis develops after a period of 6 to 12 months following irradiation. The urogram may show only slight diminution in function. In chronic radiation nephritis, there is glomerular damage, tubular atrophy, and interstitial fibrosis as well as damage to smaller arteries and arterioles. Atrophy involves the area irradiated, whether it be a portion of or the entire kidney, which is then decreased in size. The other finding is diminution in renal function which may be observed when comparison is made with the opposite normal kidney. Hypertension often develops in patients with renal damage. In some, the condition progresses to malignant hypertension which is relieved if the involved kidney is removed. The cause of hypertension in these patients is not entirely clear.

Nephrosclerosis. The term "nephrosclerosis" refers to the alteration in renal parenchyma that results from decreased arterial blood flow; therefore the condition is associated with renal ischemia. The cause may be major arterial stenosis due to a number of conditions. Other patients have small-vessel disease, and some have segmental involvement resulting in local infarction. The radiographic findings depend on the type of involvement. The infarcts produce a renal scar that appears as an irregularity indenting the renal cortical margin. The collecting system is usually normal. When the disease is uniform and widespread, the kidney decreases in size and there is also evidence of decrease in function.

Radiology in Renal Transplant Patients. In addition to arteriographic studies on potential donors, radiographic methods are used to study the collecting system, including the ureter as well as the vascular system, in transplant recipients. In the prospective donor, the arteriogram outlines anatomic variations as well as unsuspected disease involving the renal arteries. In the posttransplant period, arteriography is used in recipients who develop anuria or oliguria. Arteriographic signs of rejection are sometimes difficult to assess since no vascular abnormality may be observed, even though renal failure is severe. In the acute stage, edema results in stretching of renal vessels, and there may be minimal loss of small cortical vessels. The arterial phase is lengthened initially, and, as the process continues, the smaller arteries and cortex become poorly visualized. The lack of visualization of interlobar and arcuate arteries produces a leafless-tree appearance. In the nephrogram phase, an inhomogeneous nephrogram may be observed since many small infarcts are present. In the chronic phase, the kidney is decreased in size and there is severe loss of vessels, resulting in a pruned-tree effect.

Another late effect is renal artery stenosis which may be proximal to the area of anastomosis; renal vein thrombosis, although uncommon, may occur. Other complications include ureteral stenosis resulting in obstruction, usually at the ureterovesical junction. There may be a leak at the anastomosis with a urinoma producing a mass adjacent to the transplanted kidney and/or near the bladder. If function is satisfactory, these abnormalities are readily demonstrated by excretory urography.

TUMORS OF THE URETER

Tumors of the ureter are rare, but benign papilloma, hemangioma, benign fibrous polyps, and epithelial carcinoma may arise there. *Benign fibrous polyps* appear to be the most common of the benign tumors. The polyp is often a long, branched, smooth, intraluminal mass that may become very large, measuring up to 15 cm in length. Multiple polyps may be present. Obstruction occurs, but is not as severe as the size of the polyp would indicate. *Endometriosis* of the ureter may simulate tumor, since the lesion may invade the ureter and penetrate the mucosa; it is usually extrinsic, involving the adventitia. Obstruction may be severe enough to cause symptoms. The ureteral involvement is below the pelvic brim. Most other tumors occur in the lower one-third of the ureter. *Epithelial carcinoma* arising in the renal pelvis may implant in the ureter. The roentgen findings do not differentiate the various types. Ureteral obstruction is common, leading to hydronephrosis, and an intraluminal tumor mass may be visible in addition to the signs of ureteral obstruction. Occasionally an infiltrating carcinoma may result in local narrowing of the lumen simulating benign ureteral stricture (Fig. 20-53). In some cases there is no dilatation above the neoplasm, even though it is relatively large. The ureter apparently dilates locally as the tumor grows, so that obstruction does not develop. In these instances it is important to visualize the entire ureter in order to make the diagnosis, since the only roentgen sign is the intraluminal mass, which must be outlined by the contrast material to be seen. A localized dilatation of the ureter immediately below the tumor has been described (Fig. 20-54). When retrograde pyelography is attempted, the catheter tip may coil in this area of dilatation; its upward progress is impeded by the intraluminal mass, which is outlined when contrast material is injected. This coiling of the catheter is then a sign of ureteral tumor, since the local dilatation does not occur below the ureteral calculus unless it is very large, usually calcified, and easily detected. Tomography of the ureter at the time of urography is helpful in some instances, since ureteral tumors, particularly the papillary transitional cell type, may be multiple. These have less tendency to infiltrate than do the squamous cell tumors of the ureter. Metastases to the ureter from tumors outside of the urinary tract may cause local involvement with little or no extrinsic mass, or the ureter may be caught in a retroperitoneal mass, displaced, and narrowed. Selective arteriography is sometimes useful in identi-

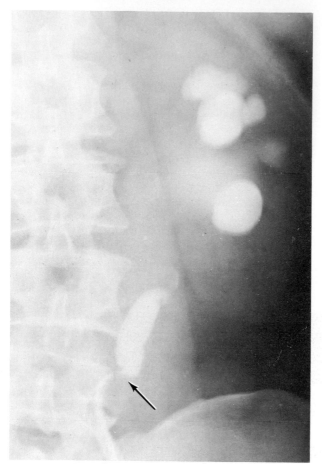

Fig. 20-53. Carcinoma of the left ureter, indicated by the **arrow,** has produced partial obstruction with hydroureter and hydronephrosis above it.

fying ureteral tumor and differentiating it from stricture, but its use in this field is limited.

OTHER URETERAL ABNORMALITIES

Ureteral Displacement. The ureter may herniate into the inguinal canal, the femoral canal, or the sciatic notch. The relationship of the ureter to these various structures usually determines the diagnosis, and there is often a portion of the bowel extending into the hernia as well. Ureters are also displaced in patients with uterine prolapse or procidentia, moving downward with the bladder and uterus, the distance depending on the severity of the abnormality. At

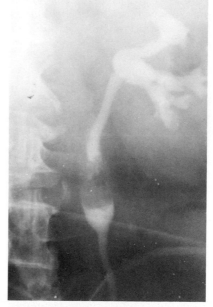

Fig. 20-54. Ureteral carcinoma. The tumor produces a filling defect that is somewhat irregular superiorly and demonstrates dilatation below the tumor.

times, there may be ureteral obstruction when these patients with uterine prolapse are in the upright position. This tends to be relieved, or partially relieved, in recumbency. Primary or secondary tumors or massive nodes may also displace one or both ureters, and sometimes will produce obstruction. Fecal impactions in the sigmoid colon may displace the ureter in a manner simulating a pelvic mass. In patients with Crohn's disease, a ureter may be caught in an inflammatory mass and displaced and/or obstructed by the accompanying fibrosis. In patients with aortic aneurysm, there may be traction displacement of one of the ureters toward the aneurysm.[96] Presumably this is an indication of retroperitoneal bleeding with resultant fibrosis causing the displacement. This medial displacement may be the first diagnostic clue to an abdominal aortic aneurysm since there may be no calcification to identify it. It is more common in fusiform than in sacular aneurysm. The maximum deviation is usually at the level of L4. The ureter on the opposite side of the aneurysm is the one drawn medially by the posthemorrhage fibrosis. The ureter on the same side may be displaced laterally by the aneurysmal mass. Pelvic lipomatosis may also result in alteration in the course of the ureters, and in some instances may produce ureteral obstruction. More common is alteration in the appearance of the bladder which is elevated and elongated vertically, the "pear-shaped" bladder.

Ureteral Calculi. As has been indicated earlier, ureteral calculi are common. Occasionally there is ureteral perforation secondary to the calculus in which case urograms demonstrate extravasation at the site of the calculus. This may lead to retroperitoneal fibrosis. At times, urographic contrast medium will show defects above and below a ureteral calculus.[4] These defects consist of a mass of cells, protein, and salts which prevents the contrast medium from reaching the stone so that the appearance tends to simulate that of a tumor. More rarely, material accumulates below the calculus, in most instances when stones are 6 mm or larger in size.

Schistosomiasis. Schistosomiasis may cause calcification in the ureteral wall as well as a medial deviation, a straight lumbar course, or a bowed appearance in the pelvis with medial and upward displacement at the level of the trigone. There may be some stasis and dilatation of the upper urinary tract, due mainly to fibrosis rather than to mechanical obstruction.

Polyarteritis. Polyarteritis may cause dilatation and nodular irregularity of the ureteral wall simulating a string of pearls.[48]

Amyloidosis. Amyloidosis may involve the ureter, causing a stricturelike defect that may partially obstruct it, producing colicky pain and hematuria as well as ureterectasis above the stricture.[72]

Primary Megaloureter. Primary or aperistaltic megaloureter appears to be a specific entity in which there is local dilatation of both ureters just above the bladder without evidence of anatomic obstruction or reflux.[98] It fails to transmit an effective peristaltic wave. Its cause is not clear. There is no upper ureteral, pelvic, or calyceal dilatation unless infection is present. Maximal dilatation is immediately proximal to the aperistaltic segment, which averages 1.5 cm in length and is relatively narrow. It may not fill on excretory urography. Video tape fluorography and fluoroscopy may be used to demonstrate the disturbed peristalsis. The peristaltic activity is normal or vigorous in the proximal dilated ureter, but peristalsis is absent in the distal ureteral segment. A bolus of contrast medium in front of the contractive wave often floods back up the ureter, but there does not appear to be any reverse peristalsis.

RETROPERITONEAL FIBROSIS

Retroperitoneal fibrosis was originally called periureteral fibrosis. The term "retroperitoneal fibrosis" is better because the disease may involve vascular and lymphatic structures in addition to the ureters. The disease is characterized by a fibrosing inflammatory process, of unknown cause, in the retroperitoneal space, which may extend from the kidneys down to the pelvic brim and spread laterally to involve the ureters. In addition to the idiopathic cases, a number have been reported in patients with migraine who have been on long-term methysergide (Sansert) therapy. In many of them, discontinuance of use of the drug causes regression of the process, but in others, the process may continue or progress. Several other drugs including phenacetin, methyldopa, and other ergot derivatives have since been implicated. Fibrosis of the orbit, duodenum, rectosigmoid, common bile duct, and pancreatic duct system has been reported in association with retroperitoneal fibrosis involving the ureters. Involvement of the splenic vein, vena cava, celiac axis, superior mesenteric artery, or iliac artery may also be associated with this condition. It is much more frequent in males than in females and is usually bilateral. The most common symptom is dull, indefinite backache. The radiographic findings may suggest the diagnosis. The normal fat lines may disappear, so that the outlines of the psoas muscle are not visible on the plain film. Intravenous urography may show delayed excretion with varying degrees of hydronephrosis or absence of excretion caused by obstruction. If the ureters opacify, local narrowing is demonstrated in which the ureters gradually taper to the area of maximum stenosis. The involved segment is often 4 to 5 cm in length and usually deviates sharply toward the midline but may not deviate. The common site of involvement is opposite the fourth and fifth lumbar vertebrae. Some slight redundancy may be observed in the ureter above the stenotic segment. Despite a rather severe degree of obstruction there is often noted a paradoxical ease of retrograde passage of ureteral catheters. Lymphangiography may be helpful in diagnosis, since lymphatic obstruction is common. Inferor vena cavography may reveal narrowing and medial displacement of the vena cava at the site of involvement.

Early recognition and surgical ureterolysis are important to preserve renal function in idiopathic disease. The vascular obstruction may be more important clinically than the ureteral obstruction in some instances.

THE URINARY BLADDER

CONGENITAL ANOMALIES

Exstrophy of the bladder is of radiologic interest only because of the wide separation of the pubic bones anteriorly at the symphysis that accompanies this defect. The symphysis is separated approximately the width of the sacrum and this leads to a rather square appearance of the pelvis (Fig. 20-55). Exstrophy consists of an absence of the anterior wall of the bladder and of the lower anterior abdominal wall. The diagnosis is made on observation, so that roentgen study is not necessary but is useful to study the kidneys and ureters, since ureteral obstruction is often associated. Wide separation of the pubic bones is also noted in some patients with epispadias.

Duplication of the *urinary bladder* is extremely rare and is usually associated with urethral duplication (Fig. 20-56). Incomplete duplication may also occur, in which a septum partially divides the bladder and a multilocular or multiseptated bladder has been described. Occasionally there may be a partial horizontal septum, sometimes resulting in an hourglass appearance. The ureters empty into the lower compartment. Cystography is often necessary to outline

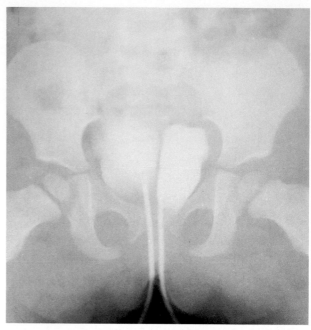

Fig. 20-56. Duplication of the urinary bladder. Cystogram outlines the duplication with each bladder drained by its own urethra.

these anomalies, but excretory urography with special films of the bladder may obviate the need for cystography.

Agenesis of the bladder is very rare and is usually incompatible with life, largely because of associated anomalies.

Congenital enlargement of the bladder with hydronephrosis and hydroureter is found in association with congenital absence or hypoplasia of the abdominal muscles, the *prune-belly syndrome.* This is a rare condition that occurs almost exclusively in males. No obstruction can be demonstrated to account for the dilatation. Associated abnormalities include nondescent of the testes, malrotation of the intestine, and, more rarely, persistent urachus, dislocated hips, clubfoot, harelip, spina bifida, hydrocephalus, and cardiac malformations. The abdomen is distended and the skin wrinkled; so the name "prune-belly syndrome" has been applied to this condition.

"Bladder ears," lateral protrusions of the bladder caused by extraperitoneal herniations through the internal inguinal ring into the inguinal canal, have been observed. They are usually observed in infants and are associated with a high incidence of clinical inguinal hernia. This is not a true bladder anomaly, but is rather a bladder deformity secondary to a large

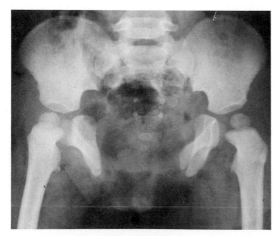

Fig. 20-55. The pelvis in exstrophy of the bladder. Note the wide separation of the symphysis pubis.

internal inguinal ring. The term "bladder ears" has been used in preference to hernia because the deformity does not usually persist beyond infancy. Roentgen findings at cystography or urography consist of anterolateral protrusion of the bladder into the inguinal canal which is usually bilateral. The protrusion is most often observed in the partially filled bladder and tends to disappear when the bladder is filled. Oblique or lateral views bring out the anterior extent of the protrusion.

The Pear-Shaped Bladder. The alteration in the shape of the bladder termed "tear-drop" or "pear-shaped" was first described in patients with pelvic hematoma, but there are a number of other abnormalities that may result in an elongated bladder with a narrow base. These include pelvic lipomatosis, hematoma, large iliopsoas muscles, enlarged pelvic nodes, lymphocysts, lymphoma and other pelvic tumors, and inferior vena cava occlusion. When the inferior vena cava is occluded, large venous collaterals compress the bladder to alter its shape.

VESICAL CALCULI

Obstruction and infection are the chief causes of vesical calculi. Many of these calculi are radiopaque and can be easily seen on plain-film roentgenograms (Fig. 20-57). Others contain small amounts of calcium and are poorly visualized on the plain film. The condition occurs largely in males.

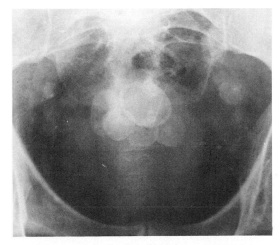

Fig. 20-57. Vesical calculi. This roentgenogram of the pelvis obtained without the use of contrast material, outlines five partially calcified bladder stones. Note their midline position.

Cystography with air or with an opaque medium can be used to outline radiolucent stones. Calculi may be single or multiple and tend to lie in the midline except when contained in a bladder diverticulum, in which case the position of the calculus depends on the site of the diverticulum. Bladder calculi must be differentiated from calcification in lymph nodes, fecaliths, calcification in uterine fibroids, and from prostatic and seminal vesicle calculi. Radiopaque bladder calculi are often laminated and very dense; when multiple, they may be faceted. Lymphnode calcification usually is higher in position and the nodes are mottled and not as uniformly dense as calculi. Uterine leiomyomas that contain calcium are often higher in position than bladder calculi and have a rather characteristic mottled appearance. Fecaliths of the sigmoid are rare but may simulate bladder calculi closely in texture and position. Oblique views and barium enema will permit differentiation. Prostatic calculi are usually multiple and produce a mottled density in contrast to the uniform or laminated appearance of vesical calculi; they are also lower in position. The same is true of calculi in the seminal vesicles. The position of bladder calculi in the midline is an important differential point.

Cystography and cystoscopy may be necessary to differentiate bladder calculi from other causes of calcification. A foreign body within the bladder may act as a nidus for deposition of calcium and other salts to form a calculus. Foreign bodies may be introduced by way of the urethra during treatment or by the patient. They also may be introduced through penetrating wounds or left in or near the bladder during surgery. The shape of the calculus then is dependent upon the foreign body, which can often be visualized on scout roentgenograms. Foreign bodies in the bladder almost invariably become encrusted with calcium.

Calculi in the prostate usually occur in the form of small granular deposits and these are visualized overlying or directly above the level of the symphysis pubis in standard anteroposterior roentgenograms of the lower abdomen. They offer little difficulty in differential diagnosis as a rule because of their position, characteristic small size, and multiplicity (Fig. 20-58).

INFLAMMATIONS OF THE BLADDER (CYSTITIS)

Acute inflammation of the urinary bladder does not produce changes that can be recognized and diagnosed on cystography. Chronic cystitis results in a

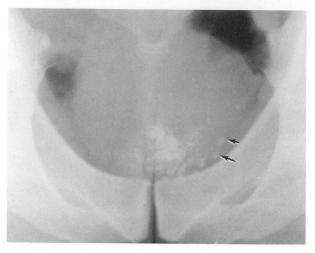

Fig. 20-58. Prostatic calculi. The mottled densities above the symphysis pubis are characteristic of prostatic calculi. Their distribution indicates probable prostatic enlargement. The calcifications on the left, which tend to parallel the pubic ramus, are phleboliths **(arrows)**.

decrease in bladder size. The wall may be smooth but sometimes is serrated and when this serration is present along with the major contraction at the dome, the so-called "Christmas-tree bladder" of chronic cystitis is formed. A bladder of this shape, also termed "pine-tree bladder," is found more frequently in association with neurogenic bladder dysfunction than with other conditions, although it may occur with any chronic bladder obstruction. Cystoscopy is a more useful method of examination in bladder infections than cystography. Various types of bladder inflammation are defined according to the gross anatomic changes found at cystoscopy and need not be discussed here.

Of interest roentgenologically is the condition know as *cystitis emphysematosa* (emphysematous cystitis). This is an inflammatory disease of the bladder in which there is gas in the vesical wall. It is caused by gas-forming bacteria. Nearly 50% of the reported cases have occurred in patients with diabetes mellitus. The gas may be present for only a short time, which probably accounts for its low reported incidence. Roentgen findings are characteristic. A ring of radiolucency outlines the bladder wall or a part of it. There is often gas within the bladder as well. The zone of gas expands and contracts with the bladder and is a transient finding unless the infection fails to respond to therapy. Some authors recommend that

an anteroposterior film of the bladder be obtained in all diabetics who have urinary infection. This bladder infection is often benign and transient, and may produce very few symptoms.

Schistosomiasis

Schistosomiasis (bilharziasis) is caused by a group of blood flukes, *Schistosoma mansoni, Schistosoma japonicum,* and *Schistosoma haematobium.* The lower urinary tract is involved mainly by *S. haematobium.* Large numbers of ova are deposited in the submucosa of the bladder wall. The wall becomes thickened and ulcerated and papillomas may be formed. In chronic disease, the distal ureters may be involved, leading to stricture, hydronephrosis, and renal damage. Calcification in the bladder wall, which occurs in chronic cases, has a characteristic appearance. When the bladder is empty, thin parallel lines of density are observed. The appearance is similar to that of the postvoiding bladder on excretory urography, in which a thin coating of opaque medium outlines the bladder wall. When the bladder is full of opaque medium, a very thin radiolucent line, representing the thickened mucosa, separates the opacified bladder lumen and the thin rim of submucosal calcification (Fig. 20-59). The ova in the bladder wall may calcify. Lower ureteral nodular involvement may produce the roentgen findings of ureteritis cystica. Bladder capacity eventually is reduced. The distal ureters may be calcified in a manner similar to that noted in the bladder. Calculi in the bladder, ureters, and kidneys are common.

Candidiasis of the Bladder

Candidiasis may involve the urinary bladder in circumstances similar to those in which the kidney is affected. There may be gas within a fungus ball giving a laminated appearance. Otherwise, the fungus balls appear as filling defects that must be differentiated from blood clot, radiolucent calculi, and tumors.

Cyclophosphamide Cystitis

Cytoxan, used in the treatment of leukemia and lymphoma, may produce a hemorrhagic cystitis with hematuria of varying degrees of severity. Blood clots within the bladder may then appear as filling defects. On cystography, minimal mucosal irregularity in addition to the clots is noted. Later, contraction and thumbprinting secondary to edema and submucosal

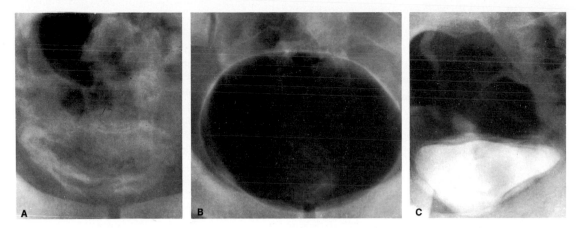

Fig. 20-59. Schistosomiasis of the bladder. **A.** Plain films showing parallel lines of calcific density in the wall of the empty bladder. **B.** Air cystogram showing a thin rim of calcium in the bladder wall. **C.** Renografin cystogram showing the thin rim of calcium separated from the lumen by a lucent line representing the thickened bladder wall.

hemorrhage are evident. Ultimately, the bladder may be markedly contracted and, very rarely, calcification may occur in its wall.

Radiation Cystitis

Large doses of radiation such as those administered in radiation therapy may produce enough necrosis of the bladder wall to result in calcification which is similar radiographically to that observed in schistosomiasis.

Cystitis Cystica

Cystitis cystica is a form of chronic disease of the bladder in which a number of small cystlike mucosal lesions are noted, mainly in the region of the trigone. In almost all instances, this condition is associated with infection, obstruction, tumor, calculi, or stasis. In children, its presence usually indicates that an associated chronic infection will be difficult to control. Radiographically, multiple filling defects are observed chiefly in the region of the trigone. The irregularity and deformity, if severe, may resemble changes observed in bladder tumor. Although the lesions may be visible on cystography, cystoscopy is the best method of examination in patients with this condition.

Cystitis Glandularis

Cystitis glandularis represents metaplasia of the bladder epithelium induced by a variety of irritants. The majority of the lesions occur in the region of the

vesical neck and trigone. They appear as irregular, rounded elevations separated by deep ridges; they are usually sharply demarcated from the normal mucosa. When they occur in the dome of the bladder, villous-like proliferations may occur, often several centimeters in size. The lesions appear to be pre-malignant ones. Because their radiographic appearance is quite similar to that in cystitis cystica, cystoscopy and often biopsy are required for definitive and differential diagnosis. The condition may also simulate bladder tumor.[31]

Malakoplakia

Malakoplakia is an uncommon chronic inflammatory disease usually confined to the bladder and renal pelvis and ureters. Rarely it may involve the renal parenchyma on one or both sides. It causes marked enlargement of the involved kidney(s) and, when renal infection with gram-negative organisms is an associated finding, xanthogranulomatous pyelonephritis and infected polycystic disease should be considered in the differential diagnosis. Malakoplakia is probably caused by an unusual histiocytic response to infection (usually *E. Coli*) and may result in renal failure when bilateral. The soft plaques formed in the bladder may not produce any recognizable roentgenographic changes on cystography.

OBSTRUCTION OF THE BLADDER

Bladder obstruction may be caused by congenital or acquired lesions. Benign prostatic hyperplasia is the most common cause. Prostatic enlargement is difficult to assess radiographically. However, when elevation of the bladder floor is accompanied by "J-shaped" or hockey-stick appearance of the distal ureters, prostatic enlargement is indicated. Prostatic carcinoma, acquired urethral stenosis, urethral valves, and neurogenic dysfunction (cord bladder) are other causes. The first change in the bladder wall resulting from obstruction is hypertrophy of the muscles. This can often be observed as a soft-tissue shadow of several millimeters thickness paralleling the opaque shadow of the inner bladder wall in excretory urography or cystography. The normal bladder wall does not ordinarily produce a visible soft-tissue shadow. As the muscle bundles enlarge they cause irregular interlacing bands known as trabeculae. The intervening depressions are called cellules (Fig. 20-60). Trabeculation becomes more prominent as obstruction continues and the cellules may enlarge until diverticula are formed. There also may be reflux of medium into one or both ureters with development of hydronephrosis (see section on hydronephrosis). It is more likely that reflux is caused by infection, however.

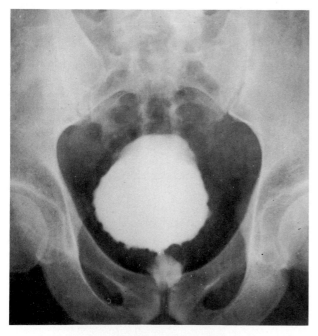

Fig. 20-60. Trabeculation of the bladder. Note the irregularity of the inferior and lateral bladder wall shown in this cystogram. The patient has had a transurethral prostatectomy with opacification of the rounded prostatic bed following the operation.

As obstruction develops the bladder may become decompensated, increasing in size and containing increasing amounts of residual urine, until it presents as a large, lower abdominal mass on physical examination and on roentgen study. The scout roentgenogram will demonstrate a large soft-tissue mass extending out of the pelvis, often displacing the bowel upward and posteriorly. Cystography will outline the large bladder with trabeculations standing out in a somewhat reticular manner, with more or less cellule or small diverticulum formation.

Cystourethrography is used to examine patients with suspected bladder or urethral obstruction as well as patients (usually children) with chronic or recurrent urinary infection. There is a great deal of controversy regarding the incidence, cause, and roentgen findings in bladder-neck obstruction. Shopfner[111] believes that a roentgen diagnosis of bladder-neck obstruction is no longer tenable, since there are changes in diameter during various stages of voiding. He also thinks that similar variation occurs in the diameter of the meatus and distal urethral segment during voiding; he has not encountered pathologic urethral narrowing. The most common abnormalities that he encountered on cystourethrography were trabeculation and cellules of the bladder which he attributes to infection. Vesicoureteral reflux, also caused by infection, was the second most common lesion. Other abnormalities include urethritis, urethral valves, bladder and urethral diverticula.

DIVERTICULUM OF THE BLADDER

A diverticulum of the bladder is a localized herniation of mucosa, usually having a narrow neck. These defects may be single or multiple and vary in size from a small cellule to a large sac having a capacity greater than the bladder itself. Chronic obstruction is a frequent cause, but some diverticula are of congenital origin. Infection is also a factor in many cases. If the diverticula are small and empty completely they are usually of no clinical significance. Large diverticula that do not empty completely, however, are often the site of infection that is fostered by stagnation. Calculus formation is also common in this type of large diverticulum and when a density resembling vesical calculus is visualized outside the usual position of the bladder, the presence of a diverticulum should be suspected and may be confirmed by means of cystography. Roentgen findings are confined to those diverticula that are noted at cystography or excretory urography unless the diverticulum is large enough to produce an actual mass shadow on a plain-film roent

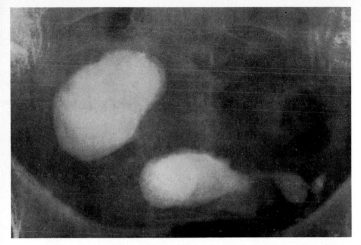

Fig. 20-61. Multiple bladder diverticula. The large opacified diverticulum on the right has a smooth wall in contrast to the trabeculation of the bladder wall. There is also a small diverticulum on the left.

genogram, and then the nature of the mass must be determined by means of cystography or cystoscopy. When the bladder is examined by means of cystography, the diverticulum is outlined by the opaque substance and its size, shape, and position, as well as the width of its neck, can be determined (Fig. 20-61). It is often of importance to assess the presence of and the amount of urinary retention in a large diverticulum and a roentgenogram obtained following voiding is usually sufficient for this purpose. If the bladder still contains enough opaque material to partially obscure the diverticulum, a second roentgenogram may be obtained following catheterization of the bladder. Occasionally a tumor may occur in a diverticulum; this lesion is often difficult to visualize, but presents as a filling defect on the otherwise smooth wall of the diverticulum. Double-contrast cystography is very useful when the presence of such a lesion is suspected.

NEUROGENIC BLADDER

Disease or injury involving the spinal cord or peripheral nerves supplying the bladder results in changes in bladder function that may produce either incontinence or retention of urine. The type of neurogenic bladder is somewhat dependent upon the lesion producing it. Usually, patients with small, spastic, trabeculated bladders have upper motor neuron lesions, but simple obstruction may cause the same appearance ("pine-tree" bladder). In theory, patients with lower motor neuron lesions have large, atonic bladders, but some have small, trabeculated bladders. The large, atonic bladder with little or no trabeculation is found in association with tabes dorsalis, diabe-

tes, or syringomyelia, but it may also be psychogenic in patients with no neurologic disease. The following findings may be observed in patients with neurogenic bladder: a trabeculated bladder with a circular or pyramidal (pine-tree) pattern; an hourglass bladder; a small, hypertonic trabeculated bladder; a large dilated hypotonic bladder without trabeculation; and variations in the contour of the vesical neck and prostatic urethra in which there may be sacular dilatation, funnel-shaped dilatation or contraction, and spasm of the bladder neck. The diagnosis of exact abnormality is difficult and is based on extensive study, including neurologic examination, cystoscopy, cystometric studies (measurement of intravesical pressures), and cystography. The cystographic study will determine vesical size, presence or absence of trabeculation, reflux into the ureters, retention or lack of it, vesical-neck dilatation, and the presence of any other associated gross anatomic changes.

VESICOURETERAL REFLUX

Infection is the most common cause of vesicoureteral reflux. It is also found in patients with obstruction in the lower urinary tract. The obstructive lesions include posterior urethral valves, urethral stricture, and median bar enlargement. Neurologic disorders which result in neurogenic bladder may also cause reflux. Congenital anomalies such as ectopic ureter and other anomalies of the distal ureter and trigone may also produce reflux.

The roentgen study used for the detection is the voiding cystourethrogram. If reflux is present it is manifested by retrograde filling of one or both ureters. The ureters may dilate considerably and there may be marked hydronephrosis associated with reflux. Any child with unexplained recurrent urinary tract infection should have a complete urologic study including cystourethrography. Since the evidence of reflux is sometimes fleeting, fluoroscopic examination is important.

Renal parenchymal scarring, either local with a single calyx blunted, or extensive involvement may be seen. In adults, about 60% of patients with reflux have extensive scarring. Mucosal striations in the pelvis and upper ureter are also observed in patients with reflux, probably the result of dilatation and infection.[61]

THE MEGACYSTIS SYNDROME

The term "megacystis" refers to a large, smooth, thin-walled bladder accompanied by vesicoureteral reflux and dilated ureters and recurrent or persistent urinary-tract infection. It is usually discovered in childhood and is much more frequent in females than in males. The trigone is usually much larger than normal and the intramural portion of the ureters is shortened and widened. The nature of the underlying disorder leading to the megacystis syndrome is not clear, but it is believed to be a congenital disproportionate increase in size of the vesical base leading to reflux and infection. Cystography demonstrates the large bladder and the large trigone with vesicoureteral reflux on one or both sides. Lalli and Lapides[70] described 21 patients who voided infrequently (*the infrequent voider*). Roentgen signs are bladder enlargement, increased bladder capacity, no evidence of obstruction, and ability to empty bladder normally. They believe that this is the same condition as the megacystis syndrome.

VESICAL TUMORS

Most malignant tumors of the bladder arise in the region of the trigone and tend to obstruct the ureteral or urethral orifices. The "benign" papilloma is the most common tumor and is often multiple, but it is so small as to be difficult, if not impossible, to visualize on cystography. This epithelial tumor is malignant or has malignant potential, thus the term "benign" is probably a misnomer; many consider it to be a grade I papillary transitional-cell carcinoma. Radiographic detection of this tumor depends upon its size. The diagnosis is best made by cystoscopy.

Malignant Tumors

Carcinoma of the bladder is usually of the transitional cell type. Cystographic finding is that of an irregular filling defect, usually at the base, often resulting in ureteral obstruction. Calcification may occur in the primary tumor and in metastases from it. The size and shape of these tumors vary widely (Fig. 20-62). Double-contrast cystography is useful for the study of the bladder mucosa in patients with intravesical tumors. Angiography using bilateral femoral artery catheterization is useful for staging bladder tumors. Cystoscopic confirmation is necessary since tumor type cannot be determined without biopsy. Occasionally the bladder may be involved by direct extension of prostatic carcinoma, rectal carcinoma, or by extension of uterine neoplasms in the female. Pelvic tumors, retroperitoneal sarcoma, and malignant lymphoma may also involve the bladder and deform it.

Rhabdomyosarcoma occasionally arises in the

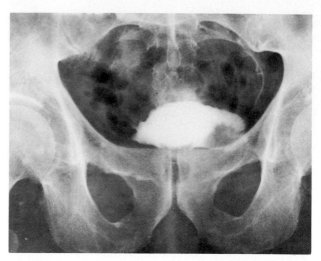

Fig. 20-62. Carcinoma of the bladder. Note the irregular filling defect in the left inferolateral aspect of the bladder.

bladder. This tumor usually presents in the first 3 or 4 years of life. It may originate in the submucosal or superficial layers, usually at the base. The tumor tends to become large enough to displace the ureters laterally and to bulge upward into the bladder to form a lobulated filling defect in it. The tumor nodules may also force their way downward into the urethra, forming a cone of dilatation in the posterior urethra. Some appear as rectal masses; others may protrude through the vulva. Urinary retention is the most common symptom. Intravenous urography often shows ureteral displacement as well as deformity and displacement of the bladder. Since there is nothing distinctive that will help in differentiating the tumor type in these patients, biopsy is necessary. Rhabdomyosarcomas comprise about 10% of malignant tumors of childhood. There is a slight male predominance. The majority arise in the bladder, but they may also arise in the prostate, vagina, spermatic cord, and broad ligament. The tumor is sometimes termed *sarcoma botryoides.*

Benign Lesions

There are a number of benign, nonepithelial tumors that may involve the bladder. They are rare and include neurofibroma, leiomyoma, fibroma, fibromyxoma, myxoma, hemangioma, pheochromocytoma, and such heterotopic types as chondroma, dermoid cysts, and rhabdomyoma. There are also several other conditions that may produce changes in the bladder, demonstrable by cystography, which resemble tumor. These include endometriosis and granulomatous disease, either involving the colon or small bowel adjacent to the bladder. Occasionally, localized cystitis glandularis and cystitis cystica may simulate bladder tumor. Roentgen findings are those of a mass which may be very large, extending into or indenting the bladder wall, with no characteristics to distinguish its cell type. In neurofibromatosis, masses may be multiple and extensive. In granulomatous disease, there may be evidence of Crohn's disease of the ileum and colon, and in patients with endometriosis, cyclic pain or hematuria may be present to suggest the diagnosis. Leukoplakia of the bladder is a cystoscopic and not a cystographic diagnosis.

Metastases to the Bladder

Three general types of metastases to the bladder may be observed: (*1*) bladder implant secondary to epithelial tumors of the kidney or ureter; (2) direct extension from primary neoplasms in the area such as from prostatic, uterine, ovarian, and colonic neoplasms; (3) hematogenous metastases from various sources such as breast, lung, or stomach and from melanoma arising at a distant site.

TRAUMA OF THE BLADDER

Rupture of the bladder may result from a direct blow to the distended bladder as a single injury or may be associated with more extensive injury such as pelvic fracture, penetrating war wounds, or gunshot wounds. Instrumentation may also cause rupture of the bladder or urethra. The rupture may be intra- or extraperitoneal. There is now a trend toward early cystographic examination to establish the diagnosis since excretory urograhy is not a very useful method of defining bladder rupture. Intraperitoneal rupture results in extravasation of urine into the peritoneal cavity and the opaque medium also enters the peritoneal cavity to outline the smooth outer wall of the pelvic and lower abdominal viscera as well as the smooth serosal surface of the pelvic walls. The actual site of rupture may not be visible on the roentgenogram because of overlapping shadows. Extraperitoneal rupture of the bladder produces a more varied pattern, depending upon the site of rupture. The medium is extravasated, outlines the tissue planes of the pelvic floor, and extends varying distances into the perivesical soft tissues in an irregular, streaky manner. At times, the differentiation between intra- and extraperitoneal rupture may be difficult. Rarely, spontaneous rupture of the bladder may occur— usually in patients with severe cystitis, extravesical infection, or malignant disease, or it may be due to overdistention secondary to mechanical obstruction or neurogenic dysfunction. Pelvic and lower abdominal trauma may also result in perivesical hematoma without rupture. Cystography will then show displacement of the bladder, which varies with the size and location of the hematoma.

FOREIGN BODIES

Foreign bodies in the bladder are usually identified on plain-film roentgenograms when they are radiopaque. Oblique and lateral views may be necessary, however, to verify the position of the foreign body in relation to the bladder. Cystography will outline radiolucent foreign bodies and demonstrate associated changes in the bladder wall. Various oblique and lateral projections are usually necessary to make certain of the location. Ultrasound is very useful in this situation. Cystoscopy is used for both diagnosis and treatment. Foreign body in the bladder is usually introduced by the patient and is therefore found in children and in adults who are perverted or psychotic. Occasionally foreign bodies are introduced at the time of surgery or instrumentation and they may also result from penetrating wounds. A foreign body may serve as a nidus for the deposition of calcium salts and the formation of a bladder calculus, as indicated previously.

HERNIA OF THE BLADDER

Bladder herniation is said to occur in 10% of all inguinal hernias in men over age 50, but large hernias with descent into the scrotum are unusual.[49] Herniation must be differentiated from diverticulum; this is usually accomplished on the basis of the hernia's location and the direction of its protrusion as well as its relatively wide mouth as compared to the diverticulum. Films with the patient in the erect and prone positions are necessary to demonstrate these findings in most patients.

URETHROGRAPHY AND SEMINAL VESICULOGRAPHY

The urethrogram is the radiographic method for examination of the urethra. It consists of injection of a relatively viscous radiopaque oil or jelly into the urethra, following which films are exposed in various projections as the occasion demands. It is used in the female to demonstrate diverticula that may be missed at cystoscopy. In the male, diverticula, strictures, abscess cavities, fistulas, and abnormalities caused by prostatic enlargement may be outlined.

Voiding Urethrography

The male urethra can be demonstrated following excretory urography by having the patient void against the partial obstruction produced by a Zipser penile clamp. High-dose urography is performed and, as soon as the urographic study is completed, oral hydration is started; the patient is asked to drink as much water as necessary to produce an urgent desire to void. The scout film is obtained with the patient in the supine, 45-degree posterior-oblique position. A Zipser penile clamp is placed at the base of the glans penis. The patient is then shown how to hold the clamp and asked to void. Voiding against a peripheral resistence slightly distends the urethra and aids in the evaluation of any abnormalities involving it. Films are obtained with the patient in both posterior-oblique positions if possible. The advantages of this method of examination are the simplicity and ease with which it is carried out and the avoidance of instrumentation. The pressure is sufficient to permit an adequate flow of the urinary stream. Before urography is started, the patient should be asked to void so that the medium is not diluted unduly by residual urine.

Seminal vesiculography is a specialized urologic-radiologic method of examining the seminal vesicles. The technique and the normal seminal vesiculogram are described by Banner and Hassler.[7]

POSTERIOR URETHRAL VALVES

Posterior urethral valves produce varying degrees of obstruction leading to infection, vesicoureteral reflux, and hydronephrosis, with more or less destruction of the kidneys unless corrected. They are found almost exclusively in males. Eneuresis is a common symptom. Symptoms and signs are bladder distention, dribbling, poor stream, and failure to thrive. At times, early signs consist of flank mass caused by urinoma, urinary ascites leading to respiratory distress, dehydrated infants in whom rapid loss of concentrating ability leads to large output of dilute urine suggesting diabetes insipidus. This group of signs should suggest the diagnosis.[85] The valves are located in the vicinity of the verumontanum. Voiding cystourethrography is the roentgen method used to demonstrate this lesion.

Roentgen findings consist of a thin membrane arising anteriorly which partially obstructs the urethra. The posterior urethra must be filled in order to distend the valve; otherwise it may not be visible. A true lateral projection is also necessary in order to identify the position of the valve. The valve stretches in sail-like fashion to obstruct the urethra. The valve itself may not be visible, but the dilatation of the prostatic urethra and a constricting ring at the vesical neck are characteristic. Rarely, anterior urethral valves may be present; obstruction with proximal dilatation similar to that in posterior valves may be present. The sail-like lucent defect may be visualized on cystourethrography.

MISCELLANEOUS CONGENITAL ANOMALIES OF THE URETHRA

Urethral diverticula may occur in males or in females. In the male, a few are congenital but most follow trauma or infection. They are readily visualized on urethrography. In the female, most, if not all, are acquired; they usually result from retention in periurethral glands. Infection and calculi may complicate urethral diverticula. Voiding urethrography usually outlines these abnormalities in the female in whom retrograde urethrography is a difficult technique.

Megalourethra in males is associated with deficient erectile tissue which allows the penile urethra to dilate.

OTHER URETHRAL DISEASES

Calculi are almost always associated with diverticula and infection in females and in males they occur largely proximal to obstruction, often in the prostatic or bulbous urethra. If the area is included on the plain or scout film, the diagnosis can usually be made radiographically.

Trauma may result in complete or incomplete urethral rupture or in urethral laceration. Urethrography may determine the diagnosis by showing extravasation of opaque medium. As a rule, when there is complete urethral rupture, no medium injected into the urethra reaches the bladder, because of retraction of the ruptured ends of the urethra.

Condyloma acuminata (venereal warts) occasionally spread into the urethra. Radiographic findings consist of varying numbers of flat verrucous filling defects. Because instrumentation is contraindicated since it may spread the disease, voiding urethrography is the method of choice in examining patients with this condition.

Urethral strictures may be caused by infection or trauma and very rarely represent a congenital anomaly in males. The site, severity, length, and associated sinus or fistulous tracts can be outlined on urethrography.

Urethral tumors are more common in females than in males. Urethrography is difficult technically and not very successful in demonstrating tumors in females, but is useful in outlining the irregularity and intraluminal masses found in the male with urethral carcinoma. Rarely, polyps may occur in the prostatic urethra of boys and are demonstrated as small, rounded or oval filling defects on urethrography.

VAS DEFERENS CALCIFICATION

Calcification of the vas deferens is occasionally present in diabetic men, rarely it occurs in nondiabetics. It probably represents a degenerative phenomenon in these patients. Roentgen findings are the presence of densely calcified bilaterally symmetrical tubular shadows about 3 mm in diameter in the low midpelvis (Fig. 20-63).

THE ADRENAL GLANDS

The adrenal glands lie upon the upper pole of the kidneys within the perirenal fascia of Gerota. The right adrenal gland is a long thin triangle or wedge while the left is wider, shorter, and is somewhat crescentic in shape. The adrenal glands are small, the combined average weight being 11 to 12 gm.

Calcification in the adrenal glands is usually an incidental finding and is of no clinical significance. The most frequent cause is believed to be hemorrhage, often associated with birth trauma or with hypoxia, severe maternal infection, hypoprothrombinemia, or increased vascular fragility. It is often present in infants born to diabetic mothers. There is a high incidence of abnormal obstetric history, including prematurity and forceps and breech deliveries, in children with adrenal calcification. Neonatal adrenal hemorrhage may be massive, unilateral or bilateral, and can be observed as a radiolucent suprarenal mass on the total body phase of excretory urography in neonates. Calcification occurs rapidly around the periphery a few weeks after the hemorrhage, then contracts slowly to the size and shape of the original

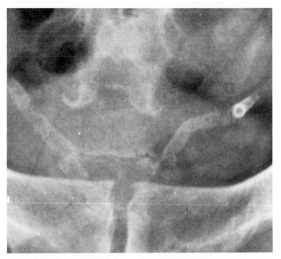

Fig. 20-63. Calcification in the vas deferens of a 45-year-old man with a history of diabetes of more than 20 years' duration.

gland. The right side is involved more frequently than the left when bleeding is unilateral. Occasionally, in adults, stippled areas of calcification are found in one or both adrenals without any signs or symptoms of adrenal insufficiency. The cause in these cases remains obscure. Oblique roentgenograms may be needed to prove the constant relationship of the calcium to the upper pole of the kidney upon which the adrenal rests. Tuberculosis of the adrenal glands (Addison's disease) results in calcification within the gland in about one-third of the patients with this disease. The calcification may outline the entire gland or appear as amorphous granular density within it.

Cysts of the adrenal glands may also contain calcium. These lesions are rare. Their incidence is 50% higher in females than in males. They occur in equal numbers on right and left sides. Approximately 20% of them contain roentgenologically visible calcification which characteristically is located peripherally, forming a thin rim of density outlining the cyst wall. When present in a suprarenal mass, the calcification is strongly suggestive of cyst when peripheral. Calcification within the mass is more suggestive of tumor. Cyst puncture is advocated by some in the diagnostic evaluation of adrenal masses, the approach being similar to that of renal cyst puncture. Cysts that do not contain calcium simulate tumor and are not visible on plain film unless they become large (Fig. 20-64).

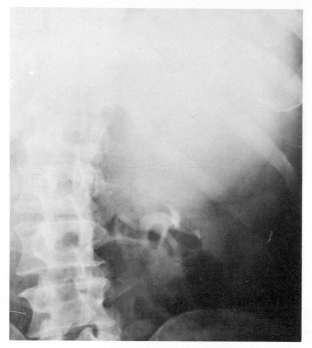

Fig. 20-64. Cyst of the left adrenal gland. Note the large mass above and partly overlying the upper pole of the left kidney. The kidney is displaced downward but is not deformed or distorted significantly.

ADRENAL CORTICAL TUMORS

Tumors of the adrenal gland are divided according to their origin into cortical and medullary types. The cortical lesions are glandular in type and are mesodermal in origin. Benign adenoma and carcinoma are the two types found. Both of these tumors as well as hyperplasia of the adrenal cortex may result in a disturbance of function of both cortex may result in a disturbance of function of both cortex and medulla. The symptoms are varied and may be caused by an excess of androgens, excess of estrogens, or excess of other hormones. Sex changes and Cushing's syndrome may be present. In some patients no hormonal disturbance is noted but this is rare. Occasionally the tumor is large enough to be visualized as a mass above the kidney. The hyperplastic gland is enlarged and retains its normal shape, whereas tumors tend to be round or oval and produce an alteration in the contour of the adrenal gland. The diagnosis of adrenal hyperplasia must be made with caution because the fat surrounding the gland cannot be differentiated from the glandular tissue. Excretory uro-

graphy is a simply and relatively safe initial step in localizing suspected adrenal tumors. The use of the large-dose method combined with tomography will reveal 70% or more of the tumors.[99] Careful technique and monitoring of the study are necessary as in the study of renal disease. CT scanning and ultrasound are the primary diagnostic methods, however. Arteriography is also used in the study of patients with suspected adrenal tumor or hyperplasia. Some have suggested that ACTH be injected prior to adrenal angiography, believing that it may increase the probability of diagnosing small adrenal cortical adenomas.[2] In some instances, aortography will clearly outline the adrenal gland and demonstrate a tumor involving it. If not, selective arteriography is necessary; some believe that a selective study should be undertaken in nearly all of these patients. Adrenal venography is now being used in the diagnosis of adrenal masses and is more reliable in detection of cortical hyperplasia than arteriography. Retroperitoneal pneumography is no longer used much, particularly in departments in which ultrasound or body CT scanning is available. The angiographic signs are similar to those of tumor elsewhere and consist of dilated and displaced vessels, tortuous vascular patterns, and arteriovenous shunts. Identification of small adrenal cortical tumors is often difficult, despite the use of the techniques mentioned. In patients with primary aldosteronism, venography may be useful in detecting a small adenoma and differentiating it from cortical hyperplasia (idiopathic aldosteronism). Scintiscanning [^{131}I] 19-iodocholesterol has been used by Conn and his associates[22, 58] to demonstrate increased radioactivity in the abnormal adrenal gland and to differentiate hyperplasia from cortical adenoma and adenocarcinoma.

ADRENAL MEDULLARY TUMORS

Medullary tumors are ectodermal in origin. They include ganglioneuroma, ganglioneuroblastoma, pheochromocytoma, and neuroblastoma. The benign pheochromocytoma often results in paroxysmal hypertension because it excretes pressor substances (catecholamines). It is usually a very vascular tumor with arteriovenous lakes and early venous filling. Because of the danger of a precipitous rise in blood pressure in patients with suspected pheochromocytoma, blood pressure and electrocardiogram are continuously monitored and phentolamine should be available for immediate intravenous injection if blood pressure rises suddenly. An injection of 5 mg phentol-

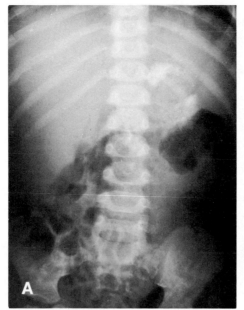 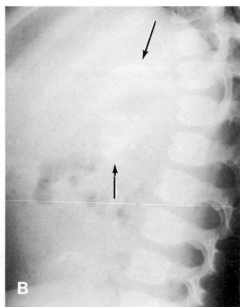

Fig. 20-65. Neuroblastoma arising in the left adrenal gland. **A.** Note the mottled calcification in the left upper abdomen, which is somewhat granular and mottled and is typical of the calcification observed in neuroblastoma. **B.** Lateral view. **Arrows** outline the extent of the large calcified mass.

amine is usually sufficient to control the blood pressure, but repeated injections may be necessary in some patients.[2] Because pheochromocytomas (about 10%) may be extra-adrenal, aortography and selective arteriography to demonstrate the blood supply of these tumors may be necessary.[128] An injection into the aorta above the celiac axis is carried out following a selective renal arteriogram that reveals no abnormality; if this also reveals no abnormality a low aortogram (to include the inferior mesenteric artery) may be obtained. If there is no evidence of a mass on either side on urography, the right adrenal is studied first because of the higher incidence of right-sided tumors and the more constant arterial anatomy. Ganglioneuroma that is also benign usually causes no symptoms. If large, these tumors may be visible on scout roentgenograms. If not, angiography, venography, or CT scan can be used.

NEUROBLASTOMA

The malignant tumor of adrenal medullary origin is the neuroblastoma, which is usually found in childhood; about one-third of these are diagnosed in children under 1 year of age, another 15% to 20% in children less than age 2, 25% in children between 2 and 5 years of age, and about 90% in those under age 8. The tumor may arise in cells of the sympathetic nervous system as well as in the adrenal medulla, so that this type of tumor may be found below as well as above the kidney. The tumor is highly malignant and may attain great size before discovery. The presence of calcification in the mass is common (about 50%) (Fig. 20-65), while in Wilms' tumor, from which it must be differentiated, there is rarely any calcium. The calcification has a fine granular or stippled appearance. Urography serves to indicate that the mass is extrarenal. The kidney may be displaced and the tumor may fill most of the abdomen. Metastases to the liver, lungs, and bone are common. The osseous metastases are often very extensive and characteristic, being of mixed lytic–blastic character. Often there is extensive involvement of the calvarium with separation of the sutures. Since this tumor may revert to benign ganglioneuroma spontaneously or during treatment, localization and treatment of the primary tumor is important.

OTHER ADRENAL TUMORS

Among tumors arising in the adrenal stroma are neuromas, fibromas, lipomas, neurofibromas, hemangiomas, myomas, sarcomas, lymphangiomas, and melanomas. All of them are extremely rare but any one may cause an adrenal mass. Tumors metastatic from other areas may also be found in the adrenal glands. Melanoma metastatic to the adrenals has been reported causing curvilinear calcifications simulating those noted in benign adrenal cyst.[120]

MISCELLANEOUS ADRENAL CONDITIONS

Adrenal abscess is very rare but it is a possible cause of adrenal enlargement in neonates. It must be differentiated from other adrenal masses such as hematoma and neuroblastoma. Total body opacification in these infants identifies the lesion as avascular and outside of the kidney but cannot differentiate hematoma from abscess.

Adrenal milk of calcium is a rare occurrence in which a suspension of calcification, resembling the milk of calcium observed in the gallbladder, accumulates in an adrenal cyst.[86]

REFERENCES AND SELECTED READINGS

1. ALBERTSON KW, TALNER LB: Valves of the ureter. Radiology 103: 91, 1972
2. ALFIDI RJ, GILL WM JR, KLEIN HJ: Arteriography of adrenal neoplasms. Am J Roentgenol 106: 635, 1969
3. ANDREWS EJ JR: The vagus reaction as a possible cause of severe complications of radiological procedures. Radiology 121: 1, 1976
4. ARNALDSSON O, HOLMLUND D: Defects in the urographic contrast medium above and below and ureteric calculus. Acta Radiol [Diagn] (Stockh) 11: 26, 1971
5. BAILEY H: Cystitis emphysematosa. Am J Roentgenol 86: 850, 1961
6. BAKER DH, BERDON WE: Use and safety of "high" dosage in pediatric urography. Radiology 103: 371, 1972
7. BANNER MP, HASSLER R: The normal seminal vesiculogram. Radiology 128: 339, 1978
8. BATSON PG, KEATS TE: The roentgenographic determination of normal kidney size as related to vertebral height. Am J Roentgenol 116: 737, 1972
9. BERDON WE, BAKER DH: The significance of a distended bladder in the interpretation of intravenous pyelograms obtained on patients with "hydronephrosis". Am J Roentgenol 120: 402, 1974
10. BERNSTEIN J, MEYER R: Parenchymal maldevelopment of the kidney. In Brennemann-Kelley Practice of Pediatrics, Vol 3, pp 1–28. Hagerstown, Harper & Row, 1969
11. BOIJSEN E, WILLIAMS CM, JUDKINS MP: Angiography of pheochromocytoma. Am J Roentgenol 98: 225, 1966
12. BOOKSTEIN JJ, ABRAMS HL, BUENGER RE et al: Radiologic aspects of renovascular hypertension. Part II. The role of urography in unilateral renovascular disease. JAMA 220: 1225, 1972
13. BOOKSTEIN JJ, MAXWELL MH, ABRAMS HL et al: Cooperative study of radiologic aspects of renal vascular hypertension. Bilateral renovascular disease. JAMA 237: 1706, 1977
14. BOSNIAK MA: Nephrotomography: a relatively unappreciated but extremely valuable diagnostic tool. Radiology 113: 313, 1974
15. BOSNIAK MA, AMBOS MA, MADAYAG MA et al: Epinephrine-enhanced renal angiography in renal mass lesions: is it worth performing? Am J Roentgenol 129: 647, 1977
16. BRODEUR AE, GOYER RA, MELICK W: A potential hazard of barium cystography. Radiology 85: 1080, 1965
17. CAFFEY J: Pediatric X-ray Diagnosis, 6th ed. Chicago, Year Book Medical, 1972
18. CAMIEL MR: Calcification of vas deferens associated with diabetes. J Urol 86: 634, 1961
19. CAPLAN LH, SIEGELMAN SS, BOSNIAK MA: Angiography in inflammatory space-occupying lesions of the kidney. Radiology 88: 14, 1967
20. CLARK RE, MINAGI H, PALUBINSKAS AJ: Renal candidiasis. Radiology 101: 567: 1971
21. CLAUS D: Systematic use of suprapubic bladder puncture for voiding cystourethrography in infants and children. Ann Radiol 18: 331, 1975
22. CONN JW, MORITA R, COHEN EL et al: Primary aldosteronism: photoscanning of tumors after administration of ^{131}I-19 iodocholesterol. Arch Intern Med 129: 417: 1972
23. COOK IK, KEATS TE, SEALE DL: Determination of the normal position of the upper urinary tract on the lateral abdominal urogram. Radiology 99: 499, 1971
24. COOPERMAN LR: Delayed opacification in congenital, multicystic dysplastic kidney, an important roentgen sign. Radiology 121: 703, 1976
25. COOPERMAN LR, LOWMAN RM: Fetal lobulation of the kidneys. Am J Roentgenol 92: 273, 1964
26. COUREY WR, PFISTER RC: The radiographic findings in renal tubular acidosis. Radiology 105: 497, 1972
27. CRUMMY AB JR, BARQUIN OP, WEAR JB JR: Renal sinus lipomatosis. J Urol 96: 127, 1966
28. CRUMMY AB JR, MADSEN PO: Parapelvic renal cyst: the peripheral fat sign. J Urol 96: 436, 1966
29. CURRARINO G: Roentgenographic estimation of kidney size in normal individuals with emphasis on children. Am J Roentgenol 93: 464, 1965
30. DALINKA MK, LALLY JF, RANCIER LF et al: Nephromegaly in hemophilia. Radiology 115: 337, 1975
31. DANN RH, ARGER PH, ENTERLINE HT: Benign proliferation processes of the bladder. Am J Roentgenol 116: 822, 1972

32. DAUGHTHRIDGE TY: Segmental, multicystic renal dysplasia. J Can Assoc Radiol 26: 149, 1975

33. DELIVELIOTIS A, KEHAYAS P, VARKARAKIS M: The diagnostic problems of hydatid disease of the kidney. J Urol 99: 139, 1968

34. DUBILIER W JR, EVANS JA: Peripelvic cysts of the kidney. Radiology 71: 404, 1958

35. EKLOF O, LOHR G, RINGERTZ H et al: Ectopic ureterocele in the male infant. Acta Radiol [Diagn] (Stockh) 19: 145, 1978

36. ELKIN M: Radiology of the urinary tract: some physiological considerations. Radiology 116: 259, 1975

37. ELKIN M, BERNSTEIN J: Cystic disease of the kidney—radiological and pathological considerations. Clin Radiol 20: 65, 1969

38. ELKIN M, MENG CH, DE PAREDES RG: Roentgenologic evaluation of renal trauma with emphasis on renal angiography. Am J Roentgenol 98: 1, 1966

39. ELLIOTT CB, JOHNSON HW, BALFOUR JA: Xanthogranulomatous pyelonephritis and perirenal xanthogranuloma. Br J Urol 40: 548, 1968

40. ERICSSON NO: Ectopic ureterocele in infants and children. Acta Chir Scand [Suppl] 197, 1954

41. FAINGOLD JE, HANSEN CO, RIGLER LG: Cystitis emphysematosa. Radiology 61: 346, 1953

42. FELSON B, MOSKOWITZ M: Renal pseudotumors: the regenerated nodule and other lumps, bumps and dromedary humps. Am J Roentgenol 107: 720, 1969

43. FISCHER HW, COLGAN FJ: Causes of contrast media reaction. Radiology 121: 223, 1976

44. FLETCHER EWL, FORBES WSTC, GOUGH MH: Suprapubic micturating cystourethrography in infants. Clin Radiol 29: 309, 1978

45. FRIEDENBERG RM, NEY C: The radiographic findings in neurogenic bladder. Radiology 76: 798, 1961

46. GELFORD GJ, WILETS AJ, NELSON D, KROLL LL: Retroperitoneal fibrosis and methysergide. Radiology 88: 976, 1967

47. GIBBONS RP, BUSCH WH JR, BURNETT LL: Needle tract seeding following aspiration of renal cell carcinoma. J Urol 118: 865, 1977

48. GLANZ I, GRUNEBAUM M: Ureteral changes in polyarteritis nodosa as seen during excretory urography. J Urol 116: 731, 1976

49. GOLDIN RR, ROSEN RA: Effect of inguinal hernias upon the bladder and ureters. Radiology 115: 55, 1975

50. GOLDMAN ML, GORELKIN L, RUDÉ JC III et al: Epinephrine renal venography in severe inflammatory disease of the kidney. Radiology 127: 93, 1978

51. GOLDSTEIN HM, MEDELLIN H, BEYDOUN MT et al: Transcatheter embolization of renal cell carcinoma. Am J Roentgenol 123: 557, 1975

52. GREEN WM, PRESSMAN BD, McCLENNAN BL et al: Col-

umn of Bertin: Diagnosis by nephrotomography. Am J Roentgenol 116: 714, 1972

53. GROSSMAN H, WINCHESTER PH, GOLSTEON WC: Neurogenic bladder in childhood. Radiol Clin North Am 6: 155, 1968

54. GWINN JL, LANDING BH: Cystic diseases of the kidneys in infants and children. Radiol Clin North Am 6: 191, 1968

55. HARRISON EG JR, McCORMACK LJ: Pathologic classification of renal arterial disease in renovascular hypertension. Mayo Clin Proc 45: 161, 1971

56. HARTMAN GW, HODSON CJ: The duplex kidney and related abnormalities. Clin Radiol 20: 387, 1969

57. HERSCHMAN A, BLUM R, LEE YC: Angiographic findings in polyarteritis nodosa. Radiology 94: 147, 1970

58. HERWIG KR, CONN JW, SCHTEINGART DE et al: Localization of adrenal tumors by photoscanning. J Urol 109: 2, 1973

59. HIMMELFARB EH, RABINOWITZ JG, KINKHABWALA MN et al: The roentgen features of renal carbuncle. J Urol 108: 846, 1972

60. HODSON CJ: The radiological contribution toward the diagnosis of chronic pyelonephritis. Radiology 88: 857, 1967

61. HYDE I, WASTIE ML: Striations (longitudinal mucosal folds) in the upper urinary tract. Br J Radiol 44: 445, 1971

62. KAHN PC: Selective venography in renal parenchymal disease. Radiology 92: 345, 1969

63. KAHN PC, WISE HM JR: The use of epinephrine in selective angiography of renal masses. J Urol 99: 133, 1968

64. KIKKAWA K, LASSER EC: "Ring-like" or "rim-like" calcification in renal cell carcinoma. Am J Roentgenol 107: 737, 1969

65. KINCAID OW, DAVIS GD, HALLERMANN FJ et al: Fibromuscular dysplasia of the renal arteries. Arteriographic features, classification and observations on natural history of the disease. Am J Roentgenol 104: 271, 1968

66. KING RL, TUCKER AS, PERSKY L: Congenital hypoplasia of the abdominal muscles. Radiology 77: 228, 1961

67. KISSANE JM: Congenital malformations. In Hepinstall RH: Pathology of the Kidney, 2nd ed., pp 69–119. Boston, Little, Brown, 1974

68. KJELLBERG SR, ERICSSON NO, RUHDE U: The Lower Urinary Tract in Childhood. Chicago, Year Book Medical, 1957

69. KOROBKIN DR, BINDER R, CLARK RE et al: Aberrant papillae and other filling defects in the renal pelvis. Am J Roentgenol 114: 746, 1972

70. LALLI AF, LAPIDES J: The infrequent voider. Radiology 92: 1177, 1969

71. LANDES RR, RANSOM CL: Presacral retroperitoneal

pneumography utilizing carbon dioxide. J Urol 82: 670, 1959

72. LEE KT, DEETHS TM: Localized amyloidosis of the ureter. Radiology 120: 60, 1976

73. LINDVALL N: Roentgenologic diagnosis of medullary sponge kidney. Acta Radiol [Diagn] (Stockh) 51: 193, 1959

74. LINDVALL N: Renal papillary necrosis. Acta Radiol [Suppl] (Stockh) 192, 1960

75. LLOYD-THOMAS HG, BALME RH, KEY JJ: Tram-line calcification in renal cortical necrosis. Br Med J 1: 909, 1962

76. LOITMAN BS, CHIAT H: Ureteritis cystica and pyelitis cystica. Radiology 68: 354, 1957

77. MARBERGER M, GEORGI M: Balloon occlusion of the renal artery in tumor nephrectomy. J Urol 114: 360, 1975

78. MCALISTER WH, NEDELMAN SH: The roentgen manifestations of bilateral renal cortical necrosis. Am J Roentgenol 86: 129, 1961

79. MCCLENNAN BL, BECKER JA: Excretory urography: choice of contrast material—clinical. Radiology 100: 591, 1971

80. MENA E, BOOKSTEIN JJ, MCDONALD FD et al: Angiographic findings in renal medullary cystic disease. Radiology 110: 277, 1974

81. MENG CH, ELKIN M: Venous impression on the calyceal system. Radiology 87: 878, 1966

82. MENG CH, ELKIN M: Angiographic manifestations of Wilms' tumor. Am J Roentgenol 105: 95, 1969

83. MILLER SM, WINSTON MC: Nephrogenic diabetes insipidus. Radiology 87: 893, 1966

84. MOELL H: Kidney size and its deviation from normal in acute renal failure. A roentgendiagnostic study. Acta Radiol [Suppl] (Stockh) 206, 1961

85. MOONEY JK, BERDON WE, LATTIMER JK: A new dimension in the diagnosis of posterior urethral valves in children. J Urol 113: 272, 1975

86. MOSS AA: Milk of calcium of the adrenal glands. Br J Radiol 49: 186, 1976

87. MURRAY RL: Milk of calcium in the kidney. Diagnostic features on vertical beam roentgenograms. Am J Roentgenol 113: 455, 1971

88. NEBESAR RA, POLLARD JJ, FRALEY EE: Renal vascular impressions. Am J Roentgenol 101: 719, 1967

89. NOYES WE, PALUBINSKAS AJ: Squamous metaplasia of the renal pelvis. Radiology 89: 292, 1967

90. OLSSON O: Studies on backflow in excretion urography. Acta Radiol [Suppl] (Stockh) 70, 1948

91. OSATHANONDH V, POTTER EL: Pathogenesis of polycystic kidneys: Type III due to multiple abnormalities of development. Arch Pathol 77: 485, 1964

92. PALMER FJ: Renal cortical calcification. Clin Radiol 21: 175, 1970

93. PALUBINSKAS AJ: Medullary sponge kidney. Radiology 76: 911, 1961

94. PALUBINSKAS AJ, CHRISTENSEN WR, HARRISON JH et al: Calcified adrenal cysts. Am J Roentgenol 82: 853, 1959

95. PAQUIN AJ JR, MARSHALL VF, MCGOVERN JH: The megacystis syndrome. J Urol 83: 634, 1960

96. PECK DR, BHATT GM, LOWMAN RM: Traction displacement of the ureter: a sign of aortic aneurysm. J Urol 109: 983, 1973

97. PETEREIT MF: Chronic renal brucellosis: a simulator of tuberculosis. Radiology 96: 85, 1970

98. PFISTER RC, MCLAUGHLIN AP III, LEADBETTER WF: Radiological evaluation of primary megaloureter. Radiology 99: 503, 1971

99. PICKERING RS, HARTMAN GW, WEEKS RE et al: Excretory urographic localization of adrenal cortical tumors and pheochromocytomas. Radiology 114: 345, 1975

100. PITT DC: Retrocaval ureter. Radiology 84: 699, 1965

101. QUELOZ JM, CAPITANIO MA, KIRKPATRICK JA: Wolman's disease. Radiology 104: 357, 1972

102. REDLIN L, FRANCIS RS, ORLANDO MM: Renal abnormalities in agnogenic myeloid metaplasia. Radiology 121: 605, 1976

103. REUTER SR, BLAIR AJ, SCHTEINGART DE et al: Adrenal venography. Radiology 89: 805, 1967

104. REYNOLDS L, FULTON H, SNIDER JJ: Roentgen analysis of renal mass lesions. Am J Roentgenol 82: 840, 1959

105. RIESZ PB, WAGNER CW JR: Unusual renal calcification following acute bilateral renal cortical necrosis. Am J Roentgenol 101: 705, 1967

106. ROBBINS JS III, MITTEMEYER BT, NEIMAN HL: The persistent nephrogram: a sentinel sign of contrast reaction. J Urol 114: 758, 1975

107. ROONEY DR: Vesicoureteral reflux in children. Am J Roentgenol 86: 545, 1961

108. SENGPIEL GW: Renal backflow in excretory urography. Am J Roentgenol 78: 289, 1957

109. SHAPIRO JH, RAMSAY CG, JACOBSON HG et al: Renal involvement in lymphomas and leukemias in adults. Am J Roentgenol 88: 928, 1962

110. SHOPFNER CE: Nonobstructive hydronephrosis and hydroureter. Am J Roentgenol 98: 172, 1966

111. SHOPFNER CE: Cystourethrography: methodology, normal anatomy and pathology. J Urol 103: 92, 1970

112. SIAO NT, SWINGLE JD, GOSSET F: Nephronophthisis. Radiology 95: 649, 1970

113. SIMON AL: Normal renal size: an absolute criterion. Am J Roentgenol 92: 270, 1964

114. STABLES DP, GINSBERG NJ, JOHNSON ML: Percutaneous nephrostomy: a series and review of the literature. Am J Roentgenol 130: 75, 1978

115. SUTTON D, BRUNTON FJ, STARER F: Renal artery stenosis. Clin Radiol 12: 80, 1961

116. SVENDSEN P, WILSON J: Adverse reaction during urography and modifications by atropine. Acta Radiol [Diagn] (Stockh) 11: 427, 1971

117. TALNER LB, GITTIS RF: Megacalyces. Clin Radiol 23: 355, 1972

118. TALNER LB, STONE RA, COEL MN et al: Furosemide-augmented intravenous urography: results in essential hypertension. Am J Roentgenol 130: 257, 1978

119. TARABULCY EZ: The radiographic aspect of urogenital schistosomiasis (bilharziasis). J Urol 90: 470, 1963

120. TWERSKY J, LEVIN DC: Metastatic melanoma of the adrenals. Radiology 116: 627, 1975

121. VESTBY GW: Percutaneous needle puncture of renal cysts. New method in therapeutic management. Invest Radiol 2: 449, 1967

122. VIAMONTE M JR, RAVEL R, POLITANO V et al: Angiographic findings in a patient with tuberous sclerosis. Am J Roentgenol 98: 723, 1966

123. WEGNER GP, CRUMMY AB, FLAHERTY TT et al: Renal vein thrombosis. JAMA 209: 1661, 1969

124. WEINTRAUB HD, RALL KL, THOMPSON IM et al: Pararenal pseudocysts. Am J Roentgenol 92: 286, 1964

125. WINOGRAD J, SCHIMMEL DH, PALUBINSKAS AJ: The spotted nephrogram of renal scleroderma. Am J Roentgenol 126: 734, 1976

126. WITTEN DM, MYERS GH JR, UTZ DC: Emmett's Clinical Urography, 4th ed. Philadelphia, WB Saunders, 1977*

127. ZANCA P, BARKER KG, PYE TH et al: Ureteral jet stream phenomenon in adults. Am J Roentgenol 92: 341, 1964

128. ZELCH JV, MEANEY TF, BOELHOBEK GH: Radiologic approach to the patient with suspected pheochromocytoma. Radiology 111: 279, 1974

* This three-volume work is a comprehensive reference and is recommended for further study of roentgen signs of urologic disease.

21

OBSTETRIC AND GYNECOLOGIC ROENTGENOLOGY

ROENTGEN DIAGNOSIS IN OBSTETRICS

There are a number of conditions arising during pregnancy in which roentgen examination of the abdomen and pelvis has been used in the past. It has been used in (1) the examination of the maternal pelvis, including pelvimetry (measurement of the pelvis), (2) estimation of the duration of pregnancy and the stage of maturity of the fetus, (3) determination of fetal death, (4) determination of fetal malformations and malpositions, (5) determination of presentation, position, and multiple pregnancy, (6) localization of the placenta, and (7) aiding localization of the fetal abdomen for intrauterine transfusions. Ultrasound, which has replaced radiography in most examinations of the fetus and placenta, is now used in the above-named situations. In view of the possible genetic effects of irradiation on the fetus as well as the mother, the roentgen examination of the pregnant woman is not to be undertaken without a firm indication for its use. Every effort should be made to avoid unnecessary irradiation of any woman who might be pregnant. Radiographic examinations that include the lower abdomen and pelvis should be performed only when there is no possibility of pregnancy unless there is urgent need for such examination. On the rare occasions when radiographs of the abdomen including the fetus are necessary, fetal irradiation can be reduced by having the patient lie in the prone position for the examination.

The use of roentgen pelvimetry is seldom necessary and guidelines should be established in order to decrease overutilization. Kelly and associates[17] proposed the following: (1) patients should be selected on the basis of individual clinical assessment, not by protocol; (2) other possible causes for delay in the progress of labor should be excluded prior to pelvimetry; (3) the possibility of inlet dystocia should be assessed by clinical or ultrasonic methods with the patient erect prior to employing pelvimetry; (4) dystocia due to fetal anomalies, placenta previa, multiple pregnancy, and fetal demise can usually be diagnosed by ultrasound without pelvimetry; (5) the magnitude of pelvic molding should be assessed in patients with low pelvimetry measurements; (6) the significance of pelvic deformities can be assessed on prior films without resort to pelvimetry; (7) induction of labor is not of itself an indication for pelvimetry; (8) presentation is not in inself an indication for pelvimetry; (9) adolescence is not in itself an indication for pelvimetry. Furthermore, normal measurements determined on roentgen pelvimetry do not necessarily indicate that a cesarean section is not needed. Roentgen pelvimetry should not be discarded, however, because it still has a place in the examination of patients in whom there is equivocal clinical evidence of cephalopelvic disproportion. In other types of roentgen examination, the dosages to the gonads are not as high as in pelvimetry; the possible harmful genetic effects to the mother and fetus must be weighed against the danger to them should the examination be omitted, and against the usefulness of the information to be obtained.

THE FEMALE PELVIS

Classification of Pelvic Types

The female pelvis has been classified by Caldwell and his associates into four major types, determined chiefly by the shape of the pelvic inlet. The characteristics of more than one of the basic types are often present in a group of intermediate types. The classification is as follows: (1) gynecoid (round), (2) anthropoid (long oval), (3) android (wedge-shaped), and (4) platypelloid (flat).

Gynecoid. This is the average pelvis found in approximately 42% of women. The inlet is round; the sacrum is usually curved posteriorly so that its anterior border presents a rounded concave contour. The sacrosciatic notch is average to wide in size; the ischial spines are small and the pelvic side walls are relatively straight. The average ratio of the anteroposterior diameter of the pelvic inlet (true conjugate) to the transverse diameter is 11 to 13. Even though this type of pelvis may be somewhat small, there is usually very little difficulty in labor due to cephalopelvic disproportion.

Anthropoid. This type of pelvis occurs in approximately 23% of white and 40% of black women. It is characterized by a long, narrow inlet; the transverse diameters of the pelvis are decreased, while the anteroposterior diameters are increased in comparison to the gynecoid type. The sacrum tends to be flatter than in the gynecoid type and the sacrosciatic notch

is usually wide and shallow. The inlet is often steeply inclined as the result of lordosis.

Android. This type occurs in approximately 32% of white and 16% of black women. It is a female pelvis in which masculine characteristics predominate. The inlet is triangular or wedge-shaped with a narrow anterior portion. The widest transverse diameter is near the sacral promontory and lies farther posteriorly than in the gynecoid and anthropoid types. The pelvic side walls tend to converge and the sacrum is flat. The sacrosciatic notch is small and the ischial spines are often large. These characteristics have led to the use of the descriptive term "funnel" pelvis. The android pelvis is a poor obstetric pelvis, and midpelvic or outlet dystocia may be anticipated frequently.

Platypelloid. The flat pelvis is characterized by short anteroposterior and wide transverse diameters. The sacrosciatic notch is wide and tends to be deeper than in the gynecoid type.

Anomalous Pelvic Types

Generally Contracted Pelvis. The shape of the pelvis including the sacral curve, inlet, and sacrosciatic notches may be normal but the measurements are all decreased.

Rachitic Flat Pelvis. The rachitic type of pelvis is rare in the United States and consists of loss of the normal concave curve of the anterior aspect of the sacrum. When the change is severe, the anterior sacrum may be convex.

Obliquely Contracted Pelvis (Naegele). This is caused by underdevelopment of the wing of the sacrum on either side. It results in considerable pelvic deformity, which is usually incompatible with normal delivery.

Transversely Contracted Pelvis. In this anomaly, both sacral wings are small or absent. This causes a marked decrease in the transverse diameter.

Other Deformities. The pelvis may be deformed as the result of injury. Generalized osseous dysplasias may also be accompanied by a considerable amount of pelvic deformity. In many of these deformities and anomalies, the birth canal is so distorted that normal delivery is out of the question, and pelvic measurements by roentgen methods are unnecessary.

ROENTGEN PELVIC MEASUREMENT

The amount of enlargement of an object measured on a roentgen depends upon its distance from the film in relation to its distance from the target of the roentgen-ray tube. This enlargement is termed "divergent distortion." All the methods of roentgen pelvimetry are directed toward correcting for this distortion or eliminating it by increasing the target–film distance. There is often no actual necessity for elaborate methods of pelvic mensuration. During the last month of gestation, a single lateral roentgenogram obtained with the patient upright may be sufficient to indicate the absence of disproportion. The fetal head frequently engages in this position even though it may be floating in the supine position. When it is engaged in the upright view and an additional anteroposterior film reveals that the pelvis is gynecoid in shape, there is no disproportion. If it is desirable to measure the anteroposterior diameters in the upright lateral view, a strip of lead notched at 1-cm intervals attached to or parallel with the intergluteal fold is used. The centimeter scale is distorted to the same degree as the anteroposterior pelvic diameters because it is the same distance from the film.

Roentgen Pelvimetry

Indications, Limitations, and Value of Pelvimetry. The guidelines listed earlier should be used when pelvimetry is contemplated. Much of the necessary information can be obtained by the use of ultrasound. It is therefore likely that radiographic pelvimetry will be undertaken much less frequently in the future than in the past.

Adequate clinical examination and measurements permit the obstetrician to classify his patients into three general groups: (*1*) group 1—pelvis adequate for normal delivery, (*2*) group 2—pelvis obviously distorted or contracted to such an extent that normal delivery is impossible, and (*3*) intermediate group —patients in whom some disproportion may exist. Roentgen pelvimetry is not indicated in groups 1 and 2 but may be indicated in the intermediate group 3 in which disproportion is suspected. The major indications are history of protracted labor in a previous pregnancy in which cephalopelvic disproportion was the likely cause, and arrest of the fetal head despite strong uterine contractions. Less strong indications are malpresentation, the elderly primigravida, and failure of the fetal head to engage in a primigravida, particularly if the external measurements are borderline.

The value of pelvimetry is limited by inability to forecast the uterine forces or the effect of the soft tissues upon the fetus. The size of the fetus must also be taken into account. The radiologist should realize that although roentgen pelvimetry yields accurate information relating to bony cephalopelvic disproportion, it does not give information regarding all of the remaining factors in labor. Therefore, in reporting the results it is important to include only the conclusions that can be based on the presence or absence of bony disproportion.

There is information to be gained in addition to the measurements of the pelvis. This includes the shape of the pelvis, the relation of the presenting part to the pelvic inlet, the position of the placenta (in many cases), and the presence of some fetal anomalies.

The roentgen measurement of the pelvis should be done while the patient is in labor for maximum information regarding the relative size of the fetal head and maternal pelvis. Both mother and fetus are exposed to irradiation in antepartum pelvimetry. Unless care is used in shielding and coning, fetal as well as maternal gonads may be included in the direct beam. Shielding can be used in the anteroposterior projection to protect the fetus, including most, if not all of the fetal head; thus the only fetal exposure is to that of scattered irradiation. The only maternal gonadal irradiation is also by scatter in the body if this method of shielding is used. Shielding can be nearly as effective in the lateral projection.[18] Actual radiation dosages differ considerably, but maternal gonadal doses of 0.090 to 0.600 R and fetal gonadal doses in the range of 0.150 R or less can be obtained if coning and shielding is effectively used.

High voltages used to reduce skin dose to the mother do not have any significant advantage so far as gonadal dose is concerned, particularly if filtration is used. The range of 60 to 70 kVp using added filtration of 2 mm of aluminum produces the best detail and is recommended for the anteroposterior projection. Higher voltages in the range of 100 to 120 kVp are needed for the lateral view.

General Considerations. Most of the numerous methods described for measurement of the pelvis are reasonably accurate. The anteroposterior diameters are readily measured because they all lie in the same plane. This plane can be determined by direct measurement on the patient because it lies in the midline. The transverse pelvic diameters are at varying distances from the film and cannot be measured directly on the patient; most of the methods have been devised to measure these diameters. The various methods of pelvimetry are described in the books and articles listed in the bibliography.

Measurement of Sagittal Diameters. Since these diameters are in the midline, measurements can be made directly using a centimeter scale. The sagittal diameters are measured on a lateral film exposed with the patient in the upright position if possible, since sagittal diameters in this position are similar to those during delivery in the supine position with the thighs and knees in flexion. A centimeter scale placed in the midline between the thighs can be used in the direct measurement of these diameters. The patient is held firmly against the table top or cassette and the centimeter scale is held parallel to the cassette and at a right angle to the central ray. Voltages ranging from 100 to 120 kVp are used.

It is also simple and accurate to use a mathematical correction factor for the divergent distortion in measuring sagittal diameters. This is based on the geometric rule that the bases of similar triangles are proportional to their altitudes. If the distance of an object (*e.g.*, one of the sagittal pelvic diameters) from the film and the distance of the target of the tube from the film are known, it is possible to calculate the actual size of the object after measuring its image directly on the roentgenogram. Since the sagittal diameters are in the midline, the distance from the symphysis to the film is measured. This can be checked by comparing it to one-half of the transverse diameter of the patient measured at the trochanters. This method of measurement is illustrated in Figure 21-1.

In pelvimetry, to simplify calculation a target–film distance of 100 cm can be used. The pelvic diameter to be measured is *CD* in the diagram; its image on the film is *AB*.

The distance of the object from the film for the anteroposterior diameters is measured on the patient at the time the lateral roentgenogram of the pelvis is obtained. Subtracting this distance from 100 gives the tube–object distance.

Measurement of Transverse Diameters. The orthometric[27] or orthodiagraphic[5] method is described here because it is simple and accurate. The anteroposterior view is obtained with the patient in the supine position with her knees flexed and thighs abducted about 90 degrees to prevent medial soft tissues from obscuring the ischial spines. The object–film distance is shortened by placing a cassette directly under the patient's buttocks. The light-beam diaphragm is adjusted to an area 10 × 4 cm in size. The

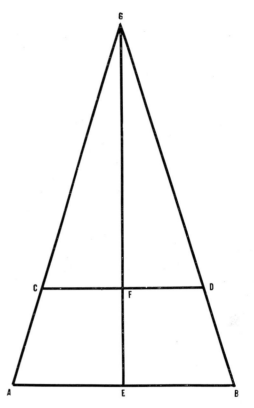

Fig. 21-1. Diagram used to indicate calculation and measurement in pelvimetry. In this diagram **GE**, target-film distance (known); **GF**, target-object distance (measured); **FE**, object-film distance (measured); **AB**, size of image on roentgenogram (measured); and **CD**, object size (to be calculated).

$$CD \times GE = AB \times GF$$
$$CD = \frac{AB \times GF}{GE}$$

tube may be angled 20 degrees cephalad, but some prefer a vertical tube angle with the patient's back arched by a pillow. The beam is centered at the upper border of the symphysis. Two exposures are made without moving the patient or the film; the tube is 5 cm to the left of the midline on one and 5 cm to the right of the midline on the other. It is essential that neither the patient nor the cassette move during the two exposures comprising the examination. To obtain the best detail, voltages in the range of 55 to 60 kVp are used with high-speed screens and rapid film.

The dose to the maternal and fetal gonads is only 0.2 mR if presentation is cephalic. The only factor producing distortion when this method is used is the difference between the tube shift (10 cm) and the length of the dimension to be measured. This results in a slight decrease in measured diameters as compared to actual diameters below 10 cm and a slight increase in measured diameters as compared to actual diameters above 10 cm. The 10-cm tube shift is used because it represents the average interspinous diameter, which is the most important transverse measurement made in this examination. The errors are very small. The correction factor is therefore small and is applied to the difference between the actual measurement (made on the film) and the tube shift (10 cm). The factor at the inlet is 1/5, at the midpelvis 1/7, and at the ischial spines 1/10. For example, the inlet measures 13 cm, the correction factor is applied to 13−10 or 3 cm; 3 times 1/5 equals 3/5 or 0.6 cm; and the actual measurement is 13−0.6 = 12.4 cm. If the interspinous diameter is 9 cm, measured on the film, the correction factor is applied to 10−9 = 1 cm; 1 × 1/7 or 0.14 cm. The actual measurement is then 9 + 0.14 or 9.14 cm.[23] When the inerspinous diameters are smaller than 8 cm, disproportion is obvious, so accurate measurement is not essential. When the diameters are over 12 cm, no bony disproportion is present, so accurate measurement of the larger diameters is not essential.

Pelvic Landmarks in Making the Measurements. The discussion of landmarks that follows refers to the diameters marked on Figures 21-2, 21-3, and 21-4.

On the lateral roentgenogram, the following measurements (Fig. 21-2) are made:

1. The sagittal (anteroposterior) diameter of the inlet—a line from the upper inner margin of the symphysis pubis to the point on the sacrum where the two iliopectineal lines intersect (*AB*).

2. The sagittal (anteroposterior) diameter of the midplane of the pelvis—a line from the lower inner margin of the symphysis through the midpoint between the tips of the ischial spines to the sacrum. If this line falls below the last fixed sacral segment, then the latter point is used as the sacral termination of the diameter (*CD*).

3. The posterior sagittal diameter (anteroposterior diameter of the outlet)—a line from the midpoint between the ischial tuberosities to the last fixed sacral segment (*EF*).

The following measurements are made on the anteroposterior roentgenogram (see Fig. 21-3):

1. The transverse diameter of the inlet—a line connecting the points of widest separation of the right and left iliopectineal lines (*AB*).

2. The interspinous diameter (transverse midpelvic diameter)—measured from the tip of one ischial spine to the other (*CD*).

3. The bituberous diameter (transverse diameter of the outlet)—measured from one ischial tuberosity to the other (*EF*). Lines are drawn downward outlining the inner aspect of the pelvic side wall on either side; the transverse distance between them is measured at the level of the ischial tuberosities. There is some disagreement in the literature regarding the range of normal pelvic measurements. Those given by Snow are listed in Table 21-1.

ULTRASOUND IN OBSTETRICS

Although diagnostic ultrasound is beyond the scope of this book, a brief discussion is warranted here since sonography is in general clinical use in obstetrics and has replaced radiologic methods to a considerable extent. Ultrasound is a form of energy consisting of mechanical vibrations produced by substances, such as quartz, that have the capability of changing mechanical to electrical energy and vice versa. These materials are termed "transducers"; the effect is called the "piezoelectric effect." The crystal is energized electrically and sends an ultrasound pulse. The return pulse or echo is received by the transducer and converted into electrical energy that can be recorded on an oscilloscope. When sound encounters a junction between two materials that have different acoustical characteristics, a sound beam may be reflected, transmitted, or refracted. The reflected sound returns to the transducer. The transmitted sound continues through the object. Refraction indicates change in the direction of the sound path when it extends from one material to another, so that it returns at a different angle than that of the incident beam. The A-scan or mode is used to measure the depth of an echo-producing boundary such as in the localization of the position of the falx cerebri. Echoes are represented as a deflection from a baseline calibrated in centimeters. This is not generally applicable to the more complex problems of scanning the pelvis and abdomen, so a multi-dimensional technique must be applied. This is termed the B-mode or scan which permits mapping of structures within the pelvis. The cross-sectional or B-scan image is built up by moving the transducer back and forth on the skin surface. The echoes are shown as dots related to the

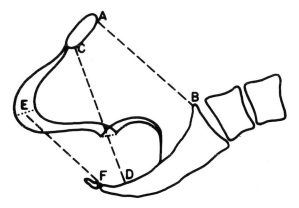

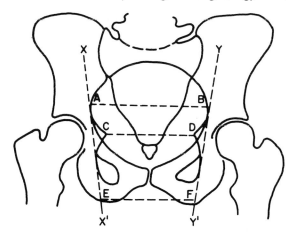

Fig. 21-2. Diagram of the pelvis indicates diameters measured on the lateral roentgenogram. **AB,** Anteroposterior diameter of the inlet; **CD,** anteroposterior diameter of the midpelvis; **EF,** posterior sagittal diameter.

Fig. 21-3. Diagram of the pelvis shows measurements made on the anteroposterior roentgenogram. **AB,** Transverse diameter of the inlet; **CD,** transverse diameter of the midpelvis (interspinous); **EF,** transverse diameter of the outlet (bituberous); x–x' and y–y' mark lateral pelvic walls.

amplitude of the echo at various anteroposterior and lateral axes. The grey scale readout uses an electronic scan convertor to store and reproduce the wide range of echo amplitudes. The image is stored in the convertor during the process and displayed on an oscilloscope screen or television video monitor. Photographs may then preserve the scans as permanent

records. The M-mode (T–M or time motion) is used in the study of motion of pulsatile structures such as the heart. The Doppler mode is based on frequency alteration caused by motion of the surface studied.

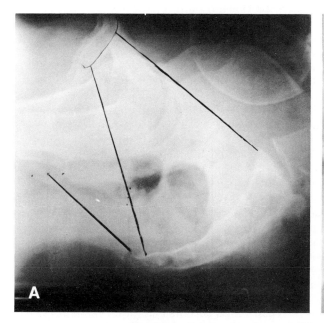

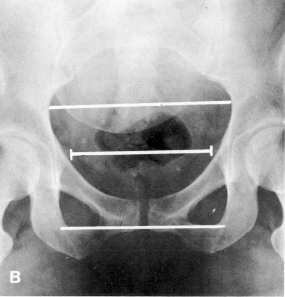

Fig. 21-4. Pelvimetry. Lateral **(A)** and frontal **(B)** projections showing the diameters indicated in Figures 21-2 and 21-3.

Table 21-1. Average Pelvic Measurements in Centimeters

	SMALL	MEDIUM	LARGE
Inlet			
Anteroposterior	Below 10.5	10.5–11.5	Above 11.5
Transverse	Below 11.5	11.5–12.5	Above 12.5
Total	Below 22.0	22.0–24.0	Above 24.0
Midpelvis			
Anteroposterior	Below 11.0	11.0–12.0	Above 12.0
Interspinous	Below 10.0	10.0–11.0	Above 11.0
Total	Below 21.0	21.0–23.0	Above 23.0
Outlet			
Posterior sagittal	Below 6.5	6.5– 8.0	Above 8.0
Bituberous	Below 9.5	9.5–10.5	Above 10.5
Total	Below 16.0	16.0–18.5	Above 18.5

(Based on Snow, W: Roentgenology in Obstetrics and Gynecology. Springfield, Ill., Thomas, 1952)

The change in frequency is related to the velocity and direction of motion with respect to the incident sound signal.

There are a number of applications of ultrasound in obstetrics. The filled urinary bladder displaces the bowel away from the uterus and allows comparison of the density of an unknown mass with that of the bladder. The applications include the following:

1. Diagnosis of pregnancy. The gestational sac can be identified as early as 5 or 6 weeks after conception. Its site can be identified.

2. Fetal growth and development. The biparietal diameter of the fetal head provides a standard for fetal growth and development from 14 weeks of gestation to term.

3. Multiple pregnancy. At about 16 weeks of gestation the fetal head and thoracic structures are identifiable so that multiple fetuses can be outlined.

4. Hydatidiform mole. This complication of pregnancy can be identified, but must be differentiated from a degenerating leiomyoma. This is usually possible since the mole is relatively transonic.

5. Hydramnios. The increased amount of amniotic fluid is readily identified.

6. Placental localization. This is usually possible by ultrasound and is the method of choice. Placental migration upward toward the uterine fundus has been observed in a number of patients so that an early diagnosis of placenta previa is not applicable later; migration toward the uterine fundus indicates that re-examination should be performed at or near term, since the placenta may have migrated away from the cervix.

7. Intrauterine fetal death. Ultrasonic methods are quite reliable in the diagnosis of fetal death.

When there is any doubt, follow-up scans may be obtained to note the presence or absence of fetal growth and of more florid signs of fetal death. Doppler instrumentation allows identification of fetal heart tones at approximately 9 weeks of gestation; the absence of fetal heart pulsation is a most accurate and specific sign of fetal death after the 14th week.

8. Fetal anomalies. Anencephaly and hydrocephaly are readily detected. In addition, a wide range of other abnormalities including hydronephrosis, hydrops, and meningomyelocele may be detected.

9. Pelvic masses associated with pregnancy. Masses such as ovarian cysts and uterine leiomyomas can be detected by ultrasound and their relationship to the uterus ascertained.

10. Ectopic pregnancy. Ultrasonography is useful in the diagnosis of ectopic pregnancy with an accuracy of over 92%. When there is an advanced, extrauterine pregnancy, the percentage is even higher.

11. Amniocentesis. The use of ultrasound for localization in amniocentesis helps to reduce the morbidity of the procedure.

12. Elective abortion. Ultrasound accurately dates the time of conception and the site of the uterus if the patient should happen to have a pelvic mass in addition to the pregnancy. Following abortion, the presence or absence of retained products of conception can be verified by ultrasound. It will also differentiate pelvic mass from pregnancy.

13. Localization of intrauterine devices used for contraception.

THE FETUS

Fetal Age and Duration of Pregnancy

Reasonably accurate estimation of fetal age is useful in a number of situations. Determination of the earliest safe date for the termination of pregnancy may be necessary in diabetics, preeclamptic states, maternal hypertension, in patients with Rh problems, in cephalopelvic disproportion, and in patients who have had previous cesarian sections. Fetal age may also be important in patients who are presumably overdue and in cases where there is discrepancy between size of the fetus and uterus or both and the given dates.

Because ultrasound has replaced radiographic methods of determining fetal age, the following discussion is largely of anatomic interest. In the early weeks of pregnancy the fetal skeleton is not visible, so that roentgen examination is of no value in determining fetal age. The skeleton is usually visible at 12 weeks. The ossification centers for the vertebral bodies are usually the first visible skeletal parts; ribs are also ossified at 12 weeks. The date and appearance of different skeletal parts can be used to estimate maturation within 1 or 2 months. Films of good quality are necessary and the various ossification centers may then be identified. For example, the semicircular canals are well outlined at the 20th week but are partially obscured by ossification around them by the 24th week and are almost completely obscured by the 40th week. The parietal bones ossify frequently by the 20th week and invariably by the 24th week. The calcaneus appears between the 24th and 26th week and the talus between the 26th and 28th week. The distal femoral epiphysis is present by the 36th to 37th week in females and in some males. The center for the upper end of the tibia appears at 38 weeks. There is individual variation, so the appearance of the various ossification centers gives only a rough approximation of fetal age.

Fetal Death

The clinical diagnosis of fetal death may be difficult to make in certain patients because of obesity, the presence of hydramnios, and other factors. In these instances, roentgenograms can be obtained to confirm the suspicion of fetal death. Ultrasound has replaced radiographic examination in suspected fetal death, but the description of roentgen signs is included here, since radiographs of the fetus may be obtained for various other reasons.

The absence of many or all of the following roentgen signs does not indicate that the fetus is living, since none of them may be present. A single, erect anteroposterior film of the mother's abdomen is obtained. This may show air–fluid levels when gas is in the fetal circulatory system and it also increases deforming pressure on the fetal skull to aid in the diagnosis of fetal death, if present. Further views may then be obtained if necessary (*e.g.,* oblique and lateral). Positive signs of fetal death are found in approximately 75% of cases. The signs are:

1. Overlapping of the bones of the skull (Spalding's sign). When the patient is not in labor, overlapping of the cranial bones is a reasonably reliable sign of fetal death. It is easily determined on films of satisfactory quality. Rarely this finding has been noted in a live infant and the sign is of no value when the patient is in labor (Fig. 21-5).

2. Unusual fetal attitude. Marked curvature of the fetal spine or abnormally sharp angulation or gibbus of the spine or of the head in relation to the body, as well as other abnormal attitudes, are suggestive signs of fetal death. Collapse of the thoracic cage may also occur. In some cases, the change is so marked that the diagnosis is certain; in others, the findings are equivocal.

3. Disproportion between the known gestation period and the calculated age. When the disproportion is marked this is a valuable sign.

4. Absence of continued fetal growth on serial roentgen examination.

5. Gas in the fetal circulatory system. This is a positive sign of fetal death when present. It appears rather early (1 to 4 days after fetal death) and remains demonstrable for 2 weeks or more. If gas is present in sufficient quantity, it is easily recognized. It is frequently observed in the hepatic vessels, where it is contrasted to the density of the liver. It is sometimes observed in the cardiac chambers, in the aorta, and in, the umbilical vessels. The mechanism of the development of gas within the circulation has not been clarified but the finding occurs in infants with marked gaseous distention of the bowel so that it is reasonable to assume that in some patients the gas enters the mesenteric veins from the distended bowel and collects in the portal system. Pneumatosis of the bowel was reported by Wolfe and Evans[37] in the cases exhibiting this sign. This would tend to support their theory of embolism. Gas has also been reported in the umbilical vessels, suggesting the possibility of gas embolism from the maternal circulation. Other investigators favor infection as the source of gas. The radiographic findings are striking and consist of linear areas of radiolucency outlining the fetal vessels, often the portal system, and occasionally outlining the chambers of the heart (Fig. 21-6).

6. The halo sign. This sign is caused by an increase in width of soft tissues between the radiolucent subcutaneous fat of the scalp and the bones of the cranial vault. In the normal fetus the subcutaneous fat of the scalp appears as a translucent line in contact with the cranial vault. There is local separation around a caput succedaneum which must be differentiated from general separation observed in the halo sign. The amount of separation varies from several millimeters to a centimeter or more. The roentgen appearance is that of a radiolucent "halo" separated from the cranial bones by several millimeters of tissue or water density. It is observed most

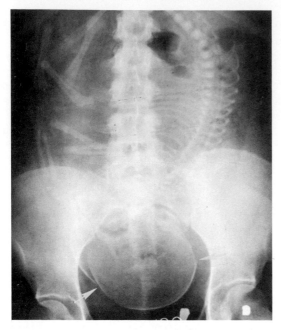

Fig. 21-5. Fetal death. This roentgenogram shows overlapping of the cranial bones (Spalding's sign). **Arrows** indicate site of overlapping.

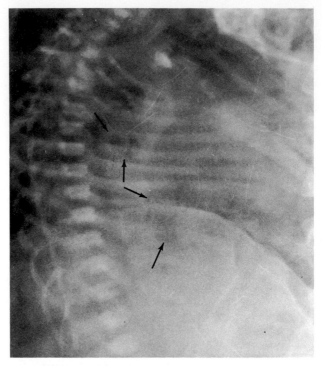

Fig. 21-6. Fetal death manifested by gas in the fetal heart **(upper arrows)** and hepatic vessels **(lower arrows)**. The gas was readily identified in the original films but is difficult to outline on these reproductions.

frequently when the fetus is at or near term, because the subcutaneous fat is readily recognized at that time.

When more than one of the above signs are present, the diagnosis is readily established. The last three are pathognomonic and when severe the first two are reliable signs, but minor alterations in attitude and questionable overlapping of cranial bones make the diagnosis difficult in some instances.

7. Amniography. Amniography may also be used to determine fetal death. Following the removal of 35 to 40 cc of amniotic fluid, a similar amount of diatrizoate or iothalamate is injected into the uterine cavity. When the fetus is alive, it swallows the amniotic fluid containing the medium. This outlines the fetal gastrointestinal tract. Films obtained in 1 hour can be checked. If the fetal gut is opacified the fetus is alive. If not, films can be obtained at hourly intervals for 3 to 4 hours. If gestation is less than 30 weeks, a 24-hour film should also be obtained, since swallowing is slow in the immature fetus. Absence of opacification of the fetal gastrointestinal tract is a reliable sign of fetal death. There are exceptions (*e.g.,* esophageal atresia) when a live infant will not have the opaque medium in the gut. When suspected fetal death cannot be determined by other methods, amniography may be used.

Fetal Abnormalities

Gross malformations of the fetus are readily demonstrated in utero by means of roentgen examination of the abdomen during pregnancy. There is usually no difficulty in the diagnosis of such conditions as anencephaly, bicephaly, and other severe anomalies on films of good quality (Fig. 21-7). Skeletal abnormalities such as osteogenesis imperfecta, Albers–Schönberg disease (osteopetrosis), severe hypophosphatasia, and rachischisis may also be detected in utero. When hydrocephalus is present to a significant degree it can usually be recognized in utero. Several, but not all of these anomalies, can be identified by ultrasound. Amniography is also used by some for detection of gastrointestinal malformations and fetal malformations such as meningocele and encephalocele. It is particularly useful in patients with unexplained polyhydramnios.

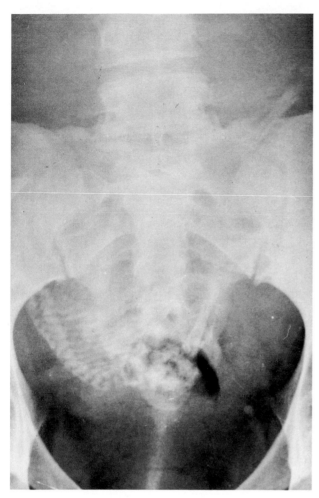

Fig. 21-7. Anencephaly. Note absence of the normal cranial vault.

Ectopic Pregnancy

Occasionally it is possible to recognize ectopic abdominal pregnancy when the fetal skeleton can be visualized roentgenographically. The diagnosis is made when the uterus is visible as a mass separate from the fetal skeleton or when the fetal skeleton is located at some distance from its normal position. The following roentgen signs have also been found in this condition:

1. Absence of the uterine shadow surrounding the fetus
2. Extension or unusual position of fetal extremities
3. Abnormally high position of the fetus

4. Fetal parts immediately beneath the anterior abdominal wall on the lateral view
5. Fetal parts overlapping the maternal spine in the lateral view
6. Transverse position, often with the back uppermost and extremities directed downward
7. Unusual fetal attitude
8. An extremity stretched down into the maternal pelvis
9. Intermingling of maternal bowel gas with fetus
10. Unusual clarity of fetal parts

These findings are suggestive, but not diagnostic, of abnormal pregnancy. When the fetus is dead, hysterosalpingography can be used to confirm the diagnosis. As indicated previously, since ultrasound is usually diagnostic, radiography need not be undertaken. In early ectopic pregnancy, ultrasound may be diagnostic when no definite abnormalities are observed on roentgenography.

Rarely it is possible to confirm the diagnosis of rupture of the uterus by correlating roentgen signs with clinical findings. This is done by visualization of the fetal skeletal parts outside the uterus or visualization of some of the parts outside of the uterus with others within it. A demonstrable uterine shadow may be absent. The fetus may be unusually high in position and free fluid may be evident in the peritoneal cavity.

The presence of hydramnios can also be recognized. The large amount of fluid surrounding the fetus causes considerable disproportion in the size of the fetus and the uterus that envelops it. Fetus papyraceous is readily recognized when it is developed enough so that fetal skeletal parts are visible. This is a dead fetus compressed to form a flattened mass of skeletal structures by a living twin. Lithopedion is a fetus that undergoes more or less calcification following death. The pregnancy is extrauterine; the fetus must survive for more than 3 months, otherwise it is absorbed. Over a long period of time, calcium is deposited in the soft tissues of the intra-abdominal fetus. The calcified mass is found long after an undiagnosed pregnancy.

Erythroblastosis

Erythroblastosis fetalis in its most severe form is manifested clinically by fetal hydrops. It is characterized by marked generalized fetal edema associated with fluid in the peritoneal, pericardial and, pleural cavities and enlargement of the heart, liver and

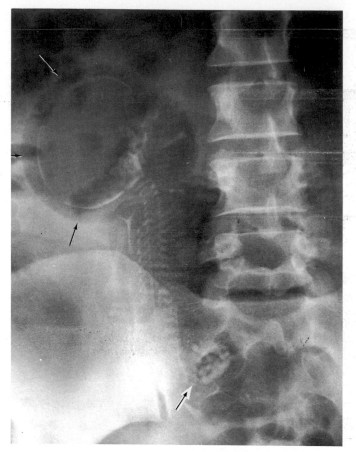

Fig. 21-8. Erythroblastosis fetalis. Fetal hydrops is demonstrated by amniography. The thick, edematous scalp is easily identified **(upper arrows).** Opaque medium in the intestine of the infant **(lower arrow)** indicates that the fetus is alive. Note the large fetal abdomen.

spleen (Fig. 21-8). It develops in utero and is accompanied by marked placental enlargement. The roentgen findings are:

1. Obliteration of the dark subcutaneous fat line as a result of edema fluid.

2. Abnormal fetal attitude or position. The severe edema results in straightening of the spine, including the neck. Also, the extremities cannot be held in flexion and tend to extend at 90 degrees to the trunk with abduction of the thighs. The resultant position is termed the "Buddha" sign.

3. Protuberant abdomen and ribs elevated to a horizontal position.

4. Enlarged placenta, which often occupies nearly half of the uterine cavity and displaces the fetus.

5. Signs of fetal death.

When these signs are present, a strong presumptive diagnosis of fetal hydrops can be made. The halo sign, previously reported in this disease, is not observed and is of no value. Ultrasound is often diagnostic and should be the initial imaging study; if equivocal, radiography may be used or follow-up ultrasound studies carried out.

Presentation, Position and Multiple Pregnancy

Fetal presentation and position are easily demonstrated by means of roentgenograms of the abdomen in frontal and lateral projections. The diagnosis of multiple pregnancy is also easily made and the position and presentation of each fetus can usually be determined without difficulty. Occasionally, persistent hyperextension of the fetal neck is observed in breech and in transverse lie. Although this may occur in Down's syndrome and hypotonia, it may also be caused by one or more loops of cord around the neck. It is also observed in the normal fetus. Therefore, it cannot be assumed to indicate serious anomaly; but caesarean section should be performed if there are signs of fetal distress to avoid the danger of cervical cord injury.

THE PLACENTA

Placenta Praevia

Roentgen examination is used in the study of patients with painless uterine bleeding in the third trimester of pregnancy. The roentgen diagnosis of placenta praevia and the localization of the placenta are fairly accurate, but ultrasound is the method of choice in the study of suspected placenta previa. Various radiographic methods are available for this examination and can be used if the occasion demands. The placenta measures approximately 20 cm in diameter and 4 to 6 cm in thickness. The inner surface is not visible because the radiographic density of the placenta is the same as that of the amniotic fluid. Its location can be surmised by the width of the soft-tissue shadow between the nearest part of the fetus and the outer uterine wall. The external surface of the uterus usually is clearly defined because of gas in the mother's intestinal tract and the intra-abdominal fat that outline the relatively dense uterus. When the fetal parts are within a few centimeters of the external surface of the uterus, the possibility of the presence of placenta in that particular area can be excluded. If there is an increase in the amount of amniotic fluid (hydramnios) the location of the placenta is difficult to determine. The placenta can be demonstrated on the lateral roentgenogram of the uterus in over 90% of pregnancies, so this projection should be obtained first.

When the placenta can be identified in this projection, no further study is necessary unless it is demonstrated to lie below the equator of the uterus. If it is not clearly outlined or is found to lie in a low position, further examination is necessary. The fetus is heavier than amniotic fluid and will sink to the lowest part of the uterus when the mother is in the upright position. Roentgen study made with the mother in this position is sometimes called the gravitational method. The bladder should be catheterized before exposing the films; having the patient void is not adequate. A small amount (30 to 40 cc) of diatrizoate or other organic iodide may be injected into the bladder if desired. The normal space between the fetal head and the opaque medium is 1 cm or less. Roentgenograms are then obtained in frontal and lateral projections with the patient in the upright position. These films will show the relative position of the presenting part of the fetus to the symphysis, the bladder, and the sacral promontory. In the normal gravid patient, the fetal head should lie equidistant from the pelvic side walls and nearly equidistant from the anterior and posterior walls of the pelvic inlet, particularly if the head is engaged. The findings are not as precise in breech presentations, but breech presentation with complete placenta praevia is rare. If the fetal head is more than 3 cm from the pubis or more than 1.5 cm from the sacral promontory when it is engaged, some degree of placenta praevia is likely (Fig. 21-9). If the head is unduly small in relation to the maternal pelvis, the range of the normal measurements is increased.

There is approximately 1 cm of soft tissue between the bones of the fetal cranium and the bladder lumen in the normal gravid patient. Any soft-tissue separation greater than this is suggestive of placenta praevia. When the patient's bladder is partially distended with contrast material the fetal head indents the dome of the bladder so that its margin forms a smooth, concave curve paralleling the curve of the fetal skull adjacent to it.

In marginal placenta praevia the mass of the placenta causes an asymmetric thickening of the space between the patient's bladder and the fetal skull. The fetal head usually extends into the pelvic inlet when

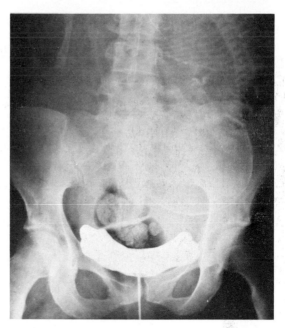

Fig. 21-9. Placenta previa. Cystogram with the patient in the upright position. Placenta previa is indicated by the eccentricity of the fetal head in relation to the pelvis and the distance of the head from the dome of the bladder caused by the presence of soft tissue between the fetal cranium and the bladder. This examination has been largely supplanted by ultrasonography.

the patient is standing, but will lie in asymmetric relationship to the symphysis pubis and sacral promontory or to the pelvic side walls, or both, depending upon the location of the placenta. The major part of the placenta may be visible above the level of the pelvic inlet in these patients.

In complete (or nearly complete) placenta praevia the fetal head often may not enter the pelvis and the thick soft-tissue mass between the fetal skull and the mother's bladder is apparent.

In summary, the roentgen signs of placenta praevia are as follows:

1. Nonvisualization of the placenta in the fundus.

2. Visualization of the placenta with the greater part of its mass noted to be below the equator of the uterus.

3. Displacement of the fetal head from the midplane of the patient's pelvis in either frontal or lateral projection with abnormal amount of soft tissue between it and the bony structures making up the pelvic inlet when the patient is examined standing.

4. Abnormally high position of the fetal head.

5. Abnormal amount of soft tissue between the fetal head and the mother's bladder when the latter is outlined by contrast material.

Methods of Placental Localization

Amniography. This examination may be used for placental localization. After removal of 30 to 40 cc of amniotic fluid, a similar amount of contrast medium (one of the organic iodides) is injected into the uterine cavity. The placenta appears as a negative shadow in the opacified amniotic fluid. Soft-tissue abnormalities of the fetus may also be recognized along with uterine deformities and tumors in the mother. Indications for the use of this procedure are limited.

Some use a combination of oily contrast medium (5 to 6 ml) and water-soluble medium when there is need to outline the fetal skin, since the oily medium coats the skin (fetography) and the fetus swallows the soluble medium, permitting visualization of its gastrointestinal tract.

Radioactive Isotope Localization. Radioactive iodinated human serum albumin (RISA = ^{131}I), ^{51}CR = labeled erythrocytes or human serum albumin, and technicium (^{99m}) = labeled human serum albumen are used for placental localization. When the placenta is anterior, lateral, or fundal in position, localization is satisfactory. When posterior, the placenta is located by exclusion. However, when the placenta is low, interpretation of results is difficult. Therefore, at present, the method is one of exclusion of placenta praevia when the placenta can be located at some distance from the internal cervical os. Using ^{131}I, a dose of 3 μCi is satisfactory. This gives a total radiation dose of 10 millirads to the mother and less than 4 millirads to the fetus. This method is not as accurate as ultrasound, which has largely supplanted it in placental localization.

Premature Separation of the Placenta

When the placenta is visible in the uterine fundus in patients with bleeding in the last trimester of pregnancy, the possibility of placenta praevia is excluded. Then the question of premature separation of the placenta arises. Occasionally there is a localized bulge of the uterus, owing to accumulation of blood when it is confined between the placenta and the uterine wall and forms a hematoma there. This does not occur frequently and is not a reliable sign be-cause a uterine fibroid or uterine asymmetry may cause similar change. Boood is not often trapped between the uterine wall and the placenta in an amount sufficient to cause local distortion. The diagnosis of this condition therefore is rarely possible by roentgen methods. However, when the placenta appears considerably enlarged and the possibility of erythroblastosis can be excluded, premature separation of the placenta can usually be inferred. The diagnosis of placental hematoma may be made by means of pelvic arteriography. The opaque medium remains in the hematoma much longer than in the normal placenta and is more homogenous than the placental sinusoids and arteries. Ultrasound may also be useful and should be employed prior to arteriography. If the diagnosis is made on the ultrasound scan, arteriography is not necessary.

Placenta Membranacea

Placenta membranacea is a rare anomaly. It is characterized by villi scattered beyond the limits of the placenta. The villi may be few in number or they may completely cover the chorion.[6] Painless antepartum hemorrhage in the third trimester suggests placenta previa. Therefore, when the possibility of the presence of placenta previa has been excluded by ultrasound, percutaneous arterial placentography carried out by way of the femoral approach may be used to make a definitive diagnosis. Small pools of contrast medium extend beyond the limits of the placenta and may envelop the fetus when the condition is extensive.

Chorioangioma of the Placenta

Cardiac failure in the newborn may occasionally be caused by large arteriovenous shunts in the fetal brain or liver, but large hemangiomas of the placenta may also act as arteriovenous fistulas and cause high output failure in the infant.[21]

Intrauterine Fetal Transfusion

Intrauterine fetal transfusion is reserved for erythroblastotic babies who would probably die in utero before attaining sufficient maturity to have a reasonable chance of survival. This type of transfusion may result in salvage of a number of such infants who can be carried until they are mature enough to be delivered. The radiologist aids the obstetrician in determining the position of the needle which is inserted into the fetal abdominal cavity

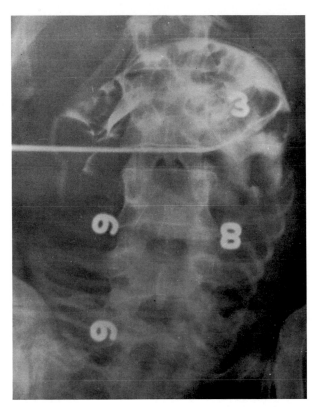

Fig. 21-10. Intrauterine transfusion. The opaque medium outlines the loops of bowel in the fetal peritoneal cavity. The needle and catheter are visualized. This indicates that the catheter tip is in the fetal peritoneal cavity.

through the maternal abdominal wall and uterus. A small amount (2 to 3 cc) of Hypaque or Renografin is injected. The pattern of the fetal abdominal cavity is characteristic (Fig. 21-10). Fluoroscopy using image intensification, or filming can be used. Markers on the abdominal wall aid in localization.

ROENTGEN DIAGNOSIS IN GYNECOLOGY

HYSTEROSALPINGOGRAPHY (HYSTEROGRAPHY)

Hysterosalpingography consists in opacification of the uterine cavity and fallopian tubes by injecting opaque contrast material into the uterus.[31] Enough pressure is applied to fill the uterus and fallopian tubes with escape of medium into the abdominal cavity when the tubes are patent. The examination

usually requires from 3 to 10 ml of contrast material. There is a considerable difference of opinion as to which of the media available is the best. Most investigators feel that water-soluble media are to be preferred to iodized oil. We use Sinografin, in which diatrizoate methylglucamine (40%) and iodipamide methylglucamine (20%) are combined. This medium is water-soluble and contains approximately 38% of iodine. It is absorbed within an hour unless there is obstruction and dilatation of the fallopian tubes, which may delay absorption for 24 hours or so. Salpix is another satisfactory water-soluble medium now in use. It contains sodium acetrizoate and polyvinyl pyrrolidone. Some prefer oily media such as Ethiodol but its absorption from the peritoneal cavity is extremely slow.

Indications. This examination has been used widely for a number of years in the study of the problem of sterility and habitual abortion in women. The opaque material outlines the uterus and tubes, indicating the presence or absence of tubal patency. Other indications for its use are not as widely accepted as those for infertility studies, but it may be used to ascertain causes of abnormal uterine bleeding, to outline anomalies, and as an aid to identification of pelvic masses and intrauterine tumors. Following sterilization by means of laparoscopy tubal electrocoagulation, it is used to determine the presence of tubal occlusion. It is also used as an aid to the diagnosis of extrauterine pregnancy when the fetus is dead.

Contraindications. Active infection of the genital tract, recent or active uterine bleeding, suspected pregnancy, genital tuberculosis, and severe systemic disease involving the cardiorespiratory system all contraindicate the use of this procedure. Risks are minimal when water-soluble media are used. There may be venous or lymphatic reflux, but this does not appear to produce morbidity; it may cause diagnostic errors, however.

Technique. The examination is usually performed jointly by the gynecologist and the radiologist. A special type of cannula that occludes the external os of the cervix and prevents escape of the material into the vagina is used. Several types of instruments are available including a vacuum cannula that does not require the use of a tenaculum. The cannula is inserted and held firmly in place. Then 3 to 10 ml of contrast medium are hand injected under fluoroscopic control using image intensification to decrease irradiation of the pelvis. The uterus and tubes can be visualized during the injection. Roentgenograms are obtained as indicated during and after injection. If there is any doubt as to whether or not there is tubal patency, delayed films may be secured. Glucagon in doses of 2 mg has been used in patients having no evidence of tubal patency.[11] This relieves tubal spasm, allowing the medium to enter the abdominal cavity and it may reduce the incidence of false positive findings in patients with infertility.

Roentgen Findings. When the tubes are patent, there is extravasation of opaque material into the pelvic portion of the peritoneal cavity. The size and shape of the uterine cavity are readily outlined and any anomalies present are easily seen (Fig. 21-11). When the fallopian tubes are occluded, th ey may be partially visualized. There may or may not be dilatation indicating hydrosalpinx. When one or both tubes are patent, the material in the pelvic peritoneal cavity is readily recognized by the fact that it outlines the peritoneal surfaces and often the loops of bowel within the pelvis. If hysterography shows no abnormality and the patient does not become pregnant, direct visualization of pelvic contents by means of culdoscopy or laparoscopy is often indicated.

Congenital Uterine Anomalies

Congenital malformations occur in approximately 1% to 2% of females. Some of them are detected on physical examination while others may be found if curettage is performed. Hysterosalpingography is a useful method of determining or confirming their presence. The müllerian ducts fuse to form the uterus and the vagina and the unfused cranial portions become the fallopian tubes. Failure of fusion results in double uterus. The term *"uterus didelphys"* indicates complete duplication of the uterus, cervix, and vagina, which is a very rare anomaly. *Partial duplication* is an intermediate anomaly. Partial duplication of the vagina in conjunction with ipsilateral renal agenesis has been reported. It may be associated with unilateral hematocolpos which may be manifested clinically by abdominal pain, pelvic mass, and menstrual irregularity. *Gartner's duct cyst,* which occurs in the lateral wall of the vagina or uterus or in the broad ligament, may also result in a unilateral mass and may be associated with ipsilateral renal agenesis. Therefore it must be differentiated from partial duplication with hematocolpos. Failure of development of one duct results in *unicornuate uterus* in which there is an elongated uterine cavity and a single fallopian tube. Complete failure of development results in uterine aplasia and incomplete development, in hypoplasia. A number of alterations in uterine shape may also occur; these include the *arcuate uterus* in which the concavity of the uterine fundus is increased. The *bicornuate uterus* is the most common anomaly, presumably caused by incomplete fusion of the superior or fundal portion of

Fig. 21-11. A. Hysterosalpingogram showing no abnormality. The uterus and fallopian tubes are well outlined. There is some opaque material in the peritoneal cavity on the right, indicating patency of the tube on that side. Some of the material on the left may also be free in the peritoneal cavity. **B.** Hysterosalpingogram. This shows rather massive backflow of the iodinated contrast material into the lymphatics and veins. Biopsy revealed secretory endometrium with some endometritis.

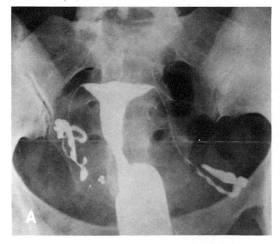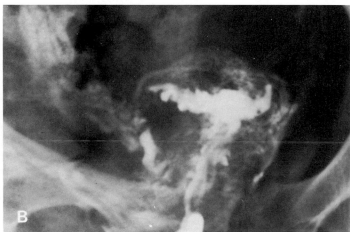

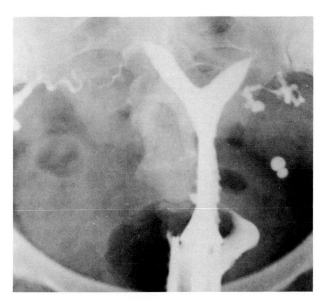

Fig. 21-12. Hysterosalpingogram showing a bicornate uterus. Note the relatively large horns as compared to the size of the uterine body.

the uterus resulting in paired uterine horns (Fig. 21-12). This anomaly varies greatly in degree. Septation of the uterus results from incomplete absorption of the median aspect of the fused müllerian ducts.

Mesonephric or Gartner's duct remnants may appear as linear diverticulumlike structures within the uterine wall extending from the region of the cervix upward and laterally toward the ovary. This anomaly is demonstrated on hysterography while Gartner's duct cysts appear as lateral vaginal masses. Alterations in uterine position, such as anteflexion and retrodisplacement, are usually found on physical examination. They may result in an unusual hysterographic appearance so that oblique and lateral views may be necessary.

Hysterography and Miscellaneous Uterine Conditions

Polypoid filling defects in the uterus may be observed on hysterography. They do not appear to be clinically significant and may represent a number of minor endometrial abnormalities. Multiple small cavities resembling diverticula may be observed in patients with *adenomyosis,* particularly when found in the upper one-half of the uterus, but cystic dilatation of cervical glands is somewhat more common and may coexist with adenomyosis.[31] Uterine leiomyomas,

particularly when they are in a subendometrial position, may cause single or multiple masslike defects encroaching upon the uterine cavity. Carcinoma of the uterus is not usually studied by hysterography but the presence of an irregular mass within the uterus should suggest the diagnosis. At times, however, endometrial carcinoma may be relatively smooth, resembling leiomyoma. When hysterography is carried out in a patient with unsuspected pregnancy, there is usually enough infiltration of the aqueous contrast medium into the substance of the decidua to produce a double outline of the uterine cavity. In these instances, if the patient is pregnant, the amniotic sac is observed as a filling defect in the uterus. Intrauterine adhesions secondary to infection or trauma are readily observed. They may appear as minimal or extensive areas of non-filling which may be smooth, irregular, round, linear, single, or multiple.

Intrauterine Device Localization

Ultrasound is used to check the position of an intrauterine contraceptive device (IUD). Poor positioning predisposes to pregnancy or expulsion of the device. Furthermore, the device may perforate the uterus and extrude into the pelvic peritoneal cavity. If the ultrasonic findings are equivocal, plain films exposed with the patient in anteroposterior and lateral positions may be helpful, but hysterography may be necessary to be certain of the position of the device. Plain-film study of patients with a Lippe's loop show widening of the loop when it has perforated the uterus and lies free in the pelvis, since the uterus tends to compress the coil of the loop when it remains in place.[9]

BEAD-CHAIN CYSTOURETHROGRAPHY AND URINARY STRESS INCONTINENCE

The radiographic method of examination of women with stress incontinence is the bead-chain cystourethrogram; this is used to demonstrate the relationship of the urethra to the base of the bladder.[34] A fine, metal, beaded chain is inserted into the bladder which is then filled with one of the organic iodide contrast materials (100 to 300 ml). Some use an opaque catheter left in place rather than a beaded chain. Films are exposed in the frontal and lateral projections with the patient upright, at rest, and straining. Two angles are measured on the film: (*1*) the posterior urethral vesical angle (PUV) which is the angle formed by a line drawn through the base of the bladder posterior to the urethra and a line drawn through the axis of the posterior urethra, and (2) the inclination angle or upper urethral axis angle which is the angle between the vertical angle and a line drawn parallel to the posterior urethra. The examination also shows the relationship of the floor of the bladder to the level of the symphysis. There is some controversy regarding normal values of the angles, the range of the PUV normal being from 100 to 160 degrees and that of the inclination angle, or the upper urethral axis angle, ranging from 30 to 45 degrees. Abnormal configurations may be divided into two main types. In type 1 the PUV angle is increased and the upper urethral angle is normal; this abnormality is correctable by vaginal repair. In type 2 the PUV angle and the posterior urethral angle are increased; this requires an abdominal repair. There is also a type 3 which is present in patients with cystocele, but these patients do not usually have stress incontinence.[34] Ala-Ketola[1] uses the change in the inclination angle and the PUV angle as criteria. He believes that a change in the inclination angle exceeding 38 degrees on straining with a PUV angle over 160 degrees indicates the likelihood of stress incontinence. Others believe that a PUV angle over 100 degrees is abnormal, suggesting stress incontinence. The descent of the bladder should be no more than 2½ cm below the upper margin of the symphysis as observed on the anteroposterior film exposed with the patient upright.

Uterine Prolapse and Cystocele

Weakness of the anterior vaginal wall with descent of the bladder or cystocele may be demonstrated during cystography. Roentgenographically the base of the bladder is projected below the level of the symphysis pubis. The pelvic floor is weakened, the uterus may also descend. If prolapse is complete, the term "procidentia" is applied. In the latter instance, the bladder may descend well below the symphysis and may be obstructed. A cystogram obtained with the patient in the upright position shows the bladder to be much below the symphysis; and often it is seen to be elongated. Uterine prolapse and cystocele are readily demonstrated on physical examination and are noted if urography or cystography is performed on these patients.

PELVIC CALCIFICATIONS

Urinary-tract calculi and appendiceal calcifications have been described in Chapter 20. Occasionally, calculi occur in a Meckel's diverticulum located in the pelvis. Phleboliths are very common. Rarely, calculi are formed in the fallopian tube; they usually result from infection and may be single or multiple. When multiple they resemble a string of beads; this appearance should suggest tubal calculi. Calcification in uterine fibroids is typical in distribution. Calcification in ovarian dermoid cysts and psammoma bodies are discussed in the section of this chapter entitled "Ovarian Cysts and Tumors." Calcification of an entire ovary and ovarian "stones" have been reported. Ovarian fibromas may contain calcium and old areas of endometriosis may calcify. The diagnosis of the presumptive site of these calcifications is made by exclusion in most instances.

PELVIC CYSTS AND TUMORS

The roentgen examination consisting of films exposed in the frontal and oblique positions may reveal abnormal pelvic masses, but, with a few exceptions, the nature of the mass cannot be established by this method. Opacification of the colon and of the urinary bladder may aid in localization of masses. Ultrasound may be useful in the evaluation of pelvic masses. Differentiation between a cyst and a solid tumor is probably ultrasound's most important contribution. Also, ultrasound may identify pelvic abscess or hematoma, but differentiation of blood from pus is impossible by this method. The finding of a "fluid level" is virtually pathognomonic of ovarian dermoid (teratoid) cyst.

Pelvic arteriography, with visualization of the uterine arteries, is of definite value in some cases.

Gynecography (pelvic pneumography) is another special examination that can be used in the examination of pelvic organs. It consists of intraperitoneal injection of 1000 to 1500 ml of nitrous oxide or carbon dioxide, followed by roentgenograms of the pelvis obtained with the patient prone and tilted about 45 degrees with the head down. The gas surrounds the pelvic organs, permitting ready visualization of abnormalities or masses involving them (Fig. 21-13). Contraindications to gynecography are the presence of pelvic inflammatory disease, peritonitis, or cardiopulmonary disorders, particularly in the elderly who cannot tolerate the head-down position. This method may be used in conjunction with hysterosalpingography to differentiate uterine from adnexal masses and for resolution of adnexal masses into tubal and ovarian components. CT scanning and ultrasound are replacing gynecography to a large extent.

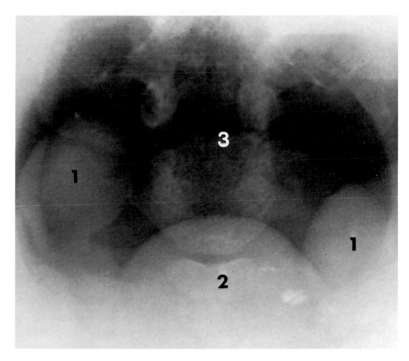

Fig. 21-13. Pelvic pneumogram. Gas within the pelvic peritoneum outlines the viscera. Numerals indicate the following: **1,** the ovaries; **2,** the urinary bladder; **3,** the uterus. These structures are normal.

Uterine Tumors

Leiomyoma. A large uterine leiomyoma produces sufficient opacity to be visible on the roentgenogram of the abdomen and pelvis and is outlined as a clearly defined, soft-tissue mass that may be smoothly rounded or lobulated. It may extend up out of the pelvis to lie in the lower abdomen. These tumors may contain calcium which assumes a characteristic mottled appearance (Fig. 21-14). The calcium may outline all or part of one or more uterine fibroids. During excretory urography, persistent uterine opacification has been observed in patients with leiomyoma. Presumably this is caused by the diffuse mass of proliferating arteries with few veins in this tumor. The contrast medium accumulates in the interstitium and capillaries. This finding is suggestive, but not diagnostic of leiomyoma. Infusion tomography of the female pelvis has been described[21] as a method of evaluating questionable pelvic masses such as leiomyomas, ovarian cysts, and solid ovarian tumors. It can be carried out in conjunction with excretory urography.

Other Uterine Tumors. Occasionally a hydatid mole may result in gross enlargement of the uterus that is readily detected on a roentgenogram of the abdomen. The diagnosis can usually be determined by ultrasound, but when this examination is equivocal, hysterography or amniography may be employed. Choriocarcinoma also causes uterine enlargement. This tumor develops after passage of a hydatid mole and less often after a normal pregnancy or abortion. It is estimated that about 2% of hydatid moles degenerate into malignant trophoblastic tumors. More than a third of chorionic malignant lesions follow moles, just under a third follow normal pregnancy, and a little less than a third follow abortion. Ultrasonography is very useful and may provide the diagnosis in these trophoblastic tumors. When findings are equivocal, arteriography may be used; also CT scanning may be helpful.

Endometrial carcinoma usually produces no changes that are evident on plain-film study, but when the lesion is advanced, uterine enlargement may be apparent. These tumors are studied by means of hysterography in a few institutions, most of which are in Europe. Carcinoma of the cervix also produces no plain-film findings until it is far advanced. Excretory urography and barium enema are used in the initial work-up. In many institutions, lymphography is used as a routine part of the pre-therapy work-up of patients with carcinoma of the cervix and endometrial carcinoma except in patients with very early lesions. Others believe that the yield of information is too low to justify its routine use.[16] Most workers

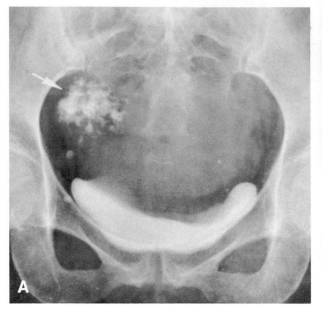

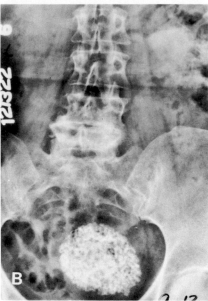

Fig. 21-14. Uterine leiomyoma. **A.** Mottled calcification characteristic of leiomyoma of the uterus is indicated by the **arrow.** The soft tissue mass above the bladder is the enlarged uterus. This film was obtained during excretory urography. **B.** Very large and densely calcified uterine leiomyoma.

agree that it is useful in advanced disease in determining the extent of metastases. It is also useful in differentiating recurrence from fibrosis following therapy. As a rule, lymphangiograms yielding positive findings are accurate and useful and indicate a poor prognosis, but those demonstrating no abnormality are of limited value. Pelvic arteriography is used by a few to aid in the staging of uterine malignant disease,[20] and pelvic venography is used somewhat more commonly since it can substantiate lymphographic diagnosis of metastasis and at times provide more information than lymphography regarding metastatic foci in the parametrial, hypogastric, and presacral regions. The use of arteriography is not as widely accepted as venography and lymphography in study of malignant disease in the uterus. Venography includes bilateral iliac venography, inferior venacavography, compression inferior venacavography for retrograde opacification of internal iliac and sacral veins, and selective ovarian venography in carcinoma of the uterine body. The place of CT scanning in patients with endometrial carcinoma is not yet determined. Occasionally leiomyosarcoma or adenocarcinoma of the endometrium may become sufficiently large for the uterus to be visible as a soft-tissue mass in the pelvis. There is no way to differentiate these masses roentgenographically.

Malignant mixed uterine tumors contain sarcomatous and carcinomatous elements. These rare tumors are manifested by uterine enlargement noted on plain-film study. About one-third contain calcium, often localized to a small area within the mass, which may suggest the diagnosis; otherwise, the tumor cannot be distinguished from other uterine masses.

ABNORMALITIES OF THE FALLOPIAN TUBES

Diverticulosis (Salpingitis Isthmica Nodosa)[35]

In fallopian tube diverticulosis, a nodular thickening of the medial third of one or both fallopian tubes is associated with a number of small diverticula which evidently represent herniation of tubal mucosa into the myosalpinx. These develop into glandlike spaces that resemble diverticula. The cause of this condition is not entirely clear, but it is probably secondary to infection. Some believe that it represents a form of adenomyosis, however. Hysterosalpingography reveals narrowing of the proximal fallopian tube with multiple, rounded filling defects varying from 2 or 3 mm to 1 cm in diameter associated with a number of small diverticulumlike outpouchings. The term "salpingitis isthmica nodosa" is applied since infection probably plays a role in most cases. The condition may result in infertility.

Hydrosalpinx

The term "hydrosalpinx" designates a rather marked dilatation of a fallopian tube usually occurring when there is obstruction in the ampulla. In contrast to this, when there is occlusion in the midportion of the tube, there is relatively minimal dilatation.

Tuberculous Salpingitis

In tuberculosis involving the fallopian tubes, usually the tubes have an irregular contour, a small lumen, and multiple strictures; at times there are excavations of the lumen or the formation of fistulas. Scarring may result in a straight or rigid luminal contour; obstruction is usually present. When treatment is effective, the hysterosalpingogram may show that the fallopian tubes have returned to their normal state.

OVARIAN CYSTS AND TUMORS

Dermoid or Teratoma

Approximately one-third of the dermoid cysts of the ovary contain some calcium, usually in a tooth or toothlike structure attached to one wall of a rounded pelvic mass. Rarely there is enough calcium in the wall of the cyst to visualize it. These dermoids vary in size and are often eccentric in position. There is

usually enough lipid material within the mass to make it relatively radiolucent and when the combination of toothlike structure within a radiolucent pelvic mass is present, the diagnosis is almost certain. In the larger percentage of ovarian dermoids in which no calcification is present, the radiolucency of the mass is a valuable diagnostic sign. The radiolucency is enclosed in a thin cyst wall that is denser than the lipid material within it. When the typical radiolucent mass is found in the pelvis or lower abdomen surrounded by the smooth and clearly defined soft-tissue wall, which is of greater density, a diagnosis of ovarian dermoid cyst can be made with reasonable certainty (Fig. 21-15). In pregnancy, the ovarian dermoid cyst may be displaced into the mid or upper abdomen or may lie deep in the pelvis, displacing the uterus upward.

Calcification in Ovarian Tumors

Psammoma bodies are frequently found on pathologic examination of papillary cystadenoma and papillary cystadenocarcinoma of the ovary. When there is enough calcification in the tumor it can be recog-

Fig. 21-15. Ovarian dermoid (teratoid) cysts. **A.** Small cyst **(arrows)** containing a tooth and a small amount of calcification in its wall. **B.** Large cyst **(arrows)** containing amorphous calcification, some of which is in the wall.

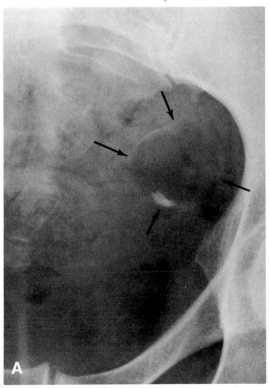
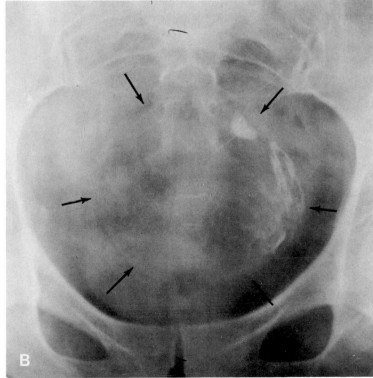

nized roentgenographically (Fig. 21-16). The psammoma bodies are small calcifications widely distributed in the tumor, giving it a more uniform type of calcification than is noted in uterine fibroids. These tumors metastasize widely and calcification may be found in the metastases, which may be scattered throughout the abdomen and chest. The calcification has been noted in metastases to peripheral nodes. The findings are typical enough to make the diagnosis or strongly suggest it in most instances (Fig. 21-17). Psammomatous calcification has also been reported in *ovarian thecoma*, but the calcification tends to be confined to a limited area. *Gonadoblastoma* may present a characteristic pattern—a small, circumscribed, dense, mottled calcification in the area of the ovarian tumor.[28]

In addition to papillary serous *cystadenocarcinoma*, metastases from pseudomucinous cystadenocarcinoma may very rarely contain calcium, often curvilinear rather than punctate and scattered.

Other Ovarian Cysts and Tumors

Ovarian cysts and tumors often attain great size before they are recognized by the patient or her physician. When large, they are readily outlined radiographically and appear as oval or rounded masses in the pelvis. They are often large enough to

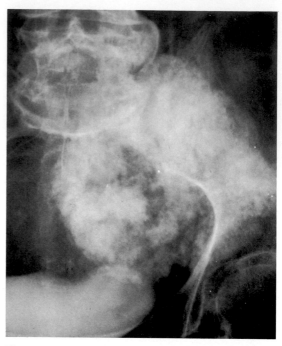

Fig. 21-17. Recurrent serous cystadenocarcinoma of the ovary. This film, exposed during an excretory urogram, shows a large irregular, densely calcified tumor in the left lower abdomen and pelvis. This represents psammomatous calcification in a recurrent tumor.

extend out of the pelvis into the abdomen and are often noted to move with change of position of the patient. They may lie directly in the midline or slightly to one side and can therefore resemble large uterine tumors. The latter do not tend to be as freely movable with change in position, however. When malignant, the ovarian tumors are often associated with ascites, which causes general increase in abdominal density; this obscures the margins of the mass and makes it difficult or impossible to identify in the roentgenogram. Occasionally large ovarian cysts may be present in the newborn. Plain films demonstrate the large mass in the pelvis which may extend upward to fill the abdomen. Total body urography demonstrates the avascularity of the mass, suggesting cyst. Ultrasound may also be used to make the diagnosis of cystic mass.

Meigs' Syndrome

This syndrome, as originally described by Meigs[22] consisted of benign ovarian fibroma associated with

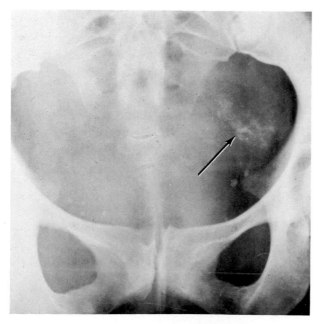

Fig. 21-16. Cystadenocarcinoma of the ovary. **Arrow** indicates calcification in this primary ovarian tumor.

ascites and pleural effusion. The fluid cleared on removal of the ovarian tumor. The designation "Meigs' syndrome" is now used by some to indicate the association of ascites and hydrothorax with any benign ovarian tumor or with low-grade or malignant ovarian tumor when the fluid clears soon after removal of the tumor. Roentgen findings are those of ascites and pleural effusion, which may be unilateral or bilateral. The ovarian tumor is small and is usually hidden by the fluid in the abdominal cavity. Exact diagnosis of Meigs' syndrome is not possible by roentgen methods.

Spontaneous Ovarian Amputation

Spontaneous ovarian amputation is a relatively rare condition in which the autoamputation of an ovary is manifested radiographically by a small, calcified pelvic mass that moves when the patient's position is changed (Fig. 21-18).[24]

THE VAGINA

Vaginography

Vaginography is used largely in infants for the detection of anomalies and foreign bodies. It consists of insertion of a small catheter into the vagina followed by

hand injection of one of the organic iodide contrast media. Films are then exposed in planes necessary to demonstrate the anomaly or the pathologic state.

Genitography

The term "genitography" is used to describe a study of all genital cavities in children with genital tract obstruction, imperforate anus, or an intersex problem. Organic iodides are used as contrast media. The intersex states have been classified and the radiographic findings described by Shopfner.[29] When the genitalia are ambiguous, the ultimate sex to be assigned should be decided before the second year of the child's life. The reader is referred to the monograph by Shopfner since such conditions and their diagnosis are beyond the scope of this volume.

Foreign Bodies

The presence of an opaque foreign body within the vagina is readily detected roentgenologically. Localization is relatively simple, using a frontal and a lateral projection. These foreign bodies are found most commonly in children. Their presence is often manifested by vaginitis, with a vaginal discharge that may be bloody. If plain films fail to demonstrate a foreign body, a small catheter may be inserted into the vagina

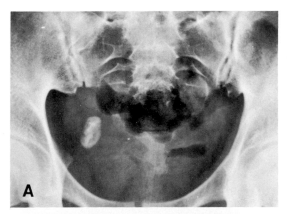

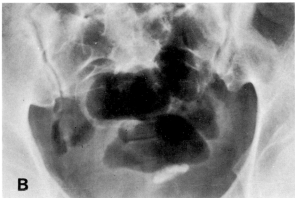

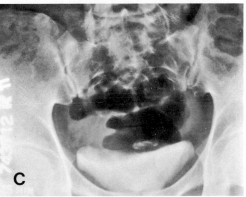

Fig. 21-18. Autoamputation of the ovary. Note the difference in position of the pelvic calcification representing an ovary in the prone **(A),** supine **(B),** and supine urogram **(C)** films.

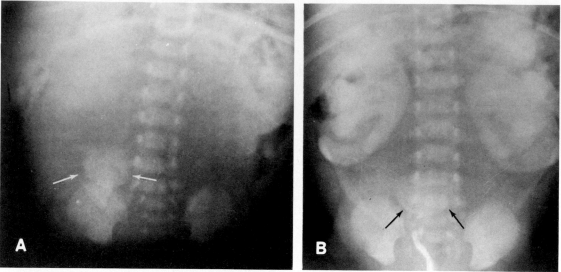

Fig. 21-19. Hydrometrocolpos. **A.** Excretory urogram. A large central lower abdominal and pelvic mass displaces the bladder **(arrows)** upward and to the right. Excretion is too poor to outline the renal pelvis and the calyces. **B.** Retrograde pyelogram shows displacement of the bladder **(arrows)** and also reveals lateral displacement of both ureters and a considerable amount of hydronephrosis.

and an opaque medium injected to outline a radiolucent foreign body. Vaginal calculi may be formed by deposition of inorganic salts around vaginal foreign bodies. Most of the so-called vaginal stones are formed in this way. Rarely, a primary calculus is formed in the vagina, presumably from deposition of urinary salts secondary to incontinence or continuous urinary leakage through a vesicovaginal fistula. At times the demonstration of a vesicovaginal fistula may be very difficult because the amount of drainage into the vagina is small. In these patients, it is sometimes useful to insert a vaginal tampon prior to obtaining an intravenous urogram. The tampon is left in place until the bladder becomes distended and then removed and radiographed. The presence of contrast material in the tampon is indicative of a fistula providing the patient has not voided or is not incontinent; in either of these instances, reflux into the vagina may cause a false positive finding.

Hydrocolpos and Hydrometrocolpos

Imperforate hymen or atresia of the vagina may lead to distention of the vagina (hydrocolpos) or of both vagina and uterus (hydrometrocolpos). This may also lead to obstruction of the urinary tract. The most consistent finding is a lower abdominal mass associated with a mass protruding from the vaginal introitus. The condition may be apparent in infancy or may not appear until puberty and the onset of menstruation. In the latter instance, hematocolpos or hematometrocolpos develops.

Roentgen findings on the plain film of the abdomen are those of a lower abdominal mass. Urograms may reveal hydronephrosis and hydroureter with distortion of the bladder and unusual separation of the lower ureters. If opaque material is injected into the vagina through the protruding vaginal membrane, the large distended vaginal and uterine cavities can be visualized. The diagnosis can be suggested when the abdominal mass is outlined and the urographic evidence of obstruction and distortion is present (Fig. 21-19).

Congenital Absence of the Vagina

This anomaly may be, but is not necessarily, associated with uterine agenesis. The uterus, when present, may be retroverted and infraperitoneal. This state is not detected on pelvic pneumography or on ultrasound. Its presence may be suspected on rectal examination when a mass is palpated and can then be confirmed by arteriography.

Transverse Vaginal Septum

A transverse vaginal septum is an extremely rare anomaly, the cause for which is not clear, since it cannot be explained on the basis of the currently accepted theories of the embryology of the vagina. It occurs high in the vagina and is usually incomplete. It can be demonstrated on vaginography.

REFERENCES AND SELECTED READINGS

1. ALA-KETOLA L: Roentgen diagnosis of female stress urinary incontinence. Acta Obstet Gynaecol Scand [Suppl] 23: 1973
2. AVNET NL, ELKIN M: Hysterosalpingography. Radiol Clin North Am 5: 105, 1967
3. BISHOP PA: The roentgenologic diagnosis of fetal hydrops. Am J Roentgenol 86: 415, 1961
4. BORELL U. FERNSTROM I: The value of the "halo sign" in the diagnosis of intrauterine foetal death. Acta Radiol [Diagn] (Stockh) 48: 401, 1957
5. BORELL U, RADBERG C: Orthodiagraphic pelvimetry with special reference to capacity of distal part of pelvis and pelvic outlet. Acta Radiol [Diagn] (Stockh) 2: 273, 1964
6. CULP WC, BRYAN RN, MORETTIN LB: Placenta membranacea. A case report with arteriographic findings. Radiology 108: 309, 1973
7. CUNNINGHAM JJ, FUKS ZY, CASTELLINO RA: Radiographic manifestations of carcinoma of the cervix and complications of its treatment. Radiol Clin North Am 12: 93, 1974
8. DIEHL J, FERNSTROM I: Radiologic pelvimetry with special reference to widest transverse diameter of pelvic inlet. Acta Radiol [Diagn] (Stockh) 4: 557, 1966
9. EISENBERG RL: The widened loop sign of Lippe's loop perforations. Am J Roentgenol 116: 847, 1973
10. GAGNON JH, ROMAN TN: Lymphography in cancer of the uterus. Aust Radiol 118: 318, 1974
11. GERLOCK AJ Jr, HOOSER CW: Oviduct response to glucagon during hysterosalpingography. Radiology 119: 727, 1976
12. GRUBER FH: Gas in the umbilical vessels as a sign of fetal death. Radiology 89: 881, 1967
13. HEAGY FC, SWARTZ DP: Localizing the placenta with radioactive iodinated human serum albumin. Radiology 76: 936, 1961
14. Hill AH: Fetal age assessment by centers of ossification. Am J Phys Anthropol 24: 251, 1939
15. ISAACS I: Roentgen pelvimetry by differential divergent distortion. Am J Roentgenol 63: 669, 1950
16. KADEMIAN MT, BUCHLER DA, WIRTANEN GW: Bipedal lymphangiography in malignancies of the uterine corpus. Am J Roentgenol 129: 903, 1977
17. KELLY KM, MADDEN DA, ARCARESE JS et al: The utilization and efficacy of pelvimetry. Am J Roentgenol 125: 66, 1975
18. KENDIG TA: Reduction of fetal irradiation in pelvimetry. Radiology 75: 608, 1960
19. LEE KF, GREENING R, KRAMER S et al: The value of pelvic venography and lymphangiography in the clinical staging of carcinoma of the uterine cervix: analysis of 105 proven cases by surgery. Am J Roentgenol 111: 284, 1971
20. LEONIDAS JC, BEATTY EC, HALL RT: Chorioangioma of the placenta. A cause of cardiomegaly and heart failure in the newborn. Am J Roentgenol 123: 703, 1975
21. LOVE L, MELAMED M, COOPER RA et al: Infusion tomography of the female pelvis. Am J Roentgenol 122: 299, 1974
22. MEIGS JV, CASS JW: Hydrothorax and ascites in association with fibroma of the ovary. Am J Obstet Gynecol 53: 249, 1937
23. MURRAY JP: Semi-orthometric pelvimetry: an appraisal. Br J Radiol 44: 524, 1971
24. NIXON GW, CONDON VR: Amputated ovary: a cause of migratory abdominal calcification. Am J. Roentgenol 128: 1053, 1977
25. ROBINS SA, WHITE G: Roentgen diagnosis of dermoid cysts of the ovary in the absence of calcification. Am J Roentgenol 43: 30, 1940
26. SAVIGNAC EM: The prenatal roentgen diagnosis of fetal hydrops. Am J Roentgenol 80: 673, 1958
27. SCHWARZ GS: An orthometric radiograph for obstetrical roentgenometry. Radiology 66: 753, 1956
28. SEYMOUR EQ, HOOD JB, UNDERWOOD PB Jr: Gonadoblastoma: an ovarian tumor with characteristic pelvic calcifications. Am J Roentgenol 127: 1001, 1976
29. SHOPFNER CE: Radiology in pediatric gynecology. Radiol Clin North Am 5: 151, 1967
30. SIEGLER AM: Hysterosalpingography, 2nd ed. New York, Medcom Press, 1974
31. SLEZAK P, TILLINGER KG: The incidence and clinical importance of hysterographic evidence of cavities in the uterine wall. Radiology 118, 581, 1976
32. STEVENS GM: Pelvic pneumonography. Semin Roentgenol 4: 252, 1969
33. STOLZ JL, FOGEL EJ: The chain cystourethrogram. Radiology 103: 204, 1973
34. TAGER SN: A new roentgen sign of fetal death. Am J Roentgenol 67: 106, 1952
35. THOMAS ML, ROSE DH: Salpingitis isthmica nodosa demonstrated by hysterosalpingography. Acta Radiol [Diagn] (Stockh) 14: 295, 1973
36. WEPFER JF, BOEX RM: Mesonephric duct remnants (Gartner's duct). Am J. Roentgenol 131: 499, 1978
37. WOLFE JN, EVANS WA: Gas in the portal veins of the liver in infants. Am J Roentgenol 74: 486, 1955

SECTION V

THE CHEST

tory in the hands of those who use them long enough to gain proficiency. The method described here is used in our department.

Contrast Material. Dionosil (3,5-diiodo-4-pyridone-N-acetic acid) is the contrast medium used most extensively. It contains 34% iodine and is available as an aqueous and an oily suspension. Since aqueous Dionosil is more irritating than Dionosil oily, we use the latter. Dionosil is rapidly absorbed and does not remain to abscure disease in the lobe or lung in which bronchography is done. This material does not break down to form free iodine and is probably the best agent now available for bronchography.

Barium sulfate suspended in carboxymethylcellulose has been advocated as a safe contrast agent for bronchography. Our experience has been limited to its use in a few patients with iodine sensitivity. It evidently causes less pulmonary reaction than any of the other agents now in use. We have had no experience with powdered tantalum, which has been used experimentally and, in a few cases, clinically.

Preparation of the Patient. The meal prior to the examination is withheld and the patient is not allowed to eat or drink for a period of 4 hours following bronchography. Premedication consisting of 100 mg of Seconal or Nembutal and 60 mg of codeine is administered an hour before the examination. If there is much bronchial secretion, 0.4 mg of atropine sulfate may be given an hour before the examination. In patients who have large amounts of sputum it is wise to employ postural drainage to decrease the amount of secretions because material in the bronchi interferes with the induction of anesthesia and with contrast filling of the bronchi.

Anesthesia. Proper anesthesia is essential for successful bronchography; the examination is almost invariably doomed to failure unless good anesthesia is attained. In infants and small children, a general anesthetic is used. This is administered by the anesthesiologist who inserts an endotracheal catheter. Under fluoroscopic control, the contrast material is then introduced into the desired lobe or segment through the catheter. In older children and adults, a local anesthetic is employed. Lidocaine hydrochloride (4% xylocaine hydrochloride) is the agent which we use. The agent is sprayed over the pharynx, hypopharynx, and tonsil areas and, after a short wait, the pharynx, pyriform sinuses, and epiglottis are swabbed with the anesthetic solution, using a long forceps and gauze sponges or cotton pledgets. As a final measure, ap-

proximately 1 ml of the anesthetic solution is dropped into the glottis by means of a curved cannula; this usually initiates severe coughing that spreads the material over the glottis and upper trachea. There is considerable individual variation in patients; some are very easily anesthetized while others are extremely refractory. It may be necessary to introduce 2 to 4 ml of lidocaine hydrochloride (4%) through the catheter into the main bronchus of the lung to be examined. An intermittent positive pressure apparatus especially adapted for administration of local anesthetics in bronchography has been developed.[32] We have had no experience with this device.

Technique of Oil Injection. When satisfactory anesthesia has been achieved, a tracheobronchial catheter is inserted into the trachea by way of the glottis. It is placed in a desired bronchus and the opaque medium can be injected directly into the bronchus. We also use the percutaneous method in which a 16-gauge needle is inserted into the trachea through the cricothyroid membrane. A catheter is threaded over a guidewire and maneuvered into the desired site in the bronchial tree.[37] When it is necessary to examine both lungs or portions of both lungs by this method, we prefer to examine one side at a time and to allow an interval of several days between the two sittings. The direct method of injection by means of a needle puncture through the cricothyroid membrane is also used in our department. A total of approximately 15 to 20 ml of contrast material is usually required to map the bronchi of one lung. The procedure is usually started with the patient in the upright or semi-upright position on the table, which is then moved into the horizontal or Trendelenberg position. The patient is rotated until fluoroscopic observation indicates that the desired filling is obtained. When local obstruction or local disease is observed during fluoroscopy, spot films are exposed. It is important that the patient breathe deeply once the contrast medium has been introduced into the desired bronchi. He or she should also be encouraged to cough a few times to aid in complete distribution of the opaque into the smaller bronchi. A lateral roentgenogram is obtained first with the examined side down, using a Bucky technique. Then an anteroposterior roentgenogram is obtained with the patient lying on the table in the supine position. The patient is turned into an oblique position and a third film is exposed using Bucky technique. For this projection the examined side is down with the opposite side elevated at a 45-degree angle. Then, with the patient in an upright position, stereoscopic posteroanterior and lateral

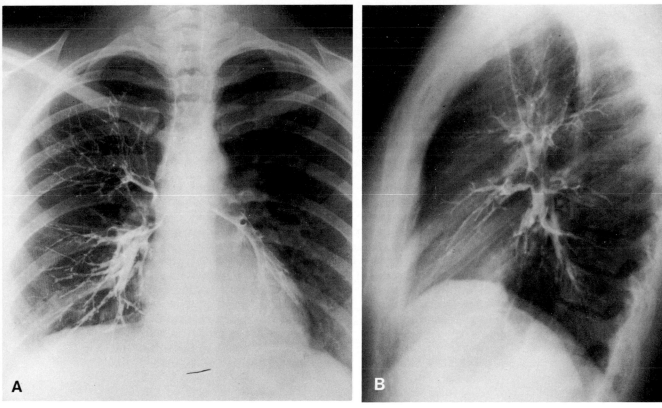

Fig. 22-3. Normal bronchographic findings. Note that the iodized oil has coated the trachea and outlines the bronchi, which branch in a treelike manner into the lungs. The peripheral bronchi are somewhat better filled in the frontal **(A)** than in the lateral **(B)** projection.

roentgenograms are obtained (Fig. 22-3). An appropriate oblique projection may also be obtained if deemed necessary. Delayed films exposed at 30 to 60 minutes after the procedure may be of value, particularly in patients in whom basal bronchiectasis is suspected but was not demonstrated on the initial films. They may also be of value when basal bronchial filling is incomplete. Following the procedure, the patient is encouraged to cough and expectorate the contrast material, using postural drainage as an aid.

Hazards

Anesthetic Reactions. The danger of anesthetic reactions can be reduced to a minimum by proper premedication and by keeping the total amount of Xylocaine used to less than 200 mg. This examination should be avoided in patients who have had previous local anesthetic reactions. Common symptoms are

dizziness, restlessness, apprehension, confusion, and convulsive twitchings progressing to convulsive seizures. Cyanosis, dyspnea, respiratory arrest, and cardiac failure may also occur. Treatment consists of administration of oxygen as soon as possible, making certain that the airway is maintained. Small doses of a short-acting barbiturate such as Pentothal sodium (Thiopental in a dose of 30 to 50 mg per minute) should be administered intravenously if convulsions occur. Artificial respiration may be necessary in the presence of respiratory failure; thoracotomy with cardiac massage may be needed if cardiac arrest occurs.

Iodized Oil Reactions. Reactions to iodized oil are infrequent and are usually allergic in type and relatively mild. Manifestations consist of bronchial asthma and urticaria; when these reactions are immediate they can be treated by the use of antihistaminic drugs. Late reactions owing to aggravations of existing inflammatory disease can be managed by administration of appropriate antibiotics. Local obstruction produced by the viscous contrast material is treated by encouraging postural drainage and cough. Oil granulomas have been reported as late complications when alveolar oil is retained but this complication is extremely rare.

Other Complications. Spread of tuberculous disease has been mentioned in the past but this is not an important factor at present with the use of antituberculous drugs and judicious timing of the procedure in relation to the activity of the tuberculous disease. Hemorrhage has also been reported but in our experience this is a rare complication and the amount of hemorrhage has never been of sufficient quantity to be a real hazard.

LARYNGOGRAPHY

Laryngography includes the study of the hypopharynx, the larynx, and the subglottic portion of the trachea. The technique consists of coating the structures to be examined with oily Dionosil. Premedication with large doses of atropine sulfate to decrease secretions is very important. We use 1 mg of atropine if the patient will tolerate it. We also use codeine to suppress the cough reflex. The pharynx and larynx are anesthetized with Xylocaine hydrochloride or Cetacaine spray or both. Then the oily Dionosil is administered by cannula over the back of the tongue. Using fluoroscopy to see that the hypopharynx and larynx are coated, spot films are exposed in lateral and frontal projections during (*1*) quiet respiration, (*2*) phonating "E," (*3*) Valsalva maneuver, and (*4*) modified Valsalva, with the mouth closed and the glottis open. Voltages in the range of 65 to 70 kV are optimal. This examination is very useful in the study of tumors of the supraglottic region and of the larynx (particularly in the evaluation of possible subglottic extension), and in determination of pyriform sinus involvement. We often use a combination of laryngography and tomography of the larynx in the study of disease in this region (Figs. 22-4, 22-5 and 22-6).

TOMOGRAPHY

Technique

Tomography is also known as body section radiography, planigraphy, laminagraphy, and stratigraphy. These terms refer to a method of radiographic examination by which it is possible to examine a single layer of tissue and to blur the tissues above and below the level by motion. This is accomplished by simultaneous motion of the roentgen-ray tube and the film cassette during the exposure by means of a connecting rod or bar. The tube and film move in opposite directions and the fulcrum of the bar or rod connecting the tube and film carrier is placed at the level to be examined (Fig. 22-7). The amount of blurring depends upon the distance of the object or tissue from the level of the fulcrum. The thickness of the plane of tissue examined is determined within certain limits by the distance traveled by the tube and film during the radiographic exposure. Zonography is a variation in which the thickness of the plane of tissue examined is increased by shortening the excursion of the tube. By raising or lowering the fulcrum one can then examine planes of tissue within the chest at various levels as desired. Most of the manufacturers of radiographic equipment also make or distribute attachments for rectilinear tomography. Special tomographic units allowing circular, elliptical, hypocycloidal, and rectilinear motion are also available. When whole-lung tomography is used, such as in a search for metastases, the anteroposterior projection is employed. Posterior oblique tomography at a 55-degree angle is preferred when the hilum is being studied. Transverse tomographic units are also available; these permit transverse axial sections rather than the usual longitudinal sections. However, CT scanners will probably replace such units. As a general role, rectilinear tomography is sufficient for most studies of the lungs and thorax. If needed, one of the other motions can be used. There is also available a multiple cassette holder that permits the simultaneous exposure of seven films so that multiple planes of thoracic tissue at 1-cm intervals can be examined on a single exposure. This reduces total radiation exposure and also decreases the time consumed in the examination, but it has not been very satisfactory in our hands.

Indications

There are many indications for tomography of the chest. It is used to outline detailed anatomy of the lung, mediastinum, or other thoracic structures in which an abnormality is observed on the chest film. It is also used to outline the vascular pattern and pulmonary pattern in diffuse processes such as emphysema, pulmonary hypertension, and pulmonary vascular anomalies. It is particularly useful in the study of patients with pulmonary tuberculosis. Cavities can be outlined that are not visible on routine roentgeno-

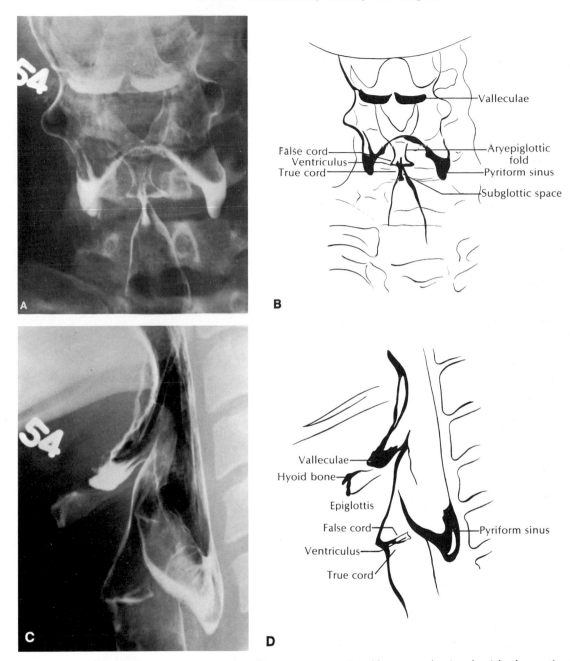

Fig. 22-4. Laryngogram. **A.** This anteroposterior film was obtained with the patient phonating "E." **B.** Diagram of **A** with anatomic structures labeled. **C.** Lateral film. **D.** Diagram of **C** with anatomic structures labeled.

grams and nodular infiltration can be more clearly defined than with any other type of examination. These studies are usually made with the patient in an anteroposterior position but lateral tomograms can be

obtained when necessary to show lesions not well seen in frontal projection. Bronchiectasis associated with tuberculosis can often be identified by means of tomography; the method is particularly useful in ex-

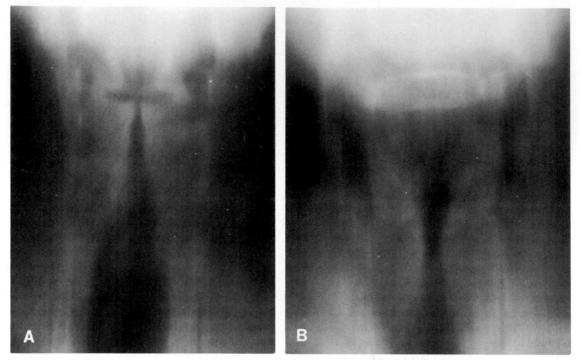

Fig. 22-5. Tomogram of the larynx. **A.** This tomogram was obtained with the patient phonating "E." Note the clear definition of the ventriculus and cords. There is subglottic stenosis of the trachea. **B.** This film was exposed with the patient performing the modified Valsalva maneuver (mouth closed, glottis open). The tracheal stenosis persists.

amining the lung compressed by thoracoplasty. In patients with bronchogenic carcinoma, the mass of the tumor can be outlined and it is often possible to visualize the site of bronchial occlusion when this is present. Tomography also is useful in detecting calcium in small parenchymal nodules (Fig. 22-8) and in the study of lung abscess. Full-lung tomography is used for the detection of pulmonary metastases in patients in whom the method of therapy is significantly altered when metastases are present. It may also be useful in studying vascular and interstitial pattern in patients with emphysema, pulmonary hypertension, or arteriovenous malformations.

PULMONARY ANGIOGRAPHY

Technique

The purpose of this examination is to outline the pulmonary arterial system. This can be accomplished in several ways. The simplest is the injection of a large bolus of contrast medium (one of the organic iodides) intravenously using a needle. Timed films then show filling of the right heart and the pulmonary arteries. Properly timed filming will also show opacification of the pulmonary veins and left heart. A major disadvantage is that filling of the desired vascular structures is less than optimal. Catheter methods include injection into the vena cava, right atrium, distal right ventricle, pulmonary artery, or, selectively, into either right or left pulmonary artery or one of their branches (Fig. 22-9). The nature of the process for which the procedure is performed tends to determine the method used. The catheter methods result in better opacification and therefore better visualization of the vessels studied. For a discussion of angiocardiography see Chapter 32.

Indications

Pulmonary angiography is sometimes used in evaluating operability of lung carcinoma. It is also used in

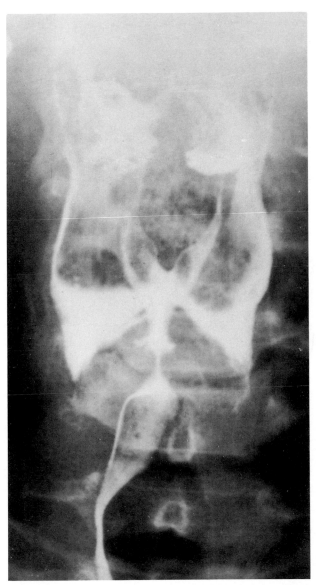

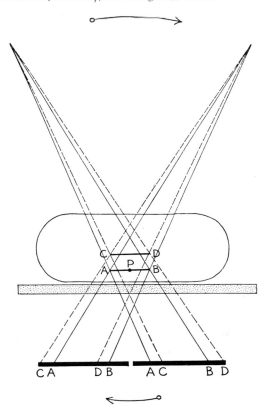

Fig. 22-7. Diagram illustrating the principles of tomography. The **upper arrow** indicates the direction of the tube shift. The fulcrum is at the level **P** on line **AB.** Note that the relationship of the projected image of **AB** remains the same on the initial and final position of the cassette, while the image of the line **CD** at some distance from the fulcrum has moved from right to left. Therefore, the tissues at the level of the fulcrum are clearly defined while those above and below it are blurred by motion.

Fig. 22-6. Laryngogram in a patient with carcinoma of the base of the tongue which had extended into the vallecula on the right. Note the clearly defined vallecula on the left side and the irregularity on the right which results from encroachment by an irregular neoplastic mass. The pyriform sinuses and glottis appear to be normal.

the study of patients with suspected pulmonary arterial or venous anomalies or diseases. Most importantly, the study of thromboembolic disease of the lungs by means of pulmonary arteriography may be

indicated. It is not used routinely, but may be needed when the diagnosis remains in doubt following roentgen and scintiscan studies and when the patient is not responding to treatment for presumed pulmonary embolism.

BRONCHIAL ARTERIOGRAPHY

This examination requires selective catheterization of bronchial arteries which is very difficult. Its use in clinical medicine is very limited.

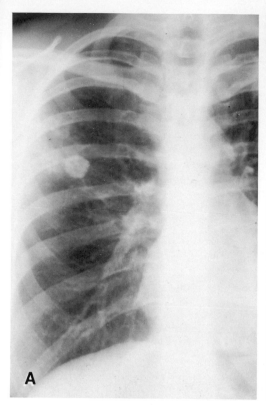
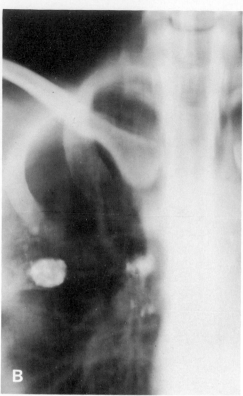

Fig. 22-8. Examples of the use of tomography. **A.** The calcified nodule on the right is clearly defined, but there is some disease above and lateral to it which is not well outlined. **B.** Definition of the large nodule is very clear and the nodular appearance of the disease above it and the homogeneous disease lateral to it are outlined to better advantage than in **A.**

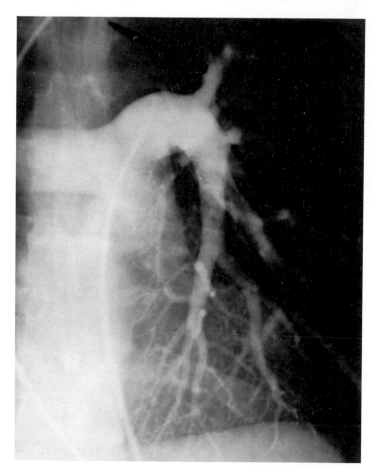

Fig. 22-9. Pulmonary arteriogram showing normal findings. This is an example of selective pulmonary arteriography. The catheter is seen to lie in the left pulmonary artery.

AZYGOGRAPHY

Azygos venography is a procedure used to outline the azygos system using the major tributaries, the intercostal veins. We use the intraosseous method, but direct catheterization by way of the femoral vein, right atrium, and superior vena cava can be accomplished.

Technique (Intraosseous Method)

A number 16 bone-marrow needle is used to hand inject 25 ml of methylglucamine diatrizoate (Renografin 60) into the marrow cavity of the eighth, ninth, or tenth rib laterally. Xylocaine is used to anesthetize the marrow space. Serial films are exposed at one per second for 6 seconds after the end of the injection. The azygos system is filled by way of the right side and the hemiazygos by way of the left side; then the azygos fills by way of communications extending across the vertebral column (Fig. 22-10).

Indications

Azygography is used in evaluating operability of lung cancer and also of esophageal cancer. It is also used in the investigation of the cause of enlargement of the azygos vein. Superior venacavography is sometimes employed in conjunction with azygography in patients with lung carcinoma. A study that fails to reveal abnormality is of little value, however, so we seldom use these studies in patients with lung tumors.

DIAGNOSTIC PNEUMOTHORAX

Diagnostic pneumothorax is occasionally used in examination of diseases of the chest. A measured amount of air or oxygen (100 to 300 ml) is introduced into the affected side and roentgenograms of the chest are obtained in desired projections. Fluoroscopy of the chest can also be carried out following injection of the gas. This method of examination is use-

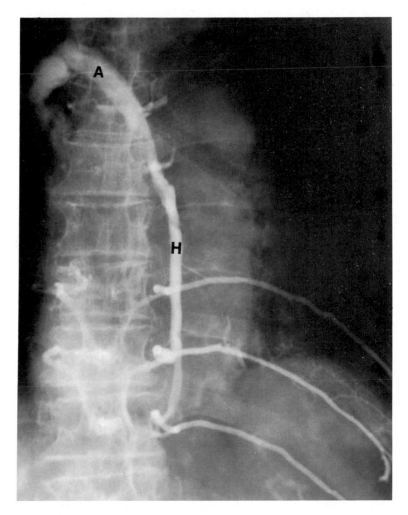

Fig. 22-10. Azygogram showing normal findings. The opaque medium was injected into the marrow cavity of the left ninth rib. There is good opacification of three intercostal veins, the hemiazygous vein **(H),** and the azygous vein **(A).** A small amount of medium is noted in the superior vena cava.

ful in differentiating the soft-tissue masses or densities in the mediastinum, chest wall, or diaphragm from intrapulmonary lesions. It can also be used in differentiating pleural disease from disease of the diaphragm. Occasionally it is necessary to use diagnostic pneumoperitoneum in conjunction with pneumothorax to differentiate lesions producing soft-tissue densities in the diaphragm from those projecting upward from the abdomen.

DIAGNOSTIC PNEUMOMEDIASTINOGRAPHY

The introduction of a gas into the mediastinum for diagnostic purposes has been used for some time, chiefly in Europe. Recently this procedure has been advocated in this country, in conjunction with scalene node biopsy. Three to 8 liters of carbon dioxide are introduced into the mediastinum through a catheter which is inserted at surgery. Films are then exposed in desired projections. Usually there is good visualization of mediastinal structures and of any mass which may be present. Tomography may also be used in conjunction with this procedure. We have had no experience with this method. It is probable that CT scanning will make this procedure unncessary in the future.

BRONCHIAL BRUSH BIOPSY

Bronchial biopsy and aspiration of bronchial secretions for microscopic study have been used in conjunction with bronchoscopy for a number of years. This method is now employed more widely in conjunction with fiberoptic bronchoscopy than in the past. Bronchoscopy allows direct examination of the bronchial tree to the subsegmental bronchi so that a biopsy specimen can be obtained directly by use of a small brush to obtain specimens for study (brush biopsy). Beyond this range, fluoroscopic control is used for obtaining brush-biopsy specimens. An estimated 75% to 85% of carcinomas of the lung can be diagnosed histologically by use of this method. Therefore, failure of a brush biopsy to yield evidence of a lesion does not exclude the possibility of carcinoma. Fennessy[15] has developed the method of transcatheter brush biopsy. The opaque, Odman type of catheter is shaped in a manner that facilitates entry into the desired bronchus. The catheter with guide wire is inserted through the pharynx, larynx, and trachea under fluoroscopic guidance. Small brushes are passed through the catheter into the lesion. Nylon-bristle brushes are used to obtain cytologic and bacteriologic specimens, steel bristle brushes to obtain tissue for viral cultures and histologic study, and a small forceps to obtain tissue.[16] Microscopic slides are then prepared immediately from the brushes. Cultures are prepared and smears made for cytologic study from material on the nylon brushes. Tissue from the steel brushes is placed in a special medium for virus culture; tissue from the steel brushes and from the forceps is fixed for histologic study. Bronchial brush biopsy is used to examine peripheral lung lesions, usually solitary, beyond the reach of the bronchoscopist and suspected of being primary lung tumors. It is also of value in diffuse lung disease, particularly in immune-deficient patients and in patients in the cancer age group who have pneumonia which resolves slowly or incompletely. It is contraindicated in patients with recent severe hemoptysis, a suspected vascular lesion, bleeding tendency, or severe dyspnea. Complications include pneumothorax, which is usually not significant, and hemorrhage, which is potentially dangerous. These complications are rare, however.

NEEDLE ASPIRATION BIOPSY

This method of examination, used largely for local lesions in the periphery of the lung, has become popular in recent years. In addition to aspiration using thin-walled, 18-gauge needles, cutting techniques are employed for obtaining histologic material. Several needles are currently available for this procedure. Trephine biopsy in which a gas-driven trephine, introduced by Steel, is preferred to any of the available needles by some workers. The major complications are pneumothorax and hemorrhage. Pneumothorax is usually easily managed, but hemorrhage occurring after any of the percutaneous procedures can be difficult to manage and has been fatal in some instances. Therefore, these percutaneous procedures are contraindicated in patients with bleeding diathesis or thrombocytopenia, a suspected vascular lesion, recent severe hemoptysis, or severe dyspnea at rest, as well as in those who cannot cooperate.[35]

XERORADIOGRAPHY AND TOMOGRAPHY

Edge enhancement and wide latitude make xeroradiography valuable in examination of soft-tissue structures. Xeroradiography is particularly useful in the examination of the pharynx and larynx. It may be used for examination of the tracheobronchial tree.[20] Endobronchial lesions and alterations in caliber of the trachea and bronchi are more easily detected than on roentgen tomography. There is more radiation exposure per tomographic "cut," but often a single xerotomogram is sufficient for making a diagnosis while several roentgen tomograms are needed for this purpose. Therefore, the total exposure may be less in xerotomography than in tomography. Peripheral lung masses may also be examined by xeroradiography. We tend to use pulmonary xerography very rarely in special situations; CT scanning is more useful in most instances.

COMPUTED TOMOGRAPHY AND DISEASES OF THE CHEST

Although the ultimate place of CT scanning in diseases of the thorax is not yet determined, it is likely that many applications will be found for the use of this modality. It has been found to be of value in identification of parenchymal pulmonary nodules, particularly at the lung periphery and below the level of the diaphragmatic dome. It is also useful in demonstrating pleural tumors and areas of pleural thickening and in the study of the mediastinum and its contents. The abnormal hilum, pulmonary cavitary disease, and diseases, including abscesses and masses, in the vicinity of the diaphragm have been studied to advantage with the use of CT scanning. It seems clear that CT scans can provide information not obtainable by any other noninvasive technique, particularly in the mediastinum.[25]

THE NORMAL CHEST

GENERAL CONSIDERATIONS IN CHEST INTERPRETATION

Interpretation of chest roentgenograms requires that the viewer first find the abnormality. It is useful to develop a method of studying the film to make certain that all areas are searched. The mediastinum including the heart, the lung fields, diaphragm, bony thorax, soft tissues of the thorax, and the subdiaphragmatic upper abdominal structures should be inspected. It is helpful for the student or trainee to compare the two lung fields interspace by interspace until he learns the normal thoroughly and can recognize variations and abnormalities. Once an abnormality is observed, interpretation of the changes follows. We find it valuable to make the initial examination of the film without knowledge of the clinical findings. Before reaching a decision, however, roentgen observations must be correlated with all of the available clinical information. Specific questions may arise, the answers to which may not be available on the chart. Additional information must then be sought from the referring physician or from the patient.

In the chapters on chest roentgenology to follow, the presentation is disease oriented. Patterns of pulmonary density of various types are observed. The terms "interstitial" and "alveolar" are used to describe the predominant pattern of pulmonary involvement. *Alveolar* or air-space disease is characterized by homogeneous density which may vary from a small area, just large enough to be recognizable, to consolidation of an entire lobe or more. The alveoli are filled with exudate, transudate, blood, or tissue which replaces the air. When the lung parenchyma is opacified by some type of fluid, the acinus may be observed as the anatomic unit that initially appears as a rosette measuring 6 to 10 mm in diameter; later, when filling is more complete, it appears to be spherical. The acinus may be defined as the lung parenchyma distal to a terminal bronchiole. As parenchymal disease progresses, individual acini are obscured by the overlapping of many opaque acini; this results in uniform density of the lung affected. Classic pneumococcal pneumonia is a good example of alveolar disease. Bronchi may become visible when such consolidation occurs; the *air bronchogram* is then observed, which indicates adjacent alveolar disease.

Interstitial disease is characterized by an increase in density of the perivascular, interlobular, and parenchymal interstitial spaces. Alveolar aeration is maintained and the interstitial tissues increase in volume. The process may be localized, as in viral pneumonia, or general as in extensive interstitial edema. The pattern may range from reticular or latticelike, to granular, to nodular, or to various combinations of these findings.

Combinations of interstitial and alveolar density may also occur. A common example of this is the patient with combined interstitial and alveolar pulmonary edema. Mycoplasmal and viral pneumonia are also frequently observed to have a combined pattern.

The localization and sometimes the recognition of pulmonary disease is dependent in many instances upon the *silhouette sign*. The term was coined by Felson, who credited Dr. H. Kennon Dunham with making the initial observations. Felson[13] defines this sign as follows: "An intrathoracic lesion touching a border of the heart, aorta or diaphragm will obliterate that border on the roentgenogram. An intrathoracic lesion not anatomically contiguous with a border of one of these structures will not obliterate that border." The principle defined above is very useful in a variety of chest conditions. Relative density is also a factor, since juxtaposed borders of similar density will produce the sign and the borders of densities that are markedly dissimilar may not be obscured.

In addition to air flow into alveoli through the bronchial system, there is peripheral communication which may explain normal or sometimes hyperaeration that may be observed distal to an endobronchial obstruction. The pores of Kohn are small (3 to 13 microns in diameter) openings in alveolar walls, lined with alveolar epithelium. Collateral air drift probably occurs through these pores. Some collateral ventilation may also occur through the canals of Lambert, which are accessory epithelial-lined tubular communications between bronchioles larger than the terminal bronchiole and the alveoli. They range up to 30 microns in diameter. There is some evidence to indicate that there are larger collateral channels, but their anatomic nature is not certain.[21]

THE ADULT CHEST

The roentgenogram of the adult chest outlines the heart, lungs, bony thorax including the ribs and thoracic vertebrae, the diaphragm, all or part of the clavicles, and all or part of the scapulas. The soft tissues making up the chest wall also are included. The thorax is divided by the mediastinum into right and left compartments, each containing an air-filled lung that is recognized by its relative radiolucency as compared to the mediastinum, chest wall, and the upper abdominal viscera. The greater part of the trachea is also shown so that most of the lower respiratory tract is visible.

The Bony Thorax

Roentgenography of the chest is undertaken primarily for visualization of intrathoracic structures, but the shoulder girdles, ribs, cervical and thoracic vertebral bodies, and sternum are often well enough outlined so that disease or anatomic variation can be readily recognized. Therefore these structures should be examined on all chest roentgenograms. The shape of the thorax varies with age and with body habitus so that the range of normal is wide. The angulation of the ribs varies considerably with body type; downward angulation is minimal in short hypersthenic individuals and maximal in asthenic patients. The intercostal spaces are numbered according to the rib above them. In describing disease in relation to intercostal spaces, the interspace must be

designated as either anterior or posterior because there is considerable difference in position of these interspaces in relation to the horizontal plane of the lung. The costal cartilages are not visible unless there is calcification within them; when calcification is present it assumes a rather characteristic mottled appearance (Fig. 22-11). The diaphragm in a normal adult is very slightly higher on the right than on the left and is at approximately the level of the posterior arc of the tenth rib or the fifth anterior rib or interspace in deep inspiration. The ribs below the level of the diaphragm are usually not as well visualized as those above it because of the greater density of the contents of the abdomen. The rhomboid fossa is an irregularly rounded indentation on the inferior surface of the clavicle near its sternal end. It marks the attachment of the costoclavicular ligament and varies

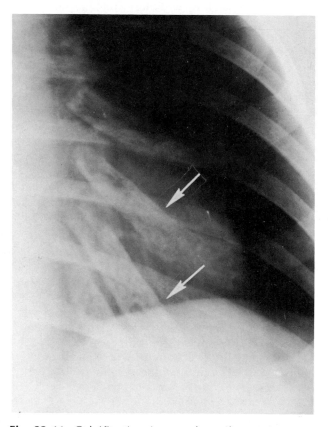

Fig. 22-11. Calcification in costal cartilages. An unusually large amount of calcification is noted in several of the costal cartilages, two of which are indicated by the **arrows.** The mottled appearance of the calcium is characteristic.

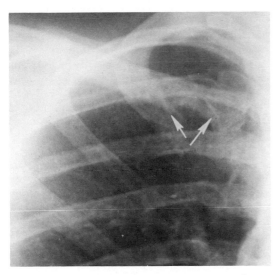

Fig. 22-12. Rhomboid fossa. **Arrows** indicate the irregular, round indentation on the inferior aspect of the clavicle.

from slight roughening that may not be visible to a deep indentation. It should be recognized on the chest roentgenogram as an anatomic variant of no clincal significance (Fig. 22-12).

The Soft Tissues

The soft-tissue structures covering the bony thorax also produce density on the chest roentgenogram and they can project over the lung and pleura in a manner that simulates disease. Skin folds in patients who have lost weight can produce linear shadows running in any direction. Breast shadows are usually not difficult to identify but do result in increase in density over the lower thorax, bilaterally. Nipple shadows may appear as rounded densities in the fourth anterior interspace or lower. They are usually bilaterally symmetric, but a film with metallic nipple markers may occasionally be necessary to differentiate them from intrapulmonary lesions (Fig. 22-13). The skin and subcutaneous tissues over the clavicles produce a faint, soft-tissue shadow paralleling the clavicles,

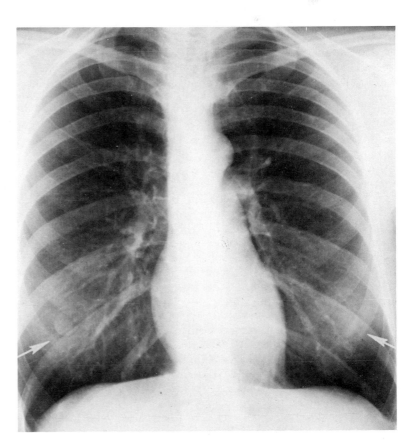

Fig. 22-13. Nipple shadows. Female with a small amount of breast tissue in whom nipple shadows appear as small rounded densities (**arrows**) in the sixth anterior interspace.

the clavicular companion shadow. This measures from 2 or 3 mm up to 1 cm in thickness, but projects beyond the lung field so that it can be identified. Soft-tissue masses or nodules projected over the lung fields can simulate pulmonary nodules. These nodules in the subcutaneous or deeper structures of the thoracic wall are usually more sharply defined than are the intrapulmonary lesions. Therefore, an extrapulmonary nodule can be suspected and a look at the patient will confirm its presence. At times lateral, oblique, or stereoscopic films must be employed to accurately localize some nodules observed on only one projection of the initial frontal and lateral roentgenograms.

The Mediastinum

Anatomic Division and Contents. The mediastinum is the space lying between the right and left pleurae in and near the median sagittal plane of the chest. It extends from the posterior aspect of the sternum to the anterior surface of the thoracic vertebrae and contains all the thoracic viscera except the lungs. It is divided into four parts, the superior, anterior, middle, and posterior mediastinum (see Fig. 22-19). The superior mediastinum lies between the manubrium sterni and the upper four thoracic vertebrae and contains structures which extend into it from below and above as well as those which traverse it and the mediastinum below it. Therefore, we often use the designations anterior, middle, and posterior mediastinum to include the length of the thorax without specific designation of superior, which contains the aortic arch and its branches as well as the innominate veins, the upper half of the superior vena cava, the trachea, esophagus, thoracic duct, thymus, lymph nodes, and various nerves some of which traverse the length of the mediastinum. If the three compartments are used to include a portion of the superior mediastinum, the anterior mediastinum is bounded above by the thoracic inlet, laterally by the pleura, anteriorly by the sternum, and posteriorly by the pericardium. It contains loose areolar tissue, the aorta and brachycephalic vessels, lymph nodes, some lymphatic vessels that ascend from the convex surface of the liver, the thymus, and the internal mammary arteries and veins. The middle mediastinum contains the heart and the pericardium, the ascending and transverse arch of the aorta, the superior vena cava and the azygos vein that empties into it, the brachiocephalic arteries, the phrenic nerves, the upper vagus nerves, the bifurcation of the trachea, the main bronchi, the pulmonary artery and its

two branches, the pulmonary veins, and adjacent lymph nodes. It is bounded in front by the anterior mediastinum and posteriorly by the posterior mediastinum. The posterior mediastinum lies behind the heart and pericardium, and extends from the level of the thoracic inlet to the twelfth dorsal vertebra. It contains the thoracic portion of the descending aorta, the esophagus, thoracic duct, the azygos and hemiazygos veins, lymph nodes, the sympathetic chains, and the inferior vagus nerves.

The Lymph Nodes. The mediastinal nodes are divided into three major groups. The anterior mediastinal nodes lie in the anterior mediastinum in relation to the innominate vein and the large arteries that arise from the aortic arch. The posterior mediastinal nodes lie behind the pericardium in the region of the descending aorta and esophagus. The tracheobronchial nodes consist of a chain of paratracheal nodes lying on either side of the trachea, the bronchial or bifurcation nodes lying between the lower trachea and bronchi, the bronchopulmonary or hilum nodes situated in the hilum of each lung, and the pulmonary nodes found in the lung substance adjacent to the larger bronchial branches (Fig. 22-14). Anatomists have recognized a greater number of lymph nodes associated with the right lung and a greater number of nodes associated with the right upper lobe bronchus than with the bronchi to the middle and lower lobes. The node adjacent to the azygos vein is termed the "azygos node." Because of its location it may become visible even when only slightly enlarged.

Roentgen Features of the Mediastinum. The trachea and main bronchi are usually visible in a chest roentgenogram of good quality. These structures lie within the mediastinum and the trachea is situated in the midline except for very slight deviation to the right at the level of the aortic arch. In infants, moderate tracheal deviation away from the side of the aortic arch (usually to the right) is common, but this is not observed in children after the age of 5 years. In older persons the trachea may curve slightly to the left above the arch and then to the right as it passes the arch. It extends from the level of the sixth cervical vertebra downward to the level of the fifth thoracic vertebra or slightly lower, where it divides into the right and left main bronchial branches. It is identified on the roentgenogram as a band of radiolucency in the midline that extends from the lower cervical region downward to the point of bifurcation. The main bronchi are somewhat smaller in diameter (Fig. 22-15). The right main bronchus continues

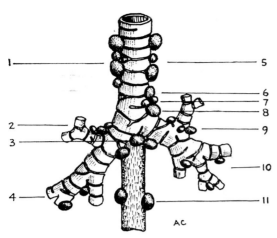

Fig. 22-14. The tracheobronchial lymph nodes. **(1)** Right paratracheal; **(2)** superior tracheobronchial on the right; **(3)** inferior tracheobronchial (bifurcation); **(4)** right bronchopulmonary; **(5)** left paratracheal; **(6)** preaortic; **(7)** nodes of the ligamentum arteriosum; **(8)** superior tracheobronchial (left); **(9)** superior bronchopulmonary (left); **(10)** bronchopulmonary; **(11)** paraesophageal.

downward more vertically than the left and divides into two main branches. The first branch is the upper-lobe bronchus, which curves sharply upward above the right pulmonary artery and is termed the *eparterial bronchus.* The continuation downward is termed the *hyparterial* or *common* (intermedius) *bronchus,* which continues as the right lower-lobe bronchus. The middle-lobe bronchus arises from the hyparterial bronchus, extending downward and laterally from its point of origin. On the left side the main bronchus is somewhat longer than on the right and forms a greater angle with the trachea. In addition to a lateral angulation it curves outward in its distal portion and divides into a lower-lobe bronchus and a left upper-lobe bronchus that courses horizontally for a short distance before dividing. A continuation of the left main bronchus downward and laterally forms the lower-lobe bronchus. It is usually possible to outline the main bronchi and portions of the upper- and lower-lobe bronchi in the normal patient. These structures have an appearance similar to that of the trachea, namely, a band of radiolucency but smaller in diameter.

In the frontal projection of the chest the mediastinum along with the sternum and thoracic spine form the dense central shadow as observed on the

normal roentgenogram. On the right side the superior margin is formed by the innominate artery or vein, below which lies the superior vena cava. The ascending aortic arch is usually not border-forming, but in cardiac diseases or aortic diseases that produce aortic dilatation it may be visualized. Immediately below the ascending aortic arch is the lung hilum. The smooth convex border of the right atrium forms the lower right mediastinal border. On the left side the left subclavian artery forms the superior aspect of the mediastinum. Below this the rounded convexity of the aortic arch is outlined. The pulmonary artery and the hilum of the left lung lie immediately below the aortic arch and the left ventricle forms most of the left lower mediastinal border, although a short segment of the pulmonary outflow tract may be visible below the hilum. In infants the thymus is often a large structure that lies in the anterior portion of the superior mediastinum and extends down into the anterior mediastinum. When visible it produces widening of the mediastinum superiorly and this widening is often asymmetric; the thymus then forms the lateral border of the superior mediastinum on both sides. Classically, the inferior aspect of the enlarged thymus forms an acute angle on one or both sides, a configuration that has been likened to a ship's sail (Fig. 22-16). It is not unusual to note some lobulation of the thymus. When such superior mediastinal

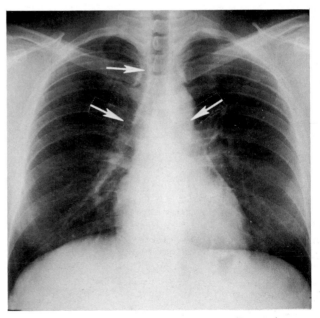

Fig. 22-15. Normal chest. The **arrows** indicate the trachea and main bronchi.

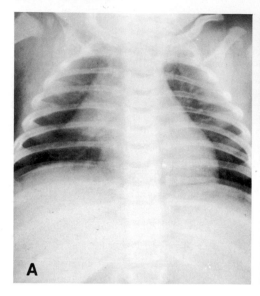
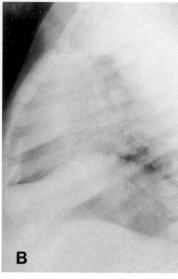

Fig. 22-16. Enlargement of the right lobe of the thymus. **A.** Note the angulation on the right which represents the sail sign. **B.** In this lateral view, an anterosuperior mediastinal density produced by the thymus is noted.

widening is present it is usually necessary to obtain a lateral projection in order to ascertain definitely that the shadow is in the anterior mediastinum and thus represents the thymus. Moderate widening of the superior mediastinal shadow is not considered abnormal in infancy; this portion of the mediastinum usually assumes its normal width during the first year of life.

The lungs approach the midline anteriorly in the anterior mediastinum. As a result the air in the lung on either side defines a vertical linear density sometimes called the anterior mediastinal line. It extends from a point near the level of the sternal angle superiorly to a point 3 or 4 inches below it. The "line" is visible on most roentgenograms of good quality. When one lung herniates across the midline, the line is displaced accordingly. The "line" thickens or diverges on either end.

The lungs also outline a "pleural" line in the paraspinal area on both sides. This is usually 2- to 5-mm thick, when measured from the lung to the lateral vertebral margin, and is often most clearly defined on overexposed high-voltage films. A pleural line is also observed on the right in the lower thorax outlining the lateral esophageal wall; this is medial to the paraspinal pleural line in the normal individual.

The hilum of the lung contains the pulmonary artery, the pulmonary veins, the bronchus, the bronchial arteries and veins, as well as lymph nodes. In the normal chest the pulmonary arteries and veins produce most of the density outlined on the roentgenogram (Fig. 22-17). The left hilum is higher in position than the right because the left pulmonary artery extends above the left main bronchus while the right pulmonary artery crosses below the right upper lobe bronchus (Fig. 22-18). In the normal person the lymph nodes in the region of the hilum do not contribute enough to the hilar density to be identified, but when enlarged or when these nodes contain calcium they can be recognized. The size of the hilum varies in the normal so that it is difficult to set a standard beyond which hilar size is abnormal. Since the size of the pulmonary vessels is related to pulmonary bloodflow, those vessels that make up the hila are increased when the bloodflow is increased and decreased in size in diseases that produce a diminution in pulmonary bloodflow. In addition to the variation in hilar size produced by the variability of caliber of the blood vessels, enlargement of hilar nodes may cause hilar enlargement; thus it is often difficult if not impossible to distinguish the cause for slight hilar enlargement. Fluoroscopy may be of some help in differentiating vascular from lymph-node enlargement. When slight node enlargement does produce alteration in the hila it is often necessary to examine progress films to determine the presence or absence of actual enlargement.

In the lateral view of the chest the four anatomic divisions of the mediastinum are well demonstrated (Fig. 22-19). The anterior mediastinum is seen as an area of relative radiolucency between the sternum and the heart. It is roughly triangular in shape, with the apex pointing downward. The internal thoracic muscle may be seen as a flat, wedgelike, soft-tissue

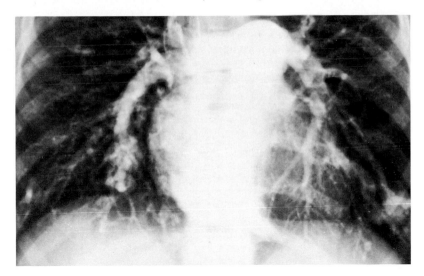

Fig. 22-17. Angiocardiogram. The right-sided heart chambers and pulmonary arteries are opacified. The radiographic hilum on the left is somewhat higher and more prominent than on the right—a normal finding. There are some basal arteriovenous malformations bilaterally.

Fig. 22-18. Normal chest. The hila are well outlined and indicated by **arrows.** The difference in height is noted. Continuations of the hilar densities can be followed in the lung fields and are noted to branch in a treelike fashion. They represent pulmonary arteries.

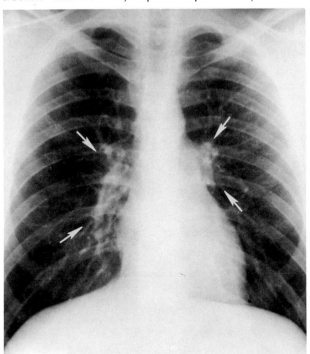

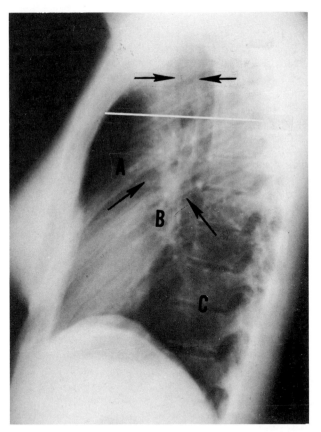

Fig. 22-19. Lateral view of chest showing divisions of the mediastinum. The superior mediastinum lies above the line extending from the sternal angle to the fourth dorsal vertebra. **(A)** The anterior mediastinum; **(B)** the middle mediastinum; **(C)** the posterior mediastinum. In the superior mediastinum the trachea is indicated by **arrows. Arrows** also indicate the region of the superimposed hila.

shadow immediately posterior to the lower sternum in the anterior mediastinum. This is more commonly observed in muscular males than in any other group. The superior mediastinum lies above it and the anterior aspect of the superior mediastinum is also radiolucent in the normal state, while the posterior portion is often somewhat opaque, owing to inability to elevate the soft parts of the shoulders and shoulder girdle enough to outline clearly this portion of the mediastinum. It is in the anterior mediastinum and anterior portion of the superior mediastinum that the enlarged thymus is noted as an area of density in infants. The middle mediastinum is clearly defined in a lateral roentgenogram, since it contains the heart and aorta. The posterior mediastinum is the area lying between the heart and the spine. It is visualized as a radiolucency of approximately the same density as that noted in the anterior mediastinum. The trachea is also visible in the lateral roentgenogram of the chest as a radiolucent structure that angles slightly posteriorly as it extends into the chest. The bifurcation is usually visible along with short segments of one or both upper-lobe bronchi. The left upper-lobe bronchus is lower than the right and is more readily outlined against the density of the left pulmonary artery which lies immediately above it. In this region an irregular, somewhat stellate density is noted that represents the vascular structures which produce the hila. The left pulmonary artery courses posterolaterally and lies above and posterior to the right pulmonary artery as viewed on the lateral film. In the examination of the mediastinum it is often of considerable value to opacify the esophagus by having the patient ingest thick barium paste. Then the relationship of the esophagus to the structures in the mediastinum can be determined and abnormalities can be clearly defined that would otherwise be very difficult to outline. The relationship of the esophagus to the trachea and its relation to the midline as well as to the heart can also be determined.

The Lungs

Lobar and Segmental Anatomy. The right lung is divided into three lobes, the upper, middle, and lower, by two fissures. The major or primary interlobar fissure separates the lower lobe from the upper and middle, while the secondary (minor) fissure separates the middle from the upper lobe. On the left side there are two lobes separated by the major interlobar fissure. The major fissures are sometimes visible in the lateral roentgenogram in the normal person and are readily visualized in this projection when there is a small amount of thickening of the interlobar pleura or small amount of fluid in the interlobar fissure. These fissures are visible in the frontal projection only when there is pleural disease or pleural thickening. The secondary interlobar fissure on the right is sometimes visible in the frontal projection in the normal individual (Fig. 22-20) and when pleural thickening is present can be easily identified in this projection as well as in the lateral view. It is horizontal and lies at the level of the anterior arc of the fourth rib or interspace. The major fissure on the right extends from the level of the fifth posterior rib downward and forward to the level of the sixth rib anteriorly, while the left major fissure is slightly more vertical and extends from the level of the third to fifth posterior ribs down to the level of the seventh rib anteriorly. The levels are somewhat variable in the normal person and in those with disease there may be marked variation in position. Occasion-

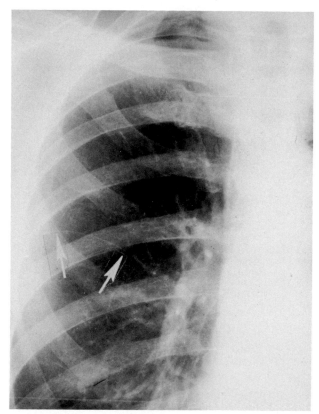

Fig. 22-20. The secondary interlobar fissure is indicated by **arrows.** It is slightly less horizontal in this patient than in the average person and its lateral aspect is higher in position than is normal.

ally, the major fissure on the right is directed slightly anteriorly into the sagittal plane in its lateral portion. It may then be visible as a "vertical" fissure line roughly paralleling the curve of the lower lateral chest wall. This is observed frequently in adults with small amounts of pleural fluid and has also been described in infants, particularly in those with cardiac enlargement.

When the major fissures are both seen in the lateral view, the left usually intersects the diaphragm more posteriorly and more vertically than does the right fissure. Not infrequently, the major fissures do not extend to the mediastinal surface of the lungs, so that lobar division is incomplete medially.

The importance of bronchopulmonary segmental anatomy has increased now that advances in thoracic surgery have made segmental and subsegmental pulmonary resection a common procedure. These segments have been classified by a number of investigators, but the classification by Jackson and Huber[23] is now in general use and will be used here. The segments and subsegments are not strictly morphological units, since arteries may cross from one segment to another and the segments contain veins that drain adjacent segments. The bronchi to these lobes and segments are not outlined on the chest roentgenogram unless they are diseased. Therefore it is necessary to use bronchography if accurate localization of a small lesion to a segment is required. By means of lateral and oblique roentgenograms along with frontal film, it is often possible to be moderately accurate in localization of pulmonary parenchymal disease without bronchography. In chronic inflammations, however, it is common to have sufficient fibrosis and contraction to distort the involved segment as well as the adjacent segments to the point that localization is not accurate without bronchography. The positions and names of the bronchopulmonary segments are given in the accompanying roentgenograms and drawings (Figs. 22-21A through F).

Roentgen Features. The normal lungs contain a considerable amount of air and since chest roentgenograms are obtained in inspiration they appear much more radiolucent than other structures making up the thorax and its contents. There is a distinct radiographic pattern that is produced largely by the blood vessels as they extend from the hilum into the lungs. The large bronchi can often be visualized as radiolucent tubes in the hilum, adjacent to which are dense smooth-walled tubes that represent the pulmonary arterial branches. These vessels branch in a treelike manner and decrease in caliber rapidly as they ex-

tend into pulmonary parenchyma. This pattern is readily visible on the roentgenogram. The pulmonary arteries lie in close relationship to the bronchi and branch and subdivide the same as the bronchi. Therefore, they lie within the pulmonary lobules. The pulmonary veins, on the other hand, have an anatomic distribution entirely separate from the bronchi. They begin at the periphery of the lobules in the pleura or interlobular septa and course to the left atrium between the lobules.

The vessels can be identified to within about 1.5 cm of the pleural surfaces of the lungs except at the apices, where the distance may be 3 cm from the pleura. In the upright position, the upper lobe vessels are smaller than those at the bases. The difference in size tends to reflect distribution of blood flow, which is greater in the lower lungs in the upright position, but tends to be nearly equal in the recumbent position. The lung fields are often divided arbitrarily into zones, depending upon the size of the vessels. The inner zone or inner one-third adjacent to the hilum contains the large main trunks. The middle zone contains intermediate-sized vessels and the peripheral one-third of the lung or peripheral zone usually contains vessels that are less than 1 mm in diameter. The pulmonary veins cannot be differentiated from the arteries in the peripheral or middle zones, but in the central zone the veins do not course near the arteries. They lie below the comparable arteries and empty into the left atrium at the lower margin of the hila. They rarely fuse into a single common trunk, so that there are usually two or more veins entering the atrium on either side. It is often difficult to outline them distinctly and differentiate them from arteries, but on tomograms they are visualized as smooth, elongated densities extending into the region of the left atrium in the lower hilum on either side (Figs. 22-22 and 22-23). Occasionally they are clearly defined on a routine frontal chest roentgenogram. This is particularly true in patients with congenital cardiac defects resulting in high-volume, left-to-right shunts. In patients with venous congestion the upper lobe veins can often be visualized as hornlike structures extending into the lower hila from the medial aspects of the upper lobes.

The pulmonary vessels at the bases are generally larger than the vessels elsewhere and, since the right medial base is better visualized than the left, the trunks stand out more clearly in this region than elsewhere in the lung fields. The anteroposterior diameter of the chest is greater inferiorly than it is superiorly and this means that more vessels are superimposed at the bases than elsewhere. This fac-

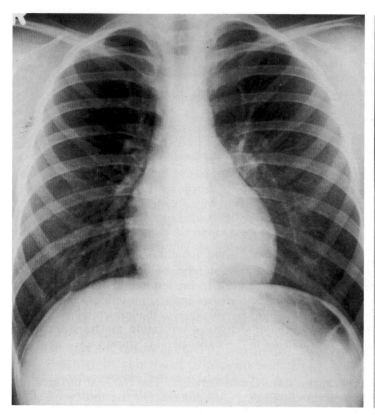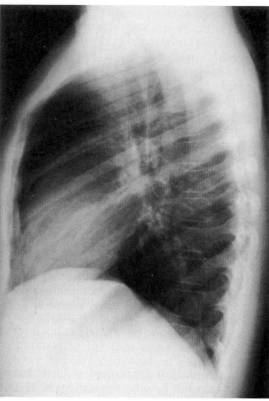

Fig. 22-28. Normal chest in a 10-year-old child. Note that the heart is somewhat globular and that the anteroposterior diameter of the chest is relatively large in comparison to the transverse diameter.

Rib irregularities from healed fractures are commonly noted and more or less calcification may be
seen in costal cartilages. This calcification varies
greatly in amount and tends to appear earlier in
women than men. Its roentgen appearance is that of
calcific density outlining the cartilage and extending
from the anterior rib edge toward the sternum.

The changes in the mediastinum with advancing
age are largely caused by alteration in the aorta and
its branches, which tend to become elongated and
tortuous. As a result the right superior mediastinal
border may become more prominent and clearly defined, because of increasing visibility of the innominate artery. The ascending arch of the aorta projects
farther to the right and causes a definite convex
shadow of soft-tissue density, the lower half of which
overlies the right hilum. Similar prominence of the
left upper mediastinum may be apparent with sclerotic changes in the left subclavian artery, and the
aortic arch tends to become increasingly prominent
(Fig. 22-29). The presence of calcification in the aor-

tic arch is common and calcification in the innominate and subclavian arteries is not rare. Pulmonary
vessels making up the roentgenographic hilar shadows may become larger, particularly when emphysema or other pulmonary abnormality results in
increased arterial pressure within the lesser circulation.

Alteration in appearance of the lung fields varies
widely with advancing age, but there is a general tendency for the vessels in the mid and peripheral zones
to be separated by hyperdistention of alveoli representing emphysema; associated perfusion decrease
results in a decrease in size of the peripheral vessels.
Pulmonary hypertension may develop; this is associated with increase in size of the vessels in the hila.
In addition, it is not uncommon to see linear shadows
produced by residues of previous inflammatory disease in one or both bases and there is a tendency for
the reticular interstitial pattern to become more pronounced. Small pulmonary parenchymal calcific foci
are common along with calcification in hilar nodes.

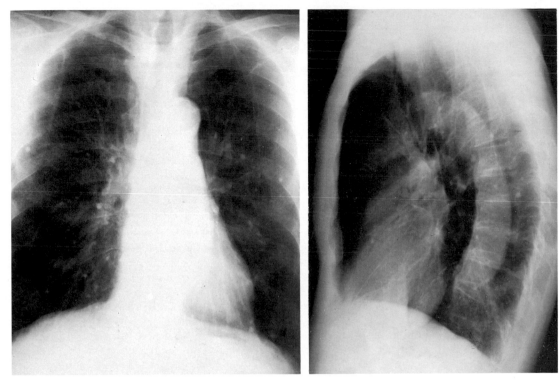

Fig. 22-29. The chest in the aged. The patient is a 71-year-old man with a considerable amount of calcification in the aortic wall, aortic dilatation, and elongation. The lungs are slightly hyperlucent. There is a little increase in the thoracic curve resulting in an increase in the diameter of the anteroposterior chest. The scattered parenchymal calcifications represent residues of previous histoplasmosis.

Apical pleural scarring producing irregular soft-tissue densities at the extreme apices is also found commonly in the aged and it is not uncommon to find one or both costophrenic sulci at least partially obliterated by previous basal pleural disease. The diaphragm tends to become lower and flatter with the alteration in the shape of the bony thorax and the appearance of senile emphysema. Irregularities of the diaphragm resulting from pleural inflammatory residuals is not uncommon. As the diaphragm becomes lower the dome becomes more horizontal and the costophrenic angles less acute.

CONGENITAL MALFORMATIONS

THE BONY THORAX

Minor developmental abnormalities are common in the ribs and are usually of no clinical significance, but should be noted and recognized as such on the roentgenogram. Cervical ribs are not uncommon and

may be very small and difficult to outline or they may be long and easily recognized as they project downward to overlie the pulmonary apex. Occasionally the transverse processes of the seventh cervical vertebra are unusually long and simulate short cervical ribs. One or both first ribs are often rudimentary in type. The most common anomaly of the remaining ribs is an anterior bifurcation, usually resulting in a broad, thin rib anteriorly that bifurcates in its anterior few centimeters. Complete fusion along the arcs of the ribs and pseudarthrosis between the ribs are other common anomalies. Intrathoracic rib is extremely rare. The anomalous rib usually arises from the posterior inferior margin of an otherwise normal rib or from a vertebral body, most often on the right side. The rib is sometimes attached to the diaphragm by a fibrous band. It projects into the pleural space and may be surrounded by lung even though its location is extrapleural. Diagnosis is suspected on viewing the chest roentgenogram and confirmed by tomography or fluoroscopy.

Anterior protrusion deformities of the sternum resulting in the so-called "pigeon breast" are usually so mild that no significant abnormality is noted on the frontal projection and only in the lateral view can the diagnosis be made. In these patients the sternum protrudes anteriorly to a greater or lesser degree. The amount of protrusion is readily apparent on the lateral roentgenogram of the chest.

Funnel-chest deformity or pectus excavatum produces changes that can usually be recognized on a posteroanterior roentgenogram. These alterations are described in Chapter 32 in the section "Funnel Chest (Pectus Excavatum)." In the lateral projection the posterior displacement of the sternum is readily discerned. Congenital midline defect in the sternum is a rare anomaly. The sternum is divided into equal halves by the fissure, which is easily recognized on the roentgenograms. Rarely, small accessory ossicles are noted immediately above the manubrium in the region of the suprasternal notch. They are termed episternal or suprasternal bones; they may be single or paired and range from a few millimeters to more than a centimeter in diameter. They may be fused to the manubrium or articulate with it; or there may be no contact with the sternum.

Scoliosis is a frequent abnormality in the thoracic spine and may be congenital. Hemivertebrae and other vertebral anomalies occur in conjunction with scoliosis and often produce it. In many instances, however, no definite anomaly is noted involving the vertebral bodies. The deformity of the thorax is proportional to the severity of the scoliosis and when marked, the anatomic alteration produced in the heart and lungs may result in alteration in cardiac and pulmonary function. Kyphosis often accompanies scoliosis and adds to the thoracic deformity. Kyphosis of the thoracic spine may also occur as an isolated deformity. It results in an increase in the anteroposterior diameter and a decrease in the vertical diameter of the thorax.

PULMONARY AGENESIS AND HYPOGENESIS (HYPOPLASIA)

Agenesis of a lobe indicates complete absence of the lobe; in aplasia, there is absence of lung tissue, but a rudimentary lobar bronchus is present. These anomalies are uncommon and are based on failure of one of the lung buds to appear in early embryonic development. The anomaly may be anatomically complete (agenesis) or there may be a small bronchus with or without a small amount of pulmonary tissue (aplasia). In hypoplasia, there is incomplete development of a lobe or lung. Roentgen findings on routine examination include a marked shift of the heart and other mediastinal structures to the involved side with decrease in size of that hemithorax; herniation of the normal lung across the midline; and evidence of increase in volume of the normal lung, which is very likely due to a combination of hyperplasia and compensatory emphysema. The right cardiac border may be indistinct if the remaining lobes fail to fill the hemithorax and do not extend to the anterior chest wall. The anterior space is then occupied by loose areolar tissue which blurs the heart border. Bronchography is necessary to visualize the bronchial tree and, on this examination, either a small bronchial stump or no bronchus at all is visualized. When an entire lung is absent, no lung is noted on the involved side except that which has herniated across the midline from the normal side. Angiocardiography can be used to outline the vascular system and will demonstrate the single pulmonary artery to the normal lung and thus confirm the diagnosis.

Pulmonary hypogenesis indicates incomplete development of the lung or a part of it and is also uncommon. All gradations from minor to severe degrees of hypoplasia may occur. Unless the anomaly is severe, there is usually very little alteration in the size of the affected hemithorax because some normal lung tissue remains; mediastinal shift along with elevation of the diaphragm on the involved side and compensatory emphysema on the opposite side all help to fill the hemithorax. This condition must be differentiated from the results of previous inflammatory disease producing fibrosis and contraction of a lobe or portion of a lobe. The evidence of previous disease may be apparent, but if not, bronchography can be used to show the bronchial distribution.

Lobar hypoplasia or agenesis may be associated with other anomalies including accessory diaphragm (Ch. 31) and partial anomalous pulmonary venous return below the diaphragm (see Ch. 32, section entitled "Partial Anomalous Venous Return").

ACCESSORY LOBES AND FISSURES

Azygos Lobe

The azygos lobe is formed when the arch of the azygos vein fails to migrate medially to lie in its normal position just above the right main bronchus. This vein remains lateral to its normal position and the small portion of the apex of the lung that lies medial to it early in development is deeply invaginated. The vessel carries two layers of visceral pleura and two layers of parietal pleura with it since it lies peripheral

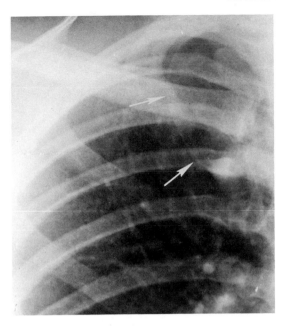

Fig. 22-30. Azygous lobe. Note the vein below the sternal end of the clavicle and the fissure **(arrows)** extending in an arc up to the pleural surface of the apex.

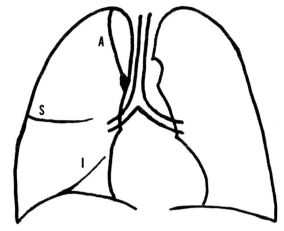

Fig. 22-31. Sketch showing position of the two most common accessory fissures: **A,** azygous; **I,** inferior accessory lobe fissure. The secondary interlobar fissure is also indicated as **S.**

to the parietal pleura. As a result, the pleural fissure is visible as a thin curvilinear line extending upward toward the apex to end at the parietal pleura of the apex. This line is usually bowed outward and its base, formed by the vein itself, is comma-shaped with the tail of the comma pointing upward toward the fissure (Fig. 22-30). The size of the azygos lobe varies but it is seldom very large. It is a common anomaly said to occur in 0.5% of the population and is usually of no significance.

The Inferior Accessory Lobe

The inferior accessory or cardiac lobe is the most common accessory lobe. The fissure may be complete or incomplete and is visualized on the posteroanterior roentgenogram as a faint line at the right medial base beginning at the diaphragm and extending upward toward the hilum. It arches somewhat with lateral convexity and there is often a very small upward projection at the diaphragmatic end of the fissure. This accessory lobe is usually supplied by a bronchus branching off the posterior basal segment of the lower lobe. The anomaly is less common on the left than on the right and is more difficult to see because it is often hidden by the cardiac shadow. It is of no

particular significance but occasionally becomes involved by disease and is then more readily identified (Fig. 22-31).

Other Accessory Lobes

The left upper lobe may be divided in a manner similar to the division on the right producing an accessory middle lobe. In these instances the interlobar fissure that divides the upper and accessory lobes is in approximately the same position as the secondary fissure on the right. This is a rare anomaly and of no clinical significance.

The posterior lobe is produced when the superior segment of the lower lobe is separated from the basal segments of the lower lobe by a horizontal fissure. This accessory lobe is rarely identified radiographically unless it is involved by disease sufficient to outline the smooth fissure separating it from the base of the lower lobe. It is somewhat more common anatomically, however, than radiographic examination would indicate.

Supernumerary bronchi are also commonly found and can be recognized roentgenographically only on bronchography, since they result in supernumerary segments rather than lobes. The most common site is the right upper lobe where the anomalous bronchus arises from the lateral aspect of the right main bronchus above the upper-lobe bronchus. Occasionally it arises from the lower right trachea, a right tracheal bronchus. Left tracheal bronchus is more uncommon, but is often of more clinical significance because it may be associated with obstructive emphysema and/or bronchiectasis. Minor variation in origin of segmental bronchi is not uncommon and displacement of a bronchus is often difficult or impossible to differentiate from a supernumerary bronchus. Numerous minor variations of bronchial segmentation have been found in all lobes and are not uncommonly visualized on bronchographic examination which is necessary to identify these bronchial variations. An entire lobe may be affected or there may be one or more segments involved (Fig. 22-32).

Absence of Fissures

Variations of interlobar fissures are relatively common, but since they occur without alteration in bronchopulmonary segmentation they produce no roentgenographic findings. In a study of 1200 lungs in cases of sudden death, Medlar[30] found the interlobar fissure on the left complete in 82% while the major fissure on the right was complete in 69% and the secondary fissure complete in only 37.7%. In the remainder the fissures were absent or incomplete.

BRONCHOPULMONARY SEQUESTRATION

Pulmonary sequestration is a congenital anomaly in which a portion of pulmonary tissue supplied by an arterial branch of the systemic circulation is sequestered from normal bronchial communication within a lobe or outside of the normal lung. Occasionally, there is a communication with the esophagus or stomach.

Intralobar sequestration of the lung or bronchopulmonary sequestration refers to a congenital anomaly in which a systemic artery arising from the lower thoracic or upper abdominal aorta extends into the lung on either side, where it supplies a portion of pulmonary tissue that is not connected with the normal bronchial tree and is therefore termed "sequestered." It is drained usually by the pulmonary venous system. This sequestered lung forms the site of a congenital cyst that may be uni- or multilocular. If it is uninfected, the lesion produces no symptoms. If it becomes infected and communicates with the bronchial tree, signs and symptoms are produced. It is almost entirely a lower-lobe lesion and usually involves the posterior basal segment of the lower lobe; the posterior segment of the left lower lobe is involved in approximately two-thirds of cases. The lesions have been found somewhat more frequently in males than in females; the ratio is approximately two to one. Occasionally, the arterial supply arises from the ascending aorta, the subclavian artery, the intercostal arteries, and, rarely, the celiac or innominate artery, and the venous drainage is into the inferior vena cava or azygos system and, rarely, into the portal system.

Roentgen findings depend upon the presence or

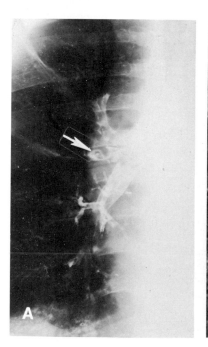
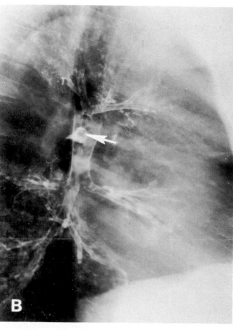

Fig. 22-32. Accessory lobe arising below the right upper lobe bronchus. This is outlined on the bronchogram, but its branches are not filled because of the presence of an intraluminal lipoma obstructing it. **Arrows** indicate the bronchus on the frontal **(A)** and lateral **(B)** projections.

absence of infection. In the patients in whom there is no infection, the condition is usually an incidental finding and presents as a round or oval mass in the posterior lung base on either side that may range up to 10 cm or more in diameter. It is usually found in the medial aspect of the lung base and occasionally a poorly defined, fingerlike projection extends toward the mediastinum from the medial aspect of the mass representing the artery supplying the tissue. When infection is present there is enough bronchial communication so that fluid levels and air are usually visible in a single cyst or in several adjacent cysts the walls of which are usually thin, if they are not obscured by infection in the adjacent lung. Even though there is evidence of bronchial communication manifested by the presence of air within the cysts, bronchography does not ordinarily demonstrate the communication. The most common finding on bronchography is that of an intralobar mass around which normal bronchial branches are draped. When there is bronchial communication as a result of infection, some of the bronchographic medium may enter the sequestered area. The lesion must be differentiated from lung abscess, acquired infected cysts, and chronic pulmonary inflammatory disease with cavitation. The asymptomatic type with no apparent connection with the bronchi must be differentiated from tumors and cysts of other origin. The location of these lesions is rather characteristic, however, and when a soft-tissue mass or an infected cyst is noted in the area, intralobar sequestration should be considered (Fig. 22-33). If this lesion is suspected, aortography is indicated. The diagnosis is established when the anomalous artery is opacified.

Extralobar sequestration results when the sequestered tissue is contained in its own pleural covering between the lower lobe and the diaphragm, within the diaphragm, in the mediastinum, or even beneath the diaphragm. This form of sequestration is drained by the vena cava or azygos venous system and occasionally by the portal system in contrast to the intralobar form which usually drains into the pulmonary venous system. It is on the left side in 90% of cases. It is asymptomatic and is therefore an incidental roentgen finding. Associated anomalies of the diaphragm are common, eventration of the diaphragm being a frequent finding. In addition to an abnormal diaphragm, a mass representing the sequestered lung may be visible. Rarely, hemorrhage into an extralobar sequestration will cause a mass to appear or to enlarge in the vicinity of the posteromedial aspect of the left hemidiaphragm.[36] Aortography can be used for confirmation when sequestration is suspected (Fig. 22-34).

BRONCHIAL (BRONCHOPULMONARY) CYSTS

Most cystic lesions of the lung are now believed to be acquired, but it is likely that the cysts occurring within the lung, lined by bronchial epithelium and resembling the bronchogenic cysts found in the mediastinum, represent congenital rather than acquired lesions. They are usually solitary and may occur anywhere within the lung. They present as rounded, clearly defined, intrapulmonary, soft-tissue masses. This lesion produces no symptoms and may be found on routine chest roentgenograms. If the cyst becomes infected and communicates with the bronchus, the roentgen findings are those of a thin-walled cavity containing gas and fluid that may be considerably obscured by inflammatory disease in the adjacent lung. The subject of cysts is discussed more fully in Chapter 24.

CONGENITAL CYSTIC ADENOMATOID MALFORMATION OF THE LUNG

This is a rare form of congenital cystic disease of the lung in which neonatal respiratory distress is often present. It usually involves a single lobe which is greatly enlarged and consists of a mass of disorganized tissue which probably represents a pulmonary hemartoma.[29] The lobe is firm and rubbery and consists of multiple cysts of varying size, with no normal bronchial or lobular pulmonary pattern. Radiologic findings are those of a pulmonary mass which displaces the mediastinum and heart and often herniates into the opposite hemithorax. The multiple cysts result in a coarse, honeycombed appearance. Irregular areas of density often outline some of the cysts and form part of the enlarged lobe. All cysts may be filled with fluid, presenting a roentgen picture of a large, solid mass. In some instances a single large cyst may be the predominant feature. Air–fluid levels may be observed. The clinical symptoms appear to be related to the size of the involved lobe. Surgical removal is necessary to allow the remaining lung to expand.

CONGENITAL PULMONARY LYMPHANGIECTASIA

This is a rare congenital disease which causes neonatal respiratory distress. The lungs are large and lobu-

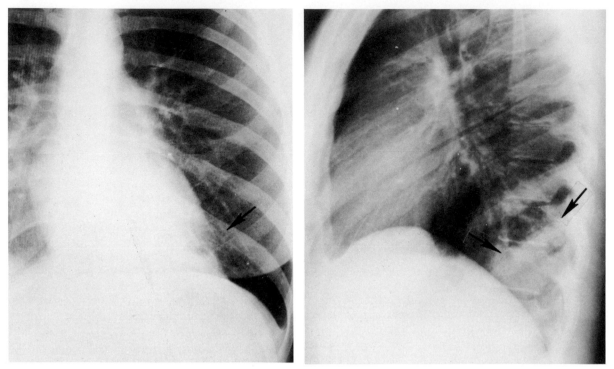

Fig. 22-33. Intralobar sequestration. The poorly defined mass at the left posteromedial base is indicated by arrows.

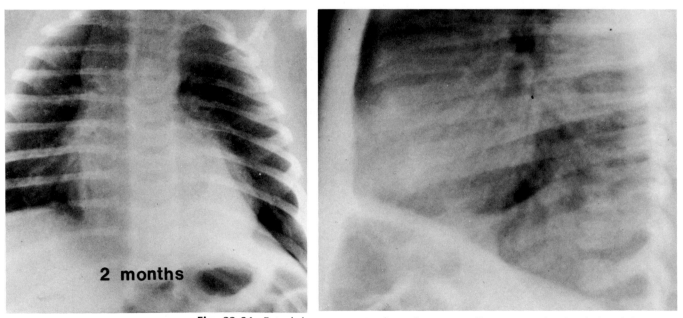

Fig. 22-34. Extralobar sequestration. A retrocardiac mass, clearly defined laterally, rests on the diaphragm posteriorly as visualized in the lateral view.

lated with prominent subpleural lymphatics which are cystic. Lobular septae are enlarged by the cystic lymphatics. Roentgen findings are those of bilateral increase in density with a reticulonodular pattern which simulates the findings in hyaline membrane disease. Kerley B-lines may be seen, caused by dilated lymphatics in interlobular septa. Most affected infants survive for only a short time. There is a milder form found in older persons in whom the major roentgen findings are related to lymphatic enlargement. Kerley's A- and B-lines are observed on the chest film. Both the severe and the milder forms may be associated with peripheral lymphangiomas.

INFANTILE (CONGENITAL) LOBAR EMPHYSEMA

Lobar emphysema in infants may not be manifest until some weeks or months after birth. Therefore, the term "infantile" or "neonatal" is probably more accurate than congenital in referring to this condition. This emphysema appears to be caused by bronchial obstruction which in turn may be produced by extrabronchial pressure, abnormality of bronchial cartilages, or redundant bronchial mucosa; in some of these patients no definite cause can be found. There is a male predominance in a ratio of 3:1. The left upper and right middle lobes are most commonly involved. The lower lobes are rarely affected. The involved lobe is greatly overexpanded and usually contains air, rendering it radiolucent. Occasionally, the involved lobe is opaque, presumably caused by intrapulmonary fluid accumulation distal to the bronchial obstruction. The fluid usually drains spontaneously, leaving the overexpanded lobe radiolucent.[12]

The roentgen findings consist of marked radiolucency in the region of the involved lobe. The volume is markedly increased resulting in depression of the hemidiaphragm on the side of involvement and displacement of the mediastinum away from it. There may be compression atelectasis of the remaining lobe or lobes. Vascular markings in the affected lobe are widely separated and small, adding to the radiolucency produced by the air trapping. Respiratory distress in affected infants often occurs during the first few days of life, and the diagnosis is usually not difficult to determine. In some instances, emergency surgery is necessary to remove the overexpanded lobe. In others, symptoms may be mild, and surgery is not required.

PULMONARY ISOMERISM

Pulmonary isomerism is an anomaly in which both lungs are similar in that both may have either two lobes or three lobes. Sometimes the anomalies are described as bilateral pulmonary right- or left-sidedness. In most instances there are associated splenic and congenital cardiac anomalies. In patients with bilateral three-lobed lungs, there may be associated congenital heart disease and abnormal visceral situs associated with asplenia, Ivemark's syndrome. In males, three-lobed lungs may also be associated with anisosplenia (large spleen and multiple accessory spleens) and congenital heart disease. Bilateral two-lobed lungs are associated with polysplenia, congenital heart disease, and abnormal visceral situs. In females, there may be anisosplenia and congenital heart disease sometimes associated with abnormal visceral situs in conjunction with bilateral, two-lobed lungs.

Corrected transposition, ventricular septal defects, common atrium, anomalous pulmonary venous connections, and bilateral superior venae cavae are the cardiovascular anomalies associated with asplenia, with pulmonary stenosis or atresia being a usual part of the cardiac abnormality. Polysplenia is often associated with azygos or hemiazygos continuation of the inferior vena cava, septal defects, anomalous pulmonary connections, and bilateral superior vena cava.[27]

APICAL HERNIATION OF THE LUNG

Herniation of the lung into the soft tissues of the neck is more frequent on the right than on the left. It is a rare anomaly probably representing a congenital defect in the costovertebral fascia which permits the upward extension of pulmonary tissue. Unless the mass increases or becomes incarcerated, no treatment is necessary, but surgical repair can be done if there are complications.[42]

REFERENCES AND SELECTED READINGS

1. ABLOW RC, GREENSPAN RH, GLUCK L: The advantages of direct magnification technic in the newborn chest. Radiology 92: 745, 1969
2. BENFIELD JR, BONNEY H, CRUMMY AB et al: Azygograms and pulmonary arteriograms in bronchogenic carcinoma. Arch Surg 99: 406, 1969
3. BERMAN EJ: Extralobar (diaphragmatic) sequestration of the lung. Arch Surg 76: 724, 1958
4. BOYDEN EA: A synthesis of the prevailing pattern of the

bronchopulmonary segments in the light of their variations. Dis Chest 15: 657, 1949

5. BOYDEN EA: The distribution of bronchi in gross anomalies of the right upper lobe, particularly lobes subdivided by the azygos vein and those containing pre-eparterial bronchi. Radiology 58: 797, 1952

6. BROWN WH: Episternal bones. Radiology 75: 116, 1960

7. CAFFEY J: Pediatric X-Ray Diagnosis, 6th ed. Chicago, Year Book Medical, 1972

8. CARTER RW, VAUGHN HM: Congenital pulmonary lymphangiectasis. Am J Roentgenol 86: 576, 1961

9. CIMMINO CV: The anterior mediastinal line on chest roentgenograms. Radiology 82: 459, 1964

10. CRUMMY AB, WEGNER GP, FLAHERTY TT et al: Azygos venography, an aid in the evaluation of esophageal carcinoma. Ann Thorac Surg 6: 522, 1968

11. DAVIS LA: The vertical fissure line. Am J Roentgenol 84: 451, 1960

12. FAGAN CJ, SWISCHUK LE: The opaque lung in lobar emphysema. Am J Roentgenol 114: 300, 1972

13. FELSON B: Chest Roentgenology. Philadelphia, WB Saunders, 1973

14. FELSON B, FELSON H: Localization of intrathoracic lesions by means of the posteroanterior roentgenogram. Radiology 55: 363, 1950

15. FENNESSY JJ: Bronchial brushing in the diagnosis of peripheral lung lesions. Am J Roentgenol 98: 474, 1966

16. FENNESSY JJ, LU CT, VARIAKOJIS D et al: Transcatheter biopsy in the diagnosis of diseases of the respiratory tract. Radiology 110: 555, 1973

17. FERGUSON CF, NEUHAUSER EBD: Congenital absence of the lung and other anomalies of the tracheobronchial tree. Am J Roentgenol 52: 459, 1944

18. FRASER RG, PARE JAP: Diagnosis of the Diseases of the Chest, Vols 1–4. Philadelphia, WB Saunders, 1978

19. GROSSMAN H, WINCHESTER PH, AULD PA: Simultaneous frontal and lateral chest roentgenograms on low birth weight infants. Am J Roentgenol 108: 550, 1970

20. HARLE TS, HEVEZI JM, ROGERS LF: Xerotomography of the tracheobronchial tree. Am J Roentgenol 124: 353, 1975

21. HEITZMAN ER: The Lung Radiologic-Pathologic Correlations. St. Louis, CV Mosby, 1973

22. HUNTER TB, KUHNS LR, ROLOFF MA et al: Tracheobronchiomegaly in an 18-month-old child. Am J Roentgenol 123: 687, 1975

23. JACKSON CL, HUBER JF: Correlated applied anatomy of the bronchial tree and lungs with a system of nomenclature. Dis Chest 9: 319, 1943

24. JACKSON FI: The air-gap technique and an improvement by anteroposterior positioning for chest roentgenography. Am J Roentgenol 92: 688, 1964

25. JOST RG, SAGEL SS, STANLEY RJ et al: Computed tomography of the thorax. Radiology 126: 125, 1978

26. KRAUSE GR, LUBERT M: Anatomy of the bronchopulmonary segments: clinical applications. Radiology 56: 333, 1951

27. LANDING BH, LAWRENCE T-WK, PAYNE VC JR et al: Bronchial anatomy and syndromes with abnormal visceral situs, abnormal spleen and congenital heart disease. Am J Cardiol 28: 456, 1971

28. LARSEN LL, IBACH HF: Complete congenital fissure of the sternum. Am J Roentgenol 87: 1062, 1962

29. MADEWELL JE, STOCKER JT, KORSOWER JM: Cystic adenomatoid malformation of the lung: morphologic analysis. Am J Roentgenol 124: 436, 1975

30. MEDLAR EM: Variations in interlobar fissures. Am J Roentgenol 57: 723, 1947

31. MICHELSON E, SALIK JO: The vascular pattern of the lung as seen on routine and tomographic studies. Radiology 73: 511, 1959

32. MOLNAR W, PRIOR JA: Anesthesia for bronchography utilizing intermittent positive pressure breathing apparatus. Am J Roentgenol 87: 836, 1962

33. NELSON WW, CHRISTOFORIDIS A, PRATT PC: Barium sulfate and bismuth subcarbonate suspensions as bronchographic contrast media. Radiology 72: 829, 1959

34. PARKER GW, STURTEVANT HN, REED JE et al: Segmental localization of pulmonary disease. Am J Roentgenol 83: 217, 1960

35. PEARCE JG, PATT NL: Fatal pulmonary hemorrhage after percutaneous aspiration lung biopsy. Am Rev Resp Dis 110: 346, 1974

36. REICHERT JR, WINKLER SS: Spontaneous hemorrhage into an extralobar bronchopulmonary sequestration. Radiology 110: 359, 1974

37. SARGENT EN, TURNER AF: Percutaneous transcricothyroid membrane selective bronchography. Am J Roentgenol 104: 792, 1968

38. SCHEFF S, LAFORET EG: The internal thoracic muscle and the lateral chest roentgenogram. Radiology 86: 27, 1966

39. SINGLETON EB, DUTTON RV, WAGNER ML: Radiographic evaluation of lung abnormalities. Radiol Clin North Am 10: 333, 1972

40. STAUFFER HM, LA BREE J, ADAMS FH: The normally situated arch of the azygos vein. Am J Roentgenol 66: 353, 1951

41. STEVENS GM, WEIGEN JF, LILLINGTON GA: Needle aspiration biopsy of localized pulmonary lesions with amplified fluoroscopic guidance. Am J Roentgenol 103: 561, 1968

42. THOMPSON JS: Cervical herniation of the lung: report of a case and review of the literature. Pediatr Radiol 4: 190, 1976

43. WEINSTEIN AS, MUELLER CF: Intrathoracic rib. Am J Roentgenol 94: 587, 1965

44. WYMAN SM, EYLER WR: Anomalous pulmonary artery from the aorta associated with intrapulmonary cysts (intralobar sequestration of lung). Radiology 59: 658, 1952

23

ACUTE PULMONARY INFECTIONS

Acute pulmonary infection may be caused by a variety of organisms. In some instances they produce a reasonably characteristic, gross pathologic pattern and, therefore, a recognizable roentgen pattern. The findings can be classified as follows:

1. Alveolar (lobar) pneumonia: This is exemplified by pneumococcal pneumonia. Alveolar exudation, which produces peripheral homogenous consolidation, spreads toward the hilum and tends to cross segmental lines. Alveolar (airspace) pneumonia is not necessarily confined to a lobe, nor does it involve an entire lobe in many instances. Therefore, the term "lobar" is a misnomer in most cases and air-space or alveolar pneumonia are preferred terms.

2. Bronchopneumonia (lobular pneumonia): This is often observed in staphylococcal infection of the lung. The disease originates in the airways and spreads to peribronchial alveoli. A variety of roentgen patterns may result, including a confluent consolidation resembling alveolar pneumonia.

3. Interstitial pneumonia: This is observed in viral and mycoplasmal infections. Often the interstitial involvement is masked by alveolar exudate. A variety of roentgen patterns are observed, but alveolar consolidation, if present, is not usually as confluent or dense as in alveolar or lobular pneumonia.

4. Mixed: A combination of alveolar, bronchopneumonia and interstitial pneumonia.

In the subsequent discussions the most common gross anatomic findings in the pneumonias of various causes as reflected in chest roentgenograms will be pointed out. However, in each instance it should be remembered that roentgen findings must be correlated with clinical and laboratory data to ascertain the correct etiologic diagnosis upon which treatment is based.

THE BACTERIAL PNEUMONIAS

Pneumococcal Pneumonia

The acute pulmonary infection caused by *Streptococcus* (formerly *Diplococcus*) *pneumoniae* is commonly termed "lobar pneumonia." However the infection does not usually involve an entire lobe and is better termed "alveolar pneumonia." There are over 82 serotypes of S. *pneumoniae*, but most of the pneumonias are caused by type 1, 3, 4, 5, 7, 8, 9, or 12. Type 8 is the most common. Type 14 causes pneumonia in children, but rarely in adults.

The organisms causing pneumococcal pneumonia are aspirated in droplets of saliva or mucus, so the lower lobe and right middle lobe are most commonly involved. The infection occurs in individuals who are otherwise healthy and frequently appears in children and adult males. The onset is sudden and the gross pathologic changes are evident early in the course of the disease, so that roentgen findings can be observed within 6 to 12 hours following the onset. Involvement begins peripherally and spreads centripetally with homogenous involvement that may cross segmental boundaries. The consolidation produced by the disease is manifested on the roentgenogram by homogeneous density. An entire lobe may be affected; more commonly only one or more segments are involved. The density usually extends to the pleural surface. A peripheral, nonsegmental, sublobar consolidation is seen when peripheral spread across segmental boundaries occurs. This tends to separate the acute pneumococcal pneumonia from the pneumonias of segmental distribution, such as those caused by bronchial obstruction by tumor. The latter disease does not ordinarily cross the barrier formed by interlobar fissures and is, therefore, clearly defined by the fissure on either the frontal or lateral projection, depending upon the lobe or segment infected (Fig. 23-1). In pneumococcal pneumonia, all of the elements in the diseased lobe except the larger bronchi are affected, resulting in complete airlessness. The larger bronchi can often be visualized as air-containing, radiolucent tubes within the otherwise homogeneous density. There is often enough pleural infection to result in elevation of the diaphragm on the affected side because of splinting, and a small amount of pleural fluid sufficient to obscure the depth of the costophrenic sulcus is not uncommon. The volume of the lobe or segment is not decreased significantly, so that the density caused by this disease can be differentiated from that produced by atelectasis, which causes considerable decrease in volume, manifested by shift of mediastinal structures to the involved side and elevation of the hemidiaphragm (Fig. 23-2). Variations in the distribution of pulmonary consolidation may occur. The spherical pattern reported in children is a rare form in which the well-circumscribed spherical consolidation may simulate a pulmonary or mediastinal mass.[19] Symptoms of an acute febrile illness preceded by a few days of mild respiratory symptoms and a rapid response to antibiotic therapy allow differentiation from other conditions such as tumor. In patients with emphysema, radiolucent blebs surrounded by consolidation may simulate cavities and, in some of these patients, the distribution of the disease is somewhat patchy or lobular simulating the distribution in bronchopneumonia. Resolution is usually fairly rapid, if there are no complications, and tends to start at the hilum and progress toward the periphery of the lobe or segment. The density becomes more irregular and patchy during resolution, in contrast to its homogeneous character earlier in the disease. Focal atelectasis often develops.

Complications are few since the disease responds well to antibiotics which are usually given at the first sign of respiratory infection. They include delayed resolution or nonresolution, empyema, and lung abscess. The roentgen findings in delayed resolution are those of persistence of density in the area, which becomes rather irregular and patchy but eventually clears. Very rarely the process clears incompletely, leaving some irregular fibrosis manifested by irregular strands of density in the segment or lobe with decrease in volume of the affected lung. The findings in empyema and lung abscess are discussed in other sections of this book.

Bronchopneumonia

Brochopneumonia (lobular pneumonia) is an acute pulmonary infection, bacterial in origin, that usually occurs as a complication of various debilitating diseases, often at the extremes of life. Therefore, it is most commonly found in the very young or very old who are afflicted with another disease. The infection is often mixed so that several pathogenic bacteria can be isolated from the sputum. The disease originates in numerous adjacent areas of the lung, resulting in scattered foci of inflammation that vary in size and shape but produce enough density to be visible on the film. The roentgen findings in bronchopneumonia are varied, since this disease may be quite localized to a single lobe or segment or may be widespread and involve all lobes. The pneumonic

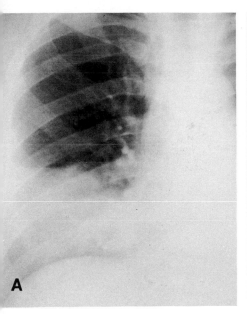
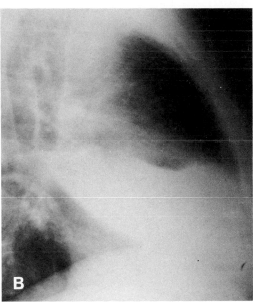

Fig. 23-1. Lobar pneumonia in the right middle lobe. Note the homogeneous density clearly defined by the secondary fissure in the frontal projection **(A)** and by the major fissure as well as the secondary fissure in the lateral view **(B).**

consolidation causes densities of varying sizes that are usually rather small, poorly defined, and are best described as "mottled." The disease may progress so that these small areas may coalesce to form large, irregular patches of density. The location is usually basal but the disease may occur anywhere in the lung fields (Fig. 23-3). It often occurs as a complication of other pulmonary disease, which may obscure the pneumonia or vice versa. It is particularly difficult to define and diagnose when it occurs as a complication

in cardiac failure with pulmonary congestion and edema, which also cause basal density. Occasionally the process may be extremely widespread and simulate miliary pulmonary disease, with small, poorly defined nodules scattered uniformly throughout both lung fields. Since bronchopneumonia produces a variety of roentgen patterns and is caused by a number of organisms, its designation is now used as a descriptive term rather than a definitive one as far as etiology is concerned. In contrast to lobar pneumonia

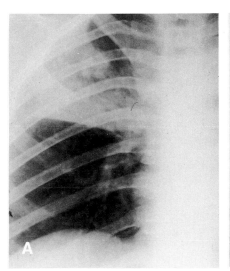
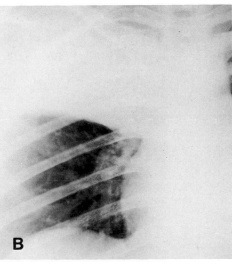

Fig. 23-2. Right upper-lobe pneumococcal pneumonia. **A.** Roentgenogram obtained the day after onset of symptoms shows the disease clearly defined by the minor fissure. Consolidation is not complete. **B.** Three days later there is complete consolidation of the right upper lobe. The upper-lobe volume is slightly reduced.

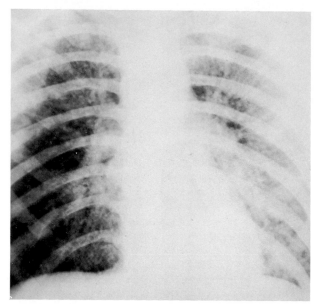

Fig. 23-3. Bronchopneumonia. Note the widespread, mottled density more severe on the left than on the right. The disease is very extensive.

it originates in bronchial airways and involves the surrounding parenchyma. As indicated, it may become confluent and then resemble alveolar pneumonia. It should be remembered that neoplasms can be masked by patchy focal pneumonia and if clinical symptoms persist unduly, progress roentgenograms as well as cytologic studies should be carried out.

Aspiration Pneumonia

Aspiration pneumonia is usually a mixed bacterial infection caused by aspiration of foreign material into the bronchial tree. The causes are numerous and range from aspiration of vomitus by a postsurgical or semicomatose patient to aspiration as a result of paresis or paralysis of the pharyngeal muscles. Tracheoesophageal fistula and various other esophageal lesions may also cause aspiration pneumonitis.

The radiographic findings vary with the extent of the disease and with its location. The right lower and middle lobes are the most frequently affected, but left lower-lobe involvement is not unusual. Irregular, poorly defined areas of increased density are visualized and may be extensive (Fig. 23-4). Early in the disease these infiltrates are focal but later they may become conglomerate. In some instances the disease is acute and clears rapidly as the patient recovers from the condition that produced the aspiration. In other instances the pneumonia results from a chronic disease and repeated aspiration leads to chronic basal pneumonitis, which causes patchy or linear basal density (Fig. 23-5). The roentgen findings are, therefore, varied and it may not be possible to differentiate this basal inflammatory disease from other nonspecific basal pneumonia and from the chronic pneumonitis associated with bronchiectasis.

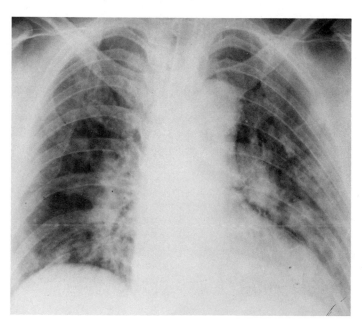

Fig. 23-4. Aspiration pneumonia. Note the scattered patchy density in the lower half of the left lung and a similar but less extensive change at the right base. This was an acute process which cleared quickly on treatment.

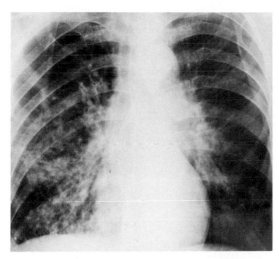

Fig. 23-5. Chronic aspiration pneumonia. The pneumonia in the parahilar areas and at the right base is somewhat more clearly defined and stringy than the acute process noted in Fig. 23-4. This patient had partial esophageal obstruction and aspirated intermittently.

However, correlation of the history with clinical and roentgen findings usually leads to the proper diagnosis.

Friedländer's (Klebsiella) Pneumonia

Friedländer's pneumonia is a confluent alveolar type of pneumonia caused by *Klebsiella pneumoniae*. The disease occurs most frequently in elderly and debilitated patients. The onset is usually sudden and the illness is often fatal within a few days. It may begin as bronchopneumonia manifested by patchy areas of increased density, usually in one or both upper lobes, but spreads rapidly to become confluent. It may involve an entire lobe. The lung tends to increase in volume, resulting in convexity of the adjacent interlobar fissure. Extensive destruction of tissues leads to abscess formation in most of these patients and the abscess cavities are typically thin-walled, if a wall can be demonstrated (Fig. 23-6). Often the confluent pneumonia surrounding the cavity obscures its actual wall. At times the necrosis is very extensive and extremely large cavitation results when the necrotic material sloughs out. Pleural effusion is common and empyema often follows the effusion. In the more

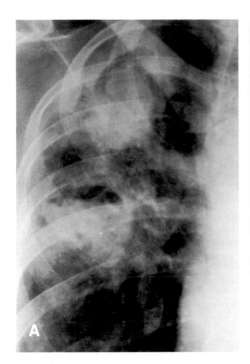

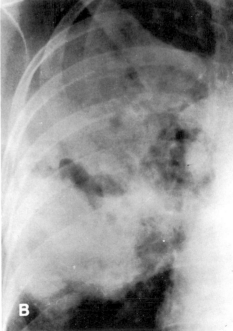

Fig. 23-6. *Klebsiella* pneumonia. **A.** The disease is extensive with evidence of cavitation in which there are masses of dense necrotic material. **B.** Ten days later, considerable advance of the disease is evident.

chronic form, the disease tends to be more patchy, the cavitation is smaller, and the lesions may closely simulate those of tuberculosis.

The diagnosis should be suspected when a rapidly progressing confluent pneumonia is observed in one or both upper lobes in which cavitation forms quickly. When the disease progresses more slowly, it is often less confluent and its distribution in one or both upper lobes plus the presence of cavities often leads to a mistaken diagnosis of tuberculosis. Bacteriologic studies are then needed for differentiation. In patients who survive, a considerable amount of fibrosis may result, leading to contraction of the lobe with secondary changes in the thorax resulting from the loss of lung volume. In this respect, the disease may resemble chronic tuberculosis.

Staphylococcal Pneumonia

Staphylococcal pneumonia may be primary in the lungs or secondary in the lungs with a primary staphylococcal infection elsewhere in the body. In the latter instance there is hematogenous spread of the organism while in the primary type the pulmonary spread is usually bronchogenic. The disease usually occurs in debilitated adults and in infants during the first year of life. The onset of the illness is usually abrupt, with severe prostration. Death may occur within 24 to 48 hours. Because some of the many areas of involvement occur adjacent to the pleura, it is not uncommon to have pleural infection with empyema and bronchopleural fistula.

In children the roentgen findings are rather characteristic and consist of dense areas of pulmonary involvement that may be segmental and local or diffuse. Consolidation rapidly spreads to involve a whole lobe (confluent bronchopneumonia); bronchi are usually obscured by exudate, so air bronchogram is not ordinarily seen in this disease. Pleural effusion, empyema, and pneumothorax are common, and pneumatoceles are often noted. Abscess formation may also occur; coalescence of small abscesses is frequent. The pneumatocele is distinguished from the abscess by its thin wall and rapid change in size. It is caused by a check-valve obstruction between the lumen of a small bronchus and adjacent interstitium and possibly a check-valve obstruction of a small bronchus in some instances. Multiple pneumatoceles may develop, usually in the first week of the disease.) They may become very large. Accumulation of fluid with air–fluid levels is common during the active phase of pneumonia. It may persist for months, but usually disappears completely (Fig. 23-7). Pleural effusion or empyema is also common in children. In adults the findings are not as characteristic. Pneumothorax and pneumatocele are rare; pleural effusion and empyema are not as common as in children. Abscesses are slightly more frequent than in children and tend to coalesce (Fig. 23-8). The disease is usually bilateral and may be diffuse and somewhat nodular, but is seldom lobar in distribution. Rapid change and lack of correlation between severity of clinical symptoms and roentgen findings is often observed. Resolution is usually slow in both children and adults. When the disease is hematogenous, septic emboli may cause multiple small abscesses and widespread, small foci of pneumonia.

Streptococcal Pneumonia

Streptococcal pneumonia, caused by Streptococcus *pyogenes* (Lancefield group A, β- hemolytic streptococcus), usually occurs following such acute infectious diseases as measles and influenza. This disease is now rare and is roentgenographically similar to staphylococcal pneumonia in the frequency of pleural involvement, including empyema if antibiotic therapy is not initiated promptly. The pulmonary involvement has a tendency to be more diffuse and interstitial in type, in comparison with staphylococcal pneumonia, with fine densities radiating outward to the periphery from the hila. The combination of rapidly developing, hazy, nodular infiltration in an acutely ill patient and subsequent cavitation in many of the areas is highly characteristic of either staphylococcal or streptococcal pneumonia, with the former more likely. However, pneumatoceles are not usually caused by streptococcal infections.

Tularemic Pneumonia

Tularemia is an infectious disease caused by *Francisella tularensis*. It is a disease of small animals and may spread to man directly from the animals. The most common mode of infection of this type is through the skin of hunters who dress small game animals. It may also be transmitted by means of tick bites and the bites of horse and deer flies. Pulmonary involvement in the form of pneumonia resulting from this organism is present in approximately 50% of humans affected. The roentgen findings are not characteristic, but some authors have reported a high incidence of oval lesions resembling an abscess without cavitation. However, others have indicated a great variability in pulmonary findings.[16] The infection

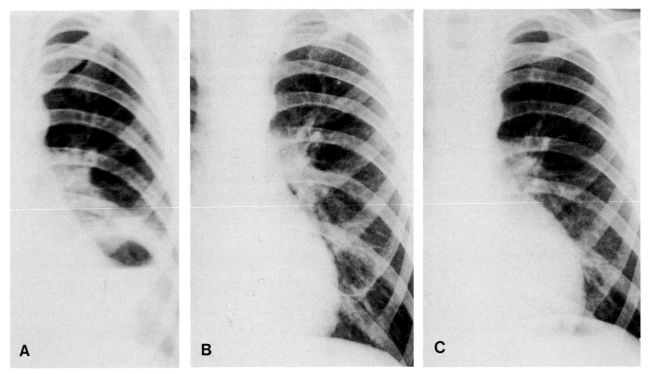

Fig. 23-7. Staphylococcal pneumonia in the left lower lobe resulting in the formation of a pneumatocele. **A.** Note the homogeneous density at the left base indicating rather extensive pneumonia. There is a radiolucent area surmounting a fluid level. The pulmonary alveolar disease surrounding the pneumatocele makes it impossible to determine the thickness of the wall. **B.** Note that the inflammatory disease has cleared nearly completely, leaving the thin-walled, cystlike pneumatocele. This film was obtained 1 month after that shown in **A. C.** The pneumatocele is no longer visible on this film obtained 3 months after the initial examination.

may produce unilateral or bilateral pulmonary inflammatory disease, which is usually poorly circumscribed. Occasionally the distribution is lobar, resulting in consolidation of an entire lobe. The infection is commonly a basal one and there is usually more disease on one side than the other so that it is asymmetric when bilateral. A small amount of pleural effusion is not uncommon and hilar lymph-node enlargement is also present in many instances. The time required for resolution varies widely. In some instances complete clearing may occur within a week or 10 days while in others the infiltrate may persist for 6 weeks. Since the roentgen picture is not characteristic, the diagnosis must be confirmed by laboratory methods. Organisms are difficult to isolate from the sputum but if the disease is suspected its presence can be proved by means of agglutination tests.

Pulmonary Brucellosis

Pulmonary involvement is uncommon in brucellosis and symptoms are usually mild. The roentgen findings are varied. Strands of density radiating outward from the hila often associated with hilar adenopathy are noted. The parenchymal infiltrates and the adenopathy may be bilateral. Pleural involvement with effusion is occasionally encountered. In other instances, widespread miliary disease is found that resembles miliary bronchopneumonia. Solitary, circumscribed, pulmonary nodules have also been described. The pulmonary roentgen changes appear quickly but tend to persist for long periods of time with very slow resolution. The diagnosis cannot be made on roentgen examination, but must depend on the results of bacteriologic studies, agglutination, and skin tests.

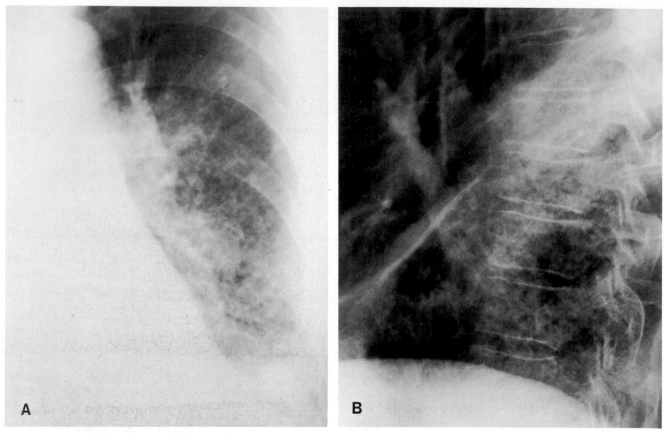

Fig. 23-8. Staphylococcal pneumonia. **A.** There is extensive disease in the left lower lobe in which there are numerous small, rounded, lucent areas representing small pneumatoceles or cavities. **B.** The lateral view shows the extensive disease in which there are a number of small, rounded, radiolucent areas.

Pertussis Pneumonia

In pertussis pneumonia, Barnhard and Kniker[1] have described central densities radiating into the pulmonary parenchyma from the hilar and low central pulmonary areas, resulting in blurring of the cardiac margins and producing an irregular appearance termed the "shaggy heart" pattern. This begins in the paroxysmal stage of the disease and extends into the resolution phase. They found the sign in 13 of a group of 32 patients who were either under 1 year of age or had serious respiratory difficulty or encephalopathy. The cause is uncertain; it may indicate a complicating bronchopneumonia. Atelectasis has also been described in older children, presumably caused by thick mucous plugs.

Pseudomonas Pneumonia

There is an increasing incidence of pneumonia caused by *Pseudomonas aeruginosa* related to increasing use of immunosuppressive drugs, antibiotics, steroids, and cytotoxic drugs. Hospitalized patients are usually involved, and there is evidence that the widespread use of positive pressure breathing apparatus is a major factor. The causative organism is extremely difficult to eradicate, once pulmonary disease is established.

Several roentgen patterns of pulmonary involvement have been described by Joffe:[12] (*1*) bilateral pneumonic consolidation, with early patchy, scattered disease progressing and coalescing to involvement of the major portions of both lungs; (*2*) extensive bilateral pneumonic consolidation with abscess formation; abscesses may be multiple and small or few and large; (3) diffuse nodular or patchy densities with or without abscess formation; and (4) unilateral pneumonia—similar to the coalescent bilateral pneumonia. Pleural effusion may occur, but is not a prominent feature of the disease.

Anaerobic Bacterial Pneumonias

A number of anaerobic organisms may cause pulmonary infection. They include, among others, *Bacteroides fragilis, Bacteroides melaninogenicus,* and *Bacteroides oralis;* members of the genera *Fusobacterium, Clostridium,* and *Eubacterium;* and the gram-positive cocci of the genera *Peptostreptococcus* and *Peptococcus.* Most of the infections are caused by a number of organisms; many are caused by aspiration of oral secretions. An alveolar type of pneumonia is usually produced which may be extensive. Abscess formation or necrotizing pneumonia are common complications. Pleural involvement with empyema is often associated with parenchymal disease. Bronchopleural fistula may complicate the disease. Anaerobic bacteria then are a prominent cause of aspiration pneumonia, lung abscess, necrotizing pneumonia, and empyema. The mortality is high in these patients; in many the natural immune responses have been suppressed, many others have leukopenia.[2]

Meleoidosis, which is due to infection with *Pseudomonas pseudomallei,* is endemic in the tropics, chiefly in India, Burma, and Ceylon. Since the Viet Nam war, sporadic cases have been reported in the United States, chiefly in Viet Nam veterans.[7] The infection may be acute or chronic. The acute form is commoner than the chronic; it is characterized by indistinct nodular disease that is often widely scattered but tends to involve the upper lobes. The nodules coalesce and cavitate in a high percentage of cases. The chronic form simulates pulmonary tuberculosis since the nodules often involve the upper lobes and cavitate in a high percentage of patients. Hilar adenopathy is uncommon and pleural effusion is rare.

Other Bacterial Pneumonias

Pneumonia due to infection with *Proteus vulgaris* is largely basal, may be alveolar or lobular in distribution, and it tends to produce cavitation. It may cause a decrease in volume of the involved lung. Pneumonia due to *Enterobacter* is multilobular, involves the lower lobes, and tends to be a mixed alveolar intersti-

tial process with lobular distribution. Rarely, *Escherichia coli* may cause pneumonia, which is usually multilobar. The alveolar pneumonia caused by this organism may result in massive cavitation occasionally. Pleural effusion is common. Pneumonic involvement may occur in *typhoid fever,* usually as a bronchopneumonia with cavitation and empyema. *Salmonella* organisms other than *S. typhosa* may produce a smilar pattern in the lung. An acute miliary pattern has also been described in salmonella bacteremia.[9] *Hemophilus influenzae* is also a rare cause of pneumonia. Roentgenographically this infection appears as an acute lower-lobe lobular pneumonia but may also appear as a more confluent lobar alveolar process. In infants, pleural effusion and empyema are common in addition to extensive alveolar disease.[27] Pulmonary involvement also occurs in patients with anthrax and bubonic plague. In anthrax pneumonia, there is often significant mediastinal lymph-node enlargement, pleural effusion, and sometimes intrapulmonary hemorrhage in addition to extensive pulmonary disease. Plague may cause a similar process. Both anthrax and plague are very rare in the United States.

Legionnaires' Disease

Legionnaires' disease, which affected nearly 200 persons at the Legionnaires' Convention in Philadelphia in July, 1976, is caused by the gram-negative bacillus *Legionella pneumophila.*[5] Clinically the acute disease is characterized by high fever, chills, and a nonproductive cough, often associated with chest pain, malaise, muscle and abdominal pain, headaches, and gastrointestinal symptoms. Since the outbreak in Philadelphia, a number of sporadic cases have been reported as well as local outbreaks of the disease in a number of areas throughout the United States. Roentgen findings are largely those of an alveolar pneumonic process which is bilateral in about one-half of the reported cases. The alveolar disease may have a lobar or lobular distribution. At times, the alveolar process appears as large, very poorly marginated, generally round or oval densities. Some of these are central and some peripheral; they may be unilateral or bilateral. The rounded lesions appear to be somewhat more common than any other roentgen manifestation. One patient has been reported in whom there was virtually universal involvement of both lungs by an alveolar process in which air bronchogram was very prominent. Cavitation, presumably a result of necrotizing pneumonia, has been reported in several patients. One patient has been reported in whom pneumatocele and spontaneous pneumothorax were manifest. Pleural effusion may occur, but its incidence is difficult to evaluate since many of the patients had complicating renal or cardiovascular disease. Most of the reported cases have been in smokers or in immunocompromised patients.

It is evident that there is a wide variety of roentgen patterns in this disease so that the diagnosis cannot be made on the basis of chest roentgenograms. However, the disease should be suspected in a patient with atypical pneumonia in whom roentgenograms show unilateral or bilateral large, poorly marginated, rounded aveolar densities which may be central or peripheral.

Pulmonary Infection in the Compromised Host

Most cases of hospital-acquired (nosocomial) pneumonia occur in patients with serious underlying disease or other predisposing factors that make them a compromised host. There are a number of organisms that are found principally in these patients who are immunosuppressed or have disease which has produced neutropenia. Diseases and organisms often associated with them include: (*1*) Acute leukemia and leukopenia—*Pseudomonas, Staphylococcus, Aspergillus,* and *Pneumocystis.* (2) Chronic lymphatic leukemia and lymphosarcoma *Pneumococcus, Staphylococcus, Cryptococcus,* and herpes viruses. (3) Hodgkin's disease—*Cryptococcus, Listeria, Pneumocystis,* and organisms causing tuberculosis and toxoplasmosis. (*4*) Myeloma and chronic myelogenous leukemia—*Pneumococcus,* gram-negative bacilli, and tubercle bacillus. (5) Renal transplants—many bacteria, *Cryptococcus, Pneumocystis,* and organisms causing toxoplasmosis, nocardiosis, and histoplasmosis. (6) Cystic fibrosis—*Staphylococcus* and *Pseudomonas.* (7) Sickle cell disease—*Pneumococcus* and *Salmonella.* (8) Drug addiction—*Staphylococcus,* mixed anaerobes, *Pseudomonas,* and *Candida.* (*9*) Hypogammaglobulinemia—gram-positive bacteria, *Pneumocystis,* and viruses. (*10*) Chronic granulomatous disease—*Serratia, Salmonella,* and staphylococci.

The organism listed first tends to be most frequent in the disease mentioned. The pulmonary findings in most of the diseases mentioned are described elsewhere. Chest roentgenology is more useful in identifying the pneumonic process and following its course than it is in suggesting the organism responsible in many of these patients.

THE VIRAL, MYCOPLASMAL, AND RICKETTSIAL PNEUMONIAS

Primary Atypical Pneumonia

The primary atypical pneumonias are caused by various strains of virus including type IV adenovirus, influenza virus, parainfluenza, and respiratory syncytial viruses. *Mycoplasma pneumoniae* (the Eaton agent) is also responsible for a significant percentage of cases. The atypical pneumonias tend to occur in epidemics, as well as sporadically, so it is difficult to obtain meaningful figures as to relative frequency of the various etiologic agents. *M. pneumoniae* and type IV adenovirus are probably the most common, however. The disease usually occurs in young adults who are in good health. It is mild and self-limited in most instances, but may be severe with widespread pulmonary lesions. Occasional fatalities have been reported. The inflammatory exudate is more interstitial than bacterial pneumonias, but alveolar exudate, which contains less cells and more fluid than in the bacterial type, may be present. The onset of symptoms is gradual and there is often a delay in appearance of visible pulmonary density on roentgen examination for 2 or 3 days.

Roentgen findings reflect the anatomic changes and are varied. Recognizable anatomic forms can be divided into several types:

1. Peribronchial type. The findings in the peribronchial type consist of streaky densities extending outward from the hilum following the pattern of the vascular markings limited to a single segment or affecting one or several lobes. Alveolar exudate may produce scattered patchy density as well as the linear shadows. This is the interstitial viral pneumonia which may also produce a widespread reticular pattern (Fig. 23-9).

2. Bronchopneumonic type. The roentgen findings are similar to those described for bronchopneumonia and may be just as widespread. Densities that are usually poorly defined and scattered may be noted in any lobe or segment and may be bilateral.

3. Segmental and lobar types. The findings are those of homogeneous density representing consolidation in a segment, several segments, or a lobe. The appearance of the consolidation is similar to that found in pneumococcal lobar pneumonia. This probably represents the pathologic process of localized hemorrhagic pulmonary edema, which may involve a segment or lobe (Fig. 23-10).

4. Extensive, severe viral pneumonia may occur in a perihilar distribution, resembling pulmonary

edema. It is often associated with pleural effusion and often is bilateral.

5. Miliary type. Widespread, small, poorly defined nodules are scattered throughout both lung fields. These patients are acutely ill and occasionally succumb to the disease. Conglomeration of the miliary infiltrates may occur to form larger densities.

6. Pleural exudation may be the predominant feature of the disease. There may also be pericardial involvement with effusion.

One or more of these gross anatomic types of the disease may be present in a patient. There is a tendency for the disease to clear in one area and spread in another, often in the opposite lung. Atelectasis is often produced by bronchial obstruction and is often lobular and focal in type. Occasionally a pneumatocele may result from check-valve obstruction and must be differentiated from lung abscess (see Fig. 23-7). Resolution is usually slow and it is common to see persistent roentgen lesions for a week or more after the clinical findings have disappeared. Occasionally the delay is considerably greater. Scattered atelectasis that is a result of obstruction by the interstitial infiltrate is a factor in the persistence of roentgen findings. Mycoplasmal pneumonia cannot be differentiated from the viral type (Fig. 23-11).

Differential Diagnosis. There are findings that help to differentiate this disease from bacterial pneumonia. They consist of the lack of pleural involvement manifested by absence of elevation of the diaphragm and absence of pleural fluid in most cases. The delay in appearance after clinical onset is also helpful. The tendency to clear in one area and spread in another is more common in this disease than in bacterial pneumonia. Bilateral involvement is more common than in bacterial pneumonias, with disease often in one lower lobe and the opposite upper or middle lobe. However, because the roentgen pattern may vary widely the diagnosis must be substantiated by clinical and laboratory findings (Fig. 23-12).

Psittacosis (Ornithosis)

Psittacosis, or ornithosis, is primarily a disease of birds and is transmitted to man by members of the parrot family. It is also found in other domesticated and wild birds and may be transmitted to man by them. The roentgen findings are similar to those in primary atypical pneumonia. The disease tends to be multifocal and is often bilateral with a tendency to change rather rapidly in appearance and distribution. A transparent reticular pattern has also been reported. Enlargement of hilar nodes may also be present. Pleural involvement is uncommon. The roentgen changes tend to persist for a long time (6 to 9 weeks) after the initial symptoms. The diagnosis is confirmed by serologic and bacteriologic studies but can be suspected when this type of infiltrate is seen in a patient who has had contact with birds.

Other Viral Pneumonias

Epidemic influenza, which is a virus disease, may be associated with virus infection of the pulmonary parenchyma in addition to involvement of the tracheobronchial tree. Roentgen signs are variable, with findings often bilateral and extensive. Especially in severe epidemics of the past, the pneumonia was often of the interstitial type with hazy, strandlike densities radiating outward from the hila. These result in a coarse appearance of the bronchovascular pattern and irregular hilar thickening. The diagnosis is often made from clinical findings during an epidemic. The roentgen changes are then largely confirmatory but roentgen examination is useful to observe the course of the pulmonary parenchymal disease. A complicating staphylococcal pneumonia may also occur, particularly in epidemics in which influenza may be severe. Most of the fatalities are caused by this complication.

Pneumonia associated with chickenpox is believed by some to be viral in origin and has been reported occasionally. It usually occurs in adults. Roentgen findings consist of widespread nodular densities associated with increase in parahilar markings and occasional enlargement of the hilar nodes. Densities are most marked in the parahilar areas and at the bases. Individual nodules are generally round but are poorly defined peripherally. There is often considerable change in the roentgen findings from day to day, since the infiltrates are transitory. Clearing is generally slow, however. In patients with fatal disease, pulmonary involvement may be virtually total, with little if any visible aerated lung. It is entirely possible for bacterial pneumonia to appear in patients with these various virus diseases and there is no way to differentiate the cause on roentgen study.

Measles is occasionally associated with pneumonia caused by the virus. Pneumonia caused by other organisms sometimes complicates measles, however, so roentgen differentiation may not be possible. The measles virus causes reticuloendothelial involvement resulting in hilar and mediastinal adenopathy. The virus may also involve the lung to produce an interstitial process that is manifested as a widespread re-

(*Text continues on p. 854.*)

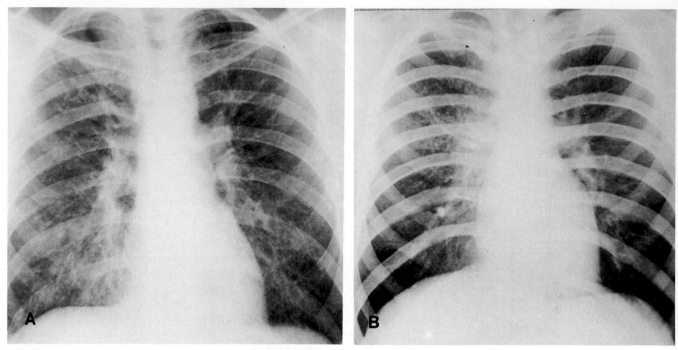

Fig. 23-9. Viral pneumonia. **A.** There is extensive interstitial disease throughout the entire right lung with similar but much less marked change on the left. **B.** There is diffuse involvement, which appears to be at least partially alveolar, confined largely to the right upper lobe in another patient.

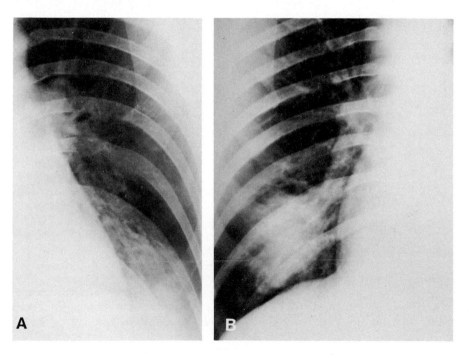

Fig. 23-10. Viral pneumonia. In these two patients, the disease is largely alveolar in type, being rather diffuse in patient shown in **A** and somewhat localized into an irregular mass-like lesion in patient shown in **B.**

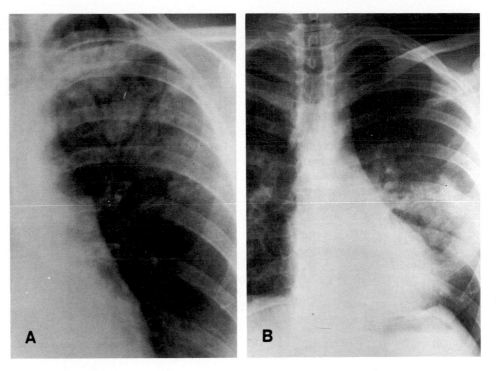

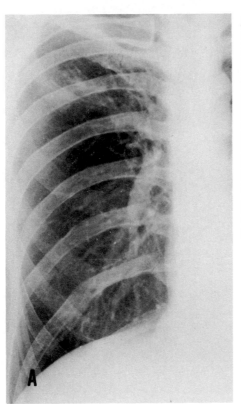

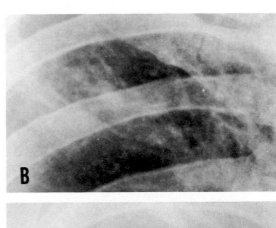

Fig. 23-11. Mycoplasmal pneumonia. **A.** The air bronchogram denotes alveolar disease, but there also appears to be some interstitial change in the upper central lung. **B.** Alveolar pneumonia is noted in the left lower lobe which is probably subsegmental.

Fig. 23-12. Viral pneumonia simulating minimal tuberculosis. **A.** Note the disease in the right subclavicular area. **B.** Close-up showing the disease in the first anterior interspace. **C.** Roentgenogram of same area shown in **B,** obtained 2 weeks later, showing complete clearing of the disease.

ticular type of reaction, with predilection for the bases. Consolidation of lung with varying degrees of atelectasis is probably a complicating bacterial pneumonia in many instances.

Pneumonic involvement may occur with a number of other viral diseases including smallpox, lymphocytic choriomeningitis, and cytoplasmic inclusion disease in infants and children. There is nothing characteristic about the roentgen appearance of the pneumonia associated with these diseases except that the pneumonia is usually bilateral and often extensive. *Cytomegalovirus* infection is the most common viral infection in immunosuppressed patients, occurring usually in patients who have had renal transplantation. *Herpes viruses* are also capable of producing pulmonary disease in compromised patients. There is nothing very characteristic in the roentgen findings although interstitial changes have been described in patients with these pneumonias; and, in patients having cytomegalovirus disease, nodules have been reported involving the outer one-third of the lungs. Lung biopsy may be necessary to establish the diagnosis.

Rickettsial Pneumonias

Q Fever. This disease is caused by a rickettsia that is an intracellular parasite considered to be intermediate between the bacteria and virus. The causative organism is *Coxiella burnetii.* The roentgen findings resemble those in pneumococcal pneumonia with a tendency to dense, homogeneous, segmental, or lobar consolidation producing a uniform roentgen density in the area of involvement. Hilar involvement and small focal lesions are uncommon. Some pleural involvement occurs in approximately one-third of these cases. This is manifested by a small amount of pleural fluid. The roentgen findings appear within 48 hours of the onset of the disease in the usual instance and resolve rather slowly so that the pulmonary consolidation persists longer than in pneumococcal pneumonia. This disease does not exhibit the migratory type of change often found in viral pneumonia. As in other pneumonias, the diagnosis depends on correlation of clinical, roentgen, and serologic findings.

Other Rickettsial Pneumonias. Pulmonary involvement has been reported occasionally in patients with other rickettsial diseases such as Rocky Mountain spotted fever and severe cases of typhus. The roentgen findings are not characteristic in these diseases, but the infiltrates are usually scattered and produce disseminated densities on the chest roentgenogram.

OTHER INFECTIONS

Lung Abscess

When an acute suppurative pulmonary infectious process breaks down to form a cavity of greater or lesser size, it is termed "lung abscess." The majority of lung abscesses are bronchogenic in origin and result from aspiration of foreign material following dental operations, surgery of the respiratory tract and elsewhere, and various conditions that produce unconsciousness. This type of abscess may also result from stasis of secretions owing to various causes and from bronchogenic carcinoma or other endobronchial tumor resulting in incomplete drainage of the bronchial tree. Anaerobic organisms are often the cause of lung abscess as indicated earlier. Hematogenous lung abscess, which is usually produced by staphylococcus and occasionally by streptococcus, has been discussed in a previous section. The abscess formation in pneumonia produced by the Friedländer bacillus has also been discussed earlier. Cavitation occurs in approximately 5% of patients with pulmonary infarction and when infected, an abscess is formed.

Because lung abscess is the result of aspiration of foreign material in many instances, it is usually found in areas in the lung that are dependent at the time of aspiration. Therefore the posterior segment of the upper lobe is the most common site, with the right side affected more than the left. The next most common sites are the superior segments of the lower lobes because these segments are dependent when the patient is in the supine position. The basal segments of the lower lobes are also commonly involved and abscess can occur in any segment of any lobe. The lesion is always peripheral in relation to the bronchopulmonary segment involved but on the frontal roentgenogram it may project in a central position. The pleura is involved adjacent to the abscess and there may be pleural effusion.

The early roentgen finding is that of consolidation producing density confined usually to one pulmonary segment. Characteristically, the lesion has a dense center with a hazy and poorly defined periphery and is often roughly spherical in shape. When bronchial communication is established, the fluid contents of the cavity are replaced, at least in part, by air and the radiolucent abscess cavity will appear within the area of disease. It is usually incompletely drained so that an air–fluid level can be outlined within it. In these cases, the fluid produces homogeneous density inferiorly when the patient is upright, which blends with the wall of the cavity. The drainage of the ab-

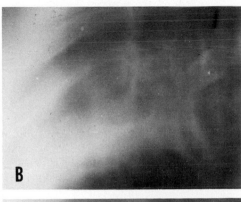
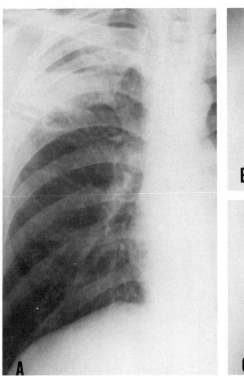
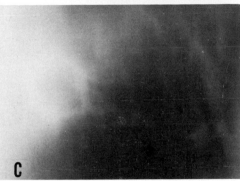
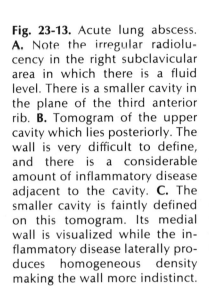

Fig. 23-13. Acute lung abscess. **A.** Note the irregular radiolucency in the right subclavicular area in which there is a fluid level. There is a smaller cavity in the plane of the third anterior rib. **B.** Tomogram of the upper cavity which lies posteriorly. The wall is very difficult to define, and there is a considerable amount of inflammatory disease adjacent to the cavity. **C.** The smaller cavity is faintly defined on this tomogram. Its medial wall is visualized while the inflammatory disease laterally produces homogeneous density making the wall more indistinct.

scess may vary so that at times it may contain more or less air. When the necrotic lung tissue has not sloughed completely, it is not uncommon to observe a crescent-shaped radiolucency due to air in the superior aspect of the partially filled cavity. In some patients, several small cavities may appear within the area and may remain as separate lesions or may coalesce to form one or more larger cavities. These may be well outlined on the routine frontal and lateral roentgenogram, but small cavities can be hidden by the surrounding pneumonic consolidation; when cavitation is suspected, tomography is indicated. It is not uncommon to see cavities on a tomogram that cannot be visualized in any other way. This examination also aids in localizing and in defining the inner and outer walls of the abscess cavity (Fig. 23-13). Tomography is also of value in differentiating lung abscess from bronchogenic carcinoma in which the central portion of the carcinoma has become necrotic and has sloughed out, leaving a central cavity. The wall of the lung abscess is usually relatively smooth on its inner aspect, whereas a carcinoma is usually irregular. In acute lung abscess the outer wall is poorly defined. As the abscess becomes more chronic the wall is thicker and its external surface more sharply marginated. Complications are much less common

now than before the use of antibacterial drugs, but empyema and spread of the infection locally or by aspiration of pus from the abscess into a more dependent portion of the lung may occur.

Differential diagnosis depends upon the stage of disease when the roentgenogram is obtained. In the early stage before excavation and communication with a bronchus has occurred, the process cannot be differentiated from that of a segmental pneumonia. However, excavation usually occurs early and the abscess cavity can then be visualized on the roentgenogram if the examination is made with the patient upright. The clinical findings of profuse, foul-smelling sputum shortly after the onset of the acute process strongly suggest lung abscess and, if the cavity is not visible on a plain film, tomography is indicated. Chronic lung abscess must be differentiated from cavitary tuberculosis, the fungal infections that produce cavitation, infected lung cyst, and bronchogenic carcinoma in which the central portion of the lesion has sloughed. This differentiation may be very difficult roentgenograhically and examination of the sputum for bacteria and fungi along with appropriate cultures are used to confirm the diagnosis. Cytologic study of the sputum and bronchial aspirates is also indicated in patients with these chronic abscesses, particularly in men over 40, because of the high incidence of bronchogenic carcinoma.

Middle-Lobe Syndrome

The middle-lobe syndrome is discussed here because the term appears frequently in the literature. It refers to recurrent pneumonitis in the right middle lobe caused by present or previous obstruction of the bronchus to this lobe. The middle-lobe bronchus arises approximately 2 cm below the origin of the upper lobe bronchus and is relatively pliable; there are nodes adjacent to it that may produce compression of this bronchus when they become enlarged. When there is sufficient compression to cause partial obstruction, pneumonitis may result. The obstruction may persist or decrease, leading to atelectasis, bronchiectasis, and chronic pneumonitis, or to temporary resolution of the process. Endobronchial disease at the site of the lymph-node compression may result in gradually increasing stenosis of the middle lobe bronchus.

The initial obstruction may be caused by any inflammatory process that produces hilar-node enlargement. This node enlargement may not be sufficient to be detected roentgenographically but when obstruction is produced, there are roentgen findings in the lung that are somewhat varied, depending upon the relative amount of pneumonitis and atelectasis. The lobe is usually decreased in size. This results in downward displacement of the secondary interlobar fissure and in increase in density below and lateral to the right hilum. This is sometimes difficult to visualize in the posteroanterior roentgenogram, although it will cause blurring of the right cardiac margin. It can usually be readily outlined on the lateral film. Then the middle-lobe will be clearly defined as a wedge-shaped or triangular area of density sharply bounded above and below by normally aerated lung. The apex of the triangle is at the hilum and the base at the anterior inferior thoracic wall. When it is not clearly defined in either projection, it can be well visualized in an anteroposterior lordotic view. When bronchiectasis is marked, the dilated bronchi may be visible in the lateral view as air-filled tubular structures within the consolidated lung. The hilar nodes producing the obstruction may contain calcium and can then be visualized. The relationship of these nodes to the middle lobe bronchus can be accurately determined by means of tomography. Collateral ventilation of the middle lobe appears to be relatively ineffective as compared to the other lobes; this may account for the persistent collapse of the middle lobe in this syndrome.

Bronchographic findings vary, depending upon the degree of bronchostenosis, the duration of the disease, and the presence or absence of bronchiectasis. There are three major bronchographic patterns that can be recognized:

1. The lobar bronchus is patent at the time of the examination and the iodized oil extends freely into the smaller bronchial branches. The bronchi are narrowed, closely approximated to one another, and surrounded by dense lung. There is no alveolar filling and no filling of the finer bronchioles. The bronchi have the appearance of the limbs of a tree completely devoid of leaves. The lobe is decreased in volume. When such a lobe is removed it will reveal chronic pneumonia or, in long-standing cases, only fibrosis and atelectasis with the alveoli completely obliterated.

2. The lobar bronchus is patent but may be concentrically narrowed at its point of origin by an inflammatory stricture. Filling of the segmental and subsegmental bronchi occurs and they are found to be dilated and involved by bronchiectasis, usually of the tubular type. Again, there is no alveolar filling and the lung surrounding the dilated bronchi is more or less solid because of atelectasis and chronic pneumonitis.

3. The lobar bronchus is more severely stenosed and little or no iodized oil will enter the lobe. The bronchus tapers gradually to a point. If any oil does extend beyond the lobar bronchus, bronchiectasis is usually apparent. Because bronchogenic carcinoma may cause somewhat similar findings, bronchoscopy, cytologic study of the sputum or the bronchial washings, or even surgical exploration may be required to make the diagnosis in this type of disease (Figs. 23-14, 23-15, and 23-16). Therefore, bronchography is now used rather rarely in the study of these patients.

Surgical removal is the usual treatment since the bronchial changes are usually irreversible by the time the syndrome is recognized.

Mucoviscidosis
(Cystic Fibrosis of the Pancreas)
and Pulmonary Infection

Mucoviscidosis is the term used to describe the generalized process of which fibrocystic disease of the pancreas is the most commonly recognized finding. It is a congenital and familial disease in which there is an abnormality involving the mucous glands. Ob-

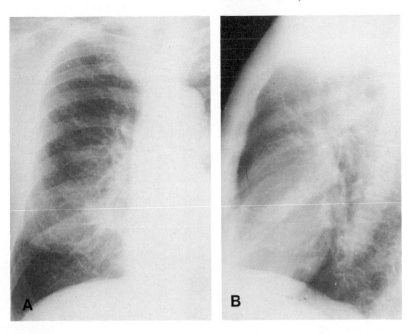

Fig. 23-14. Middle-lobe syndrome. Note the density below the right hilum **(A)** which blurs the right cardiac margin slightly. In the lateral projection **(B)**, the disease is noted to lie above the major fissure in the medial segment of the middle lobe.

struction by viscid mucus leads to atrophy and fibrosis of the gland or organ. It is probable that the condition involves all exocrine glands to some extent. The gastrointestinal changes have been described elsewhere. Pulmonary manifestations vary in degree but are almost invariably present if the child lives long enough to develop them.

The earliest roentgen change in fibrocystic disease of the pancreas is overinflation (emphysema) which is diffuse and symmetrical. This is often difficult to

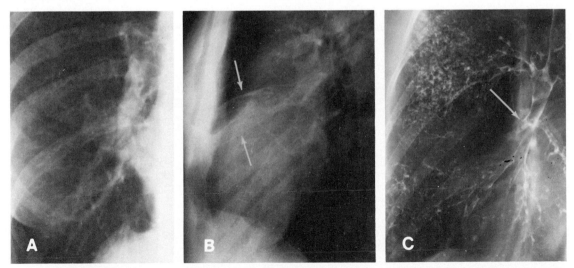

Fig. 23-15. Middle-lobe syndrome. **A.** Note the contracted middle lobe below the right hilum which obscures the central portion of the right atrial silhouette. **B.** The lateral view shows the contracted middle lobe **(arrows) C.** The bronchogram shows obstruction **(arrow)** of the middle-lobe bronchus. The upper- and lower-lobe bronchi are filled.

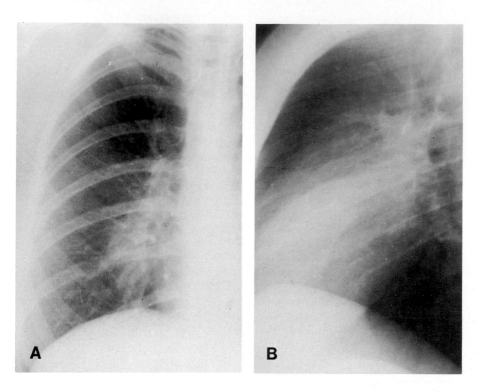

Fig. 23-16. Acute pneumonia in the right middle lobe. **A.** Note the hazy alveolar disease below the right hilum at the medial base which blurs the right cardiac margin in this area. **B.** In the lateral view the disease is clearly defined. It lies in the right middle lobe.

Fig. 23-17. Cystic fibrosis of the pancreas with chronic pulmonary disease. There is extensive involvement throughout both lungs. Rounded and oval radiolucencies indicate thick-walled bronchi, some of which are dilated, indicating bronchiectasis. There also is evidence of some overinflation, and there is bilateral hilar adenopathy.

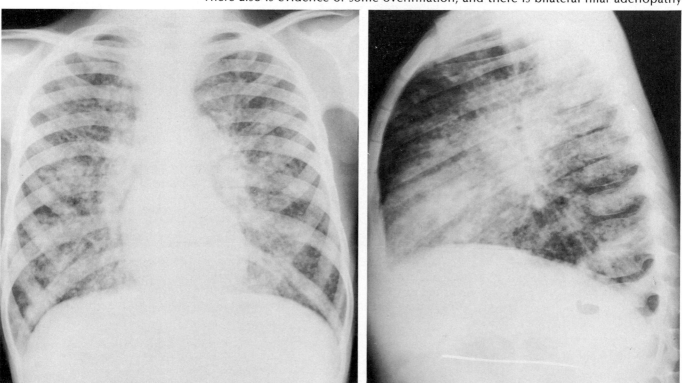

recognize in children, but films exposed in inspiration and expiration, as well as chest fluoroscopy, will indicate the distended state of the lungs and the signs of poor respiratory exchange. The degree of obstruction tends to increase to a different extent in various segments so that small areas of density resulting from focal atelectasis are visible as the disease progresses. These patients develop repeated pulmonary infection so that signs of pneumonia are superimposed. The infection is usually widespread and is peribronchial in distribution, which leads to a rather irregular, stringy accentuation of markings extending outward from the hila on both sides. This is often associated with areas of poorly defined, hazy density caused by focal areas of pneumonitis in the parenchyma. Segmental or lobar collapse may also occur and the repeated infection leads to a considerable amount of fibrosis and often to bronchiectasis. Bronchial walls are thickened. The fibrosis and inflammatory disease produces irregular stringy and patchy density. The lung between the consolidated areas is emphysematous and hyperaerated, giving a characteristic roentgenographic picture in far advanced disease (Fig. 23-17). It is often possible to suspect the presence of mucoviscidosis early in the course of the disease when emphysema, which may often be associated with small areas of focal atelectasis and which is somewhat irregular in distribution, is noted in these infants. The diagnosis can then be confirmed by the sweat test—the finding of more than 50 mEq of chloride per liter of sweat and by demonstration of decreased amounts of pancreatic enzymes in duodenal contents. An increasing number of patients live into adult life, and in these young adults, there is often a rather characteristic radiographic appearance. The disease usually involves the upper lobes with a combination of patchy, linear and nodular densities interspersed with radiolucent areas that in some instances may resemble the changes manifest in pulmonary tuberculosis. Hypertrophic osteoarthropathy has been reported in adults with cystic fibrosis.

Chronic Granulomatous Disease of Childhood

Chronic granulomatous disease of childhood[30] (CGD) is another genetically determined disorder in which pulmonary infections begin early in life and persist or recur at intervals. Leukocytes phagocytize bacteria normally but do not destroy them properly. Lobar and lobular pneumonia may occur in these patients, complicated by lung abscess and empyema.

Pulmonary involvement may resolve slowly; it may become clearly defined with sharp borders and homogeneous density. It is then termed "encapsulated pneumonia."[26]

REFERENCES AND SELECTED READINGS

1. BARNHARD HJ, KNIKER WJ: Roentgenologic findings in pertussis. Am J Roentgenol 84: 445, 1960
2. BARTLETT JG, FINEGOLD SM: Anaerobic infections of the lung and pleural space. State of the art. Am Rev Resp Dis 110: 56, 1974
3. CONTE P, HEITZMAN ER, MARKARIAN B: Viral pneumonia. Roentgen pathological correlations. Radiology 95: 267, 1970
4. DENNIS JM, BOUDREAU RP: Pleuropulmonary tularemia. Radiology 68: 25, 1957
5. DIETRICH PA, JOHNSON RD, FAIRBANK JT et al: The chest radiograph in Legionnaires' disease. Radiology 127: 577, 1978
6. EFFLER DB, ERVIN JR: The middle lobe syndrome. A review of the anatomic and clinical features. Am Rev Tuberc 71: 775, 1955
7. EVERETT ED, NELSON RA: Pulmonary melioidosis. Am Rev Resp Dis 112: 331, 1975
8. FRASER RG, WORTZMAN G: Acute pneumococcal lobar pneumonia: the significance of non-segmental distribution. J Canad Assoc Radiol 10: 37, 1959
9. GREENSPAN RH, FEINBERG SB: Salmonella bacteremia: a case with miliary lung lesions and spondylitis. Radiology 68: 860, 1957
10. HARVEY WA: Pulmonary brucellosis. Ann Intern Med 28: 768, 1948
11. HOLMES RB: Friedlander's pneumonia. Am J Roentgenol 75: 728, 1956
12. JOFFE N: Roentgenologic aspects of primary Pseudomonas Aeruginosa pneumonia in mechanically ventilated patients. Am J Roentgenol 107: 305, 1955
13. KEATS TE: Generalized pulmonary emphysema as an isolated manifestation of early cystic fibrosis of the pancreas. Radiology 65: 223, 1955
14. LEWIS EK, LUSK FB: Roentgen diagnosis of primary atypical pneumonia. Radiology 42: 425, 1944
15. MEYERS HI, JACOBSON G: Staphylococcal pneumonia in children and adults. Radiology 72: 665, 1959
16. MILLER RP, BATES JH: Pleural pulmonary tularemia. A review of 29 patients. Am Rev Resp Dis 99: 31, 1969
17. PULLEN RL, STUART BM: Tularemia: Analysis of 225 cases. JAMA 129: 495, 1945
18. QUINN JL III: Measles pneumonia in an adult. Am J Roentgenol 91: 560, 1964

19. Rose RW, Ward BH: Spherical pneumonias in children simulating pulmonary and mediastinal masses. Radiology 106: 179, 1973

20. di Sant' Agnese PA: Pulmonary manifestations of fibrocystic disease of the pancreas. Dis Chest 27: 654, 1955

21. Schultze G: Primary staphylococcal pneumonia in infants. Am J Roentgenol 81: 290, 1959

22. Southard ME: Roentgen findings in chickenpox pneumonia. Am J Roentgenol 76: 533, 1956

23. Stenstrom R, Jansson E, Wager O: Ornithosis pneumonia with special reference to roentgenological lung findings. Acta Med Scand 171: 349, 1962

24. Stuart BM, Pullen RL: Tularemic pneumonia: review of American literature and report of 15 cases. Am J Med Sci 210: 223, 1945

25. Tan DYM, Kaufman SA, Levene G: Primary chickenpox pneumonia. Am J Roentgenol 76: 527, 1956

26. Unger JD, Rose HD, Unger GF: Gram-negative pneumonia. Radiology 107: 283, 1973

27. Vinik M, Altman DH, Parks RE: Experience with Hemophilus influenzae pneumonia. Radiology 86: 701, 1966

28. Weed LA, Sloss PT, Clagett OT: Chronic localized pulmonary brucellosis. JAMA 161: 1044, 1956

29. Wiita RM, Cartwright RR, Davis JG: Staphylococcal pneumonia in adults. Am J Roentgenol 86: 1083, 1961

30. Wolfson JJ, Quie PG, Laxdal SD et al: Roentgenologic manifestations in children with a genetic defect of polymorphonuclear leukocyte function. Radiology 91: 37, 1968

24

AIRWAY DISEASES

DISEASES OF THE UPPER AIRWAY

OBSTRUCTIVE DISEASES: ACUTE

Epiglottitis. Epiglottitis commonly affects infants and young children and is usually caused by *Hemophilus influenzae.* Occasionally it may occur in adults.[12] The radiographic findings consist of swelling of the epiglottis and the structures around it, including the aryepiglottic folds, the arytenoids, the uvula, and the prevertebral or retropharyngeal soft tissues. The valleculae and pyriform sinuses may be obliterated. The amount of swelling of the surrounding structures may vary from one patient to another, but enlargement of the epiglottis is present in all. There is often some ballooning of the hypopharynx, but there is no abnormality of the glottis. The subglottic region is normal, and the lungs are not overinflated. A single lateral radiograph of the neck usually suffices to make the diagnosis in an infant or child with acute upper respiratory obstruction.

Acute Laryngotracheobronchitis (Croup). Croup is usually caused by a virus and most commonly occurs in children from 6 months to 3 years of age. The major finding on the roentgenogram is narrowing of the trachea in the subglottic area on inspiration, thickening and fuzziness of the vocal cords, and overdistention of the hypopharynx. The subglottic narrowing may change on expiration but does not ordinarily disappear. In some patients the only abnormalities are the fuzzy appearance of the thickened cords and poor definition of larynx and subglottic area. In the anteroposterior projection the glottic and subglottic areas show a somewhat fusiform or funnel-shaped narrowing on inspiration. The epiglottis and aryepiglottic folds are normal. Unlike epiglottitis, which may require tracheostomy, in croup this procedure is not ordinarily needed.

Membranous Croup. Membranous croup is a severe form of laryngotracheobronchitis probably caused by superimposed bacterial infection on the viral disease or by bacterial infection alone.[6] The disease is more severe than viral croup and tends to affect slightly older age groups. Radiographically, the subglottic obstruction may be severe, upper tracheal mucosa is thick and irregular, and detached or partially detached membranes may project into the tracheal airway, sometimes resembling foreign bodies for which they may be mistaken.

Acute Retropharyngeal Abscess. Acute retropharyngeal abscess may also cause severe obstruction. It produces a characteristic swelling of the prevertebral soft tissues posterior to the pharynx. When it is large enough to cause obstruction, the pharynx above it tends to be distended on inspiration. Other causes of thickening of the retropharyngeal tissues include tumor, hemorrhage, and the edema and hemorrhage secondary to trauma of the cervical spine. Lymphadenopathy, which may occur in association with lymphoma, chronic granulomatous disease, or histiocytosis X, and retropharyngeal tumors, such as cystic hygroma, neurofibroma, neublastoma, hemangioma, and retropharyngeal thyroid, may produce varying degrees of obstruction. In some instances the obstruction is acute while in others it is chronic. The lungs are usually normal in volume in patients with acute upper airway obstructive conditions. When a retropharyngeal mass is suspected, it is important, particularly in infants and young children, that the patients neck be extended when the lateral film is exposed, since the flexibility of the upper airway is so great that a pseudo mass or pseudostenosis may be produced if the patient's neck is flexed or incompletely extended.

OBSTRUCTIVE DISEASES: CHRONIC

Tracheal Agenesis. Absence of the trachea is a rare anomaly in which air reaches the bronchi through an esophageal communication. The anomaly is readily noted on frontal and lateral roentgenograms. It is uniformly fatal.

Laryngotracheoesophageal Cleft. This rare anomaly consists of failure of differentiation of the larynx and upper trachea from the esophagus. A common channel is observed on contrast study, with Dionosil or barium as the medium, which may be carried out following laryngoscopy and placement of an endotracheal tube. In addition to aphonia and other voice abnormalities, there may be signs of upper airway obstruction resulting in respiratory distress in the neonatal period. The cleft is minimal in some infants and extensive in others.

Congenital Laryngeal Cyst. This is another rare cause of respiratory-tract obstruction in infants.[13] Roentgen findings are those of a soft-tissue laryngeal mass occurring anywhere from the superior surface of the aryepiglottic fold to the laryngeal ventricle. This soft-tissue mass cannot be differentiated from other congenital masses such as hemangioma.

Thyroglossal Cyst. A thyroglossal cyst of the base of the tongue may cause respiratory obstruction as well as difficulty in swallowing. It is outlined as a soft-tissue mass on the lateral film.

Laryngomalacia caused by congenital aryepiglottic laxity results in supraglottic obstruction and stridor at rest which decreases or disappears when the child is excited. The obstructive soft tissue may be visible on the lateral roentgenogram of the upper airway.

Tracheal Tumors. Tracheal tumors are rare, but when present may cause varying amounts of chronic obstruction. Epidermoid carcinoma is the most common tracheal malignant lesion, but such lesions as cylindroma, lymphoma, plasmacytoma, and metastases may also occur. Papilloma may occur in the larynx or pharynx and may also involve the trachea. This lesion is probably caused by a virus, but its etiology is not entirely clear.

Tracheal Stenosis. Tracheal stenosis may result from external trauma or be secondary to intubation or tracheostomy.[8] Rarely it may be congenital. Roentgen findings are those of persistent tracheal narrowing of varying length and severity that does not change or changes very little from the inspiratory to the expiratory phase of respiration.

Tracheomalacia is another rare cause of obstruction. This abnormality should be suspected if tracheal diameter decreases by more than 50% during expiration or if it measures less than 3 mm in lateral projection. There is a wide range of normal variation, however, and the diagnosis should be made with caution. Tracheomalacia is presumably caused by weakness of the tracheal walls including the supporting cartilage and is usually associated with deficiency of cartilage plates, in the rare primary form, and in association with osseous dysplasias such as the Ellis–van Creveld syndrome. More often, it is secondary to some other abnormality of the upper respiratory tract.

Relapsing Polychondritis. When relapsing polychondritis involves the trachea, it can cause tracheal stenosis which may be severe. The narrowing is visible on frontal and lateral films of the trachea.

Tracheobronchomegaly. Tracheobronchomegaly is another rare condition that may result in chronic obstruction. On roentgenographic study the trachea and major bronchi are noted to be increased in caliber and to have an irregular, corrugated appearance caused by protrusion of the tracheal and bronchial walls between the cartilaginous rings which is sometimes termed "diverticulosis." The obstructive symptoms appear to be secondary to an inefficient cough mechanism. Most patients having this condition develop infection with associated bronchiectasis and many succumb to infection associated with respiratory failure. The tracheal width in children with this anomaly is equal to or greater than the thoracic vertebral body width, a distinct increase in diameter. On expiration or coughing, marked tracheobronchial collapse is observed.

BRONCHIAL DISEASES

BRONCHITIS

Acute Bronchitis

The term "acute bronchitis" usually refers to acute catarrhal bronchial inflammation associated with upper respiratory infection, which is not usually a severe illness when uncomplicated. There are no positive roentgen findings in this condition, but roentgenograms are useful to indicate that there is no complicating pneumonitis in patients with acute respiratory infections in whom symptoms are unusually severe.

Chronic Bronchitis

Chronic bronchial inflammatory disease may occur in patients with chronic specific pulmonary inflammatory disease. This is not considered here. We include chronic nonspecific bronchial inflammation which results in chronic cough with sputum, often of several years' duration. If etiologic factors persist, this disease progresses to pulmonary insufficiency, emphysema, and cor pulmonale. Several etiologic possibilities exist, with one or more or a combination of several of them operating in an individual patient. They include air pollution, cigarette smoking in an estimated 82%,[16] infection and hereditary weakness of bronchial walls in a few patients. Recurrent obstructive bronchitis also may be a result of gastro-esophageal reflux in children.[1] It is not uncommon to see no roentgen findings in patients with chronic bronchial disease. In these patients, the chest roentgenogram serves to exclude the possibility of other diseases which could cause the same symptoms. When the bronchitis results in thickening of bronchial walls and in peribronchial inflammation, these thick-walled structures may be visualized extending well into the parenchyma, whereas the normal bronchi within the lungs are not outlined on the plain-film roentgenogram. The visualization of these bronchi, therefore, indicates thickening of bronchial walls and peribronchial disease, which is often associated with chronic bronchitis regardless of its etiologic background. These findings are often best outlined on tomograms. Hyperinflation of the lung may also be manifested by increased lucency of the lungs and increased thoracic volume. Roentgen changes must be correlated with clinical findings. The presence of prominent basal markings does not necessarily indicate chronic bronchial disease since there is a wide variation in the normal. The roentgen diagnosis of chronic bronchitis, based on plain-film study, is therefore made with great caution.

Although there are no reliable plain-film findings in chronic bronchitis, there are reasonably reliable bronchographic signs in this disease. Small diverticulum-like projections are often observed along the inferior surfaces of the large bronchi. They represent dilated ducts of mucous glands. Distal bronchial or bronchiolar occlusions are also found. Some of them are tapering occlusions, whereas in others there is a bulbous expansion distally (bronchiolectasia). Irregularity or "beading" of the bronchial lumen may also be present. Dilatation of small bronchi on inspiration, with return to normal caliber on expiration, has been described in this disease, but we have not observed this alteration with respiration. In the absence of bronchiectasis, the presence of dilated bronchial glands, bronchiolectasia, and irregularity or beading of the bronchial lumen probably justifies the diagnosis of chronic bronchitis. Bronchography is not ordinarily used in determining diagnosis of chronic bronchitis in our department. Signs of this condition are observed in patients who are being studied for suspected bronchiectasis, or for other reasons.

Acute Bronchiolitis

The term "acute bronchiolitis" refers to the acute disease usually observed in small infants or in debilitated, elderly persons in which a widespread involvement of small bronchi and bronchioles is manifested by roentgen signs of air trapping with hyperaeration and low, flat diaphragm. The lungs appear clearer than is normal and there is very little change on expiration. This is produced by a check-valve type of obstruction of the finer bronchioles by thick secretions. As the disease progresses, focal areas of alveolar involvement are manifested by scattered small densities, which may eventually resemble a very widespread, acute, miliary type of infiltrate (Fig. 24-1). These densities appear to be caused by small areas of pneumonia around the bronchioles and by small foci of atelectasis. At times, extensive alveolar pneumonia may develop, so that there is a broad spectrum of radiographic findings. The most frequent cause appears to be respiratory syncytial virus, but other viruses including adenovirus, rhinovirus, parainfluenza virus, and, occasionally, mumps and influenza virus. In infants, *Mycoplasma pneumoniae* occasionally causes bronchiolitis. Adenovirus types 3, 7, and 21 may cause serious pulmonary infection in young children, with destruction and necrosis of bronchiolar and alveolar tissue and permanent lung damage. In addition to hyperinflation, areas of airspace pneumonic consolidation and atelectasis may be observed on the chest roentgenogram.[18]

Bronchiolitis Obliterans

Bronchiolitis obliterans results from lower respiratory tract damage, which may be caused by inhalation of toxic substance such as fumes from nitric, hydrochloric, or sulfuric acid, from talcum powder, zinc stearate, and hot gases. It may also be caused by viral infections of the respiratory tract including influenza, measles, and infections due to adenovirus.[4] As a result, the bronchioles become obstructed by masses of granulation tissue and organizing exudate. When fat-filled phagocytes accumulate behind the obstructed bronchioles, a "cholesterol" pneumonitis is produced. The clinical findings include cough, dyspnea, sputum production, fever, and malaise. Roentgenologic findings have been divided into three main categories[4]: (1) *Nodular densities* in the form of micronodular, discrete nodular, confluent nodular, or lineonodular densities. (2) *Alveolar opacities* which may be diffuse or edemalike, linear (atelecta-

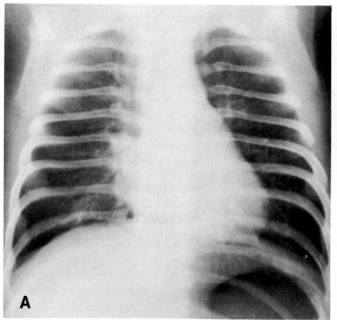
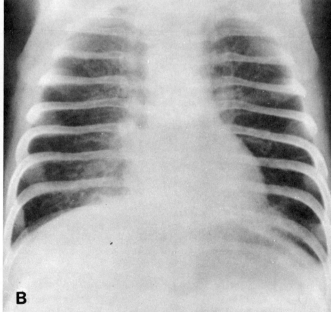

Fig. 24-1. Acute bronchiolitis. **A.** Note the relatively low diaphragm with hyperaerated lung and a small amount of density at the right medial base representing early associated pneumonia. **B.** In this film, exposed 24 hours after that shown in **A,** emphysema is shown to be slightly less marked but the pneumonia, particularly on the right side, has increased. The patient was acutely ill at the time of the first examination.

tic), or a mixed or honeycomb pattern. These patterns are usually bibasilar. In other locations the alveolar opacities take the form of lobar or segmental consolidation and atelectasis; diffuse edemalike or multiple, irregular opacities may also occur. (3) *Hyperinflation* which occurred in only two of 52 patients. The most distinctive appear to be the micronodular and lineonodular patterns similar to those in diffuse infectious granulomatous disease, occupational lung disease, or, possibly, sarcoidosis. The nodules tend to be less distinct in bronchiolitis obliterans than in the other conditions. The discrete and confluent nodular densities suggest such conditions as diffuse or localized vasculitis, multiple abscesses, or disseminated bronchioloalveolar cell carcinoma or metastases. The basilar opacities are suggestive of chronic interstitial pneumonia which may coexist in some instances. This wide variation in roentgen findings makes roentgenographic diagnosis very difficult, although it can be suspected in patients with a suggestive past history and the clinical symptoms of cough, dyspnea, sputum, fever, and malaise.

Bronchiectasis

Bronchiectasis refers to persistent dilatation of bronchi, which may vary widely in extent. It results from destruction of the elastic and muscle tissue of the bronchial walls. Descriptive adjectives such as cylindrial (tubular), varicose, saccular, and cystic are used to distinguish the various forms of dilatation. The cylindrical form of the disease is sometimes difficult to recognize, particularly when it is minimal. With progression, the bronchi tend to dilate further, making the diagnosis relatively easy on bronchography. The saccular and cystic forms are readily recognized. The disease may be local or general and is usually caused by obstruction and infection, but there is probably a congenital factor or a number of congenital factors in some instances; for example, the incidence of bronchiectasis associated with situs inversus is much greater than in the general population. The triad of situs inversus, paranasal sinus disease, and bronchiectasis is termed "Kartagener's triad" or syndrome. Bronchiectasis is also common in patients with mucoviscidosis. Immunologic defects such as agammaglobulinemia and dysgammaglobulinemia are also associated with bronchiectasis. The usual symptom of bronchiectasis is chronic productive cough, often associated with recurrent episodes of acute pneumonitis and hemoptysis.

It is often possible to make a presumptive diagnosis of bronchiectasis on plain-film study, but it must be remembered that a roentgenogram of the chest showing no abnormality does not exclude the possibility of bronchiectasis. The findings that indicate this disease are accentuation of markings in the area of disease, often with associated patchy pneumonic densities in which linear or circular radiolucencies can be outlined (Fig. 24-2). It is sometimes possible to trace a thick-walled dilated bronchus well out into the periphery when there is enough peribronchial inflammatory disease so that the air-filled bronchus is visible. When severe saccular bronchiectasis is present, oval or circular radiolucencies may be outlined (Fig. 24-3) and it is not uncommon to see fluid levels in some of the larger cystlike dilatations. There is often decrease in volume of the lobe or segment associated with the chronic inflammation that produces fibrosis and atelectasis.

The fact that the presence of bronchiectasis can be determined on plain-film study in some cases and can be suspected in others does not mean that bronchography is unnecessary in these patients. Whenever surgical intervention is planned, complete bronchographic mapping of the bronchial tree is necessary in order that the surgery can be planned intelligently. In most instances the dilatation is either saccular or cylindrical or a combination of the two (Fig. 24-4). Saccular bronchiectasis is not difficult to define but, unless there is good filling outlining the entire length of a bronchus, the presence of cylindrical bronchiectasis or the absence of it is sometimes difficult to ascertain and there is often some difference of opinion as to the presence or absence of dilatation. It is often possible to define small amounts of dilatation, however, by comparing the bronchus in question with an adjacent bronchus of a similar order.

Reversible bronchiectasis occurs in children and young adults, usually following acute pneumonia or atelectasis. In the postpneumonic group, the dilatation clears following complete resolution of the pulmonary disease. In the atelectatic group the bronchi decrease in caliber with reexpansion of the lung. Evidently the dilatation is reversible if the mucosa and musculoelastic elements of the bronchial wall are intact. The reversible disease is usually cylindrical or fusiform in type and there may be slight narrowing proximal to the dilatation caused by spasm secondary to inflammatory disease. The possibility of reversibility must be considered when surgical treatment is contemplated; a repeat bronchogram is the only accurate method of making a positive diagnosis of a return to normal.

The greatest dilatation of bronchi in nonspecific bronchiectasis is usually peripheral. In the bronchiectasis associated with pulmonary tuberculosis there is a somewhat different appearance since the

Small foci of tuberculous pneumonia are started by these bronchogenic aspirates. All of these lesions may heal, some may heal, others go on to caseation and cavitation, while still others become productive lesions resulting in the formation of a considerable amount of granulation tissue and eventual fibrosis. The fibrosis may be extensive, leading to a considerable loss in lung volume and tracheobronchial distortion.

Cavitation

The presence of cavitation in a patient with pulmonary tuberculosis is common and is often readily detected roentgenographically since the cavity is large enough to produce a distinct rounded or oval radiolucency with a moderately thick wall surrounding it. From the standpoint of management of the patient, the presence of cavitation is of great importance and it is often necessary to use a number of methods of roentgen examination to ascertain the presence of cavity and to localize it. Stereoscopic views are often of considerable value and films in lateral and oblique projections will sometimes outline cavities not clearly defined in frontal projection. It is in the detection of such lesions that tomography has its greatest use in pulmonary tuberculosis. It is frequently possible to detect cavitation on tomograms that is not suspected on any other roentgenogram.

There is wide variation in appearance of tuberculous excavation just as there is considerable variation in the appearance of the disease from one patient to the next. The cavitations all appear as radiolucent areas that vary widely in size but are generally round or oval in shape. The walls are usually moderately thick except in tension cavities, which become fairly large and may exhibit thin walls. A tension cavity develops because of a check-valve type of obstruction of the bronchus leading to it, allowing air to enter the cavity more freely than it can escape. This type of cavity may disappear very quickly when treatment is instituted because the bronchial obstruction that contributed to its size may be relieved quickly to permit the cavity to collapse. Thick-walled cavities, on the other hand, often show little tendency to close, or may close or decrease in size very slowly when treatment is instituted. In general the walls of the cavities are noted to decrease in thickness and become less distinct as the disease regresses under treatment. Fibrosis, with contraction of the previously involved lung, and emphysema may result in production of irregular or oval radiolucencies that may simulate cavities very closely. In these instances it is often difficult and sometimes impossible to differentiate between a thin-walled cavity and an area of emphysema unless the disease has been well documented by repeated roentgenograms during its course. In these patients, tomography is often of considerable value (Fig 25-6).

BRONCHIECTASIS

Endobronchial involvement in pulmonary tuberculosis is very common and leads to bronchiectasis in a number of instances. The presence of bronchiectasis in patients with tuberculosis can often be diagnosed or at least suspected on routine roentgenograms because the thick-walled bronchi filled with air stand out in contrast to the diseased lung surrounding them. In other instances a diagnosis can be made with a fair degree of certainty on tomograms, particularly in patients with far-advanced disease. Bronchography, however, remains the best method for the detection of or exclusion of the possibility of bronchiectasis associated with tuberculosis, as it is in bronchiectasis of nonspecific origin. Bronchiectasis in patients with pulmonary tuberculosis may be saccular or cylindrical and is found in the lobe or segment involved by the disease. Occasionally it will be detected in an area where there is no obvious parenchymal involvement. Presumbably the bronchiectasis was caused by tuberculous disease which has resolved to the point where no roentgen evidence remains. Therefore many investigators consider that bronchography is indicated before segmental surgery is undertaken in patients with pulmonary tuberculosis. There is some difference in the appearance of bronchiectasis in tuberculosis from that in the nonspecific type. In tuberculosis there is often peripheral obliteration and more fibrosis with greater distortion of bronchi (Fig. 25-7). We have found a very high incidence of bronchiectasis in lobes compressed beneath a thoracoplasty, which probably accounts for the persistence of tubercle bacilli in the pulmonary secretions of many of these patients. This can often be detected readily on tomography because the compressed lung serves as a contrast to the air-filled bronchi. However, in these patients, as well as others, accurate delineation and segmental distribution must be determined by bronchography.

TUBERCULOMA

The term "tuberculoma" refers to the round, focal, tuberculous lesion that may be solitary or multiple. There are many inflammatory nodules in which tubercle bacilli cannot be found. The histopathologic findings are nonspecific. They are best termed

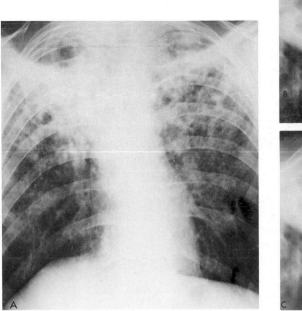
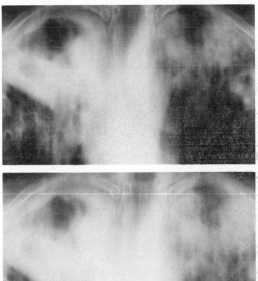

Fig. 25-6. Advanced bilateral pulmonary tuberculosis. **A.** Note the large apical cavity on the right in the supraclavicular area. The disease is very extensive in the upper half of both lungs and several suspicious radiolucent areas are noted on the left. **B** and **C.** These are tomograms of the same patient shown in **A.** The apical cavity on the right, some shift of the trachea to the right, and several small cavities on the left are evident.

Fig. 25-7. Bronchiectasis in tuberculosis. **A.** Note the dilatation of the upper lobe bronchi, which are also crowded in a patient who had had previous extensive right upper-lobe tuberculosis. There is very little alveolar filling and the distal ends of the bronchi are obstructed. The latter finding is characteristic of tuberculosis. **B.** Bronchogram in a patient with far-advanced tuberculosis of long duration. The right upper lobe is contracted and there is extensive sacular bronchiectasis, bronchial distortion, and failure of parenchymal filling.

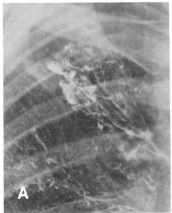
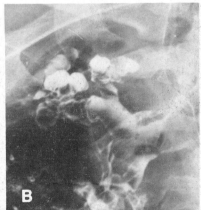

"chronic nonspecific granuloma," not tuberculoma. The tuberculous nodules vary in size from a few millimeters to 5 or 6 cm but usually range from 1 to 3 cm. They may or may not contain calcium and usually contain caseous debris. When present, calcium tends to form a more or less complete shell or ring in or near the outer wall of the nodule. It is not unusual to see several concentric rings of calcium, and a central nidus of calcium is often present. The pathogenesis is varied and the nodule may represent either the primary or reinfection type of disease. Sometimes the nodule results when a cavity is sealed by obstruction of its draining bronchus. All of these lesions are potentially dangerous, since they may contain viable tubercle bacilli for long intervals and may break down at any time with resultant dissemination of the disease. They may remain constant in size or may grow very slowly over a period of years.

The roentgen finding is that of a round parenchymal nodule. If concentric rings of calcium are visible, the lesion is almost certainly a tuberculoma or other chronic inflammatory granuloma (Fig. 25-8). If no calcium is demonstrated on the routine roentgen study of the chest, tomography is indicated. Calcium can often be seen on the tomogram when its presence is not detected on the preliminary film. If no calcification is found, there is no way to differentiate the tuberculoma or other infectious granuloma from bronchogenic carcinoma, other lung tumors, or from solitary pulmonary metastasis. In the patient with a small, solitary nodule the lesion is usually benign, particularly in the female, but resection must be considered in all patients when no calcification is present unless previous films going back over a period of years indicate that the lesion has been present for a long time and is unchanged.[16]

HEALING OF PULMONARY TUBERCULOSIS

In general, pulmonary tuberculosis heals slowly, so that it is possible by means of serial roentgenograms to follow the gross anatomic changes in the disease. Differences can be noted in the manner of healing, which very likely depend on the type of involvement and the susceptibility of the tubercle bacilli to the antituberculous drugs as well as the response of the patient. Complete resolution often occurs in some areas and it is a common observation that this is likely to occur and be most striking in patients with relatively acute disease in which the process is presumed to be largely exudative (Fig. 25-9). This accounts for the decrease in the thickness of the walls of cavities often noted in patients undergoing treatment. The exudative portion of the process making up the cavitary wall resolves, resulting in a decrease in thickness. In patients in whom the disease has progressed to the point of necrosis, complete resolution is not possible. In these patients, fibrosis with contraction of the scars results in shrinkage in the volume of the involved lobe or segment and a decrease in the size of the hemithorax. The mediastinal structures are retracted to the side of involvement. The hilum is elevated in upper-lobe disease and sometimes the diaphragm is raised. The tubercles that contain granulation tissue as well as caseation, and are often noted as poorly defined nodules, will show gradual reduction in size. The individual nodules tend to become more clearly defined on the roentgenogram, evidently also because of contraction and fibrosis. This type of lesion often is the site of calcium deposition and in some instances becomes densely calcified with the passage of time. Many of these lesions contain central areas of necrosis in which viable organisms can be found after long periods of apparent inactivity. In summary, as visualized roentgenographically, there is considerable difference in the healing process from one patient to another but it is unusual to see the disease disappear entirely (Fig. 25-10). Tomograms are very helpful in demonstrating nodular residuals that cannot be clearly defined on routine chest roentgenograms. Examination of surgical specimens has demonstrated that it is very difficult to be certain on roentgen examination that no residual disease is present.

COMPLICATIONS OF REINFECTION TUBERCULOSIS

Pleural Effusion

Because pulmonary tuberculosis is a peripheral lesion, pleural involvement is not uncommon (Fig. 25-11); effusion may be found in patients without an obvious pulmonary lesion. In some instances the density produced by the fluid obscures the parenchymal disease. In others, pleural effusion may be the only roentgen manifestation and, even when the fluid has been removed or absorbed, no definite pulmonary parenchymal focus is roentgenographically visible. In some patients the fluid disappears spontaneously or can be successfully aspirated while, in others, tuberculous empyema may result. Occasionally the pleural space may be involved by secondary infection. The tuberculous empyema is similar to the empyema of nonspecific origin in its roentgen appearance. It is usually loculated and may become very large. If present and undrained for a long period of time, calcification may occur, producing marked radiographic density outlining the wall. Bronchopleural fistula may also occur with drainage of all or part of the contents of the empyema and entrance of air into it.

Bronchostenosis

Narrowing of a bronchus may result from pressure of an enlarged lymph node that is involved by tubercu-

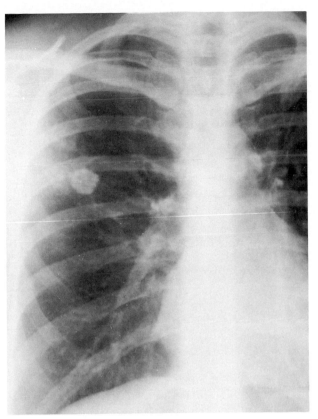

Fig. 25-8. Tuberculoma. Note the dense calcified nodule in the right midlung field. There is also a little disease noted lateral to it and above it in the lateral aspect of the second anterior interspace. Some calcified hilar nodes are noted bilaterally.

losis. This is usually found in children with primary tuberculosis. It is also caused by endobronchial inflammation and granuloma formation or fibrosis, usually in the post-primary or reinfection form of the disease. Roentgen findings are not evident until the obstruction is sufficient to cause either atelectasis or obstructive emphysema and the findings in these conditions are similar to those described in the appropriate sections of Chapter 30.

Broncholithiasis

Occasionally a calcified node adjacent to a bronchus will erode into the bronchus and the material from the node will be extruded into the bronchus. This may produce very few symptoms or it may rarely result in bronchogenic spread of tuberculous disease or hemorrhage; or the calcification may cause bronchial obstruction with emphysema or atelectasis. This complication may also occur in patients with calcified nodes secondary to lesions other than pulmonary tuberculosis. Radiographic findings vary with the situation. The calcified nodes are often visible and their relation to the bronchus can be determined by tomography or bronchography.

Tuberculous Pneumothorax

When pneumothorax complicates pulmonary tuberculosis it creates the hazard of widespread pleural involvement leading to tuberculous empyema and bronchopleural fistula, because the pneumothorax often results from rupture of a caseous subpleural

Fig. 25-9. Far-advanced bilateral pulmonary tuberculosis showing the regression resulting from treatment with antituberculous drugs. **A.** Note the extensive bilateral disease. **B.** Study made 9 months later shows great improvement. The remaining disease consists largely of fibrous strands with a few nodules in each lung.

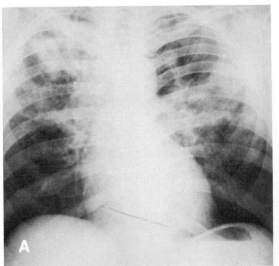
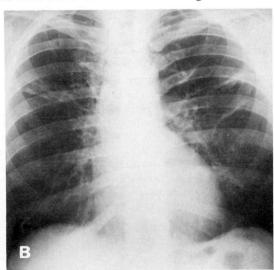

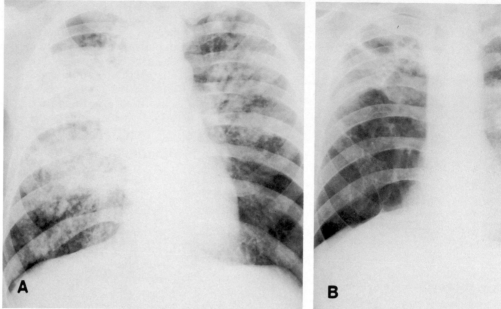

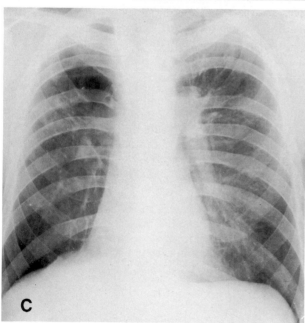

Fig. 25-10. Far-advanced pulmonary tuberculosis. **A.** Initial film showing the bilateral disease. There is a large cavity at the right apex which is rather poorly defined on this film. **B.** Nine months later, film of the right lung shows the result of treatment. The large apical cavity is more clearly defined. The upper lobe is contracted but much of the exudative disease has cleared. **C.** Sixteen months after the initial examination most of the residual disease has been resected and now the findings are those of surgical scarring in the right second anterior interspace and in the left subclavicular area.

focus into the pleural space in advanced disease. It is also possible for a small subpleural bleb to rupture leading to a simple pneumothorax that will resolve quickly without further complication. The roentgen appearance is similar to that noted in pneumothorax owing to other causes, but the tuberculous disease is visible and there may be a considerable amount of adhesive pleuritis resulting in irregular or loculated pneumothorax. This is an uncommon complication of tuberculosis.

Dissemination to Other Organs

Patients with pulmonary tuberculosis occasionally develop disease in other organs and systems such as the larynx, ileum and cecum, urogenital organs, and

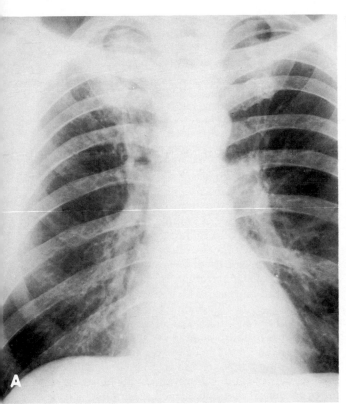
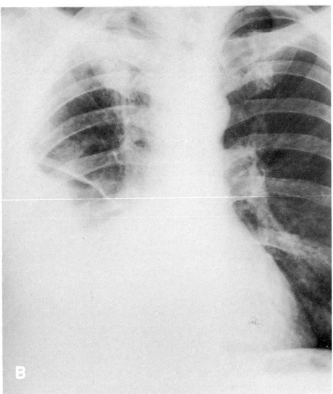

Fig. 25-11. Pulmonary tuberculosis showing the development of pleural effusion. **A.** Bilateral upper-lobe tuberculosis manifested by density which is rather homogeneous and more intense on the right than on the left. There is no evidence of pleural fluid on the right, and there was none on the left. **B.** Four weeks later a large right pleural effusion is evident. Note that the parenchymal disease has regressed slightly owing to treatment during the interval.

skeletal system. Gastrointestinal and laryngeal disease are frequently the result of contact with sputum and only rarely indicate a hematogenous spread. On the other hand, renal tuberculosis as well as skeletal involvement indicates hematogenous or lymphatic spread. These lesions are discussed under the organ or system involved.

HEMATOGENOUS TUBERCULOSIS

Hematogenous pulmonary tuberculosis includes several types of disease. When the organisms enter the bloodstream it is possible to get hematogenous involvement of numerous other organs and systems. The actual mode of dissemination is difficult to determine in any specific instance but may occur by way of the lymphatics and into the bloodstream through the thoracic duct, by direct rupture of a caseous

focus into a vessel, or by formation of a subintimal tubercle that serves as a source of organisms. The invasion of the bloodstream may occur in any stage of tuberculosis. When hematogenous dissemination develops, numerous factors have a bearing on the resultant disease. These aspects are beyond the scope of this discussion but include the following: the age of the patient, the number and virulence of the organisms entering the bloodstream, the individual and racial susceptibility, and the general health of the patient, as well as the state of allergy and immunity at the time of the invasion. Prompt treatment with antibacterial drugs, of course, alters the disease considerably in a favorable manner.

MILIARY PULMONARY TUBERCULOSIS

Two clinical types of miliary tuberculosis are recognized—acute miliary tuberculosis and subacute or chronic miliary pulmonary dissemination. Acute miliary tuberculosis follows massive bloodstream invasion, producing a severe acute illness with frequently fatal termination before the use of antituberculous drugs. In infants and children it usually results from a spread from a primary complex and produces severe clinical manifestations. In most children, however, the number of organisms is small and the host resistance sufficient to prevent miliary spread of the disease, so there are no clinical manifestations. In adults, particularly in the older age group, the disease may be very insidious and extremely difficult to recognize. Findings on chest roentgenograms depend on the size and number of miliary tubercles. The actual densities visualized on a roentgenogram are the result of superimposition of many small parenchymal lesions that create sufficient density to be recognized as a small nodule. In the typical patient the appearance is that of a fine granularity or tiny nodulation scattered uniformly throughout both lung fields. At times the lesions are rather clearly defined as innumerable fine nodules, each sharply delineated; in other patients they are less sharply outlined, with hazy margins (Fig. 25-12). In some patients with miliary pulmonary tuberculosis, no lesions can be seen on the initial chest film, but, in most instances, classical miliary pattern develops during the course of the disease.[3] There are usually some findings suggesting tuberculosis on the initial film in these patients, however. Pleural involvement is common, resulting in unilateral or bilateral pleural effusion that varies considerably in amount. Rarely, recurrent pneumothorax may complicate the disease.[7] The cause is not certain, but subpleural caseating nodules may rupture into the pleural space in some instances. The individual lesions are largely exudative and, when treatment with antibacterial drugs is effective, the widely scattered foci may disappear completely.

The differential diagnosis of miliary tuberculosis is often difficult from a roentgen standpoint because numerous other diseases produce widespread scattered and miliary type of nodulation in both lung fields. Correlation of clinical and roentgen findings is necessary in all instances. There are several acute processes that cannot be differentiated from miliary tuberculosis on a single chest roentgenogram. Miliary bronchopneumonia, which may be of viral or bacterial etiology, and bronchiolitis in children, resulting in widespread miliary nodulation, may closely resemble miliary tuberculosis. In other diseases such as sarcoidosis, the pneumoconioses, and miliary pulmonary carcinomatosis, the history and clinical course usually permit differentiation. There are a number of conditions capable of producing acute, diffuse miliary lesions in the lung. They include, in addition to those mentioned, other bacterial infections such as staphyloccal and streptococcal pneumonia, viral and rickettsial infections such as chickenpox and Q fever, mycotic infections such as histoplasmosis and blastomycosis, and parasitic infestations such as schistosomiasis. Also included are the noninfectious diseases, acute berylliosis, fat embolism, miliary hemorrhages, and acute, diffuse, interstitial fibrosis as described by Hamman and Rich. It is therefore evident that the roentgen findings must be correlated with the results of clinical and laboratory examinations and that, in many instances, serial roentgenograms, spaced over a period of days or even weeks, are necessary to establish the diagnosis.

SUBACUTE AND CHRONIC HEMATOGENOUS PULMONARY DISSEMINATION

Although hematogenous pulmonary dissemination is produced by hematogenous dissemination of tubercle bacilli, it is a somewhat different clinical entity from miliary tuberculosis in that it is often asymptomatic. Repeated small episodes may occur so that lesions, although widespread and distributed rather

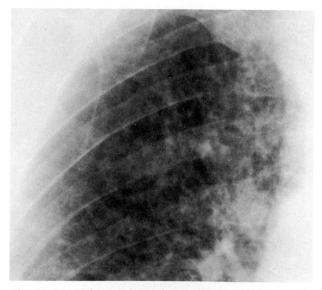

Fig. 25-12. Miliary tuberculosis. Close-up of the right upper lung in a patient with miliary tuberculosis shows the numerous, small densities along with a little increase in interstitial markings.

uniformly throughout both lung fields, are likely to be somewhat more variable in size than in the acute miliary process. When this type of dissemination is widespread, the roentgen findings are similar to those in the acute type of miliary tuberculosis, but there is considerable difference in the clinical course. In other instances the hematogenous pulmonary dissemination may be relatively localized, producing small, poorly defined, rounded or oval areas of density in a segment or lobe. Some of these nodules may regress while others may coalesce to form larger nodules and they may heal in a manner similar to that described earlier in the discussion of reinfection type of tuberculosis. In patients with far-advanced pulmonary tuberculosis and a considerable amount of cavitation there is often hematogenous spread to the lower lobes or to the opposite lung, resulting in scattered lesions that cannot be differentiated from the secondary lesions produced by bronchogenic spread of the disease.

ATYPICAL MYCOBACTERIA

There is a group of mycobacteria that may cause pulmonary disease which is similar to tuberculosis caused by *Mycobacterium tuberculosis* from the standpoint of roentgen findings. They are termed atypical, anonymous, chromogenic, or unclassified mycobacteria. The most important are *Mycobacterium kansasii* which has caused a number of pulmonary infections in the Chicago area, Dallas, Houston, and New Orleans; and the Battey strain found chiefly in the Southeast. A practical classification has been proposed by Kubica.[5] The roentgen findings are similar to those of *M. tuberculosis* infection except that there is a greater tendency to cavity formation, less parenchymal disease surrounding the cavities, and the cavity walls are thinner. Dissemination and pleural involvement with effusion are rare. The roentgen manifestations are so similar, however, that differentiation is not possible in a given patient. These organisms do not respond well to antituberculous therapy, so surgical removal is usually necessary if this is feasible.

SURGICAL MEASURES IN PULMONARY TUBERCULOSIS

Despite the undoubted value of the various antibacterial drugs now available for the treatment of tuberculosis, some patients either fail to close cavities or continue to discharge tubercle bacilli in pulmonary secretions. Others continue to have considerable residual disease after long-term treatment. These patients then become possible candidates for surgery. The surgery is usually resectional with removal of the disease.

PULMONARY RESECTION

The roentgen appearance of the chest following pulmonary resection varies with the type of resection. There is also considerable variation, depending upon the ability of the remaining lung to expand and fill the hemithorax. Immediately following lobar or segmental resection, the roentgenogram often outlines pneumothorax that varies in amount and position, depending upon the volume of pulmonary tissue removed. The diaphragm on the operated side is usually elevated and there is often a mediastinal shift to that side. A drainage tube is left in place and this is visible along with some emphysema in the lateral chest wall that often extends up into the neck. Emphysema is manifested by streaks of radiolucency within the soft tissues (Fig. 25-13). There may be some fluid in the soft tissues along with air. This produces fluid levels that may overlie the lung parenchyma. These accumulations in the wound space can usually be differentiated from loculated pockets of air and fluid in the pleural space by their position in relation to the chest wall. A segment of rib is sometimes resected and surgical section or fracture of a rib above or below the missing rib is often observed. It is not unusual to note some diffuse density at the surgical site, even on roentgenograms obtained very shortly following completion of the procedure. This is caused by a combination of edema and possibly hemorrhage at the surgical site, along with some fluid in the adjacent pleural space. The density varies considerably with the type of resection, being most commonly observed when a segmental resection is carried out. Within 24 hours there usually is fluid in the pleural space at the base and surrounding the remaining lung. The amount of pneumothorax is often decreased in that period of time. It is not unusual to observe some atelectasis in the remaining lobe that often clears within 24 hours, with resultant increase in lung volume and decrease in the size of the pneumothorax. Subsequent roentgenograms show gradual decrease in the size of the residual pneumothorax and increase in expansion of the remaining lung. The subcutaneous emphysema usually disappears in a week or 10 days. Occasionally a severe subcutaneous emphysema is noted that extends into the neck on

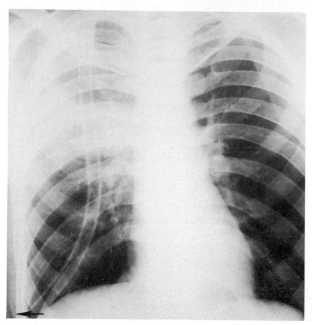

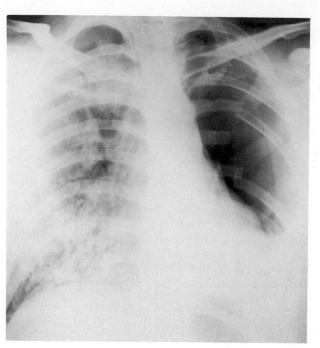

Fig. 25-13. Postoperative chest. Portable film exposed 1 day following segmental resection of the apical and posterior segments of the right upper lobe. The hazy density in the right midlung is most likely due to edema and some hemorrhage at the surgical site. The remaining lung is well expanded. The large drainage tube is easily identified. The **arrow** at the right base indicates a small amount of postoperative subcutaneous emphysema.

Fig. 25-14. Postoperative chest. A left pneumonectomy was performed 2 days before this examination was made with portable equipment. Fluid and air fill the left pleural space. Much of the density at the right base is due to iodized oil residual from previous bronchography. Note the drainage tube extending up to the vicinity of left hilum. There has been resection of the posterior arc of the sixth rib and surgical section of the fifth and seventh ribs.

both sides and into the soft tissues of the opposite hemithorax as well as into the mediastinum. This requires a longer time to clear. Eventually the pneumothorax and fluid disappear, leaving a relatively small amount of residual pleural thickening or perhaps some irregular adhesive tenting of the diaphragm manifested by local elevation of it. When segmental resection is performed and no rib is removed, it is often difficult, or impossible, to detect recognizable residues on the resected side after a period of 6 months. (See Fig. 25-10.)

Pneumonectomy is occasionally necessary in the treatment of tuberculosis and following this operation there usually is a large amount of pneumothorax noted in the immediate postoperative film along with subcutaneous emphysema as in the segmental and lobar resections. Rib removal and surgical section can also be recognized. As time goes on, fluid accu-

mulates in the hemithorax and this gradually replaces the air (Fig. 25-14). Elevation of the diaphragm and shift of the mediastinal structures to the surgical side vary considerably but are almost always present, along with some herniation of the normal lung across the midline (Fig. 25-15).

Complications may occur and can be recognized on the roentgenograms. Bronchopleural fistula is manifested by continuing pneumothorax for an unusually long period of time or by sudden increase in the amount of pneumothorax along with decrease in fluid without aspiration. When lobar or segmental resections are done, the remaining segments or lobes may collapse. These atelectatic areas are recognized as areas of increased density because of the airlessness of the pulmonary parenchyma.

The roentgen findings following pulmonary resection for disease other than tuberculosis are similar to those just described.

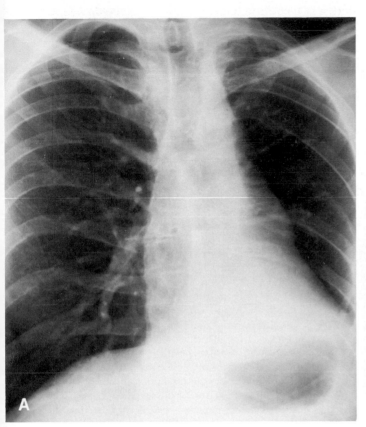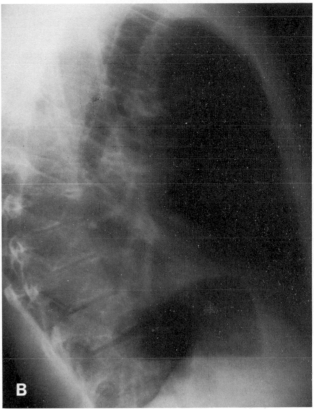

Fig. 25-15. Left pneumonectomy. Frontal **(A)** and lateral **(B)** roentgenograms show remarkable shift of the right lung into the left hemithorax through the anterior mediastinum. The heart is displaced posteriorly. The mediastinal shift and elevation of the left diaphragm are rather minimal. Radiolucency of the remaining lung is indicative of compensatory overexpansion.

OTHER SURGICAL PROCEDURES

Thoracoplasty

Thoracoplasty is an operative procedure on the chest wall in which a number of ribs are resected for the purpose of decreasing the volume of the thorax. This operation has been superseded by resectional therapy to a large extent. It was also used following pneumonectomy to obliterate the pleural space and after lobectomy or segmental resection when the remaining lung failed to expand enough to fill the hemithorax. In time there is regeneration of bone along the sites of the resected ribs, which may form a rather heavy bony plate at the operative site (Fig. 25-16). When rib regeneration is not desired the periosteum is destroyed.

Plombage

Plombage is another surgical procedure that has been used to decrease the size of the thorax. It consists of placing foreign material into a space of desired size either extrapleurally or extraperiosteally. Roentgenograms will show the site of plombage and the material used can often be visualized (Fig. 25-17). This procedure has been abandoned in favor of resection of residual cavitation or other residual disease.

Cavernostomy or Cavity Drainage

Cavernostomy is another surgical procedure formerly used in tuberculosis, often as a last resort in a patient

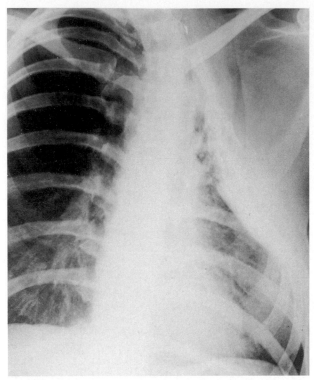

Fig. 25-16. Left thoracoplasty. This surgical procedure, which was used extensively in the pre-antituberculous drug days, is employed very seldom at present. There has been extensive resection of the upper seven ribs on the left, compressing the left upper lung. Regeneration of the ribs has formed a solid bony plate along the upper lateral chest wall. The scoliosis is a common result of thoracoplasty.

Fig. 25-17. Lucite-ball plombage. Although this procedure has been abandoned, occasionally patients are observed with the rounded lucencies representing lucite balls, usually at the apex of one hemithorax as in this patient.

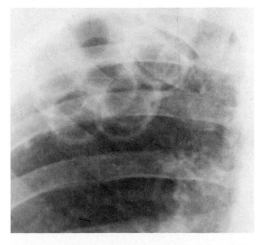

with a large cavity that could not be resected and did not drain adequately. Roentgen findings were as expected and consisted of visualization of the cavity with a drainage tube extending into it. A short overlying segment of rib was often resected and this would be visible.

REFERENCES AND SELECTED READINGS

1. BAILEY WC, BROWN M, BUECHNER HA et al: Silicomycobacterial disease in sand blasters. Am Rev Resp Dis 110: 115, 1974
2. FRIEDENBERG RM, ISAACS N, ELKIN M: The changing roentgenologic picture in pulmonary tuberculosis under modern chemotherapy. Am J Roentgenol 81: 196, 1959
3. GELB AF, LEFFLER C, BREWIN A et al: Miliary tuberculosis. Am Rev Resp Dis 108: 1327, 1973
4. GOOD CA, CARR DT, WEED LA: Positive roentgenograms plus positive sputum smears do not always equal pulmonary tuberculosis. Am J Roentgenol 81: 187, 1959
5. KUBICA GP: Differential identification of mycobacteria. VII. Key features for identification of clinically significant mycobacteria. Am Rev Resp Dis 107: 9, 1973
6. ORTBALS DW, MARR JJ: A comparative study of tuberculous and other mycobacterial infections and their associations with malignancy. Am Rev Resp Dis 117: 39, 1978
7. PEIKEN AS, LAMBERTA F, SERIFF NS: Bilateral recurrent pneumothoraces: a rare complication of miliary tuberculosis. Am Rev Resp Dis 110: 512, 1974
8. STEAD WW: The iceberg of medicine: tuberculosis. Radiol Clin North Am 3: 299, 1965

26

FUNGAL DISEASES AND OTHER CHRONIC INFLAMMATIONS

The inflammatory diseases discussed in this chapter are caused by a variety of organisms, many of which are capable of producing acute, fulminating, generalized disease in which there is associated involvement of the lungs. These organisms may also cause disease, usually chronic, limited primarily to the lungs. The diseases must be differentiated from each other as well as from pulmonary tuberculosis and occasionally from lung tumor. The ultimate diagnosis depends upon demonstration of the causative agent in bronchial secretions or in sections of the lung. In many instances this is very difficult, so that other bacteriologic studies based on immunologic reactions are required. These consist of skin tests, agglutination, complement fixation, and precipitation reactions.

The gross anatomic changes in pulmonary disease produced by these varied organisms may be similar. On the basis of roentgen examination it is often possible to indicate only that the lesion is a chronic inflammatory disease of unknown etiology. At other times it is possible to make the diagnosis with a considerable degree of accuracy on the basis of clinical findings correlated with roentgen manifestations. In the paragraphs to follow, these diseases are classified according to their etiology; brief descriptions of the major roentgen changes are given.

FUNGAL DISEASES OF THE LUNGS

ACTINOMYCOSIS

Actinomycosis is caused by an anaerobic organism, *Actinomyces bovis,* in cattle. In humans it is caused by *Actinomyces israeli,* a similar organism that occurs in rod-shaped bacterial form in the mouth and in mycelial form in infected tissues. Other actinomycetes may cause human infection; these include *A. bovis, A. naeslundi, A. ericksoni,* and *A. propionicus.* The organisms are now established as bacteria, but roentgen and clinical findings similar to those of mycotic infections justifies[39] the inclusion of actinomycosis here. The disease may affect any part of the body but is found most frequently in and about the jaw. Pulmonary infection has been said to occur in approximately 15% of patients with the disease.

However, in recent years, the incidence of pulmonary involvement has declined considerably and the classical empyema with chest-wall sinus tracts and pulmonary parenchymal disease is rarely seen. This form of the disease is characterized by its tendency to produce suppurative sinus tracts and its ability to cross tissue planes that provide a barrier to the usual infections. The roentgen findings vary greatly. The disease may be unilateral or bilateral but tends to be unilateral unless widely disseminated throughout the body. It produces a dense, confluent opacity in the affected lung in which cavitation may be present (Fig. 26-1). In the classical chest-wall disease, pleural involvement results in varying amounts of pleural thickening and fluid. Infection of the chest wall causes soft-tissue swelling and destruction of ribs with sinus tract formation; this is characteristic of advanced disease which is now observed infrequently. The parenchymal involvement may resemble an acute alveolar pneumonia in some instances.

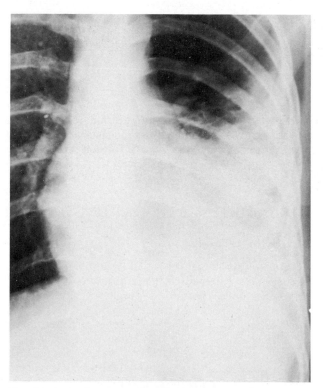

Fig. 26-1. Actinomycosis. The dense confluent consolidation in the left lower lung obscures the left hemidiaphragm and left lower cardiac border. The patient also had a chest-wall mass and sinus tracts typical of this disease.

In other cases, the disease is manifest as a local masslike density resembling bronchogenic carcinoma. Another roentgen pattern is that of a fan-shaped consolidation near the hilum or radiating from it into the superior segment of the lower lobe. When the chest-wall involvement with empyema and sinus tracts is present, the disease may be strongly suspected. Usually, however, actinomycosis must be differentiated by bacteriologic and histologic examinations from tuberculosis, from other chronic fungal infections, and from tumor.

NOCARDIOSIS

Nocardia asteroides is the most common of several species of *Nocardia* that may cause disease. It is an aerobic, gram-positive, acid-fast bacterium, formerly classified as a fungus, with finely branched hyphae. It is recognized increasingly as a secondary infection in patients with underlying chronic debilitating disease, particularly in those who have undergone therapy with immunosuppressive or cytotoxic agents or steroids. In nocardiosis, pulmonary roentgen findings consist of homogeneous segmental or lobar air-space consolidation; cavitation is common. Pleural involvement with empyema is also frequent. Single nodular lesions may also occur and may progress to cavitation. The disease is frequently bilateral. It crosses fissures and anatomic barriers, but not as frequently as does actinomycosis. The roentgen alterations in the lungs persist for long periods of time, frequently with little change unless the patient is treated with sulfonamides. *N. asteroides* is difficult to isolate in many instances so that the diagnosis is often obscure until material for histologic study is obtained by aspiration lung biopsy, transtracheal aspiration, bronchial brushing, or open lung biopsy. It is not unusual for the disease to run a protracted course with very little variation in the appearance of the pulmonary lesions and very few symptoms. Pleural involvement with empyema and extension to involve ribs with production of chest-wall abscess is not as frequent as in actinomycosis and is not ordinarily observed in nocardiosis at present. Mediastinitis with adenopathy and obstruction of the superior vena cava has been reported, however. Nocardiosis is one of the few benign diseases that cause obstruction of the superior vena cava.[32] In addition to differentiating this disease from tuberculosis, the other chronic infectious lesions of the lungs must be included in the differential diagnosis. Identification of the causative agent is necessary to confirm the diagnosis (Fig. 26-2).

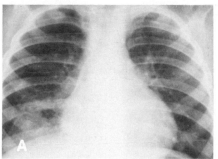 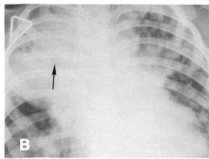

Fig. 26-2. Nocardiosis. **A.** This film shows a small amount of poorly defined density at the right base just above the diaphragm. **B.** Roentgenogram obtained 9 months later shows extensive progression of the disease with large, poorly defined nodular and patchy density in both lungs. A large homogeneous consolidation in which there is a cavity **(arrow)** is seen in the right upper lobe. There has been open drainage of the pleural space in the right upper anterolateral chest wall.

COCCIDIOIDOMYCOSIS

Coccidioidomycosis is caused by the fungus *Coccidioides immitis.*[6] It is an endemic pulmonary disease occurring in the arid southwestern part of the United States, particularly in the San Joaquin Valley in California. The initial infection produces an acute pneumonia associated with symptoms of an acute pulmonary disease including fever, malaise, headache, and cough. Erythema nodosum is a frequent clinical manifestation during the acute febrile illness and, in the San Joaquin Valley, this clinical syndrome is known as valley fever. Erythema nodosum occurs, often associated with arthralgias, at about the time the reaction to the coccidioidin skin test becomes positive. It may be the only symptom and indicates a good prognosis. Prior to this time, some patients (about 10%) develop a toxic erythema, usually in the first few days of illness. The rash is a diffuse, fine, macular erythematous reaction covering the trunk and extremities and usually occurs in children having the disease. The primary form is usually asymptomatic and may be discovered incidentally on the chest film. Roentgen findings are those of segmental pneumonitis resulting in homogeneous density that is poorly circumscribed. Hilar nodes are enlarged in about 20% of these patients, usually on the side of the alveolar disease. The roentgen findings in this type of involvement simulate those of other acute, atypical pneumonias. The pneumonia of coccidioidomycosis may be localized to one segment but wider dissemination has also been reported, with multiple areas of pneumonic consolidation. Occasionally the adenopathy in the hilar and mediastinal nodes is the

predominant feature and in these patients there may or may not be evidence of pulmonary parenchymal involvement. Multiple nodular parenchymal lesions have also been reported but are not as common as the more localized pneumonitis. Cavitation within the area of disease is not uncommon. The cavities are usually small and may disappear quickly in the primary type of infection. Occasionally, small pleural effusion is the only evidence of the disease noted on the chest roentgenogram. It occurs in about 20% of patients with coccidioidomycosis, but pleuritic chest pain has been reported in 70%; massive effusion is rare and may result from direct spread of pulmonary disease across the pleural space.

Coccidioidal pneumonia may persist for months with large areas of dense consolidation clearing very slowly. The patients are often very sick with persistent fever, prostration, chest pain, productive cough, and occasional hemoptysis. This type of the disease usually occurs in susceptible patients and occasionally in immunosuppressed patients.

Dissemination occurs rarely when the initial infection fails to become localized. This is very uncommon in members of the white race but members of dark-skinned races are more susceptible. Clinically it is a continuation and progression of the primary infection and is often manifested by exacerbation of symptoms. This miliary spread usually occurs early in the course of the disease but is sometimes a late complication of chronic pulmonary or extrapulmonary forms. Radiographic findings vary considerably from universal hematogenous spread of disease resembling miliary tuberculosis to local spread confined to the lungs. There is often bronchogenic dissemination to the opposite lung or other lobes, resulting in scattered involvement of varying extent. Large cavities may appear, along with pleural involvement leading to empyema. Associated with the extensive pulmonary infiltrates in this form of the disease there is often spread to abdominal viscera, skeletal system, lymph nodes, and sometimes to the brain and meninges. The disseminated type of involvement is usually lethal.

Residual or persistent pulmonary coccidioidomycosis results when the acute primary disease subsides without widespread dissemination. The primary disease may clear completely but when there is disease remaining within the lung it usually assumes one of three general radiographic types. These are: (1) cavitation; (2) nodules which may be single or multiple; and (3) pulmonary infiltration, which may be relatively focal and occur in a single area or in several areas. The residual type of cavitation in coccidioidomycosis often is thin-walled and may remain unchanged in size and shape for years. There usually is some fibrotic disease in the area of cavitation, but this is not always true. Studies of large numbers of patients have shown that the thin-walled cavity that was originally thought to be characteristic of the disease occurs in only 50% to 60% of patients, while the remaining cavities have relatively thick walls. Spontaneous closure of cavities occurs in about one-half of the patients. Most of the cavities are single and

in the upper lung fields, more than half are 4 cm in diameter or less. Cavitation may be complicated by secondary infection including formation of aspergillus fungus balls, pyopneumothorax when the cavity is subpleural in location, and pulmonary hemorrhage, which usually is not significant. These complications are uncommon. Cavitation in coccidioidomycosis must be differentiated from that in pulmonary tuberculosis and in other mycotic infections. This is usually not possible on roentgen examination alone, but, as a general rule, the residual cavity in coccidioidomycosis has less pulmonary infiltrate around it than is seen in pulmonary tuberculosis, since bronchogenic spread is much less common in coccidioidomycosis than in tuberculosis. This finding is important in the differential diagnosis in untreated patients with chronic pulmonary disease in which there is persistent cavitation (Fig. 26-3).

Rarely a pulmonary mycetoma (fungus ball) may be caused by *Coccidioides immitis*.[33] Arthrospores and spherules may be present along with hyphae of the mycelial phase in a pulmonary cavity. The appearance is similar to that of an aspergilloma, a much more common cause of fungus ball.

The nodular residuals of coccidioidomycosis vary considerably in size and in number. They may, or may not, contain calcium. When single, they must be differentiated from other diseases that cause solitary pulmonary nodulation, including primary broncho-

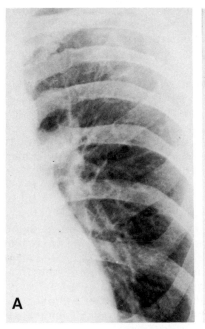
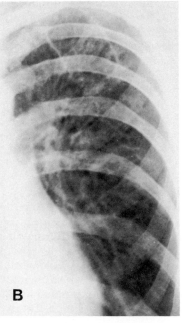

Fig. 26-3. Coccidioidomycosis. **A.** Note the cavity in the left subclavicular area. The elongated cavity has a moderately thick wall, but there is very little parenchymal disease around it. **B.** One year later, the cavity is noted to be larger, the wall thinner, and again very little other parenchymal disease is observed.

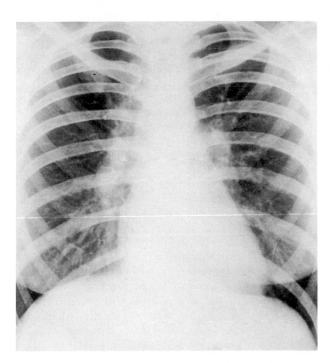

Fig. 26-4. Histoplasmosis. The parenchymal disease is minor and consists of a small amount of patchy density above the right hilum, but there is bilateral hilar node enlargement, more on the right than the left.

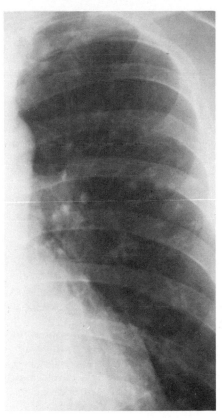

Fig. 26-5. Disseminated pulmonary histoplasmosis. Note the small, poorly defined nodules scattered throughout the left lung. The patient had been ill for several weeks.

genic tumor. When multiple, the lesions must be differentiated from other mycotic disease and from pulmonary tuberculosis. These differentiations are not possible on roentgen examination and must be made on the basis of skin tests with coccidioidin and by means of serologic studies. The infiltrative fibrotic type of residual disease is similar to the fibrotic residues of numerous other inflammations, so that there is nothing in the roentgenogram to indicate the nature of the original disease. Pleural thickening and effusion are occasionally noted as the end results of this disease, but there is nothing characteristic about these findings. Cavities are often peripheral and tend to rupture into the pleural space, resulting in empyema.

HISTOPLASMOSIS

Histoplasmosis is caused by the fungus known as *Histoplasma capsulatum.*[9] It was originally thought to be a rare and fatal disease but it is now known that

the disseminated form, which may be fatal, is only one of several types of the disease. The primary form is much more common. It is endemic in the Mississippi and Ohio valleys and along the Appalachian Mountains. In many areas, histoplasmin skin sensitivity is almost universal in the young adult lifetime residents, indicating previous infection. The disease is less common elsewhere in the United States but is found in nearly all states, as well as in Mexico and Panama.

The *primary form* of histoplasmosis is usually relatively benign and passes unnoticed in most instances (95%). The roentgen changes found in the acute benign disease are varied with single or multiple areas of pneumonic consolidation. The disease cannot be distinguished from primary tuberculosis roentgenographically. It is often segmental in distribution and may be accompanied by hilar-node enlargement. The hilar-node involvement may be more prominent than the parenchymal disease in some subjects (Fig. 26-4), particularly in children. In addition to the localized pneumonic consolidation, there is a more widespread form. Nodular lesions are scattered throughout both lung fields (Fig. 26-5). At first they are poorly defined. Later they become more clearly outlined, rounded nodules varying in size up to a centimeter. With healing, some of the nodules may disappear completely while others may gradually decrese in size and become calcified (Fig. 26-6). Calcification often occurs in the involved hilar nodes as well. Studies of large groups of people in endemic areas have shown that the amount of calcification in parenchymal nodules and in hilar nodes is greater in histoplasmosis than in tuberculosis as a general rule. The primary form of the disease may clear and leave no pulmonary residuals that can be recognized on roentgenograms. However, in others, solitary calcified parenchymal nodules with or without calcified hilar nodes may be present (Fig. 26-7). Caseous lymphadenitis is common during the primary infection. Cystlike lesions may develop in the mediastinum and become very large when liquefaction occurs in enlarged coalescent nodes. These lesions may measure 10 cm or more in diameter and may be asymptomatic, but air–fluid levels may develop within them, and there is some communication with the bronchial tree or lung. Remnants of lymph-node tissue may be observed in these cystlike lesions which tend to confirm the impression that they represent excavated lymph nodes. Miliary parenchymal calcifications scattered throughout the lungs and large "mulberry" calcified hilar nodes are usually associated with histoplasmin sensitivity rather than tuberculin sensitivity.

Symptomatic primary infection is usually found in infants and young children. In contrast to those having the more benign common form, these patients usually have cough and are often febrile for a few days, occasionally for 2 to 3 weeks or longer. Roentgen findings consist of hilar and mediastinal adenopathy with a small focal density representing air-space disease in the lung. Nodes may calcify, or occasionally may obstruct or rupture into a bronchus.

The *acute epidemic form* of histoplasmosis reported in a number of localities in the endemic regions probably represents a heavy exposure that results in more pulmonary parenchymal involvement than in the usual primary form of the disease. Very extensive bilateral lobular or nodular air-space disease may involve both lungs, and sometimes a miliary spread throughout both lungs is observed. The residuals are similar to those of the benign primary form, except that there may be more scattered, calcific, parenchymal foci in the severe acute epidemic form. It appears that reinfection may produce the acute, the chronic, or the disseminated form of histoplasmosis.

Disseminated histoplasmosis is a progressive disease with dissemination not only to the lungs but also to other organs, including the bone marrow. The course may be extremely rapid and fulminating or slowly progressive, leading to cachexia and anemia. It usually occurs in infants, in patients with compromised cellular immunity, or in those who have been immunosuppressed. Marked variation has been found in the roentgen manifestations of disseminated pulmonary histoplasmosis, ranging from widespread granular nodulations throughout both lung fields, which is the most common, to lobar type of pneumonic consolidation. Scattered involvement simulating other types of pneumonia is also noted and occasionally there is massive pleural effusion. In infants under 1 year of age the acute disseminated form is often fatal; hepatosplenomegaly is common in addition to extensive pulmonary involvement.

There is an *intermediate form* of histoplasmosis resulting in chronic active pulmonary disease and resembling reinfection tuberculosis clinically and radiographically. Cavitation along with local infiltration and nodulation similar to that noted in chronic pulmonary tuberculosis is often found. Pleural involvement, fibrosis, and contraction of the involved lobe or segment with alteration in the size of the thorax and mediastinal deviation may also be produced (Figs. 26-8 and 26-9). Histoplasmosis involving hilar nodes adjacent to bronchi may cause collapse of the middle lobe (middle-lobe syndrome) or of other pulmonary segments. It may also be the cause of broncholithiasis. In these patients with chronic active pulmonary histoplasmosis, emphysema is very common; the apical posterior segments are involved and cavitation is frequent, often persisting for long periods of time. These persistent cavities often enlarge gradually and may become very large. Disease in the adjacent lung is common, and fibrosis may become extensive.

Mediastinal involvement resulting in a chronic fibrosing process leading to superior vena caval obstruction has also been reported in this disease. The primary disease may have been quite asymptomatic, but the resultant fibrotic mediastinitis may produce pulmonary arterial and venous obstruction, and pericarditis and encroachment on the esophagus in addition to caval obstruction. Any or all of these findings may be present to greater or lesser degree. Rarely,

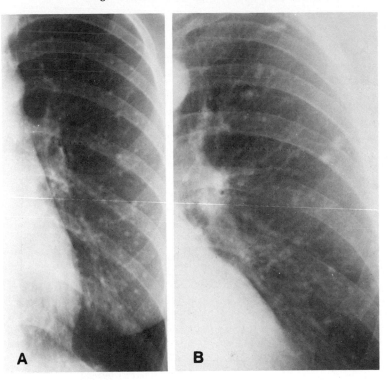

Fig. 26-6. Histoplasmosis. Examples of calcified pulmonary nodules. **A.** The nodules seen here are rather uniform in size and all are calcified. **B.** Fewer nodules but less calcification and more variation in size are noted in this film.

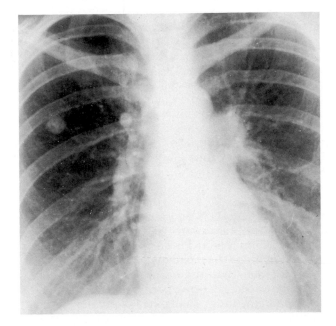

Fig. 26-7. Histoplasmosis. There is a solitary, partially calcified parenchymal nodule in the right upper lung field with several partially calcified right hilar nodes. The left hilum is also prominent and there are some enlarged nodes there.

calcification of the pericardium may result from histoplasma pericarditis.

The sole manifestation of the disease may be a solitary pulmonary nodule, the histoplasmona. This lesion may be associated with calcified hilar nodes and there may be a few satellite nodules in the lung. Calcification may or may not be present in the lesion which may vary from 1 to 3 cm or more in diameter. The calcification may be laminated, or annular, solid or stippled, and may be central with a laminated or annular peripheral ring. Skin testing, complement-fixation studies, and mycologic studies are required to differentiate this disease from pulmonary tuberculosis; occasionally both diseases may be present in the same patient.

CRYPTOCOCCOSIS (TORULOSIS)

Cryptococcosis is caused by *Cryptococcus neoformans (Torula histolytica)*. Pulmonary lesions have been reported in increasing numbers of patients with and without involvement of the central nervous system. As in other chronic pulmonary infections, several roentgen forms are found and the diagnosis cannot be made from roentgenograms alone. Three general types of radiographic change have been de-

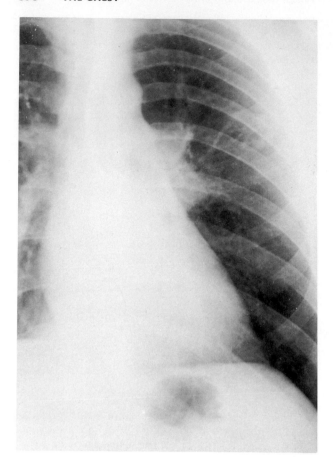

Fig. 26-8. Histoplasmosis. There are enlarged nodes in the left hilum and a little parenchymal disease in the lung lateral to the hilum which appears somewhat nodular. No other disease was observed.

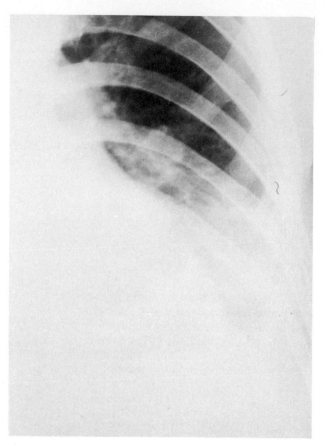

Fig. 26-9. Histoplasmosis. Note the conglomerate disease in the central and basal lung. There is also some pleural thickening and a small amount of fluid. No definite hilar enlargement is present. This is the same patient whose roentgenogram, obtained 5 years prior to this study, is shown in Figure 26-8. Slow progression of disease as illustrated here is unusual in our experience.

scribed. The first is a fairly well circumscribed, rounded mass usually occurring in the lower half of either lung field, which must be differentiated from neoplasm as well as from other chronic pulmonary granulomas. At times, multiple, closely grouped, masslike densities may be observed. The second is a pneumonic type of lesion consisting of a somewhat irregular density more likely to appear in the lower lobe than in the upper. This type of disease may be extensive, but usually is confined to one lobe; cavitation and hilar node enlargement are rare. The third type is a widespread miliary variety of nodulation often found in conjunction with severe central nervous system infection. This disease is frequently found associated with such chronic processes as Hodgkin's disease, leukemia, and lymphosarcoma, or is found to occur after steroid or antibiotic therapy.

Often the diagnosis is not made until autopsy in the patients having disseminated disease. Although the diagnosis cannot be made on the basis of roentgenographic findings, the combination of signs of meningeal irritation and pulmonary lesions resembling those described is suggestive. When the disease is confined to the lung, spontaneous resolution without treatment occurs in the majority of cases.

NORTH AMERICAN BLASTOMYCOSIS

This disease is not confined to the continent of North America and has been reported in South America, Central America, and Africa. It is caused by the yeastlike fungus, *Blastomyces dermatitidis.* Although much less common than histoplasmosis, it occurs in approximately the same geographic areas of the United States as does histoplasmosis, but extends more eastward and northward. There are two general types of the disease, cutaneous and disseminated. In the disseminated form, the portal of entry is usually the respiratory tract and 95% of the patients have some form of pulmonary involvement. The roentgen findings in pulmonary disease produced by this organism are not diagnostic. The roentgenographic manifestations are related to the clinical form of the disease.[34] In the acute form, air-space involvement causing a patchy segmental or lobar consolidation is present in the majority of patients. This is usually located in the lower lung fields. In this type, resolution usually takes place slowly and may require several months. Cavitation and miliary dissemination may complicate this acute form. There is also a severe form of acute disease in which there is bilateral exudate with the distribution resembling pulmonary alveolar edema. The onset is rapid, and the patients are very toxic.

The chronic form of the disease, which tends to occur in the upper lobe, resembles pulmonary tuberculosis. In the most common form, there is a fibronodular appearance consisting of pulmonary nodules and linear fibrotic strands (Figs. 26-10 and 26-11). Only slightly less frequent is cavitary upper-lobe disease in which the cavitary walls are moderately thick and smooth. Much less common is a masslike appearance which can closely resemble bronchogenic carcinoma (Fig. 26-12). Since these changes are similar to those noted in pulmonary tuberculosis, mycotic infections, and other chronic inflammatory diseases as well as neoplasm, the diagnosis must be based on mycologic studies.

SOUTH AMERICAN BLASTOMYCOSIS

This disease, caused by *Blastomyces brasiliensis,* is found most commonly in Brazil but has also been reported in the other South American countries. Pulmonary involvement is said to occur in 80% of the patients with the visceral type of the disease. The portal of entry is apparently the intestinal tract in this disease so that the pulmonary lesions are secondary and are widespread and nodular in type.

ASPERGILLOSIS

Pulmonary aspergillosis is rare despite the fact that fungi of the genus *Aspergillus* are ubiquitous. It is often a secondary process in patients who have been

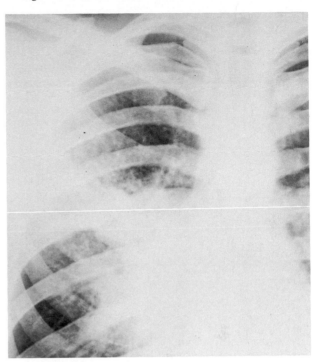

Fig. 26-10. North American blastomycosis. Note the extensive disease in the right parahilar and medial basal area as well as in the central and right lung laterally. Adjacent to the dense homogeneous involvement, a number of scattered, poorly defined nodules are observed. Roentgenographic findings in this disease are nonspecific.

treated with antibiotics and in those with debilitating disease. It does occur as a primary disease, however. Three clinical and roentgen types of the primary disease have been described:

1. An acute bronchopneumonic form with scattered multiple areas of pneumonic consolidation, some of which break down to form cavities. This disease may progress with severe invasive destructive pulmonary disease eventually leading to death. This invasive form usually occurs in infants. There is often enough hilar node enlargement to be recognized as such on the roentgenograms.

2. A more chronic and milder form than the first type. Irregular and rounded nodular infiltrates closely resembling those seen in pulmonary tuberculosis are present. The clinical course of this disease is less severe than that of tuberculosis, but the diagnosis must be made on the basis of identification of the organism in the sputum.

3. This type of aspergillosis has been described by

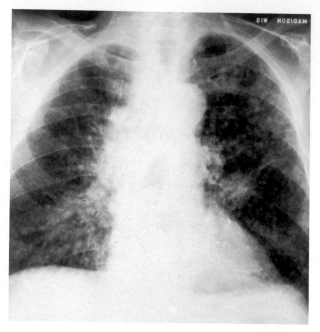

Fig. 26-11. North American blastomycosis. Numerous disseminated nodules, ranging up to a centimeter or more in diameter, are observed. On the right, either dense disease overlies the hilum or adenopathy is present, but no adenopathy is noted on the left.

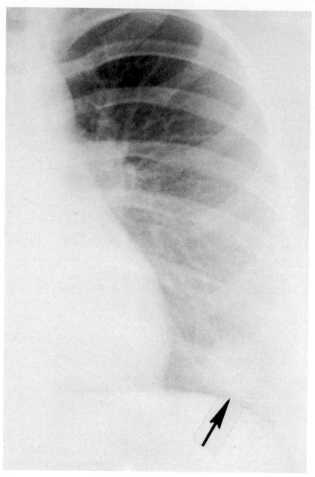

Fig. 26-12. North American blastomycosis. The large round mass at the left base resembling a tumor **(arrow)** was the only evidence of pulmonary disease in this patient. Examination after resection proved the infection to be blastomycosis.

Doub[5] in four patients in whom there were fairly widespread pulmonary nodules that at first were poorly circumscribed. These nodules became more clearly defined and eventually calcified from 2 to 4 years following the onset, leaving multiple calcified parenchymal nodules along with some calcified hilar nodes as residuals. During the acute phase there were symptoms of a respiratory infection and all the patients had some hilar-node involvement early in the course of the disease. It appears that aspergillosis may occasionally account for scattered calcified pulmonary parenchymal nodules.

Secondary aspergillosis is found in two forms, the aspergilloma (mycetoma) and a more diffuse form found in patients with severe debilitating disease and malignancies, and in those on cytotoxic drugs, steroids, or immunosuppressive agents. Patients with acute leukemia with granulocytopenia are particularly susceptible. Roentgen changes depend somewhat on the type of other pulmonary disease present. As a rule, there is diffuse consolidation with poorly defined margins in single or multiple areas. Cavitation may occur. Rarely a miliary spread throughout the lung may be observed. In these patients, the

prognosis is poor and the immediate cause of death may be aspergillosis. Since the organism is difficult to demonstrate on sputum and blood cultures, procedures such as percutaneous transthoracic aspiration may be necessary to make the diagnosis.

The aspergilloma (mycetoma) or fungus ball consists of a localized round or ovoid mass made up of aspergillus hyphae, blood, cellular debris, fibrin, and mucous, which occupies a cavity slightly larger than the mass. It is usually found in the upper lobe, probably because the primary disease, commonly tuberculosis, occurs in the upper lobe. A thin, radiolucent rim is observed surrounding the mass. This is caused by air that is between the cavity wall and the mass

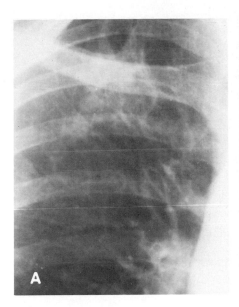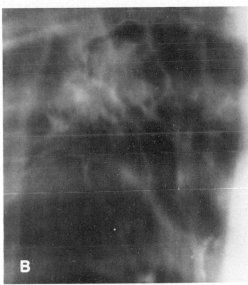

Fig. 26-13. Fungus ball. **A.** This film shows an irregular mass, somewhat obscured by the clavicle and first rib, with a little disease below it and above it. **B.** Tomogram shows a somewhat irregular cavity filled with a mass (fungus ball) separated from the wall by a radiolucent rim which is wide superiorly and medially and rather narrow laterally. The mass is not clearly defined inferiorly. There is some parenchymal disease lateral to the fungus ball.

and is virtually pathognomonic. The mass moves within the cavity. This can be demonstrated on tomography which is often helpful in the diagnosis when mycetoma is suspected (Fig. 26-13). Calcification may occur within the mass and may be extensive. Hemorrhage is common and may be severe.

It is apparent that aspergillosis can produce a wide variety of pulmonary lesions simulating other chronic inflammatory lesions and the aspergilloma can simulate tumor so that the diagnosis cannot be made on roentgen evidence alone.

Allergic (Hypersensitivity) Bronchopulmonary Aspergillosis

[22, 25] This form of aspergillosis occurs in patients with chronic bronchial asthma and is presumably caused by hypersensitivity reaction to antigens of species of the genus *Aspergillus,* chiefly *Aspergillus fumigatus.* Occasionally the organism is found in the sputum during an initial asthmatic attack or early in the course of bronchial asthma. The patients usually have fever, cough, and mucopurulent sputum, often with expectoration of mucous plugs. Eosinophilia and leukocytosis are usually present. The roentgenographic findings have been divided into transient and permanent shadows.[22] Transient shadows are: (*1*) homogeneous consolidation that may be large or small without loss of volume; (*2*) nonhomogeneous shadow or patchy consolidation; (*3*) small, circular, or nodular shadow; (*4*) atelectasis of a lung or lobe;

(*5*) bandlike and gloved-finger shadow 2 to 3 cm long and 5 to 8 mm wide, at times having a rounded end, sometimes termed a "toothpaste" shadow; (*6*) two parallel hairline shadows, with a radiolucent zone between the lines representing a normal bronchus (tram-line); (*7*) well-outlined, circular shadow with a diameter of 2 to 3 cm. The permanent shadows include: (*1*) parallel lines similar to tram-lines but with a width larger than that of a normal bronchus; (*2*) hairline ring shadow 1 to 2 cm in diameter; (*3*) decreased volume but with aeration in the segment or lobe involved; (*4*) narrowing or loss of vascular shadows; (*5*) long-line shadows. Most patients progress to varying degrees of pulmonary overinflation. The toothpaste and gloved-finger shadows represent mucous plugs in most instances. The tram-line shadows represent bronchi that are normal in diameter while parallel-line shadows represent bronchi that are increased in diameter. The ring shadow represents a dilated bronchus observed on end. Long-line shadows probably represent a wall of a bulla in some instances and pleura in others. The diagnosis is made on the basis of a history of bronchial asthma, the presence of eosinophilia, and the changing roentgenographic pattern of the lungs just described.

MONILIASIS (CANDIDIASIS)

Candida (Monilia) albicans is a yeastlike fungus, frequently present in the normal mouth, that may be occasionally mildly pathogenic for man. Since the organism is often present in the normal individual, it is difficult to document this disease. The literature is very confusing and many of the reported cases are probably examples of other diseases. However, most investigators agree that *Monilia* can produce bronchopulmonary disease, particularly in elderly or debilitated persons and in infants. Roentgen findings consist in a rather fine, mottled miliary type of nodulation associated with some prominence of pulmonary markings or, more commonly, segmental homogeneous consolidation. Cavitation, with or without a fungus ball, is rare, but is simulated when the disease involves an area of lung in which there are pre-existing emphysematous bullae. There may be some hilar-node enlargement. As in the other fungal diseases, the diagnosis must rest upon identification of the organism. The bronchial secretions rather than sputum should be examined since the organism is a normal inhabitant of the mouth.

GEOTRICHOSIS

Geotrichum is a fungus frequently found in the mouths of healthy subjects but that occasionally becomes pathogenic and causes pulmonary as well as skin and mucous-membrane infection. Pulmonary manifestations of geotrichosis are not characteristic. Irregular patchy densities are noted, often in the upper lung fields. Cavitation may develop, the cavities having rather thin walls. Hilar-node enlargement is frequent. The disease may closely resemble pulmonary tuberculosis (Fig. 26-14). *Geotrichum* has a tendency to produce an opportunistic type of pulmonary disease in severely dibilitated or immunosuppressed patients. In these patients, bronchopulmonary involvement is often extensive with air-space disease resembling extensive bronchopneumonia; often the infection is fatal. Endobronchial disease, with positive sputum cultures and no pulmonary involvement visible on chest films, may also occur in these patients. The diagnosis is based on a positive skin test plus demonstration of the organism on repeated sputum examination. The possibility of other fungal infections, as well as of tuberculosis, must be excluded by appropriate studies, since, in this disease, as in moniliasis, the organism may be saprophytic rather than pathogenic.

OTHER MYCOSES

Sporotrichosis

Sporotrichosis, produced by *Sporotrichum schenckii*, usually involves the skin, mucous membranes, and lymphatics. Occasionally, pulmonary infection may

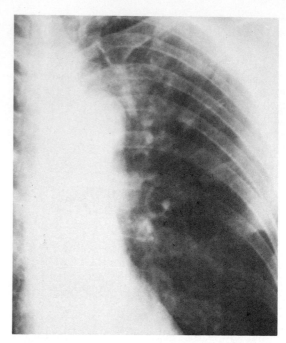

Fig. 26-14. Geotrichosis. Note the nodular disease in the left upper portion of the lung which resembles pulmonary tuberculosis. Since the disease progressed slowly, resection was undertaken proving it to be geotrichosis.

be the primary manifestation of the disease. There is nothing characteristic about the pneumonia it produces. Cavitation is often observed, however. The pulmonary infection may be local, indolent, granulomatous, and resemble chronic pulmonary tuberculosis. Also it may be suppurative and produce foci of bronchopneumonia. Scattered nodular disease has also been reported. Hilar adenopathy is common. *Sporotrichum schenckii* is sometimes found as a secondary invader in chronic pulmonary tuberculosis.

Penicilliosis

Fungi of the genus *Penicillium* are capable of producing pulmonary infection known as penicilliosis. This disease is very rare. The fungus can cause lung abscess that cannot be distinguished from cavitation produced by other organisms, so that there are no roentgen signs that would lead to the specific diagnosis.

Mucormycosis (Phycomycosis)

Mucor is a genus of fungus widely distributed in nature and is not usually pathogenic to man. It is a member of the class *Phycomycetes* along with *Absidia* and *Rhizopus*. Several cases of severe disseminated infection due to this fungus have been reported in diabetics. This infection is also found in patients with other underlying debilitating disease, such as leukemia or lymphoma. In some of these a widespread, rapidly fatal confluent pneumonia is present, which may cavitate. The hyphae tend to invade and occlude vessels. The resultant infarction leads to the cavitation. In some instances, mucormycosis may be the cause of a solitary pulmonary nodule.

DISEASES OF SPIROCHETAL ORIGIN

SYPHILIS

Involvement of the lungs in syphilis is very rare, but when this does occur it may simulate other chronic pulmonary disease symptomatically and radiographically. The diagnosis, therefore, depends upon exclusion of other diseases and upon laboratory studies as well as response to antiluetic therapy.

Roentgen Findings. Three radiographic types of pulmonary involvement have been described: (*1*) Interstitial fibrosis resulting in linear densities radiating into the lung fields from the hila. (2) A large solitary mass that may be clearly circumscribed and resemble pulmonary tumor or there may be some irregular inflammatory infiltrate surrounding it so that the lesion simulates other types of inflammatory disease. (3) Chronic lobar pneumonia with fibrosis and decrease in size of the diseased lobe. This type resembles chronic pulmonary tuberculosis.

LEPTOSPIROSIS

Leptospirosis is produced by a group of spirochetes called *Leptospira*. Several clinical forms have been described and pulmonary involvement is only a part of widespread disease in most instances. Occasionally, hemorrhagic pneumonitis is an early or striking manifestation.

Roentgenographic Findings. The hemorrhagic pneumonitis usually results in widely disseminated small areas of air-space consolidation representing hemorrhage and edema. The individual lesions are poorly defined and hazy and resemble other acute, disseminated, pulmonary inflammations. A second type of leptospirosis is characterized by a large confluent area of consolidation similar to that found in lobar or segmental pneumonia. A third type cosists of small patchy densities that resemble bronchopneu-

monia or a more linear interstitial type of disease, such as is noted in virus pneumonitis. The diagnosis cannot be made on roentgen findings and depends upon bacteriologic studies.

PROTOZOAN DISEASES

AMEBIASIS

Amebic infection of the thorax is usually secondary to gastrointestinal involvement and often is associated with hepatic amebiasis. Rarely, amebic lung abscess if found without other signs or symptoms of amebiasis.

The roentgen signs are somewhat different in the two types of disease. In the pulmonary disease without hepatic abscess, parenchymal consolidation often complicated by abscess develops well above the diaphragm. The abscess is similar to lung abscess produced by other organisms. When the abscess is evacuated into a bronchus, an air–fluid level can be demonstrated in upright views. The abscess cavity may become very large, and associated pleural effusion is not uncommon. These lesions do not respond to conventional therapy.

When the pulmonary disease or pleural disease is secondary to hepatic involvement the appearance is somewhat more characteristic. The hepatic abscess causes elevation of the diaphragm. Fluid in the pleural space on the right is common. The lower and middle lobes adjacent to the diaphragm are involved by a confluent pneumonia in which cavitation may occur. In some instances the infection is confined to the pleural space in which case an amebic empyema is formed; this is often loculated at the base. In other instances, there is a combination of pleural and pulmonary involvement with empyema and lung abscess. The diagnosis is confirmed by the presence of *Endamoeba histolytica* in the sputum.

TOXOPLASMOSIS

Toxoplasmosis is caused by the protozoan parasite *Toxoplasma*. The organism has an affinity for the central nervous system, the eyes, and the lungs. There is an infantile form of the disease in which it is not uncommon to find cerebral involvement, beginning in utero, resulting in scattered intracranial calcifications in the newborn. The disease behaves differently in the adult and involves the lungs primarily rather than the central nervous system. The roentgen findings in the lungs are similar to those noted in bronchopneumonia or viral pneumonia, namely, that of an air-space disease often with some interstitial involvement. Hilar-node enlargement is frequently associated with the pulmonary involvement. Miliary dissemination produces miliary densities not unlike those noted in other acute miliary infections. If the disease becomes chronic, it may result in scattered areas of fibrosis and in scattered nodules, some or all of which may become calcified.

PNEUMOCYSTIS CARINII PNEUMONIA

Pneumocystis carinii pneumonia is caused by *Pneumocystis carinii*, a protozoan first observed in animals and thought to be a harmless saprophyte. However, epidemics and sporadic cases of the human disease have been reported in Europe since 1945. The disease has been apparently less frequent in the United States: the first case was reported in 1955. It usually occurs in premature or debilitated infants, in infants or children with agammaglobulinemia or low gamma globulin levels, and in debilitated adults who have been on long-term steroid therapy, antibiotics, cytotoxic drug therapy, or immunosuppressive drugs. It is not infrequent in renal transplant patients.

The clinical onset may be either rapid or insidious, but there is usually a discrepancy between the physical findings in the chest, which are minimal, and the marked dyspnea and often extensive roentgen findings. Pathologic findings are those of interstitial pneumonia, with mononuclear cells infiltrating the interstitial tissues; very few polymorphonuclear cells are present. The alveoli and alveolar ducts tend to be compressed by the interstitial involvement; there is often enough obstruction to result in peripheral obstructive emphysema. Interstitial and alveolar edema may be extensive in severe disease. Simultaneous cytomegalovirus infection is very common.

The roentgen findings are sometimes characteristic. The disease begins in the hilum and spreads peripherally; ultimately, it may involve the entire lung. There is an element of linear density spreading out from the hilum. The peripheral lungs are clear and may be "honeycombed" by local areas of emphysema and small areas of atelectasis. As the disease progresses, slight generalized involvement produces rather homogeneous density spreading outward from the hila. This may progress to the point of nearly total involvement, the lungs appearing virtually airless. Hilar adenopathy does not usually occur but has been reported in several patients recently. Pleural effusion is uncommon and tends to be minimal in amount. Pneumothorax and pneumomediastinum may occur. "Atypical" or unusual roentgenographic findings are quite common in this disease. Local seg-mental and lobar consolidation, which may be bilateral and symmetrical or asymmetrical and at times mainly unilateral, have been reported. The disease may also occur with no visible radiographic abnormalities of the chest. Since the pattern may not be characteristic the disease should always be considered when persistent and extensive pneumonic disease is found in immunosuppressed adults (Fig. 26-15), posttransplant patients, and debilitated infants. In the immunosuppressed patient with fever and hypoxemia, the disease should be suspected even though the chest rentgenogram shows no abnormality.

Since *Pneumocystis carinii* cannot be cultured and the disease it causes is usually fatal if treatment is not given, some form of biopsy or bronchial brushing is often necessary to obtain material for microbiologic study if sputum examination reveals no organisms in a patient suspected of having this disease.

PLATYHELMINTH (FLATWORM) INFESTATION

ECHINOCOCCOSIS (HYDATID DISEASE)

The small tapeworm, *Echinococcus granulosus,* is found in the intestinal tract of dogs. Its larval form is the cause of hydatid cysts. The ova are ingested by man and migrate to the liver, or to the lungs, where they produce a round or oval density that may become massive. Since the cyst is readily molded as it grows, the shape may be varied, depending on its relation to the bony thorax. A wall is formed, composed of an external capsule caused by the host tissue, the pericyst. The hydatid cyst has a double wall composed of an outer thick membrane (the exocyst) and a thin inner wall of germinal cells (the endocyst). The cyst may rupture into a bronchus and empty part of its contents, in which case an air–fluid level is noted. This indicates separation of the cyst from the host tissue capsule (pericyst). When this is observed, the roentgenographic diagnosis can be made with reasonable certainty. The collapsed cyst wall may float on the fluid surface and be outlined by air above it on an upright film. This is virtually pathognomonic of hydatid disease. Rarely, rupture of the pericyst or host capsule may leave air between it and the exocyst. The crescent or meniscus sign representing the radiolucent air between the cyst and the host may then be observed, a distinctive roentgen sign of hydatid cyst. The cyst wall rarely calcifies in the lung in contrast to the hepatic lesions in which calcification is common. When the cyst ruptures

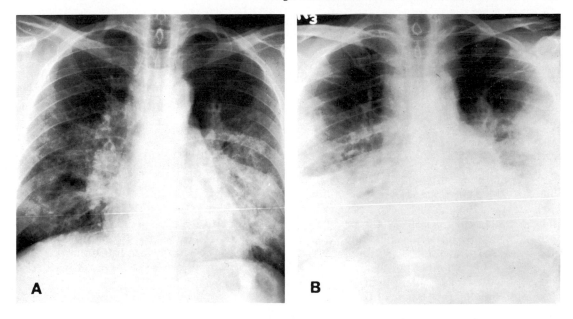

Fig. 26-15. Pneumocystis carinii pneumonia. **A.** Bilateral inflammatory disease with considerable consolidation in the left lower portion of the lung and more scattered disease at the right base. **B.** Examination 1 month later showed that, although the disease had advanced extensively bilaterally, it was confined to basal and central lung fields, sparing the upper lungs. This patient had lymphoma. We have observed wide variability in roentgenographic manifestations of this infestation.

there is a possibility of spread to other parts of the lung, giving rise to multiple, small, daughter cysts. Occasionally many small cysts are scattered throughout the lungs. Rarely the cysts may form in the pleural space or may rupture into the pleural space, resulting in pleural effusion. When calcified hydatid cysts are present in the liver and the presence of a cyst in the lung is detected, the diagnosis can be made with a considerable degree of accuracy.

CYSTICERCOSIS

Occasionally humans can develop autoinfection when they have the pork tapeworm, *Taenia solium.* In these individuals the cysticeri may be found scattered widely throughout the tissues, including the lungs, where they produce scattered soft-tissue nodular densities. When they die, calcification occurs and multiple oval or spindle-shaped calcifications measuring about 3 by 10 mm can then be noted, scattered in the lung fields and in other tissues as well. The disease, cysticercosis, is very rare in the United States.

PARAGONIMIASIS

The lung fluke, *Paragonimus westermani,* is distributed widely in the Far East, Africa, and in parts of South America, and has been further disseminated by the military.[30] Hemoptysis is a frequent symptom of infestation with this organism, along with cough and chest pain. In about one-third of those infested the organism causes an ill-defined consolidation in the lung in the form of a hazy shadow of low, uneven density. In about another one-third, the density is more homogeneous, more clearly defined, and may appear lobulated. Thin-walled, cystlike cavitation may develop within the area of consolidation. Often the cavities are multiple and have a bubblelike appearance. In some of the patients, the disease may be manifest by linear streaks that may appear within a shadow of low-density consolidation. The involved area does not usually occupy a very large volume of the lung and may be unilateral or bilateral. In two-thirds of the patients the mid zones of the lungs are involved, while in the remainder the upper and lower portions are implicated. The pulmonary disease is often not very conspicuous because of the small volume of lung involved and the low density of the disease. Pleural thickening in the interlobar fissures is also observed and fleeting densities thought to represent Löffler's pneumonia often accompany the disease. Dense linear opacities are caused by burrows of the organism which can be demonstrated by bronchography to be independent of bronchi. The burrows probably communicate with the cavities.

SCHISTOSOMIASIS

Schistosomiasis is caused by any one of three blood flukes, *Schistosoma mansoni, S. japonicum,* or *S. haematobium.* Several types of pulmonary reaction to the infestation may occur. As the larval forms pass through the lungs, an apparent allergic response produces transient mottled densities. Ova reach the lungs from the veins of the bladder, intestine, and liver where they may implant in or around the arterioles producing necrotizing arteritis and intra-arterial and peri-arterial granulomas. Either of these granulomas may obstruct the vessel. The organisms rarely may cause multiple arteriovenous fistulas.

Roentgen findings in the chronic form consist of central enlargement of pulmonary arteries secondary to pulmonary hypertension, evidence of cor pulmonale, and a rather minimal amount of interstitial fibrosis causing accentuation of reticular lung markings. At times, the appearance is more nodular, as reaction to the ova produces a local density in the interstitial tissue of the lung. The multiple arteriovenous fistulas result in cyanosis with very little change note on roentgenograms; this is a rare phenomenon. Occasionally a circumscribed nodule or mass is produced by a granulomatous mass surrounding an adult worm.

NEMATHELMINTH (ROUNDWORM) INFESTATION

A number of roundworms cause pulmonary symptoms and transitory roentgen changes in the lungs as the larvae are carried to the lungs through the veins or lymphatics. As the larvae emerge from the alveolar capillaries into the bronchial tree they produce an allergic response, usually accompanied by eosinophilia. A combination of edema and hemorrhage causes radiographic findings of patchy areas of poorly defined density scattered throughout the lungs. The changes are transitory and their extent is related to the severity of the infestation. The following roundworms are among those which cause such a reaction: *Ascaris lumbricoides, Strongyloides stercoralis, Ancylostoma duodenale,* and *Necator americanus* (hookworm disease). Opportunistic pulmonary strongyloidiasis has been reported in compromised hosts and may be fatal.[13] However, it will respond to treatment with antihelminthic agents if recognized soon enough. Filariasis due to infestation with *Filaria* or *Wuchereria bancrofti, Wuchereria malayi,* or *Loa loa* are probably causes of tropical eosinophilia. *Dirofilaria immitis* (dog heartworm) may also cause pulmonary disease in humans. Typically it produces a solitary pulmonary nodule. Because no symptoms are present, histologic examination of tissue is required to differentiate the nodule from tumor. *Trichinella spiralis* larvae usually produce no pulmonary reaction as they pass through the pulmonary circulation. In the roundworm infestations the diagnosis is made by discovery of the larvae or mature worm in the stool specimen.

TROPICAL EOSINOPHILIA

Tropical eosinophilia or pulmonary eosinophilosis is manifested by symptoms of cough, fever, lassitude, wheezing, chest pain, and sometimes dyspnea and weight loss associated with an elevation of the white blood-cell count. There is a relative and absolute eosinophilia in the peripheral blood. The eosinophilia is extreme (usually over 3000 eosinophils per cu mm of blood) and persists for weeks. Most of the reported cases originate in India, Indonesia, Sri Lanka, Pakistan, and Southeast Asia. A few have been reported in the United States and elsewhere throughout the world, largely in persons who have been in an endemic area. There have also been some cases reported in persons who have lived in India but who have been away more than a year before onset of symptoms. The disease is mild and self-limited but relapses may occur. Most of the cases are definitely caused by filarial infestation and the disease usually responds well to diethylcarbamazine, a drug effective in filariasis.[28] In other cases, the cause cannot be established.

Roentgen findings are of several types. The most common appearance is that of increased pulmonary markings extending out from the hila, associated with mottled parenchymal disease that is rather general in distribution. The hilar nodes may be enlarged. Next in frequency is the addition of areas of patchy pneumonitis to the small mottled densities. Increased markings alone are nearly as frequent, and extensive scattered involvement by a pneumonialike process is noted occasionally.

SARCOIDOSIS

Sarcoidosis, or Boeck's sarcoid, is a granulomatous disease that may affect many organs and tissues in the body. The etiology is not clear. A number of theories have been advanced but none has been proved. It is probably the result of interaction between an infective agent (not necessarily the same in all patients) and an individual with unusual immunologic responses. It is known that most patients show no reaction or only slightly positive reaction to tuberculin and 10% to 20% of patients with sarcoidosis develop frank tuberculosis. The lesion of sarcoidosis is a focal granuloma of epithelioid cells in which giant cells are usually present. Lymphocytes are generally noted around the periphery along with occasional eosinophils. The process resembles a tuberculous granuloma except that there is no central caseation necrosis. These lesions develop slowly and may resolve completely in some instances. They may also heal by a process of sclerosis leading to fibrosis and tissue distortion that may be extensive. Pulmonary involvement is frequent; the reported incidence ranges from 90% to 95%. These figures include enlargement of hilar and paratracheal nodes as well as pulmonary parenchymal lesions.

Roentgen Findings. Since sarcoidosis may be asymptomatic or nearly so for long periods of time, the roentgenographic changes produced by it are often noted for the first time in a survey film or on roentgenograms obtained as a part of an examination performed prior to entrance into the armed services or industry. It is therefore somewhat difficult to be certain that the findings observed in these asymptomatic patients represent early disease.

Roentgen findings can be classified as follows[18, 27]

1. Hilar and paratracheal adenopathy without parenchymal inolvement (Fig. 26-16). This occurs at some time during the course of the disease in over 90% of patients with sarcoidosis. Although bilateral hilar and right paratracheal adenopathy have been reported as characteristic of the disease, a recent study of 62 patients with sarcoidosis showed that bilateral adenopathy was the most common followed by adenopathy in the right paratracheal or aortopulmonary window area on the left. Over a third had a combination of bilateral hilar adenopathy, right paratracheal adenopathy, and aortopulmonary window nodes.

2. Adenopathy with parenchymal involvement. The parenchymal involvement includes a diffuse accentuation of interstitial markings resulting in a reticular pattern, a miliary nodular patern, and a reticular pattern plus miliary nodules (reticulonodular) or plus somewhat larger nodules (Figs. 26-17 and 26-18). This combination of an increase in linear interstitial shadows plus nodules, the reticulonodular pattern, is much more common than either of the changes occurring alone. An air-space or acinar type of disease may also occur in the lungs. It resembles an acute inflammatory process with poorly defined periphery and, at times, an air bronchogram. The amount of general interstitial change may be varied when associated with nodularity. There is often an inverse relationship between the adenopathy and parenchymal disease, the latter increasing while the adenopathy regresses. This does not ordinarily occur in Hodgkin's disease from which sarcoidosis must be differentiated.

3. Parenchymal involvement without adenopathy.

4. Fibrotic change progressing to pulmonary insufficiency, with cor pulmonale. There may be extensive distortion with conglomerate areas of fibrosis and emphysema. This is the late irreversible form of the disease (Fig. 26-19). It occurs in 20% to 25% of patients with sarcoidosis. It is somewhat more frequent in patients with the acinar form than in those having other forms of sarcoidosis.

5. Large nodular densities which range up to 5 cm or more in size are occasionally found (Fig. 26-20). They resemble hematogenous pulmonary metastases to some extent, but are not as clearly defined, since the periphery of the individual nodules tends to be indistinct. They may become confluent. We have also observed a unilateral solitary nodular mass that resembled primary lung tumor in one instance.

Late in the disease a somewhat cystic pattern may be observed, usually associated with extensive fibrosis which results in bullous emphysema. Pleural involvement is very rare. When present, it may cause pleural effusion and pleural thickening. It is so unusual that causes other than sarcoidosis should be sought when it occurs. Mycetoma (fungus ball) is found occasionally in pulmonary sarcoidosis. Other occasional findings include spontaneous pneumothorax and atelectasis, the latter evidently secondary to endobronchial involvement. Cavitation in one of the larger nodules may occur rarely in patients with disease manifested by large nodules. Solitary pulmonary nodule is another manifestation that is very rare. Since the roentgen findings in this disease are so varied, sarcoidosis must be considered in all asymptomatic patients with unusual pulmonary roentgenographic findings.

All these manifestations can be seen at various

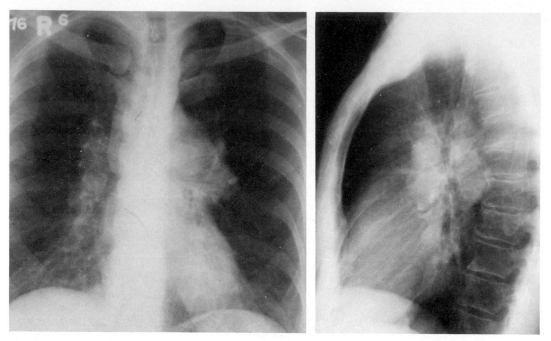

Fig. 26-16. Sarcoidosis. Hilar and right paratracheal adenopathy which is rather characteristic of sarcoidosis.

Fig. 26-17. Sarcoidosis. In this patient there is bilateral hilar adenopathy, some paratracheal adenopathy (more on the right than on the left), and moderately extensive pulmonary parenchymal involvement manifested by small, widely scattered nodules and a little increase in interstitial density.

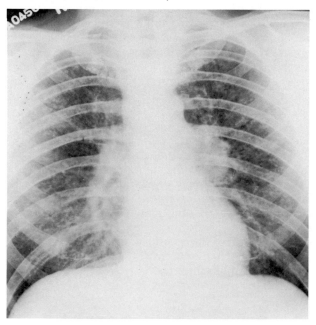

times in a single patient and the mediastinal adenopathy has been observed to regress and reappear in patients with disseminated pulmonary lesions. The node enlargement is often massive but is usually symmetric in the hila and the descriptive term "potato" nodes has been applied to the large masses. The enlarged nodes form slightly lobulated masses extending throughout the lung hilum. Characteristically there is a relatively translucent space between the mass of nodes and the cardiovascular margin. This is more apparent on the right side, where the lung hilum normally is better seen than on the left. In contrast, Hodgkin's disease, which is a frequent source of difficulty in differential diagnosis, is more likely to involve the more centrally situated nodes around the tracheal bifurcation in addition to those in the hila and the mass of nodes tends to merge with the cardiovascular silhouette.

The radiographic findings are of some prognostic significance since those patients in whom hilar and paratracheal adenopathy are observed without pulmonary parenchymal involvement often regress to complete disappearance of the large nodes over a period of months or years. Miliary nodular or reticulonodular disease with or without adenopathy also regresses completely in most patients. Steroids are

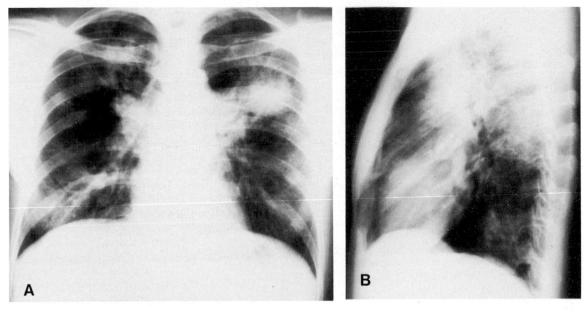

Fig. 26-18. "Alveolar" sarcoidosis. Note the hilar adenopathy and the large poorly defined areas of parenchymal involvement lateral to the left hilum in the right clavicular area and at the right base in the front view **A.** Basal disease is not very well outlined in the lateral view **(B)**.

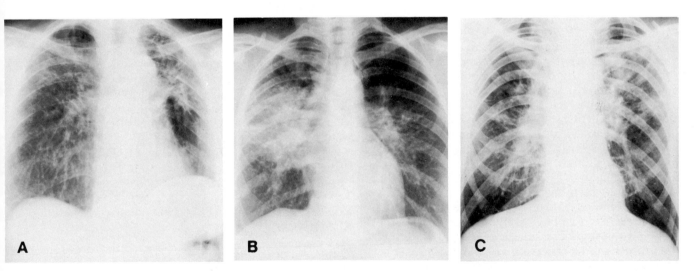

Fig. 26-19. Sarcoidosis. Extensive chronic disease in three patients. **A.** Fibrosis with elevation of the hila is evident in this patient. **B.** In this patient unusual asymmetry is noted. **C.** Hilar adenopathy persists along with extensive parenchymal involvement in the third patient.

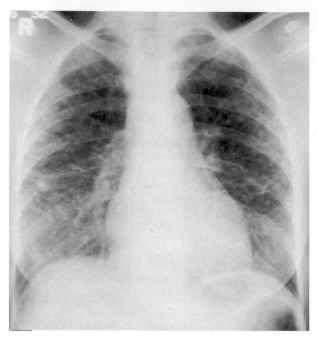

Fig. 26-20. Sarcoidosis. Example of extensive parenchymal involvement that is somewhat reticulonodular. Some of the nodules appear rather large. No evidence of hilar adenopathy is observed.

used effectively in some patients, in others the process undergoes spontaneous regression.

The roentgen diagnosis of sardoidosis can often be made with a considerable degree of certainty. The symmetry of the bilateral, hilar node enlargement along with the frequent associated enlargement of the right paratracheal and aortopulmonary window nodes is characteristic. The pulmonary parenchymal involvement is often symmetric also and this is of diagnostic importance. The discrepancy between the extensive roentgen changes and the mild symptoms is the third finding of diagnostic significance. Finally, when progress roentgenograms are available, the long and slowly progressing or regressing nature of the process can be observed. The diagnosis must be confirmed by the presence of the typical granuloma in involved nodes; therefore it is necessary to perform scalene node biopsy or a lung biopsy to secure positive proof of the disease. The fibrotic stage of the disease is probably irreversible to a certain extent, but improvement has been obtained in some patients by the use of steroids.

Differential Diagnosis. Pulmonary lesions of sarcoidosis can simulate those of pulmonary tuberculosis to such a degree that bacteriologic and histopathologic studies are required to make differentiation. It is often possible, however, to be fairly certain of the diagnosis because of the relative lack of symptoms in the patient with sarcoidosis. In differentiation between sarcoidosis and carinomatosis the wasting and weakness usually noted in patients with carcinomatosis and the presence of a known primary tumor along with clinical and roentgen findings make the diagnosis of carcinomatosis almost certain. Hodgkin's disease and lymphosarcoma may result in mediastinal lymph-node enlargement, which cannot be differentiated from that noted in sarcoidosis. However, these conditions usually produce more symptoms than does sarcoidosis and the adenopathy is not as symmetric as in sarcoidosis. The more benign types of Hodgkin's disease, however, may be relatively asymptomatic and biopsy is then necessary to differentiate the two diseases. In general the nodes are larger in Hodgkin's disease than in sarcoidosis. Other chronic pulmonary lesions such as mycotic infections, the benign pneumoconioses, and a number of conditions producing interstitial pulmonary fibrosis may result in densities in the lungs similar to those noted in sarcoidosis. In these patients all clinical data must be evaluated along with the history in order to make the differentiation. Even then it is often necessary to obtain biopsy specimens of available peripheral or scalene nodes, or of the lung. In some patients with the characteristic lesions and clinical symptoms of erythema nodosum, roentgen examination of the chest will reveal enlarged hilum nodes and, occasionally, linear and patchy infiltrations in the perihilar zones, resembling in all respects the changes of sarcoid disease. This does not necessarily indicate that the primary disease is sarcoidosis, but the combination of findings is very suggestive of this diagnosis.

REFERENCES AND SELECTED READINGS

1. BIRK M, GERSTL B: Torulosis (cryptococcosis) producing solitary pulmonary lesion. JAMA 149: 1310, 1952

2. CHAIT A: Schistosomiasis mansoni: roentgenologic observations in a nonendemic area. Am J Roentgenol 90: 688, 1963

3. CHARTRES JC: Radiological manifestations of parasitism by the tongue worms, flat worms and the round worms more commonly seen in the tropics. Br J Radiol 38: 503, 1965

4. CONANT NF, SMITH DT, BAKER RG et al: Manual of Clinical Mycology. Philadelphia, Saunders, 1954

5. Doub HP: Miliary calcification of the lung: etiologic aspects. Radiology 51: 480, 1948

6. Drutz DD, Catanzaro A: Coccidioidomycosis. State of the art, Part II. Am Rev Resp Dis 117: 727, 1978

7. Falkenbach KH, Bachmann KD, O'Loughlin BJ: Pneumocystis carinii pneumonia. Am J Roentgenol 85: 706, 1961

8. Felson B: Less familiar patterns of pulmonary granulomas. Am J Roentgenol 81: 211, 1959

9. Goodwin RA Jr, Des Prez RM: Histoplasmosis. State of the art. Am Rev Resp Dis 117: 929, 1978

10. Grossman CB, Bragg DG, Armstrong D: Roentgen manifestations of pulmonary nocardiosis. Radiology 96: 325, 1970

11. Gunderson GA, Nice CM Jr: Nocardiosis: a case report and brief review of the literature. Radiology 68: 31, 1957

12. Hammerman KJ, Powell KE, Christianson CS et al: Pulmonary cryptococcosis: clinical forms and treatment. Am Rev Resp Dis 108: 1116, 1973

13. Higenbottam TW, Heard BE: Opportunistic pulmonary strongyloidiasis complicating asthma treated with steroids. Thorax 31: 226, 1976

14. Hollingsworth G: Gumma of lung. Br J Radiol 24: 467, 1951

15. Holt JF: Roentgenologic pulmonary manifestations of fatal histoplasmosis. Am J Roentgenol 58: 717, 1947

16. Jacobs JB, Vogel C, Powell RD et al: Needle biopsy in Pneumocystis carinii pneumonia. Radiology 93: 525, 1969

17. Jacobs LG: Pulmonary torulosis. Am J Roentgenol 71: 398, 1958

18. Kirks DR, Greenspan RH: Sarcoid. Radiol Clin North Am 11: 279, 1973

19. Kunstadter RH, Milzer A, Whitcomb F: Bronchopulmonary geotrichosis in children. Am J Dis Child 79: 82, 1950

20. Lenczner M, Spaulding WB, Sanders DE: Pulmonary manifestations of parasitic infections. Can Med Assoc J 91: 421, 1964

21. Leonardi HK, Lapey JD, Ellis FH Jr: Pulmonary dirofilariasis: report of a human case. Thorax 32: 612, 1977

22. Malo JL, Pepys J, Simon G: Studies in chronic allergic bronchopulmonary aspergillosis. 2. Radiological findings. Thorax 32: 262, 1977

23. Marchand EJ, Marcial-Rojas RA, Rodriguez R et al: The pulmonary obstruction syndrome in Schistosoma mansoni pulmonary endarteritis. Arch Intern Med 100: 965, 1957

24. Mayer JH, Ackerman AJ: Sarcoidosis. Am Rev Tuberc 61: 299, 1950

25. McCarthy DS, Simon G, Hargreave FE: The radiological appearances in allergic bronchopulmonary aspergillosis. Clin Radiol 21: 366, 1970

26. McGavran MH, Kobayashi G, Newmark L et al: Pulmonary sporotrichosis. Dis Chest 56: 547, 1969

27. Mitchell DN, Scadding JG: Sarcoidosis. State of the art. Am Rev Resp Dis 110: 774, 1974

28. Neva FA, Ottesen EA: Tropical (filarial) eosinophilia. Engl J Med 298: 1129, 1978

29. Nitter L: Changes in the chest roentgenogram in Boeck's sarcoid of the lungs. Acta Radiol [Suppl] (Stockh) 105, 1953

30. Ogakwu M, Nwokolo C: Radiological findings in pulmonary paragonimiasis as seen in Nigeria: a review based on 100 cases. Br J Radiol 46: 699, 1973

31. Palayew MJ, Frank H, Sedlezky I: Our experience with histoplasmosis: an analysis of seventy cases with follow-up study. J Can Assoc Radiol 17: 142, 1966

32. Pitchenik AE, Zaunbrecher F: Superior vena cava syndrome caused by *Nocardia Asteroides*. Am Rev Resp Dis 117: 795, 1978

33. Putnam JS, Harper WK, Green JF Jr et al: Coccidioides immitis. A rare cause of pulmonary mycetoma. Am Rev Resp Dis 112: 733, 1975

34. Rabinowitz JG, Busch J, Buttram WR: Pulmonary manifestations of blastomycosis. Radiology 120: 25, 1976

35. Reeder MM: RPC of the month from the AFIP (hydatid cyst). Radiology 95: 429, 1970

36. Schwarz J, Baum GL: Fungus diseases of the lungs. Semin Roentgenol V: 1, 1970

37. Shaw RR: Thoracic complications of amebiasis. Surg Gynecol Obstet 88: 753, 1949

38. Silverstein CM: Pulmonary manifestations of leptospirosis. Radiology 61: 327, 1953

39. Slade PR, Slesser BV, Southgate J: Thoracic actinomycosis. Thorax 28: 73, 1973

40. Sullivan BH Jr, Bailey FN: Amebic lung abscess. Dis Chest 20: 84, 1951

41. Taylor AB, Briney AK: Observations on pulmonary cocciodioidomycosis. Ann Intern Med 30: 1224, 1949

27

DISEASES OF OCCUPATIONAL, CHEMICAL, AND PHYSICAL ORIGIN

THE "MALIGNANT" PNEUMOCONIOSES

The term "pneumoconiosis" refers to the group of conditions in which solid foreign substances are inhaled and stored in the lung. These conditions form a group of occupational diseases of considerable economic importance. Many foreign materials are capable of producing fibrosis leading to decrease in pulmonary function termed the "malignant pneumoconioses," while those conditions produced by substances that do not cause significant fibrosis are termed "benign." The malignant pneumoconioses include the following: (1) silicosis; (2) asbestosis; (3) talcosis; (4) bauxite fibrosis (shaver's disease); (5) coal worker's pneumoconiosis; (6) diatomite pneumoconiosis; and (7) berylliosis. (The latter condition is somewhat different from the others listed and is more properly termed "beryllium granulomatosis" or "beryllium poisoning." In addition, there is a large sensitivity factor. It is an occupational disease and is therefore related to the pneumoconioses and will be included in the present discussion.)

A number of substances may cause benign pneumoconiosis. They are: (1) coal dust (anthracosis); (2) iron oxide (siderosis); (3) barium sulfate (baritosis); and (4) tin (stannosis). Benign changes have also been reported with exposure to titanium oxide and tungsten carbide. Some of these dust diseases occur together and such terms as "anthrasilicosis" and "siderosilicosis" are then used to designate them.

SILICOSIS

Silicosis is caused by inhalation of particles of silicon dioxide that are less than 5 μ in diameter. The most active particles in producing the fibrotic reaction are those smaller than 3 μ. When these small particles are deposited in the alveoli, they are ingested by phagocytic cells. A succession of macrophages are killed, eventually resulting in formation of collagen around the area. A silicotic nodule that is relatively acellular is produced in alveoli, respiratory bronchioles, lymphatics, and lymphoid tissue. Some of them remain in the peripheral lymphoid follicles while others reach the intrapulmonary, bronchial, hilar, and paratracheal nodes. There is now some evidence to suggest that an adsorbed protein on the silica particle acts as an antigen which results eventually in an antibody reaction. This would explain the long latent period as well as progression of the disease long after the patient has been removed from exposure to silica. Silicosis is found in a large number of industries including mining, foundries, and rock drilling, as well as grinding involving the production of silica dust. The development of fibrosis requires time. Even in the most dusty occupations the average time for development of disease in workers exposed to moderate concentrations of silica is 10 to 15 years. One or 2 years of exposure are required when dust counts are unusually high. This "acute" silicosis produced by excessive exposure over relatively short periods of time may progress to severe respiratory failure and death within a year of the onset of symptoms.

Roentgen classification of silicosis and the pneumoconioses is difficult and a number of conferences and committees have presented new classifications from time to time. A classification has been published by a committee of experts under the auspices of the International Labour Office. The committee has made available a set of standardized films for comparison with roentgenograms of patients with pneumoconiosis. They have also introduced and defined standard descriptive terms. The one presented here (Tables 27-1 and 27-2) was published in 1970. The reader is referred to the original publication for information regarding it.[30]

There is now an ILO U/C 1971 International Classification of Radiographs of the Pneumoconioses[14] which should be consulted for additional information, since there are some minor changes in designation of large opacities and major changes in the system for coding pleural thickening. Of course the roentgen findings must be related to occupational history and to appropriate clinical and laboratory findings; this is true of all of the pneumoconioses.

Roentgen Observations. The earliest radiographic change produced by silicosis is slight exaggeration of the pulmonary interstitial markings. This is difficult to evaluate because many other conditions can produce the same change and the diagnosis of silicosis cannot be made on the basis of these early findings alone. Scattered pulmonary nodules are found somewhat later in the disease. At first the nodules are discrete and very small, on the order of 1 to 2 mm. At this stage, an additive effect of multiplicity is necessary to make them visible. Superimposition is probably a factor also. They are usually distributed symmetrically and widely with some tendency to spare the apices and bases. Along with the presence of the scattered nodules, there is usually enough enlargement of hilar nodes to produce a radiographically recognizable increase in hilar size. As the pulmonary nodules increase in size, they tend to become conglomerate. The conglomeration and coalescence are usually accompanied by retraction toward the hilum, leaving the periphery of the lung relatively free of nodules and emphysematous. By the time this stage is reached there is often enough emphysema present to cause a downward displacement of the diaphragm and a decrease in diaphragmatic motion on respiration. There can be a considerable variation in the relative amounts of nodulation, hilar enlargement, and emphysema. The hilar nodes may undergo fibrosis and decrease in size by the time the nodular parenchymal lesions are large enough to be readily visualized. Occasionally there is actual calcification in the silicotic nodules. This is a manifestation of long-standing disease. In addition to the more extensive classifications given earlier, which are used for industrial health purposes, the roentgen changes in simple silicosis have been classified into stages or degrees as follows:

Stage I (early nodular). Prominence or exaggeration of markings with faintly visible nodules (Fig. 27-1).

Stage II. Nodules 2 to 3 mm in size that tend to obscure linear markings (Fig. 27-2).

Stage III (Fig. 27-3). Nodules greater than 3 mm with coalescence.

The use of this classification does not indicate that the roentgen changes develop uniformly or that all patients eventually develop the lesions of third-stage silicosis. Therefore, descriptive terms such as early nodular, nodular, and conglomerate nodular are often used to describe the findings in uncomplicated silicosis. The hilar nodes are sometimes outlined because of the presence of a thin shell of calcium surrounding them. This has been termed "eggshell calcification" and when present it is very suggestive of silicosis, but this type of calcification has also been described in patients with no exposure to silica or silicates (Fig. 27-4). Rarely, an "eggshell" node may erode a bronchial wall and become a broncholith.

The diagnosis of silicosis can often be suspected on roentgen examination, but the clinical history is of great importance, since the diagnosis cannot be accurately made unless there is a history of enough exposure to silica-containing dust to produce it. Because workers in dusty industries are often followed at in-

Table 27-1. UICC/Cincinnati Classification of Radiographic Appearances of Pneumoconioses[30]

		CODES	DEFINITIONS
Small opacities	Rounded profusion		The category of profusion is based on assessment of the concentration of opacities in the affected zones. The standard films define the mid-categories.
		0/- 0/0 0/1	Category 0—small rounded opacities absent or less profuse than in category 1.
		1/0 1/1 1/2	Category 1—small rounded opacities definitely present but relatively few in number.
		2/1 2/2 2/3	Category 2—small rounded opacities numerous. The normal lung markings are usually still visible.
		3/2 3/3 3/4	Category 3—small rounded opacities very numerous. The normal lung markings are partly or totally obscured.
	Type	p q r	The nodules are classified according to the approximate diameter of the predominant opacities. p—rounded opacities up to about 1.5 mm in diameter. q—rounded opacities exceeding about 1.5 mm and up to about 3 mm in diameter. r—rounded opacities exceeding about 3 mm and up to about 10 mm in diameter.
	Extent	Lung zones	The zones in which the opacities are seen are recorded. Each lung is divided into thirds—upper, middle, lower zones. Thus a maximum of six zones can be affected.
	Irregular profusion		The category of profusion is based on assessment of the concentration of opacities in the affected zones. The standard films define the mid-categories.
		0/- 0/0 0/1	Category 0—small irregular opacities absent or less profuse than in category 1.
		1/0 1/1 1/2	Category 1—small irregular opacities definitely present but relatively few in number. The normal lung markings are usually visible.
		2/1 2/2 2/3	Category 2—small irregular opacities numerous. The normal lung markings are usually partly obscured.
		3/2 3/3 3/4	Category 3—small irregular opacities very numerous. The normal lung markings are usually totally obscured.
	Type	s t u	As the opacities are irregular, the dimensions used for rounded opacities cannot be used, but they can be roughly divided into three types. s—fine irregular or linear opacities t—medium irregular opacities u—coarse (blotchy) irregular opacities
	Extent	Lung zones	The zones in which the opacities are seen are recorded. Each lung is divided into thirds—upper, middle, lower zones—as for rounded opacities.
Large opacities	Size	A B C	Category A—an opacity with greatest diameter between 1 cm and 5 cm, or several such opacities the sum of whose greatest diameters does not exceed 5 cm. Category B—one or more opacities larger or more numerous than those in category A, whose combined area does not exceed one third of the area of the right lung. Category C—one or more large opacities whose combined area exceeds one third of the area of the right lung.
	Type	wd id	As well as the letter "A," "B" or "C," the abbreviation "wd" or "id" should be used to indicate whether the opacities are well defined or ill defined.
Other features	Pleural thickening costophrenic angle	Right Left	Obliteration of the costophrenic angle is recorded separately from thickening over other sites. A lower-limit standard film is provided.
	Other sites	1 2 3	Grade 0—not present or less than grade 1 Grade 1—up to 5 mm thick and not exceeding one-half of the projection of one lateral chest wall. A lower-limit standard film is provided. Grade 2—more than 5 mm thick and up to one-half of the projection of one lateral chest wall or up to 5 mm thick and exceeding one-half of the projection of one lateral chest wall.

Table 27-1. (continued)

	CODES		DEFINITIONS
			Grade 3—more than 5 mm thick and extending more than one-half of the projection of one lateral chest wall.
Diaphragm ill defined	Right	Left	The lower limit is one-third of the affected hemidiaphragm. A lower limit standard film is provided.
Cardiac outline ill defined (shagginess)		1 2 3	Grade 0—up to one-third of the length of the left cardiac border or equivalent. Grade 1—above one-third and up to two-thirds of the length of the left cardiac border or equivalent. Grade 2—above two-thirds and up to the whole length of the left cardiac border or equivalent. Grade 3—more than the whole length of the left cardiac border or equivalent.
Pleural calcification diaphragm walls other sites		1 2 3	Grade 0—no pleural calcification seen Grade 1—one or more areas of pleural calcification, the sum of whose greatest diameters does not exceed 2 cm Grade 2—one or more areas of pleural calcification, the sum of whose greatest diameters exceeds 2 cm but does not exceed 10 cm Grade 3—one or more areas of pleural calcification, the sum of whose greatest diameters exceeds 10 cm

Other symbols
  Obligatory
    ca —suspect cancer of lung or pleura
    co —a normality of cardiac size or shape
    cp —suspect cor pulmonale
    es —eggshell calcification of hilar or mediastinal lymph nodes
    tba—opacities suggestive of active clinically significant tuberculosis
    od —other significant disease. This includes disease not related to dust exposure, e.g., surgical or traumatic damage to chest walls, bronchiectasis, etc.
  Optional
    ax —coalescence of small rounded pneumoconiotic opacities
    bu —bullae
    cn —calcification in small parenchymal opacities
    cv —cavity
    di —marked distortion of the intrathoracic organs
    em—marked emphysema
    hi —marked enlargement of hilar shadows
    ho —honeycomb lung
    k   —Kerley's (septal) lines
    px —pneumothorax
    rl —pneumoconiosis modified by rheumatoid process
    tb —inactive tuberculosis.

From UICC/Cincinnati classification of the radiographic appearances of pneumoconiosis. *Chest 58:* 57, 1970.[30]

tervals by means of chest roentgenograms, a review of these serial films will often lead to an accurate diagnosis. Extensive roentgen findings can be present without much alteration in pulmonary function; the reverse is also true in some instances; therefore, there may be lack of correlation between roentgen appearance and pulmonary function.

SILICOTUBERCULOSIS

Silicosis appears to predispose to pulmonary tuberculosis. Massive areas of density representing conglomerate fibrosis are seen late in the course of silicosis and some believe that infection is necessary to produce these large masses. The typical location for massive conglomerate fibrosis is above and lateral to the lung hilum in the infraclavicular part of the lung field. The masses are usually bilateral and relatively symmetric in size and location. Usually the mass does not reach to the periphery of the lung field; rather a zone of emphysematous lung is to be seen lateral to the area of fibrosis, the emphysema developing as the involved lung shrinks because of the fibrosis. The typical configuration caused by these masses of fibrous tissue in relation to the central mediastinal shadow has been likened to the "wings of an angel." Atypical forms of conglomerate fibrosis are

Table 27-2. U.I.C.C./Cincinnati Classification of

Sketch Number	Quality	ROUNDED SMALL OPACITIES			IRREGULAR SMALL OPACITIES			LARGE OPACITIES	
		Type	Profusion	Zones R L	Type	Profusion	Zones R L	Type	Size
1		p	2/2	✓ ✓ / ✓ ✓		0/0			0
2		q	1/2	✓ ✓ / ✓		0/0			0
3		r	3/3	✓ ✓ / ✓ ✓ / ✓ ✓		0/0			0
4			0/0		s	2/1	✓ / ✓ ✓		0
5			0/0		t	3/2	✓ ✓ / ✓ ✓		0
6			0/0		u	2/1	✓ ✓		0
7		q	2/2	✓ ✓ / ✓ ✓		0/0		wd	B
8			0/0		t	3/4	✓ ✓ / ✓ ✓ / ✓ ✓	id	B
9		r	1/0	✓ ✓ / ✓ ✓		0/0			0
10		p	2/1	✓ ✓ / ✓ ✓	s	2/3	✓ ✓ / ✓ ✓		0
	+ ± ± U/R	p q r	0/- 0/0 0/1 1/0 1/1 1/2 2/1 2/2 2/3 3/2 3/3 3/4	Check zones involved	s t u	0/- 0/0 0/1 1/0 1/1 1/2 2/1 2/2 2/3 3/2 3/3 3/4	Check zones involved	wd id	0 A B C

not uncommon. Thus a mass of fibrous tissue may be present in one lung and not in the other; the lesions may occur in areas other than the subclavicular zones; massive fibrosis may be present with little or none of the characteristic nodulation of silicosis in the rest of the lung fields. When massive fibrosis is observed in the presence of nodular silicosis, pulmonary tuberculosis should be suspected (Fig. 27-5). Cavitation occurs in silicotuberculosis, but it is also observed in the absence of infection. Bacteriologic confirmation is necessary. This is sometimes very difficult to obtain. In the absence of positive bacteriologic findings, silicotuberculosis should be suspected when the roentgenograms reveal the large conglomerate masses in the upper lung fields, when cavitation is present, when the disease is asymmetric, and when there is a considerable amount of pleural disease. Patients with such roentgenographic findings

Radiographic Appearances of Pneumoconioses[30]

Costophrenic angle	PLEURAL THICKENING				ILL DEFINED DIAPHRAGM	ILL DEFINED CARDIAC OUTLINE	PLEURAL CALCIFICATION					Symbols	Comments
	Diffuse	Plaques	Grade	None			Diaphragm	Wall	Other	Grade	None		
0				0	0	0					0	0	0
R				0	0	0					0	0	0
0				0	0	0					0	es ax	0
0				0	0	0	L R	L R	L R	3		cp	0
0	L R		3	0	0						0	ho	0
0		L	1	0	0						0	ca	ca = mesothelioma effusion
0				0	0	0					0	bu	0
L R	L R		1	L R	3						0	0	0
L R				0	0	0					0	di tba cv	?silico-tuberculosis
0				0	0	0					0	ca k	0
0 R L	R L	1 2 3	0 if none	0 R L	0 1 2 3		R L		1 2 3	0 if none	0 ca es co od cp tba		

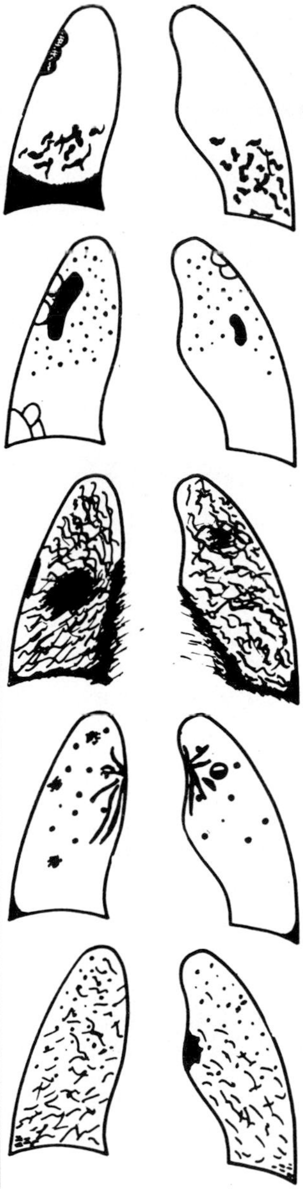

6
7
8
9
10

should be followed carefully by means of frequent chest roentgenograms and bacteriologic examination of sputum and gastric washings because of the high incidence of tuberculosis. Cavitation in conglomerate nodular silicosis is not always caused by tuberculosis, however. In one series of 182 patients with cavitation, 18% were found to be nontuberculous. In these patients the cavity results from ischemic necrosis within the conglomerate mass.

ASBESTOSIS

Asbestos, a hydrated magnesium silicate, is a fibrous mineral used as an insulator against heat and cold and as a fireproofing material. The most important, from the standpoint of pneumoconiosis, is the serpentine mineral, chrysotile (white asbestos), which is magnesium silicate. This makes up 90% of the total world production of asbestos. The other impor-

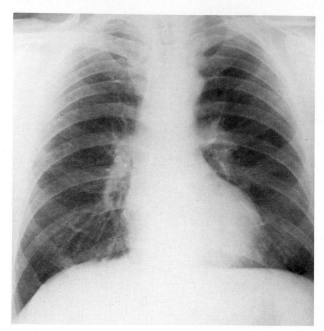

Fig. 27-1. Silicosis. There are scattered small nodules associated with minimal prominence of interstitial markings representing early nodular silicosis (category I, UICC).

Fig. 27-3. Category C silicosis. There is basal emphysema as well as conglomerate nodular disease, which is extensive in both lungs. This is the old third-stage or conglomerate nodular form of silicosis.

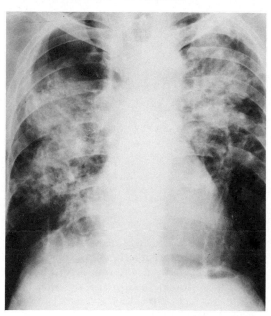

Fig. 27-2. Silicosis. The disease is more advanced than in the patient shown in Fig. 27-1. The nodules are larger, much more easily outlined, and probably more profuse. There is also hilar node enlargement. This type of silicosis is similar to that of category III, or to second-stage silicosis in the old classification.

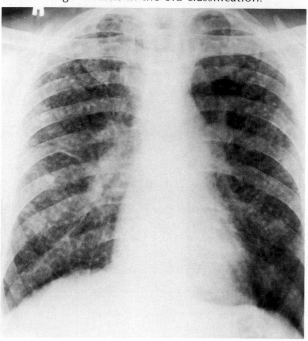

tant forms are amosite (brown asbestos), an iron magnesium silicate; anthophyllite produced largely in Finland; and crocidolite (blue), an iron sodium silicate that appears to have more carcinogenic properties than chrysotile, particularly in the causation of mesothelioma. Occupational exposure occurs in the mining industry, manufacture, and in the installation of insulating materials containing asbestos. Asbestos exposure also occurs in ship building, in the automotive industry (gaskets, brake linings, undercoating), and in the manufacture of certain "paper" products (roofing felt, flooring felt) and textiles. The mechanical irritation of the long stiff fibers when they become lodged in the lungs is believed to account, at least in part, for the fibrosis that results. The autoimmune theory has been proposed as pathogenic in this disease as in silicosis. However, there is some evidence to show that the pleural reaction is at least in part caused by mechanical irritation by the fibers that penetrate the visceral pleura. The disease does not develop unless there is a lengthy exposure, usually 10 years or more, to a fairly high concentra-

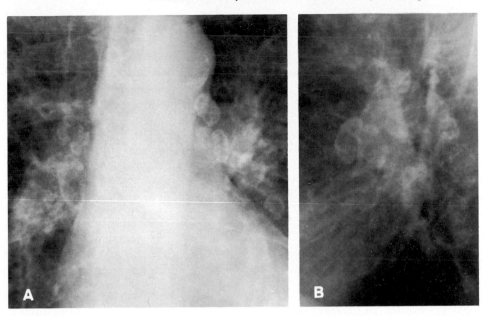

Fig. 27-4. Eggshell calcification in silicosis demonstrated in frontal **(A)** and lateral **(B)** projections.

tion of dust. When the pulmonary lesion is established, it progresses even though exposure is not continued. The clinical findings are those of progressive dyspnea that is often out of proportion to the amount of change noted on the chest films. There is often cyanosis and cough with sputum in which asbestos bodies can be detected. However, many patients with asbestos fibers in the lungs are asymptomatic. The incidence of tuberculosis is not as high as in silicosis. There is an increased incidence of carcinoma of the lungs in patients with asbestosis and an increased incidence of gastrointestinal cancer and of pleural mesothelioma has also been established. However, a recent report[12] of 36 cases of mesothelioma indicated that 19 were not associated with asbestosis. An increased incidence of peritoneal mesothelioma has also been reported in association with asbestosis.

Roentgen Observations. The fibrosis produced by the foreign material results in nonspecific accentuation of pulmonary interstitial markings extending into the perihilar regions and bases in the earliest phase of the disease. Later there is an increase in the basal fibrotic infiltrates, which usually appear stringy, irregular, and reticular, but may be nodular; a combination of the two may also occur—a reticulonodular appearance. The cardiac borders assume a shaggy appearance as a result of a combination of parenchymal and pleural disease—the "shaggy

heart" sign. Increasing fibrosis may lead to large opacities, usually when interstitial fibrosis is extensive. Lung bases are usually involved and in some instances the disease may involve the central and upper lungs as well. Cavitation and peripheral emphysema with central conglomeration as seen in silicosis does not occur. Pleural thickening, which may extend into the fissures, is common and may be the only roentgen finding; it is usually basal and bilateral. Parietal pleural plaques over the diaphragm and lower chest wall are often the only findings in asbestosis. The plaques vary in size and thickness (from 1 to 10 mm) and, because they often occur posterolaterally or anterolaterally, oblique films may be very useful in demonstrating them. They appear early as thin, local areas of pleural thickening in the lower thorax, and are often overlooked until they enlarge and become thicker. Calcification also occurs in the areas of pleural involvement. It is noted most frequently over the diaphragm in the form of a thin, curvilinear density conforming to the upper surface of the diaphragm bilaterally and is virtually pathognomonic. Bilateral pleural effusion may also occur, but the possibility of other causes must be excluded before this effusion can be attributed to asbestosis. Occasionally, areas of homogeneous density resembling pneumonic consolidation may appear. They may be unilateral or bilateral and are not necessarily symmetric. Pleural thickening is usually associated with this type of disease. When pleural thickening is

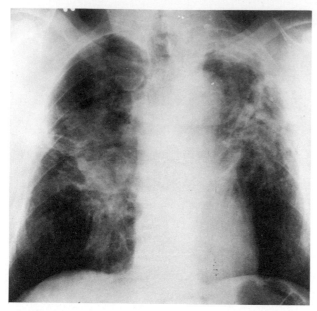

Fig. 27-5. Silicotuberculosis. Conglomerate disease is present bilaterally. Several cavities are present in the left upper lobe and tubercle bacilli were found in the sputum.

the predominant feature, a homogeneous or ground-glass appearance may result. Pulmonary emphysema is usually present and may be severe. Pulmonary hypertension leads to hilar vascular prominence, but eggshell calcification of nodes is not a feature of this disease. As in silicosis, the diagnosis is based on correlation of the roentgen with the clinical findings plus an accurate occupational history of exposure to asbestos.

TALCOSIS

Talc is a hydrous magnesium silicate in which there is no free silica. It is reported to produce a malignant type of pneumoconiosis in workers exposed to it in mining and milling operations. The roentgen findings are those of extensive pleural plaque formation. In severe cases, plaques of calcium density are deposited in and adjacent to the pleura, usually at the bases, along the cardiac borders; they sometimes extend over much of the surface of both lungs. The pleural thickening may be massive and irregular, and the calcification extensive. This can occur in other pneumoconioses but is much more common in talcosis and when present suggests the etiology of the pneumoconiosis. Pulmonary parenchymal findings

similar to those in asbestosis are sometimes observed. Emphysema is also a prominent feature of this disease. The diagnosis, as in the other pneumoconioses, is based on correlation of historical, clinical, and radiographic findings.

RARE SILICATE PNEUMOCONIOSES

Mica, a silicate containing potassium, aluminum, magnesium, calcium, and fluorine, is a rare cause of pneumoconiosis. *Kaolin* (China clay), a mixture of sand, mica, and aluminum silicate, is another rare cause of pneumoconiosis. *Cement dust* may cause a pneumoconiosis in persons exposed to high concentrations for long periods of time. Roentgen findings resemble those of silicosis or asbestosis.

BAUXITE FIBROSIS (SHAVER'S DISEASE)

Bauxite fibrosis is a form of malignant pneumoconiosis that occurs in workers exposed to fumes containing fine particles of aluminum oxide and silica used in the manufacture of synthetic abrasives. The ore, known as bauxite, is fused in furnaces.

The radiographic findings consist of fibrosis with a slight increase in interstitial markings progressing to extensive fibrotic change. Emphysematous blebs are commonly observed and spontaneous pneumothorax is not infrequent. There is often a history of repeated spontaneous pneumothorax and, in some patients, there may be considerable pleural thickening. In severe disease the strands of fibrosis radiating from the hilum become coarse and produce mediastinal widening. In these late stages, emphysema is usually marked. The diagnosis depends upon the history of exposure to the fumes of bauxite ore along with the clinical and roentgen findings. The disease is believed to be caused by the silica, but it is known that aluminum oxide can also induce pneumoconiosis under some conditions. There may be a sensitivity factor in the latter disease.

COAL WORKER'S PNEUMOCONIOSIS

This condition occurs in coal miners and also in those who work with coal elsewhere in extremely dusty conditions, such as in the hold of coal barges or ships. The condition is found chiefly in anthracite (hard coal) workers. The disabling or malignant pneumoconiosis is usually caused by silica and is, in reality, anthrasilicosis. Occasionally, a progressive form of the disease is found in bituminous (soft coal) workers; this is thought to be caused by exposure to extremely high concentrations of coal dust. This results in the accumulation of so much dust that the self-cleansing mechanism of the lung is overwhelmed and eventual damage leading to fibrosis and emphysema may take place. Roentgen findings are similar to those of silicosis and consist of a reticular or reticulonodular pattern with small granular-appearing nodules in the uncomplicated benign form. Progressive disease leading to massive fibrosis with nodules or masses that arise peripherally in the upper lung fields and tend to migrate toward the hila is termed "progressive massive fibrosis" (PMF). The characteristic appearance[32] consists of: (1) flat lateral border which is often elongated and parallels the rib cage; (2) thin mass in the sagittal plane; (3) thick-walled, eggshell calcifications within the mass; and (4) multiple satellite nodules. Cavitation may develop as a result of necrosis or tuberculosis; however, the cause is not definitely known. In some instances there may be enough silica to be a factor and, in others, it may be caused or accentuated by infection such as tuberculosis.

Caplan's Syndrome

Caplan's syndrome is the result of the combination of coal worker's pneumoconiosis and rheumatoid arthritis.[19] Roentgen findings consist of rounded, peripheral nodules, from 0.5 to 5.0 cm in diameter, that are clearly defined and may cavitate, on a background of nodular or reticulonodular pneumoconiosis. This syndrome usually occurs in those who have subcutaneous rheumatoid nodules but do not necessarily have arthritis. The pulmonary nodules may appear at intervals and often portend exacerbation of arthritis.

DIATOMACEOUS EARTH (DIATOMITE) PNEUMOCONIOSIS

Diatomaceous earth is used widely in filtration processes, as insulating material, as a catalyst carrier, and as an admixture for concrete. The crude diatomite contains amorphous silica. In certain types of processing, some of the amorphous silica is changed to crystalline silica in the form of cristobalite which produces a malignant pneumoconiosis not seen in crude diatomite workers. There is no increase in the incidence of tuberculosis in workers with this disease and there is no alteration of the course of tuberculosis.

The roentgen patterns are described as linear, nodular, or coalescent. The linear form results in accentuation of the bronchovascular pattern increasing to a reticular network of density throughout the lungs. Nodulation is very fine and granular at first; this may progress to coarse nodulation that may then progress to confluent or coalescent masses, usually appearing in the lung apices. Emphysema is often marked; bullae may rupture, leading to spontaneous pneumothorax. There is no constant progression from one stage to another as in silicosis. Hilar adenopathy is not present in this disease, and eggshell calcifications are not present in hilar nodes.

BERYLLIOSIS

Beryllium compounds are used in the manufacture of x-ray tubes, and in alloys, plastics, ceramics, and rocket fuel. Workers in industries concerned with these materials or products may be exposed to small amounts of beryllium, leading to a chronic form of beryllium granulomatosis. Workers in the beryllium-extraction industries may be exposed to larger amounts, leading to an acute pneumonitis. Laboratory research workers who have been exposed have developed the pneumonitis. The disease has also been observed in people who live in the neighborhood of plants as a result of exposure to exhaust fumes that contain beryllium.

The disease produced by inhalation of dust containing beryllium might better be termed "beryllium granulomatosis" or "beryllium poisoning" because (1) the pathologic lesion that follows is a granuloma resembling that found in sarcoidosis; and (2) relatively small exposure can produce extensive disease—this is in sharp contrast to the pneumoconioses produced by silica and the silicates (asbestos and talc), which require years of continued exposure in dusty occupations. In addition to causing pulmonary disease, beryllium results in severe reaction in other organs and tissues wherever it is lodged. There is evidently a considerable factor of individual sensitivity to this metal. Two distinct types of pulmonary disease are observed: an acute beryllium pneumonitis that develops within a few days of exposure and a chronic beryllium granulomatosis that occurs after a latent period varying from 3 months to 3 years or more after exposure.

Acute Beryllium Pneumonitis

This is a chemical pneumonitis resulting in pulmonary edema and hemorrhage. It may be fulminating if exposure has been overwhelming. Acute pulmonary edema and hemorrhage may be rapidly fatal. In the less acute form, the onset is more insidious than other types of chemical pneumonitis and tends to develop over a period of several days to 2 or 3 weeks or even months. Following the initial pulmonary edema, there is often an alveolar exudate made up largely of plasma cells leading to a severe organizing pneumonia. Hyaline membranes similar to those in viral or "uremic" pneumonitis may be present. If the disease does not terminate fatally in 2 or 3 weeks, gradual recovery tends to take place over a period of several months and may be complete. The roentgen findings in the acute process are similar to those noted in pulmonary edema. There is diffuse symmetric increase in density that is most marked in the midlung field, with poorly defined, soft shadows noted peripherally. In other instances the densities may be smaller and more patchy and tend to simulate widespread bronchopneumonia. As the patient recovers there is gradual clearing, which may be irregular, resulting in a more patchy or conglomerate nodular appearance. Complete clearing usually is slow and requires from 1 to 4 months. The history of exposure to beryllium is necessary to differentiate this disease from chemical pneumonitis and pulmonary edema resulting from other causes.

Chronic Beryllium Granulomatosis

This condition is characterized by a long latent period of 1 to 20 years after the initial exposure to beryllium of over 2 years' duration. Roentgen findings may be extensive before symptoms are marked and are somewhat variable. Fine diffuse granularity that resembles fine sand may be observed (Fig. 27-6). In other subjects, a diffuse reticular pattern plus granularity is noted. The hila are fuzzy and indistinct. In some, the lesions are larger, and distinct nodules, ranging from 1 to 5 mm in diameter, are present. Combinations may be observed. In addition, it is likely that earlier change consisting of slight increase in linear markings could be recognized if films were exposed at frequent intervals following the initial exposure. Hilar enlargement is a common finding and this in part is caused by enlargement of pulmonary vessels secondary to pulmonary hypertension leading to cor pulmonale. As the fibrosis continues, in the late stages there is some tendency to confluence, but this is much less than is noted in silicosis. Emphysema is found and may be severe. Spontaneous pneumothorax is common. There is no evidence of calcification in nodes and no pleural reaction. Tuberculosis is not ordinarily a complication so that cavitation is not present and the large conglomerate masses of density

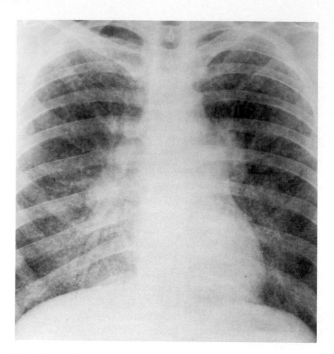

Fig. 27-6. Chronic beryllium granulomatosis. Note the massive hilar-node enlargement and granular nodularity throughout both lungs. Some of the nodules range up to 3 or 4 mm in size, particularly in the apices.

noted in silicosis are not common in beryllium granulomatosis. The diagnosis may be suspected on the roentgen examination but must be confirmed by adequate history of exposure. If history of exposure is lacking, or open to question, pulmonary biopsy and chemical determination of the presence of beryllium in the tissues are necessary.

THE "BENIGN" PNEUMOCONIOSES

There are a number of inorganic dusts that are radiopaque, may be stored in the lungs following inhalation, and produce no fibrosis or other reaction. As a result they present roentgen findings in patients with no clinical evidence of disease.

SIDEROSIS

Siderosis is a benign pneumoconiosis due to accumulation of iron oxide in the lung. It is found in electric-arc and acetylene welders, silver polishers, boiler scalers, and in grinders and burners in foundries in which there is insufficient silica to produce silicosis. The iron is inhaled as small particles or in fumes containing iron oxide produced by welding. The roentgen findings are caused by the fact that the iron accumulates in the lymphatics and interstitial tissues of the lung in sufficient quantity to produce radiographic density. No fibrosis or decrease in pulmonary function is caused and there is no predisposition to tuberculosis in these individuals.

The roentgen findings consist of discrete, sharply defined, granular densities (1 to 3 mm in size) scattered uniformly and symmetrically throughout both lung fields. The individual lesions are often more clearly defined than in silicosis and there is no tendency toward conglomeration. There is no reticular density extending from the hilum into the lung field in these patients and there is no hilar adenopathy such as is frequently observed in patients with silicosis. Other features that tend to differentiate this condition from silicosis are the absence of emphysema and clinical symptoms. The densities tend to regress and may disappear when the exposure is discontinued.

BARITOSIS

Baritosis is due to deposition of barium sulfate in the lungs of workers in barium mines. The findings are similar to those in siderosis except that the density of the barium is greater and the individual lesions tend to be larger. When exposure is heavy, roentgen signs may appear after a relatively short time (1 to 2 years). The densities disappear gradually after removal of the patient from exposure. The condition probably produces no alteration in pulmonary function. Fibrotic changes leading to diminished function have been reported, but the patients were also exposed to other dusts known to cause fibrosis.

STANNOSIS

The benign pneumoconiosis called "stannosis" is found in ore handlers and grinders, in tin-smelting workers, and in those who pack tin oxide into bags. It is caused by deposition of tin in the form of stannic oxide in pulmonary tissues. This results in a benign pneumoconiosis similar to baritosis.

PNEUMOCONIOSIS DUE TO ANTIMONY

Antimony when inhaled is sufficiently radiopaque to produce evidence of pneumoconiosis on roentgen study. It is a rare cause of a benign pneumoconiosis.

OCCUPATIONAL DISEASES RELATED TO PULMONARY HYPERSENSITIVITY

Bronchopulmonary disease caused by hypersensitivity reactions depends, to some extent, upon the size of the inhaled particles. Large particles tend to remain in the tracheobronchial tree where the hypersensitivity response is in the form of the bronchospasm or asthma. Bronchial asthma, allergic aspergillosis, usually with mucoid impaction, bronchocentric granulomatosis, and byssinosis are manifestations of this type of response. The roentgenographic findings in bronchial asthma are described in Chapter 30 and those in allergic aspergillosis in Chapter 26.

BRONCHOCENTRIC GRANULOMATOSIS

Bronchocentric granulomatosis is a distinctive lesion in which replacement of bronchial epithelium by palisaded granulation tissue is the major pathologic finding.[16] Many of the patients are asthmatics, and, in these, the granulomas contain many eosinophils, while, in the patients who do not have bronchial asthma, the granulomas contain plasma cells. The disease appears to be related to hypersensitivity and is very similar to allergic bronchopulmonary aspergillosis and mucoid impaction. The roentgen findings are also similar. There may be lobar or segmental consolidation or atelectasis; one or more large nodular or mass densities are sometimes observed. In these instances, the appearance simulates that of tumor. Small nodular or mixed nodular and linear patterns may also be seen. In some patients, more than one roentgen pattern may be observed. Bronchography in four of twenty-two patients reviewed[16] showed segmental bronchial obstruction in two, bronchiectasis in one, and atelectasis with no bronchial abnormality in the other. In this series, the lesions were unilateral in three-fourths of the patients, with upper-lobe predominance. Little radiographic difference was noted when comparing asthmatics with non-asthmatics.

BYSSINOSIS

Byssinosis is a pulmonary disease occurring in cotton-mill workers; it is sometimes called "cotton-mill fever." It appears to result from inhalation of cotton dust. Symptoms consisting of sneezing, coughing, and wheezing tend to come on in attacks related to exposure to the dust. When the patient is removed from the dusty atmosphere, the attacks subside.

Roentgen findings are nonspecific and consist of some accentuation of parahilar markings along with relatively symmetric distribution of irregular infiltrates in the form of patchy, poorly defined densities in the central lung fields. They may not appear until after the patient has had a number of acute attacks, so that there may be no roentgenographic findings early in the course of the disease. Emphysema and permanent fibrosis may result, particularly in smokers, if the patient remains in the dusty occupation. The target tissue of the antigen-antibody reaction appears to be the respiratory airways and not the alveoli, as in many of the other occupational diseases related to hypersensitivity.

BAGASSOSIS

Alveolar hypersensitivity, sometimes termed "extrinsic allergic alveolitis" or "hypersensitivity pneumonitis," indicates a response of pulmonary tissue to antigens contained in a wide variety of organic dusts in which the particles are so small that they penetrate into the most distal lung parenchyma.[8] Most of the conditions caused by such dusts are associated with specific occupations.

Bagasse is the product remaining after the juice has been extracted from sugarcane. Inhalation of this dust contaminated with *Thermoactinomyces sacchari* may cause symptomatic pulmonary disease. After an exposure of from 2 to 4 months the clinical manifestations appear in the form of an acute febrile illness with coughing and dyspnea that may become severe. The symptoms are believed to represent an antigen-antibody reaction with possible additional injury caused by the presence of the foreign bodies in lung tissue. The clinical findings usually disappear slowly when the patient leaves the dusty occupation.

Roentgen findings are those of perihilar consolidations, usually the result of prominent peribronchial markings around the hila. Occasionally a fine granular type of density is noted bilaterally and this is usually symmetric and fairly widespread. Regression is slow and the roentgen findings clear gradually in 6 to 12 months. The history of adequate exposure to the dust, along with the clinical manifestations and roentgen findings, lead to the correct diagnosis. The illness causes fever along with the nonspecific roentgen findings and must be differentiated from tuberculosis and other chronic pulmonary inflammatory diseases. Therefore it is necessary to examine and culture the sputum when there is any question as to the diagnosis.

FARMER'S LUNG

Farmer's lung, or thresher's lung, is a pulmonary disease that occurs in farm workers following exposure to moldy hay, grain, or silage, particularly in a closed area. It is the best understood of the conditions causing hypersensitivity pneumonitis. The clinical symptoms, pathology, and roentgen findings depend upon the stage of the disease, whether acute, subacute, or chronic. The acute stage is characterized by the sudden onset of intense dyspnea, cyanosis, cough, slight fever, and night sweats that usually start a few hours after exposure to moldy material. Respirations are rapid and rales are often present, but there is no typical asthmatic type of breathing. If the patient leaves the working environment the course is one of gradual improvement of clinical and roentgen findings over a period of 6 to 8 weeks; this is the subacute stage. If the patient returns to the same working environment, symptoms recur. The disease varies in severity but eventually the patient is forced to stay away from the source of the dusty material that causes it. Permanent roentgen and pathologic changes are then present which represent the chronic stage. It has been demonstrated that this is an antigen-antibody reaction, with the principal antigens being thermophilic actinomycetes, *i.e., Micropolyspora faeni,* and to a lesser extent other thermophilic actinomycetes. Histopatholgic study shows a granulomatous interstitial and alveolar pneumonitis in early cases. Later, interstitial fibrosis may result when repeated exposure has resulted in chronic disease.

Roentgen Observations. There is a considerable variation in the roentgen findings in these patients. In the acute phase there is usually a fine granular density occupying most of both lung fields. There is some tendency to spare the apices. The involvement may be so extensive that the small individual granular nodules are obscured and an acinar or alveolar pattern is observed. The hila occasionally appear thickened and poorly marginated. The disease regresses over a period of 6 to 8 weeks, often in an irregular manner so that the lesions become mottled and patchy; there is often some accentuation of interstitial markings extending outward from the hila for some time after the major part of the infiltrate has disappeared (Fig. 27-7). Eventually this interstitial type of density may also clear completely. Pulmonary function studies often indicate a definite decrease in pulmonary function even after all roentgen indications have disappeared.

In patients in whom there have been several attacks, permanent changes as shown on roentgen study are present. These consist of evidence of pulmonary emphysema and interstitial fibrosis. The latter is manifested by a general increase in interstitial markings extending from the hilum out to the periphery, often resulting in a rather coarse reticular appearance of the peripheral lung field (Fig. 27-8). These patients may become respiratory cripples.

PIGEON BREEDER'S LUNG

This disease occurs in pigeon and in other bird handlers, so that bird breeder's lung or bird handler's lung are preferred terms to designate this condition. It appears to be caused by hypersensitivity to antigens in feathers, serum, and droppings. Roentgen findings include accentuation of interstitial markings with superimposed small nodulations. In acute or severe disease, scattered areas of poorly defined, patchy density indicating alveolar exudation are observed. On biopsy, a granulomatous interstitial pneumonitis is observed. Symptoms disappear and radiographic signs clear when the patient is removed from contact with the birds and their habitat.

MAPLE-BARK DISEASE

Maple-bark disease occurs in sawmill or papermill workers exposed to the spores of the fungus *Cryptostroma corticale* which lies deep in the bark of the maple tree. Roentgen findings are similar to those of other pulmonary hypersensitivity states, namely, an increase in interstitial lung markings and nodularity producing a reticulonodular pattern in parahilar areas and lower lungs. More severe involvement results in a scattered alveolar exudate resulting in confluent pneumonia. Removal from the environment results in clearing of the process.

OTHER OCCUPATIONAL HYPERSENSITIVITY STATES

In addition to the conditions described in the foregoing paragraphs, a number of others have been reported in which pulmonary disease is caused by inhalation of material which evidently contains antigens to which the lungs react as a result of hypersensitivity. The radiographic findings in the lungs and the histopathologic manifestations are quite similar. Examples are: (1) pituitary snuff-users lung—inhaled posterior pituitary extracts used in treating patients with diabetes insipidus; (2) mushroom worker's lung; (3) malt-worker's lung; (4) sequoiosis; (5) wood-pulp worker's disease; (6) grain-weevil hypersensitivity; (7) suberosis (cork); (8) cheesewasher's lung; (9) fishmeal worker's lung; (10) coffee worker's lung; (11) lycoperdonosis; (12) alveolitis from contaminated forced-air apparatus; (13) bakelite alveolitis; (14) hypersensitivity to synthetic materials of various kinds including nylon, polyurethane, acrylic fibers, and possibly polyvinyl chloride. The mechanism of the pulmonary reaction is not clear in all of these, however. A number of other occupational diseases have also been reported including those due to sensitivity to organic chemicals such as isocynates (chiefly toluene diisocyanate) used in the manufacture of synthetic foams, synthetic rubbers, paints, and adhesives.[3]

DISEASES CAUSED BY CHEMICAL AND PHYSICAL AGENTS

HYDROCARBON PNEUMONITIS

A number of products have been implicated in hydrocarbon ingestion or inhalation or both. They include kerosene, gasoline, furniture polish, lighter fluid, cleaning fluid, and turpentine. These products are usually ingested, but some of the irritant material is also aspirated or inhaled. The aspiration is generally the most important factor in the etiology of pneumonitis. The ingested hydrocarbon is absorbed and excreted into the lungs, adding to the pulmonary injury. If vomiting occurs, some additional hydrocarbon may be aspirated. These petroleum distillates cause an acute alveolitis with exudation of leukocytes, fluid, and fibrin and a more chronic proliferative interstitial infiltration. The pathologic findings in patients who have succumbed are those of severe hemorrhagic pulmonary edema, bronchiolar necrosis, and alveolar exudation. There are sometimes few, if any, clinical signs of pulmonary involvement despite roentgen evidence of pulmonary disease.

Roentgen Observations. There is considerable variation in pulmonary roentgen findings depending upon the severity of the injury. Usually diffuse density, homogeneous or somewhat flocculent confined to the lower lobes, but in severe cases the diffuse density extends into the upper lung field as well, is manifest. When the involvement is less marked, mottled densities are noted in one or both lung fields. The individual foci are hazy and poorly defined; there may be conglomeration in some areas (Fig. 27-9). These

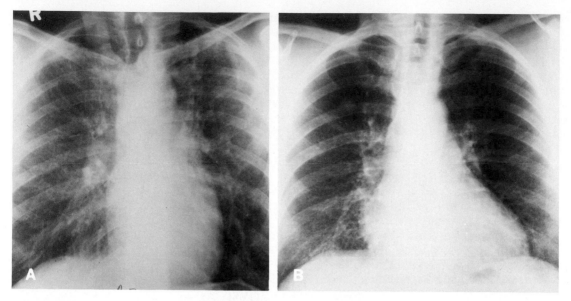

Fig. 27-7. Farmer's lung. **A.** This patient had an acute episode of cough and fever. There are some poorly defined nodularity and an increase in interstitial markings noted best in the central lung fields. **B.** The disease in this patient is manifested by some small granular-appearing nodules at the bases, best observed on the right, along with a small amount of increase in interstitial markings.

Fig. 27-8. Farmer's lung. In this patient, there was a fine granular nodularity in the lower lung fields which is not very well visualized in **A. B.** An enlargement of the right lower lung field, in which the granular appearance is quite well defined.

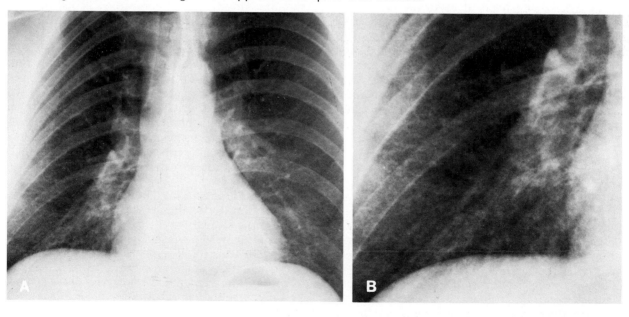

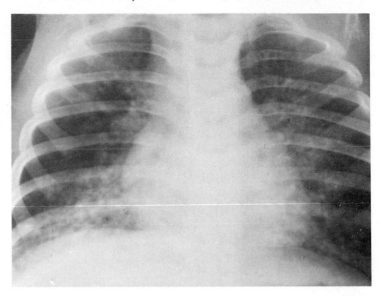

Fig. 27-9. Hydrocarbon pneumonitis (kerosene). The disease is confined to the bases of the lungs and is more marked on the right than on the left. It is a poorly defined, diffuse alveolar chemical pneumonitis.

roentgen changes develop rapidly and can be seen as early as one-half hour following ingestion. Less frequently the changes are confined to the parahilar areas, resembling pulmonary edema. Clearing of roentgen signs usually lags behind clinical improvement. Pneumatocele formation in these patients has been reported and obstructive emphysema may also occur. Rarely, pleural effusion, pneumothorax, and interstitial emphysema occur. The diagnosis is based on the history along with the roentgen manifestations described.

INDUSTRIAL AND WAR GASES

A number of irritant gases are capable of producing pulmonary changes that can be visualized roentgenographically. They include nitric fumes (which consist of five oxides of nitrogen), hydrogen sulphide, chlorine, phosgene, and mustard gas, as well as a number of other irritating gases such as ammonia, manganese oxides, zinc chloride fumes, various insecticides, fluorocarbons, and chemicals found in glue. All these gases produce pathologic changes in the lungs that vary with the intensity of exposure and the nature of the chemical. Inflammatory changes are found in the trachea and larger bronchi with minimal exposures. As the amount of exposure increases, the damage to these structures is intensified with a tendency for the process to extend farther out into the smaller bronchi and bronchioles. This results in pulmonary edema and congestion secondary to the

chemical bronchitis and bronchiolitis. If the injury is severe enough, death may result. There is often a delay in onset of clinical symptoms following exposure ranging from 1 or 2 hours to as long as 36 hours. Chest pain, cough, and dyspnea are the most common symptoms. Some of the gases are carried to the myocardium, liver, and kidneys following diffusion through the alveolocapillary membrane and may produce damage in these sites.

Roentgen Observations. Roentgen findings vary with the extent and severity of the injury. They consist of a patchy mottling, usually most marked in the perihilar areas where the lesions may be confluent (Fig. 27-10). In the central and peripheral lung fields, individual nodules may be visible that range up to 1 cm in size and are fluffy in appearance, with poorly defined edges resembling foci of bronchopneumonia but probably represent alveolar edema. The periphery of the lung fields is usually spared unless the injury has been overwhelming. When the injury has not been severe, clearing occurs rather rapidly with striking changes noted from day to day and is often complete in 10 to 14 days. During this period the lesions become more irregular and asymmetric, since small areas of atelectasis and, often, some patchy bronchopneumonia develop. The diagnosis is based on the history of exposure to noxious gas followed by the symptoms of cough and dyspnea plus the roentgen findings of pulmonary edema as described.

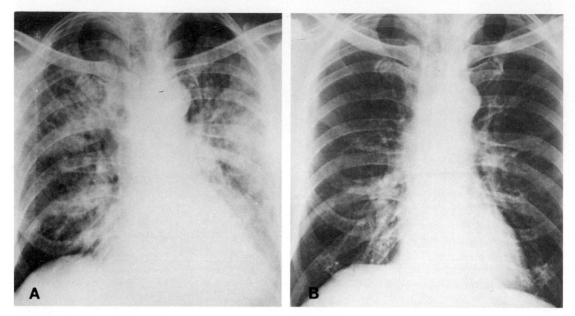

Fig. 27-10. Chemical pneumonitis. The widespread, mottled, poorly defined densities resemble, and most likely represent, pulmonary edema. Therefore a history of exposure is necessary to differentiate this condition from others producing pulmonary edema. The changes noted in **A** cleared completely, as shown in **B,** a roentgenogram obtained 3 weeks later.

SILO-FILLER'S DISEASE

It is known that nitrogen dioxide is produced in silos within a few hours to 3 or 4 days after the silo is filled. Any person entering such a confined space and remaining there is exposed to this irritating gas. Cough and dyspnea often occur immediately. Pulmonary edema in parahilar areas and at the bases may appear in a few hours. This clears rather rapidly if the patient recovers. This may be followed by a period of relative freedom or remission of symptoms for 2 or 3 weeks. There is then a second phase of illness that may be fatal or recovery may occur. This is characterized by fever, progressive dyspnea, cyanosis, and cough. The roentgen findings on films obtained during this phase consist of widespread scattered miliary densities resembling the lesions of acute miliary tuberculosis. Later these may become confluent, producing a more patchy and nodular type of appearance. The diagnosis is based upon a combination of clinical history and roentgen findings. At autopsy, patients who died a month following exposure were found to have bronchiolitis fibrosa obliterans, with each of the small densities apparently representing the typical lesion of this condition. In a patient who

died within a few hours following a similar exposure, diffuse pulmonary edema was found similar to that described in persons whose deaths were due to nitric-fume inhalation in industry.

It is, therefore, evident that exposure to nitric fumes and oxides of nitrogen can lead to pulmonary damage sufficient to cause death within a short time of exposure or symptoms may be delayed for several weeks or months, followed by a second phase of more chronic disease. It is also likely that many of these patients recover completely with no residual illness, while in others there is enough bronchial alteration to result in fibrosis and emphysema, which develop over a long period of time following the initial injury. It is also probable that other irritant gases are capable of producing a similar variety of pulmonary alteration.

CARBON MONOXIDE POISONING

Acute carbon monoxide poisoning is frequently fatal, but in a number of persons who receive sublethal doses, abnormalities may be demonstrated on chest roentgenograms. The following manifestations were found in 18 of 62 patients having acute carbon monoxide poisoning.[27] A ground-glass appearance was the most common finding; this was observed in 11. A parahilar haze was noted in 2 of these, and 4 had a combination of parahilar haze and peribronchial and perivascular cuffing, while 3 had evidence of intra-alveolar edema. All of the findings are believed to represent pulmonary edema, probably caused by tissue hypoxia and/or the toxic effects of carbon monoxide on alveolar membranes. Cardiac enlargement occurred in 4 patients, and elevation of the right hemidiaphragm in 7, usually as a later manifestation indicating hepatic enlargement. Intra-alveolar edema and parahilar haze indicated a poor prognosis; the presence of any roentgen abnormality is an indication for intensive treatment with oxygen.

PARAQUAT LUNG

The herbicide paraquat produces acute pulmonary edema and hemorrhage causing rapid death when large doses are ingested.[26, 29] When smaller amounts are taken, the patients may survive for a number of days. Roentgenographic findings consist of fine granular densities in the lower lung field which may be discrete in some areas and confluent in others. There is usually rapid progression into a pattern resembling that of severe pulmonary edema. The presence of positive roentgen findings in the chest usually indicates that a fatal amount of paraquat has been ingested. Patients who survive show a pattern of diffuse interstitial fibrosis. Pathologically there appears to be intra-alveolar fibrosis associated with pulmonary vascular disease in which there is muscularization of pulmonary arterioles; extensive fibrosis usually develops before these patients die.

RADIATION CHANGES IN THE LUNG

When tumors of the breast, lung, and mediastinum are treated with radiation, the lung tissue in the beam receives radiation in varying amounts. This is capable of causing injury sufficient to be noted radiographically and pathologically. The reaction in the lung depends on a number of factors, such as variations in the rate of treatment, port size, the presence of arteriosclerosis, and individual sensitivity of the patient. These factors alter the relationship between the total dose of radiation to the lungs and the damage produced by it. Generally there is not a direct dose or dose–time relationship. When the tissue dose is under 2000 rads, little, if any permanent pulmonary damage occurs. As a rule most patients develop permanent lung changes following a dose of 4500

rads and all have permanent damage when 6000 rads are delivered to the lung. The clinical symptoms are often minor and there may be considerable roentgen change with no symptoms. Cough and dyspnea may be present, however. During the acute phase there is a deposition of fibrinlike material in the alveoli to produce a hyaline membrane plus swelling, destruction of alveolar walls, and edema. These acute changes are often delayed for a month to 6 weeks, just as the severe acute skin reactions are delayed. Occasionally the findings may occur many months following completion of irradiation. The late changes are those of fibrosis, resulting in thickening of the alveolar walls and a decrease in the caliber of the vessels. In some patients an acute reaction may be superimposed on the late fibrosis when multiple courses of radiation are given.

These pathologic alterations are reflected in the radiographic findings. During the early acute phase when edema is a prominent feature there is a hazy, poorly defined increase in density, usually confined to the area of radiation but one that may extend for a short distance beyond it. This reaction may occur from 1 month to as long as 4 to 6 months following completion of irradiation. Most of the reaction is very likely caused by pulmonary edema but there is also some pleural reaction leading to a small amount of fluid and pleural thickening that very likely contributes. Pleural fluid in significant amounts is rare. After a time the density becomes somewhat more irregular and patchy. Strands of density develop that radiate from the hilum toward the periphery. These manifestations may clear gradually and disappear completely in a year or more, but if the original injury was severe enough there is sufficient fibrosis to cause permanent changes. These changes consist of contraction of the lung and a shift of hilar and mediastinal structures to the side or area of radiation (Fig. 27-11). Pleural thickening may appear, manifested by increased density and irregularity of the pleural surface involved. Elevation of the diaphragm and tenting of its summit may occur. Severe thoracic and pulmonary distortion may result. Chronic dry, irritating, persistent cough may be a problem in the more severely involved patients.

The diagnosis is made on the basis of the clinical history of previous radiation plus the roentgen manifestations described. There is often accompanying evidence of radiation osteitis of ribs, consisting of fractures with demineralization of ribs in the area of fracture. There is no evidence of healing for long periods of time so far as can be detected on the roentgenogram. Radiation pneumonitis must be differen-

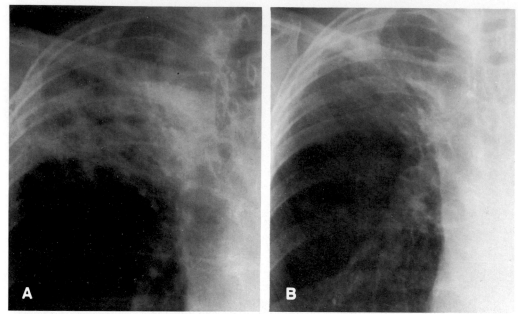

Fig. 27-11. Radiation pneumonitis **A.** Roentgenogram secured 5 months after completion of irradiation of the right upper thorax in a patient with breast carcinoma. There is a shift of the trachea and upper mediastinal structures to the right, elevation of the right hilum, and a rather diffuse, poorly defined density above the level of the anterior arc of the second rib representing a relatively acute alveolar process. **B.** This examination, made 2 years later, shows only a little strandlike density, largely confined to the clavicular and subclavicular area. The elevation of the right hilum persists, but the tracheal shift is somewhat less.

tiated from metastasis or recurrent tumor. This differentiation is often difficult, since the radiation is usually given for treatment of a tumor. In patients with breast tumor, the localization of the changes to the area of irradiation without lesions elsewhere is indicative of a radiation pneumonitis and not metastasis. The signs of shrinkage in lung volume just noted are not found in metastasis and it is rare for metastatic carcinoma to involve one lung to any significant degree without evidence of disease on the other side. The problem of recurrence or residual disease after heavy irradiation of the mediastinum for Hodgkin's disease offers a particularly difficult problem, because involvement of pulmonary parenchyma extending out along the lymphatics radiating from the hilum is found in this disease. These findings simulate the fibrotic changes resulting from radiation after treatment of hilar and mediastinal nodes. All factors, including the clinical condition of the patient, the time interval following radiation, and the progress of the lesions must be considered in these

instances. Even then differentiation is sometimes impossible. The acute pulmonary reaction must be differentiated from acute pneumonitis resulting from irritants and from bacterial infections. This can be done on the basis of clinical history plus the presence of the localized radiating strands that are common in postradiation pneumonitis.

REFERENCES AND SELECTED READINGS

1. BAGHDASSARIAN OM, WEINER S: Pneumatocele formation complicating hydrocarbon pneumonitis. Am J Roentgenol 95: 104, 1965
2. BRISTOL LJ: Pneumoconioses caused by asbestos and by other siliceous and nonsiliceous dusts. Semin Roentgenol 2: 283, 1967
3. CHARLES J, BERNSTEIN A, JONES B et al: Hypersensitivity pneumonitis after exposure to isocynates. Thorax 31: 127, 1976

4. CORNELIUS EA, BETLACH EH: Silo-filler's disease. Radiology 74: 232, 1960

5. DE NARDI JM, VAN ORDSTRAND HS, CURTIS GH: Berylliosis: summary and survey of all clinical types in ten year period. Cleve Clin Q 19: 171, 1952

6. EMANUEL DA, WENZEL FJ, LAWTON BR: Pneumonitis due to Cryptostroma corticale (maple-bark disease). N Engl J Med 274: 1413, 1966

7. FRANK RC: Farmer's lung. Am J Roentgenol 79: 189, 1957

8. FRASER RG, PARE JAP: Extrinsic allergic alveolitis. Semin Roentgenol 10: 31, 1975

9. GREENING RR, HESLEP JH: The roentgenology of silicosis. Semin Roentgenol 2: 265, 1967

10. HARDY HL: Current concepts of occupational lung disease of interest to the radiologist. Semin Roentgenol 2: 225, 1967

11. HARDY HL, TABERSHAW IR: Delayed chemical pneumonitis occurring in workers exposed to beryllium compounds. J Indust Hyg Toxicol 28: 197, 1946

12. HASAN FM, NASH G, KAZEMI H: The significance of asbestos exposure in the diagnosis of mesothelioma: a 28-year experience from a major urban hospital. Am Rev Resp Dis 115: 761, 1977

13. JACOBSON G, FELSON B. PENDERGRASS EP et al: Eggshell calcifications in coal and metal miners. Semin Roentgenol 2: 276, 1967

14. JACOBSON G, LAINHART WS (eds): ILO U/C International Classification of Radiographs of the Pneumoconioses. Med Radiog Photog 48:67, 1972

15. JIMENEZ JP, LESTER RG: Pulmonary complications following furniture polish ingestion. Am J Roentgenol 98: 323, 1966

16. KATZENSTEIN A. LIEBOW AA, FRIEDMAN PJ: Bronchocentric granulomatosis, mucoid impaction, and hypersensitivity reactions to fungi. Am Rev Resp Dis 111: 497, 1975

17. KLEINERMAN J: The pathology of some familiar pneumoconioses. Semin Roentgenol 2: 244, 1967

18. MAHON WE, SCOTT DJ, ANSELL G et al: Hypersensitivity to pituitary snuff with miliary shadowing in the lungs. Thorax 22: 13, 1967

19. MORGAN WKC, LAPP NL: Respiratory disease in coal miners. State of the art. Am Rev Resp Dis 113: 531, 1976

20. NICHOLSON DP: Bagasse worker's lung. Am Rev Resp Dis 97: 546, 1968

21. OECHSLI WR, JACOBSON G, BRODEUR AE: Diatomite pneumoconiosis: roentgen characteristics and classification. Am J Roentgenol 85: 263, 1961

22. RANKIN J, KOBAYASHI M, BARBEE RA et al: Pulmonary granulomatoses due to inhaled organic antigens. Med Clin North Am 51: 459, 1967

23. REED ES, WELLS PO, WICKER EH: Coal miners' pneumoconiosis. Radiology 71: 661, 1958

24. SANDER OA: Berylliosis. Semin Roentgenol 2: 306, 1967

25. SANDER OA: The nonfibrogenic (benign) pneumoconioses. Semin Roentgenol 2: 312, 1967

26. SMITH P, HEATH D: Paraquat lung: a reappraisal. Thorax 29: 643, 1974

27. SONE S, HIGASHIHARA T, KOTAKE T et al: Pulmonary manifestations in acute carbon monoxide poisoning. Am J Roentgenol 120: 865, 1974

28. TEPPER LB: The work history in industrial lung disease. Semin Roentgenol 2: 235, 1967

29. THURLBECK WM, THURLBECK SM: Pulmonary effects of paraquat poisoning. Chest [Suppl] 69: 276, 1976

30. UICC/Cincinnati classification of the radiographic appearances of pneumoconiosis. Chest 58: 57, 1970

31. UNGER J DEB, FINK JN, UNGER GF: Pigeon breeder's disease.Radiology 90: 683, 1968

32. WILLIAMS JL, MOLLER GA: Solitary mass in the lungs of coal miners. Am J Roentgenol 117: 765, 1973

33. ZUCKER R, KILBOURNE ED, EVANS JB: Pulmonary manifestations of gasoline intoxication. Arch Indust Hyg Occup Med 2: 17, 1950

28

CIRCULATORY DISTURBANCES

PULMONARY EDEMA

Pulmonary edema is the term used to indicate that there is an abnormal accumulation of fluid in the extravascular pulmonary tissues. There is a constant flow of fluid and proteins from the microvascular spaces (arterioles, capillaries, and venules) in the lung into the interstitial space.[19] This interstitial space includes the alveolar wall interstitium and the interlobular, perivascular, peribronchial, and subpleural connective-tissue spaces. The pulmonary lymphatics actively pump the excess microvascular filtrate into the systemic venous system. The rate of fluid and protein flow from the microvascular spaces to the interstitial spaces may increase several fold before there is a measurable increase in the extravascular fluid. When the pumping capacity of the lymphatics is exceeded, edema results. The interstitial phase of edema precedes alveolar flooding or alveolar edema. The latter is often quite abrupt and consists of rapid filling of the alveoli with fluid. Several factors are involved in the maintenance of fluid balance within the lung. The factor opposing edema within the capillary or microvasculature is the osmotic pressure; in the alveolus it is the alveolar pressure and surface tension. The factor favoring edema in the capillary is an increase in hydrostatic pressure; in the alveolus it is a decrease in alveolar pressure and surface tension. Maintenance of normal capillary permeability is also an anti-edema factor.

The most common cause of pulmonary edema is elevation of pulmonary microvascular pressure, which may be produced by a number of conditions. A secondary factor is maintenance of normal flow of lymph, which may be depressed either neurogenically or by elevation of pressure in the superior vena cava. The second major factor is an increase in permeability of microvascular walls. Alteration in the osmotic pressure in the intervascular spaces is apparently of less importance.

Pulmonary edema can then be classified into several major categories according to the primary etiologic factor. Much remains to be learned about relative importance of the various factors, however.

I. *Increased Intravascular Pressure.* Pulmonary edema caused by increased intravascular pressure occurs when the pressure increase is due to: (*1*) left heart failure; (*2*) pulmonary venous obstruction such as that due to mitral valvular disease, left atrial tumor, or, possibly, high altitude; (*3*) pulmonary venous obstruction due to other causes including mediastinal inflammatory or neoplastic disease and the rare idiopathic veno-obstructive disease of children and young adults[12]; or (*4*) neurogenic causes including brain injury, postictal edema in epilepsy and sudden increase in intracranial pressure. In some of the neurogenic cases there may be an additional factor of increased microvascular permeability secondary to hypoxemia. Whenever the pulmonary venous pressure exceeds 25 mm Hg, edema is likely to occur and Kerley's B lines have been observed at pressures of 17 to 20 mm Hg.

II. *Increased Capillary Permeability.* Pulmonary edema caused by increased capillary permeability occurs when altered permeability is due to: (*1*) toxic causes, including uremia, heroin overdose, salicylate poisoning; (*2*) noxious fumes including fumes from the oxides of nitrogen and sulfur, smoke inhalation, oxygen toxicity, as well as a variety of organic chemical fumes; or (*3*) a miscellaneous group of causes including rapid re-expansion of a lung that has been collapsed for a number of hours, possibly high-altitude edema, possibly transfusion reaction, posttraumatic fat embolism, near drowning, aspiration of liquids, postradiation edema, or circulating toxins such as snake venom and vasoactive substances such as histamine and serotonin.

III. *Combined Increased Pressure and Capillary Permeability.* In such conditions as adult respiratory distress syndrome and shock lung, a combination of increased intravascular pressure and increased capillary permeability evidently causes pulmonary edema. In several of the conditions mentioned in the foregoing paragraph (II), there may also be a combination of causes involved. In fluid overload, a combination of increase in microvascular pressure and a decrease in intravascular osmotic pressure is likely. Decreased lymphatic drainage also plays a greater or lesser role in a number of situations, and lymphatic obstruction may cause edema. Alterations in the permeability of the alveolar epithelial membrane are not well understood. There is a definite increase in permeability in the late alveolar flooding stage of pulmonary edema, however. The effect of hypoxemia also is not thoroughly understood in patients with pulmonary edema.

Clinical symptoms are varied and depend upon the associated disease or injury. When the edema is acute there is usually severe respiratory distress, but when the onset is insidious, particularly in uremia, there may be very few respiratory symptoms. There is a notable discrepancy between roentgen and physical findings in chronic pulmonary edema and in some patients with acute or subacute interstitial edema. Therefore the roentgen examination is very important. Two major roentgen patterns of edema are observed depending on the site of the transudate, namely, alveolar and interstitial.

INTERSTITIAL EDEMA

As indicated, interstitial edema precedes alveolar edema; therefore, it is necessary to be able to recognize the interstitial fluid in order to determine the presence of congestive heart failure or other cause of edema early in its course.

There are several signs of interstitial edema which are reliable as a group, particularly when correlated with the clinical findings. They are:

1. Appearance of septal lines
   a. Kerley's B lines are dense, horizontal lines which measure about 1.5 to 2.0 cm in length. They are best seen in the lower lung on oblique projection on films of good quality. They represent secondary interlobular septa thickened by fluid (Fig. 28-1).
   b. Kerley's A lines are longer and range in size up to 4 or 5 cm. They tend to be straight or slightly curved and extend from the hila or parahilar area toward the periphery. They are seen in the upper lobes and tend to appear in acute interstitial edema. Transudate in the secondary interlobular septa, largely in the upper lobes, also causes these changes.
   c. Kerley's C lines are somewhat more controversial, but appear to represent fluid in the superimposed septa.
   d. "D" lines: Kreel and associates[11] have described edema lines other than the Kerley A, B, and C lines and have designated them "D" lines. Three types have been observed: (*1*) Thick, long, often angular lines, usually anterior in the lingula and right middle lobe, overlying the heart on the lateral projection and as horizontal or vertical shadows on the frontal view. (*2*) Short and straight basal lines, usually thicker at the pleural surface associated with puckering of the pleura. On the lateral projection they resemble the pleural end of

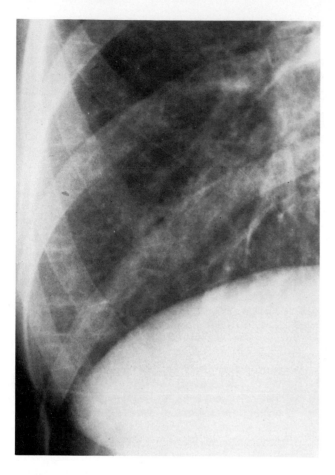

a fissure. (3) Subpleural reticular pattern of about 1 to 2 cm in diameter—detected only on autopsy-inflated lungs, not in the living. The "D" lines can be observed in patients with overt interstitial edema and are usually not observed in early subtle edema in our experience. The D-1 lines occur in areas where Kerley's B lines are inconspicuous or absent, namely, anteriorly, so they are best seen on lateral views. Also, the thick D-1 lines are usually away from alveolar edema, which tends to be posterolateral.

2. Perivascular blurring or cuffing in which the margins of the vessels become indistinct and widened beginning in the perihilar area and extending well out into the parenchyma.

3. "Hilar haze" refers to a loss of definition of large central pulmonary vessels with a slight general increase in density. This is very likely caused by interstitial edema anterior and posterior to the hilum since the central vessels do not have perivascular interstitium until they enter the lung. This is probably the phase in which the alveolar wall interstitium contains excess fluid, is very dif-

Fig. 28-1. Kerley's B lines. Close-up of the right lateral lung base in a patient with mitral stenosis and interstitial edema. The numerous transverse, short, dense lines at the periphery of the lung represent secondary interlobular septa thickened by edema fluid.

Fig. 28-2. Interstitial edema. In the roentgenograms of this patient who had rheumatic mitral disease and a grossly enlarged heart, typical Kerley's B lines are evident at both lateral bases. There are some longer, finer lines in the upper central lungs **(arrows)** which probably represent Kerley's A lines. A little parahilar haze, seen particularly on the right side, and a general increase in interstitial markings resulting in a somewhat reticular pattern, noted best in the oblique projections, are apparent. Also a small amount of pleural fluid is present on the left.

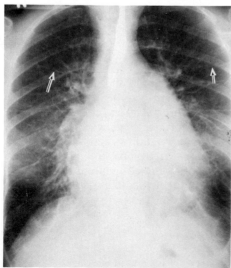
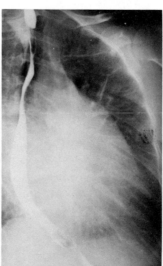
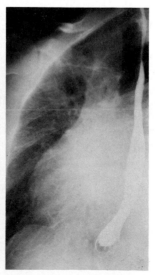

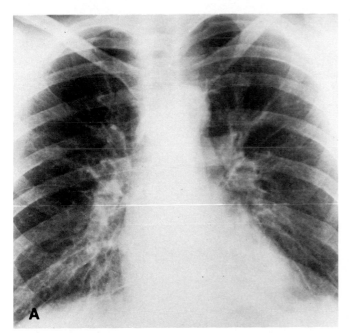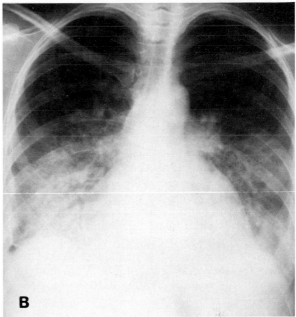

Fig. 28-3. Interstitial and alveolar edema. **A.** Interstitial edema. There is a general increase in interstitial markings, particularly in the parahilar areas and at the bases. The vessels are poorly defined, particularly at the bases, as a result of perivascular edema. Also a little parahilar haze blurring the vessels there is noted, particularly on the right. **B.** Alveolar edema. Same patient as shown in **A,** with renal failure and evidence of extensive alveolar density in the parahilar areas and at the bases. There is now some pleural fluid bilaterally. The unequal distribution of the alveolar edema is not unusual.

ficult to evaluate, and is an accessory sign at best (Fig. 28-2). It can often be best appreciated when an earlier film is available for comparison or when a film is obtained after successful treatment of the edema, it can be recognized in retrospect.
4. A diffuse, reticular pattern may be observed associated with other findings as noted in the signs described in the foregoing. This is difficult to assess but represents interstitial fluid in these patients with edema. A similar pattern may be seen in patients with widespread interstitial fibrosis, but A lines are not usually present in these. In chronic congestive failure, interstitial edema may resemble chronic interstitial thickening associated with pulmonary disease. Only after treatment of the cardiac condition brings about regression can the true nature of the process be diagnosed with certainty. Interstitial edema often occurs in combination with the alveolar type (Fig. 28-3). Interstitial edema precedes alveolar edema in these instances, but often the onset is very

rapid with massive alveolar edema overshadowing all subtle signs.
5. Subpleural edema may be observed best adjacent to the minor fissure on the right but may also be observed along the major fissures in lateral projections. Peripherally there may be enough to simulate pleural thickening.

The edema fluid accumulates first in peribronchial, perivascular, and interlobular interstitial spaces to produce the findings as noted. Edema (thickening) of the alveolar wall probably doesn't occur until later, after the other interstitial spaces are filled. Then alveolar flooding may occur if fluid continues to accumulate in the lungs.

ALVEOLAR EDEMA

The classic roentgen findings of alveolar pulmonary edema are those of bilateral densities that extend outward in a fan-shaped manner from the hilum on both sides. The peripheral lung fields are relatively clear. This includes the bases as well as the apices except in congestive failure, in which basal congestive changes and edema produce density there. Since interstitial edema precedes the alveolar form, some or all of the signs of interstitial edema may be observed. However, the alveolar edema may be so extensive that other signs are obscured. When the edema is moderate the density is somewhat patchy and mottled, but it may become quite homogeneous as the amount increases (Fig. 28-4). In the latter instance, the fluid-filled alveoli surrounding the bronchi produce contrast with the air-containing bronchi and, as a result, the bronchi are visible as linear radiolucent spaces traversing the opaque edematous area (Fig. 28-5). The density is often bilaterally symmetric or nearly so. There are many exceptions to this rule and a number of cases have been reported in which the edema was unilateral. Serial films often show rapid changes in the amount and distribution of the edema from day to day. When pulmonary edema is early and minor it may produce scattered localized densities that may simulate nodular disease (Fig. 28-6). The "nodules" are poorly defined, however, and probably represent multiple acini (the portion of lung distal to a terminal bronchiole) filled with edema fluid. Bi-

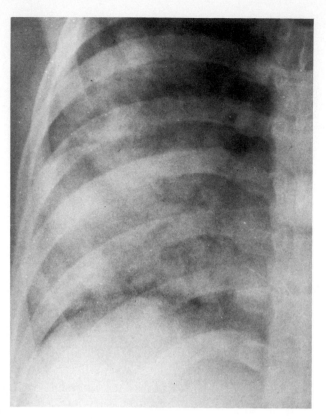

Fig. 28-5. Massive alveolar pulmonary edema. Close-up of the right lower lung to show air-filled bronchi (air bronchogram) in the otherwise dense fluid-filled lung.

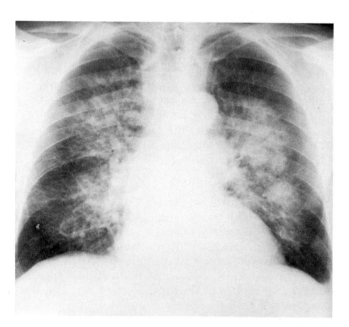

Fig. 28-4. Pulmonary edema. This is a rather typical example of alveolar edema with a fan-shaped distribution in the parahilar and mid zones of the lungs. This patient had chronic renal failure.

zarre forms may also be present with large, rather rounded areas of increased density that may actually simulate tumor. As a general rule the alveolar density is hazy and poorly defined, so that there is no difficulty in making the diagnosis. Pleural effusion is commonly associated with edema, particularly in congestive heart failure and in uremia.

Numerous reports of unusual and asymmetric distribution of edema have led to some experimental work and much speculation as to the factors involved in the distribution of edema fluid.[6] Gravity is undoubtedly a factor in many cases, but lateral views of patients who have been supine sometimes shows the fluid to be in anterior or lingular segments or in the middle lobe. Lack of peripheral edema is probably related to better peripheral drainage of lymphatics and to the increased respiratory motion of the peripheral lung acting to "pump" the fluid out. The relative lack of compliance in the central lung and in lung which

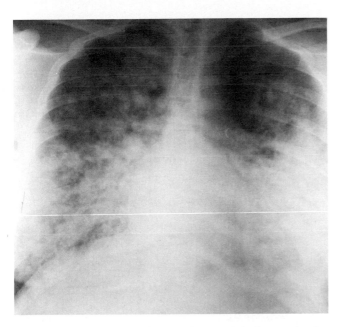

Fig. 28-6. Alveolar edema. The rounded, poorly defined densities noted best in the upper lung fields and in the right central and lower lung represent the acinar type of distribution of fluid.

has been previously diseased may also be involved. Defective lymphatic drainage favors accumulation of fluid in areas of previous disease which has resulted in scarring or decrease in compliance. Gravity definitely plays a part in most, if not all, patients with unilateral pulmonary edema. Other factors include differences in perfusion and in microvascular pressures in different areas.

There are no constantly reliable changes that will determine the cause, but in edema secondary to cardiac failure the observations of cardiac enlargement, pulmonary congestion, and pleural effusion are strong indications that the edema is the result of heart disease. Exceptions include the absence of cardiac enlargement in some patients with pulmonary edema secondary to acute coronary thrombosis, and the absence of basal congestive changes in patients with edema secondary to acute left ventricular failure. As a general rule, pulmonary edema caused by uremia (azotemic edema) produces the classic central "fluffy" density of the lungs without evidence of cardiac enlargement or pulmonary congestion. Pulmonary edema caused by inhalation of irritant gases tends to be somewhat more widespread than the other types and results in a mottled and patchy appearance extending farther to the periphery with

slightly less central involvement than is seen in uremia; it also tends to be more basal. Roentgen distribution is not characteristic, however, and the history is of great importance in arriving at the diagnosis in these patients.

ADULT RESPIRATORY DISTRESS SYNDROME (ARDS)

The term "adult respiratory distress syndrome" is used widely to describe a syndrome resulting from a number of conditions in which there is pulmonary injury. The clinical signs include marked dyspnea, increased respiratory effort, hypoxemia which is often severe, and associated cyanosis.[1, 9, 14] The basic process is probably diffuse endothelial injury in the pulmonary microvasculature causing increased permeability and pulmonary edema. Alterations in production of surfactant are proably secondary. A variety of causes have been implicated including hemorrhagic or septic shock; massive trauma, either pulmonary or general; extensive viral pneumonia; aspiration of gastric contents; drug overdose; cardiopulmonary bypass; inhalation of corrosive chemicals; smoke inhalation; hypoxemia associated with near drowning; and hemorrhagic pancreatitis. Hypovolemic shock appears to develop in most of the patients, but disseminated intravascular coagulation involving the microcirculation is a major pathogenic factor in most, if not all patients. Other factors include surfactant deficit and left ventricular failure; in some instances, oxygen toxicity and prolonged respiratory care may add to the injury.

There is a difference of opinion regarding the use of the term represented by the initials ARDS, and many would apply the etiologic terms "acute pulmonary insufficiency associated with shock, drug overdose, near drowning," and so on.

Roentgenographic findings are variable, but, in most instances, no abnormalities are noted in the first 12 hours following initiation of the syndrome. The earliest changes are those of interstitial edema, which may be associated with or followed by patchy alveolar edema causing local, ill-defined, acinar-type densities. After 24 hours or so, this may progress to more typical and massive consolidation representing extensive alveolar edema. Usually the heart is not enlarged, and there is no pleural effusion. Complications such as gram-negative pneumonias may result in multiple cavitations. Proliferative changes in the lung, which may appear as early as 2 days after the onset, are manifested as an increase in interstitial markings observed when the acute edema regresses.

The pulmonary densities are not as variable or rapidly reversible as in patients with pulmonary edema who do not have respiratory insufficiency. Finally, there is a mixed pattern of interstitial and alveolar densities usually bilateral but not always symmetrical. If the patient recovers, the changes may clear completely.

There are no signs of elevation of pulmonary venous pressure in this syndrome in that there is no redistribution of blood flow. Left ventricular failure in these patients is nearly impossible to diagnose radiographically, so the Swan–Ganz catheter is used; this provides the most dependable method now available for detecting left ventricular failure. Duration of the clinical and roentgenographic findings is quite variable in this group. In the advanced stage when respiratory insufficiency is refractory, there is usually a mixed pulmonary lesion consisting of alveolar and the interstitial densities that are bilateral, may not be symmetrical, and may be associated with cavitation if the condition is complicated by anaerobic infection. The synonyms include shock lung, posttraumatic pulmonary insufficiency, hemorrhagic lung syndrome, "stiff lung" syndrome, "solid lung" syndrome, adult hyaline membrane disease, respirator lung, congestive atelectasis, progressive pulmonary consolidation, pump lung, posttransfusion lung, transplant lung, postperfusion lung, and respiratory insufficiency associated with oxygen toxicity, fat embolism, and disseminated intravascular coagulation.

PULMONARY THROMBOEMBOLISM AND INFARCTION

Pulmonary embolism with or without infarction is a more common lesion than is generally realized. Since the majority of thromboembolic episodes cause no symptoms, they are not recognized. In addition to its occurrence as a postoperative complication and in patients with cardiac disease, pulmonary embolism occurs in a number of other conditions. The most common sources of pulmonary emboli are thrombi in the deep veins of the leg. When the embolus is very large and occludes the entire pulmonary areterial tree, death may occur very quickly. When the embolus is somewhat smaller it may or may not produce infarction but will often cause immediate symptoms of chest pain and dyspnea. There may be no symptoms or signs with small emboli. In addition to parts of thrombi, a number of other materials may act as emboli. Air embolism that may follow trauma is not usually demonstrated radiographically; it disappears very quickly if the patient survives. If it causes sud-den death the air can be demonstrated on postmortem films. Opaque contrast materials used in hysterosalpingography and in myelography occasionally enter the bloodstream and have been demonstrated in the lungs following these procedures. A few cases of barium in the pulmonary vessels following barium enema have been reported in which fatalities have occurred during the examination.

PULMONARY INFARCTION

The incidence of infarction varies in different groups of patients with pulmonary thromboembolism. In patients with chronic heart disease and congestive failure it approaches 100%, while in young, healthy individuals, complete infarct is rare unless there are complicating factors such as severe trauma. In the elderly, chronically ill who are bedridden, the incidence is in the range of 60% to 70% of those who have pulmonary emboli. The roentgenographic diagnosis is often difficult to make. The major error is usually failure to suspect infarction as the cause for abnormal roentgen findings in the chest. The roentgen signs are: (1) elevation of the hemidiaphragm on the involved side; (2) unilateral pleural effusion, usually small; (3) pulmonary parenchymal consolidation; (4) atelectasis; and (5) linear shadow(s). An infarct must be differentiated from pneumonia, edema, and atelectasis as well as other local conditions, such as infected cysts and abscesses. The lower lobes are most frequently involved, but the lesion may occur in any lobe. Elevation of the diaphragm or small pleural effusion or both may be the earliest signs of infarction. At times the shadow of the infarct may not be visible and the effusion is the only sign. It takes from 10 to 24 hours for an infarct to evolve to the point where it is visible roentgenographically. This is probably the hazy, poorly defined, edematous lesion that requires an additional 2 to 4 days and sometimes a week to form a well-defined complete infarct. Infarction of a single secondary pulmonary lobule may occur, and, since not all lobules have a pleural surface, it follows that not all infarcts have a pleural surface. Infarcts are usually aggregates of involved secondary lobules, however, so the lesion usually extends to a pleural surface. Since this may be the interlobar pleura, its shadow is not necessarily peripheral as visualized in the frontal projection. The shape of the infarct is dependent upon the location. The visceral pleura usually forms one side of the lesion and often two or three sides. The long axis of the infarct is in the plane of the longest pleural surface with which it is in contact. The actual shadow may be rounded or roughly triangular. It may assume the shape of the lingula or of the right middle lobe or may fill and obliterate a costophrenic sulcus if the lateral segment of a lower lobe is involved. Oblique views aided by fluoroscopic positioning are necessary to bring out the relationship of the lesion to the pleura in many cases. The hilar aspect of the infarct is usually described as rounded or hump-shaped rather than resembling the apex of a triangle. The appearance of a "typical" hump is unusual, if not rare, and most any shape of density may be present. The amount of associated pleural effusion is usually not great and multiple lesions may be visualized in one or both lungs (Fig. 28-7). At first the periphery of the lesion is reather hazy and poorly defined, but as time goes on it becomes more sharply outlined and as it heals it gradually becomes smaller. The size of the infarct can vary greatly, from bare visibility to the greater part of a lobe. The average size is about 3 to 5 cm. The pulmonary changes resolve rather slowly. The complete hemorrhagic necrotic infarct requires 4 weeks or more for complete resolution. When infarction is incomplete, there is no necrosis, the local findings are caused by edema and hemorrhage. This

process may clear quickly, within a week or less, and leave no residue. The complete infarct slowly decreases in size. Eventually only a linear fibrous band may remain to indicate the site of a previous infarct. The linear scar may be quite small and inconspicuous. There is often a small amount of localized pleural thickening associated with the linear density.

Linear densities in the lower lungs described in patients with embolism usually represent platelike or focal atelectasis caused by a combination of poor ventilation, narrowing of the bronchi, decreased compliance of the lung, and lack of surfactant, all of which occur in pulmonary embolism with infarction. Other causes include parenchymal fibrosis or scarring secondary to a healed or healing infarct and some probably represent linear shadows of pleural origin. Diaphragmatic splinting secondary to the pleural involvement is represented by elevation of the diaphragm. This may be the only roentgen finding in some patients. If the possibility of pulmonary infarction is kept in mind in bedridden, debilitated, or cardiac patients with sudden pleuritic type of chest pain, the presence of one or all of the signs just described should lead to the diagnosis, or at least a suspicion of

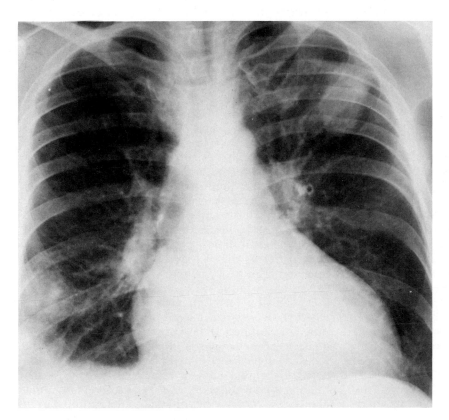

Fig. 28-7. Pulmonary infarcts. The oval density at the left apex represents an old infarct. There is a little fluid remaining in the major fissure in the region of the infarct which is now quite well circumscribed. There are two infarcts in the right base; one produces a humplike shadow obliterating the costophrenic angle and projecting above the level of the dome of the diaphragm; the other is somewhat rounded and lies above it. There is also some pleural effusion. The heart is greatly enlarged.

it, in most instances. The lack of a characteristic contour cannot be overemphasized because of the wide variety of shapes, depending on location; the size also varies greatly. It is also important to remember that infarction can occur in the absence of congestive heart disease. There may be enough fluid in the pleural space to hide the pulmonary lesion and decubitus films are of value to outline the basal lung when infarction is suspected. When the diagnosis is in doubt, progress films should be obtained since the shadow of the infarct cannot be visualized until hemorrhage and exudation have occurred. Lung scans with radioactive-tagged, macroaggregated, human serum albumin are helpful in the diagnosis of infarction when roentgen signs are present, but scanning is more useful when the chest roentgenogram shows no abnormality.

Pulmonary arteriography is the most accurate method for making the diagnosis, but selective segmental and subsegmental studies using oblique projections may be necessary to outline small-vessel involvement. The primary sign of embolism is a persistent intraluminal filling defect that may completely obstruct the involved artery. Secondary signs, helpful but not diagnostic, are areas of avascularity, focal areas of prolonged arterial filling, "pruning" or paucity of vessels, and abrupt cut off of a pulmonary artery without a visible filling defect in the lumen. This method is used if a positive diagnosis of pulmonary embolism and infarction is imperative. Its use is usually limited to patients in whom surgical therapy of any type is contemplated.

EMBOLISM WITHOUT INFARCTION

Pulmonary embolism may be massive and life-threatening. Prompt diagnosis is of utmost importance in these patients. Roentgen findings are often minimal or absent in contrast to the clinical findings in a desperately ill patient. The central pulmonary arteries may be increased in size, with sharp diminution in size of branches off the hilum and relative radiolucency of the ischemic areas. If the patient happens to have had a roentgenogram of the chest in the recent past, comparison can be very helpful (Fig. 28-8).

Secondary signs of dilatation of the superior vena cava causing some superior mediastinal widening on the right and cardiac enlargement may be helpful. At best, the diagnosis of massive pulmonary embolism can be suggested. Since embolectomy might be indicated when the patient is hypotensive and cyanotic, pulmonary arteriography is indicated to confirm the presence of large central emboli which can be surgically removed.

The diagnosis can usually be made by employing the combination of plain-film chest roentgenogram and lung scan. When serious doubt regarding the diagnosis arises following these procedures, pulmonary arteriography can be done. The angiographic signs of pulmonary embolism are: (1) the demonstration of defects in the major arteries which represent the clots (Fig. 28-9) (this is the only definitive sign); (2) "cut-off" of one or more large branch vessels with no opacification of the lung peripheral to them; (3) absent or diminished local bloodflow usually manifested by decreased arborization or truncation; and (4) prolonged arterial opacification in a local area or areas.

In embolization without infarction that is not life-threatening, plain-film findings are often very subtle and sometimes show only a normal state. The central pulmonary arteries may be dilated, but this is difficult to assess unless a comparison film is available. The dilatation may be unilateral or bilateral and probably represents the mass of the embolus. There may be a decrease in size of the arteries peripheral to the embolus; this sign is also very difficult to evaluate on a single film. Lobar or segmental hyperlucency may be present; it, too, is very difficult to evaluate. In these patients in whom the roentgenograms show normal or nearly normal states, the lung scan is virtually diagnostic. When antecedent or complicating lung disease is present, the scan is not as useful. It is in this situation that a pulmonary arteriogram may be necessary to confirm the diagnosis.

SEPTIC INFARCTION

When the embolus producing infarction contains or is made up of bacteria, septic infarction results, which leads to tissue breakdown and formation of cavity. These lesions may occur in association with subacute bacterial endocarditis or other infections in which there is septicemia. They may be single but are usually multiple. A cavity may form in an infarcted area as the result of secondary bronchogenic infection. There may be sequestration of the necrotic center of an infarct to produce cavity within infection. Usually, infection supervenes, however, and when these infarcts become infected the pneumonitis surrounding them causes further increase in density with a poorly circumscribed periphery. The roentgen appearance is that of a central cavity within a poorly defined area of increased density. When there is a typical history and other infarcts are present, the diagnosis is not difficult to determine, but in single lesions the differentiation between infarct cav-

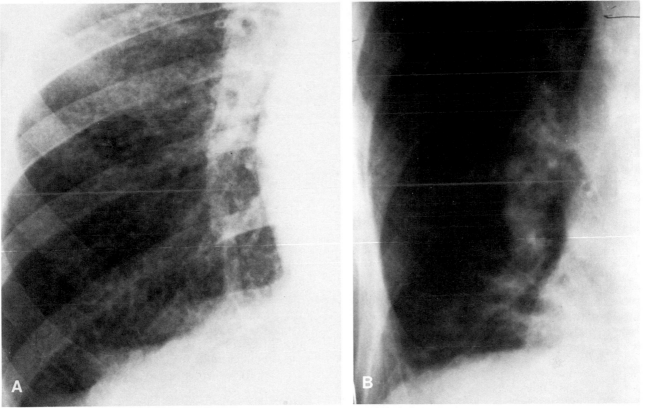

Fig. 28-8. Pulmonary embolism. The patient developed chest pain while in the hospital. **A.** Close-up of the right lower lung on admission. **B.** One week later, on film exposed 1 day after the onset of chest pain, enlargement of the pulmonary artery, which was found to be the site of a large embolus, is demonstrated. The diaphragm is elevated. The horizontal linear densities at the lung base most likely represent areas of subsegmental atelectasis. The patient did not develop infarction that could be recognized radiographically.

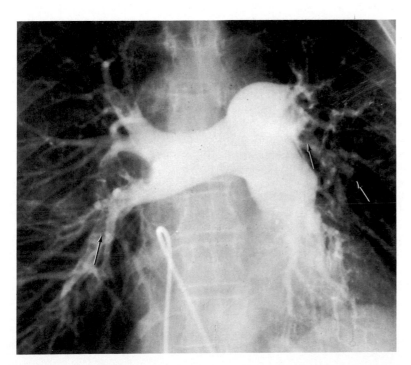

Fig. 28-9. Pulmonary emboli. This arteriogram shows several small lucencies representing emboli in the pulmonary arteries **(arrows).**

ity and cavity secondary to primary inflammatory disease is difficult, if not impossible.

POSTTRAUMATIC FAT EMBOLISM

There is experimental and some clinical evidence to show that fat embolism is very common following bone and soft-tissue injury, particularly following fractures of the tibia and femur. However, despite the fact that many severely injured patients are observed, the clinical entity and pulmonary roentgen evidence of posttraumatic fat embolism is relatively rare. It is likely that small amounts of fat may form emboli without symptoms and signs. The roentgen findings are varied, but are uniformly bilateral. They include: (1) Diffuse bilateral density which resembles pulmonary edema except that there is more basal involvement than is usually observed in edema and the involvement is more peripheral, often with relatively little alveolar density centrally. (2) Bilateral, multiple small nodular densities; often more nodules are noted in the lower lungs than elsewhere. This probably represents a somewhat lesser involvement than the more confluent homogeneous edema pattern. (3) Usually, no pleural effusion or cardiac enlargement. (4) Delayed onset, usually from 1 to 3 days following trauma. This is in contrast to pulmonary contusion with hemorrhage and edema that occurs very soon after injury. Also, contusion is usually unilateral or asymmetrical in contrast to the bilateral symmetry of fat embolism. The diagnosis can usually be made on the basis of the history of chest pain and cough 12 hours to several days following injury, along with chest roentgen findings as described. Resolution varies from 6 days to 2 weeks or more.

PULMONARY HYPERTENSION

Blood flow through the lungs and pulmonary artery pressure are dependent upon a number of factors including arterial and venous resistance, the amount of bloodflow which may be altered in various shunts, and combinations of these factors. Pulmonary hypertension may be predominantly arterial (precapillary) or venous (postcapillary) or combined. Since the roentgen changes vary with the type and the site of the major causative factors, a classification[18] of pulmonary hypertension is presented:

I. Precapillary (Arterial Hypertension)
 A. Increased resistance
  1. Obstructive: pulmonary embolism, idio-
pathic or primary pulmonary hypertension, pulmonary schistosomiasis, reverse shunts (ventricular septal defect, atrial septal defect, or patent ductus arteriosus)
  2. Obliterative: emphysema, diffuse interstitial diseases—fibrotic, granulomatous, neoplastic, or infectious
  3. Constrictive: anoxia
 B. Increased flow
  1. Large left-to-right shunts: PDA, VSD
II. Postcapillary (Venouse Hypertension)
 A. Acute: Left ventricular failure regardless of cause
 B. Chronic: Mitral valvular disease, left atrial myxoma, anomalous pulmonary venous return, mediastinal fibrosis, idiopathic or primary veno-obstructive disease.[12]
III. Combined Pre- and Postcapillary Hypertension
IV. Diffuse Pulmonary Arteriovenous Shunting Complicating Chronic Lung Disease (Simon): Emphysema—shunt syndrome

Pulmonary hypertension is defined as elevation of pressure in the pulmonary circuit above certain limits at rest or during mild exercise. These limits are generally accepted as 30 mm Hg systolic and 15 mm Hg diastolic with a mean of 18 mm Hg on the arterial side. On the venous side the upper limit is considered to be 12 mm Hg; this is applied equally to the mean left atrial pressure and to the mean capillary-wedge pressure.

Most of the diseases causing pulmonary hypertension produce an increase in pulmonary vascular resistance. In the upright chest film of the normal person, the upper zone vessels are smaller than those in the lower zones. In recumbency this difference disappears; this accounts in part for disparity between angiograms and routine films.

There are distinct radiographic differences in the pre- and postcapillary groups. The roentgen changes in pulmonary arterial (precapillary) hypertension include: dilatation of the pulmonary artery and its central branches on either side; narrowing of the peripheral pulmonary arteries, resulting in a rather sharp fall-off in size from central to peripheral arteries (Fig. 28-10); tortuosity of peripheral arteries, particularly in lower zones, observed along with a general decrease in caliber of pulmonary veins; and calcification observed in the pulmonary artery (Fig. 28-11). Cor pulmonale or pulmonary heart disease with varying enlargement of the right ventricle caused by dilata-

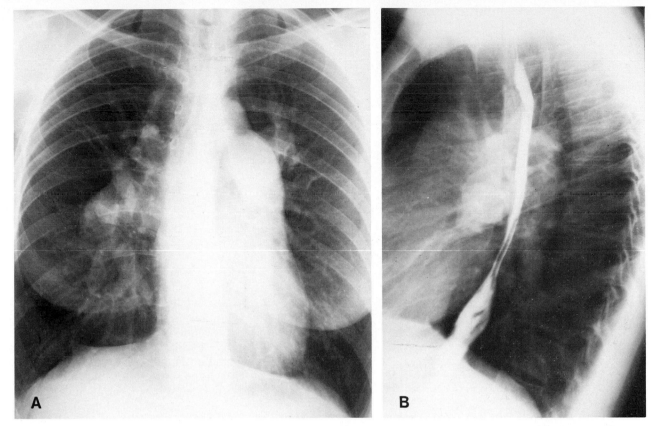

Fig. 28-10. Pulmonary arterial hypertension. The pulmonary artery and its central branches are grossly enlarged in contrast to the peripheral arteries which are small. This patient had an atrial septal defect. She developed pulmonary hypertension which resulted in reversal of the initial left-to-right shunt and was now cyanotic.

tion or hypertrophy or both is an eventual development. Signs of the underlying causative disease may be minimal, obvious, or absent. In general, increasing severity of the hypertension is accompanied by an increase in the roentgen signs, but there are exceptions, so caution should be observed in predicting pulmonary artery pressure ranges. The lungs are relatively clear unless the underlying disease has produced considerable change.

Another situation is one in which pulmonary arterial hypertension develops as systemic high-pressures are transmitted across congenital defects causing left-to-right shunts at the aortopulmonary (patent ductus) or ventricular (ventricular septal defect) level. A substantial high-pressure shunt at the aortic or ventricular level or a massive shunt at the atrial or great vein level will eventually cause a reactive sclerosis, intimal thickening, and medial hypertrophy in pulmonary arteries. This progresses to marked pulmonary arterial hypertension with resultant shunt reversal. The following roentgen signs are produced.

Fig. 28-11. Pulmonary arterial hypertension. Note the dense calcification in the pulmonary artery and ductus in this patient with patent ductus who had developed a reversal of the shunt as a result of the pulmonary hypertension.

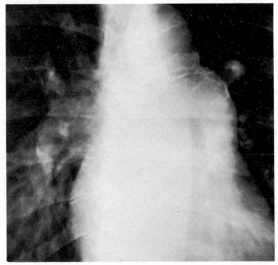

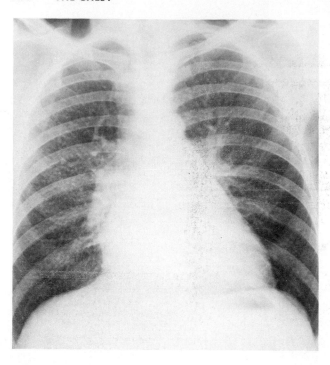

Fig. 28-12. Pulmonary venous hypertension. This patient with mitral disease demonstrates some parahilar haze and distinct difference in vessel size, the upper-lobe vessels being definitely larger than those in the lower lobe. This represents redistribution of blood flow and indicates pulmonary venous hypertension.

Fig. 28-13. Congestive failure in a patient with arteriosclerotic cardiovascular disease. **A.** Central and basal vessels are poorly defined, indicating perivascular edema. No Kerley's B lines are observed. Upper-lobe vessels are relatively prominent. Basal vessels are difficult to define because of the perivascular edema. **B.** Close-up of the right base to show the poor definition of vessels in this patient.

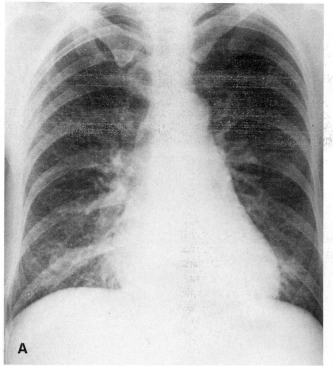

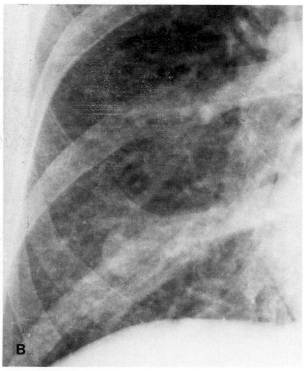

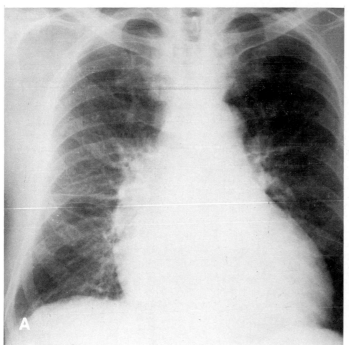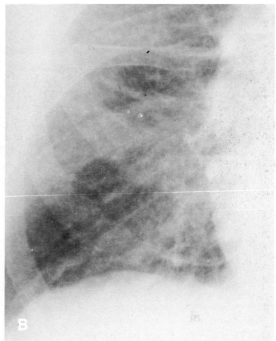

Fig. 28-14. Congestive heart failure. **A.** The heart is distinctly enlarged. There is vascular redistribution and evidence of some parahilar haze and perivascular edema noted best at the right base. **B.** Close-up of area of involvement. The individual vessels are very poorly defined. There is a hint of a little interstitial edema peripherally with short, horizontal linear densitites that are poorly defined.

1. Marked enlargement of the pulmonary artery and its central branches extending out for a short distance along the lobar arteries. Calcification is occasionally observed in the pulmonary artery.

2. Constriction of segmental and peripheral arteries to normal or smaller than normal size.

3. Normal or small pulmonary veins.

4. The heart showing alteration consistent with the initial defect. However, eventually the right ventricle may increase to become the predominant chamber (cor pulmonale).

Postcapillary hypertension is often accompanied by changes that cause a considerable increase in pulmonary density, *e.g.*, edema. Slight distention of all pulmonary veins is the earliest roentgen sign, but this is very difficult to evaluate unless comparison films are available. Constriction of the pulmonary arteries and veins in the lower zones and dilatation of the arteries and veins in the upper zones caused by redistribution of blood flow to the upper lobes are the most reliable early signs. These must be evaluated in the upright film, since there is normally some redistribution of

flow to the upper lobes in films exposed with the patient recumbent. These findings may be striking when present, but are not well defined in every patient with venous hypertension. These signs may be obliterated by pulmonary edema and congestion in left ventricular failure. The cause for the basal constriction, indicating a redistribution of blood flow, remains controversial. Mild, venous hypertension shows only the vascular constriction which may be difficult to assess (Fig. 28-12). As the venous pressure increases, additional findings of early interstitial edema can be observed; they include the appearance of Kerley's B lines and Kerley's A lines. A slight perihilar haze may be evident. Vascular margins are blurred and poorly defined and there is a general increase in interstitial markings (Figs. 28-13 and 28-14). Alveolar edema and pleural effusion appear when venous hypertension is marked and left ventricular failure occurs. Chronic postcapillary hypertension, such as that found in mitral stenosis, and left atrial myxoma result in irreversible constriction of lower-zone pulmonary vessels.

When there is a combined arterial (pre-) and venous (postcapillary) hypertension, the roentgen changes depend on the sequence of events. Mitral stenosis is a good example, with venous hypertension occurring for some time being followed by arterial hypertension. The roentgen findings are then in combination and develop as the disease develops—a summation of changes.

Chronic lung diseases such as pulmonary fibrosis and emphysema cause increased pulmonary arterial resistance resulting in pulmonary arterial hypertension. Occasionally such a patient will develop general dilatation of pulmonary arteries and veins involving all of the lung zones. This is caused by diffuse arteriovenous shunting. There may be some interstitial edema and the patients are dyspneic and cyanotic. It is postulated by Simon, Sasahara, and Cannilla,[18] that a combination of increased pulmonary resistance and left ventricular decompensation probably caused by hypoxia results in this "emphysema-shunt syndrome."

REFERENCES AND SELECTED READINGS

1. ADAMS FG, LEDINGHAM I McA: The pulmonary manifestations of septic shock. Clin Radiol 28: 315, 1977

2. BERRIGAN TJ JR, CARSKY EW, HEITZMAN ER: Fat embolism. Am J Roentgenol 96: 967, 1966

3. BOOKSTEIN JJ: Pulmonary thromboembolism with emphasis on angiographic-pathologic correlation. Semin Roentgenol 5: 291, 1970

4. FIGLEY MM, GERDES AJ, RICKETTS HJ: Radiographic aspects of pulmonary embolism. Semin Roentgenol 2: 389, 1967

5. FLEISCHNER FG: Roentgenology of the pulmonary infarct. Semin Roentgenol 2: 61, 1967

6. FLEISCHNER FG: The butterfly pattern of acute pulmonary edema. In Simon M, Potchen EJ, and LeMay M (eds): Frontiers of Pulmonary Radiology, pp 360–379. New York, Grune & Stratton, 1967

7. GOODWIN JF, STEINER RE, GRAINGER RG, HARRISON CV: Pulmonary hypertension: a symposium. Br J Radiol 31: 174, 1958

8. HEITZMAN ER, ZITER FM JR: Acute interstitial pulmonary edema. Am J Roentgenol 98: 291, 1966

9. JOFFE N: Roentgenologic findings in post-shock and postoperative pulmonary insufficiency. Radiology 94: 369, 1970

10. KEATS TE, DREIS VA, SIMPSON E: The roentgen manifestations of pulmonary hypertension in congenital heart disease. Radiology 66: 693, 1956

11. KREEL L, SLAVIN G. HERBERT A et al: Intralobar septal oedema: "D" lines. Clin Radiol 26: 209, 1975

12. LIEBOW AA, MOSER KM, SOUTHGATE MT: Primary veno-obstructive disease of the lung: clinical-pathologic conference. JAMA 223: 1243, 1973

13. MILNE ENC: Some new concepts of pulmonary blood flow and volume. Radiol Clin North Am 14: 515, 1978

14. OSTENDORF P, BIRZLE H, VOGEL W et al: Pulmonary radiographic abnormalities in shock: roentgen clinical-pathological correlation. Radiology 115: 257, 1975

15. QUINN JL: Radioisotope lung scanning. Semin Roentgenol 2: 406, 1967

16. RIGLER LG, SURPRENANT EL: Pulmonary edema. Semin Roentgenol 2: 33, 1967

17. SIMON M, POTCHEN EJ, LeMAY M: Frontiers of Pulmonary Radiology. New York, Grune & Stratton, 1969

18. SIMON M, SASAHARA AA, CANNILLA JE: The radiology of pulmonary hypertension. Semin Roentgenol 2: 368, 1967

19. STAUB NC: Pathogenesis of pulmonary edema, state of the art review. Am Rev Resp Dis 109: 358, 1974

29

TUMORS OF THE LUNGS AND BRONCHI

MALIGNANT TUMORS

Classification

The following is a satisfactory working classification of lung tumors, adapted from Liebow.[*]

    I. Primary Malignant Epithelial Tumors[6]
        A. Bronchogenic Carcinoma
            1. Epidermoid (squamous cell) 30%
            2. Adenocarcinoma 25%
            3. Anaplastic (small-cell) carcinoma 25%
            4. Large-cell carcinoma 20%
                a. Solid: with mucin
                b. Solid: without mucin
                c. Giant cell
                d. Clear cell
        B. Bronchiolar Carcinoma (bronchiolo-alveolar)
        C. Bronchial Adenoma
    II. Sarcoma
        A. Differentiated Spindle Cell Sarcoma
        B. Differentiated Sarcoma
        C. Primary Lymphosarcoma
   III. Mixed Epithelial and Sarcomatous Tumor (Carcinosarcoma)
   IV. Neoplasms of Reticuloendothelial System Involving the Lung
    V. Metastatic Tumors of the Lung

BRONCHOGENIC CARCINOMA

There has been an absolute as well as a relative increase in the incidence of carcinoma of the lung in the past 40 years that is reflected in the mortality rate. In white males the reported death rate from cancer of the lung is 25 times higher now than in 1914. Of all carcinomas this carries the highest mortality rate, but may have reached a plateau in males. The incidence and mortality rate in females is now rising, with one study showing a drop in male–female ratio from 15 to 1 in the years 1955 to 1959 to 6 to 1 in the years 1968 to 1971. Despite the advances in surgery, radiotherapy, and various combinations of

[*] Mayer, E., and Maier, H. C.: *Pulmonary Carcinoma.* New York, New York University Press, 1956, p. 74. Adapted from Liebow.[5]

chemotherapy, the overall 5-year survival rate is very low, in the range of 5% to 7%. In contrast to this, the 5-year survival rate in a small series of patients with bronchogenic carcinoma discovered in a survey of asymptomatic patients was 30%. This suggests that there is an opportunity to improve the high mortality rate in this type of cancer. Earlier diagnosis by means of roentgen examination is one way in which it may be accomplished.

The epidermoid or squamous cell neoplasm occurs predominantly in males, with a ratio of 6 or 10 to 1. They make up about one-third of all bronchogenic tumors and tend to occur in relatively old-age groups with the peak incidence at age 60. This tumor often arises in or immediately adjacent to lobar and segmental bronchi, but is occasionally peripheral. When a primary tumor is noted to invade the thoracic wall, it is more likely to be epidermoid than any other type. Necrosis with formation of cavity is also fairly common, and when a tumor of this type is found in an elderly male it is nearly always epidermoid in origin. The well-differentiated squamous cell tumor is more likely to remain confined to the bronchus of origin and adjacent nodes than the more atypical forms and the rate of growth is often less rapid in this tumor than in the others. Invasion of veins with hematogenous metastasis does occur late in the course of the disease, however.

The adenocarcinoma with an overall incidence of about 25% is the most common of the bronchogenic tumors found in the female. It tends to be more peripheral than the other types but may be central. The rate of growth is rapid; hematogenous and lymphogenous metastases occur early. This is the tumor most often observed peripherally in relatively young females. The anaplastic carcinoma, which makes up about 25% of bronchogenic tumors, often occurs centrally, with hilar enlargement and massive lymph-node metastases. This type may resemble mediastinal lymphosarcoma. It does not often form a peripheral tumor and does not usually undergo necrosis to form cavitation. The large-cell carcinomas are also anaplastic tumors and comprise nearly 20% of lung cancers. They tend to be bulky, large tumors which usually occur peripherally, grow rapidly, invade locally, and disseminate widely. Pleural involvement with effusion is common.

The alveolar- (bronchiolo-alveolar) cell carcinoma may sometimes be multifocal, but some investigators believe that it begins as a a single focus and spreads widely through the lymphatics. Two general gross pathologic types are described: (1) the tumorlike or nodular form and (2) the diffuse type, which may resemble pneumonic consolidation roentgenographically.

Bronchial adenoma is included in the malignant bronchogenic tumor group because this lesion metastasizes locally to nodes, but there is a marked difference in the clinical course and the prognosis between this tumor and bronchogenic carcinoma. The relatively good prognosis holds, even though hilar node metastases are found at surgery. The tumor occurs in a younger age group and is as frequent in females as in males. In contrast to the low survival rate in bronchogenic carcinoma, the 5-year survival rate in bronchial adenoma is 90% or more.

Roentgen Findings. The changes caused by bronchogenic carcinoma vary widely, depending upon the site of the tumor and its relation to the bronchial tree. The tumor itself may or may not be visible. When it is not visible its presence can be detected by such findings as localized emphysema, atelectasis, and inflammatory disease, all of which are secondary to the tumor within or compressing a bronchus. Each radiologic sign of bronchogenic carcinoma may occur as the only evidence of tumor or several of the signs may occur in a single patient. Any of the following may occur as the initial sign of bronchogenic carcinoma: (1) Atelectasis which may be segmental or lobar. (2) Unilateral hilar enlargement. (3) Emphysema, obstructive in type, may be segmental or lobar; this is a very rare initial sign. (4) Mediastinal mass, often simulating lymphoma; this is usually found in undifferentiated (oat cell or round cell) carcinoma. (5) Apical pulmonary density with or without rib destruction, the superior pulmonary sulcus (Pancoast) tumor. (6) Cavitation in a solitary mass; usually in squamous cell carcinoma in heavy smokers. (7) Segmental consolidation, resembling local pneumonitis which does not clear or which clears incompletely. (8) Parenchymal mass, including sharply defined peripheral nodule and poorly defined irregular nodular mass which may be surrounded by abnormal thickened vessels demonstrated on tomography.

Occasionally the initial sign may be a very poorly defined, irregular, nonhomogeneous density which may be linear and resemble a fibrotic scar. Therefore it is necessary to be suspicious of nearly every density in the lung that does not clear, or that appears in a patient with previously normal lungs, particularly if the patient is a male smoker over 40 years of age.

In addition to those listed in the preceding paragraphs a number of other roentgen signs may result from metastasis or local invasion. These consist of (1) pleural effusion, (2) hematogenous or lymphog-

an ɑ
forɱ
emp
stru
site
15).
tion
denɪ
is cc
tory
depɛ
ing ɪ
tinu

"Seɪ

Sinc
proɗ
not
sem
ther
age,
is aɩ
agin
may
nisɱ
sem
sym
Tɩ
a nc
the
lead
crea
ubri
cheɪ
terо
crea
of tɦ
is uɪ
tion
the
incr
with
mar
obst
elde

Inte

The
encɛ
lunɡ
pulr

Solita
elderɩ
preseɪ
pecteɗ
but ɱ
most
the rᴄ
or mо
dence
solitaɪ
the uɪ
these
histor
necroɪ
adeno
tate, Ƅ

Pneuɱ
of a b
flamm

enous intrapulmonary metastasis, (3) elevation of the diaphragm secondary to phrenic nerve paralysis, and (4) pleural masses with or without rib destruction.

Atelectasis. Atelectasis is probably the most common single roentgen sign of bronchogenic carcinoma. It may be segmental, lobar, or massive atelectasis of one lung. The radiographic signs of atelectasis resulting from tumor are similar to those resulting from endobronchial block from other causes. The amount of density produced varies with the size of the bronchus obstructed. It is not uncommon to find a combination of atelectasis and tumor (Figs. 29-1 through 29-4). This is most readily visualized in the right upper lobe, where the atelectasis results in elevation and concavity of the secondary interlobar fissure laterally. A convexity medially with greater density there represents the tumor mass. In these patients the inferior margin of the lobe resembles the reversed letter S. A combination of pneumonitis and atelectasis may also occur, which may cause confusion. Persistence of the shadow in spite of antibiotic therapy or failure of complete disappearance of it is strong evidence of neoplasm.

Unilateral Enlargement of the Hilum. This sign of bronchogenic carcinoma may be very difficult to evaluate when only a single roentgenogram is available. When there is a difference in the size of the hilum on the two sides, every effort should be made to obtain any previous roentgenograms of the patient that may be available. If a film of an earlier examination is obtained, a difference in hilar size between the two films is of particular significance. It is also of value to obtain tomograms through the hilum in question in an attempt to outline local bronchial narrowing produced by tumor. It is also helpful in detecting some blurring of hilar vascular detail that may be caused by tumor. Roentgenograms in inspiration and expiration should also be obtained when there is a question as to the significance of unilateral hilar enlargement, because a small amount of obstructive emphysema may be determined by this examination (Fig. 29-5).

Local Emphysema. Bronchogenic carcinoma may not cause enough obstruction to interfere with air entering the segment, lobe, or lung supplied by the bronchus, but the slight decrease in bronchial size on expiration may result in partial obstruction to the egress of air. This causes emphysema, which may precede atelectasis by a considerable period of time. It is a rare but important sign of bronchogenic carci-

noma. Films in inspiration and expiration and fluoroscopy accentuate the findings and verify the presence of obstructive emphysema. These studies should be carried out when a wheeze is detected on auscultation or the presence of local emphysema is suggested by the chest roentgenogram. When obstructive emphysema is found in a patient past middle age, bronchogenic carcinoma should be suspected. Then further studies such as tomography and bronchoscopy can be undertaken.

Mediastinal Widening. When the mediastinum is enlarged as a result of bronchogenic carcinoma, this often indicates the presence of an anaplastic type. The primary tumor is usually in a stem bronchus and rarely beyond a lobar bronchus, so that the primary tumor mass is often obscured by a large mediastinal mass. Therefore this tumor cannot be differentiated from malignant lymphoma in some patients. The tumor is inoperable when there is mediastinal invasion but may respond to irradiation and/or chemotherapy (Fig. 29-6).

Apical Density With or Without Rib Destruction. Apical density with or without rib destruction denotes the presence of a superior pulmonary sulcus tumor known as a Pancoast tumor. It is usually caused by a squamous cell type of bronchogenic tumor; occasionally other cell types may be found. The four cardinal parts of the Pancoast syndrome are: (1) mass in pulmonary apex, (2) destruction of adjacent rib or vertebra, (3) Horner's syndrome, and (4) pain down the arm. Other tumors, including metastatic carcinoma and malignant neurogenic tumor, may cause the Pancoast syndrome in addition to bronchogenic carcinoma. When only a small amount of parenchymal density is visible representing the peripheral tumor, the diagnosis of malignancy is very difficult to make because this density simulates the minor amount of pleural thickening often visualized in the apex in elderly patients. The presence of pain should lead to the strong suspicion of tumor and the other clinical findings of Horner's syndrome, loss of sensation in the forearm, and atrophy of the hand muscles that are often present make the diagnosis almost certain. The tumor often grows rapidly with early destruction of the ribs (Fig. 29-7). Special films of the apex obtained with techniques such as tomography to show bone detail may be necessary to determine the presence or absence of rib destruction. Occasionally peripheral bronchogenic carcinoma elsewhere may spread locally to produce similar roentgen findings.

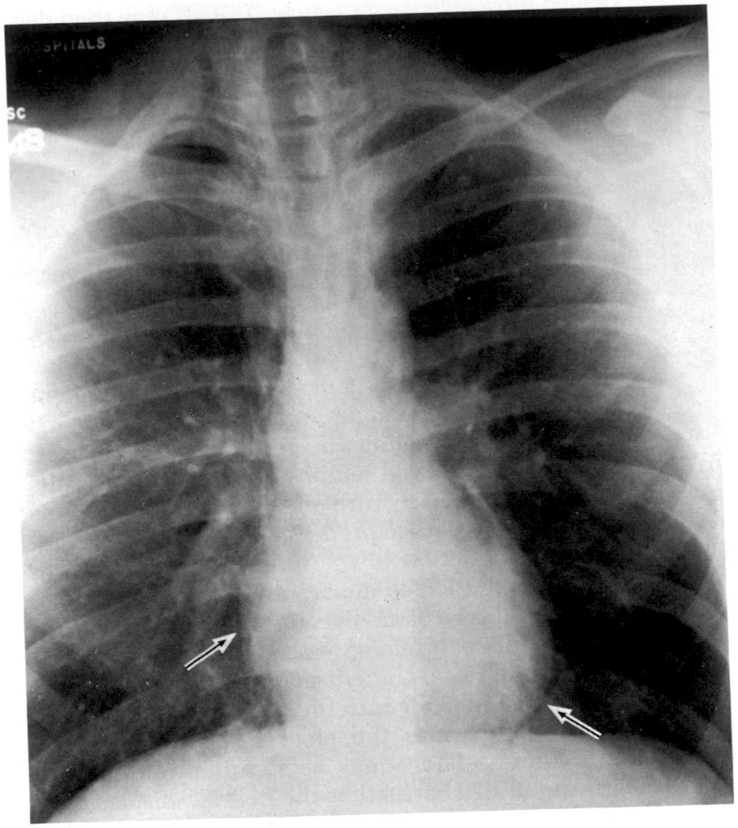

Fig. 30-5. Mediastinal and interstitial emphysema. **Arrows** indicate streaks of gas along the cardiac borders. There is also a considerable amount of streaky lucency in the superior mediastinum and lower portion of the neck. This film was obtained during an acute asthmatic attack.

easily identified in either frontal or lateral projections. Both views should be obtained when pneumomediastinum is suspected, however.

In the newborn, air may dissect from the mediastinum into the extrapleural space betwen the parietal pleura and diaphragm. The resultant accumulation may simulate pneumoperitoneum because the air is confined to the space over the diaphragm. However, the pleural line above it is not as thick as the normal diaphragm, and the air remains in the same place on supine, decubitus, and upright projections. At times, the air is interposed between the heart and diaphragm; this results in a continuous horizontal radiolucency extending across the midline between the diaphragm and the heart.[37]

Interstitial Emphysema of Thoracic Walls

Thoracic interstitial emphysema is most commonly due to thoracotomy but may also result from trauma and other causes. The amount varies considerably and, when small, the gas is limited to the side of the surgical procedure or of trauma. As the amount of gas increases it extends downward into the soft tissues of the abdomen and upward into the neck, and from there into the mediastinum, producing pneumomediastinum. Occasionally the amount of emphysema may be so great that tracheostomy is necessary to relieve respiratory embarrassment. Roentgen findings are similar to those in mediastinal emphysema secondary to pulmonary interstitial emphysema, but, in addition, there is gas in the soft tissues of the neck and thoracic wall, producing linear streaks of radiolucency. There is also evidence of thoracotomy or of trauma, which usually is sufficient to indicate the cause.

ATELECTASIS

GENERAL CONSIDERATIONS

Atelectasis is a state of incomplete expansion of a lung or any portion of it. There is a decrease or absence of air in the alveoli of the involved region. The volume is therefore diminished in the involved lung.

Atelectasis may be "active," as in obstruction, or "passive," caused by extrapulmonary pressure by fluid, air, tumor, and the like. It is always a secondary lesion and is therefore a sign of disease rather than a disease in itself. Its causes can be grouped into general categories:

1. Bronchial obstruction. This may be intrinsic, owing to tumor, foreign body, inflammatory disease, heavy secretions, or the like. Extrinsic pressure by tumor and enlarged nodes or constriction secondary to inflammatory disease may also cause it. In patients with airway obstruction, there is not always a decrease in volume caused by resorption of alveolar gas. This is because collateral ventilation or air drift may occur through the pores of Kohn (in alveolar walls) or the canals of Lambert, which extend from preterminal bronchioles to alveoli. There may be direct airway anastomoses allowing air drift. At times, air may be trapped distal to an airway obstruction, caused by collateral air drift when air can enter the obstructed segment more easily than it leaves. When bronchial obstruction is acute, there is usually some replacement of the rapidly resorbed gas by a transudate (edema fluid) that my contain varying amounts of blood.

2. Extrapulmonary pressure. This can have a variety of causes, including pneumothorax, pleural fluid, diaphragmatic elevation regardless of cause, herniation of abdominal viscera into the thorax, and large intrathoracic tumors.

3. Paralysis or paresis resulting in inability to expand a lung completely, such as is found in poliomyelitis and other neurologic disorders. In addition to the weakness of respiratory muscles per se, there is inability to raise the bronchial secretions and this may add the factor of obstruction in these patients.

4. Restriction of motion as a result of pleural disease or injury. Examples of this are chronic constrictive pleuritis, which causes decrease in volume of one hemithorax or a part thereof, so that normal expansion cannot occur. Acute conditions such as pleural infections and thoracic and upper abdominal trauma may also restrict motion and therefore produce some degree of atelectasis. In these patients there is also a factor of inability to handle secretions so that an additional obstructive element may be present.

5. Adhesive atelectasis. This refers to the nonobstructive airlessness found in patients with inactivation, decrease or loss of surfactant. Hyaline membranes may then be formed within the alveoli such as occurs in the newborn respiratory distress syndrome, in acute radiation pneumonitis, and in uremia.

6. Cicatrization atelectasis. This refers to volume loss found in patients with pulmonary fibrosis. Some prefer not to consider this a form of atelectasis, even though there is associated volume loss.

The fundamental alteration in the thorax produced by atelectasis is a decrease in volume of the lobe, segment, or lung involved. The interlobar fissure or fissures are displaced toward the airless lobe or segment. There are also roentgen signs of elevation of the diaphragm, shift of mediastinum to the side of involvement, hilar displacement, and narrowing of rib interspaces. Any of these signs may predominate in a given instance, depending on mediastinal and diaphragmatic fixation. In some patients the remaining lung on the involved side undergoes compensatory overinflation so that there is no actual change in volume of the hemithorax and few of the signs mentioned are then present. The relative airlessness of the affected portion of lung may result in an area of increased density which may be enhanced by edema, blood, and/or retained secretions. The classic ground-glass appearance is due to the density produced by airless lung plus some air in a lobe or segment anterior or posterior to it. This appearance is noted most commonly in atelectasis of the left upper lobe. The density is uniform but has a grainy character that has been likened to the appearance of ground glass. It is usually dense medially and fades off to a lesser density laterally. When atelectasis involves the entire lung, the density is complete and homogeneous. Bronchi as well as lung become airless in atelectasis caused by obstruction, so there is usually absence of the "air bronchogram." Associated with mediastinal shift there is often herniation of the opposite lung across the midline into the involved hemithorax; in chronic long-standing atelectasis this may become extensive. When the atelectasis is on the right side the height of the diaphragm is often not ascertained. There is usually enough gas in the stomach or colon to outline the left hemidiaphragm, however. The cause of the atelectasis may be evident on the film and may add to the density (Fig. 30-6).

LOBAR ATELECTASIS

Lower Lobe Atelectasis

Lower lobe atelectasis is easily overlooked, particularly on the left side where the lobe may be hidden by the heart. When there are no pleural adhesions present, the involved lobe moves medially to form ultimately a rather narrow triangle with the apex at the level of the hilum and the base at the diaphragm. In

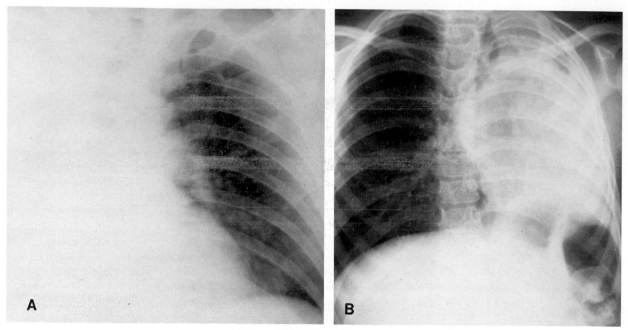

Fig. 30-6. Complete atelectasis. **A.** There is shift of the poorly outlined trachea to the right and almost complete density in the right lung. The heart is also shifted to the right. **B.** Atelectasis of the left lung. In this patient there is marked shift of mediastinal structures to the left, elevation of the left hemidiaphragm, and very little air in the atelectatic left lung.

the lateral projection the earliest sign of decrease in volume of a lower lobe is downward and posterior displacement of the major interlobar fissure. Later, as the amount of atelectasis increases, the density of the atelectatic lobe may obliterate the shadow of the posterior aspect of the diaphragm on the affected side. The signs of mediastinal shift, diaphragmatic elevation, and decrease in size of the bony thorax may be present to varying degrees or may be absent. If they are absent, there is usually enough compensatory overinflation of the upper lobe on the left or of the upper and middle lobes on the right to alert the observer to the possibility of lobar collapse. When the roentgenogram is of sufficient penetration, the triangular shadow of the collapsed left lower lobe is usually outlined behind the heart on the frontal projection.

Right Middle Lobe Atelectasis

Right middle lobe atelectasis occurs frequently; this may be complete or incomplete. It is often caused by inflammatory disease, resulting in enlarged nodes that compress the bronchus to this lobe. The obstruction may then result in inflammatory disease

within the lobe. This produces a somewhat more mottled and irregular appearance than is present in simple lobar atelectasis. When this lobe becomes atelectic, the secondary interlobar fissure moves downward and the primary fissure can be outlined in contrast to the dense lung above it on the lateral projection. The middle lobe tends to move downward and inward so that a triangular shadow appears just above the diaphragm. Its base is at the mediastinum and the apex points to the lateral chest wall. As atelectasis becomes complete, the lobe may shrink to a very small size and may be difficult to visualize clearly. The density caused by the atelectatic lobe blurs the right cardiac margin. When this blurring is noted the lateral view is confirmatory. In this view, varying degrees of collapse are readily outlined. The appearance is that of a dense triangle, the apex of which is at or near the hilum and the base points downward and anteriorly. The upper and lower borders of this dense triangle may be slightly concave.

Upper Lobe Atelectasis

In upper lobe atelectasis the roentgen appearance depends on the presence or absence of adhesions between the visceral and parietal pleurae. When adhesions are present they hold all or part of the lobe in its normal position; when there are no adhesions the lobe tends to shrink uniformly and move toward the hilum. In *right* upper lobe atelectasis the first sign is elevation of the interlobar fissure. If there are lateral adhesions the inferior aspect of the lobe becomes concave, elevating the fissure in its medial aspect, as well as producing slight increase in density of the lobe. As the amount of collapse progresses this concavity increases and the lobe shrinks to occupy the apex and upper mediastinum. Partial adherence of the lobe in one area or another may alter this general contour so that a considerable variety of form is possible. In the lateral view the major fissure tends to move anteriorly with increasing atelectasis and the upward displacement of the secondary fissure can also be outlined in this projection. The middle lobe moves upward anteriorly. The lower lobe moves upward posteriorly. Its superior segment may actually occupy the apex and rotate forward to lie in a caplike manner over the collapsed upper lobe. This is often readily outlined in the lateral projection and can be predicted by the appearance of normally aerated or hyperaerated lung at the apex above the more dense atelectatic upper lobe in the frontal projection.The signs of mediastinal and tracheal displacement toward the involved side, elevation of the right hemidiaphragm and hilum, and decrease in size of the hemithorax, resulting in narrowing of the intercostal spaces, may also occur in varying degrees; but compensatory emphysema of the middle and lower lobes may be sufficient so that none of the other signs will be present. Mediastinal displacement is usually a prominent feature when there are extensive adhesions holding the upper lobe to the lateral parietal pleura. The hilum may also be elevated and retracted to the right in such cases. When atelectasis is relatively complete and there are no adhesions, the shadow of the upper lobe tends to move toward the hilum and upper mediastinum. It may then resemble a slight mediastinal widening and occasionally may become so small that it is difficult to recognize.

Atelectasis of the *left* upper lobe is somewhat similar to that of the right upper lobe in that the lobe moves medially and anteriorly but early change is more difficult to recognize in the frontal projection because there is no secondary interlobar fissure. The ground-glass density is helpful if there is enough atelecasis and/or fluid in the lobe to produce it. In the lateral view the major fissure tends to move forward and the density produced by the collapse is noted anteriorly with the lingula occupying a position similar to that of the middle lobe on the right. The density of the partially collapsed lobe tends to be narrower inferiorly owing to the smaller volume occupied by the lingula and to extend upward and toward the periphery (Fig. 30-7). Pleural adhesions produce similar shift of the mediastinum to that noted in right upper lobe disease except that it is in the opposite direction. When atelectasis occurs in patients with chronic pulmonary inflammatory disease such as tuberculosis, there is often a considerable amount of associated pleural disease and contracting fibrosis of the lung. The lobe or segment involved is then difficult to evaluate on routine projections. In these instances, bronchography is often necessary for study of segmental anatomy.

Segmental Atelectasis

It is often possible to ascertain with a fair degree of accuracy the segment involved by segmental collapse, since the area of density produced by the atelectasis occupies the general area usually occupied by that segment in the absence of severely distorting associated pulmonary disease. By using frontal, lateral, and oblique projections as necessary, the site of the density can be clearly established and its relation to the interlobar fissures ascertained. The fissure tends to bow toward the site of the atelectasis; for example, in anterior segmental atelectasis of the right upper lobe the secondary interlobar fissure elevates centrally to indicate that the volume of this lobe has decreased and in the lateral view the density will lie anteriorly. The same rules apply for lower lobe segments but the basal segments are more difficult to identify accurately (Fig. 30-8).

Focal Atelectasis
(Platelike or Lobular Atelectasis)

When there is obstruction of a small subsegmental bronchus a small area of atelectasis may result. This produces a thin horizontal or "platelike" line that is most often seen in the basal lung fields, where it occurs frequently. These small areas of atelectasis have been referred to as platelike or lobular atelectasis. They vary in size and cannot be distinguished from small areas of fibrosis in some instances. Films exposed at frequent intervals will show disappearance or change in position of the linear areas of density and when this is evident, the diagnosis of focal atelectasis is confirmed. The amount of involved lung is small so that the finding is usually of no clinical significance. When it is observed postoperatively, however, it is an indication that aeration is incomplete and that there probably is an accumulation of secre-

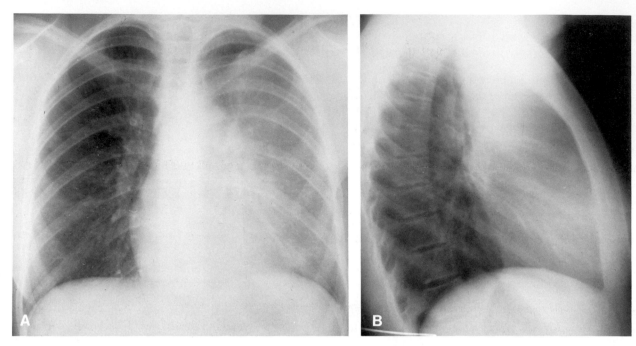

Fig. 30-7. Left upper-lobe atelectasis. **A.** Note the density on the left, which tends to fade toward the periphery. The border of the left side of the heart is blurred so that the heart is not clearly defined. **B.** Lateral view showing the density to be anterior. Note that the lower lobe extends to the apex above the partially atelectatic upper lobe. This is manifested on the frontal projection by the relatively normal aeration at the extreme left apex.

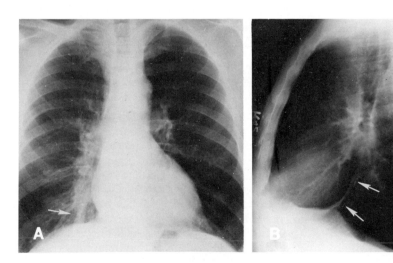

Fig. 30-8. Segmental atelectasis. There is partial atelectasis of the anterior segment of the right lower lobe producing an irregular, poorly defined density at the right medial base **(arrow in A).** In the lateral view **(B)** the density is noted to be immediately posterior to the major fissure which is bowed backward **(arrows).** Bronchogram revealed obstruction of the anterior basal segmental bronchus in this patient.

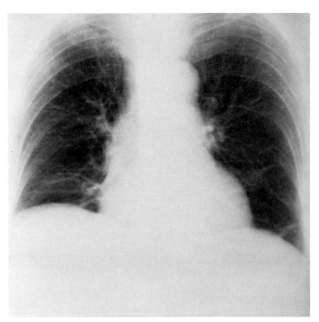

Fig. 30-9. Focal or linear or platelike atelectasis. Note the horizontal densities in both lower lung fields. These disappeared in one week. At times, linear fibrosis may occur in the lung and simulate focal atelectasis.

tions causing obstruction of some of the basal subsegmental bronchi. Restriction of diaphragmatic movement and elevation of the diaphragm are additional factors in production of this type of atelectasis (Fig. 30-9).

It is fundamental to remember that atelectasis causes an area of increased density because of airlessness or relative airlessness, usually along with some fluid, in the involved segment, lobe, or lung and that the resultant decrease in volume must be compensated by a decrease in total volume of the involved hemithorax or by an increase in volume of the uninvolved lobe or segments.

HYALINE MEMBRANE DISEASE OF THE NEWBORN (RESPIRATORY DISTRESS SYNDROME)

Hyaline membrane disease of newborn infants is characterized by increasingly labored breathing, expiratory grunting, retraction of interspaces, cyanosis, and hypercapnia. Diffuse atelectasis of the "adhesive" type is present and the terminal bronchioles are

dilated. The hyaline membrane, made up of homogeneous plasma clot, lines the bronchioles, alveolar ducts, and alveoli. The disease may lead to death by asphyxiation in the first 48 to 72 hours of life. In 90% or more of cases it occurs either in premature infants, in infants delivered by cesarean section, or in offspring of diabetic mothers. It may also occur in fullterm infants who have some condition that interferes with normal ventilation such as pneumothorax, diaphragmatic hernia, meconium aspiration, pneumonia, and birth trauma. The process is found in infants who breathe after birth, not in the stillborn. Respirations may be normal at or shortly following birth, but within a few hours dyspnea and cyanosis appear. In this disease a chest roentgenogram obtained very shortly after birth may reveal no abnormality, but abnormalities are apparent within a few hours. The disease is the result of a deficiency of surfactant in an immature lung. Histopathologic examination reveals dilated bronchioles, thick interstitial septa, collapsed alveoli, and the presence of a hyaline material lining the alveoli, the bronchioles, and the alveolar ducts. The hyaline membrane causes atelectasis of alveoli, which is accompanied by dilatation of the alveolar ducts and terminal bronchioles. Therefore the volume of the lung is not necessarily decreased, even though there is atelectasis. The hyaline membranes are the residua of pulmonary edema and are secondary to the surfactant deficiency.

Roentgen Findings. Four stages in the evolution of the disease have been described and identified radiographically. The first recognizable abnormality is an air-bronchogram pattern greater than normal. Next there is a fine miliary granularity associated with a slight increase in the reticular pattern of the lung fields. This may be so minor as to be very difficult to ascertain. The air-bronchogram pattern stands out more clearly, however. The third stage consists of a gradual progression resulting in a confluent opacification or an unequivocal dense, reticular pattern. Infants who recover show gradual clearing which is often irregular over a period of 3 to 10 days. The fourth stage is one of confluent density that may vary in extent. It is usually bilateral but it is not unusual to note some asymmetry. The roentgen pattern does not follow the described stages in each instance. The most characteristic appearance is that of a granular pattern of marked increase in density, corresponding to stage three, with associated demonstrable bronchial air shadows that are sharply outlined and extend peripherally well out into the lung fields (Fig. 30-10). There is no outward bulge of soft tissues in

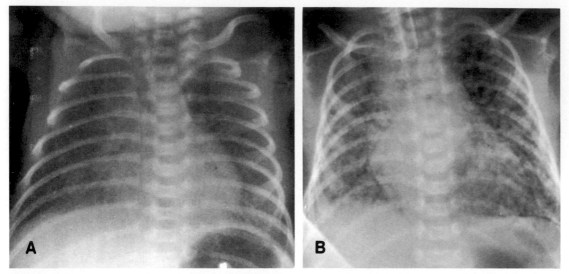

Fig. 30-10. Hyaline membrane disease (RDS). **A.** Premature infant at 2 days of age shows a rather diffuse granular and reticular density with streaks of air representing an air-bronchogram pattern noted particularly well at the bases. **B.** Three days later an endotracheal tube is in place. There is now a considerable amount of alveolar density interspersed with streaks of gas representing interstitial emphysema which is also noted along the right cardiac margin and at the left base. It is difficult to be certain how much of the density shown in this film is secondary to oxygen toxicity. The patient did not survive.

the intercostal spaces as is noted in many other conditions that cause respiratory distress.

Pulmonary interstitial emphysema may appear, usually related to positive-presssure assisted ventilation. The air trapped in the interstitium does not change much or disappear on expiration. There are elongated (1 to 3 cm) lucent areas that tend to radiate outward from the hilum. They are often somewhat tortuous. Mediastinal emphysema and/or pneumothorax may also be present.

At times the changes of hyaline membrane disease may be localized to the lower lobes, and at other times the clearing occurs first in the upper lobes when there is improvement. This suggests that upper lobes mature earlier than the lower lobes, a pattern similar to that in lambs and rabbits. Sometimes the distribution of the disease may be very uneven and atypical.[1]

In other neonatal respiratory distress syndromes caused by pulmonary disease, usually pulmonary densities are evident. However, these tend to be coarse and irregular, often bilateral but not necessarily symmetric. This pattern is usually associated with bronchopneumonia or aspiration pneumonitis.

CHRONIC PULMONARY INSUFFICIENCY OF PREMATURITY (CPIP)

This is a syndrome[34] of delayed respiratory distress in premature infants weighing less than 1250 gm. For the first 4 to 7 days following birth, these infants appear healthy. They then become dyspneic and may require oxygen. The mortality rate is 10% to 20%. Roentgen findings of hyaline membrane disease are not observed. At most, volume loss may be detected on the chest film. There appears to be a loss of compliance consistent with surfactant deficiency at a later date than in typical hyaline membrane disease.

OXYGEN TOXICITY (BRONCHOPULMONARY DYSPLASIA)

Prolonged oxygen therapy can cause pulmonary damage, and, particularly in infants with hyaline membrane disease, recognizable pathologic and radiologic changes. Northway and associates describe four stages in which the findings are somewhat characteristic.[48] In stage 1, occurring in the first 2 or 3 days, the findings are those of hyaline membrane disease. In stage 2, occurring in 4 to 10 days, opacification of lungs is marked, with a clearly defined air-bronchogram pattern. In stage 3, occurring between 10 and 20 days, the roentgen pattern is one of a spongy appearance produced by a combination of atelectasis and emphysema; there are multiple small bullae throughout the lungs. In stage 4 the bullae enlarge; this occurs in patients who survive more than a month.

In adults, prolonged exposure to oxygen may also cause pulmonary disease. There is an exudative reaction which may progress to interstitial fibrosis. Initial roentgen changes consist of a diffuse alveolar density caused by edema. Later, linear and nodular densities appear, commonly in the bases; these represent a proliferative phase. These changes occur in the adult respiratory distress syndrome, in which other pulmonary conditions may contribute to the roentgen findings.[50]

TRANSIENT RESPIRATORY DISTRESS (WET-LUNG DISEASE) OF THE NEWBORN (TRDN)

The roentgen findings in another neonatal distress syndrome, transient respiratory distress of the newborn (TRDN), have been described[65] by Swischuk. This syndrome occurs in infants delivered of diabetic mothers, in premature infants, in infants delivered by breech extraction, and those delivered by cesarean section. The distress (tachypnea) is noted early in the neonatal period and clears in 1 to 4 days. The cause appears to be incomplete or delayed clearing of alveolar fluid after birth. As a result the lungs are "wet." This is manifested radiographically by findings resembling those of alveolar edema with an air-bronchogram pattern, or, in less severe cases, interstitial edema, often with what appear to be Kerley's A lines and small amounts of pleural fluid. Minimal to moderate overaeration is common. At times, the roentgen findings may be similar to those of hyaline membrane disease, but in wet-lung disease there is progressive and rapid improvement (Fig. 30-11).[68]

WILSON–MIKITY SYNDROME

The Wilson–Mikity syndrome is another disease that produces the respiratory distress syndrome in the premature infant. Its cause remains obscure. The roentgen features are quite distinct. There is a rather coarse reticular pattern interspersed with irregularly rounded, cystlike areas of lucency. The lungs are overdistended, chiefly at the bases. This basal hyperaeration increases as the disease progresses, but coarse strands of density tend to remain in the upper lobes. Changes disappear slowly as the infant improves (Fig. 30-12). The disease tends to be chronic. Some of the babies recover over a period of months, others die of right-sided heart failure. In many reported cases, the use of oxygen therapy preceded the onset of the clinical manifestations. In these instances the disease may resemble bronchopulmonary dysplasia to a great extent radiographically. The clinical course of the two conditions is very different, however.

PNEUMOTHORAX

The presence of air or gas in the pleural cavity is termed "pneumothorax." Under normal conditions the pressure in the pleural space is less than atmospheric pressure. When this space communicates with the atmosphere, either through a defect in the parietal pleura and chest wall or through a defect in the visceral pleura, air enters the pleural space. The amount of air that enters depends upon a variety of factors, including the elasticity of the lung, the presence or absence of pleural adhesions, and the type of defect in the pleura. There are a number of conditions in which pneumothorax is sometimes observed. In the respiratory distress syndrome, pneumothorax may develop in addition to pneumomediastinum, particularly when positive-pressure respiratory assistance is used. It also occurs in patients with chronic obstructive pulmonary disease and with pulmonary histiocytosis X. It has been reported in women related to the onset of menses. Usually the right hemithorax is involved.

SPONTANEOUS PNEUMOTHORAX

The term "spontaneous pneumothorax" is usually reserved to designate pneumothorax that occurs in an otherwise healthy individual. The air enters the pleural cavity through an opening in the visceral pleura. In many instances the cause is obscure and the site of the defect not accurately localized. In some of these, pulmonary interstitial emphysema is probably the cause. In others, subpleural blebs are visible and it is presumed that rupture of one of these may introduce the pneumothorax. Once the pneumothorax is established, the course depends upon the defect in the pleura. If the defect closes promptly, the air in the pleural space is absorbed in a few days and

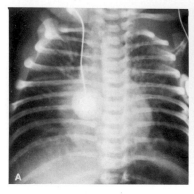
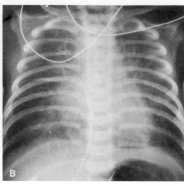
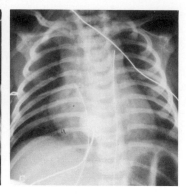

Fig. 30-11. Newborn infant with transient respiratory distress (wet lung). **A.** Shortly after birth, some central alveolar density with some linear interstitial density extending well into the lung fields is manifest **B.** Ninety minutes later, some improvement has taken place peripherally. **C.** Five hours later the lungs are clear. Such rapid improvement is characteristic of this condition.

Fig. 30-12. Wilson–Mikity syndrome in a 2-month-old child shows the typical coarse reticular pattern in which there are rounded cystlike areas of radiolucency. The disease is most clearly defined at the base of the right lung below the dome of the diaphragm.

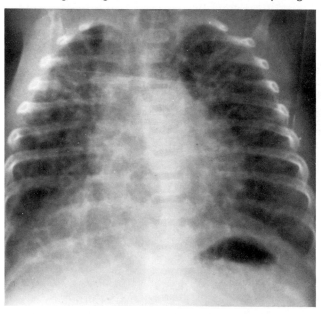

the pneumothorax disappears. If the defect remains open in a manner that allows air to enter and leave the pleural space, the size of the pneumothorax tends to remain constant provided no complications such as infection supervene (Fig. 30-13).

TENSION PNEUMOTHORAX

Occasionally there is a check-valve or one-way-valve type of defect through which air can enter the pleural space but cannot leave it. This results in a much more serious condition than spontaneous pneumothorax known as tension pneumothorax. When this occurs there is rapid or slow accumulation of air in the pleural space, resulting in complete collapse of the lung provided there are no adhesions to hold it out. This is followed by shift of mediastinal structures away from the side of the pneumothorax as well as increase in size of the involved hemithorax and depression of the diaphragm on the side of the lesion (Fig. 30-14). This condition is particularly hazardous in the newborn and, if not treated promptly, can cause death.

TRAUMATIC PNEUMOTHORAX

Air may enter the pleural space through the parietal pleura as the result of penetrating wounds of the thorax. It may also be secondary to renal surgery, sympathectomy, and other upper abdominal surgical procedures or it may be introduced through a needle at the time of thoracentesis. Trauma to the lungs or bronchi may also result in defects in the visceral pleura, causing pneumothorax. When associated with rib fractures it is often caused by a rent in the pleura produced by sharp bony spicules. There is injury to the visceral and parietal pleurae in these instances, but the air usually enters through the defect in the visceral pleura. The pneumothorax commonly

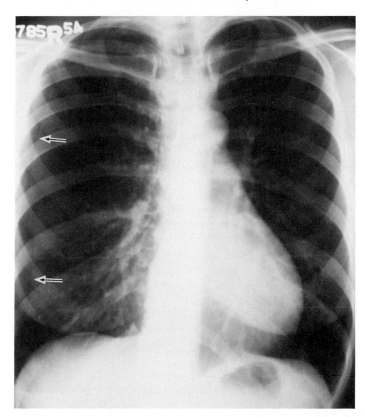

Fig. 30-13. Spontaneous pneumothorax. **Arrows** indicate the visceral pleural line of the upper and lower lobes. On the right, a small air–fluid level is noted in the posterior gutter. This is frequently present in this condition and is a helpful sign when the pneumothorax is small.

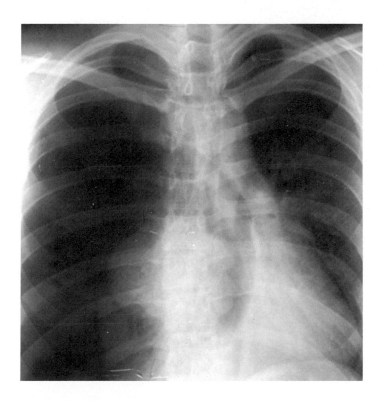

Fig. 30-14. Tension pneumothorax. The right lung is collapsed and displaced to the left. Part of it is herniated across the midline. Note complete absence of lung markings on the right and the considerable shift of mediastinal structures to the left.

seen in the newborn is very likely traumatic in origin in most instances. Pneumothorax of this type may also occur as a complication in diagnostic or therapeutic pneumoperitoneum and occasionally it follows bronchoscopy. In addition to the findings of pneumothorax, the cause may be apparent on the chest roentgenogram.

Bronchopleural Fistula

Regardless of the cause, bronchopleural fistula results in pneumothorax that usually persists for a long period of time. Tuberculosis is a common cause and the fistula can be produced by rupture of a subpleural lesion into the pleural space or by rupture of a tuberculous empyema through the pleura into the lung with subsequent formation of a fistula. Other inflammatory diseases of the lung, both acute and chronic, may also cause bronchopleural fistula with resultant pneumothorax. Other infectious diseases of the pleura producing empyema may also result in bronchopleural fistula with rupture of the empyema through the visceral pleura leading to bronchial communication.

Induced (Artificial) Pneumothorax

This pneumothorax is the result of a diagnostic procedure performed usually to differentiate intrapulmonary masses from those arising from the ribs, mediastinum, or diaphragm.

ROENTGEN CONSIDERATIONS

The presence of a large pneumothorax is identified readily on roentgen examination and in many instances, when it is secondary to disease or trauma, the cause can be established. The air in the pleural space is usually more radiolucent than the lung adjacent to it, particularly if the lung is decreased in volume, compressed, or is involved by disease that increases its density. When pleural adhesions are present, small amounts of loculated pneumothorax may be very difficult to visualilze unless lateral or oblique projections are obtained. Such spaces often contain a small amount of fluid and the presence of a horizontal fluid level indicates that gas as well as fluid is present. When the amount of pneumothorax is very small and is apical in position, its presence is indicated by visualization of a thin, smooth, curved, linear density representing the visceral pleura. Above this line no pulmonary markings are visible. Occasionally the pneumothorax is so small that its presence at the apex can only be suspected on the usual roentgenogram obtained with the patient in deep inspiration. A roentgenogram obtained during maximum expiration will aid in confirming the diagnosis, since the lung then is relatively denser than the pneumothorax. The lung decreases in volume during expiration but the pneumothorax space does not change. There is, therefore, relatively more pneumothorax in relation to lung in expiration than in inspiration and there is presumably a smaller visceral pleural surface in contact with the pneumothorax, which is easier to define. The lateral decubitus position (involved side up) with the film exposed when the patient is in expiration may be very helpful; a horizontal beam is used and the visceral pleura may be more clearly defined than at the apex where bony density (of ribs and clavicle) may make identification of pleura very difficult.[42] In tension pneumothorax the shift of mediastinal structures, compression of the lung, and depression of the diaphragm are readily visualized. When fluid is present in addition to air or gas, horizontal beam films showing an air–fluid level are diagnostic. At times, the intrapleural air is trapped in unusual positions by adhesions. Occasionally, pneumothorax may be seen in a subpulmonary position, particularly in patients with COPD and lack of lung compliance.[10] It may also be observed along the medial surface of the lung in newborn infants who are often examined in the supine position.[47] In this situation, it must be differentiated from pneumomediastinum. In young infants, it is best evaluated with anteroposterior and lateral films exposed simultaneously.

In summary, the diagnosis of pneumothorax is usually not difficult to make on roentgen examination of the chest. When the pneumothorax is small in amount a film in expiration is often of value; and, occasionally, when peripheral loculated pneumothorax is present, lateral and oblique views are needed for distinct visualization. In addition to the value of roentgenograms in making the diagnosis, progress films are used to follow its course.

Differential Diagnosis

Occasionally a peripheral emphysematous bleb or bulla may simulate a localized pneumothorax but in most instances the rounded or geometric form of its inner wall indicates the nature of the lesion and differentiates it from pneumothorax. When the diagnosis is particularly difficult, progress films are often of assistance since pneumothorax usually changes from day to day in contrast to emphysema, which is stable and changes little over long periods of time. Occasionally these emphysematous bullae become very large (tension bullae) and may displace the lung and mediastinum in a manner simulating displacement by tension pneumothorax. In these instances, differentiation cannot be made with certainty on roentgen examination alone. In patients with far-advanced tuberculosis, large peripheral cavitation, often involving the greater part of an upper lobe (usually the left), may be difficult to distinguish from pneumothorax caused by bronchopleural fistula. If serial roentgenograms are available, the progress of the lesion will indicate its nature in most instances, but there are some patients in whom the nature of the lesion remains uncertain and even at autopsy or at surgery the disease may be so extensive that the visceral pleura cannot be identified. The same type of lesion may follow other pulmonary infections but is less common.

ALTERED IMMUNITY AND THE LUNG

The immune system is composed of lymphocytes: the B- (bursa) and T- (thymic derived) cells. The B-cells secrete immunoglobulins and are responsible for humoral immunity. The immunoglobulins are: IgG, IgA, IgM, IgE, and IgD. The T-lymphocyte or T-cell is responsible for cellular immunity. The immune responses are classified into four types as follows: Type I—IgE dependent, in which the antibody is E. There is an immediate skin test; the clinical examples are extrinsic asthma and anaphylaxis. Type II—tissue-specific antibody. Antibodies are G and M. Clinical example is Goodpasture's syndrome. Type III—immune complexes. Antibodies are G and M. Clinical examples are extrinsic alveolitis produced by organic and inorganic dust and intrinsic alveolitis including collagen vascular diseases and fibrosing alveolitis. The first three are examples of humoral immune responses. Type IV—cell-mediated (delayed hypersensitivity). Clinical examples are intracellular infections, graft rejection, and cancer suppression.[55]

BRONCHIAL ASTHMA

Bronchial asthma is very common, occurs at all ages, and is characterized by wheezing, prolongation of the expiratory phase of respiration, dyspnea, and cough. It tends to appear in recurrent attacks. Early in the course of the disease there are no roentgen findings in the chest between the acute episodes. During an acute asthmatic attack there is increased radiability

of the lungs because of acute overdistention. Small areas of focal atelectasis often cause scattered patchy densities parallel to the bronchovascular markings. They are often widespread throughout both lung fields. The markings may also be thickened, particularly in the parahilar and central pulmonary zones. There is also depression of the diaphragm and decreased diaphragmatic motion that can be detected on fluoroscopic examination. In many instances no permanent radiographic changes occur. During an acute asthmatic attack, pneumomediastinum or pneumothorax may occur. This is most commonly observed in children and young adults. In patients with severe and constant asthma, roentgen changes may be permanent. These patients are subject to recurrent pulmonary infections leading to pulmonary fibrosis associated with emphysema. The roentgen findings then consist of prominence of interstitial markings in a chest that is otherwise more radiolucent than normal. The anteroposterior diameter of the chest is increased, the diaphragm is low and flat, and the ribs are often more horizontal than is normal (Fig. 30-15). The emphysema may become severe leading to formation of large emphysematous bullae and blebs peripherally. Parallel lines and tubular shadows representing thickened bronchial walls have been observed in patients with asthma, probably caused by bronchial infection. Mucous plug or impaction may also occur in asthma patients. The bronchial obstruction produced by the impaction may result in atelectasis or in an accumulation of secretions in the obstructed segment, and infection. Eventually, bronchiectasis may result; this may produce plain-film findings similar to those of bronchiectasis in nonasthmatic patients. There appears to be some predilection for the upper lobes. Roentgen findings depend on the nature of the associated pulmonary disease and, when segmental atelectasis or an apparent pneumonitis is found in an asthmatic, mucous plug or impaction should be suspected.

IDIOPATHIC PULMONARY HEMOSIDEROSIS

Hemosiderosis is a term used to indicate the presence of macrophages filled with hemosiderin which are deposited in the alveoli and interstitial tissues of the lung. Idiopathic hemosiderosis is of unknown cause, but because some immunologic mechanism is a distinct possibility the disease is discussed here. There is an injury at the level of the alveolocapillary membrane allowing the leakage of blood into the interstitial space and ultimately into the alveolar space of the lung. This is manifested by recurrent episodes

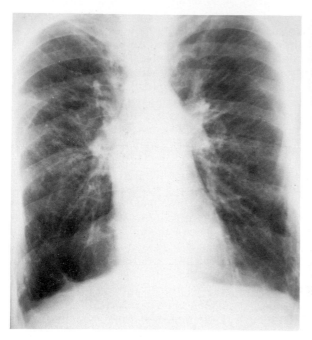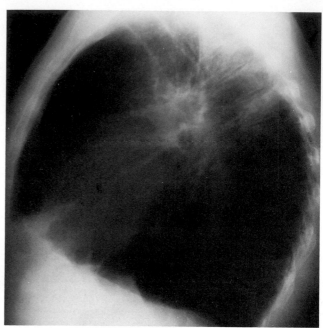

Fig. 30-15. Pulmonary changes in a 44-year-old man with a long history of bronchial asthma. Note the low, flat diaphragm, deep anteroposterior diameter of the chest, and an increase in interstitial markings throughout the lungs. The increase in central pulmonary arteries indicates arterial hypertension.

of acute illness in which dyspnea, cyanosis, and weakness along with cough, hemoptysis, and chest pain occur. The attack lasts a few days or weeks before subsiding. Recurrent episodes of bleeding ultimately produce marked roentgenographic changes. The prognosis is generally poor, although the disease may progress very slowly in some patients. It is somewhat more frequent in children than in adults. In children there is no sex predominance, but when it develops in adults, there is a preponderance of males of about 2 or 3 to 1.

The roentgen findings in the acute phase are those of alveolar hemorrhage which causes widespread, patchy alveolar densities that clear gradually over a period of days. Residual deposition of hemosiderin in the interstitium produces thickening that appears roentgenographically as an increase in interstitial markings, giving a reticular or reticulonodular appearance (Fig. 30-16). The diagnosis is made by correlating the clinical history with the roentgenographic changes. The disease must be differentiated from a number of other diseases that cause widespread interstitial change of this type.

Pulmonary Changes Following Hemoptysis

When hemoptysis occurs and blood is aspirated, the roentgen findings vary with the amount and distribution of the blood. A density comparable to that of a patch of pneumonia of similar size is produced. It is usually hazy and poorly defined and may be local or widely scattered, depending on the site(s) and amount of the bleeding. The opacity usually clears within 2 or 3 days which aids in differentiating hemorrhage from inflammatory disease. Evidence of the disease causing the hemoptysis may or may not be present.

GOODPASTURE'S SYNDROME

Goodpasture's syndrome is an autoimmune disease in which circulating antibodies against the alveolar basement membrane and against glomerular basement membrane have been demonstrated. In contrast to idiopathic pulmonary hemosiderosis, it occurs in young adults with a male predominance of 7 or 8 to 1.

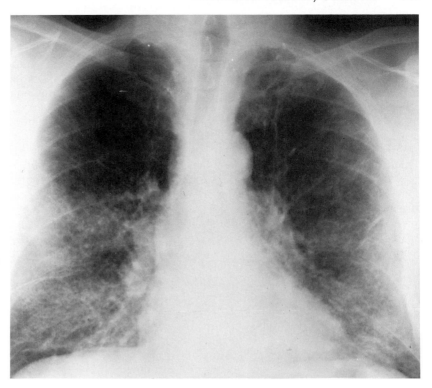

Fig. 30-16. Idiopathic pulmonary hemosiderosis in a 42-year-old man with a long history of repeated hemoptysis. Note the extensive interstitial disease which is somewhat linear in the upper lung fields and is reticulonodular in the central and basal lungs. There is pulmonary arterial hypertension manifested by large central pulmonary arteries.

The roentgen findings are related to extensive intra-alveolar hemorrhage which produces diffuse opacity of an extent proportional to the amount of bleeding. It is usually bilateral and is often more prominent in the parahilar areas and in the central and lower lungs than in the apices. If the hemorrhage stops, the blood quickly clears leaving a reticular interstitial pattern that increases as the disease progresses. Often the clearing is partial, then another hemorrhage produces additional density. Septal lines are not ordinarily observed. Adenopathy sufficient to produce recognizable hilar enlargement may be present. Pleural effusion rarely occurs. The diagnosis should be suspected when a combination of hemoptysis and renal disease occurs in a young man. The prognosis in Goodpasture's syndrome is poor.

EOSINOPHILIC LUNG DISEASE— PULMONARY INFILTRATES WITH EOSINOPHILIA (PIE)

Eosinophilic disease includes a group of disorders, sometimes termed the "PIE syndrome," in which there are five major categories: (1) Loeffler's syndrome; (2) chronic eosinophilic pneumonia or a chronic form of pulmonary infiltrates with eosinophilia; (3) chronic PIE with asthma; (4) tropical eosinophilia; (5) polyarteritis or vasculitis in association with pulmonary infiltrates which are the predominant part of the disease. There may be many manifestations in other organ systems.

Löffler's Syndrome (Transient Pulmonary Infiltration with Eosinophilia)

Löffler's syndrome consists of fleeting pulmonary infiltrations associated with eosinophilia. Usually its subjects are allergic individuals; it is believed to represent pulmonary reaction to a variety of allergens. The symptoms are usually mild and consist of cough, malaise, low-grade fever, dyspnea with occasional wheezing, mild chest pain, and metallic taste in the mouth. It is associated with an eosinophilia, that ranges from 10% to 70%, and usually with leukocytosis also. The amount of pathologic material available is small since this is a benign condition, but the findings in patients who have died accidentally consist of eosinophilic pneumonia in which the involvement is interstitial as well as alveolar and there is also some associated pulmonary edema, probably secondary to hyperpermeability of capillaries.

Roentgen Findings. The infiltrations cause poorly defined densities that may be single or multiple, unilateral or bilateral. The volume of lung affected varies considerably and the individual areas of involvement are patchy in type and usually poorly outlined. They resemble pneumonia due to other causes but are unique in that the homogeneous densities are usually periphcral and rapid change is the rule. It is not unusual to observe clearing or partial clearing in one area and progression in another area of the same lung or of the opposite lung. At times the findings remain stable for several days. When such a changing infiltrate is observed and the patient is found to have eosinophilia the diagnosis of Löffler's syndrome can be made (Fig. 30-17). A minor amount of pleural reaction resulting in small amounts of pleural effusion may occur, but the presence or absence of effusion is of no diagnostic significance.

Since similar eosinophilic pneumonias may be caused by a variety of parasitic infestations, by infections, and by drugs, the term "eosinophilic pneumonia" should be used to denote those of unknown cause. The others are better designated as eosinophilic pneumonia caused by a drug (name of drug), by infestation (name of parasite), and so on. The administration of cortisone usually produces rapid clearing of the pulmonary infiltrates and a decrease in the circulating eosinophils.

Chronic Eosinophilic Pneumonia

Chronic eosinophilic pneumonia is similar to Löffler's syndrome except that the symptoms in eosinophilic pneumonia are prolonged and the course more malignant. The disease usually occurs in women; its onset may be sudden. Its duration may extend from months to years. Episodes of weakness, weight loss, fever, cough, dyspnea, and hemoptysis may occur. Roentgen findings consist of a variety of patterns of density, some resembling confluent pneumonia, others consist of coarse, strandlike densities which may be widespread. Changes in the pulmonary disease are common as in Löffler's syndrome. Eosinophils are found in the biopsy specimen which shows interstitial pneumonia of varying degrees of severity, sometimes associated with fibrosis. There is also an elevated eosinophil count in the circulating blood. The lesions do not repond to antibiotics, but clear dramatically on steroid therapy.

Tropical eosinophila is discussed in Chapter 26.

DRUG-INDUCED HYPERSENSITIVITY DISEASE IN THE LUNGS

Pulmonary reactions to drugs are characterized by the following: (*1*) The reactions are not related directly to dosage. (*2*) A latent period is needed on initial exposure but not on readministration. (*3*) A minority of drug recipients are involved. (*4*) There is no correlation of the reaction with pharmacologic

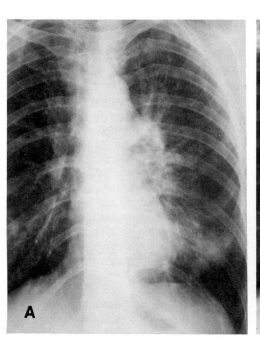
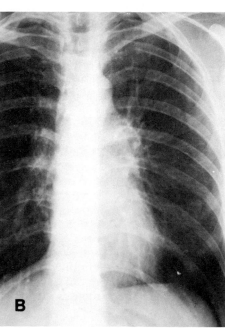

Fig. 30-17. Eosinophilic pneumonia (Löffler's). **A.** Note the poorly defined scattered infiltrate in the left central and lower lung field with a lesser amount of disease superiorly. **B.** Examination, performed 15 days later, shows that the disease has cleared. The patient had eosinophilia, eosinophils in the sputum, and was allergic.

properties of the drug. (5) Other hypersensitivity reactions such as anaphylaxis, serum sickness, urticaria, contact dermatitis, or asthma may be present. (6) Re-administration of the drug reproduces the symptoms. The hypersensitivity reactions are usually accompanied by eosinophilia and pulmonary changes that range from a diffuse alveolar pattern to a diffuse interstitial pattern or combinations of the two; the reactions may be acute or chronic. A pleuropulmonary reaction that is indistinguishable from lupus may also occur. In some, the onset of the reaction is acute with sudden chills, fever, cough, and dyspnea; in others, it may be insidious with increasing dyspnea and cough.

The radiographic features consist of (1) a diffuse, acute alveolar type of density resembling alveolar edema which varies in extent and distribution but is usually bilateral; (2) an acute, diffuse interstitial pattern resembling interstitial edema; (3) a chronic interstitial pattern; (4) a pleuropulmonary or lupus-like pattern; and (5) hilar adenopathy which may be accompanied by pulmonary changes. The drugs commonly involved are antibiotics, antimetabolites (antineoplastic agents), analgesics, anticonvulsants, and vasoactive or neuroactive substances.

Antibiotics such as Madribon (sulfadimethoxine), Prontosil (sulfachrysoindine), PAS (para-amino-salicylic acid), and penicillin may cause an acute alveolar reaction. Dilantin (diphenylhydantoin) and Mesantoin (3-methyl 5, 5-phenyl-ethyl-hydantoin) cause hilar adenopathy and a combined alveolar and interstitial pulmonary pattern (Fig. 30-18). Diuril (hydrochlorthiazide) and Methotrexate (pteroylglutamic acid) cause a similar mixed interstitial and alveolar pulmonary reaction without the adenopathy. Hexamethonium chloride, Inversine (mecamylamine), and Sansert (methysergide) produce a chronic interstitial pulmonary pattern. Reactions to Myleran (busulfan) and Cytoxan (cyclophosphamide) usually begin several months after use of the drug is initiated. The findings are those of combined alveolar and interstitial pulmonary densities. Calcifications in interstitial tissues have been reported in long-term users. Bleomycin causes a similar delayed type of reaction resulting in a linear interstitial pattern; significant residual pulmonary fibrosis occurs in a small number of patients who react to it. Fatal interstitial pneumonitis has also been reported in patients reacting to busulfan and in those reacting to bleomycin. Furadantin (nitrofurantoin) may cause either an acute or chronic interstitial reaction with some patchy alveolar density sometimes observed at the bases. D-Dimethylcysteine (D-penicillamine) may produce a diffuse miliary pattern of pulmonary density. Pronestyl (procainamide) can cause a pleuropulmonary reaction indistinguishable from that occurring in lupus erythematosus in which pleural effusion, basal pulmonary infiltrates, and sometimes pericardial effusion are manifest. The lupus pattern has been attributed to at least 25 other drugs including griseofulvin, hydralazine, isoniazid, methyldopa, propylthiouracil, reserpine, streptomycin, sulfonamides, tetracycline, and the thiazides.

Aspirin may cause asthma and sometimes pulmonary edema, especially when a large dose is taken. Procarbazine hydrochloride produces a combined alveolar and interstitial reaction, somewhat similar to reaction to busulfan. A number of other drugs in the categories mentioned earlier have also been reported as causing pulmonary hypersensitivity reactions. An example of pleuropulmonary reaction to methotrexate is shown in Figure 30-19.

The patterns described in the foregoing may vary, and hilar adenopathy may be present in some patients receiving drugs other than anticonvulsants. As a rule, the acute reactions regress rapidly when use of the drug is discontinued. The chronic interstitial changes tend to clear slowly, but in some patients, interstitial fibrosis may be permanent. The pulmonary disease has a tendency to be more severe in the bases and parahilar areas than elsewhere, but in some of these patients the distribution is universal and in others it is random.

LYMPHOCYTIC INTERSTITIAL PNEUMONITIS (L.I.P.)

Liebow and Carrington described a condition manifested by disseminated pulmonary infiltrates in patients with a history of cough, dyspnea, fever, and weight loss for long periods of time (6 months to 5 years). The cause is not clear, but some type of hypersensitivity may contribute to its development. Roentgen findings are a combination of diffuse increase of interstitial markings resulting in linear densities plus patchy nodular densities. The condition may be related to pseudolymphoma, which is a local, benign, lymphocytic infiltration of the lung characterized by the presence of true germinal centers in a mass of well-differentiated lymphocytes and other inflammatory cells. There is not roentgen similarity, since the pseudolymphoma appears as a large pulmonary mass which is often central. The margins are indistinct and an air-bronchogram pattern is usually present. The mass may resemble confluent

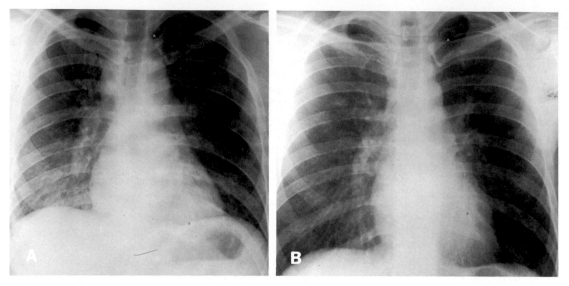

Fig. 30-18. Mesantoin sensitivity. **A.** The patient complained of cough and fever. Note the paratracheal and hilar adenopathy as well as a little basal pulmonary involvement on the right. **B.** Three weeks later, after use of the drug had been discontinued, the chest apears to be normal.

Fig. 30-19. Drug hypersensitivity. This is an example of methotrexate toxicity. **A.** This film shows a pleuropulmonary reaction with some pleural fluid on the left and interstitial pulmonary disease in the left lung field and at the right base. **B.** Examination performed 4 days later shows considerable increase in the amount of fluid and persistence of the pulmonary interstitial pattern on the left. There has been some improvement on the right. The changes cleared very slowly when the drug was discontinued.

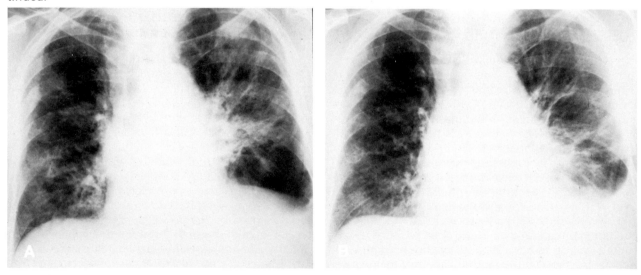

pneumonia or parenchymal tumor. Biopsy is necessary to differentiate it from other lung masses.

THE COLLAGEN-VASCULAR (CONNECTIVE TISSUE) DISEASES

The collagen diseases consist of a heterogeneous group of conditions in which involvement of connective tissue, particularly the intercellular amorphous ground substance, is the common morphologic feature. They appear to be related to hypersensitivity in some instances, but hypersensitivity is not the only cause since the tissue changes are known to be produced by a variety of dissimilar diseases. Polyarteritis (periarteritis) nodosa, rheumatic fever, rheumatoid arthritis, disseminated lupus erythematosus, and scleroderma are all members of the collagen group; Wegener's granulomatosis is related and is included by many in this group of conditions. Polymyositis, dermatomyositis, Sjogrens syndrome, and, possibly, ankylosing spondylitis are also included.[26] These diseases are related and there is a considerable amount of overlapping in the clinical findings so that lesions that are usually predominant in one entity may be seen in another. Individual cases have been reported in which four or five varieties of involvement have been present.

POLYARTERITIS NODOSA (PERIARTERITIS)

In polyarteritis nodosa the medium-sized arteries and their small branches are affected so that the lesions are often found throughout the body. Pulmonary involvement causes a variety of roentgen changes. Massive pulmonary edema may occur in patients who are acutely ill. Other pulmonary changes consist of scattered patchy densities, some of which are due to infarcts; these may excavate and cause small cavities. When present this cavitation is often multiple and it is characteristic that one cavity becomes smaller and closes while another is in the process of forming. Clearly defined or hazy nodules may appear. Some may resemble hematogenous metastases while others simulate inflammatory nodules and may raise the possibility of tuberculosis. At times the interstitial markings are increased. Basal congestion resulting in enlargement of vascular shadows and blurring of vessels is often noted and pleural effusion may occur. Enlargement of the cardiac silhouette is not uncommon. In some patients this is caused by pericardial effusion while in others there is dilatation of the heart. These pulmonary and pleural changes may

undergo rapid clearing or may progress rapidly. There is nothing characteristic about the roentgen findings, but, in a chronically ill patient with involvement of other systems, these pulmonary, pleural, and pericardial findings are suggestive of this disease. The pulmonary roentgen changes usually respond rapidly and clear following institution of steroid therapy.

RHEUMATIC PNEUMONIA

Rheumatic fever is a disease in which cardiac lesions are common and these may result in secondary pulmonary congestion and edema. The "pneumonia" seen in this disease is often caused by pulmonary edema and congestion and there is a considerable difference of opinion as to the incidence of actual pulmonary involvement in this disease. The roentgen findings of rheumatic pneumonia simulate those of pulmonary edema and congestion. They consist of hazy densities, usually in the parahilar areas and midlung fields. They may be confluent or patchy and are often associated with basal changes indicating pulmonary congestion. At times there does appear to be involvement of lungs, so that a scattered pneumonitis in the absence of cardiac failure in a patient with rheumatic fever is most likely indicative of rheumatic pneumonia. Histopathologic study is often necessary to differentiate rheumatic pneumonia from pulmonary edema and congestion, but the clinical findings, along with radiographic findings, may permit the presumptive diagnosis.

DISSEMINATED LUPUS ERYTHEMATOSUS

Disseminated lupus erythematosus is commonly found in young and middle-aged women. Pulmonary or pleural involvement of some type occurs in a high percentage of patients at some time in the course of the disease. The disease is chronic and usually fatal, but may undergo repeated remissions and exacerbations. Pleural effusion is the most common finding. The effusion is bilateral and usually small, but may be massive. Eventually, pleural fibrosis occurs following repeated episodes of pleural effusion. The diaphragm may move poorly and basal lung volume may decrease. Pericardial effusion may also occur. The pulmonary parenchymal changes are varied as in polyarteritis and range from the soft, patchy density of pulmonary edema to strandlike accentuation of bronchovascular markings. Occasionally the lesions assume a nodular appearance. Pulmonary densities are usually transitory. The pulmonary alterations

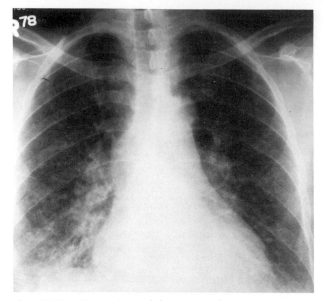

Fig. 30-20. Disseminated lupus erythematosus. Note the basal interstitial disease with a small pleural effusion on the right. This patient was a male. This disease is more common in females than in males and pleural effusion is usually a more prominent feature of the disease in the thorax.

tend to be basal in position (Fig. 30-20). In addition to pericardial effusion, pancarditis may cause enlargement of the cardiac silhouette. When the pulmonary disease becomes chronic, resulting in basal fibrosis, there is often elevation of the diaphragm and its motion is restricted. The combination of bilateral pleural effusion, pericardial effusion causing enlargement of the cardiac silhouette, and a changing bilateral pulmonary disease suggests systemic lupus erythematosus. Pulmonary changes are less frequent than pleural and cardiac involvement, but may be bizarre, with cavitation in nodules, formation of pneumatoceles, and rapid alteration. Subpleural infiltrates are common; they are probably infarcts. Pulmonary infection may be superimposed on the lung changes produced by lupus; radiographic differentiation may be very difficult.

DIFFUSE SYSTEMIC SCLEROSIS (SCLERODERMA)

Diffuse systemic sclerosis is characterized by atrophy and sclerosis of many organ systems including the skin, musculoskeletal system, and heart as well as the lungs. These conditions are discussed in the sections dealing with the gastrointestinal tract and the

soft tissues. Pulmonary manifestations occur in approximately 10% of these patients. As in the other collagen diseases a variety of lesions may be observed, but the findings tend to be more stable in this disease than in the others. The basic lesion is interstitial fibrosis, which may take the form of accentuation of interstitial markings resulting in a fine reticular pattern that becomes coarser and denser as the disease progresses. Although the lesion is usually basal at first, with slow progression, rarely it may ultimately involve the entire lung. There is often some scattered nodulation in the parahilar areas and in the bases as well. Pleural effusion may occur late in the disease, but is not a prominent feature, and pleural fibrosis is also an unusual finding. In a few patients with long-standing disease, subpleural cysts have been described that are apparently caused by a disappearance of alveolar tissues. This results in small cystic spaces, surrounded by thick fibrous walls. The apices are spared in this manifestation of the disease (Fig. 30-21). Decrease in volume of the lower lobe is characteristic of the disease. When the esophagus is involved, aspiration with the addition of basal lung changes caused by aspiration pneumonia may occur.

Mixed connective tissue disease is an overlap syndrome combining scleroderma, systemic lupus, polymyositis, and rheumatoid arthritis to varying degrees. The chest findings include basal interstitial disease

Fig. 30-21. Scleroderma. There is extensive interstitial disease chiefly in the bases and central lung fields. Apices are relatively spared. This interstitial disease is largely reticulonodular in type.

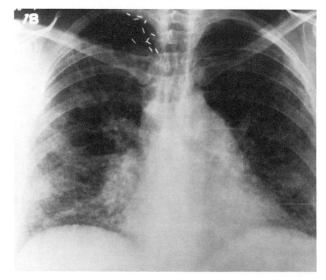

and pleural and pericardial fluid. They are similar to those of the overlap syndrome of scleroderma and systemic lupus, so that chest roentgen findings are not specifically diagnostic.

RHEUMATOID DISEASE OF THE LUNG

Rheumatoid arthritis is occasionally accompanied by pulmonary disease which is a part of the generalized involvement. The pulmonary lesions tend to occur in patients with high titers of rheumatoid factor and subcutaneous rheumatoid nodules. The most common finding in the thorax is pleuritis which is often accompanied by pleural effusion that is minimal to moderate in amount and usually bilateral. The fluid may remain for months or years with very little variation. Pleural thickening may eventually occur in these patients. The most common pulmonary change is that of an interstitial pneumonitis which produces a reticular pattern of interstitial density similar to that in idiopathic interstitial pneumonitis. The distribution of the interstitial densities may be diffuse, but at times tend to be parahilar and basal (Fig. 30-22). Occasionally the interstitial process may coalesce to form patchy areas resembling an alveolar type of pneumonitis. Rheumatoid nodules of the lung are somewhat less common than the diffuse change. They may be multiple or solitary and vary from a few millimeters to several centimeters in size. It is common to observe them in a subpleural position, and cavitation may occur.

In addition to these manifestations, a syndrome has been described in patients with coal worker's pneumoconiosis who have rheumatoid arthritis. This is Caplan's syndrome in which the patients have crops of pulmonary nodules varying from 0.5 to 5.0 cm in diameter, usually associated with exacerbation of the rheumatoid arthritis. At times, a single pulmonary nodule may be observed. This syndrome has been expanded to include asbestosis and silicosis acquired in industries other than coal mining.

Ankylosing Spondylitis

Ankylosing spondylitis is sometimes accompanied by pulmonary disease. The roentgenographic findings are those of bilateral upper lobe fibrosis manifested by small nodular and linear shadows which may coalesce to form linear and nodular opacities that may be very large. Cavitation is frequent and in many instances is associated with aspergilloma. The disease may be stable for years or may progress steadily so that extensive fibrosis results in upward retraction of one or both hila and upper lobe bronchiectasis. In

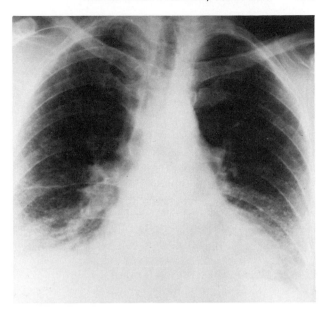

Fig. 30-22. Rheumatoid disease of the lung. In this patient there is basal interstitial disease which is quite similar to that often noted in scleroderma. Pleural effusion is a more common manifestation of rheumatoid disease of the lung.

these instances, the roentgenographic appearance is quite similar to that of chronic pulmonary tuberculosis. In addition there may be apical pleural thickening that may become extensive. These changes usually occur in patients with long-standing and extensive involvement of the spine and often involvement of the large joints as well.

POLYMYOSITIS AND DERMATOMYOSITIS

Interstitial lung disease is known to be associated with polymyositis and dermatomyositis, but with less frequency than with other collagen vascular diseases. The roentgen pattern is one of a diffuse reticulonodular interstitial process usually localized to the lung bases. In the more acute disease, there may be a mixed alveolar and interstitial pattern. Effusion rarely, if ever, occurs. The pulmonary disease resembles that of progressive systemic sclerosis (scleroderma).

SJOGREN'S SYNDROME

Sjogren's syndrome is a chronic inflammatory process characterized by atrophy of the lacrimal and salivary glands leading to decreased production of tears and dryness of the mouth. It is usually associated with rheumatoid arthritis, but systemic lupus erythematosus, dermatomyositis, and scleroderma have also been reported to be associated with this syndrome. Pleural and pulmonary manifestations are frequent and consist of an interstitial process that is reticulonodular or nodular similar to that found in rheumatoid arthritis. Pleurisy and/or pleural effusion may also occur. The pathologic change is that of a benign lymphoid infiltration. There is an associated broad spectrum of lymphoproliferative disorders ranging from extraglandular lymphocytic infiltration or lymphoid interstitial pneumonitis to pseudolymphoma and to malignant neoplasm such as reticulum cell sarcoma, lymphosarcoma, and Hodgkin's disease.

BEHÇET'S SYNDROME

Behçet's syndrome is a vasculitis resulting in aphthous ulceration of oral and genital mucosa and relapsing iritis. It occurs in young adults usually in the third decade of life. Its incidence is greater in males than females. Vascular involvement manifested by migratory thrombophlebitis may result in obstruction of the superior or inferior vena cava. Vasculitis and thrombosis involving the pulmonary arteries are rare, but since they do appear along with exacerbations of the disease elsewhere they must be considered as part of Behçet's syndrome. The pulmonary radiographic findings include fleeting bilateral alveolar densities produced by hemoptysis, which is likely a result of vasculitis. Central nervous system involvement appears to be the major cause of the high mortality (40%) observed in this disease, but massive exsanguinating hemoptysis may result from pulmonary involvement.

IMMUNOBLASTIC LYMPHADENOPATHY (ANGIOIMMUNOBLASTIC LYMPHADENOPATHY)

Immunoblastic lymphadenopathy is characterized by an acute or subacute onset of fever, generalized lymphadenopathy, and hepatosplenomegaly. In about one-third of its subjects, a history of drug ingestion is obtained and and skin rash occurs at the onset of the disease. Histologically, this condition resembles Hodgkin's disease with an infiltration of histiocytes, plasma cells, eosinophils, and immunoblasts that replace lymphocytes and efface lymph node architecture. There is also hyperproliferation of post capillary venules and amorphous interstitial deposits consist-

ing of cellular debris. In some patients the disease may evolve into a lymphoma. Although the cause is not certain, an abnormal immune state is likely. Radiographic findings consist of pulmonary densities and evidence of hilar adenopathy, mediastinal adenopathy, and pleural effusion. The pulmonary densities are varied and range from indications of diffuse interstitial lung disease to an alveolar pattern which may resemble that due to pulmonary edema and may be associated with an interstitial pattern in other parts of the lung. Superimposed infection may add to the pulmonary density and result in asymmetry. Response to steroids is dramatic in some of these patients.[73]

WEGENER'S GRANULOMATOSIS

Midline lethal granuloma is a destructive process of unknown cause, which some investigators believe is related to the collagen diseases. It is often a fatal condition in which there is extensive destruction of bony structures of the nose and paranasal sinuses. When this condition is associated with necrotizing granulomatous vasculitis of the lungs and necrotizing glomerulonephritis, which may be focal or general, the syndrome is known as Wegener's syndrome or necrotizing granulomatosis. The three main pathologic features are: (1) necrotizing granulomatous lesions of the upper respiratory tract, (2) necrotizing angiitis of arteries and veins, and (3) glomerulitis. The roentgen changes in the sinuses are those of soft-tissue density plus destruction of bone that cannot be differentiated from the destruction produced by malignant neoplasm. The granulomatous lesion of the lung, which is characteristic of the disease, may be solitary or multiple. Its size varies from 1 to 8 cm in diameter. Some of the lesions may cavitate. The cavity is usually small in relation to the size of the nodule, with an irregular inner wall, but the nodule may excavate completely leaving a thin wall, and then eventually may disappear. The outer margins of the nodules are indistinct and may have a "shaggy" appearance. When multiple, the nodules tend to be few in number, and may resemble pulmonary metastases. Occasionally a solitary mass resembling a primary lung tumor may occur. Other findings include areas of poorly defined consolidation resembling pneumonia. As in the other collagen-vascular diseases, there is nothing specific about the roentgen pulmonary changes. Pleural effusion may occur late in the disease. Rarely, an endobronchial mass may occur, resulting in atelectasis of a lobe or lung. This may be associated with pleural disease accompanied by effusion or pleural thickening. The effusion may be massive.

BRONCHOCENTRIC GRANULOMATOSIS

Bronchocentric granulomatosis is characterized by granulomatous destructive lesions of the bronchi and bronchioles. The symptoms are varied; they usually consist of cough, migratory chest pains, and recurrent "pneumonia." Some patients are asymptomatic. Radiographic changes also are varied and may be unilateral (75%) or bilateral. In some instances, pulmonary densities resembling those due to pneumonia or atelectasis are evident; in others, nodular or tumorlike masses may be seen. Cavitation in granulomas, or in asociated lung abscesses, may appear. Hilar adenopathy may be present. The lesions usually respond to steroids. The clinical course appears to be relatively benign.

PULMONARY HYALINIZING GRANULOMA

Pulmonary hyalinizing granuloma is probably caused by an exaggerated immune response. The clinical course is benign with minimal signs or symptoms. Cough, malaise, fever, dyspnea, fatigue and/or pleuritic pain may occur, however. Histologic findings in the pulmonary nodules consist of concentric hyaline lamellae with perivascular collections of lymphocytes and plasma cells. Radiographic findings are those of multiple pulmonary nodules (occasionally solitary), usually bilateral, well circumscribed, and solid. Their size ranges from a few millimeters to 15 cm in diameter. At times the lesions are irregular and poorly defined. Cavitation is not common. Most of the lesions resemble nodular pulmonary metastases. Sclerosing mediastinitis may complicate this disease.[12]

LYMPHOMATOID GRANULOMATOSIS

Lymphomatoid granulomatosis is a type of granulomatous vasculitis that resembles malignant lymphoma histologically because of prominent lymphoreticular proliferation. A necrotizing vasculitis differentiates it from lymphoma. The most characteristic radiographic appearance is that of multiple, bilateral masses that are fairly well circumscribed and resemble metastatic nodules. They are usually subpleural and may cavitate. Cavities may have thick or thin walls, sometimes with fluid levels. At times the nodules are smaller, more numerous, and poorly defined; the presence of a single, large, unilateral mass has

also been reported in patients with this disease. Hilar adenopathy may be present, and pleural effusion is occasionally observed.[38]

NECROTIZING SARCOIDAL GRANULOMATOSIS

Necrotizing sarcoidal granulomatosis is another rare type of granulomatous angiitis in which there is marked infiltration with sarcoidlike tubercles. Radiologic findings are similar to those in lymphomatoid granulomatosis except that hilar adenopathy is not ordinarily observed.

IMMUNE DEFICIENCY SYNDROMES

The immune deficiency diseases result in increased susceptibility to respiratory infections as well as infections elsewhere.[69] A number of types of deficiency states have been described. They include: (1) decrease or absence of all immunoglobulins; (2) decrease or absence of a specific imunoglobulin; (3) lack of complement; (4) inability to handle various antigens; (5) defect in leukocyte function; and (6) the presence of inhibitors of essential components of the immune system. Because findings of repeated pulmonary infection are common to many of these diseases, a specific diagnosis cannot be made radiographically.

The syndromes are classified as primary, indicating a genetic abnormality, and secondary, indicating that some disease has interfered with normal function of the immune system.

THE AGAMMAGLOBULINEMIAS

The agammaglobulinemias are deficiency states in which antibodies cannot be formed because of an absence or deficiency of gammaglobulins. The congenital form is a sex-linked recessive genetic defect transmitted by females to male offspring (Bruton's disease). Secondary agammaglobulinemia, or hypogammaglobulinemia, may be acquired as in patients with multiple myeloma, leukemia, or lymphoma. However, there is also a group in whom, although the disease is of genetic origin, it is not manifest in infancy. Repeated infections are commonly observed in the lungs in patients with the agammaglobulinemias. Infections of the paranasal sinuses and mastoids are very common; infections of the urinary tract, skin, and elsewhere also occur. The radiographic findings in the lungs are therefore those of recurrent bronchopneumonia which may lead to postinflammatory fibrotic changes and to bronchiectasis. No hilar adenopathy is present, and the decrease or absence of lymphoid tissue in the pharynx results in a large pharyngeal airway that is characteristic of these conditions in young children. This is readily observed in a lateral roentgenogram of the nasopharynx. In older children, lymph nodes and lymphoid tissue may become evident when there is hyperplasia of reticulum cells. In the acquired type of agammaglobulinemia, there may be hyperplasia of lymphoid tissue. In this situation, the mediastinal nodes may be enlarged.

DYSGAMMAGLOBULINEMIAS

The term "dysgammaglobulinemia" refers to conditions in which there is a deficiency in one or two of the immunoglobulins with normal or elevated levels of others. The patients may be susceptible to respiratory infections which are observed as repeated pneumonias and are ultimately associated with bronchiectasis, atelectasis, and fibrosis.

COMBINED IMMUNODEFICIENCIES

The basic abnormality in this group of deficiencies is cellular, but there is impairment of humeral immunity also. In severe disease, both B- and T-lymphocyte functions may be markedly depressed or absent. Children having these deficiency diseases are susceptible to viral infections in addition to bacterial, fungal, and parasitic infections.

COMPLEMENT DEFICIENCY

Patients with complement deficiency have normal antibody production, leukocyte function, and cellular immunity, but lack certain components of complement and are therefore subject to frequent infections, usually with staphylococcal or gram-negative organisms.

THE INTERSTITIAL PNEUMONIAS

The term "interstitial pneumonia," as used by Liebow and Carrington,[40] indicates a pneumonia in which the most significant or persistent component of the tissue response in the lung is in the interalveolar septa and more proximal supporting tissues. The most chronic form of the interstitial pneumonias is represented by interstitial fibrosis. In this end stage there is usually breakdown of alveolar walls in addition to fibrosis, which produces the so-called honeycomb pattern of pulmonary interstitial fibrosis. Others, including Scadding and Hinson,[59, 60] prefer the term "fibrosing alveolitis" to describe these diseases, many of which are of unknown cause. The term "pneumonia" is then restricted to denote inflammation of the lung characterized by consolidation produced by exudates filling the alveoli. Some believe that the group of idiopathic interstitial pneumonias represent inflammatory responses of the alveolar walls to injuries of different types, durations, and intensities and are thus different aspects of multifacetted "fibrosing alveolitis."

In view of the lack of knowledge regarding etiology, two partial classifications are necessary, one histopathologic, the other etiologic. Both are not mutually exclusive.

On the basis of histologic criteria and to some extent on radiographic and clinical criteria, Liebow and Carrington[40] have described the following interstitial pneumonias: (1) the classical, undifferentiated, or usual (UIP); (2) nonbacterial bronchiolitis obliterans superimposed on UIP (BIP); (3) desquamative (DIP); (4) lymphoid (LIP); and (5) giant cell (GIP).

As will be noted in the following descriptions, the interstitial pneumonias exhibit a rather wide variety of roentgenographic patterns. Because of this the differential diagnosis is based on lung biopsy with study of histologic sections. In most instances, the etiology is not clear. As indicated, many prefer the term "fibrosing alveolitis" for some of these conditions in which there is ultimately more or less interstitial fibrosis.

CLASSICAL OR UNDIFFERENTIATED INTERSTITIAL PNEUMONIA (UIP)

This disease is the result of diffuse alveolar damage from a large variety of agents, including a number of inhalants such as oxygen in high concentrations, particularly when administered by intermittent positive-pressure breathing (IPPB) machines; viruses and mycoplasma; and conditions altering immunity, such as scleroderma and rheumatoid arthritis. In some cases a genetic factor may be involved. However, the cause of most chronic interstitial pneumonias is unknown. Whatever it is, diffuse alveolar damage is produced, probably with some necrosis of alveolar epithelium and proteinacious exudates. The basement membrane is usually preserved. Hyaline membranes comprised of exudate and remnants of necrotic alveolar lining cells may be present. Interstitial infiltrations of lymphocytes and mononuclear cells are also noted in this stage. Interstitial proliferation and fibrosis eventually occur in some areas. During the acute phase, the exudates plus the swelling of alveolar cells and the interstitial infiltrate produce a roentgen picture simulating the fluffy appearance of pulmonary edema. Roentgenographic findings vary considerably, however, and in the more chronic forms of UIP the density produced is coarse and strandlike and tends to extend radially from the hilum. Small, round radiolucencies may appear and become more prominent with increasing fibrosis and destruction of the alveolar walls; this represents the honeycomb pattern of pulmonary fibrosis.

DIFFUSE ALVEOLAR DAMAGE AND BRONCHIOLITIS OBLITERANS (BIP)

When there is damage to bronchioles superimposed on the lesion of UIP, BIP is produced. Although the cause is not clear, this kind of damage can be the result of inhalation of corrosive fumes of strong acids. However, it appears to occur much more commonly as a result of a necrotizing bacterial bronchiolitis superimposed on viral pneumonia. The radiographic findings consist of streaks of flamelike density noted chiefly in the upper and central lung fields but they may occur anywhere in the lungs. This may represent UIP with superimposed bacterial infection rather than a distinct entity.

DESQUAMATIVE INTERSTITIAL PNEUMONIA (DIP)

This is an interstitial pneumonia characterized by extensive desquamation of granular pneumocytes (type II alveolar lining cells). It is associated with a mild interstitial cellular infiltration of plasma cells, lymphocytes, and eosinophils and with some septal and pleural edema. These desquamated cells and large aggregated macrophages may fill the bronchioles as well as alveoli. As in the other diseases affecting the alveolar walls, the cause is not certain, but in many an immunologic mechanism is a factor.

Roentgenographic findings consist of bilateral basal shadows which often are hazy and may have a ground-glass appearance. As the disease progresses, the basal density increases. The pattern is variable, however, with more density in upper than in lower lung fields in some patients. In many of our patients, the disease has been widely scattered with pulmonary densities of varying configuration, often with a mixed interstitial and alveolar pattern (Fig. 30-23). Rapid response to steroids usually occurs, but, in some instances, the disease may progress to a non-specific, honeycomb pattern of fibrosis with loss of pulmonary volume.

LYMPHOID INTERSTITIAL PNEUMONIA (LIP)

In lymphoid interstitial pneumonia there is massive and widespread infiltration of both lungs by lymphoid tissue which resembles lymphoma very closely histologically. The history is that of a very chronic interstitial pneumonia, however. The infiltration is interstitial in the interalveolar septa and in the peribronchiolar and perivenous spaces. Local lymph nodes and extrapulmonary tissues are not involved. The infiltrate is a mixture of small lymphocytes, plasma cells, and occasional large mononuclear cells, with the small lymphocytes predominating. Radiographic changes are variable and range from bilateral diffuse, nodular infiltrates to peripheral densities which may be linear or branching, sometimes appearing rather poorly defined and conglomerate. Some of the peripheral linear densities resemble Kerley B-lines. As the disease progresses, alveoli are compressed and obliterated by dense, linear opacities. The disease is usually bilateral but not necessarily symmetrical. Ultimately, fibrosis may lead to some honeycombing. This pneumonia does not respond to steroids and tends to progress slowly. At times the infiltrate can be relatively local, producing a rather conglomerate-appearing, poorly defined, masslike density.

GIANT CELL INTERSTITIAL PNEUMONIA (GIP)

This unique interstitial pneumonia is characterized by the presence of intra-alveolar giant cells and an interstitial infiltrate that is predominately lymphocytic. The giant cells are very large and may nearly fill an alveolus. Clinically, the condition is manifest by cough and dyspnea; there may be some weight loss and fever. Roentgen findings are varied. A confluent nodular process may be present in one or both lungs and in either upper or lower lobes. Sometimes, mottled nodular densities and strandlike or streaklike densities extending from the hilum to the periphery of the lung may be noted.

DIFFUSE PULMONARY FIBROSIS OF UNKNOWN ETIOLOGY

Fibrosis of the lungs may result from a number of diseases. These include infections such a tuberculosis, the fungal diseases, bronchiectasis, the collagen-vascular and other diseases with altered immu-

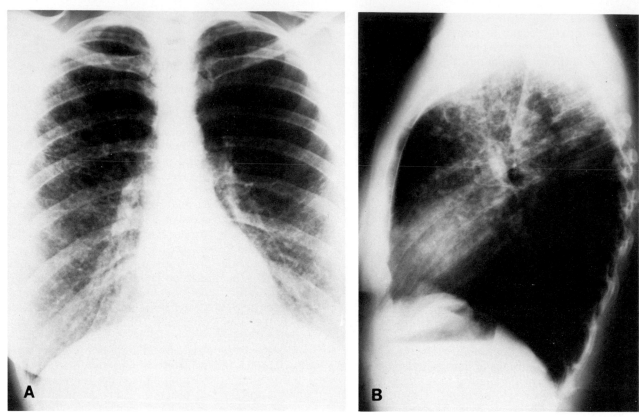

Fig. 30-23. Desquamative interstitial pneumonia (DIP). Note the widespread, somewhat stringy, interstitial disease which is noted best at the bases in the frontal projection **(A)** and in the upper lung field in the lateral projection **(B)**. In our experience there has been no characteristic roentgenographic pattern in this disease.

nity, the malignant pneumoconioses, and others. The cause can sometimes be ascertained in this group if clinical history, physical findings, laboratory findings, and roentgen alterations are correlated. The roentgen manifestations of these diseases are discussed in the appropriate section. There is a large group of conditions in which fibrosis may be localized or scattered and in which there is no evidence of cause, a nonspecific fibrosis of obscure etiology. As more knowledge is gained regarding histopathology of the lung, however, it is likely that the number of patients placed in this category will decrease. The roentgen findings are those of an increasing thickening of interstitial lung markings that is often more prominent in the bases than elsewhere. This produces a fine reticular pattern that gradually becomes coarser. If there is a considerable amount of associated emphysema, a honeycomb pattern may be observed. In other instances, a more linear pattern is produced

which at times may be associated with a fine nodular or granular pattern. Secondary pulmonary hypertension may develop, resulting in a gradual increase in the size of the pulmonary artery and its hilar branches, as well as evidence of right ventricular enlargement. The roentgen changes develop over a period of years or many months. The etiology is never determined; even at autopsy the findings can only be described as those of nonspecific fibrosis (Fig. 30-24).

HAMMAN–RICH SYNDROME (DIFFUSE INTERSTITIAL PULMONARY FIBROSIS)

This disease, originally described by Hamman and Rich, is characterized by an insidious onset of general malaise, fever, occasional dry cough, chest pain, and dyspnea, which soon becomes severe. The pa-

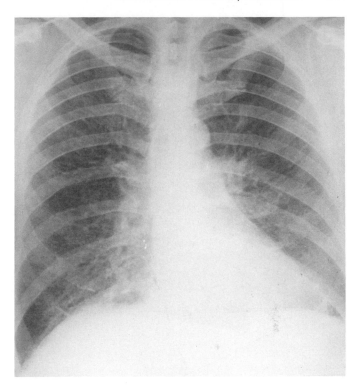

Fig. 30-24. Diffuse pulmonary fibrosis. The interstitial change is very extensive in this patient in whom there was nothing in the history to indicate the cause. Lung biopsy revealed diffuse pulmonary fibrosis of unknown cause.

tients usually die in 1 to 6 months of pulmonary insufficiency. The disease may also be subacute or chronic, with slow progression for a number of years. Respiratory insufficiency and right-sided heart failure occur and recurrent infections are common in the late stage of the disease. Microscopic examination shows marked fibroblastic proliferation in the alveolar walls often associated with edema and an infiltration of lymphocytes and plasma cells. The presence of eosinophils has been noted by several investigators. Later the fibroblastic proliferation results in extensive thickening of alveolar walls and interstitial tissues, causing severe respiratory dysfunction leading to death.

This condition probably is one of several histopathologic responses of the alveolar walls to injuries of different types, durations, and intensities. Therefore, it is related to the other interstitial pneumonias (fibrosing alveolitis). More accurate classification of these conditions will be possible when the etiologic factor(s) can be determined, and the cause of variations in pulmonary response are better understood. The term "Hamman–Rich syndrome" should probably be confined to signify the acute, diffuse alveolar fibrosing disease that leads to death in less than a year.

Roentgen Findings. Early in the disease there is slight increase in pulmonary interstitial markings and slight decrease in diaphragmatic motion that can be noted fluoroscopically or on roentgenograms obtained when the patient is in inspiration and expiration. As the fibrosis progresses the interstitial markings become more prominent, resulting in thick linear shadows extending outward from the hila and a reticular pattern of increased density in the peripheral lung fields. The change is not necessarily symmetric but is usually bilateral. In far-advanced disease there is extensive strandlike thickening with considerable lucency surrounded by the thick strands resembling a coarse honeycomb or cystic pattern. The volume of the lung decreases progressively (Fig. 30-25). Because the roentgen findings are not characteristic, the diagnosis must be based on clinical manifestations with the history of rapidly progressing dyspnea plus failure to find any definite cause. Lung biopsy is necessary to make the diagnosis, particularly in patients with subacute or

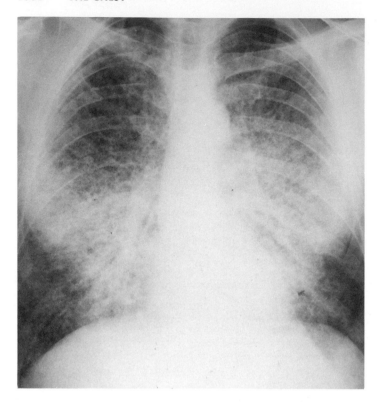

Fig. 30-25. Hamman–Rich syndrome. The pulmonary biopsy showed changes compatible with this syndrome. There is marked accentuation of interstitial markings which is stringy and strandlike and is confluent in some areas. It is associated with some peripheral emphysema.

chronic disease in whom the clinical course is of no particular diagnostic value. Some investigators believe that this condition is based on sensitivity but exact etiology has not been proved. There is enough variation in the reported cases to suggest that there may be a variety of causes.

LUNG DISEASE IN NEUROFIBROMATOSIS

Fibrosing alveolitis or interstitial pulmonary fibrosis occurs in about 20% of patients with neurofibromatosis who are over 30 years of age. The pulmonary disease in these patients does not become manifest until adult life. The cause is not known, but there probably is a genetic influence. Radiographic findings consist of linear interstitial density that is bilateral and tends to be basal. Large upper-lobe bullae also are part of the disease which produces relatively minor dyspnea.[67]

AMYLOIDOSIS

Amyloidosis is usually classified into the primary and secondary types. The secondary type is found in patients with chronic inflammatory disease, such as chronic osteomyelitis, bronchiectasis, and tuberculosis. It also develops in patients with rheumatoid arthritis and in those having malignant neoplasms; it is much more common than the primary type.[70] Amyloid is deposited in the spleen, liver, adrenal glands, and kidneys secondary to the chronic inflammatory disease or malignancy. In the primary form of the disease the amyloid is typically deposited in the heart, gastrointestinal tract, lungs, muscle, and skin. Primary amyloidosis is rare. It develops in patients with plasma-cell abnormalities, such as multiple myeloma, and in patients with abnormal immunoglobulins, but the cause is unknown. There is pulmonary involvement in 30% to 70% of patients with primary amyloidosis. Amyloid is made up of a protein matrix consisting of fragments of immunoglobulin polypeptide chains. Its chemistry is not fully understood. This material is deposited in the alveolar walls and around the interalveolar capillaries as well as in the walls of the smaller blood vessels in the lung when pulmonary involvement is present. The myocardium is affected in approximately 70% of patients with the primary form of the disease. Deposits may also occur in bronchial and tracheal wall.

The patterns of amyloid deposition can be classified into three major types: (*1*) tracheobronchial in which amyloid deposition in the wall results in a diffuse thickening and distortion of the tracheobronchial tree; (2) nodular pulmonary in which single or multiple parenchymal nodules are produced by masses of amyloid that increase very slowly in size; and (3) diffuse alveolar septal in which amyloid is deposited in interstitial tissues, often perivascular, but also in alveolar walls and septa.

Roentgen Findings. The roentgen findings in the tracheobronchial form of amyloidosis are related to obstruction causing atelectasis or overinflation. Bronchial distortion, tracheal irregularity, and luminal narrowing can be observed on bronchography. The nodular form consists of single or multiple masses that can become calcified or may cavitate. The alveolar septal form may show a miliary nodular or reticulonodular pattern. There may also be a form resembling diffuse fibrosis with radiating strands extending outward from the hilum into the central lung fields. In the alveolar septal type there is often associated pleural effusion that may appear, regress, and then reappear. Pleural deposits may cause pleural thickening in these patients. There is also deposition of amyloid in hilar and mediastinal nodes with a gradual increase in the hilar size and blurring of mediastinal borders. As the disease progresses, the radiating strands increase and, in some instances, fine granular or more coarse nodular lesions develop. Calcification and bone formation may be observed in the pulmonary lesions and in the hilar and mediastinal nodes. The bone formation is peculiar and resembles spikelike pieces of broken glass. The roentgen progression is accompanied by increasing dyspnea. This generalized type of involvement must be distinguished from other chronic diseases that cause interstitial fibrosis. It may resemble sarcoidosis. The nodular form of the disease consists of one or more homogeneous masses that may be somewhat lobulated and resemble primary lung tumor closely; the local form is usually found in elderly men. The prognosis is poor in the tracheobronchial and the alveolar septal forms of the disease. Decreasing pulmonary volume and respiratory insufficiency are observed in the alveolar septal form and obstruction is noted in the tracheobronchial form.

HISTIOCYTOSIS X

Eosinophilic granuloma is the most benign of a group of diseases of unknown cause referred to as histiocytosis X (synonyms: generalized xanthomatosis, lipid histiocytosis, lipid granulomatosis, reticuloendothe-

liosis). Hand–Schüller–Christian disease and Letterer–Siwe disease are closely related to eosinophilic granuloma. Letterer–Siwe disease occurs in infants; it is acute and often rapidly fatal. Hand–Schüller–Christian disease occurs in older children and is more benign, while eosinophilic granuloma occurs in young adults and is often localized and benign. Eosinophilic granuloma has been found as a lesion occurring only in the lung with increasing frequency. In some patients (about 20%) the typical bone lesion has been associated with the pulmonary disease, but in others the lung appears to be the sole site of involvement.

The roentgen manifestations of pulmonary histiocytosis X are reasonably characteristic. Generalized involvement is noted, manifested by an increase in linear markings along with small nodular lesions on the order of 1 to 3 mm in size. These nodules are rather poorly defined, with hazy borders (Fig. 30-26A). They may be scattered generally throughout the lungs but tend to be somewhat more pronounced in the upper lung fields (Fig. 30-26). The disease may regress spontaneously. It may progress, with increasing interstitial involvement. The appearance is then that of a somewhat reticulonodular pattern of increased markings with small foci of cystlike rarefaction, resulting in a honeycomb lung (Fig. 30-26B). There is no hilar adenopathy and usually no pleural involvement.

In eosinophilic granuloma the patient is asymptomatic or has relatively few symptoms and the lesions clear slowly. Because the roentgen findings are not characteristic and simulate those of other chronic interstitial pulmonary disease, the diagnosis must be based on clinical manfestations plus the presence of the typical roentgen changes observed in bone. Lung biopsy is necessary, but the diagnosis can be suspected in asymptomatic young patients with extensive pulmonary disease and no adenopathy or pleural involvement. Diabetes insipidus may be present and is helpful in making the diagnosis. A history of repeated spontaneous pneumothorax in a patient with the above pulmonary findings is also suggestive of histiocytosis X.

GAUCHER'S DISEASE AND NIEMANN-PICK DISEASE

Gaucher's disease is due to an inborn error of metabolism in which there is an accumulation of glucosylceramide in reticuloendothelial cells. The lung may be involved with roentgen findings of interstitial disease manifested by a diffuse reticulonodular or mil-

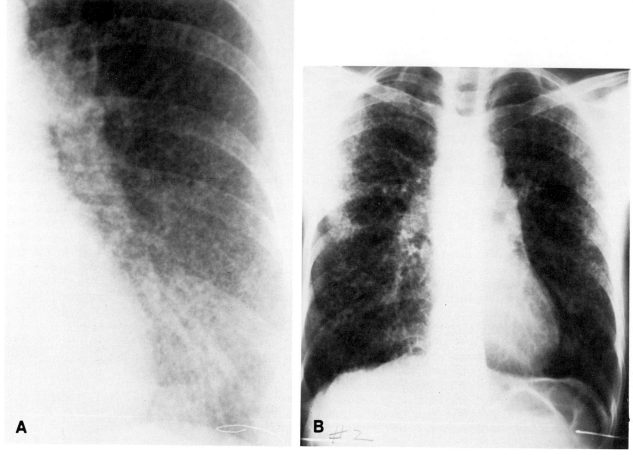

Fig. 30-26. Pulmonary histiocytosis X. **A.** The patient, a 40-year-old woman, had extensive pulmonary involvement consisting largely of tiny nodules and very few cyst-like areas as shown in this close-up view. **B.** In another patient with chronic disease, a considerable amount of fibrosis has produced a "honeycomb" lung, noted best in the lateral aspect of the left central and upper lung. Elsewhere there are small granular-appearing nodules. There is a little emphysema with blebs at the left apex.

iary pattern of pulmonary density.[72] *Niemann–Pick disease* is a related lipid storage disorder of phospholipid metabolism. Pulmonary involvement causes diffuse nodular disease with linear strands producing a honeycomb effect or a coarse reticulonodular pattern on the roentgenogram of the chest. Basal Kerley-B lines may also be present, and there may be some pulmonary calcifications.[35]

PULMONARY TUBEROUS SCLEROSIS AND LYMPHANGIOMYOMATOSIS

Tuberous sclerosis is a hereditary disease characterized by mental deficiency, seizures, adenoma sebaceum (acneform rash) on the face with butterfly distribution, and hamartomatous tumors that may affect various parts of the body, including the central nervous system, liver, spleen, kidneys, and bones. The pulmonary form of tuberous scleroisis usually occurs in adults in whom there is no mental deficiency and no clinical evidence of central nervous system damage even though calcifications are noted intracranially. Several patients have been reported in whom chest roentgenograms revealed a reticular or reticulonodular pattern throughout both lung fields, resembling the changes noted in other interstitial diseases of the lungs. In some patients the reticular pattern is rather coarse and the small radiolucencies produced by the cystic lesions vary from 1 or 2 mm to 1 cm in diameter, a honeycomb pattern. These cysts may occur subpleurally and rupture to cause spontaneous pneumothorax. Pulmonary volume does not decrease as in many interstitial diseases and may be increased in some patients. Pleural effusion may occur in addition to the pulmonary changes. It may be unilateral or bilateral. The effusions are usually large, tend to recur, and are chylous.

Lymphangiomyomatosis (lymphangiomyoma, muscular hyperplasia, muscular cirrhosis) is a rare disease of young women in which there is an overgrowth of atypical smooth muscle along the lymphatics of the lung. There may also be involvement of the extrapulmonary thoracic lymphatics and abdominal lymphatics. The disease is sufficiently similar to tuberous sclerosis to warrant an assumption by some authorities that it is a forme fruste of tuberous sclerosis. Others believe that there are enough differences to make the diseases separate entities. Radiographic findings that are often observed late in the course of lymphangiomyomatosis are similar to those in tuberous sclerosis. Recurrent spontaneous pneumothorax

may occur before any pulmonary abnormalities are visible on the chest roentgenogram. The earliest pulmonary findings are those of a diffuse pattern of tiny opacities described as reticulonodular, granular, miliary, or interstitial (Fig. 30-27). Later, a coarser reticular pattern is observed, often with septal lines. Eventually, a honeycomb pattern is seen but its appearance is more delicate than the usual honeycomb pattern noted in end-stage interstitial disease. The lungs tend to increase rather than decrease in volume. Chylous effusions may occur similar to those in tuberous sclerosis.[9, 64, 66] Although the diagnosis depends upon lung biopsy, the disease may be suspected in young women having chylous pleural effusions and repeated spontaneous pneumothorax with or without a fine reticulonodular pulmonary interstitial pattern and progressive enlargement of lung volume. In most interstitial lung disease, the pulmonary volume is diminished.

Fig. 30-27. Lymphangiomyomatosis in a young woman. A rather fine reticular interstitial pattern is noted best in the right central lung field in the frontal **(A)** and in the upper lungs in the lateral **(B)** projection. The lung volume was increased in this patient. Note the low flat diaphragm in the lateral view.

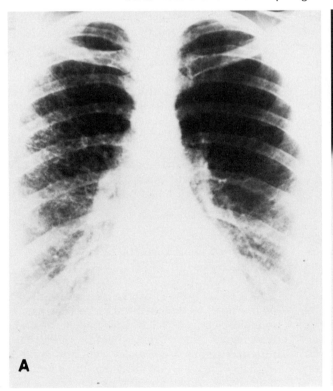
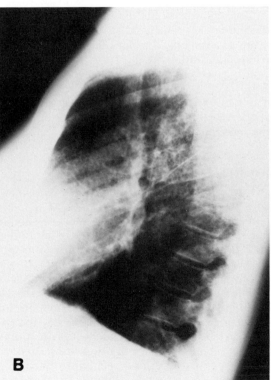

PULMONARY ALVEOLAR MICROLITHIASIS

This rare disease is characterized by the presence of small calcium-containing bodies in the alveoli of the lung. The cause is not known but there is a high familial incidence, indicating that there is a hereditary factor. The disease is asymptomatic for long periods of time but eventually dyspnea appears, followed by cough, cyanosis, and right-sided heart failure. Because of the late appearance of symptoms the disease is usually first discovered on routine chest roentgenography.

Roentgen Findings. The appearance of the chest in this disease is characteristic. There is widespread uniform distribution of fine sandlike particles of calcific density, which are usually less than 1 mm in diameter. They are uniform in size and there is no tendency to conglomeration. When extensive, some of the tiny calcifications may overlap and be difficult to define as individual particles. Overexposed or Bucky films are of value in visualizing them, particularly when the disease is far advanced. The density is often great enough to obscure the heart and mediastinal outlines as well as the diaphragm. In some patients, the pulmonary density is so great that the pleura appears as a negative or black-line shadow instead of a white one, and even the heart may appear radiolucent in contrast to the extensive pulmonary calcification.[31] There is no other disease that resembles this condition since these tiny particles are calcific and are denser than particles of comparable size in any of the miliary diseases.

FAMILIAL DYSAUTONOMIA (RILEY–DAY SYNDROME)

Familial dysautonomia results from dysfunction of the autonomic nervous system. It is a familial congenital disorder transmitted as an autosomal recessive trait that occurs in children and young adults, usually of Jewish extraction. Clinical findings consist of defective (decreased) lacrimation, excessive perspiration, blotchy skin, drooling, emotional instability, motor incoordination, hyporeflexia, and indifference to pain. Death is usually due to pulmonary disease. The pulmonary findings are related to bronchial hypersecretion and resultant obstruction that often leads to infection. Pulmonary manifestations sufficient to produce roentgen changes on the chest film occur in approximately two-thirds of the pa-

tients. Early changes consist in diffuse accentuation of markings resulting from interstitial infiltration. Patchy bronchopneumonia is common and often persists for long periods of time. The repeated episodes of pneumonia accentuate the findings and may produce areas of homogeneous density scattered in the lung fields; these areas appear and disappear. Atelectasis of a lobe or segment is common and tends to persist for several weeks. The right upper lobe is frequently involved. Bronchiectasis is not commonly found. The pulmonary disease is usually more focal and not as widespread as in cystic fibrosis of the pancreas, but there is some similiarity in the roentgen findings of these two diseases.

POLYCYTHEMIA

Polycythemia may be secondary to anoxia in a variety of chronic pulmonary diseases and in congenital heart disease. In these instances it is a compensatory phenomenon and there are no pulmonary roentgen findings indicating its presence. Polycythemia vera or primary polycythemia is a hematologic disorder characterized by hyperplasia of the red bone marrow, resulting in an increase in circulating red blood cells and in leukocytosis. In these patients, vascular engorgement results in prominence of vascular shadows in the lung fields. Basal fibrosis resulting in increased basal markings is sometimes noted along with changes suggesting basal congestion. Discrete rounded densities in the midzones of the lungs that are believed to represent venous thromboses have also been reported; they vary in size and appear and disappear in a few weeks. These findings are not diagnostic, but when pulmonary vascular distention is present without cardiac or pulmonary disease evident to account for it, the diagnosis can be suggested.

CHRONIC PNEUMONITIS OF THE CHOLESTEROL TYPE

This is a rare type of chronic interstitial inflammation of the lung in which the exudate consists of large mononuclear cells filled with cholesterol and cholesterol esters. These cells are noted to infiltrate the interstitial tissues and alveolar walls and to fill the alveoli. The etiology is not clear and the disease does not appear to be related to lipid pneumonia of the aspiration type. This disease is sometimes called "endogenous lipid pneumonia" and deposits are often found associated with chronic pulmonary diseases that produce bronchial obstruction. For example, it may occur in chronic bronchial obstruction by an endobronchial neoplasm or in bronchiolitis obliterans with diffuse alveolar damage (BIP). It may also occur in the absence of obstruction in slowly resolving pneumonias, the "inflammatory pseudotumor."

Roentgen Findings. In the obstructive types, the signs of BIP or of an obstructive tumor may be observed. In the nonobstructive type, the disease is characterized by a single confluent homogeneous density that may be lobar or segmental in distribution. There is usually a decrease in the volume of the lobe affected by the disease. The process extends to the pleura and the medial border is clearly defined. Hilar node enlargement may occur, and pleural fluid or pleural thickening is often present. The absence of endobronchial block and the fact that only a part of a segment is involved in the segmental type of disease are factors in favor of cholesterol pneumonitis over tumor. The disease is more compact and clearly defined than lipid pneumonia and its distribution, with the lesion extending to the pleura, is unlike that in lipid pneumonia.

LIPID PNEUMONIA

Lipid pneumonia is the term used to designate the granulomatous and fibrotic changes resulting from aspiration of various organic or inorganic fatty materials. In adults, the most common cause is the use of mineral oil taken for the treatment of constipation. Frequent or continued use of oily nose drops can also cause this condition and, rarely, it occurs after bronchography. In children it is caused by aspiration of cod liver oil and, in some instances, milk fats probably produce the condition in infants. Lipid pneumonia also occurs in achalasia (see Ch. 15, section on achalasia). Inhalation of burning animal fats has also been reported as a cause of lipid pneumonia.[49] As the result of aspiration of lipid materials, an inflammatory process is produced that results in consolidation of pulmonary parenchyma. Large phagocytes containing lipid material are noted in the alveoli and in the interstitial tissues. Chronic inflammatory cells may also be present within the alveoli. As the disease progresses, a considerable amount of fibrosis develops that causes contraction of the involved lung, compression of the alveoli, and often compression and obliteration of the bronchi. These pathologic changes

result in abnormalities that can be outlined on chest roentgenograms.

The roentgen findings are of two general types, diffuse and nodular. In the diffuse type there are scattered areas of increased density that are usually at the bases but may involve the right middle lobe and the superior segment of the lower lobe as well. Occasionally the condition involves the upper lobes. The individual lesions are usually poorly defined, with the density fading off into normal lung radiolucency. The lesions are not unlike those found in other types of aspiration pneumonitis but tend to be more linear with a fine granular and linear pattern (Fig. 30-28B). There is also reduction in volume of the affected lobe. Serial films show that the infiltrate in this condition persists with little change over a long period of time, in contrast to the changes noted in bacterial and viral pneumonias which resolve leaving little, if any, residual density. In some of these patients, as lipid pneumonitis progresses, the area involved may decrease in size because of fibrosis. At times there may be persistent, irregular, patchy densities scattered in one or both lungs which resemble chronic nonspecific inflammatiory disease. In the absence of a suggestive history, lung biopsy is the only method of diagnosis.

The nodular type of disease may also be unilateral or bilateral and probably results from a local conglomeration of the diffuse type. The area of density varies considerably in size but may reach 8 to 10 cm in diameter. It appears as a mass, usually oval or rounded in shape. The periphery of the nodule is usually irregular but occasionally becomes very smooth, so that the lesion may resemble a cyst or tumor (Fig. 30-28A). This lesion is also known as an oil or lipid granuloma. In some patients the right middle lobe is involved, being contracted and completely airless with its bronchus obstructed by inflammatory reaction.

Lipid pneumonitis produces less symptoms than does comparable involvement by an infectious process. This is of help in differentiating it from infectious disease. Serial examinations also show more stability of this lesion than in most of the lesions it may simulate. The nodular disease may resemble bronchogenic carcinoma or other intrapulmonary tumor and in some instances thoracotomy and biopsy are the only methods of differentiation. If a history of ingestion of mineral oil or the use of oily nose drops can be obtained and the roentgen findings described are also associated with the presence of lipid-containing phagocytes in the sputum, the diagnosis can be made with considerable degree of accuracy.

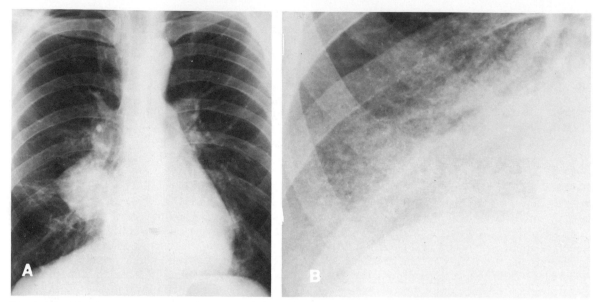

Fig. 30-28. Lipid pneumonia. **A.** This represents the nodular type of lipid pneumonia. There is a large mass in the right medial base. Another mass, of similar size, behind the heart was best noted on a tomogram. **B.** Diffuse type of lipid pneumonia in which there is a rather marked increase in density at both lung bases. This film is a close-up of the right base to show the strandlike increase in density along with the somewhat nodular disease.

PULMONARY ALVEOLAR PROTEINOSIS

This disease was described by Rosen, Castleman, and Liebow in 1958.[57] It is characterized by the presence in the alveoli of PAS-positive (periodic acid-Schiff stain) proteinaceous material rich in lipid. The exact nature of the material has not been determined; it appears to be produced by septal lining cells which slough into the lumen and become necrotic. Cellular infiltrate and reaction are absent or minimal. The cause is not known; inhalation of some of the newer chemical agents used in sprays and the like has been suggested, along with an infectious agent antigenically allied to *Pneumocystis carinii*. In some instances, the disease is associated with immunoglobulin deficiency and the incidence appears to be increased in patients with lymphoma or a hematologic malignant lesion.[8] The disease occurs in adults who are in the age range of 20 to 50 years, but may occasionally be observed in children. It appears to be a new disease, since no examples of it were observed before 1955. It often runs an insidious course characterized by malaise, cough, dyspnea, and weight loss. Physical findings are minimal and gross roentgen abnormality

may be observed in patients with few symptoms. The course of the disease may also be variable; in a few patients it is rapidly progressive, leading to pulmonary insufficiency with cyanosis, clubbing of the fingers, and death caused by the progressive loss of pulmonary function or intercurrent infection. Secondary fungal infection is the cause of most deaths in this disease. *Nocardia* is the most common of these organisms, but *Candida, Mucor,* and *Cryptococcus* may also be the cause. In other patients the symptoms may regress, with partial clearing of pulmonary changes; occasionally the disease may clear completely. Tracheobronchial lavage of the involved lobes with saline solution has been used with definite improvement in some patients. Steroids are ineffective and their use is contraindicated.

The roentgen findings at the height of the disease are those of perihilar densities simulating pulmonary edema. The infiltrate appears to radiate from the hila chiefly to the bases; it is indistinct or "soft" and may have a somewhat irregular pattern resembling nodularity. There are variations of this pattern; at times the disease appears to be unilateral and it need not be perihilar; it is predominantly basal and central, however. A number of cases have been reported in which

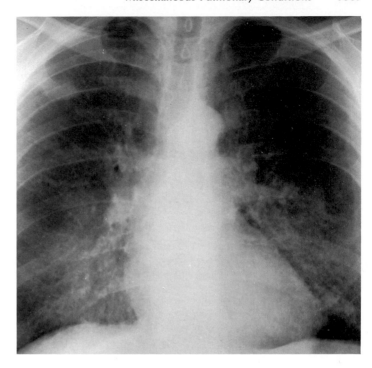

Fig. 30-29. Pulmonary alveolar proteinosis. There is bilateral basal involvement medially. It is somewhat confluent on the right and indistinct on the left. The medial basal distribution of the disease is characteristic but is not always present.

distribution of the alveolar density was quite atypical, so the disease must be kept in mind when alveolar densities persist in an afebrile, relatively asymptomatic patient. (Fig. 30-29). Roentgen findings change slowly and when clearing occurs there may be some residual fibrosis. The diagnosis can be suspected on the basis of clinical and roentgen findings. The presence of PAS-positive material in the sputum is diagnostic, but, if it is not obtained, lung biopsy may be necessary to establish the diagnosis.

NEAR-DROWNING

When a patient is recovered from the water in a state of apnea and subsequently revived, pulmonary changes occur which are evidently caused by hypoxia or a combination of aspiration of water and hypoxia. In "dry" near-drowning, there is enough laryngospasm to prevent inhalation of water and the pulmonary changes are secondary to hypoxia. Recovery rate is highest in this group. In "wet" near-drowning, water is aspirated in varying amounts and may contribute to the clinical and roentgen findings. In experimental animals, sea water, being hypertonic, increases pulmonary alveolar fluid and leads to

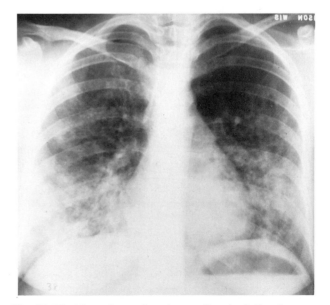

Fig. 30-30. Near drowning. Immediately following resuscitation there were no abnormalities noted on the chest film. This film, exposed 3 hours later, shows bilateral density with a central and basal distribution resembling alveolar edema. The upper lungs are relatively clear.

hypovolemia; while hypotonic fresh water is absorbed quickly leading to hemodilution and hemolysis of red cells. Clinically and radiographically, no clearly defined differences have been reported in humans who have aspirated water.[27] Pulmonary edema and hemorrhage have been observed histopathologically in drowning victims, and the roentgen findings in the near-drowning patient resemble those of pulmonary edema of varying degrees of severity. There may be a delay in appearance of roentgen changes for several hours. The findings consist of bilateral, poorly defined, alveolar densities which may be very extensive and confluent, sparing the periphery (Fig. 30-30). In other patients the involvement is less marked and tends to be reticulonodular and poorly defined. Clearing is usually rapid and is complete in 2 to 6 days. As the process resolves, the appearance changes from that of alveolar edema to a pattern resembling interstitial edema. Aspiration of foreign material may complicate the picture by causing atelectasis and pulmonary infection. When recovery is delayed, pulmonary infection is usually found as a complication. Pneumothorax and pneumomediastinum are complications of resuscitation efforts.

REFERENCES AND SELECTED READINGS

1. ABLOW RC, ORZALESI MM: Localized roentgenographic pattern of hyaline membrane disease. Am J Roentgenol 112: 23, 1971
2. American Thoracic Society: Definitions and classification of chronic bronchitis, asthma and pulmonary emphysema. Am Rev Resp Dis 85: 762, 1962
3. BAGHDASSARIAN OM, AVERY ME, NEUHAUSER EBD: A form of pulmonary insufficiency in premature infants. Pulmonary dysmaturity? Am J Roentgenol 89: 1020, 1963
4. BRETTNER A, HEITZMAN ER, WOODIN WG: Pulmonary complications of drug therapy. Radiology 96: 31, 1970
5. BRODY JS, LEVIN B: Interlobar septa thickening in lipid pneumonia. Am J Roentgenol 88: 1061, 1962
6. BRUTON OC: Agammaglobulinemia. Pediatrics 9: 722, 1952
7. BRUWER AJ, KIERLAND RR, SCHMIDT HW: Pulmonary tuberous sclerosis. Am J Roentgenol 85: 748, 1956
8. CARNOVALE R, ZORNOZA J, GOLDMAN AM et al: Pulmonary alveolar proteinosis: its association with hematologic malignancy and lymphoma. Radiology 122: 303, 1977
9. CARRINGTON CB, CUGELL DW, GAENSLER EA et al: Lymphangioleiomyomatosis. Physiologic-pathologic-radiologic correlations. Am Rev Resp Dis 116: 977, 1977
10. CHRISTENSEN EE, DIETZ GW: Subpulmonic pneumothorax in patients with chronic obstructive pulmonary disease. Radiology 121: 33, 1976
11. DULFANO MJ, DIRIENZO A: Laminagraphic observations of the lung vasculature in chronic pulmonary emphysema. Am J Roentgenol 88: 1043, 1962
12. ENGLEMAN P, LIEBOW AA, GMELICH J et al: Pulmonary hyalinizing granuloma. Am Rev Resp Dis 115: 997, 1977
13. ESPOSITO MJ: Focal pulmonary hemosiderosis in rheumatic heart disease. Am J Roentgenol 73: 351, 1955
14. FEINBERG R: Necrotising granulomatosis and angiitis of the lungs and its relationship to chronic pneumonitis of the cholesterol type. Am J Pathol 29: 913, 1953
15. FLEISCHNER FG, BERENBERG AL: Idiopathic pulmonary hemosiderosis. Radiology 62: 522, 1954
16. GAENSLER EA, GOFF AM, PROWSE CM: Desquamative interstitial pneumonia. Engl J Med 274: 113, 1966
17. GENEREUX GP: Lipids in the lungs: radiologic-pathologic correlation. J Can Assoc Radiol 21: 2, 1970
18. GLUECK MA, JANOWER ML: Nitrofurantoin lung disease. Am J Roentgenol 107: 818, 1969
19. GOMEZ GE, LICHTEMBERGER E, SANTAMARIA A et al: Familial pulmonary alveolar microlithiasis. Radiology 72: 550, 1953
20. GREENSPAN RH: Chronic disseminated alveolar diseases of the lung. Semin Roentgenol 2: 77, 1967
21. GREER AE: Mucoid impaction of the bronchi. Ann Intern Med 46: 506, 1957
22. HAMMAN L, RICH AR: Acute diffuse interstitial fibrosis of the lungs. Johns Hopkins Med J 74: 177, 1944
23. HAMPTON AO, BICKHAM CE JR, WINSHIP T: Lipoid pneumonia. Am J Roentgenol 73: 938, 1955
24. HEITZMAN ER, MARKARIAN B, DELISE CT: Lymphoproliferative disorders of the thorax. Semin Roentgenol 10: 73, 1975
25. HODGKIN JE, BALCHUM OJ, KASS I et al: Chronic obstructive airway diseases. Current concepts in diagnosis and comprehensive care, JAMA 232: 1243, 1975
26. HUNNINGHAKE GW, FAUCI AS: Pulmonary involvement in the collagen vascular diseases: state of the art. Am Rev Resp Dis 119: 471, 1979
27. HUNTER TB, WHITEHOUSE WM: Fresh-water, near-drowning. Radiological aspects. Radiology 112: 51, 1974
28. HUTCHINSON WB, FRIEDENBERG MJ, SALTZSTEIN S: Primary pulmonary pseudolymphoma. Radiology 82: 48, 1964
29. JENSEN KM, MISCOLL L, STEINBERG I: Angiocardiography in bullous emphysema: its role in selection of the case suitable for surgery. Am J Roentgenol 85: 229, 1961
30. JOFFE N: Roentgenologic findings in post-shock and postoperative pulmonary insufficiency. Radiology 94: 369, 1970

31. KINO T, KOHARA Y, TSUJI S: Pulmonary alveolar microlithiasis. Am Rev Resp Dis 105: 105, 1972

32. KIRKPATRICK R, RILEY CM: Roentgenographic findings in familial dysautonomia. Radiology 68: 654, 1957

33. KOGUTT MS, SWISCHUK LE, GOLDBLUM R: Swyer-James syndrome (unilateral hyperlucent lung in children). Am J Dis Child 125: 614, 1973

34. KRAUSS AM, KLAIN DB, AULD PAM: Chronic pulmonary insufficiency of prematurity (CPIP). Pediatrics 55: 55, 1975

35. LACHMAN R, CROCKER A, SCHULMAN J et al: Radiological findings in Niemann-Pick disease. Radiology 108: 659, 1973

36. LACKEY RW, LEAVER FY, FARINOCCI CJ: Eosinophilic granuloma of lung. Radiology 59: 504, 1952

37. LEVIN B: The continuous diaphragm sign. A newly-recognized sign of pneumomediastinum. Clin Radiol 24: 337, 1973

38. LIEBOW AA: Pulmonary angiitis and granulomatosis. Am Rev Resp Dis 108: 1, 1973

39. LIEBOW AA, CARRINGTON CB: The eosinophilic pneumonias. Medicine (Baltimore) 48: 251, 1969

40. LIEBOW AA, CARRINGTON CB: The interstitial pneumonias. In Simon M, Potchen EJ, LeMay M (eds): Frontiers of Pulmonary Radiology. New York, Grune & Stratton, 1969

41. LILLARD RL, ALLEN RP: The extrapleural air sign in pneumomediastinum. Radiology 85: 1093, 1965

42. MACEWAN DW, DUNBAR JS, SMITH RD et al: Pneumothorax in young infants—recognition and evaluation. J Can Assoc Radiol 22: 264, 1971

43. MACKLEM PT, THURLBECK WM, FRASER RG: Chronic obstructive disease of small airways. Ann Intern Med 74: 167, 1971

44. MACKLIN CC: Transport of air along sheaths of pulmonic blood vessels from alveoli to mediastinum: clinical implications. Arch Intern Med 64: 913, 1939

45. MARTELL W, ABELL MR, MIKKELSEN WM et al: Pulmonary and pleural lesions in rheumatoid disease. Radiology 90: 641, 1968

46. MILNE ENC, BASS H: The roentgenologic diagnosis of early chronic obstructive pulmonary disease. J Can Assoc Radiol 20: 3, 1969

47. MOSKOWITZ PS, GRISCOM NT: The medial pneumothorax. Radiology 120: 143, 1976

48. NORTHWAY WH JR, ROSAN RC, PORTER DY: Pulmonary disease following respirator therapy of hyaline-membrane disease. Bronchopulmonary dysplasia. N Engl J Med 276: 357, 1967

49. OLDENBURGER D, MAUERER WJ, BELTAOS E et al: Inhalation lipoid pneumonia from burning fats. JAMA 222: 1288, 1972

50. PETTY TL, ASHBAUGH DG: The adult respiratory distress syndrome. Chest 60: 233, 1971

51. PREGER L: Pulmonary alveolar proteinosis. Radiology 92: 1291, 1969

52. REID LM: Correlation of certain bronchographic abnormalities seen in chronic bronchitis with pathologic changes. Thorax 10: 199, 1955

53. Report of the conclusions of a Ciba guest symposium: Terminology, definitions and classification of chronic pulmonary emphysema and related conditions. Thorax 14: 286, 1959

54. ROBBINS LL, SNIFFEN RC: Correlation between the roentgenologic and pathologic findings in chronic pneumonitis of the cholesterol type. Radiology 53: 187, 1949

55. ROBERTS SR JR: Immunology and the lung: an overview. Semin Roentgenol 10: 7, 1975

56. ROGERS LF, PUIG AW, DOOLEY BN et al: Diagnostic considerations in mediastinal emphysema. A pathophysiologic-roentgenologic approach to Boerhaave's syndrome and spontaneous pneumomediastinum. Am J Roentgenol 115: 495, 1972

57. ROSEN SH, CASTLEMAN B, LIEBOW AA (with collaboration of ENZINGER FM, HUNT RTN: Pulmonary alveolar proteinosis. N Engl J Med 258: 1123, 1958

58. SANDLER BP, MATTHEWS JH, BORNSTEIN S: Pulmonary cavitation due to polyarteritis. JAMA 144: 754, 1950

59. SCADDING JG: Diffuse pulmonary alveolar fibrosis. Thorax 29: 271, 1974

60. SCADDING JG, HINSON KFW: Diffuse fibrosing alveolitis (diffuse interstitial fibrosis of the lungs). Thorax 22: 291, 1967

61. SIMON G: Radiology and emphysema. Clin Radiol 15: 293, 1964

62. SOSMAN MC, DODD GD, JONES WD et al: Pulmonary alveolar microlithiasis. Am J Roentgenol 77: 947, 1957

63. STERN L, FLETCHER BD, DUNBAR JS et al: Pneumothorax and pneumomediastinum associated with renal malformations in newborn infants. Am J Roentgenol 116: 785, 1972

64. STOVIN PGI, LUM LC, FLOWER CDR et al: The lungs in lymphangiomyomatosis and in tuberous sclerosis. Thorax 30: 497, 1975

65. SWISCHUK LE: Transient respiratory distress of the newborn (TRDN): a temporary disturbance of a normal phenomenon. Am J Roentgenol 108: 557, 1970

66. VALENSI QH: Pulmonary lymphangiomyoma, a probable forme frust of tuberous sclerosis. Am Rev Resp Dis 108: 1411, 1973

67. WEBB WR, GOODMAN PC: Fibrosing alveolitis in patients with neurofibromatosis. Radiology 122: 289, 1977

68. WESENBERG RL, GRAVEN SN, MCCABE EB: Radiological findings in wet-lung disease. Radiology 98: 69, 1971

69. WILLIAMS JL, MARKOWITZ RI, CAPITANIO MA et al: Immune deficiency syndromes. Semin Roentgenol 10: 83, 1975

70. WILSON SR, SANDERS DE, DELARUE NC: Intrathoracic manifestations of amyloid disease. Radiology 120: 283, 1976

71. WOLFSON SL, FRECH R, HEWITT C et al: Radiographic diagnosis of hyaline membrane disease. Radiology 93: 339, 1969

72. WOLSON AH: Pulmonary findings in Gaucher's disease. Am J Roentgenol 123: 712, 1975

73. ZYLAK CJ, BANERJEE R, GALBRAITH PA et al: Lung involvement in angioimmunoblastic lymphadenopathy (AIL). Radiology 121: 513, 1976

31

DISEASES OF THE PLEURA, MEDIASTINUM, AND DIAPHRAGM

fer
obs
of
lun
flui
uni
trik
The
ins
viei

Lor

Ple
late
incl
mo:
her
diar
fiss
viei
fiss
fror
ing
vex
con
ova
tun
out
tair
tene
in t
bor
ent
terl
crea
proj
tify
loct
gen
mer
cen
viev
are
enc
is a
mas
face
lem
pror
the
thor

THE PLEURA

PLEURAL EFFUSION

General Considerations

The pleural space is lined by a smooth serous membrane that is lubricated by a small amount of serous fluid. This fluid is absorbed as fast as it is secreted so that an excess does not accumulate. Except for this thin layer of lubricating fluid, the pleural surfaces are in contact; therefore the pleural space is a potential one in the normal person. The formation of excess fluid is caused by many conditions, a number of which are serious diseases either involving the lungs primarily or as a secondary manifestation of systemic disease. The causes include infections by many types of bacteria of which the tubercle bacillus (*mycobacterium tuberculosis*) is one of the most frequent. Infections caused by viruses, rickettsia, parasites, or fungi may also cause effusion. Massive pleural effusion has been reported in children with coccidioidomycosis; this suggests a severe form of the disease. Malignant tumors of the lung, mediastinum, and chest wall and metastatic tumors may also cause pleural effusion that is often bloody or blood-tinged. In lymphoma, pleural effusion, which may be chylous, is not common but indicates a poor prognosis when it occurs. Diseases that cause lymphatic obstruction and produce hypoproteinemia as well as cardiac failure and pulmonary infarction are also accompanied by pleural effusion in many instances. Accidental and surgical trauma produce effusions that are often bloody or blood-tinged. Massive pleural effusion, usually on the left side but sometimes bilateral, may complicate pancreatitis. The fluid contains high levels of amylase and of protein and tends to recur following thoracentesis. Small pleural effusions are common following upper-abdominal surgery.[20] They tend to disappear spontaneously and do not represent a significant complication even though a number are exudates. Spontaneous esophageal rupture (Boerhaave's syndrome) is rare but may be followed by pleural effusion. A significant number of effusions occur in patients with immunologic abnormalities such as systemic lupus erythematosus, Wegener's granulomatosis, and rheumatoid disease. In some patients the cause cannot be found.[33]

1011

Summary

Pleural fluid causes a homogeneous density that does not vary with the type of fluid. In the upright chest roentgenogram obtained in the frontal projection, several hundred cubic centimeters of fluid may be present without producing any roentgen change, but much smaller amounts, ranging from 25 (or less) to 100 cc, can be detected when lateral decubitus views are obtained. As the amount of fluid increases it gradually obscures the diaphragm and lower lung field and, when large, tends to depress the diaphragm also and displace the mediastinum to the opposite side. Free fluid is concave superiorly, owing to capillary action, unless air or gas is present, in which case a straight, horizontal gas–fluid level is present. Loculated fluid may simulate tumor but recumbent, lateral, and decubitus views plus progress roentgenograms to show the rapid changes that often occur are usually sufficient to make the proper diagnosis. Pulmonary disease may alter pulmonary elasticity and lead to atypical accumulations of free pleural fluid.

The use of CT scanning may be of importance in the future in localizing small loculated effusions and pleural plaques, but its place has not yet been established. Ultrasound may be valuable in localizing and identifying loculated pockets of fluid or pus.

INFLAMMATORY DISEASES

Acute Pleuritis

Acute infection of the pleura results in a serofibrinous inflammatory reaction that causes some pleural thickening and edema. This produces density that can sometimes be recognized radiographically, provided that the area of involvement is situated in a region in which the thickness of the pleura can be determined. This condition is associated with considerable pain, resulting in some fixation of the thorax and decrease in diaphragmatic motion as well as elevation of the diaphragm; in some instances these may be the only roentgen signs. A correlation of history, clinical findings, and roetgen findings indicates the diagnosis. A small amount of pleural effusion may result and, if it is large enough in amount, it can be recognized also. The diagnosis of acute fibrinous or serofibrinous pleurisy is not ordinarily difficult to make on clinical examination but chest roetgenography is of value in excluding the possibility of other disease even though the small area of pleural thickening or fluid associated with it may not be visible.

Chronic Pleural Thickening

Chronic, nonsuppurative pleural disease may be caused by a variety of bacteria; tuberculosis is among the most common causes. Pleuritis of tuberculous origin is often localized to the apex of the lung. The apical pleural thickening or cap may not indicate previous tuberculosis, however. In some instances, there is thickening of the visceral pleura plus fibrosis of subpleural lung which is nonspecific.[29] Its incidence increases with age, so that nonspecific infection of the subpleural lung associated with some ischemia may be the cause in some cases. Chronic pleuritis results in pleural thickening manifested by soft-tissue density between the inner aspect of the ribs and the adjacent lung. The inner surface is often irregular. The amount varies from a very thin linear band to a large amount of homogeneous density, representing grossly thickened fibrotic pleura. In other instances, pleural thickening may extend along the lateral chest wall to the base and occasionally may surround the entire lung, resulting in gradual fibrotic contraction leading to decrease in size of the involved hemithorax, along with the homogeneous density produced by the thickened fibrotic pleura. It is not uncommon to find large, thick, calcium plaques in the pleura in these patients. Occasionally a shell of pleural calcification may encase large portions of the lung and may also extend into the interlobar fissures. It is manifested by irregular linear plaques of density that are more opaque than the soft-tissue density produced by thick pleura alone (Fig. 31-5). Other organisms that produce chronic granulomatous inflammatory disease may cause similar changes.

When extensive bilateral pleural thickening is present, particularly if linear calcific plaques are visible in the diaphragmatic pleura, asbestosis or talcosis is nearly always the cause. Talcosis is uncommon, while asbestosis is a relatively common condition. Noncalcified local pleural thickening is somewhat more frequent than are the extensive changes just described. These pleural plaques may be quite thin and inconspicuous. Apical involvement is rare in asbestosis, and costophrenic angle obliteration is also rare. Calcification is usually a late finding in asbestosis and is most frequently observed in the parietal pleura of the diaphragm. Calcific plaques may also occur along the mediastinal pleura and along the lower lateral chest wall (parietal pleura) bilaterally. They are usually seen as linear or irregular plaques which are not very thick in contrast to the heavy, irregular plaques that may occur in chronic inflammatory disease. Parenchymal pulmonary involvement

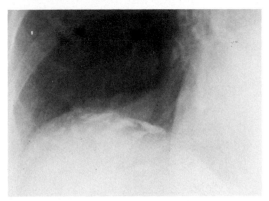

Fig. 31-5. Pleural calcification. Note the dense linear masses of calcium in the diaphragmatic pleura. No basal pulmonary disease is present.

need not be roentgenographically visible in asbestosis.

In many instances, small amounts of pleural thickening are noted along one or both thoracic walls in patients with no history of antecedent disease, so that the cause cannot be established. Often this may be caused by asbestosis in patients who may not have a history of working in an industry in which known exposure has occurred.

Unilateral pleural thickening with calcification is nearly always secondary to inflammatory disease or to trauma with calcification in a hematoma. It is not infrequent to observe obliteration of a costophrenic sulcus in patients who previously have had pneumonia with associated pleuritis. Pleural infection results in more or less obliteration of the pleural space as a result of fibrous adhesions between the visceral and parietal layers. These adhesions are recognized roentgenographically by their effect on adjacent structures as well as by visualization of the bandlike density representing them. Adhesions over the diaphragm often produce small, local tentlike elevations of the diaphragm. Similar distortion may be caused by contraction of local pulmonary lesions, however. Adhesions between the pleura and pericardium can sometimes be recognized roentgenographically by small spikelike irregularities of the outline of the pericardium. When sizable pneumothorax is present, the presence of adhesions can be readily detected since the lung pulls away from the parietal pleura if there are no adhesions.

Empyema

Thoracic empyema, or pyothorax, is an inflammatory disease of the pleura with suppuration that results in

an accumulation of pus in the pleural space. A number of organisms may cause this disease, including *Mycobacterium tuberculosis*. Staphylococcal pneumonia is frequently complicated by empyema. It is likely that any organism capable of causing pulmonary infection may also produce empyema and the latter is usually, but not always, a complication of the former. Roentgenograms outline the empyema as a mass that may vary in size from a large lesion that obscures most of the lung to a relatively small loculated mass along the chest wall or in an interlobar fissure. Postpneumonic empyemas usually occur along the posterior pleural space or within an interlobar fissure. Anterior empyema from this cause is very rare. There need not be evidence of associated pulmonary disease. If present, the type of alteration in the lungs resulting from the disease may aid in determining the cause of the empyema. In the acute stage there is usually some inflammation in the lung adjacent to the empyema cavity and this results in fuzzy irregularity of the margin. The fluid may not be loculated early in the disease. In the more chronic empyema the pulmonary inflammatory reaction may subside so that the mass is more clearly defined and sharply demarcated from the adjacent aerated lung (Fig. 31-6).

Fig. 31-6. Massive loculated pleural density. **Arrows** indicate some linear calcification in the pleura. This large loculation was found to represent a chronic empyema.

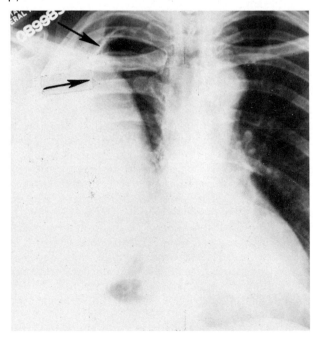

Air or gas within the empyema causes a fluid level and indicates communication with a bronchus or with the skin surface. The pleural infection is usually peripheral, with one part of the empyema adjacent to the costal pleura. It can be localized roentgenographically or fluoroscopically and aspirated if there is doubt as to the diagnosis.

TUMORS OF THE PLEURA

Benign Tumors

Pleural-based tumors include lipoma, fibroma, fibromyxoma, hemangioma, chondroma, and neurofibroma; these tumors actually originate in the chest wall and project into the thorax. The fibrous pleural mesothelioma is the only benign tumor that originates in the pleura. It is localized and may be pedunculated and move in relationship to other thoracic structures. It may be lobulated, usually arises from the visceral pleura (75%), and its pleural origin may not be obvious because there may be an acute angle between it and the chest wall. When pedunculated, the appearance may change markedly; this can be observed particularly well at fluoroscopy. The pleural-based or chest-wall tumors may become very large and produce large, smoothly rounded or lobulated densities, the internal aspects of which are clearly outlined by the air-filled lung. The outer aspects blend into the chest wall and often produce some widening of the intercostal space and rib erosion or deformity to indicate that they are primary chest-wall tumors. At times it is necessary to differentiate them from tumors arising in the lung. Diagnostic pneumothorax is then of value. It will clearly outline the relationship of the lung to the mass.

Primary Malignant Tumors

Diffuse pleural mesothelioma is usually malignant; its relationship to asbestos exposure has been well documented. These tumors are usually unilateral but may spread to the pericardium or opposite pleural surface late in the course of the disease. They arise in the pleura, often in the interlobar fissures, and extend rapidly to involve a large part of the pleural space. The roentgen findings consists of a somewhat scalloped-appearing mass involving the pleura. It is often extensive when first observed, and may surround the entire lung (Fig. 31-7). Earlier, an irregular nodular or scalloped pleural mass may be observed. Pleural effusion is common and may obscure the tumor.

Effusion may be the first sign of the tumor and

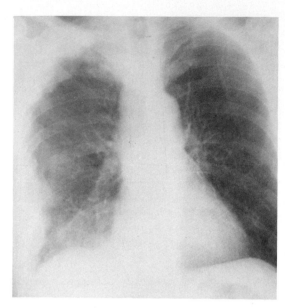

Fig. 31-7. Malignant mesothelioma of the pleura on the right. Note the irregular lobulated pleural density representing the tumor. There is very little pleural effusion.

may be massive in the presence of a relatively small mass arising in the pleura. When massive effusion is present, mediastinal shift toward the contralateral side may not occur because of fixation of the mediastinum by tumor. Fluid tends to reaccumulate rapidly following thoracentesis. When extensive, these tumors may block the lymphatics sufficiently to result in accumulation of interstitial fluids in the lungs, so that severe interstitial edema is observed. The major differential problem is metastatic malignancy with extensive pleural involvement. If the fluid is drained and pneumothorax induced, the tumor may be visible. Even then, the appearance simulates that of pleural thickening and loculated fluid associated with the pleural disease so that diagnosis usually depends upon biopsy.

Local mesothelioma occasionally may be malignant, although it is usually considered benign. Radiographically, the only sign suggesting malignancy is rib erosion caused by invasion of the chest wall.

Metastatic Tumors

Metastatic pleural tumors occur much more frequently than the malignant primary neoplasms. The actual pleural tumor in many instances is very small and forms tiny nodules in the visceral or parietal pleura that are not visible roentgenographically.

Bloody pleural effusion is common so that the major roentgen finding is often that of pleural effusion. There may be direct extension into the pleura from a chest-wall metastasis in which rib is also involved. Then a soft-tissue, chest-wall mass and irregular rib destruction indicate that there is a malignant neoplasm present to account for the pleural effusion and mass projecting into the pleural space. The history of primary tumor elsewhere is of great importance in making the roentgen diagnosis. In our experience, breast carcinoma is the most common cause of pleural metastases, but the primary tumor may arise in the lung, pancreas, ovary, colon, or other sites of adenocarcinoma. Lymphoma may also invade the pleura. Plasma cell myeloma involving ribs often results in a chest-wall mass, displacing and sometimes invading the pleura.

Fibrin Bodies

Fibrin bodies or fibrin balls are made up of masses of fibrin that resemble tumor within the pleural space. They form in patients with fibrinous pleuritis with effusion and are usually obscured by the fluid during formation, but when the fluid is removed by means of thoracentesis or is absorbed they become apparent. They were commonly observed in patients with pulmonary tuberculosis who were treated with pneumothorax. They often complicated the effusion that developed during artificial pneumothorax when that was used as a method of collapse therapy. The roentgen findings are those of rounded or oval, single or multiple masses usually appearing at the base, often partially obscured by pleural effusion or becoming visible after the effusion has been drained or absorbed. Alteration of the patient's position may result in displacement of these bodies; when this is observed, the diagnosis is almost certain. However, occasionally a pedunculated tumor such as a fibrous pleural mesothelioma may change position in a similar manner. It may disappear spontaneously, but may persist for years.

THE MEDIASTINUM

INFLAMMATORY DISEASES

Acute Mediastinitis

Acute inflammations of the mediastinum most commonly arise following injury of the esophagus caused by ingestion of sharp foreign bodies that penetrate the esophagus, or instrumentation of the esophagus. When esophageal rupture is suspected, it can be confirmed quickly by the demonstration of extravasation of ingested contrast material into the mediastinum or pleural space. Occasionally inflammation extends into the mediastinum from infections involving the sternum, spine, anterior chest wall, and mediastinal lymph nodes, and rarely from infections originating in the anterior neck and in the subdiaphragmatic area. These infections may result in the formation of abscesses that may rupture into the esophagus, tracheobronchial tree, or pleural space. This may cause a rapid change in the mediastinal contour as well as a sudden clinical change. When antibiotics are given early following an esophageal injury, actual abscess formation is uncommon so that the incidence of mediastinal abscess is now relatively low. The roentgen findings are those of a diffuse increase in density and widening of the mediastinum to both sides of the midline in the region of involvement. If the process extends downward from the neck from a retropharyngeal abscess, roentgenograms of the neck obtained in lateral projection often show the soft-tissue mass displacing the pharynx and trachea anteriorly. When the infection has resulted from esophageal injury it is not uncommon to observe a small amount of mediastinal emphysema manifested by streaks of radiolucency. If an abscess becomes chronic, it may be large and clearly defined so that its appearance may simulate that of mediastinal tumor. It is not unusual to have enough pleural reaction to produce effusion (Fig. 31-8). The diagnosis is made on the basis of correlation of roentgen findings with the clinical history. A rapid accumulation of blood, chyle, or edema fluid may also cause acute mediastinal widening. The history and clinical findings are usually helpful in differentiating these.

Chronic Mediastinitis

Granulomatous Mediastinitis. Tuberculosis and actinomycosis may produce a chronic granulomatous infection in the mediastinum. Other organisms are less commonly involved. The roentgen findings are not characteristic and may be very minor unless chronic mediastinal abscess is formed. In the latter event, the abscess produces a mass shadow that is usually found in the posterior mediastinum. This lesion may be impossible to differentiate from mediastinal tumor. Occasionally diffuse mediastinal inflammation caused by histoplasmosis results in enough fibrosis to produce obstruction of the superior or inferior vena cava and in these patients roentgen findings may be minimal. There may be an associated pulmonary involvement. Enlargement of mediastinal

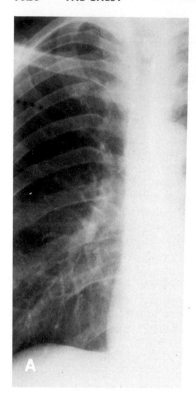

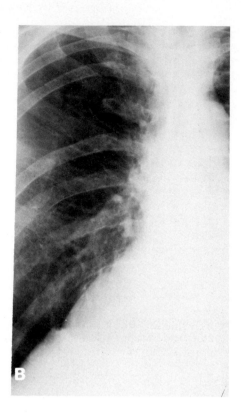

Fig. 31-8. Acute mediastinitis. **A.** No mediastinal abnormalities are noted in this preliminary examination. **B.** Examination performed 2 weeks following resection of an esophageal neoplasm. The patient had developed an acute febrile illness. Now the mediastinal border on the right is indistinct superiorly. There is some widening and the infection resulted in mediastinal pleuritis with loculated pleural fluid producing the mass density at the right medial base.

nodes is common early in the disease. These nodes may decrease in size and disappear in the chronic phase, however. In other patients they may calcify and may gradually increase in size. If they are adjacent to the superior vena cava, they may produce caval obstruction many years after the initial infection.

Fibrous (Sclerosing) Mediastinitis. Occasionally, signs of superior caval obstruction will appear with no antecedent history of pulmonary, esophageal, tracheal, or pharyngeal disease. These signs evidently may be caused by a number of conditions, including subclinical histoplasmosis, other infections, and an idiopathic fibrosis similar to that noted in retroperitoneal fibrosis. Nocardia may occasionally cause mediastinitis with caval obstruction and rarely sarcoidosis is responsible. The most common cause is bronchogenic carcinoma while lymphoma is the next most common cause. Masses are usually observed in the presence of these tumors, however. Venography can be used to demonstrate venous obstruction. The clinical findings must be correlated with radiographic findings to determine diagnosis. Surgical exploration may be necessary to confirm it.

Inflammatory Diseases of the Mediastinal Lymph Nodes

In nearly all infectious diseases of the lungs and bronchi there is histopathologic involvement of the mediastinal nodes, but most of these diseases do not usually cause enough enlargement to be of roentgen importance. There are chronic pulmonary inflammatory diseases, however, in which there is sufficient enlargement of hilar and mediastinal nodes to produce recognizable density on chest roentgenograms.

Acute Nonspecific Lymphadenopathy. Some enlargement of the hilum shadow is often present in pneumonia but is so minimal that it usually escapes detection or is obscured by the pulmonary infection. Lung abscess is frequently accompanied by hilar and/or mediastinal adenopathy. Rarely, infectious mononucleosis is associated with mediastinal adenopathy. Occasionally an infected node may undergo suppuration, leading to acute mediastinitis or mediastinal abscess.

Chronic Inflammations. Occasionally, lymph nodes are enlarged in patients with chronic suppurative disease of the bronchi and in some patients with mucoviscidosis, leading to recognizable hilar enlargement which is often poorly defined and is associated with the accentuation of basal markings and patchy pneumonitis often found in bronchiectasis. A number of fungi are capable of producing pulmonary disease and they also involve the hilar nodes, resulting in enlargement. Adenopathy is most commonly found in the acute phase of coccidioidomycosis and histoplasmosis and may be present in other fungal diseases, such as actinomycosis and blastomycosis. In these diseases the pulmonary infection produces changes that have been described in the previous sections relating to these infections. This involvement of hilar and mediastinal nodes often leads to calcification in the nodes, which requires 1 or 2 years to develop. It is most commonly observed in histoplasmosis.

Primary tuberculosis is associated with mediastinal lymphadenopathy. The enlargement of hilar or paratracheal nodes may or may not be associated with a visible parenchymal lesion. Characteristically, in primary tuberculosis a single group of nodes is involved. If more than one group is affected, one group is usually considerably larger than the other. The roentgen findings are those of a somewhat lobulated hilar enlargement with the outline of the hilum being moderately fuzzy and indistinct. A visible parenchymal lesion may be present. When the acute phase is over, the borders of the hilum become more distinct and nodes gradually decrease in size. Calcification is often noted after a year or more; complete resolution may require several years.

All these chronic inflammatory diseases that involve the lungs, as well as the mediastinal nodes, must be differentiated from one another by appropriate skin tests and bacteriologic studies as indicated in Chapters 25 and 26. Node enlargement is noted in a variety of diseases of the lungs, including some of the pneumoconioses. In these patients the pulmonary lesions are usually predominant.

Massive mediastinal lymph-node enlargement has been reported occasionally in patients without other disease. The large nodes simulate mediastinal tumors or malignant lymphomas. Biopsy reveals a nonspecific chronic lymphadenitis.

Sarcoidosis. Sarcoidosis is usually associated with mediastinal lymphadenopathy sufficient to produce recognizable enlargement of hilar and mediastinal lymph nodes at some time during the course of the disease. This is discussed in Chapter 26 under the heading "Sarcoidosis."

Other Causes of Mediastinal Node Enlargement. *Giant mediastinal lymph node hyperplasia (Castleman's disease)* is an asymptomatic, idiopathic, massive adenopathy usually appearing as a solitary mass most commonly in the middle or posterior mediastinum. The mass becomes extremely large but does not calcify. *Benign lymphoid hyperplasia* may be associated with abnormalities of the immune system such as hypergammaglobulinemia. *Angioimmunoblastic lymphadenopathy* involving the mediastinal nodes represents a lymphoproliferative disorder. It responds to corticosteroid therapy.

The three disorders just described must be differentiated from disseminated malignant disease by laboratory methods and by biopsy in some instances.

TUMORS AND ALLIED LESIONS

There are a number of structures within and extending through the mediastinum. Tumors and cysts may arise from any of them. There is a definite correlation between location within the mediastinum and the histologic type. Table 31-1 lists the lesions in order of incidence and site of relative frequency.

In addition to routine roentgenograms in frontal and lateral projections it is often necessary to obtain oblique projections and to examine the patients fluoroscopically in order to obtain as much information as possible. Esophagrams, tomograms, angiograms, or retrograde aortograms may be needed in some cases. The place of CT scanning has not been completely determined, but it appears that it will become of increasing importance in the evaluation of the mediastinum. Its usefulness in locating obscure lesions and in determining relative tissue density and extent of mediastinal tumors as well as in the investigation of abnormal plain-film findings has already been demonstrated. When the mass is localized in relation to other mediastinal structures and its dynamic characteristics are determined by fluoroscopy (pulsation or lack of it, movement or lack of it on respiration and swallowing), it is often possible to be reasonably certain of the diagnosis. In other instances, thoracotomy is necessary to make the histologic diagnosis as well as to remove the mass.

Tumors of the Mediastinal Lymph Nodes

Lymphoma. The lymphomas commonly involve the hilar and mediastinal lymph nodes and often cause massive enlargement of them. The involvement is characteristically bilateral and the nodes affected produce mass shadows corresponding to their location.

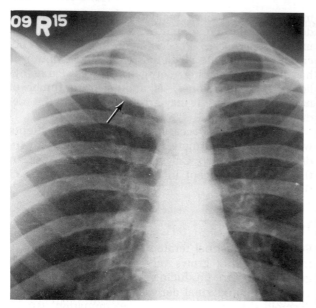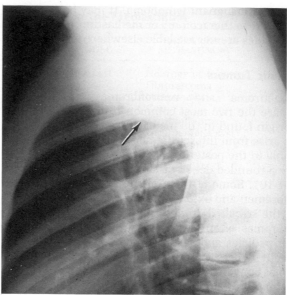

Fig. 31-10. Neurofibroma. Note the smooth outline of the tumor and its posterior location **(arrows),** evident on the lateral view **(arrows).** Since it extends to the apex of the right thoracic cavity, it must lie posteriorly.

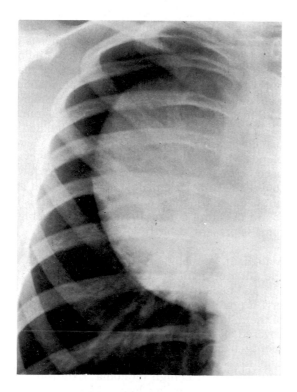

Fig. 31-11. Ganglioneuroma. Large right posterior mediastinal mass with a vertical diameter greater than transverse diameter, a characteristic of this tumor.

Prognosis is poor in malignant teratoma of the mediastinum.

Seminoma is another malignant tumor that may arise in the mediastinum (from aberrant germ cells). This rare tumor is found in young adult men. The roentgen study reveals a lobulated anterior mediastinal mass often extending to both sides of the midline. This tumor may or may not cause symptoms. The prognosis is generally good.

Mediastinal Cysts

All the mediastinal cysts appear as rounded or oval mass lesions that are smooth and clearly defined. They tend to change slightly in shape with alteration in position and with respiration. Fluoroscopy is helpful in determining motion, alteration on position change, and the absence of expansile pulsations in these cysts.

Bronchogenic Cyst. Cysts of bronchogenic origin are lined with ciliated columnar epithelium and are

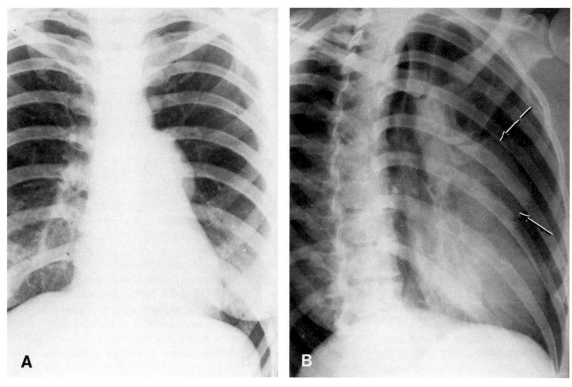

Fig. 31-12. Mediastinal dermoid cyst. **A.** Frontal view showing a mass projecting to the left just below the transverse aortic arch. The mass obscures the left pulmonary artery and the left hilum. **B.** In the right anterior oblique view the mass is seen to lie anteriorly **(arrows).** There is no calcification within it or in its walls.

usually asymptomatic. They commonly occur in the superior and middle mediastinum near the trachea and in the region of the carina but may be found anywhere in the mediastinum (Fig. 31-13). They range considerably in size. All are clearly defined and are not lobulated. They may compress or displace the bronchi and/or trachea in children, resulting in symptoms. In adults they do not usually compress or displace these structures and are ordinarily asymptomatic. Rarely, "milk of calcium" is observed within the cyst.

Gastroenteric Cyst (Duplication). Gastroenteric cysts probably represent small local duplications of the intestinal tract. They contain secretory cells and may grow to a large size early in life. They produce symptoms because of pressure on mediastinal structures and are often discovered during infancy, usually before the child is 2 years old. They appear as large rounded or oval densities in the posterior mediastinum near the esophagus and usually extend to

one side of the midline (Fig. 31-14). They are related to neurenteric cysts but have no connection to the neural canal. Many are associated with vertebral anomalies and other abnormalities such as meningocele, intestinal malrotation, and esophageal atresia; congenital heart disease may also be present. They are also related to bronchopulmonary foregut malformations but usually have no connection with the gastrointestinal tract. Partial pericardial defect may accompany the type that is more closely related to bronchopulmonary foregut malformation.

Neurenteric Cyst. This is a rare mediastinal cyst[24] which appears to be formed from a remnant of the neurenteric canal that forms an evanescent communication from the gut through the dorsal midline structures to the dorsal surface of the embryo, the neural canal. The lesion consists of a mediastinal cystic mass that may be continuous with a duplication or giant diverticulum of the intestinal tract and

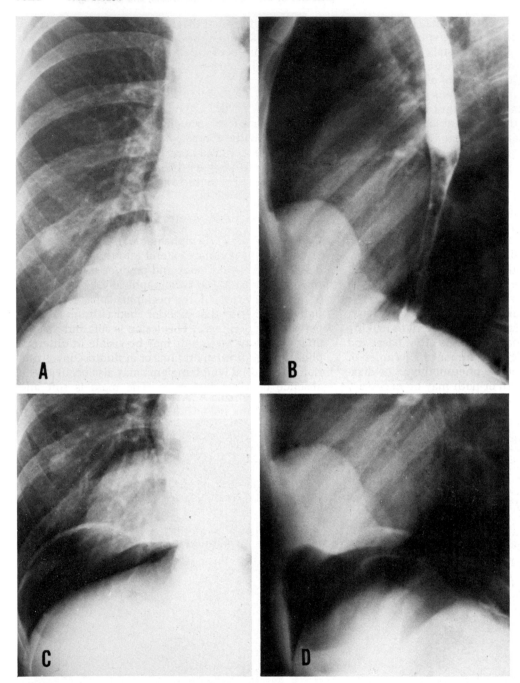

Fig. 31-16. Pericardial cyst. Mass of water density is noted at the cardiohepatic angle in **A.** In **B** its anterior location is confirmed. Studies made following diagnostic pneumoperitoneum **(C and D)** show the mass to be above the diaphragm. Foramen of Morgagni hernia usually occurs in the same position.

spongy, so that it does not ordinarily displace or compress the trachea.

Intrathoracic Thyroid. This is a relatively common tumor, noted in the anterior and superior mediastinum, which is usually connected by an isthmus of tissue to the thyroid gland in the neck. This isthmus is often wide enough to be recognized roentgenographically so that the connection between the intrathoracic mass and the thyroid is demonstrated. Even if the tumor is bilateral, it is usually eccentric enough to produce tracheal deviation and often compression; this becomes a significant finding for the diagnosis of intrathoracic goiter. The lateral view often shows posterior displacement of the trachea as well. It is not uncommon to observe calcification within the mass. The intrathoracic thyroid often moves on swallowing but may be fixed. Occasionally it may produce a mass in the posterior mediastinum behind the trachea, almost always on the right side. The mass of thyroid tissue may also extend far downward into the inferior aspect of the anterior mediastinum. We have observed one patient in whom the goiter encircled the esophagus in a manner that simulated leiomyoma. The mass may reach great size without producing symptoms. Even though the mediastinal thyroid is posterior in position, there is usually some displacement of the trachea as well as the esophagus. This is helpful in making the diagnosis (Fig. 31-17). Brachiocephalic vessels may be displaced or compressed. When the reaction is positive, scans using radioactive iodine (^{131}I) are diagnostic; but there may be no function, so a negative scan does not exclude the possibility of intrathoracic thyroid.

Parathyroid Adenoma. This tumor is usually found in the anterior aspect of the superior mediastinum or

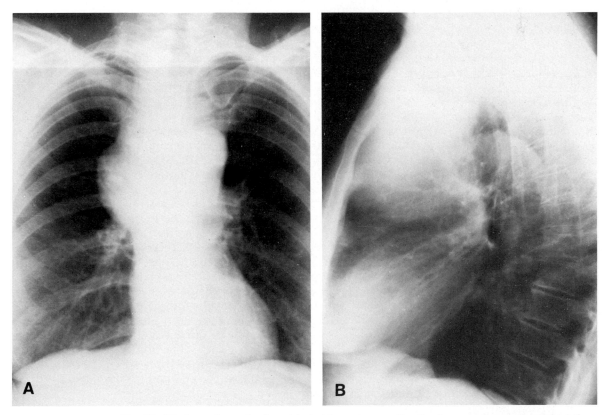

Fig. 31-17. Intrathoracic thyroid. **A.** Note the mediastinal mass above the right hilum with widening of the superior mediastinum which extends up into the neck. The trachea is displaced somewhat to the left. **B.** The lateral view shows the anterior position of the mass and posterior displacement of the upper trachea. The patient was asymptomatic.

in the anterior mediastinum. It is usually eccentric and presents to either side. It tends to be relatively small. There is nothing diagnostic about the appearance of the mass as visualized on the roentgenogram. When renal lithiasis or bone lesions of hyperparathyroidism are present in association with an anterior mediastinal mass, the diagnosis of parathyroid adenoma is reasonably certain. Often no mediastinal mass will be visible in patients having a parathyroid adenoma; in this instance, angiography with selective catheterization of the inferior thyroid artery may be helpful in determining the diagnosis. Selective catheterization of neck veins for parathormone may lateralize but not localize the adenoma. It is likely that in the future, CT scanning will play a major role in the examination of these patients with hypercalcemia.

Thymic Tumors. The normal thymus lies in a retrosternal position largely behind the manubrium, but in children, in whom it is often large, it may extend well down into the retrosternal space anterior to the heart. The retrosternal line formed by the anterior mediastinal pleural reflections is seen above the heart on the lateral view of the thorax. There is usually some soft tissue between the sternum and this line which ranges from 2 or 3 mm to a maximum of 8 mm in length. The thymic shadow in infants and children tends to obliterate the line. If there is more than 8 mm between the line and the sternum, the posssibility of abnormalities such as tumor, internal mammary artery, vein or node enlargement, and hematoma must be considered in adults and older children. However, a large normal thymus may persist into the mid teens and cannot be differentiated from other anterior mediastinal masses. Rarely the thymus may be in an aberrant position, such as behind the trachea or adjacent to the base of the heart, and occasionally it may be in the posterior mediastinum. The only finding that might suggest the diagnosis is a change in size and shape of the mass on inspiration and expiration.

Benign Lesions. The *benign thymoma* is located in the anterior mediastinum at the level of the junction of the heart and great vessels. It grows slowly and may become very large. At times the tumor is in the midline and may be difficult or impossible to visualize in the frontal projection, but is readily visible in oblique or lateral views. Mottled calcification is occasionally noted within it. Myasthenia gravis is found in 50% of patients with thymoma. Of the patients with myasthenia gravis, about 15% have thymic tumors. The patient with myasthenia gravis should be examined for thymic tumor because of this relationship. It is likely that CT scanning will be helpful in making the diagnosis when a thymic mass is not observed on chest films.

Thymoma may be cystic and contain calcium which outlines the wall and suggests the cystic nature of the tumor. Its location is similar to that of the solid type of thymoma (Fig. 31-18). There is no way to be certain that a thymic mass is benign or malignant on roentgen examination, however.

Thymolipoma is an uncommon benign fatty tumor that originates in the atrophic thymus. It usually becomes very large and is asymptomatic. The presence of this tumor may be suggested when a large, fatty, anterior mediastinal mass is observed in an asymptomatic adult.

Malignant Lesions. Early in its development, the thymic malignant tumor resembles benign thymoma in appearance and location. It grows rapidly, however, and is invasive, so that the margins become blurred. It often becomes very large, extends to both sides of the midline, and then resembles malignant lymphoma. It spreads by direct invasion, and sometimes there may be implantation of tumor on the adjacent pleura or pericardium. The tumor may be carcinomatous or sarcomatous.

Intrathoracic Meningocele. Intrathoracic meningocele is a herniation of the meninges laterally to cause a posterior mediastinal mass. It is rare and is usually mistaken for the more common posterior mediastinal neurofibroma. Diagnosis is made readily on myelography if the lesion is suspected, since the opaque medium will enter the meningocele when the patient is positioned properly. Kyphoscoliosis frequently accompanies this abnormality, and its presence may aid in suggesting the diagnosis. An intrathoracic meningocele is often associated with neurofibromatosis (von Recklinghausen's disease). There may be erosion about the intervertebral foramen through which the meninges protrude and skeletal defects are commonly associated with it. These meningoceles may be single or multiple and unilateral or bilateral. The diagnosis can be made when the presence of this lesion is supected and confirmed by myelography.

Mediastinal Lipomatosis Caused by Steroids. The use of long-term, large-dose steroid therapy in renal transplantation and in treatment of various chronic diseases may result in deposition of fat in the mediastinum. The patients usually manifest Cushing's syndrome, often with fat deposition in supraclavicular

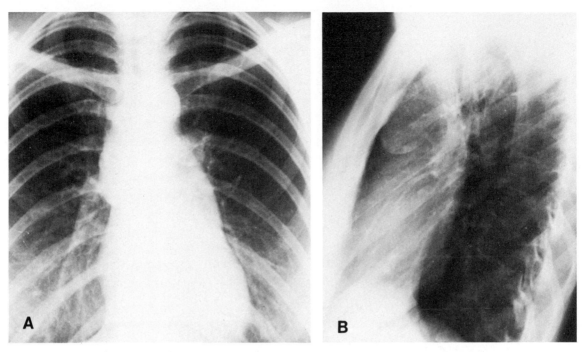

Fig. 31-18. Thymic cyst. In the frontal projection **(A)** a mass is seen in the right upper mediastinum. This extends downward below the level of the inferior branch of the right pulmonary artery. Its upper extent is not clearly defined. In the lateral view **(B)** the mass is noted to lie anteriorly and, again, its upper extent is not clearly defined. There is a little calcification inferiorly causing a slightly mottled appearance of the smooth lower margin.

and epicardial areas as well as in the mediastinum. The condition is important only in that it must be differentiated from other conditions that may cause mediastinal widening. Roentgen findings consist of mediastinal widening which is relatively radiolucent and poorly defined when compared to other superior mediastinal masses (Fig. 31-19). The trachea is not compressed or displaced, and excess epicardial fat may also be present.

Miscellaneous Masses. Benign tumors such as lipoma, fibroma, chrondroma, and hemangioma occur rarely within the mediastinum. There is nothing characteristic about the roentgen appearance of a lipoma or fibroma. The chondroma may contain a considerable amount of irregular calcification that helps to identify it. Hemangioma often is a poorly defined, widespread mass and may contain small rounded calcifications that represent phleboliths. When the latter are present, the diagnosis can be made with a reasonable degree of certainty. Most hemangiomas

occur in the anterior mediastinum. They tend to be clearly defined in the anteroposterior projection but are often difficult to outline in the lateral projection. Varices or venous aneurysms involving mediastinal veins may cause asymptomatic mediastinal widening. Desmoid tumors arising in the chest wall may project into the mediastinum but more commonly are pleural based and tend to resemble fibrous pleural mesotheliomas. Rarely, pheochromocytoma may occur in the thorax; its posterior location is similar to that of neurogenic tumor. Otherwise unexplained hypertension plus the mass should lead to the suspicion of this tumor. Fibrosarcoma and other sarcomas arising in the mediastinal soft tissues are extremely rare and there is nothing characteristic about their radiographic appearance.

Extramedullary hematopoiesis may occur in a number of diseases in which there is chronic anemia. It has also been reported in Paget's disease of bone. Occasionally, the heterotopic bone marrow may develop in the paravertebral region of the thorax, pre-

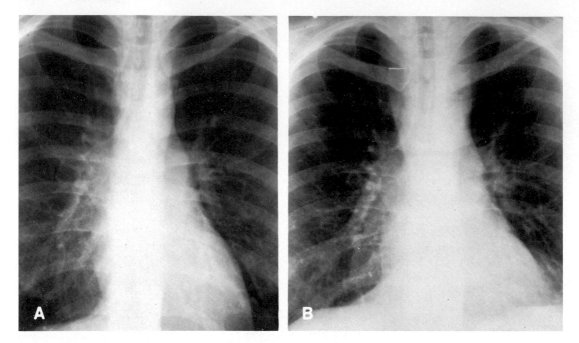

Fig. 31-19. Mediastinal lipomatosis. The patient, an 18-year-old girl, had a renal transplant and was on long-term steroid therapy. **A.** Initial chest film. **B.** Film obtained 1 year later shows mediastinal widening superiorly which is very poorly defined. There is more epicardial fat at the apex and the cardiohepatic angle than was present earlier.

senting as a posterior mediastinal mass that may be very large. It may be unilateral or bilateral and may extend for some distance along the spine in the posterior mediastinum. Lobulation is usually present. It is believed to represent extruded bone marrow that results from progressive lysis of the cortex of ribs or vertebrae by the hyperactive marrow cells. Continuity with the marrow space may be lost, and longitudinal growth occurs in the extrapleural paraspinal space producing the elongated, lobulated paraspinal masses. The diagnosis can be suspected if the patient has a history of anemia of long duration.

Occasionally, esophageal diverticula may attain large size and appear as mediastinal masses. There is usually enough air within them so that a gas–fluid level is demonstrated, indicating the type of lesion. An esophagram will readily outline and define this type of lesion. In achalasia (cardiospasm) of the esophagus this organ becomes grossly dilated and may simulate mediastinal tumor.

Paraspinal abscess secondary to tuberculosis or other chronic infection of the thoracic spine often produces a shadow that may simulate tumor. The ab-

scesses are usually somewhat spindle-shaped and the density produced merges with the normal paraspinal shadow above and below the mass. Lateral and oblique projections that outline the vertebral bodies and intervertebral discs usually indicate the cause for the lesion, since varying amounts of destruction of one or more vertebral bodies, along with narrowing of the intervening intervertebral disc space, are common findings. There is also calcification within the abscess in many instances. Tumors of the thoracic spine may produce masses but their location is usually clearly defined in lateral views so that there is no difficulty in differentiation between these lesions and mediastinal tumor.

Mediastinal hematoma may also produce a mediastinal mass. Usually there is a history of trauma or of recent surgical procedure so that presumptive diagnosis can be made. Rapid changes in the size of the mass are characteristic when they occur. This is discussed further in Chapter 32.

Cardiac disease and lesions of the great vessels within the mediastinum are discussed in the chapter on cardiovascular diseases. Mediastinal emphysema

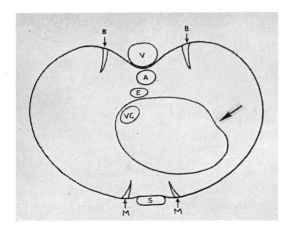

Fig. 31-20. Diagram to show the normal openings and areas of potential weakness in the diaphragm. The sketch is drawn viewing the diaphragm from above downward. The vertebral body **(V)** and the sternum **(S)** are labeled for orientation purposes. The letters represent the following: **B**, foramen of Bochdalek; **A**, aorta; **E**, esophageal hiatus; **VC**, the opening for the inferior vena cava; **M**, the foramen of Morgagni (potential opening). The attachment of the pericardium to the diaphragm is also sketched **(arrow).**

and mediastinal pleural effusion are discussed in the sections on emphysema and on pleural effusion respectively.

THE DIAPHRAGM

The diaphragm is a muscle of respiration that separates the thorax from the abdominal cavity. The muscle fibers of the diaphragm originate from the xiphoid process and the eighth to twelfth ribs and insert into the central tendon. Posteriorly, the diaphragmatic crura arise from the vertebral bodies and extend down as far as the third lumbar body. The central tendon lies somewhat anterior to the mid thorax and roughly parallels the anterior chest wall. The muscle fibers anteriorly are relatively short and posterolaterally are two to three times longer, so that the major muscle mass is in the posterior aspect of the diaphragm. The position of the diaphragm is described in Chapter 22. There are a number of openings in it through which structures such as the esophagus and aorta pass to enter the abdomen (Fig. 31-20). The superior surface of the diaphragm is readily visualized in the roentgenogram of the normal chest because it is clearly outlined by the radiolucent lung above it. Its lower margin is often visible on the left, at least in part, because there is usually some gas in the fundus of the stomach and gas or fecal material in the splenic flexure of the colon that define its undersurface. On the right side, the liver is of comparable density so that the undersurface of the diaphragm cannot be visualized unless pneumoperitoneum is present. The right diaphragm is usually one interspace higher than the left. In full inspiration the dome of the right leaf of the diaphragm is at the ap-

proximate level of the tenth rib posteriorly, the left is at the level of the eleventh rib posteriorly. Using the anterior ribs as landmarks, the dome of the right diaphragm lies between the level of the fifth rib and the level of the sixth interspace measured on the standard 6-foot roentgenogram obtained with the patient in moderately deep inspiration. It tends to be higher in hypersthenic and in obese patients and may be lower in asthenic subjects. The height of the diaphragm appears to be related to the position of the apex of the heart rather than to the position of the liver; *e.g.*, the low hemidiaphragm is on the side of the heart.

MOTION OF THE DIAPHRAGM

Asynchronous motion is common, and there is often more excursion on the left than on the right. Average range of motion is 3 to 6 cm, but it can be increased by training. In patients with emphysema, the motion range is often less than 3 cm. On rapid inspiration that is induced by a rapid inspiratory "sniff," there is often a minimal temporary paradoxical motion, usually on the right. Then the hemidiaphragm moves downward normally. The momentary paradoxical motion is normal. With the patient in a lateral decubitus position, the dependent hemidiaphragm is high, and excursion is greatly enhanced. This position may be helpful in assessing diaphragmatic weakness and significant paradoxical motion.

FUNCTIONAL DISTURBANCES OF THE DIAPHRAGM

The most common disturbance of the diaphragm is hiccough (singultus). This consists of sudden diaphragmatic contraction associated with closure of the glottis. It is either local in origin, caused by irritation of the diaphragm, or central, in which case it may be produced by encephalitis, uremia, or brain tumor. Occasionally it is hysterical in origin. Attacks are usually very short, but occasionally paroxysms may last for months or years. Radiography is of indirect value only if it may serve to identify the irritating lesion producing the contraction. Fluoroscopy can be used to determine the severity of the contraction and to determine whether one or both hemidiaphragms are involved.

Tonic contraction or splinting of the diaphragm often results when basal pleuritis, subphrenic abscess, or trauma has produced diaphragmatic injury. In any of these instances there is greater or less elevation of the diaphragm, which may be bilateral but is usually unilateral, and may be confined to one portion of a hemidiaphragm. Chest roentgenography outlines the height of the diaphragm and fluoroscopy will reveal the amount and location of the limitation of motion.

PARALYSIS AND PARESIS OF THE DIAPHRAGM

When the diaphragm is paralyzed, it is elevated by intra-abdominal pressure that is greater than the thoracic pressure. The amount of elevation varies considerably and it may be unilateral or bilateral. When paralysis is complete on one side, paradoxical motion is usually visible at fluoroscopy. This means that during inspiration the paralyzed hemidiaphragm rises while the normal hemidiaphragm descends; during expiration the normal hemidiaphragm rises and the paralyzed one descends. This paradoxical motion can be accentuated by having the patient sniff. This causes a rapid but shallow inspiration. In paresis of the diaphragm there may or may not be elevation visible on chest roentgenograms, but a lag in contraction of the involved hemidiaphragm is readily visible fluoroscopically and this is also accentuated by having the patient sniff. Normally there may be a slight difference in motion on the two sides. In our experience, the left diaphragm moves slightly more rapidly than the right on deep, rapid inspiration. When there is much difficulty in determining relative diaphragmatic motion on the two sides, fluoroscopy with the patient in the lateral decubitus position is helpful, since motion on the dependent side is augmented and comparison is easier with greater excursion.

EVENTRATION OF THE DIAPHRAGM

"Eventration of the diaphragm" is the term used to describe an abnormal elevation of the diaphragm. It is thought to result from a deficiency of muscular development that may be general or local. The local form may be bilateral, but bilateral general eventra-tion is very rare. There is some difference of opinion as to the cause of eventration. Some observers believe that there is a deficiency of nervous as well as of muscular tissue. The diagnosis is based upon observation of the elevated diaphragm on a chest roentgenogram. There is no disease or tumor visible to produce the elevation and at fluoroscopy the hemidiaphragm involved is usually observed to move. The movement may be normal or diminished and paradoxical motion can be observed on rapid inspiration in some instances. It is often difficult to differentiate from hernia and from phrenic paralysis or paresis. When eventration is left-sided, the fundus of the stomach or the splenic flexure of the colon lies adjacent to the undersurface of the diaphragm in both frontal and lateral projections (Fig. 31-21). There is often a long fluid level in the gastric fundus when the patient is in the upright position. The afferent and efferent limbs of the stomach or colon are widely separated in eventration, but are together or nearly so in congenital or acquired hernia, being constricted at the hernial opening.

Localized Eventration

Local weakness of the diaphragm with upward protrusion of the liver is the most common manifestation of localized eventration. It usually occurs on the anteromedial aspect of the right diaphragm through which a portion of the right lobe of the liver bulges. This has been termed the "anteromedial hump of the liver." The smoothly rounded appearance of the bulge is usually characteristic, but, if the bulge simulates tumor, pneumoperitoneum or preferably liver scan will make differentiation possible. In our experience, primary or metastatic hepatic tumor does not cause this type of local elevation. Local eventrations may occur elsewhere, particularly posteriorly, where upward displacement of the kidney may produce a rounded mass density simulating tumor. This probability should be considered when the mass is comparable in size to the upper pole of the kidney. When suspected, intravenous urography can be used to outline the kidney and determine its relationship to the diaphragm.

DIAPHRAGMATIC DISPLACEMENTS

In addition to the elevation of the diaphragm noted in eventration, paralysis, and paresis, a number of intrathoracic and intra-abdominal conditions may result in elevation of the diaphragm. On the right side, tumors and cysts of the liver, subphrenic abscess, and right renal tumors may elevate the diaphragm

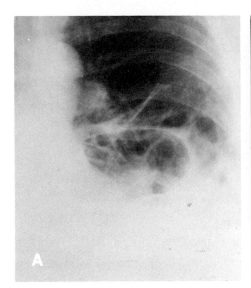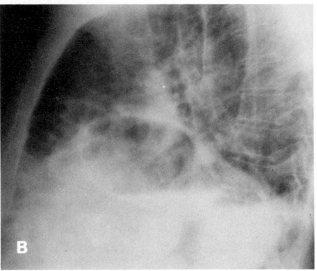

Fig. 31-21. Eventration of the diaphragm. The dome of the diaphragm is difficult to visualize in the frontal projection **(A)** because of changes in the basal lung on the left. It is more clearly defined in the lateral view **(B)** and is noted to be elevated. Since the patient experienced respiratory symptoms secondary to poor diaphragmatic function, surgical repair was carried out, and the diagnosis of congenital eventration confirmed.

generally or locally. On the left side the causes include enlargement of the spleen, left renal tumors, and dilatation or tumors of the stomach and of the splenic flexure of the colon. Ascites, obesity, large intra-abdominal tumors, and pregnancy may result in bilateral elevation. Intrathoracic diseases that decrease pulmonary volume cause elevation on the side involved. These include pulmonary fibrosis, chronic pleural disease, and atelectasis. The elevation may be relatively uniform or rather irregular. The amount depends upon the severity of the lesion producing it.

Irregularity of the diaphragm superiorly is often secondary to previous pulmonary inflammatory disease. This is termed "tenting" or "adhesive tenting" and is often associated with basal pulmonary fibrosis and obliteration of the costophrenic sulcus.

The diaphragm is displaced downward by lesions that produce an increase in thoracic volume, such as large intrathoracic neoplasms, massive pleural effusion, pulmonary emphysema, and tension pneumothorax. Massive pleural effusion may actually cause inversion of the left diaphragm, displacing the kidney, spleen, and stomach downward. This inversion may produce a pseudomass in the left upper abdominal quadrant which disappears when thoracentesis and removal of pleural fluid is accomplished (Fig. 31-22).

DIAPHRAGMATIC TUMORS

Primary diaphragmatic tumors are rare and may be benign or malignant. The most common benign tumor is lipoma, but numerous other benign tumors have been reported; they include fibroma, chondroma, neurofibroma, angiofibroma, and angioma as well as congenital cysts. The malignant tumors are all sarcomas; fibrosarcoma is the most common but others such as fibromyxosarcoma, fibroangioendothelioma, undifferentiated sarcoma, myosarcoma, hemangioendothelioma, hemangiopericytoma, leiomyosarcoma, or mesenchymoma may occur. Malignant tumors predominate in a ratio of 3:2 over benign tumors arising in the diaphragm. These tumors produce basal masses that usually project above the normal rounded density produced by the diaphragm. They may be smooth or lobulated and vary considerably in size. When the tumor is on the left it may project downward to encroach on the gastric air bubble. The limits of the tumor may then be outlined inferiorly as the tumor projects into the stomach and superiorly as it projects above the diaphragm. It is often necessary to use diagnostic pneumoperitoneum to differentiate a tumor of the diaphragm from an intra-abdominal mass and diagnostic pneumothorax to differentiate it from a mass arising in the basal

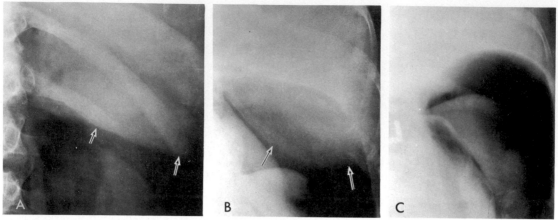

Fig. 31-22. Inversion of the diaphragm caused by massive left pleural effusion. **A.** This film shows the mass in the left upper quadrant which was continuous with massive left pleural effusion **(arrows). B.** Pneumoperitoneum shows the inverted diaphragm projecting downward into the abdominal cavity **(arrows). C.** Pneumoperitoneum following thoracentesis shows the diaphragm to have assumed its normal upward convexity. There is still a moderately large, left pleural effusion that obscures the lower lung on the left.

lung. Roentgen studies serve only to identify a mass. Since the various cell types produce no characteristic findings, surgical exploration is usually indicated when a tumor is found in the diaphragm.

DIAPHRAGMATIC HERNIAS

Esophageal Hiatal Hernia

Herniation of all or part of the stomach through the esophageal hiatus into the thorax produces a mass shadow at the left medial base that is often visible on the frontal roentgenogram. Not infrequently, gas and fluid within the thoracic portion of the stomach make the diagnosis apparent on plain-film roentgenograms; if not, the lesion can be readily identified by means of a barium swallow. This examination also serves to identify the occasional diverticulum of the esophagus in this region and to differentiate the esophageal lesions from pulmonary cyst or abscess as well as from diaphragmatic tumor.

Morgagni Hernia

Hernia of Morgagni is a rare diaphragmatic hernia that may result in a basal mass shadow, usually in the region of the cardiohepatic angle since it occurs mainly on the right (Fig. 31-23). This type of hernia through the retrosternal "foramen" of Morgagni

(space of Larrey) on either side of the midline is usually small and often contains omentum, but occasionally a portion of bowel may lie within the hernial sac. In the latter instance, it may be possible to make the diagnosis on routine roentgenographic study of the chest, but further studies are usually required for the smaller hernias. These studies include barium enema examination, which may show upward angulation of the midtransverse colon when the hernial sac contains omentum. The pyloric end of the stomach and proximal duodenum may also be displaced upward toward the diaphragm. In some instances, pneumoperitoneum may be necessary to make a diagnosis. Rarely, the liver may herniate through the foramen of Morgagni into the thorax in infants and young children. This is usually accompanied by partial obstruction of the inferior vena cava. Inferior vena cavography demonstrates the kinking and partial obstruction.

Bochdalek Hernia

The pleuroperitoneal hiatus or foramen is posterolateral in position, but in large, congenital hernias arising in this area, the hiatus may be very large, with absence of much of the involved hemidiaphragm. In such instances, most of the abdominal viscera may be in the thorax, leading to severe pulmonary hypoplasia. The presenting complaint may then be neonatal

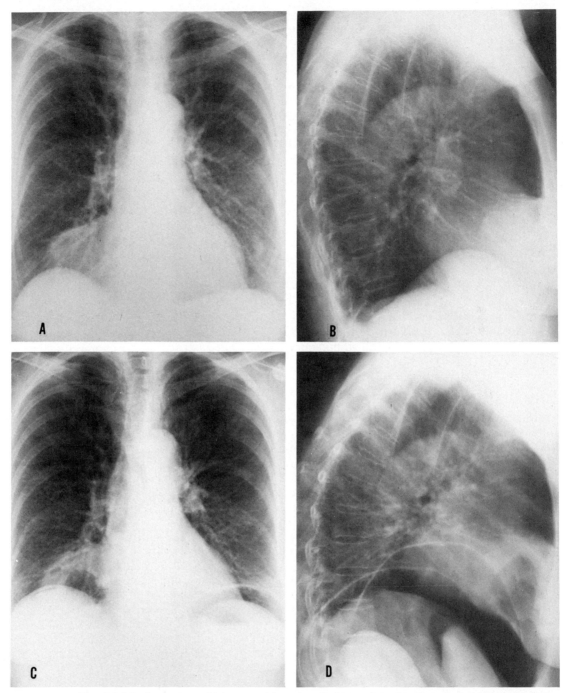

Fig. 31-23. Foramen of Morgagni hernia. **A.** Frontal projection shows a mass at the cardiohepatic angle. **B.** The anterior location of the mass is noted. **C.** Following diagnostic pneumoperitoneum, air is seen to extend up into the thorax through a defect in the diaphragm. Since surgery was not performed the presence of hernial sac was not confirmed nor was its possibility excluded.

respiratory distress. These hernias usually occur on the left side. In contrast to the foramen of Morgagni hernias, true pleuroperitoneal hiatal hernias do not have a hernial sac. This is because the abdominal contents enter the thorax before the space between the septum transversum and the pleuroperitoneal membrane is closed.

Herniation through the pleuroperitoneal foramen of Bochdalek is often large, and loops of bowel can be visualized and identified so that differential diagnosis is not difficult. When the hernia is smaller and does not contain gas-filled bowel, the diagnosis is more difficult to make. Occasionally the left kidney projects upward through a weak area in the posterior portion of the left hemidiaphragm and may be mistaken for tumor. The high position of the kidney can sometimes be determined on the chest roentgenogram; if not, intravenous urography can be used to make the diagnosis. The roentgen findings vary with the amount of herniation. Gas-filled bowel is recognized within the thorax when the defect is on the left. The liver may also extend into the thorax when the defect is on the right. The remaining diaphragm is often visible; oblique and lateral views will often demonstrate the site of the defect.

Traumatic Hernia of the Diaphragm

Traumatic rupture of the diaphragm usually results from severe crushing types of injury to the abdomen, thorax, or both. The diaphragm may be ruptured completely with defects in the parietal pleura and peritoneum. Then there is no hernial sac. In other instances, either the pleura or peritoneum may form a sac. The left diaphragm is involved in 95% of cases. The roentgen signs in this condition vary with the extent of the rupture and depend upon upward displacement of abdominal content. At times, no abnormality is observed. There may be elevation of the hemidiaphragm or apparent elevation, since herniated viscera may parallel the diaphragm on both frontal and lateral projections. This "elevation" may change in shape with change in position, however; in these instances it is strongly suggestive of hernia. Apparent normal diaphragmatic motion does not exclude the possibility of hernia. Recognizable bowel shadows may be visible in the thorax and sometimes in the pericardial sac. Administration of barium by mouth and by rectum to identify the relationship of the gastrointestinal tract to the diaphragm usually confirms the diagnosis. Both loops of gut are kept close together by the diaphragm surrounding the rupture, so that ordinarily there is no problem in differentiation from eventration. Since there may not be immediate herniation of abdominal viscera into the thorax, serial films are sometimes necessary. Occasionally the traumatic rupture of the diaphragm is followed years later by a traumatic hernia. The roentgen findings are similar to those in the immediate type of post-traumatic herniation. Oblique and lateral views often permit localization of the defect. There may be partial or complete obstruction of the involved gut, either with or without vascular compromise in both immediate and delayed herniation. Hemothorax or hydrothorax may also be present. The combination of a high left hemidiaphragm and splenic flexure obstruction in a patient with history of trauma is very suggestive. Right-sided rupture, which may be more common than reported figures would indicate, also may cause diaphragmatic elevation with partial or total herniation of the liver and intrathoracic fluid. Diagnostic pneumoperitoneum may be necessary to confirm the diagnosis. A high index of suspicion when diaphragmatic abnormality is observed in a patient who has suffered thoracoabdominal trauma is necessary to suggest, then confirm, the diagnosis. Immediate surgery is necessary in many instances.

Epicardial Fat Pads

Localized fat deposits are often present at the cardiac apex and in the cardiohepatic angle. Those at the apex are usually readily identified. When the amount of fat is unusually great it can produce a mass in the cardiohepatic angle that simulates foramen of Morgagni hernia or diaphragmatic tumor. Deposits of fat are usually of less density than are the adjacent heart and diaphragm but this difference in density is small and not entirely reliable since the omentum, frequently present in foramen of Morgagni hernia, is of similar density. It is probable that small foramen of Morgagni hernia is sometimes the cause of the shadow, but this is usually asymptomatic and the differentiation is then of no clinical importance. The fat pads tend to occur in obese patients and, when a fat pad is present in the cardiohepatic angle, there is usually a fat pad at the cardiac apex. The association of these densities is of some diagnostic importance.

ACCESSORY DIAPHRAGM

Accessory diaphragm, sometimes termed "duplication of the diaphragm," is very rare and usually occurs on the right side. It consists of a sheet of fibrous and muscular tissue, which represents a par-

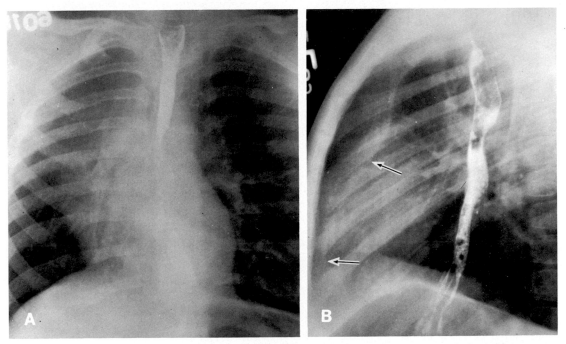

Fig. 31-24. Accessory diaphragm on the right. **A.** Note the mediastinal shift to the right with poor definition of mediastinal structures on the involved side. There is also hazy density in the medial aspect of the upper half of the right hemithorax. **B.** The lateral projection shows a somewhat curved line resembling an anteriorly displaced major fissure except that it extends down to the diaphragm anteriorly **(arrows).** An aortogram showed an anomalous artery originating below the diaphragm supplying a portion of the right lower lobe.

tial duplication, extending from the anterior aspect of the normal diaphragm, upward and posteriorly, to insert along the fifth to seventh rib. It parallels the major fissure and usually extends into it to separate the lower lobe from the upper and middle lobes. It is usually attached to the pericardium medially and has a medial hiatus. Pulmonary anomalies associated with accessory diaphragm include partial fissure anomalies, aplasia or hypoplasia of a lobe, partial division of the lower lobe by the anomalous diaphragm, and anomalous pulmonary vascular supply including lower lobe venous drainage into the inferior vena cava, the scimitar syndrome, and anomalous arterial supply to the lower lobe from the aorta. This complex of anomalies is sometimes called the "venolobar syndrome."

Roentgen findings include shift of mediastinum to the involved side because of hypoplasia, lack of clarity of the mediastinum on the same side with hazy den-

sity of the central lung field. On the lateral view the accessory diaphragm may be visible; it resembles the major fissure but extends to the diaphragm and is more anterior in position than the normal fissure (Fig. 31-24). Bronchography may show the lobar hypoplasia and angiography may demonstrate the anomalous arterial supply and venous drainage that often accompanies this anomaly.

Cysts of the Diaphragm

Intradiaphragmatic cysts usually represent extralobar sequestration in which aberrant lung tissue is enclosed within the diaphragm. The left hemidiaphragm is involved in about 90% of cases. Occasionally, a coelomic cyst may be found in the diaphragm. Roentgen findings of a diaphragmatic mass are similar to those produced by benign diaphragmatic tumors.

REFERENCES AND SELECTED READINGS

1. BERNE AS, HEITZMAN ER: The roentgenologic signs of pedunculated pleural tumors. Am J Roentgenol 87: 892, 1962

2. CAMPBELL JA: The diaphragm in roentgenology of the chest. Radiol Clin North Am 1: 395, 1963

3. COLLINS JD, BURWELL D, FURMANSKI S et al: Minimal detectable pleural effusions. Radiology 105: 51, 1972

4. DAVIS VE, SALKIN D: Intrathoracic gastric cysts. JAMA 135: 218, 1947

5. DAVIS WS, ALLEN RP: Accessory diaphragm: duplication of the diaphragm. Radiol Clin North Am 6: 253, 1968

6. FEIGIN DS, FENOGLIO JJ, McALLISTER HA et al: Pericardial cysts. Radiology 125: 15, 1977

7. FINBY N, STEINBERG I: Roentgen aspects of pleural mesothelioma. Radiology 65: 169, 1955

8. FLEISCHNER FG: Atypical arrangement of free pleural effusion. Radiol Clin North Am 1: 347, 1963

9. FREIDMAN RL: Infrapulmonary pleural effusions. Am J Roentgenol 71: 613, 1954

10. HANSEN KF: Idiopathic fibrosis of the mediastinum as a cause of superior vena caval syndrome. Radiology 85: 433, 1965

11. HESSEN I: Roentgen examination of pleural fluid. Acta Radiol [Suppl] (Stockh) 86, 1951

12. HUTCHINSON WB, FRIEDENBERG MJ: Intrathoracic mesothelioma. Radiology 80: 937, 1963

13. INADA K, KAWAI, K, KATSUMURA T et al: Giant lymph node hyperplasia of the mediastinum. Am Rev Tuberc 79: 232, 1959

14. KATZ S, REED HR: Unusual pleural effusions. Radiology 45: 147, 1945

15. KEEGAN JM: Hemangioma of the mediastinum. Am J Roentgenol 69: 66, 1953

16. KEIRNS MM: Tumors of the diaphragm. Radiology 58: 542, 1952

17. KIRKLIN BR, HODGSON JR: Roentgenologic characteristics of diaphragmatic hernia. Am J Roentgenol 59: 77, 1947

18. LAXDAL OE, McDOUGALL H, MELLEN GW: Congenital eventration of the diaphragm. N Engl J Med 250: 401, 1954

19. LEIGH TF: Mass lesions of the mediastinum. Radiol Clin North Am 1: 377, 1963

20. LIGHT RW, GEORGE RB: Incidence and insignificance of pleural effusion after abdominal surgery. Chest 69: 621, 1976

21. LULL GF JR, WINN DF JR: Chronic fibrous mediastinitis due to Histoplasma capsulatum. Radiology 73: 378, 1959

22. MAIER HC: Lymphatic cysts of the mediastinum. Am J Roentgenol 73: 15, 1955

23. MEIGS JV, CASS JW: Hydrothorax and ascites in association with fibroma of the ovary. Am J Obstet Gynecol 33: 249, 1937

24. NEUHAUSER EBD, HARRIS GBC, BERRETT A: Roentgenographic features of neurenteric cysts. Am J Roentgenol 79: 235, 1958

25. PAUL LW: Diseases of the mediastinum. Radiology 40: 10, 1943

26. PAUL LW: Basal mass shadows in chest roentgenograms. Tex Med 52: 1, 1956

27. PINCKNEY L, PARKER BR: Primary coccidioidomycosis in children presenting with massive pleural effusion. Am J Roentgenol 130: 247, 1978

28. PRICE JE JR, RIGLER LG: Widening of the mediastinum resulting from fat accumulation. Radiology 96: 497, 1970

29. RENNER RR, MARKARIAN B, PERNICE NJ et al: The apical cap. Radiology 110: 569, 1974

30. ROSENBLUM D, NUSSBAUM A, SCHWARTZ S: Partial obstruction of the inferior vena cava by herniation of the liver through the foramen of Morgagni. Radiology 68: 399, 1957

31. SENGPIEL GW, RUZICKA FF, LODMELL EA: Lateral intrathoracic meningocele. Radiology 50: 515, 1948

32. SIMONDS B, FRIEDMAN PJ, SOKOLOFF J: The prone chest film. Radiology 116: 11, 1975

33. STOREY DD, DINES DE, COLES DT: Pleural effusion. A diagnostic dilemma. JAMA 236: 2183, 1976

34. SWINGLE JD, LOGAN R, JUHL JH: Inversion of the left hemidiaphragm. JAMA 208: 863, 1969

32

THE CARDIOVASCULAR SYSTEM

METHODS OF EXAMINATION

Roentgen study of the heart and great vessels is an essential part of the examination of patients suspected of having disease involving these structures. In some conditions the diagnosis can be made by means of roentgen methods alone, but it is important to recognize that roentgenographic and fluoroscopic studies form only a part of the complete examination and that the findings must be correlated with clinical history, physical and electrocardiographic findings, and sometimes with angiocardiographic and catheterization studies to obtain a complete picture of cardiovascular disease. On roentgen examination, the size and shape of the heart can be determined in various projections and indications of diseases of the pulmonary artery and aorta may be visualized. In addition, the roentgenogram furnishes a permanent record of the cardiac size and shape.

ROENTGENOGRAPHY

Roentgen study of the heart usually requires a minimum of four projections: posteroanterior, left anterior oblique at approximately 60 degrees, right anterior oblique at approximately 45 degrees, and lateral. The films are exposed at a 6-foot distance, with the patient in the upright position and in moderately deep inspiration. Magnification resulting from divergent distortion is minimized by obtaining posteroanterior and anterior oblique views to place the heart closer to the film (the anterior chest is adjacent to film). A left lateral view (with the left side adjacent to film) also tends to minimize magnification. We use a barium suspension to outline the esophagus as an aid in determining position and size of the aortic arch and left heart chambers when necessary.

FLUOROSCOPY

Fluoroscopy is an adjunctive method for examination of the heart. It is useful for determination of the amplitude and direction of pulsation in varying degrees of rotation. The presence of calcification within the heart can be determined more readily by fluoroscopy than by any other means. Examination of the pulmonary vessels can also be accomplished. The examination is used only when it is important to study motion of the heart or great vessels, and to determine the presence of calcification in the heart. In our department, its use has declined considerably in the study of congenital heart disease because many of the patients require more definitive studies such as cardiac catheterization and/or angiocardiography and ultrasonography.

The procedure used in fluoroscopy varies with the indication for the examination as well as with the individual examiner. It is necessary to study chest roentgenograms prior to fluoroscopy. The examination should be systematic and the patient should be examined in frontal, both oblique, and lateral projections. It is sometimes of value to fluoroscope patients in the recumbent as well as in the upright position; a thick, micronized barium suspension can be used to outline the esophagus.

There are several disadvantages in cardiac fluoroscopy, one of the most important of which is the amount of radiation to which the patient is exposed. This can be kept to a minimum by observing the rules described in Chapter 22. The second disadvantage is distortion. Because the distance between the target of the x-ray tube and the patient is short, there is considerable enlargement of the cardiac silhouette and distortion of other thoracic structures. This can be decreased by using longer distances between target and the patient and by using a small shutter opening, producing the central-beam effect. The third disadvantage is lack of permanent record. This is obviated to a certain extent by the use of spot films exposed during fluoroscopy and by roentgenograms obtained following this procedure. We prefer to study roentgenograms on each patient before doing fluoroscopy, in order to thoroughly understand the diagnostic problems involved, which helps to save fluoroscopic time.

ANGIOCARDIOGRAPHY

This method of contrast cardiac visualization has been used widely for examination of patients with all types of cardiac and pulmonary diseases (Fig. 32-1). The technique and indications are discussed briefly in Chapter 22. The method is used in the diagnosis of congenital and acquired cardiac disease. Selective angiocardiography in which a small amount of opaque medium (an organic iodide) is injected into a specific chamber or vessel during cardiac catheterization is used extensively.

Coronary Arteriography

Selective catheterization of the coronary arteries followed by injection of a contrast medium (one of the organic iodides) is used in combination with cineradiography or rapid filming to visualize the coronary arteries. Details of technique are beyond the scope of this volume.

Retrograde Aortography

This examination consists of the injection of one of the organic iodides into the aorta through a catheter introduced into one of its major branches and placed into a desired position in the proximal aorta. The examination has a place in the investigation of patients with certain diagnostic problems relating to the aortic arch.

It is used in infants with congestive heart failure in whom there is evidence of a left-to-right shunt and in whom patent ductus arteriosus is suspected. Coarctation of the aorta in infants may also cause congestive heart failure and the lesion can be defined by aortography. In adults, aortography is used to define anomalies of the aortic arch and its branches as well as in the study of the aortic valve and the coronary arteries. It is also useful in patients with masses adjacent to the aorta in whom aneurysm is a possibility and in patients with suspected dissecting hematoma or traumatic aneurysm.

Tomography

This method of examination has also been described in Chapter 22. Its use in the study of the heart and great vessels is very limited. Calcification in coronary vesssels has been identified and calcification in the mitral valve has also been visualized on tomograms. The method has been used in the study of coarctation of the aorta. All these studies have been on an investigative basis and the examination is not generally used in clinical study of the cardiovascular system.

Ultrasonic Investigation of the Heart

The use of ultrasound in examination of the heart has increased greatly in the past 10 years, and it is now well established as a diagnostic tool. Ultrasonic investigation is a noninvasive study that permits detection of valvular motion, chamber size, and chamber motion. It is used to assess the mitral valves in mitral stenosis and mitral regurgitation and in assess-

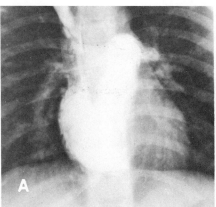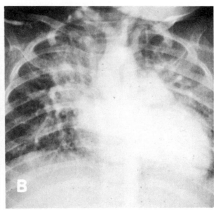

Fig. 32-1. Angiocardiogram—normal findings. **A.** Filling of the right side of the heart. Some medium is in the superior vena cava and can be seen entering the right atrium. The right ventricle is partially obscured by the atrium. Note relative radiolucency of the left side of the heart. The pulmonary outflow tract and artery are well visualized but there is no opacification of the branches of the pulmonary artery as yet. **B.** This is a later phase in a younger child to show filling of the left side the heart. The left ventricle is clearly defined, making up the left lower cardiac border. The aorta and its brachiocephalic branches are outlined. The left atrium is well filled and is noted to overlie the root of the aorta with the appendage projecting to the left above the ventricle. A considerable amount of the medium remains in the pulmonary vascular system.

ment of mitral valvotomy. It is also used in the detection of aortic regurgitation and stenosis, but is of less value in the examination of the tricuspid valve. It is of value in the study of the hypertrophic cardiomyopathies both with and without associated subaortic stenosis and in the study of the congestive type in which there is chamber dilatation. With ultrasound, left ventricular diameter and outflow configuration can be determined; also qualitative assessment of right and left ventricular size is possible. The size of the left atrium can be measured with reasonable accuracy and left atrial myxomas or other intra-atrial tumors can be detected. Ultrasound is also useful in the investigation of congenital heart disease, particularly the patients with hypoplastic left-heart syndrome, those with double-outlet right ventricle, and those having right ventricular volume overload. In addition, it is an accurate method of determining the presence of pericardial effusion.

DETERMINATION OF CARDIAC SIZE

The size of the heart is related to body weight and height as well as to surface area, sex, and age. A number of methods of correlation of these factors with cardiac size, as measured on the roentgenogram, have been described. It is unfortunate that in the borderline cases in which determination of possible cardiac enlargement is most needed, the mathematical formulas are most faulty since there is a normal variation of approximately plus or minus 10%. Numerous factors such as thoracic deformities and pulmonary and abdominal diseases that elevate or depress the diaphragm affect the size of the cardiac silhouette. Because the line between the normal and the abnormal size cannot be sharply drawn in an individual patient, most of the methods of measurement are chiefly of statistical value. These methods are usually based on direct measurement on teleoroentgenograms. The most commonly used are: (1) measurement of transverse diameters; (2) measurement of surface area; and (3) cardiothoracic ratio. The transverse diameter of the heart is the sum of the maximum projections of the heart to the right and to the left of the midline, the measurement being made with care not to include epicardial fat or other noncardiac structures (Fig. 32-2). The diameter can then be compared with the theoretical transverse di-

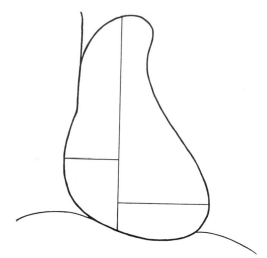

Fig. 32-2. Sketch showing the method of measuring the transverse diameter of the heart. The sum of the horizontal projections from the vertical line is the transverse diameter.

ameter of the heart for varius heights and weights as described by Ungerleider and Clark.[64] Surface area estimations based on artificial construction of the base of the heart and of the diaphragmatic contour of the heart have been worked out by Hodges and Eyster.[28] Nomograms showing relationship of the frontal area of the heart as predicted by height and weight to the measured area using the long and broad diameters of the heart have been described by Ungerleider and Gubner.[65] A nomogram used for measuring children's hearts has been reported by Meyer.[44] The cardiothoracic ratio is the ratio between the transverse cardiac diameter and the greatest internal diameter of the thorax, measured on the frontal teleoroentgenogram. This is the easiest and quickest method of measurement of cardiac size; an adult heart that measures more than one-half of the internal diameter of the chest is considered enlarged. The method is gross and inaccurate, since the cardiothoracic ratio varies widely with variations in body habitus. It can be used as a rough estimate of cardiac size, however.

These are a few of the many methods described; there are a number of objections to each of them. The objections are largely to the use of such methods in borderline cases, because the numerical exactness of the various measurements is not matched by the reliability of the method. Most of the measurements are relatively simple and easy to apply and do serve as a basis for discrimination between hearts that are obviously normal and those obviously enlarged. They are accurate enough for most statistical studies.

Ultrasonography is now used widely in determination of cardiac size and wall thickness. Cardiac chamber size can be determined with considerable accuracy by ultrasonic methods and increases or decreases in chamber size can be determined by serial examination; ventricular wall thickness can also be measured.

THE NORMAL HEART

THE ADULT HEART

The heart and its major vessels occupy the middle mediastinum and produce a uniform density that is readily recognized on the roentgenogram. The density of the great vessels and of the blood within the heart is comparable, so that the contours of the silhouette are visible in contrast to the adjacent radiolucent lungs. The inferior cardiac border is of density comparable to that of the diaphragm and often is not clearly defined. On the right side the shadow of the liver below the diaphragm blends into that of the heart, but on the left side there is often enough air in the stomach immediately below the dome of the diaphragm to outline the left inferior border of the heart. Marked individual variations are noted in the relationships inferiorly so that in some persons the inferior border is difficult or impossible to define while in others it is clearly outlined. The heart lies two-thirds to the left of the midline and one-third to the right in the average normal person.

The Posteroanterior Projection

In the posteroanterior projection the right side of the heart border is divided into two segments. The lower segment is usually convex and represents the lateral border of the right atrium. This segment is often separated from the upper border by an indentation. The upper segment is nearly vertical in the young adult and is usually formed by the superior vena cava. In older adults, the aorta tends to dilate and elongate so that the right upper border becomes more convex. The convexity represents the right lateral aspect of the ascending aortic arch. In asthenic persons with vertical heart, it is sometimes possible to outline the reflection of the pericardium down to the inferior vena cava. It appears as a small, straight or slightly concave downward continuation of the convex shadow of the right atrium. On the left side there are usually three visible segments. The uppermost is rounded and convex laterally. It represents the aortic knob, or transverse aortic arch. The descending aorta may also form a portion of the left border, particularly in the persons with vertical hearts. The left lateral wall of the aorta can often be followed downward behind the heart, in the left paraspinal area nearly to the diaphragm, particularly on overpenetrated films. Immediately below the aortic knob is another short segment, the contour of which varies considerably. It represents the pulmonary artery and occasionally its left main branch. In most normal adults it is straight or slightly convex. Considerable prominence of the pulmonary artery is a common finding in normal young women and should not be considered abnormal. The left pulmonary artery passes over the lower portion of the left main bronchus and the proximal left upper lobe bronchus, and the main pulmonary artery arises just below the level of the left main bronchus. There is some variability, but the left auricular appendage usually forms a short segment of the left border of the heart below the pulmonary artery. It is likely that in some persons a portion of the distal right ventricular outflow tract may be border-forming in this area. The left ventricle forms the remainder of the left cardiac margin including the apex and is by far the largest segment. The contour of this border is usually dependent upon the habitus of the person. It tends to be relatively straight and descends sharply in the asthenic individual while in the hypersthenic person it is convex and angles outward considerably. There is thus a considerable range between the extremes of vertical and transverse cardiac configuration. There has been some difference of opinion, but the wide use of angiocardiography has demonstrated rather clearly that the left auricular appendage normally does not project beyond the left ventricle along the left border of the heart. In patients with disease resulting in enlargement of the left atrium, the appendage may project to the left of the ventricle and produce a convexity immediately below the level of the pulmonary artery. The amount of this change varies with the amount and type of left atrial enlargement. These various segments can usually be identified on the roentgenogram and alterations aid in the diagnosis of various cardiovascular abnormalities. The cardiac apex usually forms the lower left border of the heart and is usually at or near the level of the dome of the diaphragm; it is somewhat angular, with the apex of the angle rounded (Fig. 32-3). A shadow that is less than the density of the heart often extends lateral to it. This is the apical fat pad.

The Right Anterior Oblique Projection

In this projection the person being examined is rotated to his or her left 45 degrees so that the right anterior chest wall is nearest the cassette and the left posterior chest wall is nearest the tube. In this projection the left or most anterior cardiac border consists of the ascending aortic arch, the pulmonary artery, pulmonary conus (conus infundibularis) or outflow tract of the right ventricle, and a portion of the left ventricle, from above downward. If the subject is rotated more than 45 degrees, an increasing amount of the left border is made up of right ventricle accompanied by a decrease in the left ventricular contribution to this border. The posterior (right) contour in this projection is formed by the left atrium, right atrium, and a short segment of the inferior vena cava from above downward. These contours are outlined in Figure 32-4. This projection is useful in detecting enlargement of the left atrium and in determing the prominence of the pulmonary outflow tract and artery.

The Left Anterior Oblique Projection

In this projection the subject is turned to his or her right about 60 degrees so the left anterior chest is nearest the cassette while the right posterior chest is nearest the tube. In this projection the anterior (right) contour is formed by the ascending aorta, the right atrial appendage, right atrium, and occasionally the right ventricle from above downward. In most instances the right atrium forms the lower anterior border in this projection, however. The posterior (left) contour is formed by the left atrium above and the left ventricle below. Occasionally the shallow indentation representing the atrioventricular groove can be outlined in this projection. The contours are indicated in Figure 32-5. The left anterior oblique view is also used in examination of the aorta, since the arch is "opened," with very little overlapping.

The Lateral Projection

In the lateral projection the anterior contour of the cardiovascular silhouette is formed by the ascending aorta, the pulmonary artery, the pulmonary outflow tract, and the right ventricle from above downward. The posterior silhouette is formed by the left atrium and left ventricle from above downward. The contours are indicated in Figure 32-5, except that slight rotation into the lateral projects the right ventricle

(*Text continues on p. 1049.*)

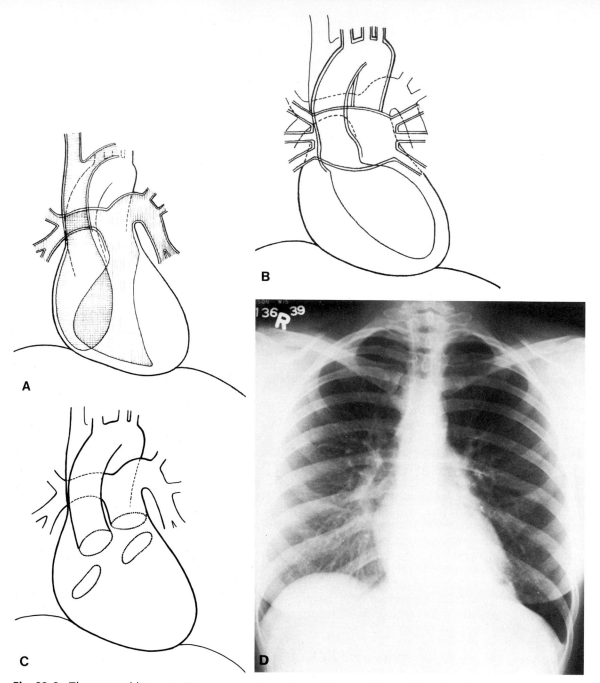

Fig. 32-3: The normal heart. **A.** Diagram to show the relative position of the chambers of the right side of the heart in the anteroposterior projection. Horizontal lines outline the vena cava and right atrium. Vertical lines outline the right ventricle and the pulmonary artery and its major branches. The position of the aorta is also indicated. **B.** The left side of the heart in frontal projection. Note that the left ventricle forms most of the left border of the heart. The position of the left atrium in the diagram is slightly above its usual position. **C.** Sketch to show approximate position of valves in the frontal projection. The mitral valve is above to the left of the tricuspid. Aortic and pulmonic rings are noted at the root of their respective arteries. **D.** Roentgenogram showing the normal cardiovascular silhouette. There are many variations as indicated in the text. (From Dotter, CT, Steinberg I)

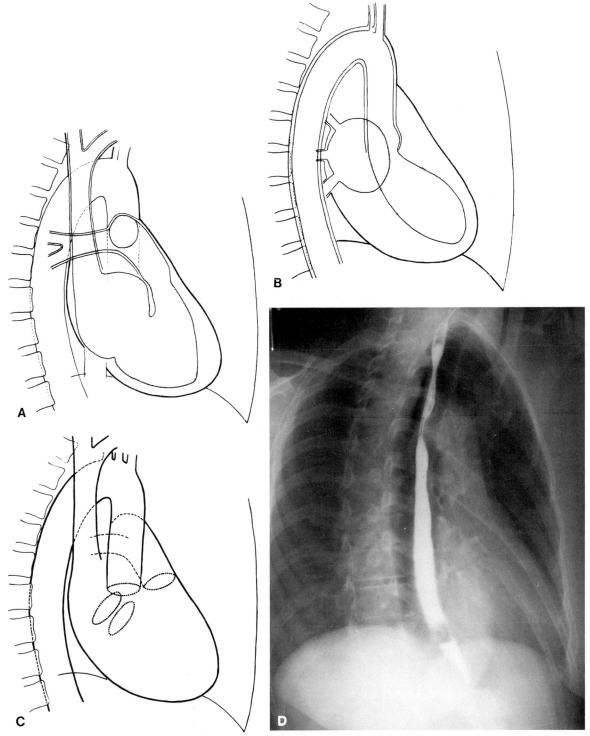

Fig. 32-4. The normal heart in the right anterior oblique projection. **A.** The right side of the heart. The vena cava, right chambers, and pulmonary arteries are outlined by vertical lines. **B.** Left side of the heart. Note that the left atrium forms the left upper posterior contour, and the apex of the left ventricle forms the lower anterior contour. **C.** Sketch to show the approximate position of the valves in the right anterior oblique position. The mitral valve is posterior to the tricuspid. Aortic and pulmonic rings are noted at the roots of their respective arteries. **D.** Roentgenogram in this position showing the normal cardiac configuration. Barium in the esophagus tends to outline the posterior cardiac border below the carina. (From Dotter CT, Steinberg I)

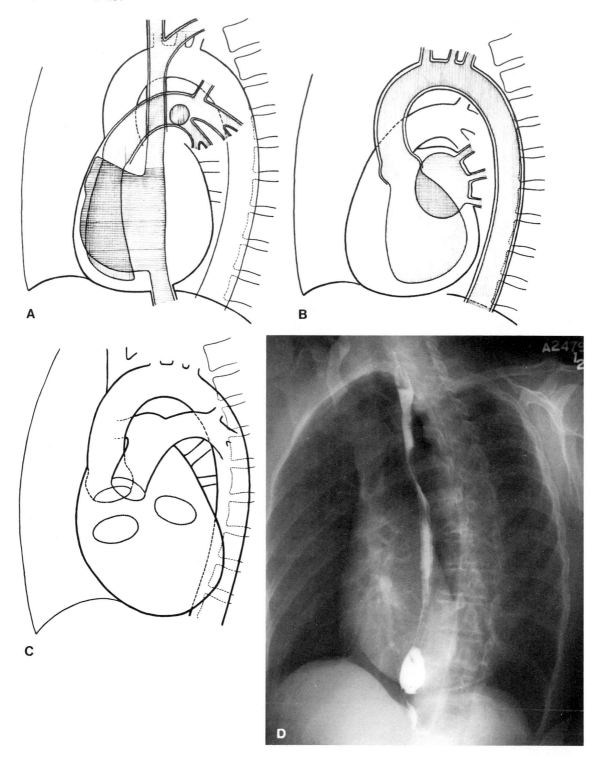

anteriorly to form the lower anterior contour (Fig. 32-6).

THE HEART IN INFANCY AND CHILDHOOD

At birth the right ventricle is relatively large and is approximately the same size as the left ventricle. During early life the left ventricle grows more rapidly than the right and its wall becomes thicker. The heart is globular in shape in the newborn and extends to the right almost as far as it does to the left in contrast to the adult heart, two-thirds of which lies to the left of the midline in the average normal person. In addition to the globular shape noted on the frontal projection in infants, the chambers and great vessels are not clearly defined. There is great variability in the size and shape of the heart in the newborn and during the first few weeks of life. Therefore the diagnosis of cardiac enlargement should be made with caution. There is often more prominence in the region of the pulmonary artery and right ventricular outflow tract than in the adult and the aortic knob is not readily visible in the newborn and in the young infant. It is sometimes important to determine the position of the aortic arch in infants. Often there is a very slight local displacement of the trachea away from the side of the arch, which is helpful in these situations. There is frequently enough thymic enlargement so that the cardiac base and great vessels are obscured. As a rule the heart maintains its globular shape for the first 6 months of life. Then it begins to descend in the thorax and, as it does, the long axis shifts from horizontal to a more oblique and then to an obliquely vertical position. This is a gradual process and when the child is 5 to 7 years of age the silhouette approaches that of the adult heart, although the ascending aortic arch and knob are not as prominent as they will become later.

As in the adult, the general contour of the heart is related to body habitus. This becomes apparent in the 5- to 10-year-old child.

Measurements of cardiac size in children show that the size of the heart in relation to the thoracic size is somewhat greater than in adults. This is particularly true when the cardiothoracic ratio is used as an indication of relative heart size. The long axis of the heart tends to be more horizontal in infants and children than in adults so the cardiothoracic index ranges from an upper limit of 0.65 in the first year to 0.50 in the fifth year and from then on until the early teens the ratio is in the range of 0.50. Measurements of the heart in children are subject to the same errors as indicated in the discussion on heart size in the adult, and there is the additional factor of inability to control the depth of respiration in infants and young children.

THE NORMAL AORTA

The border-forming contours of the aorta have been mentioned in the foregoing and are outlined in Figures 32-3 through 32-5. The right lateral contour of the ascending aorta is partially border-forming in adults with aortic dilatation or elongation. The medial border of the ascending aorta is not visible in the frontal projection, but the superior and lateral borders of the aortic knob are visualized as the upper left margin of the cardiovascular shadow and, in older adults, a portion of the descending aorta may be border-forming just below the aortic knob. It is often possible to outline the descending aorta even though it is not border-forming. It appears as a slightly convex, linear shadow extending downward, overlying the left upper cardiac silhouette. In the right anterior oblique view the upper anterior portion of the cardiovascular silhouette is formed by the ascending aorta.

◀Fig. 32-5. The normal heart in the left anterior oblique projection. **A.** The right side of the heart. The vena cava and right atrium are outlined by horizontal lines. The right ventricle and outflow tract along with the pulmonary artery are outlined by vertical lines. The aortic arch is also indicated. This is a somewhat exaggerated left oblique projection and differs very little from the lateral. Note that the anterior contour is made up of the right atrium and ventricle. **B.** The left side of the heart. The left atrium is outlined by horizontal lines, the left ventricle and aorta by vertical lines. The pulmonary artery is also indicated. **C.** Sketch to show approximate position of the valves in the left anterior oblique position. The mitral valve is posterior to the tricuspid, and the aortic and pulmonary rings are noted at the roots of these arteries. **D.** The left anterior oblique roentgenogram shows the normal cardiac contour in this projection. The esophagus, outlined by barium, is normal. (From Dotter CT, Steinberg I)

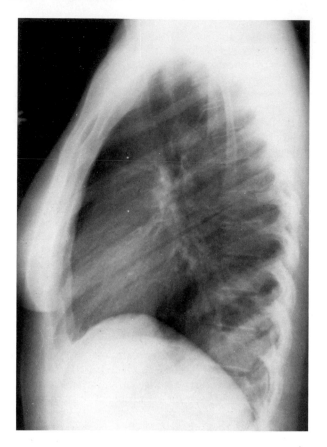

Fig. 32-6. The normal heart shown in the lateral roentgenogram. The contours are described in the text and are similar to those seen in Fig. 32-5.

In this view the descending arch and part of the thoracic aorta can often be outlined posterior to the cardiac silhouette. In the left anterior oblique view the aortic arch is more clearly defined. Again the ascending arch forms the upper anterior portion of the cardiovascular silhouette, and the transverse and descending portions of the arch, as well as the remaining thoracic aorta, are often visible in this projection. The aorta is often clearly defined in older adults in whom arteriosclerotic changes have resulted in deposition of calcium in the aortic walls. With the development of arteriosclerosis associated with advancing age the aorta becomes elongated so that the ascending arch becomes more prominent and its silhouette more convex. The aortic knob also becomes prominent and larger in diameter and there is often considerable tortuosity of the aorta, which is the result of elongation.

Numerous methods of aortic measurement have been described. They are subject to the same errors as the various mathematical formulas used in determining cardiac size. The measurements are most faulty in the borderline group in which accurate determination is most necessary. There is a gradual decrease in diameter of the aorta as it is more distant from the heart so that the ascending portion of the arch is the widest, followed by the transverse, the descending, and the lower thoracic aorta. Dotter and Steinberg measured the inner diameter of the aorta by means of angiocardiography and observed a wide range. In 100 patients the diameter of the ascending aorta ranged from 16 to 38 mm with an average of 28.6 mm. Measurements elsewhere showed comparable wide ranges.

In addition to visualization of the aorta on roentgenograms obtained in various projections, this structure is occasionally studied by means of fluoroscopy. It is usually not difficult to identify because of its typical pulsation and appearance. Aortography is often used when localized density continuous with the aorta cannot be differentiated from aortic aneurysm on the roentgenograms.

THE PERICARDIUM

The pericardium is a closed endothelium-lined sac that envelops the heart. It consists of a visceral layer covering the heart and a parietal layer reflected to form a continuous sac. It contains 15 to 25 cc of clear fluid. The parietal pericardium fuses with the diaphragm below and the mediastinal pleura laterally and anteriorly, except in the sternal area, where there is no pleura. The reflection of the parietal pericardium occurs in a line that begins at the superior vena cava above its junction with the right atrium on the right side and continues to the left over the anterior aspect of the ascending aorta to the pulmonary artery, which is covered by pericardium nearly to the level of the ligamentum arteriosum. Posteriorly the pericardium extends up as far as the proximal superior vena cava and down to the inferior vena cava. The pericardium cannot be visualized roentgenographically in the normal person. The apical fat pad frequently seen at the left cardiodiaphragmatic angle lies between the parietal pericardium and a reflection of the parietal pleura as it extends downward and laterally to cover the diaphragm in this region. A similar situation exists on the right and a fat pad is occasionally noted in the cardiohepatic angle.

ENLARGEMENT OF THE HEART

GENERAL CARDIAC ENLARGEMENT

General cardiac enlargement may be caused by disease that produces a toxic effect on the myocardium and weakens it, and by conditions that cause an increase in the work load on the heart. This load is usually on a single chamber at first, and when it fails a second chamber becomes enlarged; eventually all chambers may be enlarged. In the latter type of disease, therefore, single or double chamber enlargement may predominate while in the conditions producing toxic myocarditis there is more likely to be uniform generalized cardiac enlargement.

The roentgen appearance of the heart in generalized myocardial disease varies considerably, but the lateral contours on both sides often become more convex inferiorly and the normal slight alterations in the contour indicating the various segments are often effaced. The transverse diameter is usually increased more than the vertical diameter. Evidence of pulmonary congestion manifested by prominence and poor definition of pulmonary basal vascular markings may also be present. At fluoroscopy, pulsations are diminished and in extreme cases are so poor as to be difficult to define. When single or multiple chamber enlargement is present, the cardiac contour often shows characteristic changes that can be recognized roentgenographically.

LEFT VENTRICULAR ENLARGEMENT

When there is an increased work load on a cardiac chamber, the muscle fibers elongate in response to the added work and dilatation results. When this load is maintained over a period of time the dilatation is followed by hypertrophy, which is represented by actual increase in the size of the individual muscle fibers. The initial dilatation that precedes hypertrophy is the means by which heart muscle increases its ability to work. When the work load becomes great there is secondary dilatation that results from failure of the heart muscle to do its work adequately. This type of dilatation indicates cardiac decompensation and failure. Hypertrophy of the heart muscle is a clearly defined pathologic finding, but the roentgen changes are often minimal or absent, making it difficult to determine in many instances. Hypertrophy may cause alteration in cardiac shape, however. This is usually a rounding of the contour of the ventricle involved. Little if any change in size results when hypertrophy is present without dilatation. On the other hand, dilatation causes an increase in size and may also alter the shape of the cardiac silhouette. The ventricles may be divided into two functional components, the inflow tract and the outflow tract. The blood flows into the left ventricle from the left atrium through the mitral valve that lies posterior and somewhat caudad to the aortic valve. The inflow tract extends from the valve along the posterior wall of the left ventricle and posterior half of the septum to the apex. The outflow tract is anterior and extends from the apex along the anterior half of the septum and anterior portion of the lateral ventricular wall. Any disease that causes an increased work load on the left ventricle may cause enlargement of this chamber. This is manifested first by elongation of the outflow tract. This produces an increase in the length of the left ventricular segment making up the left lateral cardiac contour as visualized roentgenographically. The second sign of enlargement of this tract is rounding of the contour of the left ventricle. As a result of this enlargement downward and to the left, the cardiac apex may extend below the dome of the diaphragm. Enlargement of the inflow tract of the left ventricle, which follows that of the outflow tract, produces posterior enlargement best outlined on the roentgenogram obtained in the left anterior oblique projection. This posterior enlargement has led to the use of the angle of clearance between the left ventricle and spine in the left anterior oblique position as a criterion for left ventricular enlargement. The angle of clearance of the left ventricle is the angle through which the patient must be rotated to his right from the posteroanterior position into the left anterior (or right posterior) oblique position to clear the posterior silhouette of the left ventricle from the thoracic spine. The angle is measured at the point where these structures do not quite overlap. There is so much normal variation, however, that the specific angle of 55 degrees, which is often quoted, is very likely too high in some individuals and too low in others. In addition to the enlargement downward and to the left as well as posteriorly, disease resulting in increased left ventricular work may result in concentric hypertrophy of this chamber. This indicates that the ventricle is hypertrophied without significant dilatation so that there is very little actual enlargement. The hypertrophy is manifested roentgenographically by rounding of the left ventricular contour and apex as visualized in the frontal projection. Enlargement of the left ventricle is demonstrated in the posteroanterior, lateral, and left anterior oblique projections.

The most marked enlargement of the left ventricle is caused by hypertension and aortic insufficiency.

Other lesions that produce enlargement of this chamber are aortic stenosis, mitral insufficiency, coarctation of the aorta, arteriovenous shunts that may be intracardiac or extracardiac, arteriosclerotic cardiovascular disease, and hyperthyroidism.

RIGHT VENTRICULAR ENLARGEMENT

The right ventricle is enlarged in persons having diseases that increase the work of this chamber. These diseases include a number of pulmonary diseases as well as primary vascular disease in the pulmonary arteries that results in pulmonary hypertension. Stenosis of the pulmonary valve or infundibulum and other congenital cardiac lesions, such as truncus arteriosus and septal defects, may also result in enlargement of this ventricle. Mitral valvular disease is also a common cause. When enlargement occurs, the outflow tract is the site of the earliest dilatation. This extends from the apex of the right ventricle to the pulmonic valve and includes the anterior wall along with the upper half of the interventricular septum. The inflow tract that extends from the tricuspid valve to the apex includes the lower half of the interventricular septum, the disphragmatic wall of this ventricle inferiorly, and the lower part of its outer wall anteriorly. Enlargement of the outflow tract of the right ventricle results in lengthening of the anterior ventricular wall, which is manifested radiographically by prominence of the distal right ventricle or pulmonary conus, resulting in an anterior bulge in the upper anterior cardiac contour just below the pulmonary artery noted in the right anterior oblique projection. There is often associated enlargement of the pulmonary artery, which adds to the anterior prominence of the upper border of the heart in this projection. When this occurs there is more prominence and convexity of the pulmonary artery segment in the frontal projection than is normal. This results in straightening or convexity of the left upper cardiac contour below the aortic knob. When the enlargement of the right ventricle becomes greater, the heart tends to be rotated to the left (counterclockwise as viewed from the front) so that the conus of the right ventricle may become border-forming, and in the right anterior oblique projection the anterolateral bulge in the region of the outflow tract of the right ventricle reduces the size of the retrosternal space between the upper cardiac border and the sternum. The pulmonary artery also contributes to this narrowing. There is also noted a fullness superiorly in the retrosternal space in the lateral projection. When the inflow tract of the right ventricle enlarges, the diaphragmatic portion of this ventricle is increased in length and this results in an anterior rounding or bulge in the right ventricular area as visualized in the left anterior oblique projection. This enlargement may also displace the left ventricle posteriorly and elevate the cardiac apex. The latter is a common finding in infants and children with congenital cardiac disease resulting in right ventricular enlargement. When right ventricular dilatation is associated with enlargement of the left ventricle, the differentiation and evaluation of the relative size of each chamber are often very difficult to make.

LEFT ATRIAL ENLARGEMENT

Rheumatic mitral valvular disease has been the most common cause of left atrial enlargement. It also occurs in other diseases such as congenital cardiac lesions resulting in intracardiac shunts, and in left ventricular failure. The left atrium lies posteriorly and does not form any part of the cardiac contour as visualized in the frontal projection in the normal subject. Small amounts of enlargement are often entirely posterior and the earliest radiologic sign is displacement of the esophagus posteriorly and slightly to the right. This can be demonstrated on a chest film exposed following the oral administration of barium to outline the esophagus. In the normal person, the esophagus is relatively straight as visualized in this right anterior oblique projection and a small amount of atrial enlargement produces a localized posterior bulge in the region of the atrium that lies just below the level of the carina. As this chamber becomes larger, it enlarges to the right and left as well as posteriorly. The left auricular appendage may then project beyond the left ventricle to produce a localized convexity or straightening of the left cardiac border just below the pulmonary artery segment. The atrial appendage is usually relatively larger in patients with rheumatic heart disease than in those with comparable left atrial enlargement secondary to other diseases. This enlargement causes the contour change often termed the "mitral silhouette" in which the appendage produces a considerable convexity of the left upper cardiac margin just below the level of the pulmonary artery. The enlargement to the right may be sufficient to make the right border of this chamber extend beyond the upper aspect of the right atrium and the superior vena cava, resulting in a double contour on the right as visualized in the frontal projection. There may also be a visible double contour on the right when the left atrium does not project beyond the right atrial border. This is caused by the increased density of the large left atrium. Elevation of the left main bronchus may also be visible and when the enlargement reaches this stage, the mass of this chamber is often large enough to produce an oval localized density that can be seen through the heart in the frontal projection. When enlargement is massive, the left atrium may form most of the right cardiac contour and part of the left upper cardiac contour in the frontal projection. Rarely the left atrium projects only to the left when it enlarges. In the left anterior oblique projection, enlargement of the left atrium produces a posterior bulge just below the left main bronchus. This is a relatively constant and sensitive indicator of enlargement of this chamber provided that the proper obliquity of approximately 45 degrees is obtained.

Westcott and Ferguson have described a method for measuring left atrial size on lateral films. This method depends on clear visualization of the right pulmonary artery since it relies upon a line drawn downward from the anterior wall of the right pulmonary artery parallel to the barium-filled esophagus. The anteroposterior diameter is measured from this line to the anterior esophageal wall. The anterior wall of the right pulmonary artery indicates the level of the anterior wall of the left atrium and the anterior esophageal wall outlines the posterior atrial margin. Westcott and Ferguson found the normal diameter of the left atrium to be in a range of 25 to 42 mm for men 25 years of age and 17 to 38 mm for women of the same age. The male mean is 30.04 plus or minus 3.9 mm and the female mean is 28 plus or minus 3.9 mm. This correlated well with echocardiographic measurements in the study.[67]

A method for measuring the left atrial diameter on the frontal film has been described by Higgins and associates.[27] In this method, measurement is made from the midpoint of the curvilinear margin of the double density produced by the left atrium on the right side to the midpoint of the inferior wall of the left bronchus. By this method the diameter of the left atrium was found to be less than 7 cm in 96% of normal persons and greater than 7 cm in 90% of patients with left atrial enlargement as determined on echocardiography. The method is not very reliable in children, however. It is simple to obtain and permits comparison of left atrial size in patients with mitral valvular disease. Measurements were not corrected for magnification.

RIGHT ATRIAL ENLARGEMENT

The right atrium is enlarged in atrial septal defect, tricuspid stenosis and insufficiency, and in right ventricular failure. The right auricular appendage enlarges first and enlargement of the right atrium can be suspected when there is a bulge or prominence in the right atrial segment in the left anterior oblique projection. This bulge represents the auricular appendage and occasionally enlargement of this appendage produces actual angulation between it and the right ventricle in the left oblique projection. When the body of the atrium enlarges, it produces enlargement of the lower right cardiac contour to the right with increased convexity of this contour. Marked increase of this chamber produces great enlargement to the right in the frontal projection and a local prominence to the right and posteriorly as visualized in the right anterior oblique projection. In this view the local enlargement lies just above the diaphragm and below the area in which the left atrium is visible when it is increased in size. Slight enlargement of the right atrium is very difficult to detect radiographically, particularly when other chambers are enlarged as in severe rheumatic valvular disease with chronic congestive failure.

CONGENITAL HEART DISEASE

Accurate diagnosis of the nature of congenital cardiac malformations is now imperative because surgical techniques are available for the cure of a number of lesions and palliation of others. The radiographic methods are a very important part of the examination of patients with congenital defects, but accurate diagnosis depends upon correleation of all clinical and laboratory findings. There are wide variations in the roentgen findings in any single defect because of the wide range of severity of single or multiple defects. For example, septal defects may be small and produce little shunting of blood and very little alteration in the appearance of the cardiovascular silhouette; they may be very large and accompanied by a large shunt and marked changes in the cardiovascular silhouette. The same is true of the defects that produce cyanosis and a broad spectrum of physiologic and anatomic alteration is possible for each defect. The typical findings in the various defects will be described. The differential diagnosis of many of these lesions is difficult to make and it is helpful to classify the defects into those that produce cyanosis and those that do not. These can then be subdivided according to the radiographic appearance of the pulmonary vessels and to the presence or absence of cardiac enlargement. These differentiations are listed in Table 32-1. By using this approach, each defect can be placed in a relatively small group and special studies can then be made to differentiate the members of that group. Comprehensive review of all con-

Table 32-1.   Common Congenital Cardiac Defects

CYANOTIC	NONCYANOTIC
Increased pulmonary vascularity	
Transposition of great vessels	Patent ductus arteriosus
Patent ductus (malignant) with reversed flow	Interventricular septal defect
Eisenmenger's complex	Interatrial septal defect
Interatrial septal defect with reversed flow	Lutembacher's syndrome
Decreased pulmonary vascularity	
Tetralogy of Fallot	
Truncus arteriosus	Ebstein's anomaly
Pulmonary stenosis plus interatrial septal defect	
Tricuspid atresia	
Ebstein's anomaly	
Normal pulmonary vascularity	
	Coarctation of the aorta
	Pulmonary stenosis—occasionally
	Aortic stenosis
	Endocardial fibroelastosis
	Ebstein's anomaly
Heart enlarged	
Transposition of great vessels	
Eisenmenger's complex	Coarctation (infantile type in failure)
Truncus arteriosus	Interatrial septal defect
Tricuspid atresia	Interventricular septal defect
Pulmonary stenosis with interatrial septal defect	Fibroelastosis
Ebstein's anomaly	
Heart not enlarged or slightly enlarged	
Tetralogy of Fallot	Patent ductus
Tricuspid atresia	Pulmonary stenosis
	Aortic stenosis
Variable	
	Interatrial septal defect
	Interventricular septal defect

genital defects is not within the scope of this volume. Selective angiocardiography is the most useful radiologic method for the diagnosis of the congenital cardiac diseases.

CYANOTIC DEFECTS

Tetralogy of Fallot

The tetralogy of Fallot consists of two fundamental defects: (1) pulmonic stenosis and (2) high interventricular septal defect. The third and fourth alterations described in this tetralogy are secondary to these and consist of the aorta overriding the ventricular septum with dextro-position, and hypertrophy of the right ventricle. The pulmonic stenosis causes an elevation of pressure in the right ventricle; the septal defect and overriding of the aorta allow blood from the right ventricle (venous blood) to be shunted directly into the general circulation. This right-to-left shunt from the right ventricle into the aorta results in cyanosis owing to unsaturation of the arterial blood. In addition to the abnormalities originally de-scribed, other anomalies often occur in combination. The most common is a patent foramen ovale. True atrial septal defect is less common; when this defect is present, the term "pentalogy of Fallot" is sometimes used. A right-sided aortic arch is present in about 25% of patients with tetralogy. Extracardiac anomalies consisting of malformations of the aortic arch system are also common. Rarely, such abnormalities as stenosis of peripheral pulmonary arteries, partial anomalous venous return, absence or hypoplasia of the pulmonary valve, persistent common atrioventricular canal, and tricuspid insufficiency may be associated with tetralogy of Fallot. The pulmonic stenosis is usually infundibular in type. The infundibulum is usually constricted into a long, narrow channel and there may be an associated valvular stenosis. Valvular stenosis alone is unusual in tetralogy, however. When this occurs there may be some poststenotic dilatation of the pulmonary artery that alters the configuration of the left cardiovascular border. Occasionally the stenosis is localized to the proximal infundibulum, the ostium infundibuli. When this occurs the infundibulum dilates to a greater or lesser extent, forming a "third" ventricle. The degree of stenosis varies from a very slight narrowing to pulmonary atresia. In the latter instance, which is very rare, the aorta forms a pseudotruncus and the pulmonary blood supply is through the bronchial arteries or through a patent ductus arteriosus and pulmonary arteries. The roentgenographic findings vary with the degree of pulmonic stenosis and the amount of shunt.

Roentgen Findings.

Heart Size. The heart is usually within the normal limits of size and may appear to be somewhat smaller than the average normal. Appreciable cardiac enlargement in this condition is unusual unless the patient survives into adult life. The right ventricle hypertrophies, but usually does not dilate.

Pulmonary Artery. The pulmonary artery segment, as visualized in the frontal projection, is small and this results in concavity of the upper left cardiac margin in the region of this segment. The degree of concavity is dependent upon the degree of stenosis and varies from marked concavity to a pulmonary artery segment that cannot be distinguished from the normal. In the occasional patient with stenosis of the ostium infundibuli the dilated infundibulum may produce a convexity in the left side of the heart border at and just below the level of the left main bronchus, which represents the distal right ventricle. When poststenotic dilatation of the pulmonary artery is present, in patients with valvular stenosis, there is slight convexity rather than concavity in the region of this artery.

Pulmonary Vascularity. There is a decrease in pulmonary vascularity, resulting in decrease in the size of the vessels making up the hilum on both sides, and relative avascularity of the lung fields. This is an indication of decreased pulmonary bloodflow. In severe stenosis and in patients with pseudotruncus, the branching of the dilated bronchial arteries may produce a brushlike appearance, with small vessels of uniform caliber in contrast to the decreasing caliber of pulmonary arteries usually noted. In patients with minimal defects resulting in the so-called "acyanotic" tetralogy, the vascularity is normal or nearly so.

Heart Shape. The enlargement of the right ventricle results in elevation of the apex and a rounded configuration of the lower left cardiac margin. In the left anterior oblique projection the right ventricular enlargement produces rounding of the anterior cardiac contour and, when the enlargement is great, the left ventricle is elevated and displaced posteriorly so that the left or posterior cardiac border has a convex prominence in its central portion well above the diaphragm. This represents the left ventricle in an abnormal position, sometimes termed the "left ventricular cap." There is also noted unusual radiolucency in the region of the pulmonary artery that lies below and within the arch of the aorta. This is sometimes termed the "aortic window." In the right anterior oblique projection there may be rounding of the anterior cardiac contour in the region of the right ventricle, with decrease in the region of the distal pulmonary outflow tract and pulmonary artery segment. In the lateral view there is anterior and upward bulging of the heart, tending to fill the retrosternal space superiorly.

The Aorta. The findings in the right aortic arch that occur in approximately 25% of patients consist of absence of aortic shadow on the left and presence of a vascular shadow on the right at the aortic level. This is readily detected in adults and in older children, but in infants the aortic arch may not be visible. The superior vena cava is displaced laterally, however, and the resulting convex density in the right upper mediastinum may suggest the aortic position. Sometimes barium in the esophagus is helpful along with visualization of the trachea, where an indentation on the right may identify the site of the aortic arch. The aorta is enlarged in rough proportion to the amount of right-to-left shunt.

Other Findings. Occasionally there is poststenotic dilatation of the main pulmonary artery, as has been indicated, so that the pulmonary artery is normal or slightly larger than normal. Also the presence of a "third" ventricle may alter the silhouette as noted previously. It is apparent then that the appearance of the heart in tetralogy varies from one in which there is very little deviation from the normal to one in which there is marked alteration (Figs. 32-7 through 32-9).

Angiocardiography. Angiocardiography outlines the right ventricle and shows immediate filling of the aorta from the right ventricle, often with little if any shunt into the left ventricle. The site of stenosis is usually outlined, particularly in the right anterior oblique or lateral view. Pulmonary artery size is also defined.

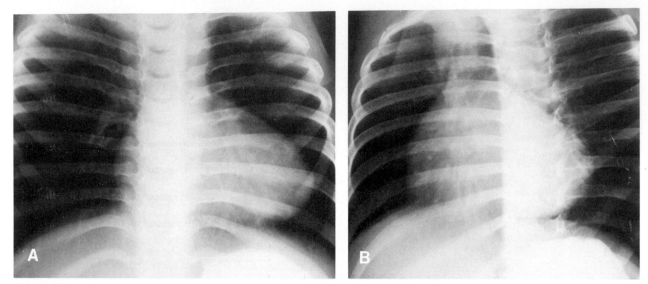

Fig. 32-7. Tetralogy of Fallot. Severe tetralogy in a 6-month-old child. Note the concavity in the left upper cardiac border, the elevation of the apex, and the relative avascularity of the hila and lung fields **(A)**. The left anterior oblique projection **(B)** shows the prominence of the chambers of the right side of the heart as well as the elevation of the apex and the avascularity.

Fig. 32-8. Tetralogy of Fallot. Moderately severe tetralogy in an 11-year-old child. Note the round apex and the prominence of the right border of the heart in the left anterior oblique projection. The diminution of vascularity is minimal.

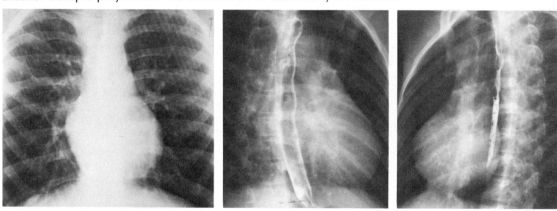

Pulmonary Stenosis with Intact Ventricular Septum and Atrial Right-to-Left Shunt (Trilogy of Fallot)

In this entity the atrial defect is usually a patent foramen ovale. Cyanosis appears when right atrial pressure has increased enough to cause a right-to-left shunt through the patent foramen ovale or atrial sep-tal defect. This often occurs early in life but may be delayed.

Roentgen Findings

Heart Size. The heart is moderately to markedly en-larged, with elevation of the apex indicating right ventricular enlargement. The aorta is usually normal in size and the arch is on the left side.

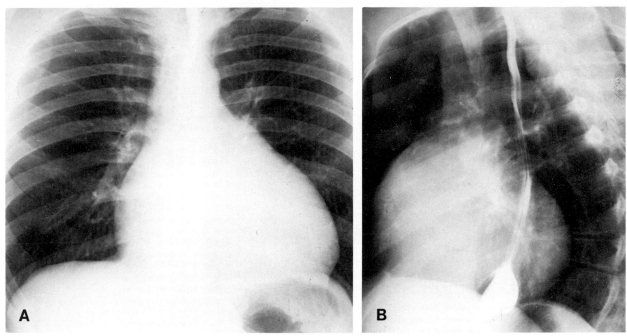

Fig. 32-9. Tetralogy of Fallot in a man, age 35, with moderate cyanosis. **A.** Note that the heart is enlarged but the hilar vessels are small, and there is scanty vascularity in the lungs. There is no concavity in the region of the main pulmonary artery. **B.** In this left anterior oblique projection, the marked prominence of the cardiac silhouette anteriorly indicates the massive enlargement of the right side of the heart.

Pulmonary Artery. Poststenotic dilatation of the main and left pulmonary artery results in prominence of the pulmonary artery segment in the frontal and oblique projections but is not always present. Poststenotic dilatation occurs with valvular stenosis, which usually occurs in this condition. Infundibular stenosis may result as a secondary change when muscular hypertrophy occurs in the infundibulum, or it may be primarily responsible for the high right ventricular pressure which occurs in an estimated 10% of patients. If stenosis is of infundibular type, there is a small pulmonary artery distal to the narrowing (Fig. 32-10).

Pulmonary Vascularity. Pulmonary vascularity tends to be decreased but may appear normal when the stenosis is not marked.

Heart Shape. The silhouette is that of right atrial and right ventricular enlargement; poststenotic dilatation results in prominence of the pulmonary artery. The left atrium may be enlarged. The apex is elevated and

the right ventricle prominent in the left anterior oblique and frontal projections.

Angiocardiography. Angiocardiography is a valuable examination in this condition and films exposed in rapid succession after caval or right atrial injection will show the defect at the atrial level, with a jet of opaque material propelled through the defect rapidly filling the left atrium, left ventricle and then the aorta. This results in rapid opacification of the left atrium and ventricle along with opacification of the right chambers and simultaneous, or nearly simultaneous, opacification of the pulmonary artery and aorta. The pulmonary stenosis may be directly visible in some cases. The poststenotic dilatation frequently present is also readily recognized on the angiocardiogram. Selective right ventricular injection is best to show the enlarged right ventricle associated with muscular hypertrophy. The pulmonary valve is usually thickened and often dome-shaped, with a jet of opaque medium crossing the valve into a moderately dilated pulmonary artery. The infundibulum is

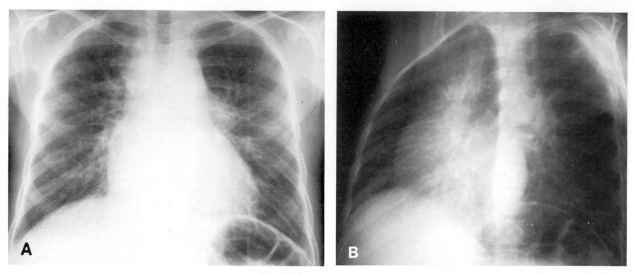

Fig. 32-10. Pulmonary stenosis with interatrial septal defect. The stenosis was severe, and the lungs were supplied by bronchial arteries to a great extent. This accounts for the absence of normal hilar vessels noted particularly on the right. The brushlike arteries that are present represent bronchial arteries which supplied the lungs. Frontal **(A)** and left anterior oblique **(B)** projections.

long and smooth and shows rather marked change in diameter from systole to diastole in contrast to the findings in tetralogy of Fallot.

Complete Transposition of the Great Vessels

The relative positions of the pulmonary artery and the aorta are reversed in complete transposition. This would result in two closed circulations because the blood from the lungs enters the left atrium by way of the pulmonary veins and goes from there into the left ventricle and through the pulmonary artery back to the lungs. The systemic venous return enters the right atrium, goes into the right ventricle, and out through the aorta back into the systemic circulation. Since this situation is incompatible with life, complete transposition must be accompanied by other anomalies allowing intra- or extracardiac shunts. These consist of patent ductus arteriosus and interatrial and interventricular septal defects. Ventricular septal defect occurs in less than one-half of patients while some type of interatrial defect is usually present. It may be a small atrial septal defect or a patent foramen ovale. The ductus arteriosus may be patent. Rarely, anomalous pulmonary venous return shunts blood from the lungs to the right side of the heart.

This anomaly is more frequent in males than females in a ratio of two or four to one. Prognosis is poor, with an estimated 90% mortality in the first year of life.

Roentgen Findings. *Heart Size.* The heart is usually normal or nearly normal in size at birth and for the first 2 weeks of life. Then increasing size leads to definite enlargement in most patients in a few weeks. Nearly all of these infants have enlargement by the age of 2 months.

Heart Shape. Both ventricles are enlarged and the general contour of the heart is oval or egg-shaped. The right ventricle is usually enlarged to a greater extent than the left. The shape of the heart in the lateral and left anterior oblique positions tends to be round, and as the obliquity is increased, the vascular pedicle tends to become larger in its transverse diameter. In the frontal projection, however, the base usually produced by the great vessels is narrow. Furthermore, the absence of normal thymic tissue accentuates this finding. The thymus may also be small or absent in other severe congenital heart conditions and in infants with severe, stressful, noncardiac disease.

Pulmonary Artery and Aorta. There is narrowing of the shadow of the great vessels in the frontal projection, the result of a more anteroposterior course of the aorta that arises anteriorly and tends to course directly backward. This produces a widening of the shadow of the great vessels in the oblique projections, because the vessels that are superimposed in the frontal projection are separated by the obliquity. Since the pulmonary infundibulum is not normally formed and the pulmonary artery lies nearer the midline than normal, the convexity usually formed by the infundibulum and pulmonary artery is not present, and in some instances a distinct concavity is noted in the left upper cardiac border. The outline of the aortic arch is absent. (Fig. 32-11.)

Pulmonary Vascularity. Pulmonary vessels are enlarged and prominent and may pulsate in a hyperactive manner as visualized fluoroscopically. Occasionally there is pulmonic stenosis associated with transposition. This results in a decrease in size of the pulmonary vessels. Because the heart is not as large and the contour is not abnormal, the diagnosis of transposition with pulmonic stenosis may be very difficult to make.

Angiocardiography. Venous angiocardiographic findings consist of filling sequentially of the right atrium, the right ventricle, and of an anteriorly placed aorta from the right ventricle. There is usually very poor opacification of the pulmonary artery and the shunt that makes this condition compatible with life may be visualized. If an atrial septal defect is present it is usually apparent, with rapid opacification of the left atrium. Patent ductus may be demonstrated. Interventricular septal defect is very difficult to define. The enlargement of the right-sided heart chambers can also be noted on the angiocardiogram. There tends to be some difference in relationship of the great vessels, ranging from a pulmonary artery that lies posterior and slightly to the left of the aorta to one which lies directly posterior or rarely directly to the left of the aorta.

Selective, right-ventricular angiocardiography is somewhat more satisfactory than a venous injection, particularly in outlining ventricular septal defect and the pulmonary artery.

Tricuspid Atresia

Tricuspid atresia with hypoplasia or aplasia of the right ventricle is associated with several other malformations in order that circulation may be sustained. The tricuspid valve is atretic and there is hypoplasia or absence of the right ventricle. Edwards and associates[12] classify these anomalies based on the relationship of great vessels and the presence or absence of pulmonary stenosis. In type I the great vessels are normally related and there are: (*1*) coexistent tricuspid and pulmonary atresia; (*2*) a narrow

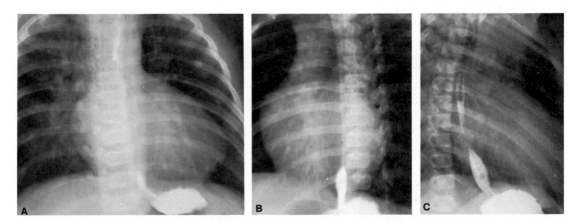

Fig. 32-11. Transposition of the great vessels. **A.** Frontal projection. **B.** Left anterior oblique projection. **C.** Right anterior oblique projection. There is cardiac enlargement. The large pulmonary vessels are best seen in the right hilum and central lung. The apex is elevated, indicating right ventricular enlargement. The vascular pedicle is narrow in the frontal projection and broad in both oblique views. This is characteristic of transposition.

septal defect between the left ventricle and the infundibular portion of the right ventricle, a small vestigial right ventricle, and a small pulmonary artery (this is the most common form); or (3) a large interventricular septal defect with valvular stenosis and normal pulmonary artery. Rarely, transposition of great vessels occurs in this form. In type II, transposition of the great vessels without pulmonic stenosis occurs, and there is essentially a common ventricle. Rarely, this anomaly is found without transposition. As indicated, in type I there is some type of right ventricular or pulmonary artery obstruction. In these patients, an atrial septal defect is present so that the blood flows into the right atrium, is shunted across the septal defect to the left atrium, and then to the left ventricle. The blood is then distributed to the lungs by way of an interventricular septal defect and hypoplastic right ventricle through the pulmonary artery to the lungs. If the right ventricle or pulmonary artery is atretic, then the blood must get to the lungs by way of a patent ductus.

Tricuspid Atresia with Pulmonary Stenosis

Roentgen Findings. *Heart Size.* The heart is usually enlarged, but there is considerable variation; at times the enlargement is slight and in others it is marked.

Heart Shape. The heart is often boot-shaped and may resemble the silhouette of tetralogy of Fallot. The right heart border is relatively straight or flat and may not extend to the right of the spine. The pulmonary artery segment is concave. The left atrium may be enlarged; when enlargement is present this is a helpful diagnostic sign. The right atrium is usually somewhat enlarged and may be markedly enlarged. Evidence of left ventricular preponderance on the electrocardiogram is often necessary to make certain that the left ventricle is enlarged, because right ventricular enlargement can rotate the heart and produce a similar silhouette. The left side of the heart border is rounded with apparent elevation of the apex, simulating the elevation associated with right ventricular enlargement. The change in the contour of the heart commonly described to indicate absence or hypoplasia of the right ventricle is not often found in this condition. This change consists of diminished convexity or actual concavity of the right lower heart border in the frontal projection and of the anterior inferior border in the left anterior oblique view. The

reason for the absence of this sign is that the right atrium enlarges to the extent that it fills the deficit resulting from right ventricular absence or hypoplasia.

Pulmonary Artery. There is concavity in the region of the main pulmonary artery in the frontal projection. It may be extreme, so that the junction between the aorta and the upper left ventricular silhouette is angular.

Pulmonary Vascularity. Pulmonary vascularity is usually decreased, unless there is complete transposition of the great vessels. When that is present, vascularity is normal or increased.

The Aorta. The aorta is generally enlarged.

Angiocardiography. This examination is useful in establishing the anatomic diagnosis in tricuspid atresia. The findings are those of large right atrium below which is a triangular radiolucent notch, representing the defect caused by absence of filling of the right ventricle. A shunt from the right to the left atrium is observed, resulting in rapid opacification of the left side of the heart. The size of the pulmonary vessels is demonstrated, but the root of the pulmonary artery, the site of stenosis, and the right ventricular chamber may be difficult to outline.

Tricuspid Atresia Without Pulmonary Stenosis

As has been indicated, this form of the anomaly is usually associated with transposition of the great vessels and a common ventricle.

Roentgen findings consist of gross cardiac enlargement, narrowing of the great vessels at the base, indicating transposition, and some left atrial enlargement. Pulmonary vascularity is greatly increased. Correlation with electrocardiographic findings of left ventricular preponderance in a cyanotic child with hypervascularity is very suggestive of the diagnosis.

In patients with transposition and tricuspid atresia, the right atrial appendage may lie to the left of the aorta and the pulmonary artery and behind the great vessels. It projects above the left atrial appendage. The term "juxtaposition of the atrial appendages" is used to describe this anomaly which produces a large bulge high on the left cardiac border that is quite characteristic and suggests the diagnosis.

Tricuspid Stenosis

Congenital tricuspid stenosis is very rare and is usually combined with other congenital cardiac defects. The only consistent roentgen finding is hypovascularity of the lung fields. The enlargement of the right atrium present in these patients may not be readily recognized. In some cases, the appearance simulates that of tetralogy of Fallot. No consistent roentgen appearance has been described.

Ebstein's Anomaly

This malformation consists of downward displacement of the tricuspid valve far into the right ventricle. The upper portion of the right ventricle is incorporated into the right atrium. As a result the ventricle is small and the atrium is large. The myocardium proximal to the abnormally placed valve is thin and the large right atrium is unable to empty itself properly. Cyanosis is often present in this disease because venous blood is shunted from the right to the left atrium through an interatrial septal defect that is usually present. If there is no intracardiac shunt no cyanosis is produced.

Roentgen Findings. The heart is usually greatly enlarged and the lungs are hypovascular. The right atrium and ventricle are the chambers involved. Enlargement to the right with a shoulderlike prominence of the right upper cardiac enlargement is characteristic. There is often enlargement of the left upper cardiac contour in a more sloping manner, caused by enlargement of the outflow tract of the right ventricle. This gives the heart a square or boxlike shape with a narrow vascular pedicle and a small aortic arch (Fig. 32-12). When this is found, along with hypovascularity of the lung fields and a small aorta, the roentgen diagnosis can be made with reasonable certainty, particularly when correlated with electrocardiographic findings. Therefore, angiocardiography may not be needed. On venous angiocardiography, the large right atrium fills and empties slowly through the foramen ovale into the left atrium and through the tricuspid valve into the right ventricle. The right side of the heart remains opacified for an unusually long period of time. Selective injection of contrast medium into the right ventricle will identify the level of the tricuspid valve and will show tricuspid insufficiency when present. Occasionally there is an associated pulmonic valvular stenosis which may be defined by this examination. In these patients, there

may be a considerable right-to-left shunt manifested by marked hypovascularity. In those patients without a shunt, pulmonary vascularity is normal.

Total Anomalous Pulmonary Venous Return

In this anomaly the pulmonary veins empty into the right atrium by one of several pathways. The most common is a left innominate vein. Others empty (*1*) directly into the coronary sinus, (2) directly into the right atrium, (3) through a large vein into the right superior vena cava, (4) into a persistent left superior vena cava, (5) into the portal vein, ductus venosus or inferior vena cava below the diaphragm, or, (6) occasionally into the azygos vein or hepatic vein. The latter type occurs predominantly in males. In the patients with the persistent left superior vena cava or vertical vein the blood flows upward in this vein for a short distance to the level of the superior aspect of the aortic arch and then flows to the right, in the left innominate vein, which unites with the superior vena cava on the right. When all the pulmonary venous blood is returned to the right side of the heart, a right-to-left shunt is needed to be compatible with life. The most common anomaly is atrial septal defect or patent foramen ovale. As a result of this combination of defects, the right heart is overloaded and becomes enlarged while the left heart and aorta are relatively small. Cyanosis is usually present but may not be severe.

When the anomalous venous return is above the diaphragm, the pulmonary venous pressure is moderately increased, and minimal pulmonary edema is often present. In total anomalous venous return below the diaphragm, there is usually a greater increase in venous pressure and severe pulmonary edema is common.

Roentgen Findings. In total anomalous venous return above the diaphragm, the heart is enlarged. The enlargement is right-sided although this may not be readily apparent. Pulmonary vessels are prominent, owing to the increased bloodflow in the lesser circulation. When there is a persistent left vena cava, or left vertical vein with total anomalous pulmonary venous connection to the left innominate vein, there is characteristic figure-of-eight deformity of the cardiovascular silhouette. The upper limbs of the "eight" are formed by the vena cava on the right and the vertical vein on the left. They are dilated and form convexities on either side above the heart (Fig. 32-13). The blood flows upward in the vertical vein,

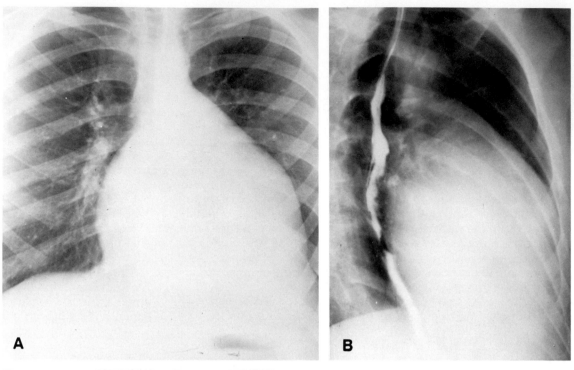

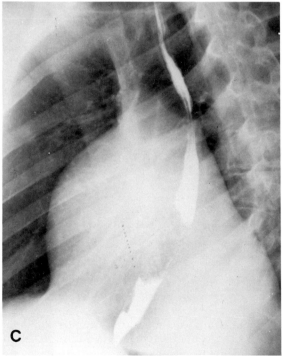

Fig. 32-12. Ebstein's anomaly. The heart is greatly enlarged. Massive enlargement of the right atrium in the left anterior oblique projection is noted. Frontal **(A)** right anterior oblique **(B),** and left anterior oblique **(C)** positions.

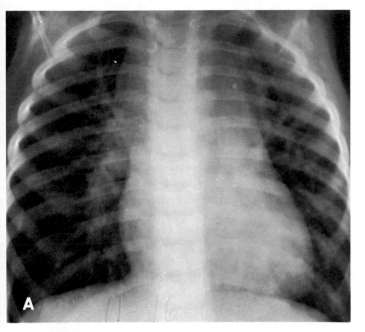

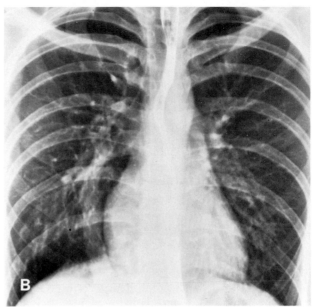

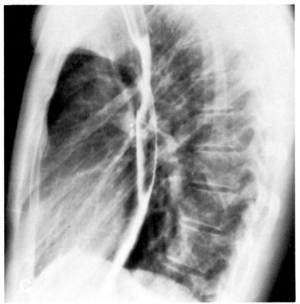

Fig. 32-13. A. Total anomalous pulmonary venous return. This is a reasonably typical example of a figure-of-eight deformity with the large veins forming a convexity on either side in the upper mediastinum. The pulmonary vascularity is not very well seen in this illustration but was distinctly increased. **B.** Partial anomalous pulmonary venous return (Scimitar syndrome). Note the hypervascularity and the large vessel paralleling the border of the right side of the heart and extending below the level of the diaphragm. **C.** This vessel is seen posteriorly. It somewhat overlies the vertebral bodies in the lower thorax. This vein emptied into the inferior vena cava. There is also an azygous fissure in this patient.

across to the right, and into the superior vena cava. In the occasional patient in whom the veins drain into the right superior or inferior vena cava, they may be visualized on the plain-film roentgenogram. Tomography will often outline the abnormal vessel to good advantage. The aorta is small and hypoplastic and the pulmonary artery is often enlarged to the extent that its upper border forms a horizontal shelf immediately below the hypoplastic aortic arch. Angiocardiography can be used to establish the diagnosis, but when the figure-of-eight is present, along with the evidence of enlargement of pulmonary vessels, the diagnosis can be made with reasonable certainty on plain films alone. The thymic shadow may produce a figure-of-eight sign and must be differentiated. This "snowman" or "figure-of-eight" is often not apparent in the first few weeks of life. The lateral view may then be helpful, since the shadow of the anomalous vertical vein or left superior vena cava is denser and has a sharper anterior border than the shadow of the thymus. Most of the other sites of return show no characteristic vascular pattern, but since there is a bidirectional shunt, cyanosis and pulmonary hypervascularity are both present. There is right-sided cardiac enlargement with no evidence of left atrial enlargement. When the anomalous venous return is into the coronary sinus, this structure dilates and may cause a local identation on the anterior aspect of the barium-filled esophagus.

Total anomalous pulmonary venous return below the diaphragm presents a different roentgen picture. The heart is usually normal in size and shape, but the lungs are abnormal. The findings are of pulmonary vascular congestion and edema. The vascular changes resemble those seen in adults with venous hypertension secondary to mitral valvular disease, except that the hilar vessels are not prominent in these infants. This association of normal-sized heart and roentgen and clinical evidence of congestive failure in a cyanotic male infant with no heart murmurs is highly suggestive of the diagnosis. Angiocardiography can then be used to demonstrate the draining vein extending below the diaphragm.

Partial Anomalous Venous Return

The most common partial anomalous venous connection is to the right atrium. This results in a left-to-right shunt of modest proportions which usually does not cause symptoms and is often found upon study of patients with atrial septal defect. Roentgen findings are similar to those of atrial septal defect and include pulmonary arterial enlargement and hypervascularity related to the size of the shunt. A rare combination of hypoplasia of the right lung and anomalous right pulmonary venous return into the inferior vena cava is termed the "scimitar syndrome" because the anomalous vein is visible as a curved shadow in the right lower lung. There may also be other associated anomalies such as accessory diaphragm, sequestration, and hepatic herniations. The term "congenital pulmonary venolobar syndrome" has been used to describe this combination of anomalies, some of which may be absent in a given patient.

Partial anomalous drainage of the left upper lobe may be by way of an anomalous vertical vein that produces a left paramediastinal density lateral to the aortic knob with a smooth, curvilinear border outlined against the lung. This appearance is similar to that of the left side of the "snowman" sign observed in total anomalous pulmonary venous return, but the anomaly causes no symptoms and the finding is often incidental. Tomography may be used for better definition of the density.

Persistent Truncus Arteriosus

There are four types of this rare anomaly in which there is only one large arterial trunk that overrides the ventricular septum. The pulmonary artery may arise (type I) as a branch of the common trunk. This is the most common type (48%) and carries the worst prognosis. A second form consists of separate origin of pulmonary arteries from the dorsal wall of the truncus (29%). In a third form, one or both pulmonary arteries arise independently from either side of the truncus (11%). In these anomalies, the pulmonary vascularity is usually increased. A fourth form consists of absence of the pulmonary artery with a truncus arteriosus that supplies the lungs by way of the bronchial arteries or other collateral vessels (12%). There is marked decrease in pulmonary vascularity in this type.

Roentgen Findings. The truncus is usually large and produces a convexity in the region of the ascending arch. There is often prominence of the peripheral pulmonary vessels despite a concavity in the region of the main pulmonary artery. The heart is usually enlarged. Right ventricular enlargement predominates, resulting in elevation of the cardiac apex that may be striking, so that the silhouette resembles that of severe tetralogy of Fallot except that it tends to be larger in truncus. In the fourth type and in pseudotruncus the ascending aortic arch is prominent and the pulmonary artery segment is concave, and the pulmonary vascularity is markedly diminished and the bronchial arteries that supply the lungs are visualized as small vessels extending outward in a fine brushlike pattern from the hila on both sides. The comma-shaped pattern of the pulmonary arteries is absent in these patients. The shape of the heart is often significant in the frontal position. There is a sharp right-angled junction between the vascular pedicle on the left and the upper left ventricular border, or an acute angle may be present. Right aortic arch is present in about 25% of these patients. Angiocardiography demonstrates opacification of the large truncus from the large right ventricle and shows the pulmonary artery filling after the truncus has filled. In the fourth type and in pseudotruncus the appearance is similar to that in severe tetralogy on the angiocardiogram.

OTHER CYANOTIC DEFECTS

Transposition of the Taussig–Bing Type

This is a variant of transposition in which the aorta arises from the right ventricle while the pulmonary artery overrides the ventricular septum. A high ventricular septal defect is present. When this defect is above the crista supraventricularis and is closely applied to the origin of the pulmonary trunk, it represents the Taussig–Bing type of transposition. Another type is one in which the ventricular septal defect is below the crista supraventricularis, remote from the pulmonary valve. In the latter, the left ventricular bloodstream is directed toward the aorta, while in the Taussig–Bing type the left ventricular bloodstream is directed to the pulmonary artery. This results in enlargement of the right ventricle and atrium. The pulmonary artery is dilated but its branches are often diminished in size as compared to the large main vessels. This is the result of vascular changes that cause pulmonary hypertension.

Roentgen Findings. There is cardiac enlargement, primarily owing to the enlarged right ventricle. This is associated with enlargement of the pulmonary artery segment and hilar vessels. The midzone pulmonary vascular channels may be full but become small when pulmonary hypertension develops. There may be left atrial and left ventricular enlargement as well. On plain films the two types cannot be differentiated. In the Taussig–Bing type, angiocardiography shows immediate filling of the aorta from the right ventricle with relatively poor filling of the pulmonary artery and its branches from this chamber. The pulmonary trunk is wider than the aorta. The aortic and pulmonary valves are at the same horizontal level and are superimposed in the lateral view.

When the septal defect is below the crista supraventricularis there is better filling of the pulmonary artery from the right ventricle. The valves are on the same horizontal plane or the pulmonary valve may be slightly higher than the aortic. Similar lateral superimposition is noted.

Congenital Heart Disease in the Neonatal Period

According to Gyepes and Vincent,[23] there are nine congenital heart lesions that commonly produce cyanosis or distress in the first 2 weeks of life that may be life-threatening and require emergency diagnostic studies. They are: (1) pulmonary atresia or severe pulmonic stenosis with intact ventricular septum; (2) pulmonary atresia or severe pulmonic stenosis with ventricular septal defect; (3) Ebstein's malformation; (4) tricuspid atresia; (5) transposition of the great arteries; (6) syndrome of coarctation of the aorta; (7) total anomalous pulmonary venous return with obstruction; (8) hypoplastic left heart syndrome; and (9) severe coarctation of the aorta. These lesions are grouped into three categories related to cardiovascular pathophysiology. Group I is characterized by decreased pulmonary blood flow; pulmonary atresia, tricuspid atresia, Ebstein's malformation, and pulmonary atresia with ventricular septal defect are included in this group. Intense cyanosis occurs early and usually, in this group of patients, there is a severe hypoplastic right ventricle incapable of dilatation. About 20% have a normal right ventricle which, however, is dilated; and when the right ventricle is dilated the right atrium may also be dilated. Group II consists of lesions with increased blood flow; transposition of the great arteries and the syndrome of coarctation of the aorta are included in this group. Group III consists of lesions with severe pulmonary venous congestion; this group includes total anomalous venous return, hypoplastic left heart, and severe coarctation with intact ventricular septum. In the coarctation syndrome in which there is a ventricular septal defect associated with severe coarctation, the ventricular shunt volume becomes greater than in patients with isolated ventricular septal defect, and failure typically occurs when the patient is under 2 weeks of age.

The chest roentgenogram in the posteroanterior projection may be very helpful, particularly in differentiating the groups. In group I, in which decreased pulmonary blood flow results in decreased vascularity, it is likely that the patient has pulmonary atresia, severe stenosis, or Ebstein's anomaly. If gross enlargement of the right atrium can be detected, Ebstein's anomaly is likely. If the heart is only moderately enlarged or normal, the combination of pulmonary atresia or stenosis plus ventricular septal defect, or pulmonary atresia or stenosis with intact ventricular septum and a hypoplastic right ventricle is likely.

In tricuspid atresia, the heart may be normal or slightly enlarged. In some instances, there is discrete enlargement of the right atrium in these patients.

In the second group in which there is normal or moderately increased pulmonary arterial pattern, transposition of the great arteries or coarctation syndrome are the most likely. If the heart is oval or egg-shaped, transposition is likely, while infants with coaractation syndrome have a combination of a large heart, increased pulmonary blood flow, plus some degree of pulmonary venous congestion. Identification of the site of the coarctation is usually not possible in this age group.

In the third group in which there is cardiomegaly and pulmonary venous congestion, it is likely that the infant has either severe coarctation of the aorta or some form of the hypoplastic left-heart syndrome. When the heart is normal or slightly enlarged in these infants with pulmonary venous congestion, it is likely that total anomalous pulmonary venous return with obstruction is present. Although these diagnoses or differentials can be suggested, the severity of the problem is such that emergency cardiac catheterization and angiocardiography are usually necessary. The procedures are usually shortened, and only crucial diagnostic information is sought.

Hypoplastic Left Heart Syndrome

This syndrome consists of hypoplasia of the left ventricle associated with a number of anomalies including aortic valvular stenosis or atresia, an atretic aortic arch, and/or mitral stenosis or atresia. As has been noted, the hypoplastic left heart syndrome is one of the causes of congestive failure in the first week of life, usually within 2 or 3 days following birth. Roentgen findings consist of progressive cardiomegaly, increased pulmonary vascularity caused by venous congestion, and a somewhat globular-appearing heart. Failure is often impossible to control, with death occurring in the first week of life.

Other Anomalies

A number of other rare anomalies may be associated with cyanosis. They include the trilocular heart, the bilocular heart, atrioventricularis communis, and a number of others, often associated with obstruction to pulmonary flow. The roentgen findings are not characteristic in these conditions, but the heart is usually enlarged in all of them.

NONCYANOTIC DEFECTS

The cardiovascular anomalies to be discussed in this section consist of defects that cause left-to-right shunts under ordinary circumstances and of other anomalies, chiefly involving the valves. The shunting of blood from left to right is dependent upon the pressure gradient across the defect. The pressure is usually higher on the left side so that the shunt is maintained from left to right, but when pulmonary hypertension is caused by the lesion, the pressure in the right-sided heart chambers may exceed that on the left. Then the shunt is reversed and cyanosis or arterial unsaturation develops. The roentgen diagnosis of this group of congenital anomalies often rests in part upon differentiation between right and left ventricular enlargement. The criteria for enlargement of these chambers described in the sections on "left ventricular enlargement" and "right ventricular enlargement" may be useless in these patients because enlargement of one chamber may simulate that of another. Therefore differentiation cannot be made on plain-film study alone and radiographic findings must be correlated with clinical, electrocardiographic, angiocardiographic, and catheterization data. In patients with left-to-right intracardiac shunts, pulmonary inflammatory disease is common. Obstruction with lobular, segmental, and even lobar atelectasis may be found. These findings may be of significance when the cardiac silhouette does not suggest the type of congenital anomaly. The large pulmonary artery associated with left-to-right shunts plus a large left atrium may cause complete atelectasis of the left lung. The bronchus is evidently compressed between the artery and the atrium in these cases. The result is a small, opaque, left hemithorax.

Patent Ductus Arteriosus

The ductus arteriosus serves to shunt blood into the systemic circulation from the pulmonary artery in intrauterine life and is patent at birth. Functionally the ductus apparently closes very early in life and anatomic closure is usually complete in 2 months but is sometimes delayed up to 6 months and rarely for a year. The ductus arises near the origin of the left pulmonary artery and empties into the aorta just distal to the left subclavian artery. Occasionally a right-sided ductus is found.

Roentgen Findings. The findings on the routine frontal, oblique, and lateral roentgenograms are not always diagnostic, particularly in infants and young children, and must be correlated with clinical data. The left atrium and left ventricle are enlarged and there is enlargement of the aorta proximal to the ductus. The pulmonary artery and peripheral pulmonary vessels are enlarged. The findings are roughly parallel to the amount of left-to-right shunt. In patients with small shunts, no detectable cardiovascular abnormalities may be noted radiographically.

Heart Size. Slight cardiac enlargement is present in about half the patients; in large shunts, a considerable amount of enlargement may be present.

Heart Shape. There may be enough left atrial enlargement to produce recognizable displacement of the esophagus in the right anterior oblique projection. Left ventricular enlargement is also present, causing elongation of the left border of the heart in the frontal view and rounding of the left ventricular silhouette in the left anterior oblique projection. Continued increase in pulmonary bloodflow may result in some degree of pulmonary hypertension, which in turn causes right ventricular enlargement.

Pulmonary Artery. The most consistent finding in patent ductus arteriosus is enlargement of the pulmonary artery segment. This produces convex prominence in the region of the segment in the frontal projection (Fig. 32-14).

Pulmonary Vascularity. The vascularity in the hila and lung fields is increased. Measurement of pulmonary arteries is ordinarily not very useful in the detection of enlargement since there is a wide range of normal. However, the diameter of the right descending pulmonary artery has been found to be nearly that of the trachea in children over 2 years of age.[10] When a left-to-right shunt was present, the artery diameter was never less than that of the trachea in a study of 102 children with left-to-right shunts. In 90% of a group of 112 normal children these structures measured the same or varied within 2 mm. Measurement of pulmonary arteries may be used to corroborate the subjective impression of arterial enlargement. A shunt is unlikely if the diameter of the descending artery is smaller than that of the trachea.

The Aorta. The aorta is often enlarged (Fig. 32-15). There may be a slight bulge of the left aortic wall below the prominent knob indicating minor enlargement in this region. This represents the infundibulum of the patent ductus. It is not a frequent sign in children and is not diagnostic, since similar slight convexity can occur in patients without patent ductus. Rarely there is calcification at the aortic end of the ductus in adults; it has not been reported in children. Occasionally the ductus itself is visible as a small convexity between the aortic knob or transverse arch and the pulmonary artery.

Angiocardiography. This examination is often disappointing but may show reopacification of the pulmonary artery from the aorta and slight enlargement of the left heart chambers. The demonstration of the local aortic enlargement at the site of the ductus or of a ductus diverticulum is helpful but not conclusive. A transient local defect in the opacification of the pulmonary artery at the site of the ductus, owing to a jet of nonopacified blood shunted through the ductus, is diagnostic when visualized.

Retrograde Aortography. This examination is much more useful than angiocardiography. The opaque material is injected directly into the aorta and the opacified blood traverses the ductus and outlines the pulmonary artery and its branches.

Patent Ductus with Right-to-Left Shunt

This is sometimes termed a "malignant ductus." The flow is reversed when the pulmonary arterial pressure exceeds that in the aorta. Normally the pulmonary arterial systolic pressure is much lower than systemic arterial pressure. In wide patent ductus arteriosus the pulmonary and systemic arterial pressures are equal. Equalization depends on a large-volume, left-to-right shunt. Pulmonary arterial disease may eventually develop to the point where pulmonary arterial resistance is greater than systemic resistance. When this degree of pulmonary hypertension is reached, the ductus acts as a safety valve for the lesser circulation. A right-to-left shunt is created so that cyanosis becomes apparent in the lower extremities but may not be present in the upper extremities. As a result of the pulmonary hypertension, the right ventricle becomes enlarged and the main pulmonary artery is often increased further in size along with the vessels in the hila, while the vessels in the central and peripheral lung fields are relatively small. This difference in size of proximal and peripheral pulmonary vessels is reliable only when it is unequivocal, however. There may be calcification in the pulmonary artery and aorta adjacent to the ductus as well as in the ductus in these patients. Isolated calcification in the pulmonary artery may occur in association with pulmonary valvular ste-

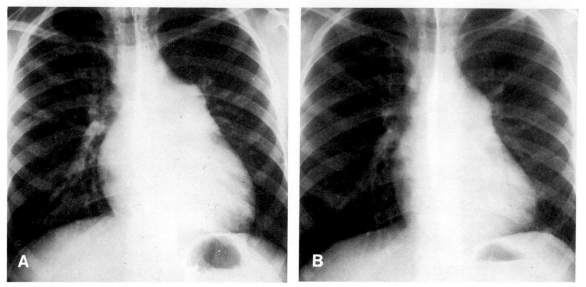

Fig. 32-14. Patent ductus arteriosus. **A.** Moderate cardiac enlargement, considerable prominence of the pulmonary artery resulting in convexity of the left upper cardiac border below the aortic arch, and hypervascularity noted best in and adjacent to the right hilum. **B.** This film obtained 1 year after ligation of the ductus shows diminution in heart size and pulmonary vascularity without much change in the size of the main pulmonary artery.

Fig. 32-15. Patent ductus arteriosus in a 12-year-old boy. The aorta is large and indents the esophagus in both frontal **(A)** and right anterior oblique **(B)** views. The main pulmonary artery is enlarged, and there is moderate hypervascularity. The slight indentation of the esophagus below the carina noted in the oblique view indicates left atrial enlargement, and there is probably a little left ventricular enlargement as well.

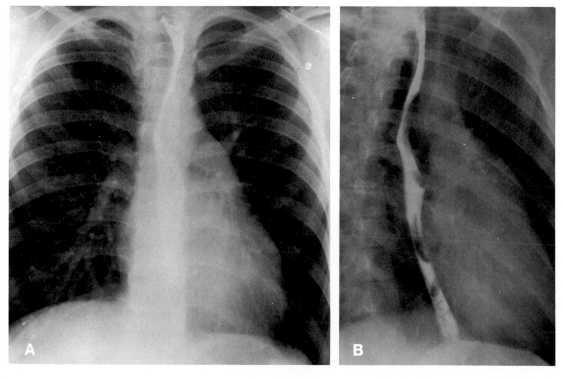

nosis, pulmonary artery aneurysm, and Eisenmenger's syndrome, as well as with patent ductus arteriosus. However, when calcification occurs in the pulmonary artery and the adjacent aortic arch, the combination is suggestive of patent ductus with or without reversal of flow.[47] This is particularly true in females younger than 40 years of age. The left atrium tends to decrease in size when the shunt is reversed in these patients with patent ductus arteriosus.

Interatrial Septal Defect

Atrial septal defects are among the most frequent congenital heart lesions. There are several types. The most common is a patent foramen ovale that is large enough to result in a shunt. When there is a defect at the fossa ovalis, it may be termed an "ostium secundum defect." Persistent ostium primum is a defect at the base of the atrial septum. There may also be a high atrial septal defect which is usually associated with anomalous pulmonary venous return from the right lung. As a result of the defect there is free communication between the two atria, permitting a shunt. The anatomic location of the defect is not as important as its size and the difference in atrial pressures; these factors determine the amount of blood shunted across the defect. Since left atrial pressure is usually higher than the pressure in the right atrium, the shunt is from left to right. As a result, the pulmonary bloodflow is increased and this increases the amount of right ventricular work.

Roentgen Findings
Heart Size. The heart is usually slightly enlarged, but may be normal in size.

Heart Shape. Enlargement of the right ventricle and atrium occurs and may be typical enough to be recognized, but differentiation between right and left ventricular enlargement is not always possible. The left atrium is not enlarged.

The Pulmonary Artery. This artery is enlarged and may be markedly increased in size, causing a large convexity that may partially obscure the smaller aortic knob. The size of the pulmonary artery segment in this anomaly is usually larger than in the other two common anomalies that produce left-to-right shunts, patent ductus arteriosus, and ventricular septal defect (Fig. 32-16).

Pulmonary Vascularity. The hilar and pulmonary vascularity is also increased.

The Aorta. The shunting of blood away from the left side of the heart into the lesser circulation results in decreased flow through the aorta. The aorta tends to be smaller than normal in size. This may readily be visualized, particularly in adults, but in infants and small children aortic size is often difficult to determine.

Angiocardiography. Angiocardiography is used occasionally to visualize the shunt and indicate its size and location.

Atrial Septal Defect with Right-to-Left Shunt

Pulmonary hypertension may occur, causing a reversal of the shunt when the right atrial pressure exceeds that in the left atrium. It is caused by organic changes in pulmonary arteries resulting in increasing vascular resistance. Arterial unsaturation occurs and cyanosis may then be observed. The right-sided heart chambers become more enlarged, particularly the right ventricle. The pulmonary artery also increases in size and there may be a marked decrease in size of peripheral pulmonary arteries, a sign of pulmonary hypertension. This may result in a considerable difference in diameter of central and peripheral pulmonary arteries.

Atrial Septal Defect with Mitral Stenosis (Lutembacher's Syndrome)

This rare condition consists of atrial septal defect combined with either congenital or acquired mitral stenosis. It results in a greater increase in right ventricular work load than does an uncomplicated atrial septal defect of similar size because the increased left atrial pressure results in an increased left-to-right shunt. It causes extreme enlargement of the pulmonary artery; this is the characteristic feature noted on the roentgenogram. The heart is generally enlarged and pulmonary vascularity is increased. The right ventricle and atrium are considerably enlarged and there may be some enlargement of the left atrium.

Angiocardiographic findings in this condition are similar to those in atrial septal defect. A jet of opaque medium crossing the plane of the septum from the left atrium to the right atrium is diagnostic of atrial septal defect. The mitral stenosis may also be demonstrated. There are other indirect angiocardiographic signs that may aid in the diagnosis. They consist of (1) enlargement of the right atrium and ventricle along with the pulmonary artery, (2) reopacification of the right side of the heart following left-sided opa-

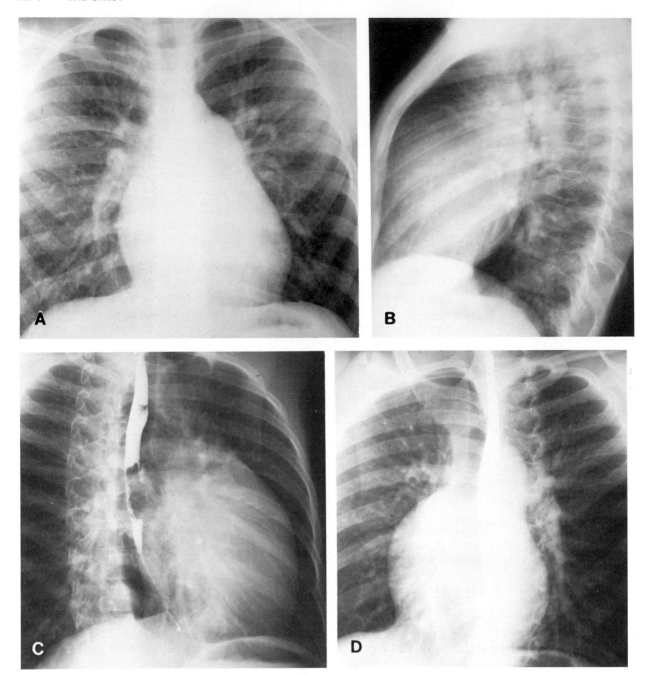

Fig. 32-16. Atrial septal defect. Note the enlargement of the right ventricle and pulmonary artery; the lung fields are hypervascular. Frontal **(A)**, lateral **(B)**, right anterior oblique **(C)**, and left anterior oblique **(D)** projections.

cification, and (3) dilution in the right atrium when a large shunt is present.

Ventricular Septal Defect

This is the most common of the congenital cardiac diseases. Defects may occur low in the septal wall but more commonly the defect is high. When the opening occurs high and adjacent to the mitral and tricuspid valves, it may involve the atrial septum and result in the defect known as atrioventricularis communis. Ventricular septal defect results in a left-to-right shunt because the left ventricular pressure is usually higher than the pressure in the right ventricle. As in the atrial septal defects, the size of the shunt is determined by the relationship of pressures on the two sides of the shunt and the size of the defect. There may be very little change in the size and shape of the heart when the defect is small and there is not much shunt. If a sizable shunt is present, there will be alterations that can be visualized on the chest roentgenogram.

Roentgen Findings. The left ventricle and left atrium are enlarged, along with the right ventricle. The right ventricle increases in size as pulmonary arterial pressure rises. It is often difficult to determine which ventricle predominates. The aorta is normal in size.

Heart Size. The heart may be normal in size but is often enlarged.

Heart Shape. Ventricular work is increased on both sides so that both ventricles may enlarge. The left ventricle often enlarges first. There may be left atrial enlargement resulting in recognizable displacement of the esophagus by this chamber in the right oblique and lateral projection (Fig. 32-17).

The Pulmonary Artery. This vessel is enlarged and prominent.

Pulmonary Vascularity. Hilar and peripheral pulmonary vascularity is increased when the shunt is large.

The Aorta. The aorta is normal in size.

Angiocardiography. Angiocardiography shows a shunt of opaque material across the defect from the left into the right ventricle. Cardiac catheterization is a reliable diagnostic method in the study of this anomaly. Selective angiocardiography can be used to localize the site of the defect.

Ventricular Septal Defect with Right-to-Left Shunt

Occlusive pulmonary vascular changes develop in patients with ventricular septal defect, leading to reversal of the shunt when the pulmonary arterial pressure exceeds the systemic pressure. The term "Eisenmenger's complex" has been used in the past to indicate this complication of shunt reversal with cyanosis developing in adolescence or in adult life.

Roentgen findings are those of cardiac enlargement, usually biventricular and moderate in amount. The pulmonary artery segment and central hilar vessels are very large, with disproportionate decrease in midzone and peripheral arteries indicating pulmonary hypertension. (Fig. 32-18). When there has been a small left-to-right shunt or a right-to-left shunt from early childhood, the heart is not as large and the arterial disproportion is minimal. In the latter type, plain-film study may reveal very minor changes or changes resembling those of isolated pulmonic stenosis.

Persistent Common Atrioventricular Canal (A–V Communis)

This defect may vary from the complete form in which there is a low atrial septal defect, a high ventricular septal defect, and clefts in mitral and tricuspid valves to a lesser form in which the tricuspid valve is normal, or one in which the ventricular septum is intact and the tricuspid valve is normal.

As in other left-to-right shunts, the roentgen findings depend upon the magnitude of the shunt and the presence or absence of pulmonary hypertension. Cardiac enlargement, usually biventricular, is present along with hilar prominence and peripheral hypervascularity. As a rule the heart is larger than in patients with atrial or ventricular septal defect. (Fig. 32-19.) There may be left atrial enlargement. The aorta tends to be small. If pulmonary hypertension develops, the changes are similar to those noted in ventricular septal defect with right-to-left shunt.

Pulmonic Stenosis

The term "pulmonis stenosis" is usually used to refer to the two types of this condition, namely, valvular and infundibular stenosis. Of the two, the former is the more frequent when pulmonary stenosis occurs as an isolated lesion. Occasionally supravalvular stenosis may occur.

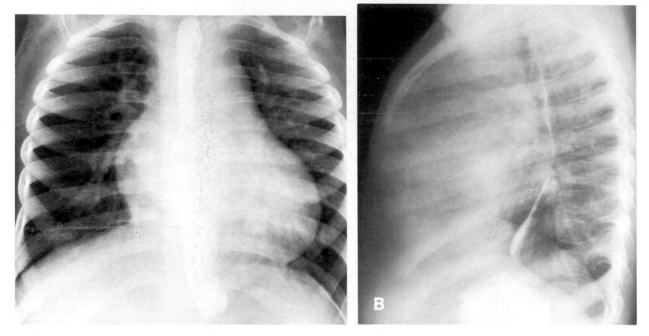

Fig. 32-17. Ventricular septal defect in a 16-month-old child. The heart is enlarged, and there is some hypervascularity in the lung fields. The posterior displacement of the mid esophagus noted in the lateral projection **(B)** indicates some left atrial enlargement. The size of the aorta is very difficult to assess in a child of this age.

Fig. 32-18. Ventricular septal defect with a right-to-left shunt and evidence of pulmonary hypertension. The heart is generally enlarged and there is great enlargement of the pulmonary artery and central hilar vessels in contrast to peripheral hypovascularity. Right ventricular enlargement is manifested by prominence of the distal right ventricle in the right anterior oblique projection **(B)** and of the right side of the heart in the left anterior oblique projection **(C)**.

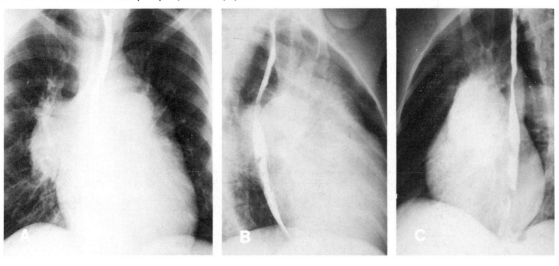

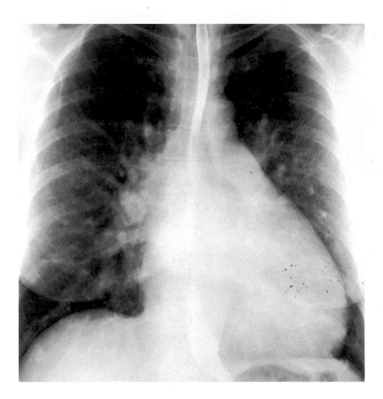

Fig. 32-19. Persistent common atrioventricular canal. Note the gross cardiac enlargement and hypervascularity, particularly marked in the central lung fields. The enlargement appears to be biventricular.

Roentgen Findings. In a number of patients no recognizable abnormality is noted. The characteristic findings in valvular stenosis are right ventricular enlargement and prominence of the pulmonary artery in a patient with normal or slightly decreased peripheral pulmonary vascularity. The right atrium is sometimes enlarged. Isolated infundibular stenosis is rare.

Heart Size. The heart may be normal in size but is enlarged in about half of these patients.

Heart Shape. The enlargement is right-sided and results in a rounded, right lower cardiac contour in the frontal projection and rounding of the right upper cardiac border in the left anterior oblique projection. The apex may be elevated and blunted. The outflow tract of the right ventricle is often prominent in the right anterior oblique projection.

Pulmonary Artery. The most characteristic finding is enlargement of the main pulmonary artery, resulting in convexity of the left upper cardiac margin below the aortic knob. This enlargement of the main pulmonary artery is due to poststenotic dilatation. The dilatation involves the pulmonary artery and the left pulmonary artery which result in prominence of the arterial silhouette in the left hilum. The right pulmonary artery may be dilated, but this vessel is hidden by mediastinal density. Therefore, the size of hilar vessels tends to be asymmetric in contrast to the symmetry often observed in pulmonary hypertension, and is a helpful differential diagnostic sign. Poststenotic dilatation ocurs in valvular stenosis (Fig. 32-20). In infundibular and supravalvular stenosis, the pulmonary artery is not prominent, and there may be no roentgen findings indicating cardiovascular disease.

Pulmonary Vascularity. The large main artery is associated with normal size of the vessels in the lungs and in the right hilum. The pulsation in the left pulmonary artery may be increased as observed fluoroscopically, while pulsation in the right pulmonary artery is usually decreased.

Angiocardiography. Angiocardiography may demonstrate enlargement of the right atrium and ventricle, as well as outline the actual site and degree of pulmonic stenosis along with the poststenotic dilatation of the pulmonary artery.

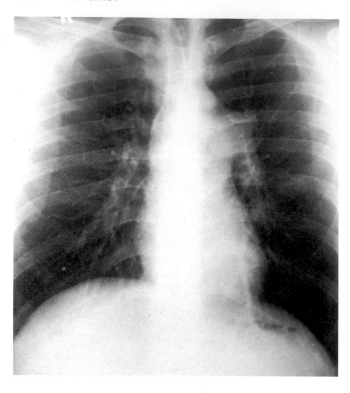

Fig. 32-20. Valvular pulmonic stenosis in a 23-year-old man. Note the great enlargement of the pulmonary artery and the proximal aspect of the left pulmonary artery resulting in large hilar vessels on the left in contrast to the small hilar vessels on the right.

Aortic Stenosis

Congenital aortic stenosis may be valvular, supravalvular or subvalvular. The valvular type of stenosis is more common than subaortic stenosis of the ventricular outflow tract, and supravalvular stenosis is quite rare. The valve may be bicuspid, but, more commonly, there is a single cusp with a single commissure. Usually the bicuspid valve is not stenotic, but there is a tendency to acquire calcification and to become stenotic.

Roentgen Findings. Poststenotic dilatation of the aorta usually occurs in valvular stenosis. The dilatation is characteristically located in the ascending aorta and results in increased convexity of the right lateral aspect of the ascending aorta. It may be more clearly defined in the left anterior oblique than in the frontal projection. The transverse arch or aortic knob is not enlarged. Left ventricular hypertrophy and dilatation also occur in this condition and result in increased prominence of the left ventricle in the left oblique projection and enlargement of the heart downward and to the left. The heart is usually not greatly enlarged. In nearly half of our patients (in whom the stenosis was minimal to moderate) no de-

tectable roentgen abnormalities were found except for the slight prominence of the ascending aorta. When present, the findings are characteristic. Subaortic stenosis is particularly difficult to diagnose roentgenographically because, in idiopathic hypertrophic subaortic stenosis, there is little if any poststenotic dilatation and in the membranous type of stenosis there is often no poststenotic dilatation and the left ventricular hypertrophy is often minimal. The pulmonary artery, right side of the heart, and pulmonary vascularity are normal. In membranous, subaortic stenosis, there is a discrete, fibrous membrane below the aortic valve. This anomaly results in poststenotic dilatation in about 50% of the patients. It is associated with other abnormalities in descending order of frequency: thick aortic valves, aortic insufficiency, ventricular septal defect, dilated sinuses of Valsalva, coarctation of the aorta, and mitral insufficiency.[3]

Corrected Transposition of the Great Vessels

There are two major components in this anomaly: (*1*) transposition of the origins of the aorta and pulmonary artery, so that the aortic root is anterior and to the left of the pulmonary artery; and (*2*) inversion of the ventricles with their accompanying atrioventricular valves. There is also inversion of the coronary arteries. Venous blood then enters the right atrium and flows through a bicuspid (mitral) valve into the anatomic left ventricle and to the lungs through the posteriorly placed pulmonary artery. Arterial blood returns from the lungs into the left atrium and flows through a tricuspid valve into the anatomic right ventricle and to the general circulation through an anteriorly placed left-sided aorta.

When this lesion occurs alone, no functional circulatory abnormality is present and no symptoms occur. In the majority of these patients, however, there is an associated cardiovascular anomaly. Septal defects, especially ventricular, are the most common of these, and mitral valve anomalies are common. Pulmonic stenosis is also frequent.

The roentgen appearances depends on the associated defects. However, there are signs caused by the anomalous position of the great vessels which may be quite characteristic. The ascending aorta often forms the upper left border of the heart and may produce a slight convexity, a long straight line, or a very slight concavity of this border (Fig. 32-21). The pulmonary artery does not form a part of the left border, but may indent the esophagus below the normal position of the aortic indentation. In some of these patients, the outflow tract of the right ventricle is directed to the right, resulting in greater perfusion of the right lung and enlargement of the right pulmonary artery and it major branches. The right hilar vessels may then be much more prominent than the left. Angiocardiography can be used to confirm the diagnosis. The anomalous position of the great vessels is readily determined.

Endocardial Fibroelastosis

Endocardial sclerosis, congenital subendothelial myofibrosis, congenital idiopathic hypertrophy of the heart, prenatal fibroelastosis, fetal endocarditis, endocardial dysplasia, and elastic-tissue hyperplasia are all synonyms of endocardial fibroelastosis. The disease is probably congenital or developmental in origin, although the cause is not definitely known. It is manifested by marked endocardial thickening that involves the left ventricle. The endocardium is thickened by fibrous and elastic tissue without evidence of inflammation. The myocardium is usually markedly hypertrophied, and the left ventricle is dilated but is occasionally small—the contracted form of fibroelastosis, usually associated with aortic stenosis. Valves are often involved by contracture, thickening, and

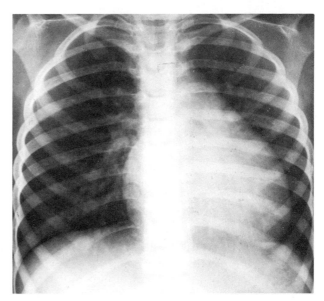

Fig. 32-21. Corrected transposition of the great vessels. Note the slight convexity of the left upper cardiovascular border produced by the ascending aorta. No aortic shadow is noted on the right. There was an associated atrial septal defect with a very small left-to-right shunt.

sometimes adhesions of the leaflets. The mitral valve is the most commonly and the most severely affected and mitral regurgitation is common. The patients usually show no evidence of heart disease at birth and may develop normally for a variable period of time. Then symptoms begin and progress rapidly. They consist of dyspnea and evidence of congestive failure that may lead to death in a very short time. In others the process appears to develop more slowly and the patient survives for some length of time.

Roentgen Findings. The heart is usually enlarged and may be markedly so. It tends to be globular in shape and there is often evidence of pulmonary congestion indicating failure. The involvement of the mitral valve produces left atrial and ventricular enlargement. This can be recognized by the characteristic posterior displacement of the esophagus, bulging of the left upper cardiac border, double contour on the right, and enlargement of the left ventricle downward and to the left. Pulmonary venous congestion may be present as well as pulmonary edema. When the history is reasonably typical and these radiographic findings are noted, the diagnosis is fairly certain. In many instances the diagnosis is made largely

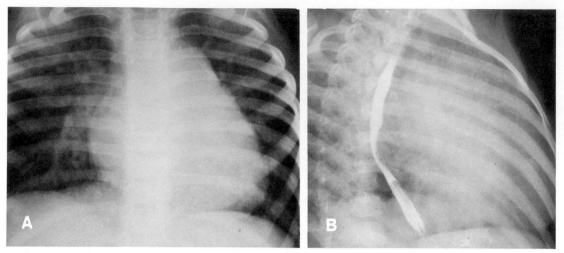

Fig. 32-22. Endocardial fibroelastosis. **A.** There is general cardiac enlargement and some evidence of pulmonary congestion. **B.** In addition to the generalized backward displacement of the esophagus by the large heart, there is local displacement caused by enlargement of the left atrium. The patient was found to have mitral valvular involvement producing stenosis.

by the exclusion of the possibility of other diseases (Fig. 32-22). A difference in pulsation may be observed fluoroscopically as a result of the predominant left ventricular involvement. The right ventricle pulsates normally, whereas the left ventricular pulsation is decreased or absent.

Coarctation of the Aorta

This congenital malformation consists of an area of constriction in the aorta. It varies in degree from slight stenosis to atresia. The most commonly associated abnormality is bicuspid aortic valve, which is found in about 85% of patients with coarctation. Two general types, or groups, are recognized. The most common is the type in which the site of constriction is at or distal to the ductus arteriosus. The constriction develops early in intrauterine life, resulting in stimulus to the formation of collateral circulation to the lower·body. As a result the infant is born with some collaterals and there is no change in the circulation when the ductus closes. The other general group, termed the "preductal type," consists of constriction proximal to the ductus. The coarcted segment is usually longer than in the other form and this lesion is often associated with other congenital cardiovascular anomalies. In this type there is no stimulus to the development of collateral circulation for the lower extremities during intrauterine life because

blood from the pulmonary circulation is shunted into the descending aorta through the ductus. This preductal or infantile type, usually associated with other defects, such as ventricular septal defect or atrial septal defect, is termed the "coarctation syndrome." After birth the ductus closes and the pulmonary bloodflow to the descending aorta is shut off, causing a sudden increase in left ventricular work. This often results in decompensation before collaterals are developed. If the patent ductus persists in coarctation of the preductal type, it results in cyanosis of the lower extremities with normal oxygenation of the head and upper extremities. Associated cardiac anomalies may result in intracardiac right-to-left shunt; then desaturation is generalized. In the infantile type the roentgen findings are not characteristic. The heart is often grossly enlarged and there is evidence of pulmonary congestion. When coarctation results in congestive cardiac failure in infants, the roentgen and clinical findings are usually not diagnostic. Then retrograde aortography may be used to make the diagnosis.

Roentgen Findings. The signs in the adult type (postductal) are usually characteristic enough to permit the diagnosis of coarctation on routine roentgen studies.

Rib Notching. Rib notching is an important radiologic sign. It is caused by dilatation and tortuosity of the intercostal arteries which serve as collaterals between the proximal aorta, through the internal mammary, and the aorta distal to the coarctation. It is almost universally present in adults but may not be demonstrated in children in the first 5 or 6 years of life. The sign consists of an irregular, scalloped appearance of the inferior margins of the ribs that is usually most common and readily outlined in the fourth through the eighth ribs. The third rib is sometimes involved but the first and second are rarely notched. The irregularity is usually bilateral, but it is not necessarily symmetric (Fig. 32-23). A number of other causes for rib notching have been described. They include subclavian artery obstruction, superior caval obstruction with long-standing venous engorgement, arteriovenous fistula of the intercostal vessels, aortic valvular disease, and tetralogy of Fallot. In this group of diseases the rib notching is often local and almost invariably unilateral.

The Aorta. The appearance of the aorta may be characteristic. The ascending arch is wide, producing convexity on the right side while the aortic knob or transverse aortic arch is small. Normally the left contour of the descending aorta can be visualized as a straight or gently convex line extending downward from the knob until it is obscured by the shadow of the heart below the hilum. In coarctation, a small indentation may be visible just below the knob that represents the actual site of coarctation. This is often associated with convexity below the coarctation site representing poststenotic dilatation. The appearance is that of two convexities, one representing the aortic knob and the second representing the dilated aorta distal to the coarctation. In other patients the actual indentation is not visible but the normal, clearly visualized, left aortic border is discontinuous. In the frontal projection, when the esophagus is filled with barium, there may be two clearly defined indentations on its left border, one above and one below the coarctation, which is sometimes termed the "reverse-3 sign." There is often enough dilatation of the left subclavian artery to result in convexity or prominence of the left superior mediastinal contour; this is often noted to be continuous with the shadow of the aortic knob. In the left anterior oblique projection, the notch and dilatation below it may be visible and the esophagus is often displaced by the dilated aorta immediately below the coarctation, as noted previously. This displacement is to the right and slightly anteriorly and is definitely below the transverse aortic arch (Fig. 32-24). Congenital nonstenotic "kinking" of the aorta has also been described that may

cause roentgen changes in this artery resembling those of coarctation. The other roentgen findings are absent, however, and there is no clinical evidence of coarctation.

Heart Size and Shape. The heart may be normal in size and shape but the left ventricular work load is increased; eventually left ventricular hypertrophy and dilatation result in enlargement of this chamber. The left atrium may also be enlarged. In infants with the coarctation syndrome and cardiac failure the heart is relatively larger and there is evidence of pulmonary venous congestion as well as arterial hypervascularity since the associated anomaly such as patent ductus arteriosus and interventricular septal defect result in a left-to-right shunt. It is difficult to ascertain how much of the change is secondary to shunting and how much to congestive failure in these infants who often go into failure a week or two after birth.

Angiocardiography. This method is not ordinarily employed for the diagnosis of coarctation.

Retrograde Aortography. This examination is more useful than angiocardiography and clearly defines the coarcted segment as well as the aorta and its branches above and below it.

Kinking of the Aortic Arch (Pseudocoarctation)

Kinking or buckling of the aortic arch is sometimes termed "pseudocoarctation" because it simulates coarctation roentgenographically. No aortic constriction is present, however. The abnormality is presumably caused by a short, taut ligamentum arteriosum; but since this does not account for the elongation of the arch that may be observed in this condition, a more likely cause is variation in normal differential growth rate of the aortic arch segments in early development.

Roentgen findings are somewhat variable, depending on the amount of elongation. The high aortic arch casts a round or crescentic shadow projecting to the left in the superior mediastinum, which may simulate a mediastinal tumor. Below this a second convexity projects to the left. The latter represents the arch at and distal to the kink and may be more dense than the upper shadow. In other patients the appearance is that of an unusually large aortic knob with an abrupt indentation at its inferior margin and a second convexity immediately below it caused by actual dila-

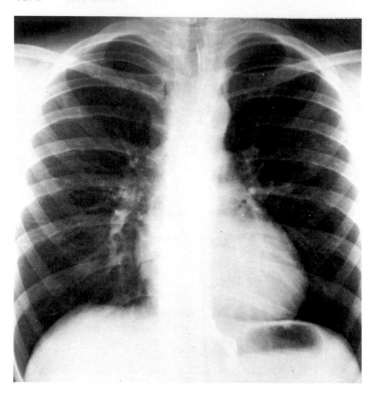

Fig. 32-23. Coarctation of the aorta in a 10-year-old girl. There is very clearly defined rib notching which is very helpful in determining the diagnosis since the site of the coarctation is not demonstrated, nor is there a very clearly defined area of poststenotic dilatation.

Fig. 32-24. Coarctation of the aorta. In this patient the rib notching is relatively minor. The aortic knob is small but there is a dilatation below it representing poststenotic dilatation of the aorta (retouched) (arrow). In the left anterior oblique projection **(B)** the esophagus is seen to be displaced slightly by the dilated aorta below the coarctation.

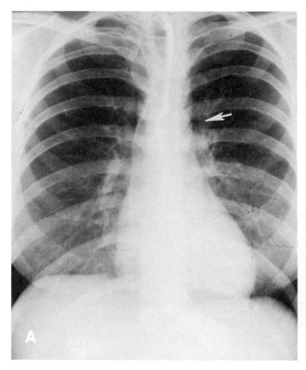
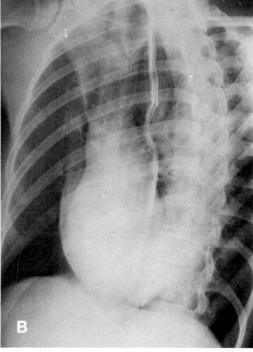

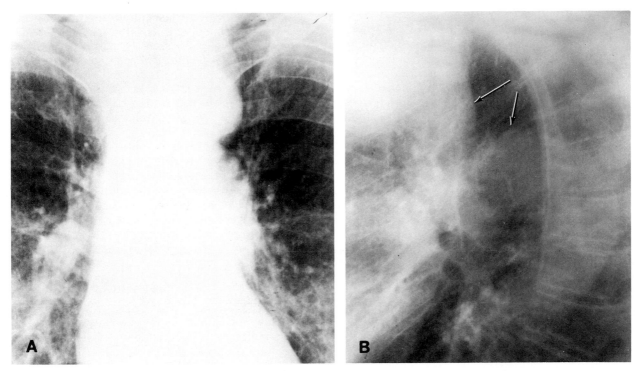

Fig. 32-25. Pseudocoarctation of the aorta. **A.** The transverse aortic arch is high, and there is a very large, broad convexity of the aorta to the left below the arch. **B.** The severe kinking is demonstrated in the lateral view **(arrows).**

tation of the aorta distal to the kink. Either or both of the shadows may indent the esophagus. The left anterior oblique and lateral views are usually diagnostic, since the indentation at the site of buckling can usually be identified (Fig. 32-25). Tomograms in these projections may aid in the diagnosis. There is no left ventricular enlargement or rib notching.

Aneurysm of the Sinus of Valsalva

The aortic sinuses are three dilatations in the root of the aorta just above the aortic valves. They are named according to their corresponding aortic valve cusps, the right, left, and posterior. The right and left coronary arteries originate in or above the corresponding sinus of Valsalva and the posterior sinus is sometimes termed the "noncoronary sinus." Aneurysm is a rare congenital anomaly, usually involving the right aortic sinus. This sinus lies adjacent to the ventricular septum and occasionally a fistulous tract develops into the right ventricle. Rupture into the right atrium has also been reported. When this occurs, the size of the right heart increases and the left-to-right shunt created results in an increase in size of the pulmo-

nary artery and its branches. When the aneurysm remains confined to the sinus, there is usually no alteration of the cardiovascular silhouette, but there may be some calcification in the aneurysm wall. However, in the acquired type of aneurysm caused by cystic medial necrosis with or without Marfan's syndrome, there is usually aortic regurgitation leading to left ventricular enlargement and general dilatation of the ascending aorta. Aortic dissection is a frequent complication. The most common roentgen finding in any acquired type of aneurysm of the sinus of Valsalva is a local bulge of the right anterolateral cardiac contour. Aortography can be used to define the site and size of the aneurysm. Rarely, aneurysmal dilatation of all the sinuses of Valsalva may be associated with coarctation of the aorta.

Anomalous Left Coronary Artery

In this anomaly the blood supply to the myocardium is affected because the left coronary artery arises from the pulmonary artery. As a result the left ventricle dilates early in life, leading to marked cardiac enlargement. The roentgen findings are not characteristic, but the large heart is visualized and there is often evidence of pulmonary congestion. Although the left ventricle is enlarged, the signs commonly associated with enlargement of this chamber are not necessarily present. When a large collateral vessel forms, the blood flows into the pulmonary artery through the anomalous coronary, a left-to-right shunt. Angiocardiography is necessary to make the diagnosis.

Rotation Anomalies of the Heart

The literature on classification and descriptions of various rotation and alignment anomalies is voluminous and somewhat confusing. Rosenbaum's classification[51] of cardiac alignments based on patterns of bloodflow is presented because of its consistency with current embryologic thought, and its relative simplicity and precision. His definitions are indicated in Table 32-2. The possible courses of bloodflow are given in Figure 32-26.

Using these definition and combining them with the positional designations, a description of cardiac alignment includes designation of the ventriculotruncal alignment (*e.g.*, isolated ventricular inversion, inverted transposition, etc.), and a secondary indication of: (*1*) the presence of situs solitus or situs inversus, and (*2*) a left-sided or right-sided heart. The abdominal visceral situs (situs solitus indicates the stomach is on the left; situs inversus indicates the stomach is on the right) indicates the position of the atria according to Rosenbaum[51] except in rare instances of isolated gastric inversion. Elliott, Jue, and Amplatz,[13] and others, believe that atrial position is more consistent with the side of the aortic arch. If the right atrium is on the side opposite the stomach and on the same side as the liver, nearly all of the possible alignments can be determined with good biplane an-

giocardiograms. A few exceptions include the abnormalities associated with asplenia and polysplenia as well as some cases of common atrium. Although Rosenbaum's classification is not in common use, it is valuable in defining the four fundamental ventriculotruncal alignments (Fig. 32-27). Figure 32-28 outlines the possible variations in abdominal situs and cardiac position and their relation to ventriculotruncal alignments.

Dextrocardia with situs solitus is nearly always associated with severe congenital cardiac malformation. Dextrocardia that is a part of complete situs inversus, a mirror image of the normal, nearly always has a normal ventriculotruncal alignment. When the heart is right-sided as a result of pulmonary, diaphragmatic, or spinal abnormalities, there are usually no associated cardiac malformations.

ANOMALIES OF THE AORTIC ARCH AND ITS LARGE BRANCHES

The embryologic development of the aortic arch and its branches is complex. Six pairs of aortic arches develop in the embryo of man but not all are present at the same time. They originate anteriorly in the aortic sac, which represents the proximal portion of the developing aortic arch. They course backward on both sides to join the dorsal aorta, which is bilateral. The arches develop in the fifth week and their transformation occupies the sixth and seventh weeks of fetal development. The first and second arches disappear early. The dorsal aorta at these levels persists as part of the internal carotid and the third arch persists as the proximal part of the common carotid artery on either side. The external carotid arteries arise as separate buds from the aortic sac and later transfer their origins onto the third arches. The fourth arch persists on both sides. The left forms the permanent or left-sided aortic arch while the right side forms the innominate artery. The fifth arches are transitory and disappear without a trace. The sixth arches arise from each dorsal aorta and extend across to the primitive pulmonary artery on either side to form the ductus arteriosus. The connection is lost on the right but persists on the left until after birth, when it closes to form the ligamentum arteriosum. Early in development the dorsal aorta fuses below the arch to form a single descending aorta.

Left Aortic Arch with Right Descending Aorta

In this anomaly the left aortic arch arises normally and passes backward to the left of the trachea and

Table 32-2. Definitions

Right and left ventricles and atria	Denotes morphology only; no functional or positional connotation
Inversion	Relationship between ventricles and feeding atria
	Noninverted: RV* fed by RA, and LV fed by LA
	Inverted: RV fed by LA, and LV fed by RA
Transposition	Aorta arises from RV anterior to pulmonary artery which arises from the LV

* RV, right ventricle; LV, left ventricle; RA, right atrium; LA, left atrium. (Rosenbaum HD: The roentgen classification and diagnosis of cardiac alignments. Radiology 89: 466, 1967.)

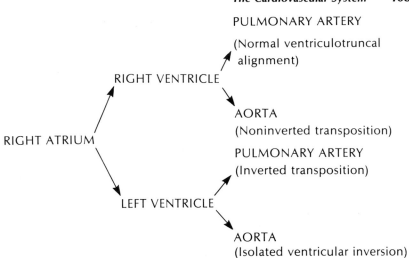

Fig. 32-26. Possible courses of blood flow from the right atrium. (Rosenbaum HD: The roentgen classification and diagnosis of cardiac alignments. Radiology 89: 466, 1967)

Fig. 32-27. Diagrams of four fundamental ventriculotruncal alignments in situs solitus. Relationships are reversed in situs inversus. (Rosenbaum HD: The roentgen classification and diagnosis of cardiac alignments. Radiology 89: 466, 1967)

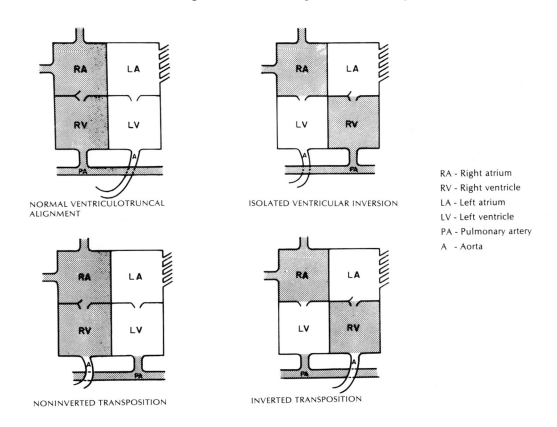

NORMAL VENTRICULOTRUNCAL ALIGNMENT

ISOLATED VENTRICULAR INVERSION

NONINVERTED TRANSPOSITION

INVERTED TRANSPOSITION

RA - Right atrium
RV - Right ventricle
LA - Left atrium
LV - Left ventricle
PA - Pulmonary artery
A - Aorta

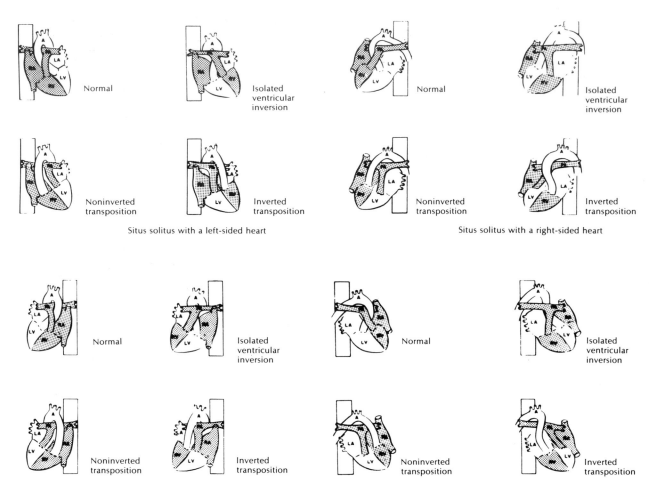

Fig. 32-28. The four fundamental ventriculotruncal alignments in situs solitus and situs inversus, both with a right-sided heart and with a left-sided heart. Note that the alignments of situs solitus with the right-sided heart are identical to those seen with situs solitus and the left-sided heart. The only difference is the location of the cardiac apex. Similarly, the alignments for situs inversus and a left-sided heart are identical to those seen in situs inversus with a right-sided heart. (Rosenbaum HD: The roentgen classification and diagnosis of cardiac alignments. Radiology 89: 466, 1967)

esophagus and crosses to the right side of the mediastinum behind the esophagus where it continues as the right descending aorta. There is a left-sided aortic knob, absence of the aortic shadow below it on the left, and indentation on the posterior aspect of the esophagus; often the descending aorta is visualized to the right of the midline.

Right Aortic Arch

There are five types of right aortic arch, classified according to arrangement of arch vessels.[55] Type I right aortic arch, or mirror-image branching, is the more common of the mirror-image types. The first branch is the left innominate artery, followed by the right common carotid and the right subclavian. The aortic arch is to the right of the trachea and esophagus and descends on the right. This is the type usually associated with tetralogy of Fallot or truncus arteriosus and rarely with tricuspid atresia. The aortic knob can usually be identified on the right. It displaces the superior vena cava to the right and often produces a slight local deviation of the trachea to the left. When the esophagus is opacified, slight displacement to the left is often observed.

The second type is a rare type of mirror-image branching in which the left innominate artery is the first major branch, the right common carotid is the second, and the right subclavian is the third. The left ductus arteriosus extends from the upper descending aorta to the left pulmonary artery, forming a vascular ring. An aortic diverticulum may be present at the aortic origin of the left ductus. The arch descends on the right. This is a rare cause of a vascular ring, formed by the right arch on the right side and the ligamentum or ductus on the left, which extends from the pulmonary artery posteriorly and to the right behind the esophagus where it joins the proximal descending aorta. Radiographic findings include the evidence of right aortic arch; barium study of the esophagus will show a posterior indentation produced by the ligamentum or ductus arteriosus.

Type III right aortic arch is one in which four vessels originate from the arch in the following order: left common carotid artery, right common carotid artery, right subclavian artery, and an aberrant left subclavian artery, which arises from the upper descending aorta. In this anomaly the aorta may descend either to the right or to the left of the spine. There are two variations. In one, the aorta ascends to the right of the trachea and esophagus, and the arch passes to the left behind the esophagus and usually descends on the left side (Fig. 32-29). The left sub-

clavian takes origin from the left posterior diverticulum of the distal aortic arch. In this variation, there is a large retroesophageal arch. A left ductus arteriosus may extend from the aortic diverticulum to the left pulmonary artery completing the vascular ring (Fig. 32-30). In the other variation, the aorta ascends and descends to the right of the spine. The left subclavian artery arises from the descending aorta and courses obliquely behind the esophagus to reach the left arm, thus the retroesophageal vessel is smaller since it represents only the left subclavian artery. This type with the aberrant left subclavian artery is the most common of all types of right aortic arch and is often encountered as an incidental finding on routine chest film. The incidence of associated congenital heart disease is very low, in the range of 5% in these patients. Chest-film findings are those of the aortic mass to the right side of the trachea, often indenting it. The arch is often higher in position than the normal left arch. On the lateral film, the retroesophageal aorta may be visible as a round mass displacing the trachea anteriorly; also it will be noted to displace the esophagus anteriorly if the esophagus is filled with barium. The descending aorta may be seen coursing inferiorly on the left side.

In type IV right aortic arch the left innominate artery is aberrant, arising as the third branch from the distal right arch and passing behind the esophagus, then dividing to form the left common carotid and subclavian arteries. The vascular ring is formed by the right arch, the retroesophageal innominate artery, and the left ductus arteriosus. In this anomaly, which is very rare, the right common carotid is the first branch and the right subclavian is the second. Chest-film findings include the evidence of right aortic arch with posterior compression of the esophagus produced by the aberrant left innominate artery.

In type V right aortic arch the left common carotid, the right common carotid, and the right subclavian arteries arise from the arch in that order. The left subclavian is connected to the left pulmonary artery by the left ductus arteriosus and has no connection to the aorta (isolation of the left subclavian artery). This anomaly is also uncommon. The chest-film findings include a right aortic knob and descending aorta and there may also be signs of cyanotic congenital heart disease which is frequently associated with this malformation, the most common of which is tetralogy of Fallot. There is no vascular ring. In some of these patients, there is a subclavian steal syndrome in which this artery is supplied by the left vertebral artery.

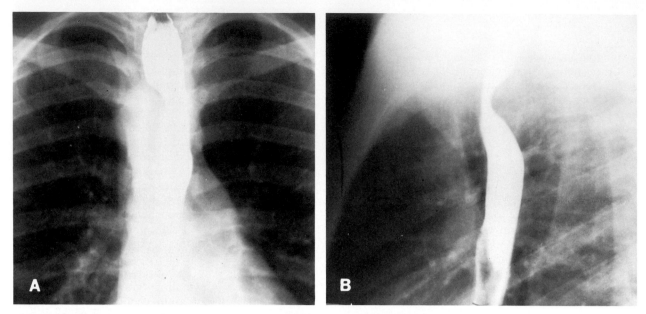

Fig. 32-29. Right aortic arch. **A.** In the frontal view no arch is noted on the left, and there is a vascular shadow on the right resembling the transverse aortic arch which indents the esophagus. **B.** In the lateral view there is posterior indentation of the esophagus indicating that the arch turns to the left and, in this patient, descends on the left.

Fig. 32-30. Right aortic arch with a left patent ductus forming a vascular ring that resulted in moderate dysphagia. **A.** In the frontal projection the aortic knob is absent on the left and the aorta is noted on the right where it indents the right lateral aspect of the esophagus. it also descends on the right. Some indentation is noted on the left lateral aspect of the esophagus slightly below the level of the aorta. **B.** Spot film exposed during fluoroscopy showing the esophageal narrowing clearly outlined. The ductus arteriosus crossed behind the esophagus from below upward, producing the well-marked posterior indentation noted. The ductus was ligated and sectioned, relieving the patient's symptoms.

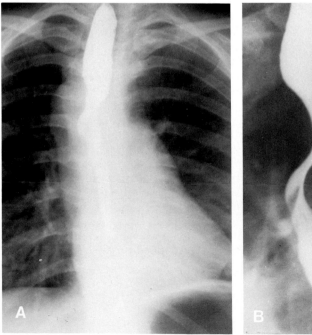
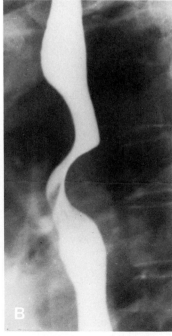

Cervical Aortic Arch

Cervical aortic arch is a rare congenital anomaly in which the ascending aorta extends higher than usual so that the aortic arch is in the neck.[45] The incidence of right and left arches is approximately equal and the branching of the great vessels may vary from one patient to another in this condition. The plain-film findings consist of absence of the normal aortic arch in the thorax, an apparent cutoff of the tracheal air column in the superior mediastinum, a mass on either side caused by the arch that displaces the trachea, and superior mediastinal widening on the side of the descending aorta. The origin of the anomaly is uncertain since it may represent failure of descent of an otherwise normal fourth arch or persistence of one of the higher arches as the aortic arch.

Other Anomalies of the Aortic Arch and Its Large Branches

The innominate artery may arise more distally than normal and cross anterior to the trachea from left to right. It produces slight indentation and occasionally may cause respiratory distress in infants. Similar anterior indentation and compression may be caused by the left carotid artery when it arises more proximally than normal and must cross from right to left anterior to the trachea.

Anomalies Forming Vascular Rings

Double Aortic Arch. The double aortic arch comprises a large group of anomalies in which there are many variants. The fundamental defect results from persistence of both the right and the left aortic arches that encircle the trachea and esophagus and often produce partial obstruction of these structures. Either or both of the arches may function and may be comparable in size or one may be larger than the other. The aorta may descend on either the right or the left side and anomalous origins of one or more of the great vessels often accompany this anomaly. The roentgen and fluoroscopic findings consist of evidence of compression of the trachea and esophagus by an encircling vascular ring (Fig. 32-31). The double arch produces densities on either side of the midline that may be symmetric. Angiocardiography has limited value but, if necessary, aortography can be used to define the vascular ring.

Aberrant Right Subclavian Artery. This is the most common of the anomalies of the great vessels. The right subclavian originates as the most distal of the branches of the arch and reaches the right side by coursing obliquely upward and to the right, usually behind the esophagus. This defect is often asymptomatic but may be asociated with other cardiovascular anomalies. The major roentgen finding is an oblique indentation of the posterior aspect of the esophagus above the aortic arch, which extends upward and to the right. It is usually outlined best in the lateral and left anterior oblique projections. Fluoroscopic examination with barium swallow will outline this defect and its effect on the esophagus.

CONGENITAL ANOMALIES OF THE PULMONARY ARTERY AND ITS BRANCHES

Agenesis of the Pulmonary Artery

This is an uncommon anomaly in which there is absence of one pulmonary artery. It is associated with an anomalous systemic arterial blood supply to the lung that arises either from the aorta or from one of its major branches. The anomaly is often associated with other congenital anomalies of the cardiovascular system. Occasionally the systemic artery supplying the involved lung is very large; this results in a large arteriovenous shunt that may eventually cause cardiac failure. The high pressure in this anomalous system is believed to be the cause of hemoptysis, the most common symptom of the condition.

Roentgen Findings. The roentgen findings are characteristic enough to make the diagnosis or make one strongly suspect it in most instances. The involved hemithorax is smaller in size than is normal. In addition to the difference in size of the bony thorax, the hemidiaphragm is often elevated and mediastinal structures are shifted to the affected side. There is often some herniation of the normal lung across the midline anterior to the aorta. The normal shadows of the pulmonary arterial branches in the hilum and in the lung are absent and the vessels that are visible form a relatively fine reticular vascular pattern caused by the branching bronchial arteries. The result is an absence of the hilum shadow or an inconspicuous one. Tomography is very useful to define clearly the difference in the hilar vessels on the two sides. Bronchography outlines the normally branching bronchial tree and excludes the possibility of atelectasis, while angiocardiography can be used to define the main pulmonary artery and its remaining branch and to show the lack of filling on the opposite side (Fig. 32-32). Agenesis of a lobe, or lobes, may occur in conjunction with agenesis of the pulmonary

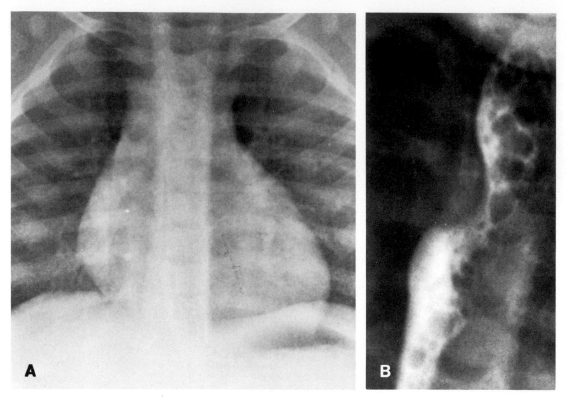

Fig. 32-31. Double aortic arch. **A.** Note the very slight deviation of the trachea to the left in this 6-month-old infant with feeding problems. The vascular shadow on the right at the level of the aortic arch is somewhat larger than on the left. **B.** Spot film with barium in the esophagus shows the indentation on the right to be higher and larger than the one on the left which is smaller and lower, lying just above the left bronchus.

Fig. 32-32. Agenesis of the right pulmonary artery. **A.** Frontal chest film shows a marked shift of the heart and mediastinal structures to the right. The branches of the right pulmonary artery are absent so that no hilar vessels are visible and the entire right lung shows very little vascularity. **B.** The angiocardiogram shows the main pulmonary artery and its left branch. Note that the right pulmonary artery is absent.

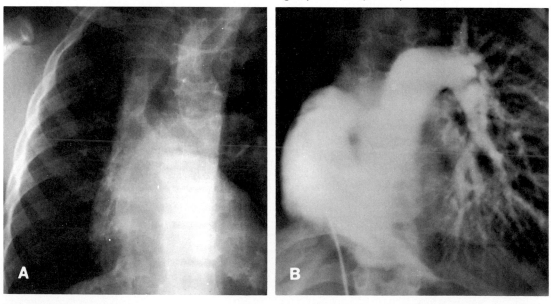

artery. Hypoplasia of one pulmonary artery may result in similar but somewhat less marked roentgen findings. Unless the hypoplasia is relatively severe, however, it is unlikely that the diagnosis can be made without the use of angiocardiography.

Congenital Absence of the Pulmonary Valve

Congenital absence of the pulmonary valve is a rare malformation. It is usually associated with tetralogy of Fallot and occasionally with ventricular septal defect, but it may occur as an isolated anomaly. Roentgen findings in patients with associated anomalies include dilatation of one or both pulmonary arteries. The dilatation may be of such magnitude that wheezing due to obstructive emphysema on one or both sides is usually present. To and fro murmurs along the left sternal border and absent or diminished pulmonary second sounds are common. Absence of the pulmonary valve without associated anomalies produces much less dilatation of the pulmonary arteries centrally, so that respiratory distress is not produced. Varying amounts of right ventricular dilatation and hypertrophy alter the shape of the cardiac silhouette. Bronchography demonstrates the bronchial compression caused by the large artery.

Aberrant Left Pulmonary Artery

This anomaly, termed "pulmonary sling," consists of a distal origin of the left pulmonary artery. The origin may be from the right pulmonary artery or from the distal main pulmonary artery.[25] The aberrant artery passes over the right main bronchus, then passes backward and to the left between the trachea and esophagus to the left hilum. If it compresses the right main bronchus, obstructive symptoms result in respiratory distress. Roentgen findings include evidence of obstructive emphysema on the right, a low, small left hilum, and, on the lateral view, a round mass indenting the barium-filled esophagus, the key finding in this condition. Dysphagia is not usually present. The anomalous artery may also produce a right-sided mediastinal mass, particularly if it causes no symptoms and is observed in the older child or in an adult. There is sometimes decreased vascularity of the left lung. Pulmonary angiography will confirm the diagnosis.

Aberrant Vascular Connection Between Right Pulmonary Artery and the Left Atrium

This is a very rare anomaly. It causes cyanosis and clubbing of fingers and toes.[35] The distinctive roentgen finding is that of a small rounded mass which, on frontal projection, is seen overlying the mid right atrium and protruding to the right beyond it; the lateral and inferior border is clearly defined. On the left anterior oblique projection, the density is seen to overlie the lower anterior aspect of the left atrium; again its inferior border is clearly defined. The diagnosis can be confirmed by right-sided angiocardiogram.

Pulmonary Arteriovenous Malformations

A pulmonary arteriovenous malformation is a congenital vascular anomaly, sometimes termed a fistula or aneurysm (we prefer the term "arteriovenous malformation") through which a relatively large amount of nonoxygenated blood flows; therefore the lesion represents a right-to-left shunt and is associated with varying degrees of unsaturation of the arterial blood. The malformations are usually multiple and occur more frequently in the lower lobes than elsewhere. Because the caliber of the vessels within the mass varies, there is no quantitative correlation between the size of the anomaly and the amount of shunt. The pulmonary lesions may be accompanied by hemangiomas or telangiectases elsewhere and are then a part of a generalized angiomatous process. Since these are right-to-left shunts which may be quite large, the filtering effect of the pulmonary capillary circulation is lost and any embolic process arising in the systemic venous system may result in systemic embolization. For example, brain abscess is among the complications.

Roentgen Findings. The malformation is represented by a round, oval, or lobulated mass or several masses, usually in the lower lobes. The lesion is clearly defined and it is often possible to see a large pulmonary artery extending from the hilum to the lesion and another vessel, the pulmonary vein, extending from it to the region of the left atrium. If large vessels can be demonstrated going to it and draining it, the diagnosis should be strongly suspected. Tomograms are useful in outlining the blood supply and in clearly defining the lesions. When one is visualized, it is wise to look carefully for others since they are often multiple. At fluoroscopy, active pulsations may be visible in the malformation itself as well as in the pulmonary artery supplying it. It may be possible to demonstrate a decrease in size during the Valsalva experiment (expiration against closed glottis) and an increase in size of the lesion when the intrathoracic pressure is reduced (Müller maneuver). At times, the malformations may appear as nodules (single or

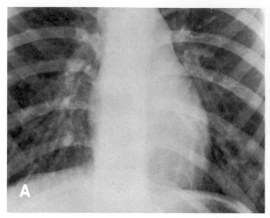 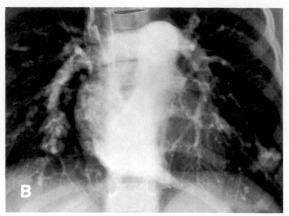

Fig. 32-33. Multiple pulmonary arteriovenous malformations. **A.** In the frontal chest film, numerous large vessels are seen extending from the hila down to the bases with an irregularity lobulated, clearly defined mass in the left base just above the diaphragm. At the right medial base there are many vessels resulting in an increase in density. **B.** In the angiocardiogram the right side of the heart and pulmonary arteries are noted to be filled, clearly defining the large basal arteriovenous malformations.

multiple) in patients in whom no such lesions have been seen in the area previously. This may present a very difficult diagnostic problem, since primary or metastatic tumor is then a consideration. Tomography may reveal feeding and draining vessels. Pulmonary arteriography is used to confirm the finding before surgical removal and also to determine the presence of smaller lesions that cannot be outlined on routine roentgenograms (Fig. 32-33)

Diffuse Pulmonary Hemangiomatosis

Diffuse pulmonary hemangiomatosis is a rare condition in which the lungs are the major sites of multiple hemangiomas that occur primarily along the bronchi, arteries, veins, and within the septa as well as in the pleura.[52] Hemangiomas may also occur in other sites such as the spleen and the thymus. Radiographic finding are those of diffuse, interstitial disease simulating fibrosis in children who have a history of repeated pleural effusions, often bloody, as well as pulmonary infections usually with hemoptysis. Thrombocytopenia and anemia develop and eventually dyspnea and cyanosis appear associated with increasing interstitial disease and bloody pleural effusion. Prognosis is poor.

Pulmonary Varices

Pulmonary varix is another rare anomaly in which the arteries are normal and there is no capillary

shunting.[5] In the venous phase, the veins feeding the varix (or varices) are seen to be filling at the same time as normal veins are filling, but there is delay in emptying of the varix, which drains directly into the left atrium. This anomaly should not be confused with pulmonary arteriovenous malformations which cause right-to-left shunting of blood. Plain-film findings are those of densities resembling dilated, tortuous vessels, usually in the parahilar area. Pulmonary angiography will confirm the diagnosis.

Pulmonary Artery Coarctations

A wide variety of pulmonary coarctations have been reported. The stenosis may involve the pulmonary artery above the valve and either or both of its main branches. Multiple peripheral stenoses involving many segmental arterial branches may also occur. The stenosis may be sharply localized or involve a relatively long segment of the affected artery. The coarctation may be unilateral or bilateral and is associated with valvular pulmonic stenosis in 60% of these patients. Supravalvular aortic stenosis also may be associated with pulmonary artery coarctations.

Roentgen findings are varied and depend upon the location of the stenotic lesion, its length, and the presence or absence of poststenotic dilatation. In the central types, poststenotic dilatation may result in an increase of the hilar vascular shadow. When the stenosis involves a long segment of either the right or left pulmonary artery or both, the hilar vascular shadow may be decreased, often with distinct increase in vessel size a short distance from the central hilum. In patients with multiple peripheral stenoses, the poststenotic dilatations may produce a nodular vascular pattern in the parahilar region unilaterally or bilaterally. When such findings are present, the diagnosis can be suspected. Pulmonary arteriography is needed for definitive diagnosis and, in many instances, the lesions are discovered on arteriographic study performed for identification of other lesions or conditions.

Idiopathic Enlargement of the Pulmonary Artery

Dilatation of the pulmonary artery in diseases of the heart and lungs has been described. Occasionally, marked dilatation of the pulmonary artery occurs as an isolated finding. This is sometimes termed "congenital aneurysm." The dilatation may extend into the left main branch for a short distance and occasionally into the right branch. When all clinical and laboratory studies, including cardiac catheterization, fail to demonstrate a cause, occasionally this enlargement probably represents a true congenital aneurysm. The diagnosis is made by exclusion, however, since there are many known cardiac and pulmonary diseases that can result in considerable dilatation of the pulmonary artery. The only roentgenographic finding is prominence in the region of the artery, resulting in convexity and enlargement of the artery segment as seen in the frontal projection. The enlargement can also be observed in oblique and lateral views. The diagnosis is made with caution since it is one of exclusion and cannot be made on the basis of roentgenographic findings alone.

The pulmonary artery is often prominent in childhood and early adult life. The convexity produced by the pulmonary artery is moderately enlarged, with no sign of cardiac or pulmonary disease on roentgenographic examination. Examination reveals no cause for it and the vessel evidently decreases in size because the finding is uncommon in older adults.

ACQUIRED VALVULAR CARDIAC DISEASE

MITRAL STENOSIS

Acquired mitral valvular disease usually results from rheumatic heart disease. Mitral stenosis is most common but there is often some degree of mitral insufficiency. The left atrium must empty itself against increased resistance caused by the mitral stenosis and the chamber enlarges. The increased pressure is reflected back through the lesser circulation to the right ventricle. This results in changes in the pulmonary vessels and in the right side of the heart.

Roentgen Findings. The appearance of the cardiovascular silhouette in mitral valvular disease is often characteristic (Fig. 32-34). There are alterations caused by left atrial enlargement. This may be the only change in the cardiac silhouette for some time. There is often enough stenosis to ultimately cause right ventricular enlargement and enough insufficiency to cause some left ventricular enlargement. There are also pulmonary vascular alterations which will be described. The signs of left atrial enlargement are: (*1*) Convexity of the left upper cardiac margin below the level of the left main bronchus. This represents enlargement of the auricular appendage (Fig. 32-35). In patients with a transverse heart the only alteration may be a straightening of the left upper cardiac margin in contrast to its usual slight concavity below the pulmonary artery. (2) A double contour or double convexity occurring on the right. The atrium may be large enough to be border-forming on the right side in which case a double convexity is visible. When it is not border-forming it is often of sufficient density to be identified within the right atrial border, forming a more dense convexity within the longer, right atrial convexity. (3) Sufficient posterior enlargement of the atrium to enable it to be seen as an area of increased density within the cardiac margins on either side below the level of the carina. (4) Elevation of the left main bronchus. (The findings through 4 are observed in the frontal projection.) (5) In the lateral and right anterior oblique projections, displacement of the esophagus, which is outlined with barium, posteriorly and sometimes slightly to the right by the enlarged atrium. This results in a posterior convexity of the esophagus in this region. (6) In the left anterior oblique projection, visualization of the enlarged atrium just below the left bronchus.

Calcium is often deposited in the mitral valve and in the mitral annulus. This may be somewhat difficult to demonstrate on roentgenograms of the chest but is usually easily seen fluoroscopically. The valvular calcification generally indicates mitral stenosis, while calcium in the mitral annulus may not necessarily be associated with valvular abnormality. The latter has a somewht elliptical shape.

Calcification in the left atrium is occasionally observed in patients with mitral stenosis. The calcium may be in the atrial wall or within a thrombus at-

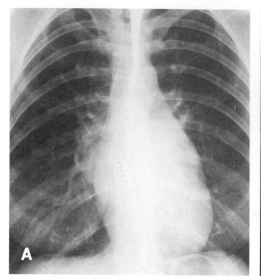

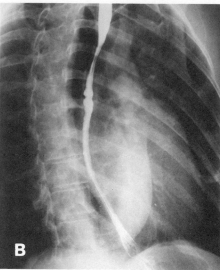

Fig. 32-34. Mitral stenosis. **A.** There is a double convexity on the right and a prominence of the left upper cardiac border. These signs indicate left atrial enlargement. The overall cardiac size is normal. Note the scarcity of pulmonary vessels at the bases despite sizeable hilar arteries. **B.** The right anterior oblique view shows posterior displacement of the esophagus by the enlarged left atrium. There is also noted some prominence of the outflow tract of the right ventricle manifested by some convexity of the upper cardiac border on the left. The vascular redistribution indicates pulmonary venous hypertension.

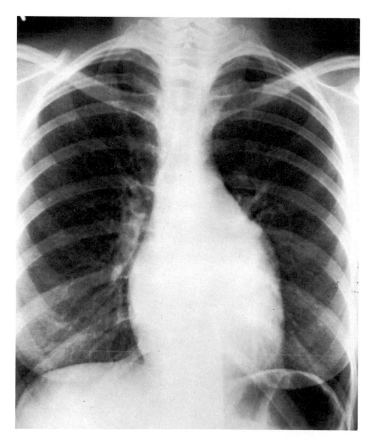

Fig. 32-35. Mitral stenosis. In this patient the left atrium is very large and the appendage produces a marked local bulge below the left pulmonary artery in the upper left cardiac margin. Vascularity is approximately equal in the upper and lower lung fields.

tached to the wall. When calcification in the atrium is suspected but not positively identified on the chest film, fluoroscopy can be used to confirm the diagnosis. When the calcification is in the atrial appendage, it is usually associated with mitral stenosis. Calcification in the wall of the atrium as well as in the appendage often indicates severe stenosis.

If the disease results in pulmonary arterial hypertension, eventually the right ventricle enlarges and the signs of an increase in size of this chamber are observed. Enlargement of the central pulmonary arteries is helpful in calling the attention of the observer to the likelihood of right ventricular enlargement.

As has been indicated, there are alterations in pulmonary vascular pressure which tend to cause progressive pulmonary changes. Initially there is some venous hypertension. The first sign is that of slight general venous distention or engorgement that is difficult to assess. It is most readily identified when earlier films are available for comparison. As the hypertension becomes more marked there is constriction of the lower-lobe arteries and veins and distention of the upper-lobe vessels resulting in a reversal of the usual pattern in which the lower-lobe vessels are more prominent (Fig. 32-36). Most of the blood flow is then maintained through the upper lobes. This alteration in the vascular pattern is usually readily identified early, but in long-standing chronic venous hypertension there may be enough interstitial change to obscure the vascular findings. As the venous pressure increases, more fluid escapes into the perivascular tissues and the lymphatics become dilated. This causes the appearance of Kerley's B lines, which are short, dense lines representing interlobular septa extending to the pleural surface. They are observed in the lower lung fields and are at right angles to the pleural surface (Fig. 32-37). They do not bifurcate and are often observed best on oblique films. Interstitial edema fluid causes the density. The deep septal lines, Kerley's A lines, may also become visible. They are about 2- to 5-inches long, tend to be straight and extend outward and upward in a somewhat fanlike manner from the upper hilar area into the periphery of the upper lung field. Kerley's C lines also represent interstitial structures or lymphatics within the interstitial structures. They tend to be transient and difficult to visualize but cause a fine spiderweb or reticular pattern throughout the lung. In chronic venous hypertension associated with chronic passive congestion, deposits of hemosiderin are added to the other causes for prominence of the septal lines.

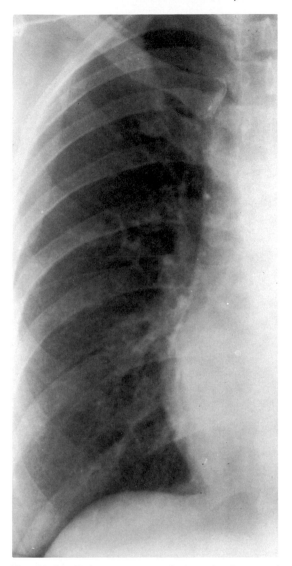

Fig. 32-36. Pulmonary vessels in mitral stenosis. The lower lung vessels are constricted and appear to be smaller than the vessels in the upper lung.

Eventually pulmonary arterial hypertension may occur. This results in dilatation of the main pulmonary artery and its branches centrally, which is associated with a constriction of arteries in the midlung and peripheral lung zones. These findings are then superimposed on those of chronic venous hypertension and right ventricular hypertrophy.

Pulmonary hemosiderosis secondary to mitral disease is a frequent pathologic finding but is not commonly recognized as such on chest films. It consists

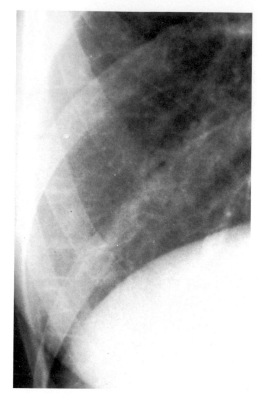

Fig. 32-37. Kerley's B lines. This close-up view of the right lateral lung base of a patient with mitral stenosis shows short, horizontal, dense lines representing interstitial edema.

of a deposition of blood pigments in the interstitial tissues. When the amount is sufficient the deposits are visible roentgenographically as fine granular or miliary shadows throughout the lungs (Fig. 32-38). They may become large enough to produce nodular densities ranging from 2 to 5 mm in diameter. Then the appearance of the lungs may resemble that noted in miliary tuberculosis or early nodular silicosis. The associated findings of mitral disease are usually obvious, however, so that there is no difficulty in making the differential diagnosis.

Pulmonary ossification or calcification is an uncommon finding in mitral stenosis. It is usually found in the lower lobes and produces multiple opacities resembling the calcified lesions of histoplasmosis scattered widely in the lung bases.

MITRAL INSUFFICIENCY

Mitral insufficiency is often associated with mitral stenosis. This valvular defect increases the left ventricular work load and leads to dilatation and hyper-

trophy of this chamber. It is manifested by enlargement of the heart downward and to the left with lengthening and rounding of the left lower cardiac contour. The left atrium is also enlarged and causes the signs described previously for enlargement of this chamber. Pulmonary congestion develops as in mitral stenosis. Often it is impossible to differentiate mitral stenosis and insufficiency. Relative mitral insufficiency commonly occurs in diseases that produce left ventricular dilatation. Its presence, although suspected, may be difficult to detect radiographically in many of these cases. Acute mitral insufficiency caused by ruptured chordae tendinae may occur as a result of bacterial endocarditis, rheumatic endocarditis, blunt trauma, or myocardial infarction. Idiopathic or spontaneous rupture may also occur. Usually there is an abrupt onset or sudden increase in dyspnea in a patient with existing cardiopulmonary disease. The chest film reveals pulmonary edema, moderate to no enlargement of the left atrium, and little if any cardiac enlargement.

COMBINED MITRAL DISEASE

In many instances there are gross changes indicating a double lesion, while in others the findings are sufficiently characteristic to warrant the diagnosis of mitral stenosis without significant regurgitation. There is a third group in which differential diagnosis is difficult to make on roentgen study. As a rule, the left atrium is larger in combined stenosis and insufficiency than in stenosis alone. There should be left ventricular enlargement when insufficiency is present, but this may be very difficult to detect. The posterior curve of the enlarged left atrium in the right anterior oblique projection tends to be longer in insufficiency than in isolated stenosis. Rheumatic heart disease also causes aortic stenosis and insufficiency that result in left ventricular enlargement. These lesions must be kept in mind in addition to mitral insufficiency when left ventricular enlargement is present (Fig. 32-39). When surgery is contemplated in patients with mitral valve disease, cardiac catheterization is used to assess pulmonary arterial and venous pressures as well as to define the amount of stenosis or insufficiency or both present. Selective angiocardiography may be used in conjunction with catheterization to assess the amount of regurgitation, the severity of the stenosis, and the pliability of the valve.

AORTIC STENOSIS

Rheumatic heart disease has been the most common cause of acquired aortic stenosis. However, it may de-

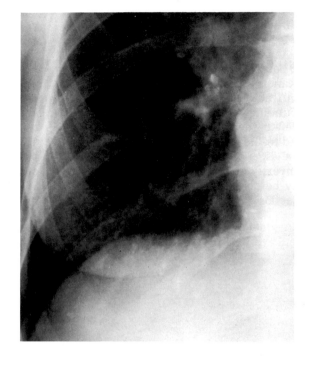

Fig. 32-38. Hemosiderosis in a patient with mitral stenosis. Close-up view of the right lower lung field shows numerous small, granular-appearing nodules that developed over several years of observation.

Fig. 32-39. Combined mitral stenosis and insufficiency. Marked cardiac enlargement with massive enlargement of the left atrium noted on the frontal **(A)** and right anterior oblique **(B)** projections. There is also marked prominence of the pulmonary outflow tract. Note the paucity of basal vessels.

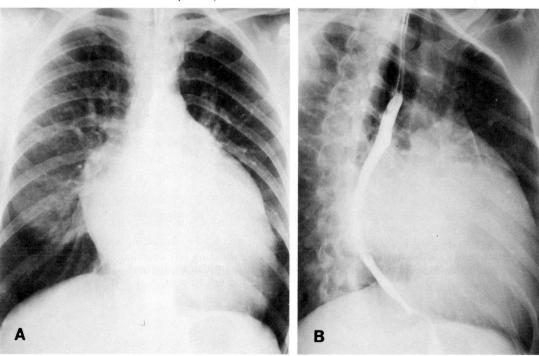

thoracoplasty, pulmonary artery disease such as arteriosclerosis that elevates the pressure, chronic pulmonary inflammatory disease such as pulmonary tuberculosis, the pneumoconioses, and suppurative diseases such as chronic bronchiectasis. Pulmonary emphysema of the chronic type is also a common cause. Usually the diseases cause changes in peripheral arteries and arterioles or there is a primary disease of these vessels that leads to pulmonary hypertension. There is some controversy regarding pathogenesis in some of the conditions. In addition to the findings described in the following paragraphs, pulmonary changes caused by the underlying disease may be present.

Roentgen Findings. The heart is not necessarily enlarged and in the frontal projection is often vertical in type and appears small and round. There is prominence of the pulmonary artery segment in the left upper silhouette along with prominence of the arteries in the hilum on both sides. The pulmonary infundibulum is enlarged along with the pulmonary artery. This is manifested by convex prominence of the pulmonary outflow tract and infundibular segment noted in the right anterior oblique projection. There is a discrepancy between the caliber of pulmonary arteries; the hilar arteries are enlarged and the midzone and peripheral arteries are either normal or smaller than normal in diameter. In some instances there is a rapid and striking diminution in caliber of arteries in the parahilar areas. Not infrequently, the vascular changes must be used to suggest the diagnosis, since the cardiac silhouette may not be typical. When right ventricular hypertrophy is marked, there may be some increased convexity of the lower right anterior cardiac silhouette noted in the left anterior oblique projection and the apex may be elevated and rounded. There is no enlargement of the left atrium or left ventricle in this condition. Pulmonary emphysema is often present and may be severe. When the ventricular enlargement becomes great there may be sufficient anterior protrusion and convexity to result in decrease in the retrosternal space anterior to the base of the heart as viewed in the lateral or extreme left anterior oblique projection. In addition, marked enlargement of the pulmonary outflow tract may produce a longer convexity in the region of the pulmonary artery segment than is normally outlined.

In patients with severe thoracic deformities or marked pulmonary disease, the disease causing the increase in pulmonary artery pressure may distort the heart to the point where chamber enlargement cannot be ascertained but the enlargement of the

pulmonary artery is usually visible. In order to determine the diagnosis, correlation with clinical history, physical findings, and electrocardiographic findings should be made, but when they are typical the roentgen findings are reasonably reliable.

Acute cor pulmonale is found in massive pulmonary embolism, pulmonary edema, tension pneumothorax, the other conditions which cause acute hypoxia or anoxia. The various conditions are discussed under the pulmonary disease in question.

THE HEART IN THORACIC DEFORMITIES

Kyphoscoliosis

The heart is usually displaced to the side opposite the convexity of the dorsal spine and when the convexity is to the right, the right side of the heart border is often obscured by the shadow of the lower thoracic vertebrae. When the thoracic deformity is marked there is often rotation and torsion sufficient to interfere with cardiac function. In these patients there is so much deformity of the heart produced by the thoracic change that normal landmarks are altered and evaluation of chamber size and identification of chambers is very difficult.

Funnel Chest (Pectus Excavatum)

This deformity consists of depression of the sternum, which may be severe, and results in displacement of the heart backward and to the left. On the lateral view the position of the sternum is easily recognized so that the diagnosis is made without difficulty in this projection. In the frontal view there are several radiographic signs that are diagnostic when present. They consists of the following: (1) Sharp downward angulation of the anterior arcs of the ribs with the degree of slant roughly proportional to the amount of depression. (2) Displacement of the cardiac shadow to the left with some convexity in the left upper border so that the silhouette suggests mitral disease with enlargement and prominence of the left atrial appendage. (3) Indistinct border of the right side of the heart. The border is often obscured by the thoracic spine. (4) Decreased density of the heart with more severe deformity, owing to the decrease in its anteroposterior diameter. In these patients the lower thoracic spine is more readily visible than in the normal person. (5) Increased density and cloudiness of the medial aspect of the right lung base. This is caused by some compression of the underlying lung and is accentuated by the visibility of pulmonary vessels that are often hidden by the right lower cardiac bor-

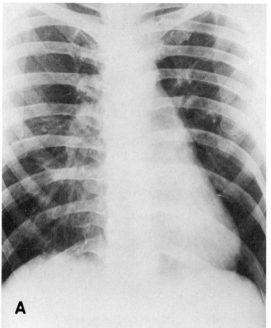
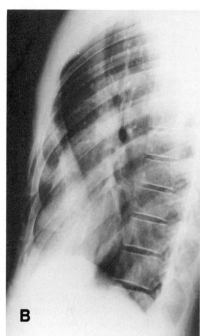

Fig. 32-46. Funnel-chest deformity. **A.** Most of the signs described in the text are present, including prominence of the left upper cardiac border, shift of the heart to the left, slight increase in density below the right hilum, failure to visualize the border of the right side of the heart, and accentuation of the downward angulation of the ribs. **B.** The lateral view shows the marked posterior displacement of the lower sternum.

der. (6) Some straightening of the normal rounded curve of the thoracic spine or actual reversal of the curve in some instances. (7) Occasional backward displacement and compression of the heart between the sternum and thoracic spine so that there is actual widening with an increase in the transverse diameter to the right as well as to the left. Most of these signs are usually present so that the diagnosis of this deformity in the frontal projection is not difficult to make. The differentiation from mitral valvular disease in this projection is important, however (Fig. 32-46). Fixation of the sternum to the central tendon of the diaphragm may result in paradoxical cardiac enlargement during inspiration in children with pectus excavatum. The diaphragm pulls the lower sternum posteriorly as it moves downward in inspiration, reducing the space between the spine and sternum and flattening the heart so that it appears wider and thus larger in the frontal projection.

DISEASES OF THE MYOCARDIUM

CARDIOMYOPATHY

The cardiomyopathies[59] have been divided pathophysiologically into three main groups: (*1*) Conges-

tive myopathy. This group includes idiopathic myopathies, the majority of which occur with a known systemic disease such as infectious, postpartum, or connective tissue disease, or with a neuromuscular myopathy. (*2*) Constrictive myopathy. This includes those conditions that simulate constrictive pericarditis, including infiltrative lesions of the myocardium and endocardium, such as endomyocardial fibrosis and endocardial fibroelastosis, either of which may also present as a congestive myopathy. (*3*) Obstructive myopathy. The clinical manifestations suggest an obstructive valve lesion. Included in this category is idiopathic, hypertrophic, and subaortic stenosis (hypertrophic obstructive cardiomyopathy), and malignant infiltration of the myocardium by tumors.

The roentgen manifestations of these diseases are not specific, but there is usually cardiac enlargement that may be massive. The enlargement is usually caused by dilatation of all the chambers. The contractility of the heart is decreased so that, at fluoroscopy, marked diminution of pulsation is noted. The transverse diameter often increases more than the longitudinal diameter. The heart appears broad and normal contours are effaced. Even though the heart may be markedly enlarged, there may be no signs of failure.

In these patients the differentiation from pericardial effusion is often difficult.

Infectious Myocarditis (Cardiomyopathy)

In infectious myocarditis the degree of cardiac dilatation is proportional to the severity of muscle damage, and there may be rapid progression to gross generalized enlargement of the heart augmented by some pericardial effusion which is often present. The amount of effusion is often small. The roentgen findings of generalized enlargement of the cardiac silhouette are similar regardless of the infectious agent. However, in parasitic disease, such as hydatid myocarditis, calcification may occur.

Anemia

In severe anemias there may be considerable cardiac enlargement. Correction leads to regression to normal unless there has been a great deal of muscle damage. Radiographically, the enlargement tends to be general with some pulmonary artery prominence.

Postpartum Cardiomyopathy

Postpartum cardiomyopathy is rare but when heart failure develops for the first time in the postpartum period, cardiomyopathy is a likely diagnosis.

Connective-Tissue Diseases

In systemic lupus erythematosus, polyarteritis, or scleroderma, a cardiomyopathy, often associated with pericardial effusion, may be present. In rheumatoid arthritis, there is a slightly greater tendency to involvement of the endocardium and the aortic and mitral valves than in any of the three conditions just mentioned.

Alcoholic Cardiomyopathy

Alcoholism may result in cardiomyopathy with severe myocardial damage and gross enlargement of the heart in some patients. In others with less severe myocardial damage, the findings are not as great and recovery may be complete, unlike the prospects for the more severe group in whom the prognosis is poor. Roentgen findings of cardiac enlargement vary with the severity of the disease. Thiamine deficiency may be a factor so that it is possible that there is a combination of causes in some of these patients.

THE CONSTRICTIVE MYOPATHIES

The constrictive myopathies include infiltrative lesions of the endocardium and myocardium, such as endocardial fibroelastosis and myocardial fibrosis. The findings in endocardial fibroelastosis have been described earlier in this chapter. Endomyocardial fibrosis is found most often in the tropics and may be right- or left-sided and, in some patients, both ventricles are involved. Roentgen findings are those of cardiac enlargement with evidence of right atrial dilatation. Often pericardial effusion is present making chamber identification difficult. The right ventricle is small, but the outflow tract and pulmonary arteries are large. When the left ventricle is involved, pulmonary venous hypertension and mitral incompetence result in an appearance simulating that of mitral valvular disease. In the biventricular form, the right-sided features tend to dominate, but there is usually evidence of enlarged upper-lobe pulmonary veins in contrast to pulmonary oligemia observed in isolated right-sided disease.

OBSTRUCTIVE CARDIOMYOPATHY

Obstructive cardiomyopathy includes hypertrophic obstructive cardiomyopathy or idiopathic hypertrophic subaortic stenosis. The muscle hypertrophy may be patchy so that no outflow tract obstruction is produced. There may then be no alteration in the cardiac configuration. When there is outflow tract obstruction producing increased left ventricular workload, the heart may enlarge, and secondary mitral insufficiency may develop so that the mitral configuration is produced. There is usually no significant poststenotic dilatation of the aorta so that, unless the mitral valve is involved, the only finding is that of left ventricular enlargement. Therefore, the diagnosis is usually made by angiocardiography.

The Heart in Beriberi

Vitamin B$_1$ (thiamine) deficiency resulting in beriberi is uncommon in the United States, but is occasionally encountered. The roentgen findings are those of cardiac dilatation that may be diffuse and symmetric producing generalized enlargement of the cardiac silhouette. The right ventricle is occasionally damaged more markedly than the myocardium elsewhere, resulting in dilatation of the pulmonary artery and of the right ventricle and atrium. Pericardial effusion may be present and contribute to the enlargement of the cardiac shadow. Successful treatment results in prompt regression of the enlargement and reabsorption of pericardial fluid.

The Heart in Diseases of the Thyroid

Hypothyroidism. Hypofunction of the thyroid gland resulting in myxedema causes general dilatation of the cardiovascular silhouette. Pericardial effusion is common in myxedema and may contribute part, if not all, of the increase in cardiac size. Some patients with "myxedema heart" have been shown to have massive pericardial effusions that have contributed to most of the enlargement. In treated patients with myxedema, the heart returns to normal quickly, but, in chronic myxedema heart disease, return to normal may require many months of treatment.

Hyperthyroidism. The heart of a patient with hyperthyroidism is hyperactive. The pulse pressure is usually high, resulting in an increased amplitude of pulsation as visualized fluoroscopically. The cardiac configuration is not characteristic, but cardiac enlargement is frequently present. The enlargement may be left ventricular with rounding and elongation of the left ventricular border; but often the right ventricle is mainly affected and the pulmonary artery and right ventricular outflow tract are enlarged. Some investigators believe that right ventricular enlargement is more characteristic of this disease than is left ventricular enlargement. It is generally agreed that there is cardiac enlargement in severe hyperthyroidism and that the size of the heart decreases when the disease is controlled, but may not return to normal because of extensive myocardial damage.

CARDIAC INJURIES

Blunt cardiac injury may be suggested when chest films reveal fracture of the sternum or evidence of soft-tissue injury in the precordial area. Contusion of the myocardium often occurs with no external evidence of chest injury, and may simulate myocardial infarction, including the formation of posttraumatic ventricular aneurysm. Rupture of papillary muscle or chordae tendinae may occur, resulting in acute mitral insufficiency manifested by acute pulmonary edema with a heart of normal size.

Penetrating injuries may result in death before the patient can be treated, but occasionally various types of wounds result in hemopericardium without

enough tamponade to cause immediate death. The roentgen signs are similar to those of pericardial effusion described in the section on diseases of the pericardium. In addition, the injury that produces the hemopericardium may cause hemothorax or pneumothorax. Occasionally, metallic foreign bodies such as bullets can penetrate the heart wall or go through it into one of the cardiac chambers without causing death. They are readily visualized and may be localized by fluoroscopy. The motion of the opaque foreign body can be used as an aid in identifying its position. When the projectile is within a cardiac chamber, a considerable amount of movement is usually visualized in a somewhat irregularly circular or pendulous type of motion, while a projectile imbedded in the myocardium moves in a more uniform manner. Whenever foreign bodies are found within the heart or in its wall, study of the heart shortly before surgery is important since the foreign body may move out through the aorta into the systemic circulation when on the left side or into the lesser circulation when on the right. Occasionally small opaque foreign bodies such as lead shot have been observed to move through the venous system to the heart.

TUMORS OF THE HEART

Primary cardiac tumors are rare. Benign and malignant neoplasms can occur, however, and such tumors as fibroma, myxoma, rhabdomyoma, and rhabdosarcoma have been described, along with primary tumors of vascular origin. The most common benign tumor is the myxoma. It is found in the left atrium in about 75% of cases, arising from the atrial septum near the foramen ovale. Most of the remainder arise in the right atrium. Ventricular myxoma is rare. The tumor is usually pedunculated and may cause intermittent obstruction at the mitral valve. When it occurs in the right atrium, it may obstruct the tricuspid valve. Roentgen findings in myxoma may then resemble those of mitral or tricuspid stenosis, depending upon the site of origin. Left atrial myxoma can be suspected when there is roentgen evidence of mitral stenosis with no previous history of rheumatic fever, an inconstant and changing murmur, and embolic phenomena occuring without atrial fibrillation (Fig. 32-47). Right atrial myxoma results in roentgen findings suggesting tricuspid stenosis or Ebstein's anomaly; here, too, the murmur is inconstant and embolic (pulmonary) phenomena occur. About 10% of atrial myxomas calcify enough

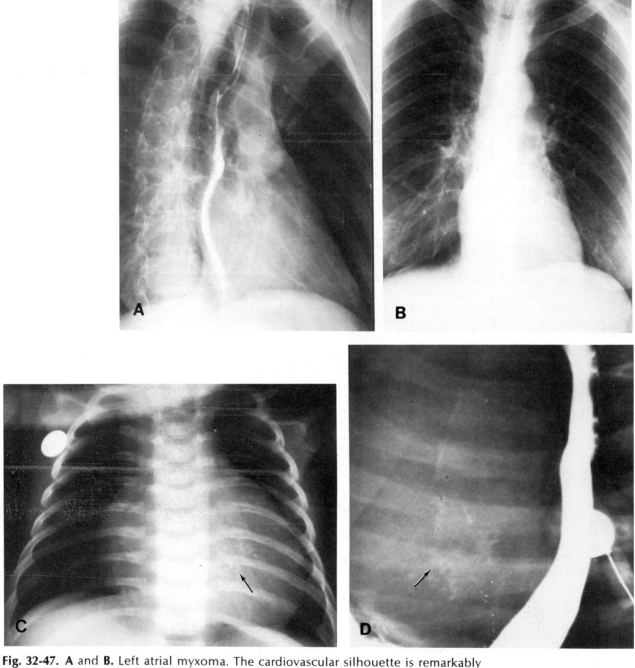

Fig. 32-47. A and **B.** Left atrial myxoma. The cardiovascular silhouette is remarkably similar to that of mitral stenosis including slight constriction of basal vessels in the lungs. Note the definite posterior displacement of the esophagus by the enlarged atrium in the right anterior oblique view **(B). C** and **D.** Calcified left ventricular tumor in a 7-week-old infant. In the frontal projection **(C)**, the arrow points to the site of the tumor. Spot film with barium in the esophagus **(D)** shows mottled calcification in the intraventricular tumor **(arrow).**

to be visible at fluoroscopy. Right atrial myxoma does not interfere with valvular function as often as myxoma of the left atrium. Therefore the right atrial tumor tends to be larger than the left before causing symptoms. Angiocardiography is useful in outlining the intracardiac tumor. The other benign tumors tend to be intramural and include fibroma, hamartoma, rhabdomyoma, and lipoma. Most involve the left ventricular wall. They tend to produce cardiac enlargement, to calcify (20%), and usually occur in children.

Rarely, intraventricular hematoma may calcify and resemble intracardiac tumor. Symptoms depend on the size and mobility of the hematoma. Its location, usually in the right ventricle, can readily be observed at fluoroscopy. Echocardiography is very useful in the study of intracardiac tumors.

Malignant tumors such as rhabdomyosarcoma or fibrosarcoma are very rare and usually arise in the ventricular walls, while angiosarcoma apparently arises most commonly in the right atrial wall. Angiocardiography is required to make the diagnosis. Masses projecting from the outer cardiac surface may produce bizarre cardiac shapes, but the diagnosis may be suspected on roentgen examination, however. Diagnostic pneumopericardium or pneumothorax may be of value in demonstrating the site of a bizarre mass that appears to be intimately associated with the heart.

Metastatic myocardial tumors are much more common than the primary tumors. Cardiac involvement by lymphoma and various carcinomas often results in pericardial effusion. Therefore the roentgen findings may be caused by hemopericardium. An irregular cardiac mass occurring alone (or associated with hemopericardium) in a patient with known Hodgkin's disease, lymphoma, or carcinoma virtually indicates myocardial metastasis.

Pericardial tumors, like those of the heart muscle, are rare. Of the primary tumors, the benign and malignant form are about equal in number, but metastatic pericardial tumors are more common than the primary ones. Fibroma, fibrosarcoma, benign and malignant mesothelioma, vascular tumors such as hemangioma and lymphangioma, teratoma, thymoma, leiomyoma, hamartoma, and intrapericardial bronchial cyst may arise in the pericardium. All are rare and cannot be differentiated radiographically. They may cause pericardial or pleural effusion. The major radiographic feature of the tumor itself is alteration of the cardiac contour which varies with the size and shape of the mass.

ACQUIRED DISEASES OF THE AORTA

ARTERIOSCLEROSIS OF THE AORTA

A certain amount of alteration in the apperance of the aorta with advancing age is secondary to loss of elasticity. The change consists of elongation and dilatation; it eventually occurs in all persons who live long enough. As a result of these anatomic changes, the configuration of the aortic arch changes roentgenographically. The ascending arch becomes more prominent, resulting in more convexity of the right upper cardiac margin. The aortic knob on the left side becomes more prominent and somewhat enlarged. The descending aorta curves to left in the posteroanterior view and then back to midline or even to the right side before passing through the diaphragm. In the left oblique view and in the lateral projection, the arch of the aorta is noted to swing in a wider arc so that it often angles forward and upward, then backward, resulting in widening of the area between the limbs of the arch, which is termed the "aortic window." The descending aorta may curve far backward to overlie the thoracic spine in the lateral view.

In arteriosclerotic disease of the aorta, the manifestations of elongation and dilatation occur earlier in life and plaques of calcium are often visualized in the transverse aortic arch. The amount of calcification varies considerably. The plaques are noted as dense linear shadows and are most commonly seen in the aortic knob but may be extensive throughout the aorta distal to the transverse arch, so that the entire wall of this structure may be outlined by calcium in extreme instances (Fig. 32-48). Aortic arteriosclerotic disease per se may not be significant unless complicated by dissection or aneurysm, but it is often associated with arteriosclerotic disease elsewhere, e.g., in the carotid, renal, and coronary arteries, which may cause morbidity and mortality. Atheromatous fibrous plaques consist principally of an accumulation of intimal, smooth muscle cells loaded with lipid, chiefly cholesterol. The cells are also surrounded by lipid and by collagen elastic fibers. These cells and extracellular material cover a large deeper deposit of free extracellular lipid intermixed with cell debris. The plaque may become altered as a result of hemorrhage, calcification, cell necrosis, and/or mural thrombosis. The most distinct characteristic of this complicated lesion is the presence of calcification. This is the type of lesion that often becomes associated with occlusive disease. The latter usually occurs at the site of bifurcation or of arterial fixation.

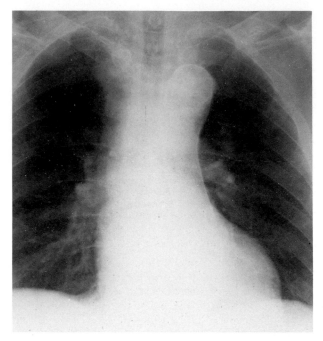

Fig. 32-48. Arteriosclerotic disease of the aorta. Note the extensive calcification in the thoracic aorta. The aorta is slightly dilated, elongated, and tortuous. The patient also had extensive generalized arteriosclerosis.

Large arteries such as the carotid, renal, femoral, and coronaries may be involved by disease severe enough to produce occlusion. Angiography is used to outline these lesions. Discussion of the technique and findings is beyond the scope of this volume.

Takayasu's Arteritis

Takayasu's arteritis was initially called "pulseless disease." It involves the aorta and its branches as well as the pulmonary arteries in an extensive manner.[6] Peripheral arteries are not usually involved. It is a disease of young women with a female to male ratio of about 8 to 1. Most of the patients are under 30 years of age. Although its etiology is not definitely known, it probably represents an autoimmune disease in which granulation tissue destroys the media of the large vessels; inflammatory cells are also present. As the inflammatory reaction subsides, scar tissue in the arterial walls causes marked thickening resulting in luminal narrowing and occlusion. Plain films show widening of the aorta with irregularity of aortic contour and aortic calcifications that are linear and may involve short or long segments of the aortic arch or the descending or the abdominal aorta. Aortic

insufficiency resulting from dilatation of the aortic root is present in 10% to 20% of the patients. The aortic valve is normal. Rarely, aortic dissection may occur in this disease. When the pulmonary arteries are involved the roentgen findings may be those of pulmonary hypertension with prominence of the central pulmonary arteries. Partial occlusions of the branches may result in hypovascularity in the involved areas, which may be difficult to define roentgenographically, but the possibility should be kept in mind in young women with a dilated, irregular aorta containing calcium.

SYPHILITIC AORTITIS

Luetic aortitis produces alterations that can often be recognized radiographically before clinical signs of specific aortic involvement are present. Circumscribed dilatation of the ascending aortic arch may occur and be recognized as enlargement of this portion of the aorta before the signs of aneurysm appear, but, since similar dilatation may occur in arteriosclerosis and in aortic stenosis (poststenotic dilatation), this finding cannot be considered as pathognomonic. The dilatation in arteriosclerotic disease is usually more diffuse than in luetic aortitis. Calcification in the wall of the ascending aortic arch is a more reliable sign of luetic aortitis. It is manifested by a thin, curvilinear shadow of calcific density in the outer wall of the ascending aorta that may be visible in the frontal projection but is often more readily visualized in the left anterior oblique and lateral projections. This is in contrast to the calcification in arteriosclerotic disease that is noted in the transverse aortic arch. Calcification may occur in the ascending aortic arch in arteriosclerosis, but this is usually found in elderly patients in whom the disease is severe. Furthermore, the plaques are thicker and more irregular than the somewhat thin linear shadows noted in syphilis. On pathologic examination of the aorta in arteriosclerosis, calcification is often found in the ascending aorta but it is most prominent in the inner wall of the arch and may not be roentgenographically visible. Late syphilis is now so rare that it can be assumed that most patients with calcification in the ascending aorta have advanced arteriosclerotic disease. However, aneurysms of the ascending aorta are frequently found in association with vascular syphilis.

AORTIC ANEURYSM

An aneurysm is a circumscribed area of localized widening in the wall of a blood vessel. Some dilatation of the aorta occurs in arteriosclerosis and there is no sharply limited differentiation between simple dilatation and an aneurysm. The latter term is usually reserved to designate a clearly defined local area of cylindrical or saccular enlargement. Aneurysms involving the ascending aortic arch in the past were often of syphilitic origin, particularly when saccular in type, but connective-tissue disorders with medial necrosis such as in Marfan's syndrome may also be associated with aneurysm. Aneurysms of the descending aorta may be arteriosclerotic in origin; rarely their origin is mycotic, traumatic, or congenital. Roentgen and fluoroscopic studies usually are sufficient to make the diagnosis.

Local aneurysms of the descending thoracic aorta often produce no symptoms and are detected as incidental findings on chest roentgenograms. They usually project from the posterolateral aspect of the mid or lower descending thoracic aorta to appear as left-sided masses. They are usually of arteriosclerotic origin, but other lesions causing aneurysms may be present.

Roentgen Findings. Aneurysm results in a mass shadow continuous with the aortic silhouette that varies considerably in size and shape from one patient to another. It is not unusual to note widening of the superior mediastinum above the arch on the right when the aneurysm involves the ascending aorta, caused by aneurysm of the innominate artery. The mass of the aneurysm in the ascending aortic arch usually projects to the right while that of the descending arch projects to the left in the frontal plane. Occasionally the communication between the aorta and the aneurysm is very narrow (pedunculated aneurysm). Then the aneurysm may project in a direction not usually observed in the more common saccular lesion. The relationships should be studied in the lateral and in the oblique projections. Barium in the esophagus is used to show the relationship of the aortic mass to the esophagus in fluoroscopic and roentgen examinations. The lesion is most clearly defined in the left anterior oblique projection in the usual instance. Occasionally there may be more than one saccular aneurysm with an area of fusiform dilatation between them. It is often possible to make the diagnosis of aneurysm on roentgenographic evidence alone, but fluoroscopy is useful in detecting the amount of pulsation. When the differentiation between aortic aneurysm and mediastinal mass due to other cause cannot be made roentgenographically, fluoroscopy is of value in demonstrating the relationship of the mass to the heart and aorta and determining the presence of expansile pulsation which usually indicates that the lesion is an aneurysm. Occasionally, however, a tumor may partially surround the aortic arch in such a manner that it may actually exhibit expansile pulsation. Furthermore, when there is a considerable amount of thrombus within an aneurysm, pulsation may be markedly dampened or absent. When there is any doubt in such a patient, aortography can be used to make the differential diagnosis. Arteriosclerotic aneurysms usually occur in the abdominal aorta but may occur in the arch and descending portion of the thoracic aorta. They are generally smaller than those of luetic origin and often show calcification. Rarely, there may be erosion of bone secondary to aortic aneurysm. When the ascending arch is involved the erosion occurs along the posterior aspect of the sternum; erosion through this bone has been described. Aneurysms of the distal arch may erode one or more of the dorsal vertebral bodies. The bone erosion is a manifestation of the syphilitic type of aneurysm in most, if not all, instances. The vertebrae involved have a scalloped appearance because the discs resist the erosion. The vertebral bodies are then concave anteriorly. Retrograde aortography may be necessary to differentiate aneurysm from other mediastinal masses (Fig. 32-49).

TRAUMATIC ANEURYSM OR HEMATOMA

Rupture of all layers of the aorta caused by trauma usually leads to exsanguination and sudden death. When the adventitia is spared and rupture is incomplete, the patient may survive. Survival in others is evidently dependent upon mediastinal hematoma which may temporarily prevent exsanguination. An infolding of the media may then result in a false aneurysm with a connective tissue wall. The usual site of such rupture is in the aortic arch, immediately distal to the left subclavian artery at the site of the ligamentum arteriosum. The disruption is often circumferential and the ruptured layers may retract. The roentgen findings in the acute phase consist in evidence of hematoma in the vicinity of the aortic arch, manifest by widening of the mediastinum in that area which also obscures the aorta. This is an important finding in this condition. Slight deviation of the trachea to the right also appears to be a significant finding; it was present in all eight patients at our hospital, as reported by Flaherty and associates,[18] including one in whom the mediastinum did not appear to be widened. Extrapleural hemorrhage may cause an apparent apical pleural thickening or mass, another significant plain-film finding when present. Hemorrhage into the pleural space and lung is common and there may be evidence of rib or sternal fracture.

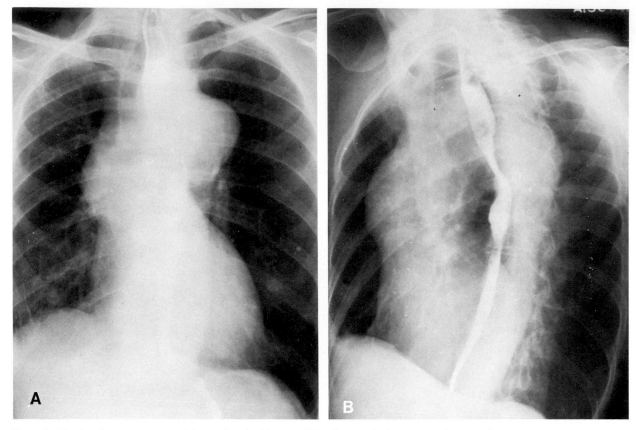

Fig. 32-49. Aortic aneurysms. Note the fusiform dilatations of the ascending and transverse portions of the aortic arch in both frontal **(A)** and left anterior oblique **(B)** projections.

Pneumomediastinum and pneumothorax may occur but are not of particular diagnostic significance. When these signs are present in a patient who has suffered severe thoracic trauma, traumatic aortic fracture should be suspected.

A chest film should be obtained in all patients having severe deceleration accidents in order to detect aortic injury. Since the traumatic dissections and pseudoaneurysms are unstable and may rupture, prompt diagnostic and surgical measures are necessary. Because multiple arterial injuries involving major arch branches may be present, the innominate, carotid, and subclavian arteries should be examined at the same time. Percutaneous transfemoral arteriography is usually the method of choice used to confirm the diagnosis (Fig. 32-50). Surgical repair may then be carried out. When no corrective measures are taken and the patient survives with a traumatic aneurysm of the aorta or one of its major brachyce-

phalic branches, in time the diffuse mediastinal density clears leaving a more or less clearly defined mass which represents the false aneurysm. Calcification develops in the wall in most of the lesions as they become chronic. Expansile pulsation is not necessarily present, because of the organized thrombus in the wall. The diagnosis can usually be made on the basis of the roentgen findings in a patient who has a history of previous thoracic trauma. Aortography can then be used to confirm the diagnosis and localize the site of origin (Fig. 32-51).

DISSECTING ANEURYSM

Dissecting aneurysm of the aorta begins at the site of an intimal tear, usually within the first 5 cm of the ascending aorta, although the dissections are related to degenerative disease of the media. The cause of the initial rupture or tear is not clear in most patients.

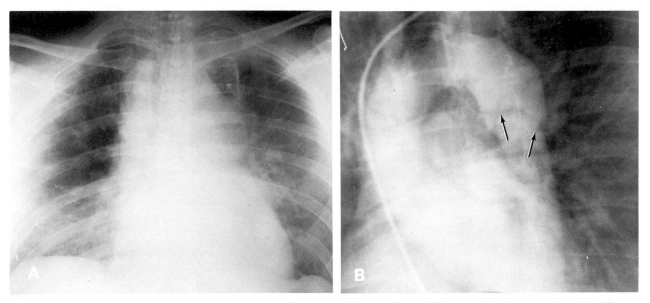

Fig. 32-50. Traumatic fracture of the aorta. **A.** This examination, made a few hours after injury, shows widening of the superior mediastinum, loss of clear definition of the transverse aortic arch, and deviation of the trachea to the right. On the initial film there also appeared to be downward displacement of the left main bronchus. **B.** Forward aortogram with a catheter in the right ventricle shows aortic dilatation distal to the left subclavian artery with infolding of the disrupted aortic wall **(arrows);** below this the caliber is normal.

Fig. 32-51. Chronic traumatic fracture of the aorta. **A. Arrows** indicate the mass in the vicinity of the transverse and upper descending aorta. Note the thin curvilinear calcification in the wall of the mass. **B.** Aortogram shows the false aneurysm. A thin infolding of the aortic wall is also observed **(arrows)**.

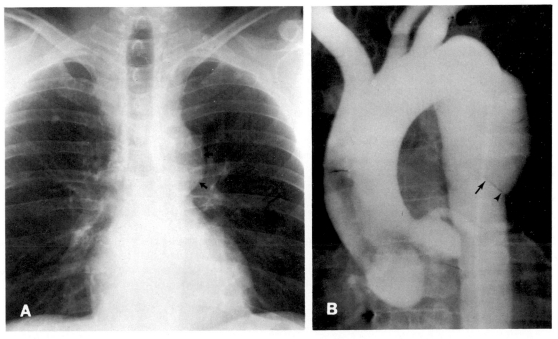

Dissection produces a false channel which may be so thin that there is virtually no dilatation. In such an instance, the term "aneurysm" is a misnomer. DeBakey's classification is widely accepted since it is useful in the angiographic diagnosis and management of dissections.[26] In this classification dissecting aneurysms are divided into three types: Type I—the dissection begins in the ascending aorta and extends through and beyond the aortic arch, often to the common iliac arteries. Type II—the dissection is limited to the ascending aorta. This is most commonly observed in Marfan's syndrome. Type III—the dissection begins in the thoracic aorta distal to the subclavian artery and extends for a variable distance proximal and distal to the original site. The common sites of the intimal defects are in or adjacent to the sinus of Valsalva and in the descending aorta near the ligamentum arteriosum. Dissection or rupture may also start at the site of an atheromatous plaque, and in this instance the abdominal aorta is the more common site. The condition ends fatally in a few hours or days in most patients. In about 10%, there is a "reentry" into the abdominal aorta at the bifurcation or into one of the iliacs. This permits the dissection to decompress and the patient may live for months or years. The roentgen diagnosis is often difficult to make and the findings must be correlated with the clinical history of severe pain that usually occurs at the site of dissection, along with pallor and, often, shock. There may be widening of the aorta extending from the site of dissection distally and, occasionally, proximally. This can be most readily appreciated when a chest roentgenogram obtained prior to dissection is available for comparison. Roentgenograms obtained on successive days may show extension of the area of widening and when this is observed in a patient with a typical clinical history and findings, the diagnosis of dissecting aneurysm is almost certain. When the false channel is very thin, there may be little, if any, increase in the apparent width of the aorta. When the false channel is wide, there may be some displacement of the trachea to the right, and displacement of the esophagus by the dissection may be visible on an esophagram. In the patients with extensive arteriosclerosis in whom calcification in atheromatous plaques is visible, it is sometimes possible to outline the inner wall of the aorta by means of this calcification and to note the great thickening formed by the dissecting aneurysm because the outer wall is readily visible against the radiolucency of the lung. This is not an absolute sign, however, because circumferential neoplasm and periaortic fat may cause an apparent thickening of the wall. Pleural effusion is a common accessory finding. It usually occurs on the left side. Occasionally, recognizable enlargement of the branches of the aorta can be demonstrated, since dissection not infrequently extends into the walls of these vessels. When such enlargement is present it is of considerable diagnostic significance. Since the patients are often desperately ill, making roentgen examination difficult, the use of this method of study is limited in many instances. In patients in whom the diagnosis is suspected early in the course of the disease, surgical measures may be warranted. In these instances, aortography may be used to confirm the diagnosis. Angiography may determine the site of the initial tear, the extent of the dissection (false channel), the amount of deformity or narrowing of the true channel, and involvement of aortic branches.

DISEASES OF THE PERICARDIUM

PERICARDIAL EFFUSION

The pericardium is a thin membrane that is not ordinarily recognized as a separate structure since it is of the same density as the adjacent heart. It is relatively inelastic and conditions that produce rapid accumulation of fluid within it may compress the heart enough to produce severe alteration of cardiac function leading to death. This occurs most commonly as the result of hemorrhage secondary to trauma. Roentgenograms are not usually obtained during this acute situation.

In chronic or subacute pericardial effusion, roentgen changes are produced when the amount of fluid reaches 400 or 500 ml. Smaller effusions up to 300 ml are not ordinarily diagnosed, since they produce no significant alteration in the contour of the cardiovascular silhouette. This slow accumulation of fluid may reach massive proportions without producing tamponade.

Roentgen Findings. There is an increase in size of the cardiac silhouette that depends upon the amount of fluid present. The shape of the cardiovascular silhouette is also altered. With moderate amounts of fluid, the enlargement is generalized and the cardiohepatic angle appears more acute than is normal. As the amount of fluid increases there tends to be disproportionate enlargement of the heart inferiorly in the transverse diameter as compared to the increase in the vertical diameter. Demonstration of rapid progression, or regression, of these findings is a most valuable sign in roentgen diagnosis (Fig. 32-52). At

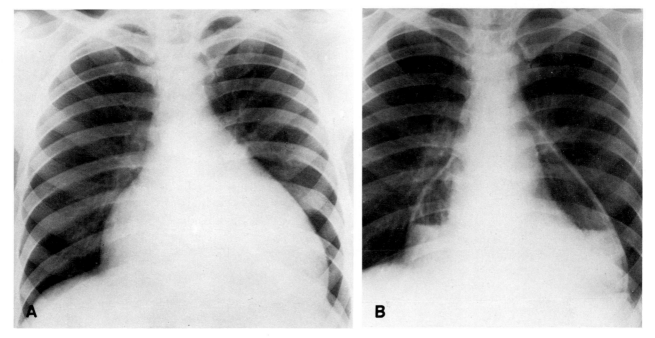

Fig. 32-52. Pericardial effusion. **A.** The cardiac silhouette is grossly enlarged. The lung fields are quite clear and there is no evidence of pleural effusion. Two months earlier the heart size had been normal. **B.** This film was exposed following pericardial tap. Some fluid was removed, and air was injected to determine the thickness of the pericardial wall since there were leukocytes in the fluid. Note that the wall is several millimeters thick.

fluoroscopy the pulsations are dampened or obliterated and there is some alteration in contour of the heart noted between the upright and the recumbent positions. This finding is often equivocal, however. Large effusions also tend to obliterate the normal segments noted on either side and the cardiac enlargement is noted to extend to the right as well as to the left. Dilatation of the heart in myocardial failure can produce a silhouette that simulates that of pericardial effusion. Furthermore, in these patients the amplitude of pulsation is also small owing to the myocardial weakness so that differentiation is very difficult. Mellins, Kottmeier, and Kiely[43] found experimentally on dogs that fluid accumulated anteriorly, laterally, and superiorly, but not posteriorly in the pericardial space. As a result, pericardial fluid dampened the cardiac pulsations anteriorly but not posteriorly. This sign was noted on a few patients and may be of value. Cineradiography in the lateral projection may show dampened or absent anterior pulsations and normal pulsations manifested by motion of the barium-filled esophagus posteriorly. There

is a layer of epicardial fat beneath the visceral pericardium that may be visible and thus outline the cardiac borders. In our experience, this is most frequently seen over the lower two-thirds of the left cardiac margin extending over the inferior aspect of the heart, but usually not to the right of the midline (Fig. 32-53). We use a combination of fluoroscopy with image intensification and cine to detect this layer of fat. If fat can be demonstrated, this finding is of definite value, if it cannot be demonstrated this is of no assistance. When differentiation between pericardial effusion and enlargement resulting from other cause cannot be determined in any other way, angiocardiography can be used to define the inner wall of the cardiac chambers and thus indicate the presence of effusion. Venous angiocardiography may also be used. A measurement of the combination of right atrial wall and pericardial thickness over 5 mm should indicate the presence of effusion. Blood-pool scanning using technetium[99]-labeled albumin may be employed, but this method is not as accurate as venous angiocardiography. Thickening of the right

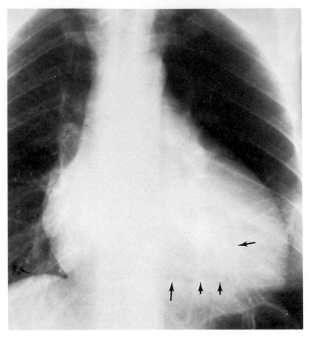

Fig. 32-53. Large pericardial effusion. The epicardial fat line was easily observed on cineradiography and at fluoroscopy. It was faintly observed on this roentgenogram **(arrows)**. It lies well within the silhouette and is indicative of the presence of a large pericardial effusion.

atrial wall may result in a false positive sign of the presence of pericardial fluid obtained by these methods, however. Pericardial tap can also be done as a diagnostic and therapeutic procedure and, if necessary, air can be injected to determine the thickness of the parietal pericardium as well as the actual heart size. Films can then be exposed in various projections to outline the heart borders and pericardium. Ultrasonography is very useful in the detection of pericardial effusion and has largely replaced other methods.

ADHESIVE AND CONSTRICTIVE PERICARDITIS

Adhesive pericarditis without constriction is usually of little clinical significance. Adhesions between the pleura and pericardium may result in some irregularity of the cardiac silhouette in the neighborhood of the adhesions. The cause of constrictive pericarditis is often obscure although a number of possibilities exist, including infection and trauma. Whatever the

cause, the amount of pericardial fibrous-tissue reaction may reach the point where constriction occurs. The visceral and parietal pericardium is adherent and also contracted. The basic abnormality is the inability of the ventricles to fill normally, resulting in diminution of stroke volume. Venous pressure is elevated. When this occurs there may be severe clinical symptoms but the radiographic changes are minimal. The heart is often normal or small, and engorgement of the great veins may be evident. At fluoroscopy the diminished pulsations may be apparent. Calcific plaques often occur in the thickened pericardium and are readily visible. At times the heart is nearly encased in a calcific shell. Occasionally there is actually ossification that follows the calcification. When calcification is present in a patient with clinical signs of constrictive pericarditis, the diagnosis is not difficult to determine; but when no calcification is present, roentgen findings are often equivocal. Calcification is present in about 50% of patients with constrictive pericarditis. However, the presence of pericardial calcification does not necessarily indicate significant constriction. The classic finding is that of a quiet heart with clinical signs of failure. The heart may be enlarged, however. Hepatic enlargement and ascites may be evident on abdominal examination. The symptoms of severe cardiac amyloidosis with noncompliant myocardium are similar to those of constrictive pericarditis, but there is usually more cardiac enlargement in amyloidosis than in constrictive pericarditis.

PERICARDIAL TUMORS

The most common mass lesion of the pericardium is the pericardial or clear-water cyst that has been described in Chapter 31 under the heading "Pericardial Cyst." Primary pericardial tumors are rare and produce localized enlargements of various sizes and shapes that cannot be differentiated from cardiac tumors unless pneumopericardium is used. Occasionally, sarcoma or mesothelioma arising in the pericardium can surround the cardiac shadow and produce enlargement of it. The pericardium is much more frequently involved by metastatic tumor and the presence of pericardial and pleural effusion may obscure the actual lesion. Hodgkin's disease not infrequently involves the pericardium and malignant melanoma occasionally metastasizes to the heart and pericardium. CT scanning and ultrasonography are now being used in patients with pericardial masses. The ultimate place of these methods has not yet been determined. The associated presence of masses elsewhere in the thorax is helpful in making the diagnosis. In the presence of a solitary pericardial or cardiac mass, thoracotomy may be necessary to confirm the diagnosis.

"SPONTANEOUS" PNEUMOPERICARDIUM

This is a rare condition for which there are a number of causes. Left subphrenic abscess may penetrate the pericardial portion of the diaphragm, resulting in infection with pus and often gas within the pericardial sac. Direct extension of esophageal carcinoma may produce a similar situation. Occasionally, congenital diaphragmatic hernia may occur through a defect in the pericardial portion of the diaphragm. In this situation, gas-filled loops of bowel may be noted within the pericardial sac. Traumatic hernia of abdominal contents into the pericardial sac has also been reported. Gas-filled loops of intestine may also be visible within the pericardium in this condition.

CONGENITAL PERICARDIAL DEFECTS

The majority of congenital pericardial defects are on the left side. They vary from a small defect overlying the pulmonary artery to absence of the pericardium on the left; the parietal pleura is also involved, so that there is no barrier between the heart and the left lung. The defects occur predominantly in males with the ratio of 3 to 1. Associated anomalies include patent ductus arteriosus, atrial septal defect, bicuspid aortic valve, pulmonary sequestration, bronchogenic cyst, and diaphragmatic hernia. One or more of these are found in about 30% of patients with partial defects. The roentgen findings in complete absence of the left pericardium are characteristic enough to make the diagnosis or strongly suggest it. The heart is shifted to the left. The left border of the heart is flattened as the heart extends to the left over the dome of the diaphragm. The pulmonary artery segment is long and more sharply defined than usual and there is a radiolucent portion of lung between the aorta and pulmonary artery which provides the contrast necessary for the clear definition. The left ventricular segment is also distinct and clearly defined. In the lateral view the pulmonary artery may be more distinct than usual. Diagnostic pneumothorax can be used to confirm the diagnosis; the air extends into the pericardial sac. Partial defects may permit herniation of the left auricular appendage to produce a bizarre appearance of the left upper cardiac silhouette. Right-sided defects permit unusually clear visualization of the great vessels including the

aortic root; lung tissue may herniate medial to the superior vena cava to clearly outline this vessel. Protrusions of the heart, usually the atria, through surgical defects in the pericardium are not uncommon. This possibility must be kept in mind when an unusual bulge or protrusion is noted in the postoperative period. Following surgery or major chest injury, acute cardiac herniation with incarceration causing obstruction of the superior vena cava may occur. Roentgen findings are usually diagnostic.

CARDIAC PACEMAKERS

There has been increasing use of permanent cardiac pacemakers in recent years.[56] The roentgenographic appearance and characteristics of pacemakers used commonly has been described by Walter.[66] The power source and generator are assembled together and coated with a silicone rubber; these are buried in the subcutaneous tissues of the chest wall. The pacemaker leads are also coated with silicone. A soft-tissue tunnel is created to provide for their passage to the external surface of the myocardium or, more commonly, to the venous system for entry of transvenous pacemakers. Epicardial electrodes are sutured in place while the transvenous electrodes are placed at the apex of the right ventricle. Since the power source, the leads, and the electrodes are readily observed radiographically, their position can be determined, and, in case of malfunction, follow-up studies may be useful. When the leads are not long enough, the electrodes may be displaced from the right ventricular apex into the high right ventricle or right ventricular outflow tract, or into the right atrium or inferior vena cava. Initial malpositioning can also be detected. Occasionally, the right ventricle is perforated by the electrodes projecting anterior to the cardiac wall. Fracture of the leads may be detected, usually at the fixation point in the myocardium when epicardial leads are employed, and at points of flexion over the margins of the clavicle or ribs when the transvenous type of leads are used. Some fractures are subtle and can be demonstrated only with oblique views or with the patient in multiple positions during inspiration and expiration. The pacemaker generator is sometimes rotated by the patient, thereby pulling the electrodes out of position. Malplacement in the coronary sinus occurs occasionally, and, in this case, the electrodes lie posteriorly instead of in their normal anterior position in the right ventricular apex. Battery failure can sometimes be detected by the presence of free mercury, which is radiopaque, in the radiolucent electrolyte areas that become indistinct and somewhat opaque.

REFERENCES AND SELECTED READINGS

1. ABRAMS HL, KAPLAN HS: Angiocardiographic Interpretation in Congential Heart Disease. Springfield, IL, Thomas, 1956

2. AMPLATZ K, LESTER RG, SCHIEBLER GL, et al: The roentgenologic features of Ebstein's anomaly of the tricuspid valve. Am J Roentgenol 81: 788, 1959

3. BALTAXE HA, MOLLER JH, AMPLATZ K: Membranous subaortic stenosis and its associated malformations. Radiology 95: 287, 1970

4. BANDOW GT, ROWE GG, CRUMMY AB: Congenital diverticulum of the right and left ventricles. Radiology 117: 19, 1975

5. BARTRAM C, STRICKLAND B: Pulmonary varices. Br J Radiol 44: 927, 1971

6. BERKMEN YM, LANDE A: Chest roentgenography as a window to the diagnosis of Takayasu's arteritis. Am J Roentgenol 125: 842, 1975

7. BERKOFF HA, ROWE GG, CRUMMY AB et al: Asymptomatic left ventricular aneurysm. A sequela of blunt chest trauma. Circulation 55: 545, 1977

8. BRUWER AJ: Posteroanterior chest roentgenogram in two types of anomalous pulmonary venous connection. J Thorac Surg 32: 119, 1956

9. CAREY LS, EDWARDS JE: Roentgenographic features in cases with origin of both great vessels from the right ventricle without pulmonary stenosis. Am J Roentgenol 93: 269, 1965

10. COUSSEMENT Am, GOODING CA: Objective radiographic assessment of pulmonary vascularity in children. Radiology 109: 649, 1973

11. DAVIS GD, KINCAID OW, HALLERMANN FJ: Roentgen aspects of cardiac tumors. Semin Roentgenol 4: 384, 1969

12. EDWARDS JE, CAREY LS. NEUFELD HN, LESTER RG: Congenital Heart Disease. Philadelphia, Saunders, 1965

13. ELLIOTT LP, JUE KL, AMPLATZ K: A roentgen classification of cardiac malpositions. Invest Radiol 1: 17, 1966

14. ELLIS K, LEED NE, HIMMELSTEIN A: Congenital deficiencies in the parietal pericardium. Am J Roentgenol 82: 125, 1959

15. EPSTEIN BS: Calcification of the ascending aorta. Am J Roentgenol 77: 281, 1957

16. EYLER WR, ZIEGLER RF, SHEA JJ, et al: Endocardial fibroelastosis: roentgen appearance. Radiology 64: 797, 1955

17. FIGLEY MM: Accessory roentgen signs of coarctation of the aorta. Radiology 62: 671, 1954

18. FLAHERTY TT, WEGNER GP, CRUMMY AB, et al: Nonpenetrating injuries to the thoracic aorta. Radiology 92: 541, 1969

19. GAY BB Jr, FRANCH RH, SHUFORD WH, et al: The roentgenologic features of single and multiple coarctations of the pulmonary artery and branches. Am J. Roentgenol 90: 599, 1963

20. GOETZ AA, GRAHAM WH: Aneurysm of the sinus of Valsalva. Radiology 67: 416, 1956

21. GOTT VL, LESTER RG, LILLEHEI CW, et al: Total anomalous pulmonary return. An analysis of thirty cases. Circulation 13: 543, 1956

22. GYEPES MT, VINCENT WR: Severe congenital heart disease in the neonatal period. Am J Roentgenol 116: 490, 1972

23. HARRIS EJ: Aneurysms of the sinus of Valsalva. Am J Roentgenol 76: 767, 1956

24. HARRIS GBC, NEUHAUSER EBD, GIEDION A: Total anomalous pulmonary venous return below the diaphragm. Am J Roentgenol 84: 436, 1960

25. HATTEN HP JR, LORMAN JG, ROSENBAUM HD: Pulmonary sling in the adult. Am J Roentgenol 128: 919, 1977

26. HAYASHI K, MEANEY TF, ZELCH JV et al: Aortographic analysis of aortic dissection. Am J Roentgenol 122: 769, 1974

27. HIGGINS CB, REINKE RT, JONES NE et al: Left atrial dimension on the frontal thoracic radiograph: a method for assessing left atrial enlargement. Am J Roentgenol 130: 251, 1978

28. HODGES PC, EYSTER JAE: Estimate of transverse cardiac diameter in man. Arch Intern Med 37: 707, 1926

29. JÖNSSON G, SALTZMAN GF: Infundibulum of patent ductus arteriosus—diagnostic sign in conventional roentgenograms. Acta Radiol [Suppl] (Stockh) 38: 8, 1952

30. KEATS TE, KREIS VA, SIMPSON E: The roentgen manifestations of pulmonary hypertension in congenital heart disease. Radiology 66: 693, 1956

31. KEATS TE, STEINBACH HL: Patent ductus arteriosus. A critical evaluation of its roentgen signs. Radiology 64: 528, 1955

32. KERLEY P: Lung changes in acquired heart disease. Am J Roentgenol 80: 256, 1958

33. KLATTE EC, CAMPBELL JA, LURIE PR: Aortic configuration in congenital heart disease. Radiology 74: 555, 1960

34. KRABBENHOFT KL, EVANS WA: Some pulmonary changes associated with intracardiac septal defects in infancy. Radiology 63: 498, 1954

35. KRAUSE DW, KUEHN HJ, SELLERS RD et al: Roentgen sign associated with an aberrant vessel connecting the right main pulmonary artery to the left atrium. Radiology 111: 177, 1974

36. LESTER RG, ANDERSON RC, AMPLATZ K, et al: Roentgenologic diagnosis of congenitally corrected transposition of the great vessels. Am J Roentgenol 83: 985, 1960

37. LEVIN B, BORDEN CW: Anomalous pulmonary venous drainage into the left vertical vein. Radiology 63: 317, 1954

38. LEVIN B, RIGLER LG: Rib notching following subclavian artery obstruction. Radiology 62: 660, 1954

39. LEVIN B, WHITE H: Total anomalous pulmonary venous drainage into the portal system. Radiology 76: 894, 1961

40. LODWICK GE: Dissecting aneurysms of the thoracic and abdominal aorta. Am J Roentgenol 69: 907, 1955

41. LODWICK GS, GLADSTONE WS: Correlation of anatomic and roentgen changes in arteriosclerosis and syphilis of the ascending aorta. Radiology 69: 70, 1957

42. McCORD MC, BAVENDAM FA: Unusual causes of rib notching. Am J Roentgenol 67: 405, 1952

43. MELLINS HZ, KOTTMEIER P, KIELY B: Radiologic signs of pericardial effusion. Radiology 73: 9, 1959

44. MEYER RR: A method for measuring children's hearts. Radiology 53: 363, 1949

45. MONCADA R, SHANNON M. MILLER R et al: The cervical aortic arch. Am J Roentgenol 125: 591, 1975

46. PAUL LW, RICHTER MR: Funnel chest deformity and its recognition in posteroanterior roentgenograms of the thorax. Am J Roentgenol 46: 619, 1941

47. POCHASZEVESKY R, DUNST ME: Coexistent pulmonary artery and aortic arch calcification. Am J Roentgenol 116: 141, 1972

48. REICH NE, WITTER M: Roentgenographic visualization of the coronary arteries. Am J Roentgenol 77: 274, 1951

49. ROEHM TU Jr, JUE KL, AMPLATZ K: Radiographic features of the scimitar syndrome. Radiology 86: 856, 1966

50. RONDEROS A: Endocardial fibroelastosis. Am J Roentgenol 84: 442, 1960

51. ROSENBAUM HD: The roentgen classification and diagnosis of cardiac alignments. Radiology 89: 466, 1967

52. ROWEN M, THOMPSON JR, WILLIAMSON RA et al: Diffuse pulmonary hemangiomatosis. Radiology 127: 445, 1978

53. SCHINZ HR, BAENSCH WE, FROMMHOLD W, GLAUNER R, UEHLINGER E, WELLAUER J: In RIGLER LG (ed): Roentgen Diagnosis, Vol IV, 2nd ed. New York, Grune & Stratton, 1970

54. SCHWEDEL JB: Clinical Roentgenology of the Heart. New York, Harper & Row, 1946

55. SHUFORD WH, SYBERS RG: The Aortic Arch and Its Malformations. Springfield, IL, Thomas, 1974

56. SORKIN RP, SCHUURMANN BJ, SIMON AB: Radiographic aspects of permanent cardiac pacemakers. Radiology 119: 281, 1976

57. STEINBERG I: Anomalies (pseudocoarctation) of the arch of the aorta. Am J Roentgenol 88: 73, 1962

58. STEINBERG I, FINBY N: Roentgen manifestations of unperforated aortic sinus aneurysms. Am J Roentgenol 77: 263, 1957

59. STEINER RE: The roentgen features of the cardiomyopathies. Semin Roentgenol 4: 311, 1969

60. STEVENS GM: Buckling of the aortic arch (pseudocoarctation, kinking): a Roentgenographic entity. Radiology 70: 67, 1958

61. SUSSMAN ML, JACOBSON G: Critical evaluation of roentgen criteria of right ventricular enlargement. Circulation 11: 391, 1955

62. SWISCHUK LE: Plain Film Interpretation in Congenital Heart Disease. Philadelphia, Lea & Febiger, 1970

63. TORRANCE DJ: Demonstration of subepicardial fat as an aid in the diagnosis of pericardial fluid or thickening. Am J Roentgenol 74: 850, 1955

64. UNGERLEIDER HE, CLARK CP: Study of transverse diameter of heart silhouette, with prediction table based on teleroentgenogram. Am Heart J 17: 92, 1939

65. UNGERLEIDER HE, GUBNER R: Evaluation of heart size measurements. Am Heart J 24: 494, 1942

66. WALTER WH III: Radiographic identification of commonly used pulse generators—1970. JAMA 215: 1974, 1971

67. WESCOTT JL, FERGUSON D: The right pulmonary artery—left atrial axis line. Method for measuring left atrial size on lateral radiographs. Radiology 118: 265, 1976

68. WYMAN SM: Congenital absence of a pulmonary artery. Radiology 62: 321, 1954

69. WYMAN SM: Dissecting aneurysm of the thoracic aorta: its roentgen recognition. Am J Roentgenol 78: 247, 1957

SECTION VI

THE FACE, MOUTH, AND JAWS

33

THE ORBIT AND EYE

Roentgen examination of the orbit and eye is used to detect and localize foreign bodies, to detect the presence of tumor within the orbit, and to determine what effect, if any, this tumor has on the bony orbital wall. Orbital size and shape, calcifications within the orbit and globe, and fractures of orbital walls may also be visualized. Special studies such as venography and arteriography may be used to detect vascular anomalies as well as tumors. CT scanning is used for the study of exophthalmos, orbital masses, orbital trauma, unilateral papilledema, and visual field defect, among other things.[14] Ultrasonography is used for detection of masses and foreign bodies and for measurement of the optic nerve, of extraocular muscles, of the globe, and of tumors or other abnormalities within the globe.[1, 16, 17] The optic canal is examined to determine its size in the presence of alteration caused by disease or by tumor involving the optic nerve.

ROENTGEN METHODS

As a general rule the orbits are examined by means of posteroanterior and lateral views (Fig. 33-1). Additional projections may be used, depending upon the problem. If the presence of an opaque foreign body is suspected, localizing procedure usually is preceded by a scout roentgenogram in frontal and lateral projection to determine the presence of the suspected foreign body and its general location. Bone-free films are sometimes made, using small dental films to outline foreign bodies in the anterior chamber of the globe. The simplest method to determine whether a foreign body is intra- or extraocular is to make a double exposure in the lateral projection with the patient looking up, then down. If the head is immobilized properly, a double image of the foreign body on the film is presumptive evidence that it is in the globe. Slight motion is possible if it is lodged in one of the ocular muscles. Therefore, the method carries some chance for positive error but is simple and, in the absence of suitable localizing equipment, is useful. The optic canals are examined by means of a specialized technique. Views of both canals are obtained in order to compare the two sides. An example of the

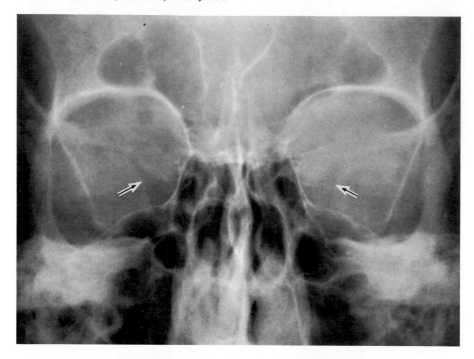

Fig. 33-1. Normal orbit. The bony orbital rims are clearly defined. The bony walls are thin resulting in radiolucency. The superior orbital fissures are indicated by **arrows.**

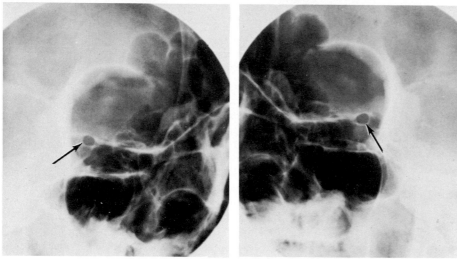

Fig. 33-2. Normal optic canals. Arrows indicate the clearly defined, corticated optic canals.

projection is shown in Figure 33-2. Tomography of the optic canals is useful in patients with suspected disease in this region. It is also used in the diagnosis of destructive, sclerotic, or traumatic changes in the orbital walls.

Orbital Pneumography and Contrast Orbitography. These methods have been abandoned in favor of the noninvasive techniques, ultrasonography and CT scanning, because these latter procedures are noninvasive and carry no appreciable risk.

Orbital Venography. The ophthalmic veins are opacified by hand injection of an organic iodide into the frontal vein, angular veins, or by means of retrograde catheterization of the inferior petrosal sinus. Serial filming in frontal, lateral, and basal projections then outlines the ophthalmic veins. These veins are more constant in location than the arteries, so venography is more accurate than arteriography in localizing intraorbital masses. The risk is minimal in frontal vein venography, particularly if jugular compression is not used. Inferior petrosal sinus venography is more dangerous because of the risk of rupture of the sinus. Although orbital venography has been replaced by the noninvasive techniques to a great extent, it is still useful in patients with questionable cavernous sinus or posterior opthalmic vein thrombosis, those with venous malformations, and in patients in whom CT scans are inconclusive, unsatisfactory, or fail to reveal suspected lesions.

Ophthalmic Artery Angiography. In this method of examination the contrast medium (organic iodide) is injected selectively into the internal carotid artery and the examination is timed for best visualization of ophthalmic arteries, capillaries, and veins. This examination has been replaced as that used for the study of proptosis by CT scanning, but it is still used in patients with suspected vascular anomalies causing proptosis. Subtraction techniques are very helpful in the study of ophthalmic vessels.

Tomography. Tomography is very useful in the evaluation of a number of orbital lesions, particularly in excluding the possibility of nonorbital causes of exophthalmos. Coronal, axial, and lateral projections are employed, depending on the problem. The coronal view is most useful in the detection of expanding lesions, such as blow-out fractures, and in the demonstration of lacrimal-gland tumors. The axial projection is also used in patients with suspected expanding orbital tumors as well as in those with ethmoid sinus masses or suspected orbital-wall fractures. The lateral projection may be needed to supplement either of the two frontal views in blow-out fracture and in suspected frontal or ethmoid mucocele. Circular or hypocycloidal motion is preferable to linear tomography in most instances.

Computed Tomography (Fig. 33-3 and 33-4). Computed tomography has replaced orbitography and has largely replaced arteriography and venography. Axial projections paralleling the optic nerves are used but may be augmented by coronal sections. Thin sections (4 mm) are preferred because they produce greater detail, particularly at the orbital apex.[14] The method is used in the study of inflammatory disease. Graves' disease, vascular abnormalities, orbital injuries, orbital tumors, and such intraocular conditions as retinoblastoma and intraocular foreign bodies. It is also valuable in the study of masses in the region of the lacrimal gland.

Ultrasonography. Ultrasonography was first employed in the study of intraocular abnormalities such as retinal detachment, tumors, and foreign bodies; its usefulness in these conditions is now well established. It is also of value in the study of unilateral exophthalmos, and particularly in optic nerve lesions. It may also be useful in the examination of inflammatory diseases of the lacrimal gland.

Measurement of Interorbital Distance. The interorbital distance in the growing child as well as in the adult is of some importance, since there are a number of congenital disorders in which ocular hypertelorism or hypotelorism are an important part. Hansman[11] has presented standards for interorbital distances in males and females to age 24 (Tables 33-1 and 33-2). The distance was measured on sinus films taken on an angle board with the patient's nose and forehead touching the cassette and the tube in a vertical position. Focal film distance was 28 inches. The subjects were healthy and presumably normal.

In addition to Greig's syndrome, hypertelorism is found in a number of conditions including craniostenosis, craniofacial dysostosis, mandibulofacial dysostosis, achondroplasia, Bonnevie–Ullrich syndrome, and in some patients with cleft palate. Hypotelorism may be found in such disorders as arrhinencephaly and Marchesani's syndrome.

Orbital Asymmetry. In unilateral supraorbital fibrous dysplasia the orbit is small and the homolateral frontal sinus is often small. Small orbit and small sinus, when present, are helpful signs in differentiating this lesion from meningioma in which there also may be extensive bone thickening but no change in orbital or sinus size. The orbit may be distorted and often is small and unusual in shape in patients with neurofibromatosis, unilateral coronal craniosynostosis, chronic juvenile subdural hematoma of the temporal fossa, enucleation of the eye in childhood (small orbit), and paranasal sinus hypoplasia (large orbit).[4]

(*Text continues on p. 1125.*)

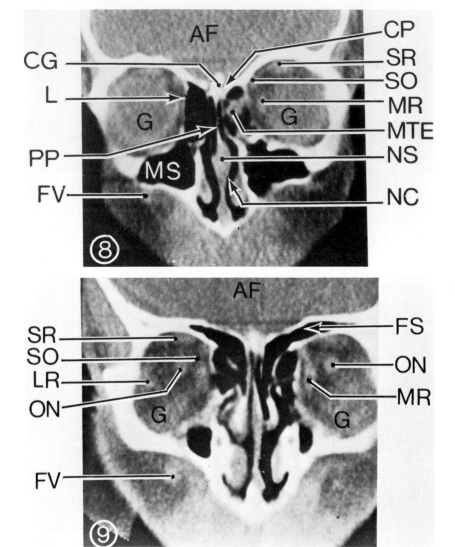

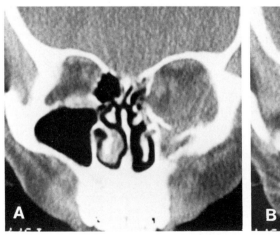
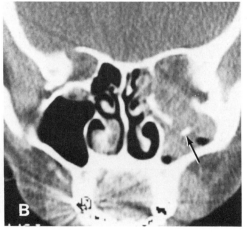

Fig. 33-3. Coronal CT scans through the orbit. **Section 8** through the globes. **Section 9** behind the globes. **AF,** Anterior cranial fossa; **CG,** crista galli; **CP,** cribriform plate; **FS,** frontal sinus; **FV,** facial vein; **G,** globes; **L,** lamina papyracea; **LR,** lateral rectus muscle; **MR,** medial rectus; **MS,** maxillary sinus; **MTE,** membrane thickening in the ethmoid sinus; **NC,** nasal cavity; **NS,** nasal septum; **ON,** optic nerve; **PP,** perpendicular plate; **SO,** superior oblique muscle; **SR,** superior rectus. (Hesselink JR, et al: Computed tomography of the paranasal sinuses and face: Part I. Normal anatomy. Journal of Computer Assisted Tomography 2: 559–567, Nov, 1978)

Fig. 33-4. Coronal CT scans in the examination in orbital injuries. **A** and **B.** These scans demonstrate blow-out fractures of the floor and medial wall of the left orbit. **B.** A fragment of bone is displaced into the left antrum **(arrow).** Also noted is some protrusion of soft tissue into the ethmoid sinuses. (Hesselink JR, et al: Computed tomography of the paranasal sinuses and face: Part II. Pathological anatomy. Journal of Computer Assisted Tomography 2: 568–576, Nov, 1978)

Table 33-1. Percentile Standards for Interorbital Distance as Measured on Sinus Roentgenograms for Girls

AGE	N	MINIMUM	10TH	25TH	50TH	75TH	90TH	MAXIMUM
0-6	95	1.200	—	—	—	—	—	2.160
1-0	96	1.230	—	—	—	—	—	2.270
1-6	100	1.290	1.514	1.632	1.733	1.854	1.988	2.290
2-0	99	1.330	1.567	1.682	1.784	1.905	2.039	2.330
2-6	100	1.340	1.616	1.726	1.823	1.949	2.084	2.370
3-0	98	1.360	1.657	1.764	1.859	1.992	2.130	2.390
3-6	100	1.430	1.696	1.801	1.892	2.032	1.173	2.450
4-0	102	1.460	1.729	1.837	1.929	2.070	2.215	2.480
4-6	98	1.570	1.763	1.873	1.968	2.109	2.252	2.523
5-0	97	1.620	1.790	1.906	2.007	2.146	2.288	2.530
5-6	97	1.650	1.817	1.936	2.043	2.183	2.324	2.560
6-0	98	1.690	1.842	1.964	2.078	2.218	2.362	2.636
6-6	98	1.730	1.868	1.992	2.111	2.254	2.398	2.680
7-0	96	1.750	1.896	2.021	2.144	2.288	2.431	2.703
7-6	94	1.770	1.923	2.053	2.174	2.320	2.459	2.730
8-0	94	1.790	1.949	2.087	2.207	2.352	2.487	2.758
8-6	92	1.830	1.970	2.118	2.237	2.379	2.513	2.803
9-0	89	1.860	1.989	1.140	2.270	2.409	2.542	2.840
9-6	89	1.860	2.015	2.159	2.292	2.433	2.568	2.880
10-0	88	1.880	2.044	2.180	2.313	2.458	2.596	2.900
10-6	89	1.900	2.076	2.207	2.332	2.481	2.620	2.940
11-0	84	1.930	2.102	2.234	2.359	2.510	2.649	2.998
11-6	82	1.940	2.128	2.262	2.389	2.541	2.679	3.000
12-0	82	1.980	2.148	2.284	2.419	2.573	2.710	3.050
12-6	80	1.990	2.174	2.308	2.445	2.602	2.742	3.110
13-0	76	2.020	2.196	2.328	2.466	2.623	2.766	3.110
13-6	74	2.050	2.216	2.350	2.484	2.638	2.782	3.130
14-0	73	2.080	2.228	2.363	2.498	2.646	2.786	3.130
14-6	71	2.080	2.235	2.375	2.513	2.656	2.792	3.150
15-0	68	2.100	2.243	2.385	2.524	2.668	2.803	3.150
15-6	66	2.115	2.255	2.399	2.538	2.683	2.820	3.150
16-0	64	2.120	2.275	2.416	2.547	2.693	2.833	3.150
16-6	59	2.080	2.293	2.430	2.556	2.699	2.841	3.155
17-0	58	2.130	2.306	2.442	2.563	2.704	2.847	3.160
17-6	51	2.135	2.309	2.448	2.573	2.714	2.856	3.165
18-0	49	2.140	2.309	2.453	2.581	2.724	2.865	3.170
18-6	47	2.140	2.310	2.457	2.587	2.733	2.874	3.175
19-0	46	2.140	2.314	2.459	2.588	2.738	2.882	3.180
19-6	43	2.135	2.314	2.459	2.587	2.742	2.887	3.191
20-0	42	2.130	2.318	2.460	2.587	2.743	2.890	3.200
20-6	37	2.136	2.323	2.462	2.585	2.740	2.889	3.200
21-0	35	2.143	2.333	2.466	2.584	2.738	2.888	3.200
21-6	32	2.149	2.332	2.463	2.583	2.733	2.884	3.200
22-0	32	2.120	2.326	2.458	2.579	2.722	2.869	3.200
22-6	28	2.138	2.312	2.450	2.573	2.707	2.842	3.200
23-0	24	2.148	2.293	2.444	2.569	2.693	2.814	2.880
23-6	20	2.142	2.270	2.439	2.573	2.690	2.802	2.886
24-0	19	2.141	2.256	2.437	2.583	2.698	2.806	2.898
24-0	18	2.143	—	—	—	—	—	2.912
25-0	18	2.145	—	—	—	—	—	2.915

Hansman CF: Growth of interorbital distance and skull thickness as observed in roentgenographic measurements. Radiology 86: 87, 1966.

Table 33-2. Percentile Standards for Interorbital Distance as Measured on Sinus Roentgenograms for Boys

AGE	N	MINIMUM	10TH	25TH	50TH	75TH	90TH	MAXIMUM
0–6	91	1.230	—	—	—	—	—	2.160
1–0	94	1.230	—	—	—	—	—	2.270
1–6	95	1.250	1.524	1.651	1.773	1.920	2.063	2.290
2–0	95	1.270	1.578	1.700	1.822	1.971	2.114	2.360
2–6	96	1.290	1.631	1.748	1.866	2.013	2.157	2.390
3–0	92	1.350	1.680	1.795	1.909	2.056	2.201	2.393
3–6	93	1.400	1.725	1.839	1.953	2.099	2.246	2.470
4–0	95	1.420	1.760	1.877	1.994	2.143	2.292	2.530
4–6	95	1.420	1.795	1.916	2.035	2.187	2.337	2.570
5–0	94	1.450	1.830	1.952	2.073	2.229	2.382	2.620
5–6	93	1.520	1.864	1.989	2.110	2.270	2.427	2.650
6–0	91	1.520	1.896	2.022	2.143	2.308	2.466	2.730
6–6	91	1.560	1.925	2.050	2.173	2.342	2.501	2.750
7–0	89	1.570	1.957	2.076	2.199	2.371	2.537	2.840
7–6	91	1.620	1.991	2.103	2.226	2.400	2.573	2.890
8–0	93	1.640	2.025	2.132	2.256	2.429	2.607	2.860
8–6	92	1.680	2.049	2.161	2.284	2.456	2.634	2.950
9–0	92	1.720	2.069	2.187	2.310	2.480	2.656	2.950
9–6	93	1.730	2.089	2.211	2.333	2.506	2.685	2.990
10–0	92	1.750	2.114	2.236	2.357	2.534	2.716	3.080
10–6	89	1.800	2.139	2.262	2.385	2.564	2.752	3.080
11–0	88	1.920	2.164	2.288	2.412	2.592	2.780	3.160
11–6	86	1.870	2.191	2.315	2.440	2.617	2.807	3.180
12–0	84	1.860	2.220	2.344	2.468	2.643	2.834	3.100
12–6	78	2.000	2.251	2.375	2.498	2.674	2.868	3.123
13–0	78	2.050	2.278	2.405	2.529	2.704	2.904	3.160
13–6	78	2.050	2.304	2.433	2.560	2.735	2.938	3.220
14–0	74	2.080	2.328	2.460	2.590	2.760	2.964	3.250
14–6	70	2.090	2.353	2.489	2.622	2.789	2.993	3.250
15–0	70	2.180	2.374	2.515	2.650	2.817	3.024	3.320
15–6	69	2.180	2.392	2.537	2.672	2.847	3.059	3.330
16–0	68	2.190	2.407	2.553	2.697	2.868	3.084	3.372
16–6	66	2.180	2.422	2.570	2.713	2.884	3.096	3.390
17–0	65	2.180	2.438	2.586	2.723	2.894	3.101	3.430
17–6	64	2.205	2.447	2.599	2.733	2.903	3.107	3.464
18–0	62	2.230	2.454	2.608	2.741	2.915	3.119	3.490
18–6	56	2.230	2.454	2.612	2.750	2.924	3.131	3.505
19–0	55	2.230	2.456	2.616	2.759	2.937	3.148	3.520
19–6	50	2.230	2.463	2.622	2.768	2.952	3.169	3.535
20–0	45	2.230	2.469	2.629	2.778	2.971	3.196	3.550
20–6	40	2.230	2.468	2.633	2.788	2.993	3.224	3.560
21–0	37	2.230	2.461	2.638	2.806	3.014	3.247	3.570
21–6	33	2.230	2.460	2.643	2.822	3.033	3.265	3.570
22–0	29	2.370	2.470	2.653	2.830	3.041	3.269	3.570
22–6	28	2.384	2.477	2.651	2.835	3.043	3.271	3.573
23–0	26	2.400	2.479	2.651	2.836	3.043	3.269	3.577
23–6	23	2.400	2.476	2.647	2.839	3.053	3.276	3.580
24–0	23	2.400	2.472	2.647	2.843	3.059	3.273	3.583
24–6	22	2.400	—	—	—	—	—	3.587
25–0	21	2.400	—	—	—	—	—	3.590

Hansman CF: Growth of interorbital distance and skull thickness as observed in roentgenographic measurements. Radiology 86: 87, 1966

INTRAOCULAR FOREIGN BODIES

Before any special methods are used to localize radiopaque foreign particles in the eye, roentgenograms in frontal and lateral projections are necessary to make certain that the foreign material is visible and can be identified on the radiographic localization films. More than sixty techniques for localization have been described.[6] If the presence of a foreign body is detected on the scout films, then special localization can be undertaken. An early method in use in the United States is the method of Sweet[22] for which special apparatus and charts are available. It is a triangulation method, the details of which are available in standard texts dealing with roentgen technique. Problems with eye motion and swelling of the eyelid diminish the accuracy. Contact-lens methods in which metal reference points are used and held in place by a vacuum are hazardous when the eye has been traumatized and in patients with narrow-angle glaucoma. A silicone contact lens has been developed[3] in which a vacuum is not required. The lens is applied by an ophthalmologist, and patient positioning and filming are supervised by the radiologist. The lens method has proved to be quite accurate. If no foreign body is found on plain-film study in a patient with positive clinical findings, ultrasound B-scan may reveal the foreign body. CT scanning may also identify a foreign body of low radiographic density. Ultrasonography is also used to localize foreign bodies in relation to the structures within the globe. If necessary, it can be used during surgery performed for removal of the foreign body. When a small, semiopaque, foreign body is suspected in the anterior chamber, the bone-free type of examination can be used.

CALCIFICATIONS WITHIN THE ORBIT AND GLOBE

HYPERCALCEMIA

Calcification within the conjunctiva and cornea has been described in patients with hyperparathyroidism and hypervitaminosis D, evidently secondary to the associated hypercalcemia. Radiographically, these calcifications appear as faint annular shadows that can be localized to the cornea and conjunctiva in tangential views of the anterior globe. The bone-free type of examination can be used to demonstrate the calcium.

RETINOBLASTOMA

Retinoblastoma is a glioma of the retina that occurs chiefly in infants and children. There are other diseases, including inflammations, which simulate this tumor clinically and make its differentiation difficult. Because early removal of the eye is necessary to effect cure, roentgen signs that assist in making the diagnosis are important. There is stippled or mottled calcification in the globe that is almost pathognomonic of retinoblastoma (Fig. 33-5). It is found in approximately 75% of patients so that its absence does not exclude the possibility of retinoblastoma. Calcifications have also been reported in intracerebral metastases from retinoblastoma. In addition to the calcification, a soft-tissue mass may be noted within the orbit. The tumor may extend along the optic nerve to produce enlargement of the optic canal which can be visualized roentgenographically, and, when the tumor spreads beyond the nerve, irregular erosion of the optic canal may develop.

OTHER CALCIFICATIONS

1. Calcium deposits occasionally occur in the cornea, associated with degenerative processes there.
2. In hypermature cataracts, calcification may be visualized in the lens. This results in a typical, small, rounded, calcific density located within

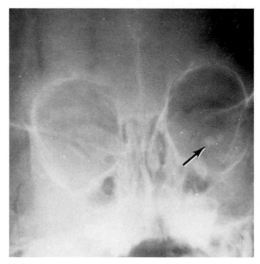

Fig. 33-5. Calcification in the globe in a patient with retinoblastoma **(arrow).**

the globe in the position of the lens (Fig. 33-6). Calcification may also occur in congenital cataract and, therefore, may be seen in children.

3. Intraorbital hemangioma and orbital varices may be recognized by the presence of round, calcified phleboliths.

4. Calcification also occurs in intra- and extra-orbital hemorrhage following trauma.

5. Retrolental fibroplasia may also cause calcification in the globe.

6. Calcification and ossification may occasionally occur in degenerative diseases of the choroid and produce a curvilinear density conforming to the shape of the globe.

7. Rarely, calcification and ossification may occur in the vitreous, producing a localized central shadow or a diffuse or irregular shadow of calcific density peripherally in the globe.

8. Globe degeneration, phthisis bulbi, may be acompanied by nodules and plaques of calcium in the lens and globe (Fig. 33-7).

9. Ocular phacoma may contain nodular calcification.

10. Meningioma, neurofibroma, and epidermoid and dermoid tumors may contain enough calcium to be visible on orbital radiographs.[15]

THE OPTIC CANAL

GENERAL CONSIDERATIONS

The optic canals are examined by means of special posteroanterior projections in which the beam is parallel to the long axis of the canal. Both canals are examined for comparison in most instances. Special devices are available to hold the patient's head and to insure proper angulation, which is about 37 degrees off the sagittal plane toward the side examined and 31 degrees caudad to a line from the outer canthus of the eye to the external auditory meatus. Tomography may be of value in patients in whom no abnormality is visible on the standard projection. Films can be exposed perpendicular to the long axis of the canal or in the axial projection, parallel to it, using the basal (submentovertex) position, or both of these may be used if necessary. CT scanning is now employed extensively in the examination of the optic canals because it reveals the extent of soft-tissue masses as well as the bony walls. The canal is approximately 7 mm in length. The canals are not always bilaterally

symmetric but they are usually nearly the same size. Their margins are very clearly defined. The normal optic canal measures approximately 5 mm in its greatest diameter on the roentgenogram. Any diameter over 7 mm or under 4 mm is considered abnormal. Changes in diameter caused by pathologic processes may be less than the normal variation, so that comparison with the opposite canal is imperative. The canal attains its adult size early in life, when the individual is between the ages of 3 and 5 years. The canal is slightly oval at either end, the long axis is roughly horizontal at the cranial end and vertical at the orbital end, and the midportion is round. In the standard view, the orbital end is visible, since its walls are denser. Rarely, the canal is divided, with an upper opening for the optic nerve and a lower one for the ophthalmic artery. Narrowing of the canal may be congenital in patients with craniofacial dysostosis (Crouzon's disease) and in those with oxycephaly; the deformity may be so severe as to cause blindness in some of these patients. Acquired narrowing may be caused by Paget's disease or fibrous dysplasia, or may be secondary to trauma, osteopetrosis, or pycnodystosis.

TUMORS INVOLVING THE OPTIC CANALS

Tumors usually cause enlargement of the optic canals. In neurofibromatosis, involvement of the optic nerve on one side or the other may result in marked enlargement. The walls are usually smooth, even when considerable enlargement is present. Retinal glioma may extend posteriorly along the optic nerve to enlarge the optic canal. A normal-sized canal does not exclude the possibility of the presence of a tumor involving the nerve, however. Glioma arising in the brain and extending anteriorly along the optic nerve may also enlarge this canal. Meningioma may extend from the globe into the cranial vault, or vice versa, resulting in enlargement of the optic foramen. In addition, meningioma usually evokes a hyperstotic response and causes a dense bony thickening that may actually narrow the foramen. Rarely, inflammatory disease may enlarge the canal. Arteriovenous malformations and opthalmic artery aneurysm may erode and enlarge it. Extrinsic lesions may also cause changes in the optic canals. The optic strut which forms the lateral and inferior wall is affected by conditions that enlarge the superior orbital fisssure. Sphenoid sinus lesions may cause erosion of the medial wall. The roof may be eroded and thinned by an increase in intracranial pressure.

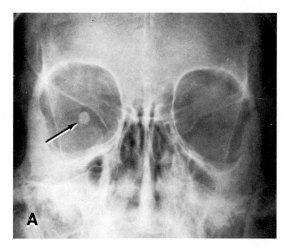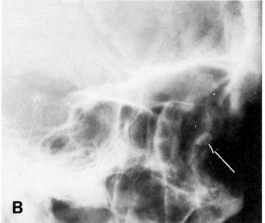

Fig. 33-6. Cataract with calcification of lens in right eye. The small rounded calcific density seen in the frontal **(A)** and lateral **(B)** projections represents calcification in the lens **(arrows).**

Fig. 33-7. Phthisis bulbi. There is a local plaque of calcium inferiorly with faintly visualized, curvilinear calcifications extending to either side appearing to be in the wall of the globe.

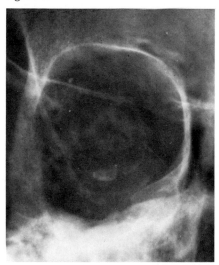

THE SUPERIOR ORBITAL (SPHENOIDAL) FISSURE

The superior orbital fissure is bounded below by the greater sphenoid wing and above by the lesser sphenoid wing. It is bounded medially by the body of the sphenoid and by the orbital plate of the frontal bone laterally. It is usually readily visualized in standard posteroanterior views of the orbits. It is oblique; its wide medial end is posterior and the more narrow lateral end is anterior and slightly superior to the medial end. The wide end is at the apex of the orbital pyramid, and is below and lateral to the optic canal. The third, fourth, and sixth nerves, the ophthalmic division of the fifth, the ophthalmic veins, the nasociliary nerve, and the sympathetic root of the ciliary ganglion all pass through the wide medial portion of the fissure. All of these structures may be involved by a disease process in this region. Infection; tumors arising locally such as orbital tumors, meningiomas, and metastatic tumors, and aneurysm of the anterior half of the intracavernous portion of the carotid artery are among the conditions that may affect the orbital apex. The fissure is widened by aneurysm at this site; often there is also erosion of the under surface of the anterior clinoid and partial or complete erosion of the optic strut that separates the fissure from the optic canal. Enlargement may also be produced by masses within the orbit that extend through the fissure. Extrinsic sinus masses may also erode and enlarge the fissure, but usually major signs of the sinus mass and the bone destruction are produced by these masses.

THE INFERIOR ORBITAL FISSURE

The inferior orbital fissure forms an angle with the superior orbital fissure which is open laterally. It lies between the greater sphenoid wing superiorly and the orbital surface of the maxilla inferiorly and connects the orbit with the pterygopalatine fossa. The orbital branches of the sphenopalatine ganglion and a venous plexus extend through it. This is not often examined by roentgen methods, but a special view obtained posteroanteriorly at 25 degrees caudad to the canthomeatal line with the central ray on the glabella will outline the fissure adjacent to the postero-superior aspect of the maxillary sinus on either side.

TUMORS OF THE ORBIT

A number of tumors and inflammatory lesions may result in intraorbital mass that may produce some radiographic changes in the bony walls of the orbit. Plain films may then be sufficient to determine the site and cause of the mass (Fig. 33-8). When there are clinical signs of an intraorbital mass without definitive plain-film findings, CT scanning of the orbit is employed, sometimes preceded by ultrasonography. These intraorbital masses often are difficult clinical problems and require cooperative effort of the ophthalmologist, the neurosurgeon, and the radiologist in the complete study of the patient.

Among the masses that may produce exophthalmos without bone changes are lacrimal-gland tumors, hemangiomas, inflammatory granulomas, neurofibromas, dermoids and epidermoids, optic nerve gliomas, rhabdomyosarcomas, orbital varices, metastases, melanomas, lymphosarcomas, histiocytosis X, pseudotumors, hematomas, pseudolymphomas, meningiomas, and fibromas. Many of them may cause bone changes early, and others cause bone changes late in their development if at all.

There are other masses which usually cause bone change that can be recognized radiographically; in some instances the diagnosis can be made on plain-film study with reasonable certainty. Among the diseases that usually cause bone changes are inflammatory disease of paranasal sinuses with spread to the orbit, mucocele of frontal sinus with orbital involvement, carcinoma of sinus with orbital spread, meningioma, dermoid cyst, aneurysm, ossifying fibroma, fibrous dysplasia, posttraumatic meningocele, various sarcomas, and, in some instances, neurofibromatosis. The tumors listed exibit changes in the orbital walls similar to those produced in other areas. The hyperostotic changes in meningioma are characteristic of that type of tumor. Meningioma arising primarily within the orbit is rare, but may cause enlargement of the optic canal, local hyperostosis, and calcification in the optic nerve sheath producing a rim of density around the nerve in the optic canal view and parallel lines in the axial view. Typical stippled or cloudlike

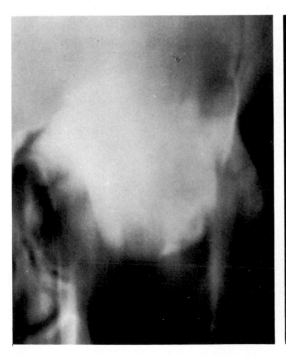
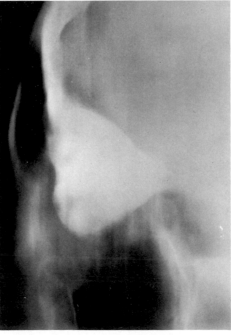

Fig. 33-8. Orbital osteoma. Note the large, dense tumor mass arising in the roof of the left orbit and projecting downward. These tomograms outline the dense mass.

calcification may be present in some. In neurofibroma, enlargement of the optic foramen is a helpful diagnostic sign; this tumor is also capable of producing great orbital enlargement and distortion. Dermoid cyst or cholesteatoma may also result in orbital enlargement and distortion as well as erosion and decalcification of the bony orbital walls. When malignant tumor is present, bone invasion may result in destruction of orbital walls; this is particularly true of carcinoma extending from adjacent sinuses. The destruction is manifested by disappearance of bone in an irregular manner without sclerosis. Tumors of the lacrimal gland may cause erosion or destruction of

bone in the orbital roof adjacent to the gland, which lies in a shallow fossa that indents the superior aspect of the orbit laterally. Slowly expanding benign tumors, such as mixed tumors, may enlarge the fossa without invasion of bone. Malignant tumors tend to invade and either destroy the bone or cause sclerosis of the fossa and adjacent orbital rim.

Pseudotumor of the orbit is the term applied to chronic inflammatory conditions that may appear as a mass in the region of the lacrimal gland, or an intraconal mass causing painful proptosis, which may be diffuse or multifocal. The lesion is usually visible on the CT scan but may be very difficult to differenti-

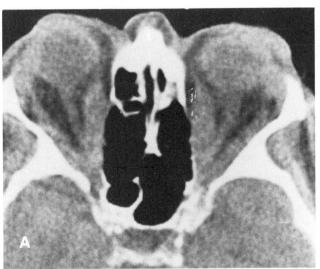

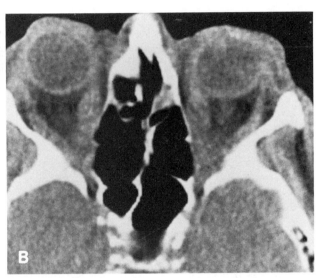

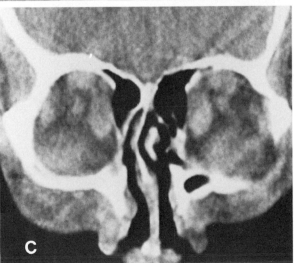

Fig. 33-9. Graves' disease. This illustrates the use of CT scanning. **A** and **B** are transverse scans showing the exophthalmos and the thickening of the extraocular muscles. The coronal scan **(C)** also shows the thick muscles in this section which is behind the globe. (Courtesy Dr. J. R. Hesselink, Boston)

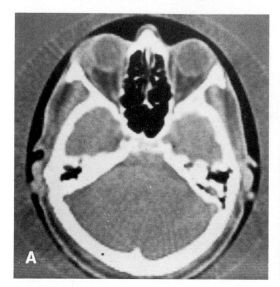
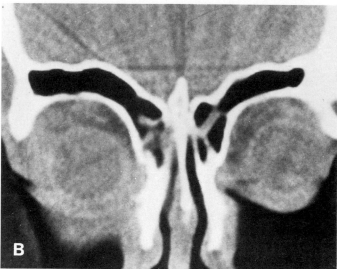

Fig. 33-10. CT scan in a patient with pleomorphic adenoma of the lacrimal gland. The transverse **(A)** and coronal **(B)** scans demonstrate a soft-tissue mass in the temporal quadrant of the right orbit displacing the globe medially and inferiorly. In **A** the center is slightly lower in absorption and contains cystic fluid. (Hesselink JR: Radiology 131: 143–147, 1979)

Fig. 33-11. CT scan in a patient with acute dacryoadenitis involving the lacrimal glands. There is swelling of the left gland and adjacent orbital soft tissues including the lateral rectus muscle, particularly in its anterior aspect. No organism was cultured, but the patient responded to antibiotic therapy. (Hesselink JR: Radiology 131: 143–147, 1979)

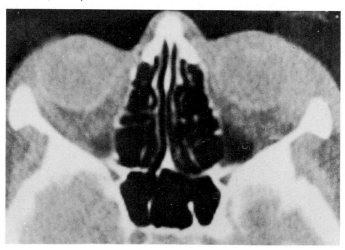
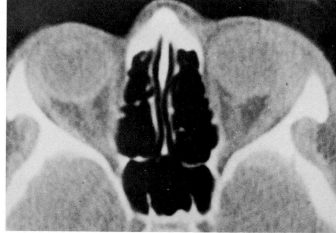

ate from orbital tumors. *Graves' disease* occasionally may be associated with unilateral exophthalmos so that intraorbital mass may be suspected. The major roentgen finding is enlargement of extraocular muscles which can be detected on CT scan (Fig. 33-9). There may be contrast enhancement which is suggestive of tumor since the enhancement and attenuation patterns are often difficult to correlate with histopathology.

Rare nontumorous causes of exophthalmos include traumatic orbital pneumatocele, which is acute and may be diagnosed on plain-film study, orbital pseudomeningocele, and orbital encephalocele.

THE LACRIMAL PASSAGES

The lacrimal passages extend from the puncta in the medial aspect of the eyelids to the inferior nasal meatus. Radiographic methods may be used to study them. An iodine-containing contrast material is injected into the lower canaliculus and films are exposed in frontal and lateral projections (dacryocystography). The water-soluble media are now preferred over Lipiodol which was used for a number of years. The examination is used chiefly in localizing the site of obstruction of the nasolacrimal duct. Tomography may be useful in the examination of fine bony structures in this area. CT is very useful in the study of masses involving the lacrimal gland and surrounding structures[13] (Figs. 33-10 and 33-11).

REFERENCES AND SELECTED READINGS

1. ARGER PH: Orbit Roentgenology. New York, John Wiley & Sons, 1977
2. BINET EF, KIEFFER SA, MARTIN SH et al: Orbital dysplasia in neurofibromatosis. Radiology 93: 829, 1969
3. BONFIELD RE, WAINSTOCK MA: A silicone contact lens for intra-orbital foreign body localization. Radiology 109: 593, 1973
4. BURROWS EH: Orbitocranial asymmetry. Br J Radiol 51: 771, 1978
5. DAVIS LA, DIAMOND I: Metastatic retinoblastoma as a cause of diffuse intracranial calcification. Am J Roentgenol 78: 437, 1957
6. ERKONEN W, DOLAN KD: Ocular foreign body localization. Radiol Clin North Am 10: 101, 1972
7. ETTER LE: Detailed roentgen anatomy of the orbits. Radiology 59: 489, 1957
8. FLEISCHNER FG, SHALEK SR: Conjunctival and corneal calcification in hypercalcemia: roentgen findings. N Engl J Med 241: 863, 1949
9. HANAFEE WN, DAYTON GO: The roentgen diagnosis of orbital tumors. Radiol Clin North Am 8: 403, 1970
10. HANAFEE WN, SHIU PC, DAYTON GO: Orbital venography. Am J Roentgenol 104: 29, 1968
11. HANSMAN CF: Growth of interorbital distance and skull thickness as observed in roentgenographic measurements. Radiology 86: 87, 1966
12. HARTMANN E, GILLES E: Roentgenologic Diagnosis in Ophthalmology. Philadelphia, Lippincott, 1959
13. HESSELINK JR, DAVIS KR, DALLOW RL et al: Computed tomography of masses in the lacrimal gland region. Radiology 130: 563, 1979
14. HILAL SK, TROKEL SL: Computerized tomography of the orbit using thin section. Semin Roentgenol 12: 137, 1977
15. LLOYD GAS: The radiology of primary orbital meningioma. Br J Radiol 44: 405, 1971
16. LLOYD GAS: Radiology of the Orbit. London, WB Saunders, 1975
17. LLOYD GAS: The impact of CT scanning and ultrasonography on orbital diagnosis. Clin Radiol 28: 583, 1977
18. MERRILL V: Atlas of Roentgenographic Positions, Vol II. St. Louis, Mosby, 1967
19. NEWTON TH: Roentgen appearance of lacrimal gland tumors. Radiology 79: 598, 1962
20. POTTER GD, TROKEL S: Tomography of the optic canal. Am J Roentgenol 106: 530, 1969
21. ROBERTS WE: The roentgenographic demonstrations of glass fragments in the eye. Am J Roentgenol 66: 44, 1951
22. SWEET WM: Improved apparatus for localizing foreign bodies in the eyeball by the roentgen rays. Arch Ophthalmol 38: 623, 1909
23. WHEELER EC, BAKER HL Jr: The ophthalmic arterial complex in angiographic diagnosis. Radiology 83: 26, 1964

34

THE SINUSES AND MASTOIDS

THE PARANASAL SINUSES

The roentgen examination of the paranasal sinuses is an essential part of the study of these structures. Diseases affecting them cause alterations in the normal radiolucency of the sinuses that can be detected on roentgenograms.

METHODS OF EXAMINATION

Standard Positions

There are a number of special views for demonstrating the various paranasal sinuses. The technical details are described in the text on radiographic technique[11] and will not be discussed here. If possible, roentgenograms of the sinuses should be obtained with the patient in the upright position in order to demonstrate fluid levels when they are present. Techniques for the various projections should be standardized so that films of comparable density are obtained. Some techniques call for a stationary grid or Potter–Bucky diaphragm while others specify a nongrid technique with cones to confine the beam to the area of the sinuses. The standard positions that we use are: (1) The occipitomental or Waters' projection in which the maxillary antra are particularly well defined. This view is also used in trauma cases for examination of the facial bones (Fig. 34-1). (2) The occipitofrontal or Caldwell position, which is of particular value for visualizing the frontal and ethmoid sinuses. The upper aspect of the maxillary antra is also well outlined (Fig. 34-2). (3) The lateral position, chiefly for viewing the sphenoid and frontal sinuses (Fig. 34-3). (4) The occipitosubmental position with the mouth open, primarily used to demonstrate disease in the sphenoid sinuses but maxillary and frontal sinuses are also fairly well visualized (Fig. 34-4). (5) The submentovertical with 15-degree cephalad angulation to give a clear definition of the sphenoid and posterior antra including the pterygoid plates (Fig. 34-5). A number of other projections may be used to solve problems in any patient.

Special Methods

Contrast Studies. Dionosil, oily, may be introduced into the paranasal sinuses by the displacement tech-

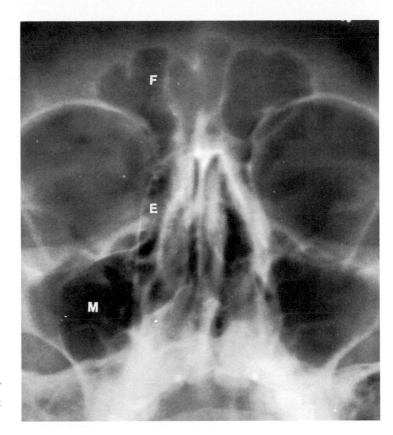

Fig. 34-1. Normal sinuses as seen in Waters' projection. **F,** Frontal sinus; **E,** ethmoid cells; **M,** maxillary sinus.

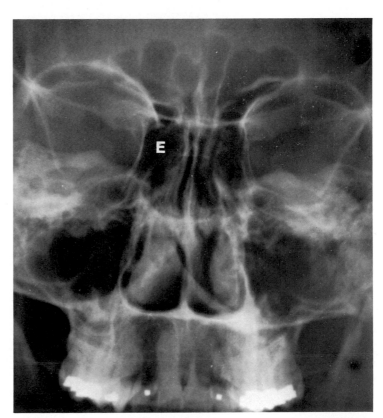

Fig. 34-2. Normal sinuses as seen in the occipitofrontal or Caldwell position; **E** indicates the ethmoid cells on the right.

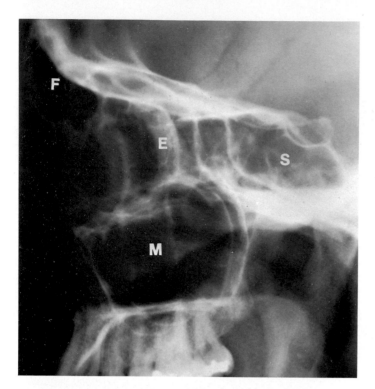

Fig. 34-3. Normal sinuses on lateral view. **F,** Frontal sinuses; **E,** ethmoid cells; **S,** sphenoid sinus; **M,** maxillary antra.

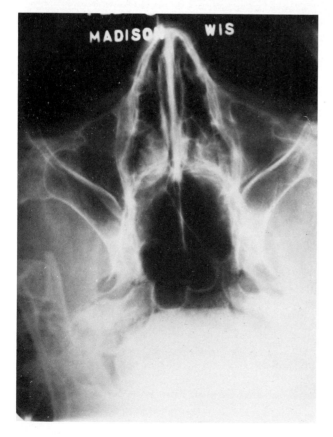

Fig. 34-4. Normal sinuses. The occipitosubmental open-mouth position shows the sphenoid sinuses just above the soft-tissue mass density of the tongue and below the maxillary alveolus. In this patient the right sphenoid sinus is considerably larger than the left. The maxillary antra are also quite well outlined in this projection.

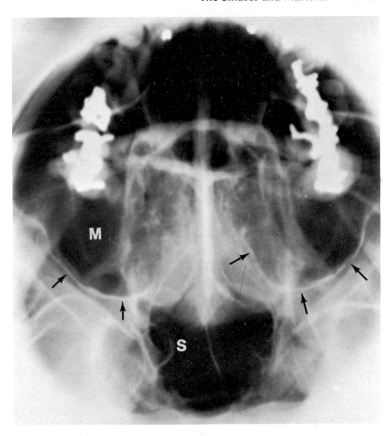

Fig. 34-5. Normal sinuses. Submentovertical (basal) projection. **M,** Maxillary sinus; **S,** sphenoid sinus. **Arrows** outline the posterior walls of the maxillary sinuses which are well visualized in this projection.

nique of Proetz or it can be injected by direct antral puncture. The latter method is preferred. Once the iodized oil is within the desired sinus or sinuses, roentgenograms can be obtained in the routine projections and in any additional projections deemed necessary to obtain desired information. This method is not used in our department.

Tomography. This method is used extensively in the examination of paranasal sinuses to outline foreign bodies, to determine the presence and extent of bone involvement by tumor, and to determine the extent and location of fractures of the bony walls of the sinuses and nasal bones. It is now an essential part of the radiographic study of the sinuses. Various projections may be used as indicated by the problem at hand; these include lateral, coronal, and sometimes an axial or half-axial projection.

Computerized Tomography (Figs. 34-6 and 34-7). Although computerized tomography has been in use for a relatively short time, it appears that it is valuable particularly in demonstrating the extent of soft-tissue masses expanding or eroding the sinus walls. It clearly defines posterior, superior, orbital, and infratemporal extent of tumors, but as yet does not differentiate soft-tissue masses of benign origin from those of malignant origin.

Whenever there is a questionable area of bone destruction in a patient with a sinus shown to be opaque on the routine roentgen examination, tomograms and/or computerized tomography should be used to confirm or disprove the presence of bony involvement.

THE NORMAL SINUSES

The paranasal sinuses are paired cavities lined by mucous membrane (mucoperiosteum) that arise as outpouchings from the nasal fossa and extend into the maxillary, ethmoid, sphenoid, and frontal bones. They are named according to the bones in which they develop.

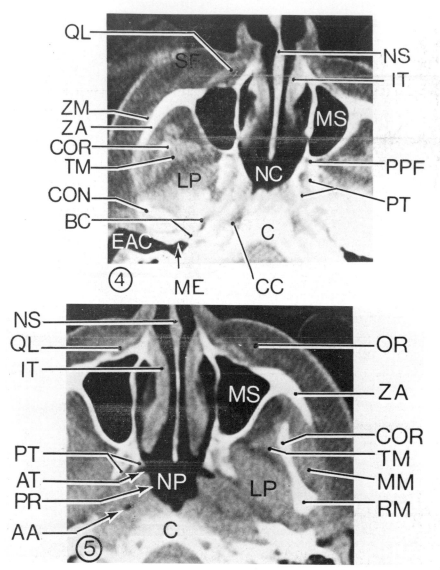

Fig. 34-6. Transverse CT scans of the maxillary sinuses. **Section 4.** Level of the mentomaxillary sinus. **Section 5.** Level of the inferior maxillary sinus. **AA,** air in the auditory tube; **AT,** opening of the auditory tube; **BC,** bony canal of the auditory tube; **C,** clivus; **CC,** carotid canal; **CON,** condyle; **COR,** coronoid process; **EAC,** external auditory canal; **IT,** inferior turbinate; **LP,** lateral pterygoid muscle; **ME,** middle ear cavity; **MM,** masseter; **MS,** maxillary sinus; **NC,** nasal cavity; **NP,** nasopharynx; **NS,** nasal septum; **OR,** orbicularis oculi; **PPF,** pterygopalatine fossa; **PT,** pterygoid plates; **PR,** pharyngeal recess; **QL,** quadratus labii superioris; **RM,** ramus of the mandible; **SF,** superficial fat; **TM,** temporalis muscle; **ZA,** zygomatic arch; **ZM,** zygomaticus major. (Hesselink JR; Journal of Computer Assisted Tomography 2: 559–567, 1978)

Maxillary Sinuses

The maxillary antra are the first of the paranasal sinuses to appear in fetal life. They arise as outpouchings from the anterior recess of the middle meatus. At birth they are small, vertically ovoid cavities located in the maxilla on either side of the midline. They usually contain a jellylike material and are not clearly defined roentgenographically at birth. Aeration is often incomplete for a week or 10 days after birth and may be incomplete for a month or more. At times, aeration is not complete for 6 months after birth. These sinuses develop gradually and at 1 year the outer wall of the antrum is medial to the infraorbital foramen; at 2 years it extends to the level of the foramen. The growth in the transverse diameter is nearly completed at 8 years of age and most of the later growth takes place in the vertical and anteroposterior diameters. Growth is usually complete at 12 years. When fully developed, each sinus is shaped by the body of the maxillary bone. It is considered to have a roof, a floor, and three walls—the nasal, facial,

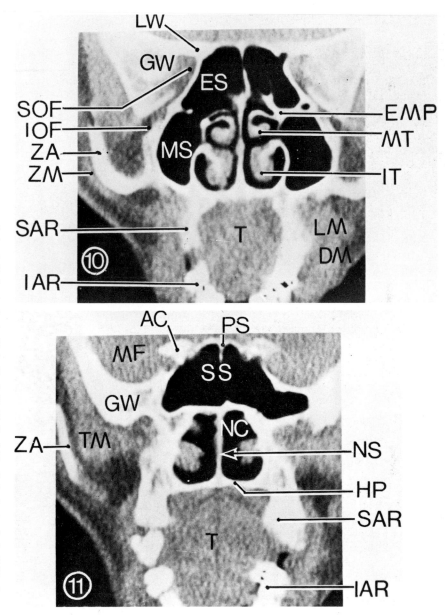

Fig. 34-7. Coronal CT scans. **Section 10.** Through the ethmoid and maxillary sinuses. **Section 11.** Through the sphenoid sinus. **AC,** Anterior clinoid process; **DM,** depressors of the mouth; **EMP,** ethmoidomaxillary plates; **ES,** ethmoid sinus; **GW,** greater wing of the sphenoid; **HP,** hard palate; **IAR,** inferior alveolar ridge; **IOF,** inferior orbital fissure; **IT,** inferior turbinate; **LM,** levators of the mouth; **LW,** lesser wing of the sphenoid; **MF,** middle fossa; **MS,** maxillary sinus; **MT,** middle turbinate; **NC,** nasal cavity; **NS,** nasal septum; **PS,** planum sphenoidale; **SAR,** superior alveolar ridge; **SOF,** superior orbital fissure; **SS,** sphenoid sinus; **T,** tongue; **TM,** temporalis muscle; **ZA,** zygomatic arch; **ZM,** zygomaticus major. (Hesselink JR: Journal of Computer Assisted Tomography 2: 559–567, 1978)

and infratemporal. The floor is often irregular since the alveolar process of the maxilla is immediately below the sinus and some of the teeth may project with their bony and periosteal coverings into the floor of the sinus. Complete or incomplete bony or membranous septa occasionally divide the antrum into two or more compartments.

Frontal Sinuses

The frontal sinuses are usually present at birth but cannot be identified because they are incompletely aerated and lie adjacent to the anterior ethmoid cells in the orbital plate of the frontal bone. They communicate with the middle nasal meatus by means of the nasofrontal duct. These sinuses can usually be identified by the end of the first year following birth but may not be visible until the child is 2 years of age, when they have extended up into the vertical plate of the frontal bone. They can then be differentiated from the anterior ethmoid cells. These sinuses are often asymmetric and vary widely in size. They may extend high into the vertical portion of the frontal bone and backward into the orbital plate. They gradually increase and reach their extent of growth when the child is 10 to 12 years of age. Complete and incomplete division into compartments by septa is common. Agenesis of one or both frontal sinuses is quite frequent.

Ethmoid Sinuses

The ethmoid sinuses consist of two groups of cells lying on either side of the midline in the ethmoid bone, where they form the medial wall of the orbit and the lateral wall of the upper half of the nasal cavity. They vary from 3 or 4 up to 18 or more in number. The frontal anterior ethmoids open into the frontal recess, the infundibular anterior cells open into the ethmoid infundibulum, and the bullar anterior cells open above the ethmoidal bulla. The posterior ethmoid cells usually communicate with the superior or supreme nasal meatus. The ethmoids may extend into the adjacent maxillary, frontal, sphenoid, and palatine bones; their distribution varies considerably. Some of the ethmoid cells are present at birth but are often poorly aerated and difficult to visualize. These sinuses enlarge at about the same rate as the maxillary antra and are usually fully developed when the child is 10 to 12 years of age. The ethmoid cells often extend into the frontal, nasal, maxillary, sphenoid, and palatine bones. In congenital absence of a frontal sinus, there is frequent development of an ethmoid cells on the affected side. It is usually impossible to differentiate an underdeveloped frontal sinus from an ethmoid cell in the frontal bone.

Sphenoid Sinuses

The sphenoid sinuses lie in the body of the sphenoid bone and communicate with the sphenoethmoid recess in the posterior superior portion of the nasal cavity. They are not ordinarily visible at birth. Pneumatization begins anteriorly in the third or fourth year of age and progresses posteriorly into the sphenoid bone below the sella turcica. The sphenoid sinuses not infrequently extend posterior to the sella turcica upward into the dorsum. These sinuses, although superimposed, are most readily outlined in the lateral projection. Their development is somewhat slower than that of the remaining sinuses and their growth continues into young adult life. In the first 4 years of life these sinuses develop in the cupolar recess of the nasal cavity. Pneumatization extends posteriorly in the next 8 years, and from age 12 to 20 the migration extends posteriorly to the level of the dorsum sellae and sometimes extends into it. There is a wide variation in sphenoid sinus development. In some persons (1%), pneumatization is rudimentary or conchal in the anterior portion of the sphenoid, but not beyond the planum sphenoidale; in 40%, development is presphenoidal in which the sinus extends to the level of the anterior wall of the sella; and in about 60% development is postsphenoidal in which the sinus extends posteriorly to the level of the dorsum sellae and sometimes into the dorsum.[5] There may also be extension into the greater wing, the pterygoid process, the lesser wing, and the rostrum of the sphenoid bone. Since aplasia is very rare, if the sphenoid sinuses are not visible by age 10, disease should be suspected.

Normal Roentgen Appearance

The normal sinuses are radiolucent because of the air content; the radiability of the maxillary antra is usually comparable to that of the orbits. Variations in thickness of the bony walls of the sinuses may alter the density to a moderate degree. This is particularly true of the frontal sinuses in which the frontal bone may be relatively dense. In the interpretation of roentgenograms of the sinuses the variation in bone density and in thickness of overlying soft tissues must be considered. The normal lining membrane of the sinuses is invisible on the roentgenogram and the bony walls are distinct and clearly defined. Any increase in density involving one or more sinuses must be examined carefully to exclude the possibility of changes caused by normal soft-tissue structures. Care must be taken in interpreting variations of aeration in the sinuses in infants because the mucosa is often redundant and aeration incomplete in the normal infant, particularly in one less than 1 month of age. Furthermore, the frequent asymmetry of the sinuses must be kept in mind.

INFLAMMATORY DISEASES
Acute Sinusitis

Acute inflammatory disease involving paranasal sinuses results in swelling of the lining membrane.

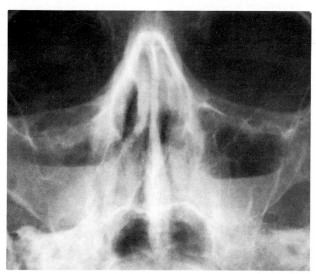

Fig. 34-8. Waters' view of the sinuses showing fluid levels in the maxillary antra in this patient with bilateral acute maxillary sinusitis.

There is often retention of the fluid in the sinus also. The maxillary antra are most commonly affected and, in the present of disease affecting the other sinuses, the changes in the antra are often more marked than those elsewhere. The disease may be unilateral or bilateral. Fluid is manifested by fluid levels when roentgenograms are made with the patient upright (Fig. 34-8). The levels are noted particularly in the maxillary antra and frontal sinuses and occasionally in the sphenoids. In patients who cannot assume an upright position, horizontal-beam films may be exposed with the patient recumbent and appropriate projections obtained in order to define fluid levels. The presence of some air in addition to fluid is required to demonstrate a fluid level. When there is a problem in positive identification of a fluid level, the patient's head can be tilted and another horizontal-beam film obtained for confirmation. A loss of translucency resulting in a hazy, diffuse opacity is observed as the result of thickening of the lining membrane and the presence of inflammatory exudate. The mucosal swelling may be manifested by a soft-tissue density lining the bony walls of the sinus if it is not sufficient to cause complete diffuse type of density. In the acute disease there is no alteration in the bony walls. The roentgen findings should be correlated with clinical findings in these patients because some swelling of the lining membrane may persist after an infection has subsided. It is also possible

to have an acute process with very little swelling of the mucosa so that no detectable roentgen findings may be present.

In the interest of decreasing radiation and cost to the patient, a Waters' view may be obtained in suspected maxillary sinusitis (see Fig. 34-8). If this film shows no abnormality, no further views are necessary. If some opacity or other abnormality is observed, the remaining films of the series can be obtained.

Chronic Sinusitis

Chronic sinusitis may follow the acute phase or represent a more slowly developing process that is subacute or chronic from its inception. The roentgen findings are due to thickening of the mucosa that results in soft-tissue density of varying thickness lining the sinus or sinuses involved. Fluid levels may also be present in the patients with chronic sinus disease. The thickening of the membrane is usually more clearly defined and less hazy than in more acute disease. In chronic sinusitis the additional finding of some thickening or sclerosis of the bone forming the wall of the sinus may be observed (Fig. 34-9). This is found more commonly in the frontal sinuses than elsewhere. In chronic sinusitis, as a general rule the maxillary antra are the most commonly affected; the ethmoids are often involved as well. When the frontal sinuses are infected, almost invariably sinusitis affects the ethmoid cells, but the ethmoids may be infected without involvement of the frontal sinuses. The sphenoids are less frequently the site of disease, but when they are the posterior ethmoids are almost invariably involved. Rarely, infection may lead to osteomyelitis of the sinus wall. This is more commonly associated with involvement of the maxillary antrum secondary to dental infection than it is with sinusitis. When this osteomyelitis occurs there is usually clouding of the sinus and an irregular moth-eaten type of destruction of the bony sinus wall in the area of involvement; dense sequestra are often present. Prior to the use of antibiotics, acute frontal sinusitis occasionally led to the development of acute osteomyelitis of the frontal bone. This is a rare lesion at the present time.

Occasionally the sinuses may be involved by such chronic inflammatory diseases as tuberculosis, syphilis, actinomycosis, and other bacterial and fungal infections. The roentgen findings are not specific. There is evidence of chronic sinus disease in these patients, with or without destruction of bony walls. Occasionally it is possible to suspect certain orga-

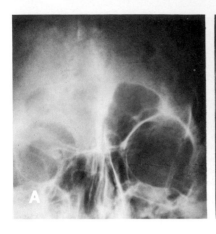
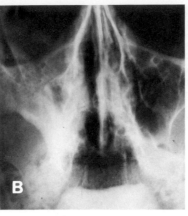

Fig. 34-9. Chronic right frontal and maxillary sinusitis. **A.** Occipitofrontal projection showing clouding in the right frontal sinus along with considerable sclerosis of its bony walls. Contrast this with the normal radiolucency and normal bony walls of the left frontal sinus. **B.** There are changes in the right maxillary antrum similar to those in the right frontal sinus, with extensive bony sclerosis and clouding of the sinus. Note the normal appearance of the left maxillary antrum in contrast to the right.

nisms, *e.g., Actinomyces, Mucor,* and other fungi, because they characteristically cross tissue boundaries and destroy bone. Diagnosis of the specific organism is made on bacteriologic study of material from the infected sinus. However, when bone is destroyed, biopsy is essential, since the possibility of malignant disease cannot be excluded by radiographic means, and tumor may be present in addition to infection.

Scleroma (Rhinoscleroma)

This rare disease is evidently caused by *Klebsiella rhinoscleromatis;* it often starts in the nose and progresses down the respiratory tract. Roentgen findings are those of thickening of the nasal septum and intranasal soft-tissue masses which often occlude the nares. Sinuses are often opaque and, in advanced disease, extensive destruction of the bony sinus walls may be present. The disease may progress down the respiratory tract to the larynx, leading to laryngeal or subglottic stricture.

CYSTS AND TUMORS

Mucous Cyst (Retention Cyst)

A mucous cyst is a secretory retention cyst caused by obstruction of a mucous gland, usually within the maxillary antrum. This results in gradual enlargement with formation of a cyst most often in or near the floor of the antrum but it may be formed anywhere in the sinuses. It appears as a smooth, rounded soft-tissue opacity usually projecting from the floor of the antrum. It is usually small but rarely may become large enough to occupy most of the sinus (Fig. 34-10). Mucous cysts usually indicate

that there has been infection in the sinus but they are asymptomatic and are often incidental findings. They are lined by columnar epithelium.

Serous (Nonsecreting) Cyst

This cyst arises in the connective tissue of the sinus mucosa. It has no epithelial lining and usually lies on the floor of the maxillary antrum. It is the most common antral cyst and is usually not associated with other abnormality of the affected sinus. Like the mucous retention cyst, it is usually small and never enlarges to the point where it erodes the sinus walls. Roentgenographically it cannot be differentiated from mucous retention cyst.

Mucocele

Mucocele consists of a fibrous tissue sac lined by low cuboidal or stratified columnar epithelium. It is produced by obstruction of a sinus ostium. It occurs commonly in the frontal sinuses and with somewhat less frequency in the ethmoids. It is rare in the maxillary antra and in the sphenoids.

Roentgen Findings. The increased pressure within the mucocele caused by accumulation of secretions results in enlargement of the sinus, causing gradual erosion of bony walls. As a result of the destruction of bone, the mucocele is often as radiolucent as an air-filled sinus. The degree of radiolucency of the lesion depends upon the degree of destruction of bony sinus walls (Fig. 34-11). The enlargement of the sinus as a result of the expanding mucocele causes loss of the normal scalloped sinus margin, and the normal soft tissue making up the wall of the sinus is obliterated. The lesion is usually unilateral and the difference be-

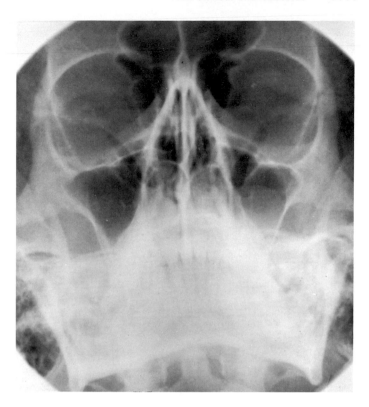

Fig. 34-10. Retention cyst in the floor of the left maxillary antrum. Note the clearly defined, smoothly rounded superior border silhouetted against the air in the maxillary sinus.

Fig. 34-11. Mucocele of the right ethmoids. This tomogram shows a large radiolucency in the ethmoid area on the right in which no cell walls are visible. The mucocele has enlarged into the medial aspect of the orbit where the thin wall is outlined by **arrows** (retouched).

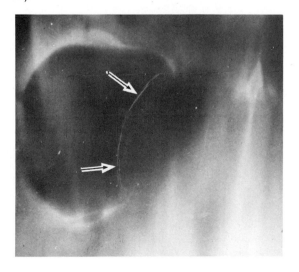

tween the normal and abnormal sinus is readily apparent. Mucocele of the sphenoid sinus is rare, but the enlargement of this sinus may erode the sellar floor, extend anteriorly into the ethmoid area, and erode the superior orbital fissure or optic canal. It may also extend posteriorly to erode the dorsum sellae, posterior clinoid process, and clivus. Visual loss, diplopia, exophthalmos, or lateral displacement of the globe may occur. In some instances, misdiagnosis of pituitary tumor has led to craniotomy or radiotherapy. This makes accurate diagnosis very important. Tomography is of particular value in mucocele of the sphenoid or ethmoid areas, since the thin expanded wall may be clearly defined (see Fig. 34-11). This results in a correct diagnosis and proper treatment. Hypocycloidal or circular tomography is used in preference to linear in these patients. Computerized tomography may be the procedure of choice in the future.

Rarely there is a sclerotic change in the bone forming the margins of the mucocele. Calcification in a mucocele is sometimes found and may be very dense, but this is also rare.

Polyposis and Allergic Disease

Allergic conditions which involve the upper respiratory tract are often associated with polyposis. Polyps consist of edematous masses of mucous membrane with some myxomatous changes; most of them are secondary to allergy. They are usually found in the nasal cavity and when present are often associated with polyps in the maxillary antra. They may also occur in sphenoid, ethmoid, and frontal sinuses, but are more difficult to demonstrate roentgenographically in these locations. In the antra they produce soft-tissue densities, projecting from the sinus wall, that may be single or multiple and may fill the entire sinus, causing general cloudiness. The density caused by these masses is similar to that caused by mucous retention cysts, but polyps are often associated with polyps in the nose so that there is loss of aeration of the nasal cavities. As a general rule, both maxillary sinuses are involved with multiple, small mucosal masses. There is often some associated thickening of the mucosal lining of the antra and sometimes of the frontal sinuses. It is not unusual to have complete clouding or opacity of one or both antra, and fluid levels may be present. The roentgen observations should be correlated with the clinical findings in these patients.

Benign Tumors

Tumors of Soft-Tissue Origin. Fibroma, neurofibroma, papilloma, and angioma may occur in the wall of the maxillary antrum. They are rare, usually small, and cannot be differentiated from cysts. Epidermoid tumors (cholesteatomas) may rarely arise in the frontal or maxillary sinuses. Their pathogenesis is somewhat controversial, but most of them are evidently acquired. Occasionally they become large and their slow growth gradually expands the sinus. This produces atrophy and sometimes complete destruction of one or more bony walls in a manner similar to that caused by mucocele. When this occurs, these tumors may resemble mucoceles to the point where they cannot be differentiated roentgenographically. Similar gross enlargement is sometimes seen with other benign tumors; biopsy is necessary to differentiate them.

Inverting papilloma usually arises in the lateral wall of the nasal cavity but may arise in the maxillary or sphenoid sinus. This tumor may become large, expanding and thinning the bony walls in a manner similar to that of mucocele. Also, it may be mistaken for antral carcinoma with bone destruction. It usually occurs in men over 40 years of age.

Tumors of Bony Origin. Osteoma is a relatively common tumor that usually arises in the frontal and much less frequently in the ethmoid sinuses. Rarely it is found in the maxillary or sphenoid sinuses. The roentgen findings are characteristic and consist of a rounded or lobulated mass of bony density. The tumor is usually small but may become moderately large and is readily recognized because of its ivorylike density similar to that of cortical bone (Fig. 34-12). Occasionally osteochondroma may arise in the wall of the sinus; this tumor may become large, resulting in pressure with erosion and atrophy of bone. If calcification does not occur within the tumor it cannot be distinguished from other slowly growing soft-tissue masses such as a large fibroma or mucocele; however, calcification is often present within it. The calcification has a mottled appearance similar to calcification occurring in osteochrondroma elsewhere. If this is visible, the diagnosis can be made with a reasonable degree of certainty. Occasionally a hemangioma occurs in the wall of a sinus. Its appearance resembles the striated appearance of hemangiomata occurring in the bones of the cranial vault. Paget's disease of the skull may extend to involve sinus walls,

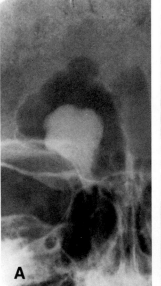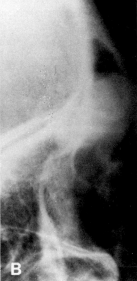

Fig. 34-12. Osteoma of the right frontal sinus. Note the ivorylike density in the floor of the right frontal sinus. Occipitofrontal **(A)** and lateral **(B)** projections.

and fibrous dysplasia may also involve sinus walls as well as other facial bones. These lesions are discussed more fully in Chapters 2 and 8.

Malignant Tumors

Sarcoma. Fibrosarcoma occasionally occurs in the sinuses, usually in the maxillary antrum, and causes destruction of the walls of the sinus in addition to the production of a soft-tissue mass. From the radiographic standpoint it cannot be distinguished from carcinoma. Myxosarcoma may also occur and has an appearance similar to that of fibrosarcoma on the radiograph.

Carcinoma. Carcinoma may arise in any of the paranasal sinuses but is much more common in the maxillary antrum than elsewhere. Occasionally the ethmoids are the site of origin while the frontal and sphenoid sinuses are rarely involved. The roentgen findings are caused by the dense appearance of the mass of the tumor plus irregular destruction of bone. The tumor may be very large, obliterating the airspace and causing soft-tissue density beyond the sinus. The destruction of bone is irregular with no evidence of sclerosis (Fig. 34-13, 14). It is entirely different from the smooth, pressure atrophy type of defect that results when large benign soft-tissue tumors involve the sinuses. Tomography is of value in outlining the extent of destruction. We use tomography in addition to the standard projections in virtually every patient with clinical findings suggesting sinus carcinoma. Computerized tomography tends to outline the extent of bone destruction and soft-tissue mass very completely and will likely be the method of choice in the examination of patients with suspected sinus carcinoma in the future. (Figs. 34-15 and 34-16).

When a carcinoma arising in a sinus extends into the nasal cavity it may occlude the ostia of the other sinuses and lead to infection involving them. A malignant tumor primary in the nasal cavity is prone to obstruct the ostia of the sinuses on that side. In either event, the roentgen signs of uniformly clouded sinuses on one side (unilateral pansinusitis) with normal sinuses on the other may be encountered. This observation always raises the question of a tumor as the causative agent and necessitates careful clinical and additional roentgen investigation for such a lesion.

Miscellaneous Tumors. Plasmocytoma or plasma cell myeloma may arise in the sinuses producing bone de-

struction and soft-tissue mass similar to that caused by carcinoma. Metastatic tumors may involve the bones of the sinuses and produce destruction and soft-tissue mass that is visible radiographically. Tumors of the pituitary, as well as chordoma that may arise in the region of the clivus, may project into the sphenoid sinus and produce soft-tissue density there. The appearance of the sella and of the clivus usually indicates the site of primary disease. Cysts and tumors of dental origin involve the lower jaw as well as the floor of the maxillary sinuses and are discussed in Chapter 35.

MISCELLANEOUS CONDITIONS

Syndromes with Sinus Abnormality

Gorlin and Sedano[8] have tabulated a number of syndromes involving the paranasal sinuses. These are described briefly in the following six paragraphs

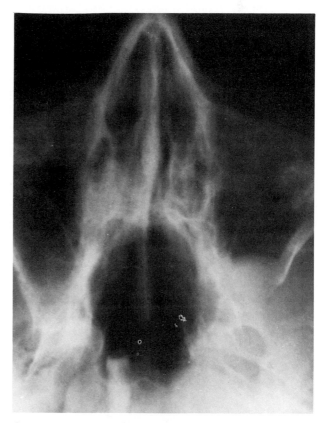

Fig. 34-13. Carcinoma of the left maxillary antrum. Note the soft-tissue mass in the floor of the antrum with destruction of the bony wall of the floor.

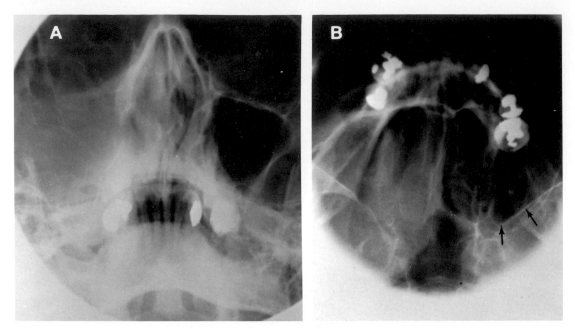

Fig. 34-14. Carcinoma of the right maxillary antrum. **A.** Waters' view shows a soft-tissue mass filling the antrum and destroying its walls. **B.** Submentovertical view shows the mass on the right. The **arrows** indicate normal lucency of the left maxillary antrum in contrast to the right. The tumor has extended posteriorly into the pterygoid plate which is partially destroyed.

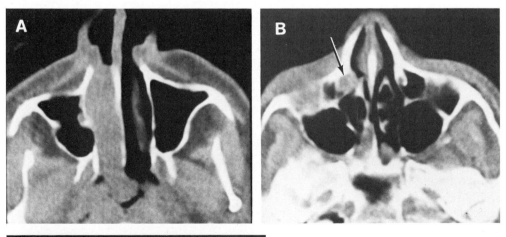

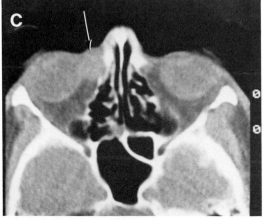

Fig. 34-15. Transverse CT scans of a malignant melanoma of the left side of the nose. The tumor extends up the nasolacrimal duct to involve the left orbit. **A.** Note the large soft-tissue mass in the nasal cavity, which appears to have bowed the medial wall of the maxillary antrum somewhat laterally and has thinned it in its posteromedial aspect. **B. Arrow** indicates the mass in the nasolacrimal duct. **C.** This scan through the orbits shows the tumor in the inferomedial aspect of the orbit **(arrow).** (Hesselink JR: Journal of Computer assisted Tomography 2: 568–576, 1978)

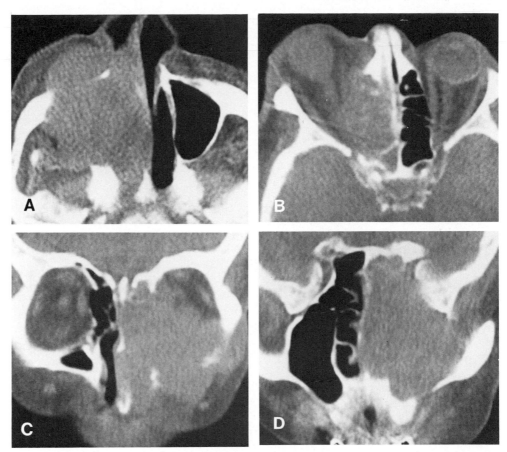

Fig. 34-16. Transverse **(A** and **B)** and coronal CT scan **(C** and **D)** showing a large carcinoma of the left maxillary sinus. In **A,** note the mass that has largely destroyed the walls of the sinus, filled the nasal cavity, and extended posteriorly into the pterygopalatine fossa and anteriorly into the orbit. In **B** the scan is through the orbits. The mass is noted to encroach on the posteromedial aspect of the orbit and to have destroyed the ethmoid cell walls. The extent of the tumor in the coronal views **(C** and **D)** into the ethmoid area and orbit is readily appreciated. (Hesselink JR: Journal of Computer Assisted Tomography 2: 568–576, 1978)

since the roentgen examination of the sinuses may suggest the diagnosis.

Gardner's Syndrome. This syndrome includes (1) multiple polyposis of the colon; (2) multiple osteomas in sphenoid and ethmoid sinuses, frontal bone, maxilla, and mandible as well as the calvarium; and (3) epidermoid inclusion cysts of the skin and fibromas, lipomas, and desmoid tumors of the skin.

Cleidocranial Dysostosis. In this condition, aplasia or hypoplasia of clavicles is present; the paranasal sin-

uses are often absent or underdeveloped; anomalies of teeth and calvarium occur.

Maxillonasal Dysplasia. In this condition, aplasia or hypoplasia of anterior nasal spine of maxilla occurs, and uni- or bilateral hypoplasia of frontal sinuses is found.

Pycnodysostosis. Sinus films may show frontal sinuses absent, other sinuses are hypoplastic or absent, and increased radiopacity is evident at the base of the skull. Dwarfism, osteopetrosis, partial agenesis of terminal phalanges, cranial anomalies such as persistence of fontanelles and open cranial sutures, frontal and occipital bossing, and hypoplasia of the angle of the mandible are also found."

Progeria. Sinus examination shows hypoplasia of maxilla and mandible with crowded teeth, the frontal sinuses often are absent, and the other sinuses are hypoplastic.

Craniometaphyseal Dysostosis and Craniodiaphyseal Dysostosis. In both of these conditions there is severe overgrowth of bone in the frontal bone, maxillae, and basal skull resulting in encroachment upon, or obliteration of, paranasal sinuses. There are differences in long bone involvement in the two conditions, but both show considerable sclerosis of long bones.

Midline Lethal Granuloma

This disease is often associated with generalized necrotizing granulomatous vasculitis. The etiology is not definite but it is most likely a hyperimmune reaction involving the nose and paranasal sinuses. Visceral changes may or may not be present. There are granulomatous masses in the nose and sinuses that result in roentgen clouding and complete obliteration of the airspace; this is followed in time by extensive destruction of bone. The bone and cartilage in the nose and the medial walls of the maxillary antra are most frequently involved but the remaining sinuses may also be affected. When there is associated visceral disease, the changes often progress more rapidly than when the midline facial tissues are the only site of involvement. There is a relationship of this disease to Wegener's granulomatosis. They both appear to be autoimmune in origin. Wegener's syndrome includes pulmonary and renal lesions in addition to the involvement of the upper respiratory tract.

Trauma

Fractures of the bony walls of the paranasal sinuses are not uncommon and are usually associated with fractures of the other facial bones or base of the skull. The signs of fracture are irregular linear defects, often with jagged overriding edges and depression or displacement of bony walls. The involved sinus is usually clouded, with loss of aeration secondary to edema and hemorrhage into the lining membrane or into the sinus itself. Facial bone fractures are discussed in Chapter 35.

Foreign Bodies

Foreign bodies may gain access to the sinuses by direct trauma such as gunshot wounds. Dental roots may be displaced into the antrum during extraction. Roentgenograms obtained in various projections or tomograms will outline the foreign body and ascertain its relationship to the sinus. Foreign bodies within the nasal cavities can also be localized provided they are dense enough to be visible on the roentgenogram.

THE MASTOIDS

The roentgen examination of the temporal bone in which the mastoid cells are located is important in the diagnosis of middle-ear and mastoid diseases. Prime prerequisites for roentgen interpretation of mastoid disease are films of good technical quality in proper projections.

METHODS OF EXAMINATION

There are several projections used in the examination of the mastoids. They should be standardized technically so that films of good quality are available on each patient. There have been numerous projections described; most are useful if properly carried out. We use the following in our routine examination of the mastoids:

1. Schüller (or Runstrom), a lateral projection with the tube angled 30 degrees caudad.
2. Mayer, an axial projection in which the patient's head is angled 45 degrees toward the side to be examined and the tube is angled 45 degrees caudad.
3. Chamberlain–Towne, an anteroposterior projection in which the tube is angled caudad (we use a 30-degree angle).
4. Chausse III, an anteroposterior projection with the patient's head rotated 15 degrees away from the side to be examined and the tube rotated 30 degrees caudad.

On all of the anteroposterior projections the caudad angles are in relation to the canthomeatal line. Good coning is essential to quality examinations. Both mastoids are always included on the examination so that the two sides can be compared. Tomography is of considerable value in examining the mastoid. The ossicles of the middle ear can also be studied by means of tomography and this method is also essential in the study of the inner ear, facial canal and internal auditory canals.

When we refer to tomography of the mastoid and petrous pyramid, we mean that multidirectional equipment is essential. We use equipment capable of hypocycloidal, circular, and elliptical motion in addition to linear and zonographic techniques. Hypocycloidal motion is superior to the circular and elliptical motions for fine detail of the middle and inner ear; however, it depends on an excellent technologist and careful monitoring of the films as the study progresses. As a rule we begin with sections obtained at 2-mm intervals, and after the radiologist has checked these, we expose as many intermediate 0.5- or 1.0-mm films as needed. These methods are used in study of trauma as well as in disease of the middle ear particularly when there is seventh nerve involvement. Because there is a radiation dose to the cornea approaching 10 R in petrous tomography, eye shields and precise coning are advisable to reduce the corneal radiation.

THE NORMAL MASTOIDS

The temporal bone is an extremely complex structure that contains the external auditory canal and the middle and internal ear as well as the vestibular appa-

ratus. The bone consists of three parts: (*1*) the squamous or squamozygomatic, (*2*) the tympanic, and (*3*) the petrous or petromastoid. Mastoid cells are found in the squamous as well as in the petrous portion of the temporal bone. The relationship of the mastoid cells to the adjacent structures is illustrated in Figures 34-17 through 34-20.

Development of the Mastoids

The mastoid cells develop as saclike extensions from the mastoid antrum which is invariably present at birth. The process begins in the first year of life and is usually complete by puberty, but some increase in size of the cells may occur well into adult life. There is considerable variation in the amount of pneumatization in the normal mastoid. When pneumatization is complete and involves the mastoid process and the lateral aspect of the petrous and the squamous portion of the temporal bone, the mastoid is called pneumatic in type. Occasionally the antrum is very large—mega-antrum.[9] Rarely pneumatization is very extensive with cells extending into the parietal and occipital bones. When pneumatization is incomplete with only small, thick-walled cells formed immediately above and posterior to the tympanic cavity the mastoid is diploic in type (Fig. 34-21). The mastoid is sclerotic in type when there is no pneumatization

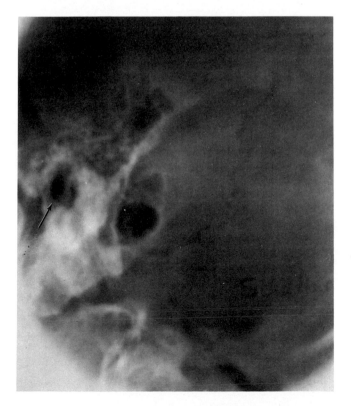

Fig. 34-17. Normal mastoid as seen in the Schüller projection. The external auditory canal **(arrow)** lies directly posterior to the manibular condyle and fossa.

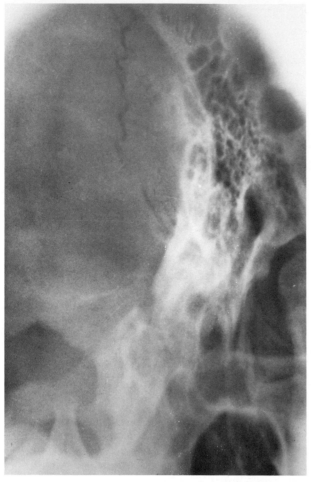

Fig. 34-18. Normal mastoid as viewed with the patient in the Mayer position. In this projection the bony bridge adjacent to the mastoid aditus is clearly defined.

and the bone is dense and eburnated. Intermediate degrees of pneumatization are frequent. There is a difference of opinion as to the cause of the sclerotic type; some believe that failure of development is genetic while others think that it is caused by infection in infancy. Most believe that early infection inhibits pneumatization, so that some of the diploic and sclerotic types are acquired.

In addition to the parts of the ear, there are vascular and nerve structures that can be visualized. Their location is of considerable importance if surgery is necessary. The lateral venous sinus forms a groove that curves downward posterior to the mastoid. When the mastoid is diploic or sclerotic in type, this groove is well outlined; but when it is pneumatic in type the sinus groove is sometimes difficult to define. The location of emissary vessels if present is also important. The mastoid emissary vein is commonly seen and is usually found midway between the mastoid tip and the genu, or curve, of the lateral sinus (see Fig. 34-21). Using tomography in both sagittal and frontal planes, the facial canal through which the seventh nerve courses, can be seen. This is important in trauma, tumors, and infection in the region of the middle ear. Tomographic anatomic detail of the middle and inner ear are beyond the scope of this volume. The interested reader is referred to the references listed at the end of this chapter.[6, 14, 20, 21, 23]

INFLAMMATORY DISEASES

Acute Mastoiditis

Mastoid infection usually follows otitis media and is secondary to the middle-ear infection. In early otitis

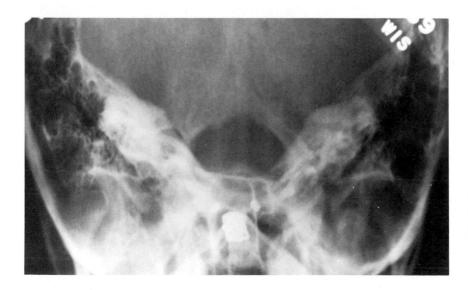

Fig. 34-19. Normal mastoids as seen in the Chamberlain–Towne projection. The internal auditory canals and petrous pyramids are outlined in this position.

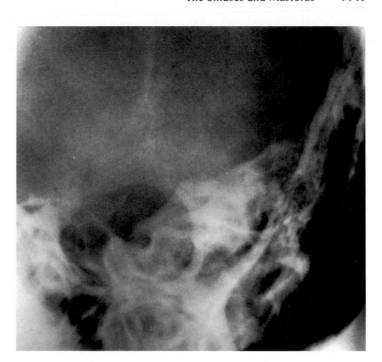

Fig. 34-20. Normal mastoid as seen with the patient in the Chausse III position. The petrous pyramid and tip are well outlined in this projection.

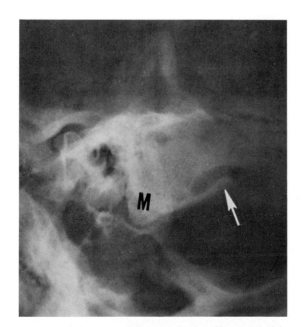

Fig. 34-21. Diploic mastoid. Very few cells are visible adjacent to the mastoid antrum. Elsewhere the mastoid is diploic. **Arrow** indicates an emissary vein. The mastoid process **(M)** is dense because of a lack of pneumatization, but there is no sclerosis. This type should not be mistaken for a diseased mastoid.

media it may be possible to observe a slight increase in haziness or density in the middle-ear cavity. When the infection extends to the mastoid the normal translucency of the mastoid air cells is slightly decreased, resulting in slight cloudiness unless the infection is minor and recovery is rapid. The change is minimal and this diagnoisis should be made with great caution. When the infection in the mastoid continues for a time, edema and hyperemia result in thickening of the lining of the cells in the region of the mastoid antrum. This is noted radiographically as a loss of the normal clear outline of the cells plus a slight increase in density. The change at this stage is minor, and comparison with the normal side is the basis of the diagnosis. The disease may spread to the remaining cells so that the process becomes more generalized. The roentgen findings are then more generalized with a loss of the shadow of the ossicles and poor definition of all mastoid cells. The next change is absorption of bone that is manifested radiographically by loss of some of the cell walls with thinning and poor definition of others. The earliest signs of bone destruction are usually observed in the cells surrounding the attic. If the process continues further with suppuration and complete breakdown of cell walls, a mastoid abscess is formed. This is manifested by an area of radiolucency which begins in the epitympanic recess (attic) above and posterior to the tympanic cavity. The abscess may also extend to the tip of the mastoid process and from there into the soft tissues in the posterior aspect of the neck (Bezold's abscess). The infection may spread upward and medially into the petrous portion of the temporal bone or to the tegmen tympani and occasionally may destroy the tegmen to form an epidural abscess. Acute mastoid abscess is an uncommon finding now that a number of antibiotics are available for treatment of acute otitis media. These antibiotics may mask symptoms in some patients in whom roentgen examination shows that the destructive inflammatory process is advancing. It is, therefore, important to correlate the clinical and roentgen findings.

Chronic Mastoiditis

In chronic infection the changes in the mastoid are similar to those in other bony structures involved by infection. When the disease is low-grade and of long duration, bone production causes thickening and sclerosis of mastoid cell walls. When the infection is of suppurative type the cell walls are destroyed and an abscess is formed.

Roentgen Findings. The affected mastoid is dense and the few cells that may be visible in the region of the antrum often have thickened bony walls. The marked density in chronic low-grade infections may obscure the radiolucency caused by an abscess; tomograms are indispensable in the examination of densely sclerotic mastoids in which abscess is suspected. When abscess is present, it produces an area of poorly defined radiolucency in a mastoid in which there is evidence of sclerotic change elsewhere. The defect caused by cholesteatoma is similar and cannot be differentiated from that of an abscess. The clinical history and examination must be correlated with roentgen findings in these situations.

Cholesteatoma

Cholesteatoma is an accumulation of cellular debris in the mastoid that develops when the tympanic membrane is perforated and the epithelium of the external auditory canal extends into the middle ear. It is the result of chronic mastoid disease. The accumulated material tends to destroy cell walls and create an irregularly rounded or oval cavity within the sclerotic infected mastoid. The patients usually give a history of long-continued discharge of pus from the ear.

Roentgen Findings. The cholesteatoma is noted radiographically as an area of radiolucency in the region of the mastoid antrum that may be very large. There is evidence of chronic mastoid infection with sclerosis and thickening of any cell walls that may be visible. Tomography is essential in the examination of the middle ear when cholesteatoma is suspected. The early lesion begins in the region of the attic. Its inferolateral wall, the scutum (spur), is usually the site of the earliest evidence of bone destruction in osteitis and cholesteatoma (Fig. 34-22). As the cholesteatoma enlarges, it causes an enlarging cavity in the mastoid antrum (Fig. 34-23). Occasionally there is an unusually large mastoid antrum in the normal person which may be unilateral. On standard projections differentiation from cholesteatoma may be very difficult, but on tomography no destruction of ossicles is evident and the scutum (spur) is intact in these persons. The cholesteatoma usually has a smooth wall which may be very clearly defined, however (Fig. 34-24).

Petrositis

The pneumatization of the mastoid often extends well into the petrous portion of the temporal bone. Therefore, the cells in the petrous apex may be infected along with cells in the mastoid process and those adjacent to the tympanic cavity. The roentgen findings in the early stages of petrositis are similar to those of acute mastoiditis. These consist of loss of clear bony detail. Positive diagnosis cannot be made at this stage and must await evidence of decalcification and destruction of bone in the petrous tip. At times, the petrous tip may be completely destroyed. Petrositis may follow mastoidectomy and should be kept in mind in a postmastoidectomy patient in whom symptoms recur. Occasionally the infection is chronic and low grade; then the roentgen findings simulate those of chronic sclerotic type of mastoiditis with increase in density of the tip of the petrous bone. The basal and Stenvers' views are of particular value in addition to tomography in this condition and the abnormal side can then be compared with the normal. The disease is uncommon (Fig. 34-25).

The Postoperative Mastoid

The interpretation of disease in the mastoid following mastoidectomy is difficult. Cell walls may be partially removed and still be visible so that residual disease in intact cells is simulated. The postoperative absence of cells may also closely resemble cholesteatoma. It is

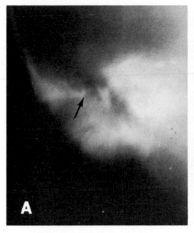
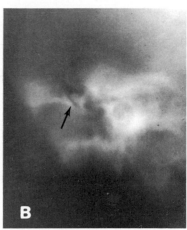

Fig. 34-22. Early osteitis and cholesteatoma. **A.** Tomogram shows destruction of the scutum (spur) **(arrow).** Note the wide separation between the ossicles and the base of the spur that remains. **B.** Tomogram of the opposite ear (reversed for easy comparison) showing a normal spur **(arrow)** and the relationship of this structure to the ossicles that are immediately medial to it.

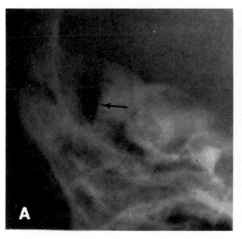
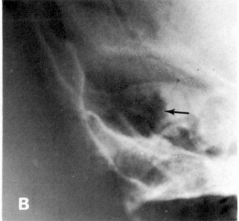

Fig. 34-23. Cholesteatoma. **A.** Chamberlain–Towne view showing a defect in the mastoid antrum caused by a large cholesteatoma **(arrow). B.** Coned Stenvers projection of the same patient shown in **A.** The defect **(arrow)** is much more clearly defined in this projection than in the Chamberlain–Towne view.

Fig. 34-24. Cholesteatoma. **Arrow** indicates the area of destruction of cell walls at the site of the cholesteatoma. There is a moderate amount of sclerosis and less pneumatization on this side than on the normal left side.

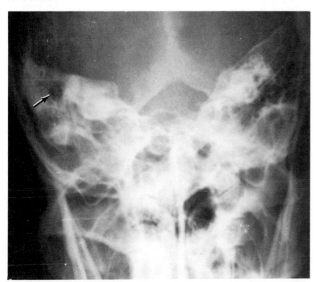

essential, therefore, that the radiologist be advised of previous surgical procedures on the mastoid in order to avoid unnecessary error in interpretation of findings.

The extent of the surgical cavity as well as the extent of remaining cells can be outlined. Occasionally, bony sequestra may be observed; they are most clearly defined on tomography. The detection of residual disease is very difficult after mastoidectomy, and follow-up studies may be required to demonstrate change produced by continuing infection.

FRACTURES OF THE TEMPORAL BONE

Fractures of the temporal bone can be classified into longitudinal (85%) (parallel to the long axis of the pyramid) and transverse (9%) (perpendicular to the long axis of the pyramid). Occasionally there are combined fractures. The longitudinal fracture is much more frequent than the others and results

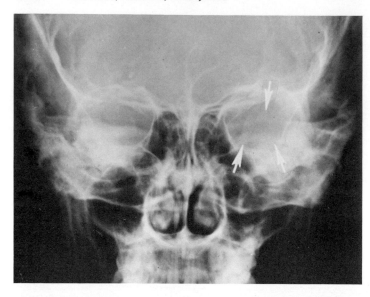

Fig. 34-25. Petrositis. The right side is normal. On the left side there is extensive destruction of the petrous tip as the result of infection involving it **(arrows).**

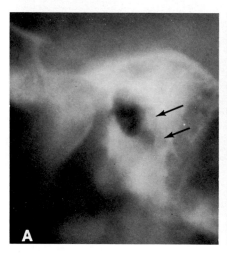

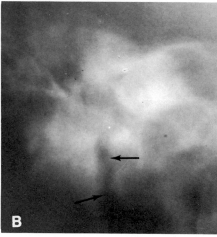

Fig. 34-26. A. Longitudinal fracture of the temporal bone. This lateral tomogram shows the fracture line in the anterior wall of the external auditory canal which continues posteriorly coursing downward as well as posteriorly **(arrows). B.** Transverse fracture of the temporal bone. This frontal tomogram shows a wide fracture **(arrows).** The patient shown in **A** and the one shown in **B** both had seventh nerve involvement with recovery after surgery.

when force is applied to the mandibular condyle or to the temporoparietal portion of the skull. It originates in temporal squamosa, extends medially along the external auditory canal into the tegmen tympani, then anteriorly along the carotid canal to the foramen lacerum. This is usually associated with bleeding from the ear, otorrhea, and conductive hearing loss. It may originate posteriorly in the occipital bone, cross the petrous pyramid through the jugular fossa, the labyrinthine capsule, and the carotid canal. In this type, there is neurosensory hearing loss and facial paralysis caused by eighth nerve or labyrinthine trauma. Although standard views of the mastoid should be obtained, it is always advisable to se-

cure tomograms in the patient with suspected fracture of the petrous pyramid. As a rule, since lateral tomograms are of more value than frontal views in longitudinal fracture, these should be obtained first (Fig. 34-26 A). We usually obtain frontal tomograms as well, particularly if no fracture can be seen on the lateral tomograms or on the standard films. The transverse fractures, which are much less common, are usually visualized best on anteroposterior tomograms (Fig. 34-26B).

Ossicle dislocations, which are often associated with longitudinal temporal bone fracture, are best seen on the lateral projection. Lateral tomography is necessary in order to confirm the presence of an abnormality suspected on viewing the standard projections, or to detect dislocations not visible on other films. Rarely, we use submentovertex tomograms when a fracture is suspected.

TUMORS

Benign Tumors

Benign tumors of the middle ear and mastoid are rare. Occasionally, osteoma arises in the mastoid process and results in radiographic findings of a dense mass of solid cortical bone in or attached to the mastoid process. Rarely, hemangiomas arise in the middle ear and result in destruction of mastoid cells because of pressure erosion. This results in radiolucency in the region of the tumor. Evidence of hypervascularity in the area, consisting of prominent vascular channels in the bone adjacent to the mastoid process and enlargement of the emissary vein, may suggest the diagnosis. The glomus jugulare tumor (chemodectoma) is the most common benign soft-tissue tumor arising in the temporal bone. It arises in the vicinity of the tympanic branch of the ninth cranial nerve in the adventitia of the jugular bulb. Its counterpart, the chemodectoma of the middle ear, is called glomus typanicum. The radiographic findings are not typical. The tumor grows slowly and destroys the cell walls by pressure erosion. When this occurs,

radiolucency can be outlined at the site of involvement. Angiography may be helpful in localization and retrograde injection of the jugular vein may help to determine jugular bulb involvement. The temporal bone including the petrous pyramid can also be involved by eosinophilic granuloma (histiocytosis X) which more commonly involves the flat bones of the skull. It is a purely destructive, clearly defined lesion which may be extensive. Eighth-nerve neuroma and meningioma are described in Chapter 11.

Malignant Tumors

Carcinoma occasionally arises in the middle ear or in the external auditory canal and extends into the antrum and mastoid process. The roentgen findings are those of destruction of bone, which is similar to bone destruction by malignant invasion elsewhere (Fig. 34-27). The process is one of osteolysis without reactive sclerosis; the soft-tissue mass associated with it can also be demonstrated on the roentgenogram.

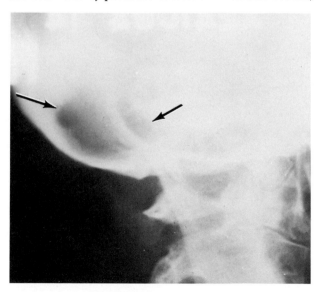

Fig. 34-27. Carcinoma that arose in the middle ear on the right and has destroyed much of the bone in the mastoid process as well as in the lateral aspect of the petrous pyramid **(arrows).**

REFERENCES AND SELECTED READINGS

1. BECKER JA, WOLOSHIN HJ: Mastoiditis and cholesteatoma: a roentgen approach. Am J Roentgenol 87: 1019, 1962
2. BRUNNER S: Infection of the temporal bone and its complications, including cholesteatoma. Semin Roentgenol 4: 129, 1969
3. COMPERE WE, VALVASSORI G: Radiographic Atlas of the Temporal Bone. St. Paul, American Academy of Ophthalmology and Otolaryngology, 1964
4. ETTER LE: Opacification studies of normal and abnormal paranasal sinuses. Am J Roentgenol 89: 1137, 1963
5. FUJIOKA M, YOUNG LW: The sphenoidal sinuses: radiographic patterns of normal development and abnormal findings in infants and children. Radiology 129: 133, 1978
6. GADO MH, ARENBERG IK: Radiological visualization of the vestibular aqueduct. Radiology 117: 621, 1975
7. GEIST RM, MULLEN WH: Roentgenologic aspects of lethal granulomatous ulceration of midline facial tissues. Am J Roentgenol 70: 566, 1953
8. GORLIN RJ, SEDANO HO: Syndromes involving the sinuses—congenital and acquired. Semin Roentgenol 3: 133, 1968
9. HERZON F, ANTOINE JE: Mega-antrum. Ann Otol Rhin Laryngol 85: 408, 1976
10. KASEFF LG: Tomographic evaluation of trauma to the temporal bone. Radiology 93: 321, 1969

11. MERRILL V: Atlas of Roentgenographic Positions, Vol III. St. Louis, Mosby, 1967

12. POTTER GD: Chausse III position. Semin Roentgenol 4: 116, 1969

13. POTTER GD: Trauma to the temporal bone. Semin Roentgenol 4: 143, 1969

14. POTTER GD, GOLD RP: Radiographic analysis of the skull. Med Radiog Photog 51: 2, 1975

15. ROBINSON AE, MEARES BM, GOREE JA: Traumatic sphenoid sinus effusion. An analysis of 50 cases. Am J Roentgenol 101: 795, 1967

16. ROSENDAL T, EWERTSEN H: Roentgen examination of the temporal bone for cholesteatoma. Acta Radiol [Suppl] (Stockh) 37: 431, 1952

17. SAMUEL E: Inflammatory diseases of the nose and paranasal sinuses. Semin Roentgenol 3: 148, 1968

18. SAMUEL E, LLOYD GAS: Clinical Radiology of the Ear, Nose and Throat. Philadelphia, Saunders, 1978

19. TARP O: Tomography of the temporal bone with the polytome. Acta Radiol [Suppl] (Stockh) 51: 105, 1959

20. VALVASSORI GE: Otosclerosis. Otolaryngol Clin North Am 6: 379, 1973

21. VALVASSORI GE, BUCKINGHAM BA: Tomography and Cross Sections of the Ear. Philadelphia, Saunders, 1975

22. WIGH R: Mucoceles of frontoethmoidal sinuses; analysis of roentgen criteria. Radiology 54: 579, 1950

23. WORTZMAN G, CONRAD ADK, FARKASHIDY J: Temporal bone: a tomographic-anatomic study. J Can Assoc Radiol 28: 95, 1977

24. ZIZMOR J, NOYEK AM: Cysts and benign tumors of the paranasal sinuses. Semin Roentgenol 3: 172, 1968

25. ZIZMOR J, NOYEK AM: Tumors and other osseous disorders of the temporal bone. Semin Roentgenol 4: 151, 1969

26. ZIZMOR J, NOYEK AM: An Atlas of Otolaryngologic Radiology. Philadelphia, Saunders, 1978

35

THE TEETH, JAWS, AND FACIAL BONES

The roentgen examination of the teeth is used by the medical profession largely to determine the presence or absence of infection involving the teeth and jaws. There are certain changes in the alveolus that result from generalized disease, and examination of the teeth is helpful in these conditions as well. Tumors arising on the alveolar ridge, tongue, or other intraoral sites may involve the bony alveolus. Roentgen examination is used to look for and follow the progress of such tumors.

Specific techniques for dental radiography include intraoral dental roentgenographic study and the panoramic type of extraoral examinations. Two general intraoral methods of examination are used, the intraoral dental and occlusal. The standard intraoral films are placed in position and held there by the patient while the exposure is being made. A total of 14 of these small films are exposed as a complete dental survey. These exposures should include the crowns and roots of all the teeth. The occlusal film is larger and is also employed as an intraoral film. It is used most widely in patients who are edentulous in a search for retained root fragments or local infection of the alveolus. It is also useful in the examination of small cysts or tumors of the alveolar ridge and jaw. Panoramic devices save time and radiation exposure. The Panorex and the more sophisticated orthopantomograph and GE-3000 are used in this country (see Fig. 35-11). These devices rotate during filming around a fixed head position. A single exposure may be used to survey all of the teeth as well as the jaws. In our experience, because dental detail is not as good as in dental films, we use the panoramic devices for the examination of the mandible and maxilla and as a screening examination of the teeth. The panoramic methods reduce radiation exposure considerably, from a dose of about 15 rads for a full-month dental survey with two bite-wing exposures to about 3 rads for a panoramic exposure, plus bite wings. Lead-lined cones are effective in reducing skin exposure in dental radiography, however. The mandible is examined by means of special views in frontal and lateral oblique projection. The temporomandibular joints also require special techniques and are examined with the mouth opened and closed. Films of the normal as well as the abnormal joint are usually obtained for comparison purposes. Tomography is of considerable value in the examination of the temporomandibular joints.

THE NORMAL TEETH

The teeth appear in two sets. The first are termed "deciduous" or "temporary" teeth. There are 20 deciduous teeth, 10 in each jaw and 5 in each quadrant. They are named from the midline as follows: central incisor, lateral incisor, cuspid, first molar (premolar), and second molar (premolar). In the adult jaw there are normally 32 teeth; 8 in each quadrant named as follows from the midline: central incisor, lateral incisor, cuspid, first bicuspid, second bicuspid, and first, second, and third molar. Examples of these teeth are shown in Figures 35-1 through 35-3.

Each tooth consists of a crown and a root. The junction between them is called the neck or cervix. The roots lie in sockets in the alveolar process of the jaw and are attached by alveolar periosteum. There are a number of variations in density noted on dental radiographs. Listed in decreasing order of density they are as follows: (1) metal crowns and fillings; (2) enamel of the teeth; (3) dentine; (4) cementum; (5) cortical bone; (6) cancellous bone; and (7) medullary spaces, canals, foramina, and soft tissues. The crown of the tooth is therefore slightly denser than the root and within each tooth is a narrow radiolucency termed the "root canal." Immediately surrounding each tooth is a radiolucent space representing the alveolar periosteum (periodontal membrane). Adjacent to this is a thin, dense structure composed of compact bone called the lamina dura (Fig. 35-4).

The mandible or lower jaw is composed of two equal halves united at the symphysis anteriorly. Each half consists of a body extending from the midline backward in a roughly horizontal direction and a ramus at somewhat less than a right angle so that the ramus is nearly vertical. It articulates with the base of the skull by means of a condylar process that projects upward from the posterior aspect of the ramus. The other upward projection anteriorly is termed the "coronoid process." The lower teeth are set in the alveolar process. The upper teeth are set in the alveolar process of the maxilla. The lower aspect of the maxillary antrum is visible on dental films of the upper teeth. The mental foramen appears as a radiolucency below and between the lower bicuspids. The mandibular canal extends forward, parallel to the alveolar ridge, and is a radiolucency that should not be mistaken for disease (Fig. 35-5). There are a few structures in the maxilla that should also be mentioned. The intermaxillary suture is observed in children and often in young adults. It appears as a midline radiolucent suture extending from the alveolar crest between the upper central incisors back to the posterior aspect of the palate. It may be interrupted in some areas. It has cortical margins that are smooth or slightly irregular. Usually there is no difficulty in differentiating it from a fracture. The incisive foramen (anterior palatine foramen) varies in size from a slit near the sagittal plane of the maxilla near the level of the apices of the central incisors to a rather large round or oval foramen, usually clearly marginated and occasionally appearing somewhat bilobed. The radicular cyst, from which it must be differentiated, maintains its relation to the dental root in contrast to the foramen (see "Chronic Rarefying Osteitis with Cyst Formation" under section entitled "Periapical Infections" in this chapter).

DENTAL INFECTIONS

DENTAL CARIES

The presence of a cavity may escape detection by clinical methods of examination and yet be readily visible on a roentgenogram. Regardless of their cause, dental caries may lead to foci of infection involving the periapical tissues of the jaw and are, therefore, important lesions. On the roentgenogram a carious area is radiolucent and appears as an area of decreased density that is usually slightly irregular and may occur anywhere on the crown of a tooth or in its neck (Fig. 35-6).

Pulp Changes

The dental pulp contains the blood supply and nerve supply of the tooth. The cellular elements include odontoblasts and mesenchymal cells capable of differentiating into odontoclasts. Therefore, irritation caused by a number of external stimuli including occlusal wear, dental caries, and minor trauma may lead to formation of calcifications (pulp stones) or thickening of the walls of the pulp chamber. There may be resorption with pulp chamber enlargement when infection is severe; this is caused by metaplasia with formation of osteoclasts.[18]

PERIAPICAL (PERIRADICULAR) INFECTIONS

All the periapical inflammatory lesions represent chronic disease when they are advanced enough to

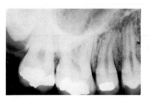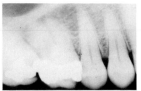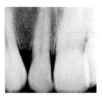

Fig. 35-1. Examples of teeth in the upper jaw. From left to right: partially outlined unerupted third molar, second molar, first molar, second bicuspid, first bicuspid, partially visualized second molar, first molar, second bicuspid, first bicuspid, partially visualized cuspid, remainder of the cuspid, lateral incisor, central incisor. Note the radiolucency representing the floor of the maxillary antrum. There are metallic restorations (fillings) in the molar teeth.

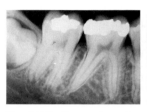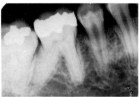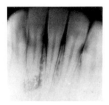

Fig. 35-2. Examples of teeth in the lower jaw. From left to right: partially visualized and unerupted third molar, second molar, first molar, partially visualized second bicuspid, partially visualized second molar, first molar, second bicuspid, first bicuspid, lateral incisor, central incisor, central incisor, lateral incisor, cuspid. Note fillings in the molar teeth.

Fig. 35-3. Examples of developing teeth. The unerupted permanent teeth are noted in the alveolus with some resorption of the roots of the deciduous teeth. **A.** Upper incisors. **B.** Lower bicuspid and molars.

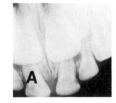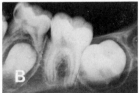

Fig. 35-4. Lower molar teeth. The **arrow** indicates the lamina dura surrounding the dental root. The bony alveolus extends to the neck of the tooth. The crown is above it and the roots are embedded in the bone. The dental root canal is represented by the thin radiolucent line extending into the dental root. The alveolodental periosteum (periodontal membrane) forms a radiolucent line between the lamina dura and the dental root.

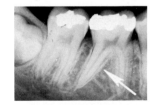

Fig. 35-5. Mental foramen. The arrow indicates the foramen. The mandibular canal extends posteriorly from the foramen in this edentulous mandibular alveolus.

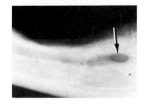

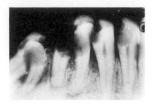

Fig. 35-6. Dental caries. Note the multiple radiolucent defects in the crowns of the teeth, particularly the first and second molars, and to a lesser extent in the bicuspids.

produce roentgen changes. Chronic infection around the apex of a dental root is manifested by several changes that can be recognized and classified. At times the division into the various types of roentgen pattern is difficult. The lesions may occur in the absence of clinical signs, which makes radiographic examination doubly important. Usually the infection follows the death of the pulp; bacteria pass through the root canal into the periapical tissues.

Chronic Alveolodental Periostitis. This condition may be caused by occlusal trauma as well as by infection. It results in some thickening of the periosteum (periodontal membrane) at the apex of the root and is manifested on the roentgenogram by increased width of the radiolucent space between the lamina dura and the dental apex. The lamina dura is usually intact but may be thinned and partially resorbed (Fig. 35-7A).

Chronic Rarefying Osteitis and Granulation Tissue (Periapical "Granuloma"). This represents the second stage of periapical infection in which there is de-

struction of bone adjacent to the apex of the tooth. The resultant space is filled with granulation tissue. Roentgenographically there is a radiolucent zone, usually with clearly defined margins, which is located at the dental root apex. The lamina dura is usually destroyed but the bony margin of the radiolucent zone is clearly outlined (Fig. 35-7B). It should be realized that a granuloma, cyst, and abscess may be similar roentgenographically and that they cannot be differentiated in many instances.

Chronic Rarefying Osteitis with Abscess (Periapical Abscess). This is the stage of the disease in which there is actual suppuration. A radiolucent zone is noted around the apex of the tooth in this condition and the margin is somewhat irregular and poorly defined but may be sclerotic in disease of long duration. The lamina dura is destroyed in the area of the disease (Fig. 35-7C).

Chronic Rarefying Osteitis with Cyst Formation (Radicular or Root Cyst). Proliferation of squamous cells frequently found in granulation tissue about a dental root apex is stimulated by chronic inflammation. This mass of epithelial cells breaks down to form a cystlike cavity that gradually enlarges, owing to slow constant pressure produced by the cellular proliferation. Eventually a cyst wall is formed by dense fibrous tissue. Roentgen findings are those of a radiolucent area around the apex of one or more teeth, which may be rather large. The margins are clearly defined, often with a thin layer of compact bone clearly outlining the cyst. A large cyst may expand the bone and displace contiguous teeth (Fig. 35-8).

At times the various manifestations of periapical infection are difficult to classify into one of the groups

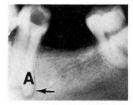 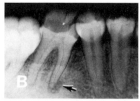 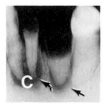

Fig. 35-7. Periapical infections. **A.** Alveolodental periostitis. The **arrow** indicates an increase in radiolucency between the dental apex and the lamina dura. This tooth is also carious. **B.** Chronic osteitis with granulation tissue. The **arrow** indicates destruction of bone adjacent to the apex of the root of the first molar. Note that the crown is carious. **C.** Periapical abscess. The **arrows** indicate an abscess resulting in considerable destruction of bone around the apices of the involved teeth.

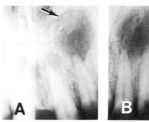

Fig. 35-8. Radicular (root) cyst. **A.** Note the large rarefied area extending into the alveolus from the root of the lateral incisor. The cyst is moderately well circumscribed with a clearly defined margin **(arrow). B.** Slightly different view in which the cyst overlaps the apex of the adjacent cuspid **(arrow).** Note the small abscess or granuloma involving the first bicuspid. All of the crowns are carious.

named in the foregoing, but should be recognized as lesions caused by infection; that is, they represent a focus of infection that must be managed by dental surgery.

ALVEOLAR (PERIODONTAL) INFECTIONS

The earliest clinical manifestation of infection involving the alveolar tissues surrounding the teeth is that of gingivitis. The process begins with an accumulation of bacterial plaques on dental surfaces which cause loss of the supporting structures, since there is bacterial invasion of the gingival margins from the plaques. The accumulation of calculus above and below the gingival margin may play a role, but its relation to gingivitis is not clear. The infection progresses to the alveolodental periosteum, where chronic periostitis is produced. This results in absorption and destruction of bone surrounding the teeth (alveolar recession) (periodontitis). When the process involves a single tooth and extends downward toward or to the apex it is called the vertical type of alveolar periostitis. If it is more generalized and results in destruction of the alveolar septum between several teeth, it is termed the horizontal type of periostitis (alveolar recession) (periodontitis).

Roentgen Findings. The roentgen changes parallel the destructive process. At first there is some widening of the radiolucency between the root and the lamina dura at the neck associated with some loss of the alveolar process. In the vertical type, the radiolucency around a single tooth increases. This indicates thickening of the periodontal ligament (membrane) and early bone involvement leading to loss of bony support and loss of the lamina dura. In the horizontal type, the alveolar ridge gradually disappears between the teeth until there is loss of bony support for several teeth. From the roentgen standpoint, the presence of pus in these pockets of infection cannot be ascertained, but when the alveolar destruction is marked there usually is a considerable amount of local sepsis. Dense projections often appear at the neck of the affected teeth which represent calculus. Occasionally, root resorption occurs, resulting in loss of the root in one or more areas. This is manifested on the roentgenogram by an area of irregular radiolucency indenting the normally smooth surface of the involved root (Fig. 35-9A, B, and C).

Hypercementosis (Exostosis of the Dental Root). Cementum that is somewhat denser than cortical bone is produced and accumulates around the root of an affected tooth, usually a permanent one, to cause this abnormality. The upper bicuspids and lower first molar are the most commonly affected. Roentgen findings are those of an enlarged, bulbous, dense root that may be rather bizarre in shape. The relationship of the lamina dura to the root does not change; it covers the abnormal root as in the normal state.

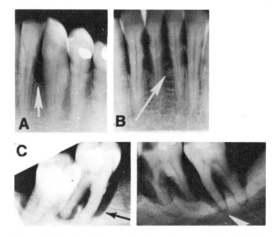

Fig. 35-9. A. Vertical alveolar periostitis (periodontitis). Note loss of bone extending between the roots of the lateral incisor and cuspid in the lower jaw **(arrow).** The process is localized in this patient. **B.** Horizontal alveolar periostitis (periodontitis). The alveolus has been destroyed to a comparable extent throughout the incisor area **(arrow).** The density surrounding the necks of the teeth represents calculus. **C.** Examples of severe alveolar periostitis with pockets extending nearly to the apices of the involved teeth **(arrows).**

DENTAL TRAUMA

Minimal trauma is a frequent occurrence, and there are no roentgen findings. If the pulp is damaged, it may be stimulated to lay down calcified scar tissue which may fill the pulp chamber. Root resorption may also result from minor trauma. These changes can be observed roentgenographically. Trauma to a deciduous tooth may injure and thus impair the developing permanent tooth. The enamel may be hypoplastic in some; in others, there is failure of narrowing of the pulp chamber, caused by degeneration of the pulp which cannot form dentin; therefore, a wide pulp chamber in an adult may be the result of childhood trauma. The opposite may also occur, *e.g.,* self-obliteration of the pulp by excess dentin deposition.

Various types of trauma that are important in children are described. Complicated crown fracture or crown-root fracture exposes the pulp. This makes prognosis poor for saving the tooth. In uncomplicated crown or crown-root fracture, the dentin is not exposed and prognosis is better. The root fracture that is usually missed clinically can be detected radiographically, but tomography may be required. Other complications of dental injury in children are failure of union, traumatic bone cyst, and apical cyst.

DENTAL MANIFESTATIONS OF GENERALIZED DISORDERS

Intraoral dental films in addition to outlining the teeth also include the alveolar process of the mandible, which may reflect changes in certain systemic diseases.

ENDOCRINE AND METABOLIC DISORDERS

Hypopituitarism. Delayed dentition along with delay in osseous development is characteristic of hypopituitarism and dental films will show the delay in development as well as the small underdeveloped jaw. There is also a delay in loss of primary teeth and development of permanent teeth. The teeth are normal in size.

Hyperpituitarism. In acromegaly and giantism there is an overgrowth of the mandible making the teeth more widely separated than normal. The tongue is large and may protrude past the anterior teeth or past both teeth and lips. It also narrows the pharyngeal airway and may obliterate the valleculae. The greatest mandibular growth is in the incisor area. Rami

may be normal or short. Roentgen study is helpful in differentiating this type of overgrowth from that associated with other conditions that produce abnormal enlargement of the jaw.

Hypothyroidism (Cretinism). Delayed development of the teeth that occurs in this condition is associated with underdevelopment of the jaw. Primary teeth remain for several years after the normal time for exfoliation, and there is a comparable delay in appearance of permanent teeth.

Hypoparathyroidism. Hypoplasia of the enamel occurs when the onset of the disease is early in life, before the enamel is completely formed. Hypoplasia of the dentine may also occur if the hypoparathyroidism occurs before the dental roots are developed. This is manifested by short underdeveloped roots.

Hyperparathyroidism. There is thinning or loss of the lamina dura noted on dental roentgenograms along with marked decalcification of the alveolus. Dental films of the upper jaw also demonstrate a loss of the clearly defined outline of the bony floor of the maxillary antrum that is also a result of decalcification (Fig. 35-10). In severe disease, cystlike rarefactions may appear in the mandible. Following successful removal of the tumor causing the parathyroid hyperfunctition, the alveolus tends to return to normal and the lamina dura reappears. This disease is now discovered at a relatively early stage in many instances, so there may be no radiologic changes observed in the alveolus.

Cushing's Syndrome. Moderate decalcification of the alveolus is noted on the dental roentgenogram in this condition along with partial loss of the lamina dura. As a result this structure is sometimes difficult to

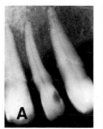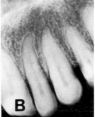

Fig. 35-10. Hyperparathyroidism. **A.** Note the absence of the lamina dura of the teeth. There is also loss of bone density in the alveolus and some alveolar periostitis. **B.** Normal teeth with normal lamina dura and alveolar density.

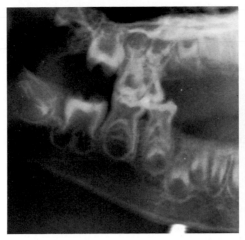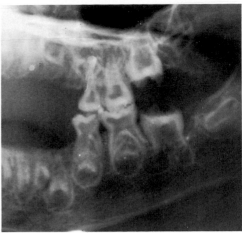

Fig. 35-11. Hypophosphatasia in a 2-year-old child. Panorex film of the teeth and jaws. All deciduous teeth have been lost except the premolars. The roots are small and the pulp cavities are very large.

outline, but there are usually some areas in which it can be observed.

Diabetes Mellitus. In severe diabetes, particularly in children, dental infection is a problem so that periapical as well as periodontal disease is commonly present and may be severe. These changes are readily outlined on dental roentgenograms but are not present in all patients and are nonspecific.

Hypophosphatasia. There is loss of alveolar bone, enlargement of pulp chambers of root canals, and a decrease in thickness of the enamel and dentine. As a result the roots are thin with wide pulp cavities. Deciduous teeth are lost early because of absence of cementum without early eruption of permanent teeth (Fig. 35-11). Mild forms of the disease may have no dental findings.

DEVELOPMENTAL DISORDERS

Midline Facial Clefts. In cleft lip and cleft palate, there are dental anomalies ranging from deformity and malposition of some upper central teeth, to the presence of supernumerary teeth, to absence of a number of teeth. The films outline the osseous deformity as well as the dental alterations. A number of other isolated anomalies of the jaws and teeth are clearly defined on occlusal films or on panoramic films of mandible and maxilla. They include congenital hypoplasia and hyperplasia of the mandible, and unilateral hypoplasia of the face.

Osteogenesis Imperfecta. The characteristic dental alteration in this condition is replacement of the pulp canals by dentine, resulting in teeth that are uniformly dense. The finding of absent root canals is first observed in the incisor and the first molar teeth, which are the earliest to develop completely.

Dentinogenesis Imperfecta. This is an autosomal dominant trait that is unrelated to osteogenesis imperfecta. The deciduous and permanent teeth are brown and wear away rapidly. Dental roots are small and conical; small molars have single roots. The root canal may be very small, partially obstructed, and pulp is diminished or absent.

Osteopetrosis. The dense, ivorylike bone characteristic of this disease is noted in the alveolus; the roots of the teeth are often incompletely developed.

Achondroplasia. There is delay in dental development in this condition that is readily observed on roentgenograms of the teeth. Many of the teeth remain unerupted into adult life.

Ectodermal Dysplasia. This disease is characterized by partial or complete absence of hair, sweat glands, and teeth. The degree of dental abnormality ranges from complete dental aplasia to congenital absence of a few of the deeth.

Chondroectodermal Dysplasia (Ellis–van Creveld). This disorder is characterized by dysplasia of fingernails, short stature caused by shortening of the tubular bones, polydactyly, carpal fusion, and dental abnormalities. Congenital cardiac abnormality may also be present. There is usually a decreased number of teeth which are widely spaced and peg-shaped. Malocclusion is frequent; the mandible is always hypoplastic and the undersurface often markedly concave (antegonial notching).

Cleidocranial Dysostosis. Abnormal dentition and abnormality of the jaws is very frequent in this condition. There is often a delay in appearance of the teeth, with numerous supernumerary teeth. Permanent teeth are frequently malposed and fail to erupt. There is absence of or hypoplasia of the clavicles and anomalies of the cranial bones; numerous wormian bones are common.

Unilateral Hyperplasia of the Face. The teeth develop prematurely on the hyperplastic side of the face so that films of the jaws showing the difference in development of the teeth may permit early diagnosis of this rare condition. The jaw is deviated to the normal side, and malocclusion is common.

Mandibulofacial Dysostosis (Treacher–Collins Syndrome). The teeth may be malposed, widely separated, hypoplastic, displaced; and malocclusion is common in this syndrome in which there is hypoplasia of the facial bones, particularly the zygoma and mandible. Cleft palate, absence of palatine bones or high palate, and underdevelopment of paranasal sinuses and mastoids may also be observed on roentgenograms of the facial bones.

Other Anomalies. There are a number of other developmental disorders in which abnormality occurs, but most are very rare. They include Rutherfurd's syndrome in which deciduous teeth are unerupted and absorb with permanent teeth visible below them. This is evidently caused by gingival hyperplasia to an extent that eruption of the teeth is prevented. Oculomandibulodyscephaly (Hallermann–Streiff syndrome) is another rare condition in which teeth are malformed, erupt early and irregularly, and may be erupted at birth. The palate is high and narrow, and there is hypoplasia of the mandible.

Dental and jaw abnormalities may also occur in *dysosteosclerosis* in which there is dental hypoplasia and the permanent teeth fail to erupt. Sclerosis of bone is noted in the base of the skull, ribs, and vertebral bodies. *Micrognathia* may be congenital and is associated with a number of syndromes; it is sometimes acquired and secondary to trauma or infection. In juvenile rheumatoid arthritis, the mandible is often underdeveloped and a rather deep local notch may be observed on the undersurface of the mandibular body, just anterior to the angle (gonion). There

is also a congenital form of notching (antegonial) which is a uniform concavity of the entire undersurface of the body of the mandible. Radiotherapy of the jaw in childhood may cause dental anomalies and hypoplasia, depending on age of the child and radiation dose. Other causes of dental and jaw abnormalities include achondroplasia, the mucopolysaccharidoses, chondrodystrophia calcificans congenita, hypotelorism, hypertelorism, Marchesani's syndrome, Marfan's syndrome, and mental deficiencies of various types including mongolism. The list is virtually inexhaustible; it is beyond the scope of this book to include all of them.

MISCELLANEOUS DISORDERS

Eosinophilic Granuloma (Histiocytosis X) of Bone. This lesion not infrequently involves the jaw, resulting in destruction of the area of bone affected, with no visible reaction. It is not unusual to observe the bone destroyed so completely that teeth are left with no visible bony supporting structure; the so-called "floating" teeth. The bony lesions may be solitary or multiple within the mandible and may involve other bones. There are several other diseases that may destroy the mandible in a similar way; they include reticulum cell sarcoma, lymphosarcoma, metastatic neuroblastoma, and Ewing's tumor. The teeth may appear to "float," but there are often soft-tissue changes and other signs that tend to make the diagnosis.

Acrosclerosis and Scleroderma. There is an increase in the thickness of the alveolodental membrane, resulting in uniform widening of the radiolucent space between the dental roots and the lamina dura. The uniform widening of this space in all the teeth differentiates acrosclerosis and scleroderma from inflammatory disease of the alveolus.

Osteomalacia. The decalcification caused by this disease is noted in the alveolus. The lamina dura is also involved and is absent in some areas but can usually be visualized in others.

Rickets. A deficiency of vitamin D may cause dental disturbances as well as the classic skeletal abnormalities. Hypoplasia of the enamel is frequently observed, since the disease usually occurs in young children and infants. When the onset is late as in rachitis tarda, the development of the dental roots may be retarded. This is caused by defective dentine and cementum which may result in poor attachment of the teeth and lead to periodontal infection. The pulp chambers are abnormally large.

Renal Osteodystrophy. The dental findings are similar to those of hyperparathyroidism, with demineralization of the alveolus and loss of the lamina dura. In the child, delayed dental development is also observed.

Infantile Cortical Hyperostosis. This disease frequently involves the mandible causing soft-tissue swelling, pain, and varying amounts of periosteal new-bone formation. It is described in Chapter 8, under the heading "Infantile Cortical Hyperostosis."

CYSTS AND TUMORS OF THE JAW

There are many lesions in the mandible that may cause a local radiolucent defect. Some of these are clearly defined by a sclerotic rim of bone, while others may have indistinct borders. There is so much similarity between benign cysts and tumors and low-grade malignancies in the jaw that roentgen findings are often equivocal. In such instances, biopsy must be performed. It is worthwhile to describe these lesions, however, because there are a number of them that can be clearly distinguished roentgenographically.

DENTAL CYSTS

Radicular or Dental Root Cysts. These cysts are the result of chronic periapical infection and have been described in the section on "Periapical Infections." The cystic cavity is clearly defined and usually unilocular. The relationship of the radiolucent cystic structure to the dental root is important in the differential diagnosis. This is the most common "cyst" of the jaw, all others are relatively rare.

Follicular Cysts. This type of cyst arises in relation to a tooth follicle. Three forms may occur, depending upon the cyst content. These are the (1) dentigerous, (2) simple follicular (primordial), and (3) cystic odontoma.

The most common type of follicular cyst is the *dentigerous cyst* formed about the crown of a tooth. It develops about an unerupted, malposed tooth. Characteristically, it produces a sharply marginated, expansile, rarefied area with a formed or incompletely formed tooth projecting into the cavity along one side.

Roentgen examination shows the large rarefaction, usually in the molar area, which causes expansion of the mandible. Its edges are clearly defined and there is a tooth or a part of a tooth projecting into the radiolucent cyst (Fig. 35-12). These cysts may occur in the maxilla as well as in the mandible.

The *simple follicular (primordial) cyst* is rare; it arises from the epithelium of the enamel before development of the tooth, so that it is roentgenographically similar to the dentigerous cyst, except that there is no tooth associated with it. Since these follicular cysts are related to the developing teeth, they are usually found in patients under the age of 15 years. Occasionally this type of cyst may originate in a supernumerary tooth bud, in which instance it can occur in a patient with a full complement of teeth.[13] Simple follicular cysts tend to occur in the third molar region of the mandible.

Cystic odontoma is a follicular cyst that contains a mass of rudimentary teeth or a mass of very dense material that may be amorphous.

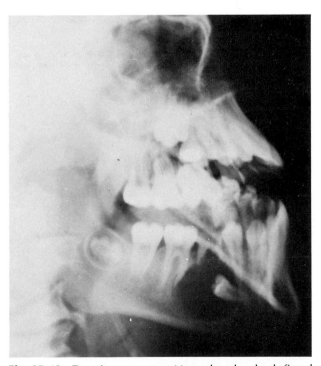

Fig. 35-12. Dentigerous cyst. Note the clearly defined radiolucent cyst in the mandible that has resulted in erosion of the root of the second bicuspid and first molar. The small tooth projecting into it is typical, and, when this is present, a positive diagnosis can be made.

Odontogenic Keratocyst. This cyst may occur as a solitary lesion but may be associated with the basal-cell nevus syndrome. Because the cyst resembles a primordial cyst radiographically the diagnosis must be made histologically. The recurrence rate is high, up to 50%, therefore it should be differentiated from a primordial and from a dentigerous cyst.

Calcifying Epithelial Odontogenic Cyst. According to Gorlin,[5] who first described it, this cyst occupies an anomalous position between cyst and neoplasm. Most of them occur in the mandible and are situated either centrally (75%) or on the gingiva causing superficial erosion of bone. Roentgen findings are those of a central lucent lesion with scattered, irregular foci of calcification. The margins are clearly defined, but there is no limiting area of sclerosis. The cyst is apparently benign but is locally aggressive.

Basal Cell Nevus Syndrome. This is an hereditary disorder manifested by multiple, basal cell epitheliomas of the skin, cysts of the jaws, and skeletal anomalies which include short fourth metacarpal, rib anomalies, vertebral anomalies, and ectopic calcifications in soft tissues. The cysts in the jaw are usually symptomatic before the skin changes are noted and appear to be either a odontogenic keratocyst or a simple follicular or dentigerous cyst.

ODONTOGENIC TUMORS

Ameloblastoma (Adamantinoma): The adamantinoma is a slowly growing tumor that is malignant, since local recurrence with eventual widespread local involvement may occur. It arises from the anlage of the enamel organ. It is usually found in older children and young adults of ages varying from 10 to 35 years. It may occur in either jaw but is more common in the mandible than the maxilla. The tumor may be divided into numerous compartments by bony septa. The roentgen findings are those of a central tumor producing destruction of bone and the dental roots as well as expansion of the cortex through which numerous complete or incomplete trabeculations pass to give the appearance of multicystic mass (Fig. 35-13). Occasionally the tumor is unilocular with no trabeculation. There is no attempt at new bone formation but the mass is clearly defined by a smooth-appearing bony wall. The recurrent or more malignant form is more invasive and its limits are not clearly defined. The unilocular adamantinoma may resemble a radicular cyst or simple follicular cyst. The polycystic

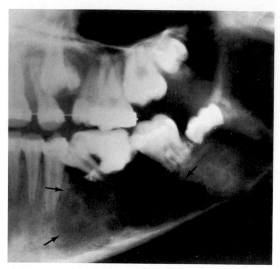

Fig. 35-13. Ameloblastoma. This tumor in the body of the mandible is reasonably well defined **(arrows).** It has destroyed the bone in the premolar and molar areas and appears to be somewhat multicystic anteriorly.

type may resemble a central giant cell tumor and radiographic differentiation is not absolute.

Adenomatoid Odontogenic Tumor. This tumor is benign. It is twice as frequent in females as in males, and usually occurs before its subject is 30 and often before 20 years of age. It occurs commonly in the anterior maxilla, related to an unerupted tooth. Roentgen findings are those of a small (under 2 cm) radiolucent area, usually clearly defined. It contains foci of calcification that may rarely be extensive.

Calcifying Epithelial Odontogenic Tumor (Pindborg Tumor). This tumor arises from odontogenic cells but is unlike the ameloblastoma.[11] Amyloid, which subsequently calcifies, is deposited in this tumor which usually occurs in the premolar-molar area of the mandible in association with an impacted or unerupted tooth. As the tumor develops around the crown of an unerupted tooth, it resembles a dentigerous cyst. However, as it increases in size, the periphery becomes poorly defined and calcifies in an irregular pattern which eventually resembles that of an osteosarcoma.

Complex (Complex Composite) Odontoma. This is a single mass made up of two or more of the solid dental tissues, including enamel, dentin, pulp, and cementum. Roentgenographically it is a densely opaque mass of malformed dental elements in either jaw, surrounded by a thin radiolucent line similar to the periodontal membrane. There is condensation of bone surrounding the mass resulting in an encapsulated appearance. The most common sites are the upper central incisor and the lower molar areas. Complex odontomas are usually found when the patient is in childhood, are asymptomatic except that a mass is produced that may become very large.

Compound (Compound Composite) Odontoma. This is similar to the complex odontoma except that the dense mass is composed of a bundle of dwarfed misshapen teeth, which are recognizable as teeth. It is found most often in the cuspid area with equal frequency in maxilla and mandible.

Odontogenic Fibroma (Fibromyxoma). This evidently arises from dental tissue and may be associated with an unerupted tooth. Radiographically it is a multicompartmented, cystlike rarefaction, with fine trabeculations that may be angular. Thinning of the cortex is present in large lesions. At times the lesion is unilocular and associated with an unerupted tooth. Then it cannot be differentiated from dentigerous cyst since roentgen appearances are identical. When the posterior maxilla is involved, the tumor may extend into and fill the antrum.

Cementoma (Periapical Cemental Dysplasia). Cementoma usually occurs in the mandible and is often multiple. It begins in the periapical region with proliferation of connective tissue of the periodontal membrane; in this stage it resembles a periapical granuloma or root cyst. The second stage is one in which the fibrous tissue is converted into a calcified cementumlike substance. This dense mass then develops within the cystlike space. There may be some associated hypercementosis of the adjacent dental root.

Central Cementifying Fibroma. This fibroma occurs in young adults, more commonly in the mandible than in the maxilla. It grows slowly and may expand bone. Roentgen findings are variable; there may be a dense or radiolucent 3- to 5-cm lesion that is well circumscribed but may expand bone. The density, or lack of it, depends on the amount of calcified material (cementum) in the lesion.[5]

Static bone cavity (Stafne Cyst). This is an asymptomatic cystlike lesion of the posterior mandible anterior to the angle.[15] It is a medial concavity of the mandible that may be related to salivary gland hyper-

trophy. Radiographically it appears as a small (usually less than 3 cm), ovoid, cystlike lucency that is clearly defined by a narrow border of sclerotic bone. Unlike most other cysts or cystlike lesions, it lies below the mandibular canal. It may be bilateral.

NONODONTOGENIC CYSTS AND TUMORS

Incisive Foramen Cyst (Anterior Palatine Foramen Cyst). As indicated earlier, the normal incisive foramen may vary considerably in size, so that the roentgen diagnosis of a cyst in this foramen must be made on the basis of the clinical history of a slowly enlarging mass either in the anterior palate or protruding into the nose, associated with a midline cyst which usually has clearly defined borders of condensed bone. Since incisive foramen cysts are benign, their course can be followed if there is any doubt as to the diagnosis. Rarely, a median mandibular cyst may occur; its appearance is similar to that of the incisive foramen cyst except for location.

Solitary Bone Cyst of the Mandible. This cyst is probably caused by trauma to the developing mandible. It is lined by connective tissue and may contain blood, serosanguineous fluid, or blood clot. The roentgen findings are those of a radiolucency which may be quite large, but poorly defined and with an irregular wall. There may be thinning and expansion of the cortex. These cysts arise in the cancellous bone of the medullary canal. In the posterior mandible the large cysts tend to extend into the alveolus between the dental roots. They occur in young adults and appear to regress spontaneously. The relationship of this lesion to *aneurysmal bone cyst* is not clear.

Aneurysmal Bone Cyst. An aneurysmal bone cyst occurs very rarely in the mandible. As in aneurysmal bone cyst elsewhere, it tends to be a cortical lesion that expands the bone locally. It has the appearance of a trabeculated lytic cavity projecting blisterlike from the bone in a manner that may suggest a soap-bubble. There may be marked expansion and thinning of the cortex. Its relation to trauma is not entirely clear, nor is its relationship to reparative giant cell granuloma.

Benign Giant Cell Reparative Granuloma (Benign Giant Cell Tumor). There is controversy as to how this lesion should be classified, but it is probably a nontumorous reparative process. The origin may be central or peripheral; when peripheral the tumor originates in the alveolar soft tissue and may produce a smooth, pressure defect of the bone on the alveolar crest, but does not invade bone. The central type may be unilocular and expansile, and may resemble a large cyst, except that there is no condensation of bone forming the wall of the defect. The other form is multilocular. It may also expand the cortex and deform and displace adjacent teeth. The borders are not clearly defined by condensation of bone; this type cannot be differentiated from ameloblastoma on radiographic examination.

Osteoblastoma. Osteoblastoma is another rare tumor that may involve the mandible. It is a tumor of young adults (under 30 years of age). When the lesion is less than 1 cm in diameter, it is termed "osteoid osteoma." When it occurs in the mandible, its roentgen appearance is that of a spherical ossified tumor surrounded by a clear radiolucent halo which in turn is surrounded by smooth, dense bone. Osteoblastomas occur adjacent to a dental root and may engulf it.

Fibrous Dysplasia of the Jaw. The alveolar areas of one or both jaws may be involved by fibrous dysplasia as local or as part of general disease. This is not a true tumor but does cause expansion of the cortex in the area involved. It characteristically involves a considerable extent of bone and may occur in both the mandible and maxilla in the same patient. The roentgenographic findings consist in the appearance of an expanding bone lesion which may be extensive. At times, the lesion may be uniformly dense with a ground-glass appearance in which normal trabeculations are not seen. Some of these lesions are radiolucent with irregular trabeculations giving them a multicystic appearance. At times the disease may be localized, with a reasonably well-circumscribed area of mandibular expansion in which there are mottled areas of density and rarefaction. In some cases, a mixture of increased and decreased density is present. The teeth are not usually displaced or resorbed.

OTHER BENIGN TUMORS

Cherubism. This is a familial disease characterized by symmetric swellings of the mandible caused by a rather massive, fibrous tissue proliferation which expands the cortex. The tissue proliferation is centered in the region of the angle and extends to the ramus and body. The maxilla may also be involved occasionally. The swelling appears in early childhood (at about the age of 3 years) and is more common in males than females. Roentgen findings consist of expansive areas in the mandible that are bilaterally symmetric. The cortex may be very thin and there

are no teeth in the involved areas. These radiolucent expansile lesions are usually multiloculated and bilaterally symmetrical. Abnormal dentition with wide separation, poor development, or absence of teeth is common in the mandible, but there is more variability in the maxilla and the upper teeth may be normal (see also Ch. 2).

Torus Palatinus and Torus Mandibularis. *Torus palatinus* is an exostosis arising at the margins of the palatal processes at the median palatal suture, usually bilaterally. The radiographic signs are those of a moderately flat mass of cortical bone density projecting downward from the palate, often somewhat lobular with a midline groove (Fig. 35-14). *Torus mandibularis* is a similar dense exostosis projecting from the medial aspect of the anterior mandible. It is usually bilateral and there may be multiple masses with a somewhat lobulated appearance. The torus is significant only if it becomes large enough to interfere with speech or with dental function.

Miscellaneous Benign Tumors. *Osteoma* of the jaw may occur and resemble osteoma elsewhere. Multiple osteomas are not uncommon. As in other bones, they may be flat and broad based, or somewhat pedunculated and are more common in the mandible than in the maxilla. Osteomas of the jaws and other bones are associated with multiple polyposis of the colon, multiple epidermoid cysts, and desmoid tumors in Gardner's syndrome, a rare familial condition. Occasionally *ossifying fibroma* may occur in the mandible or in the maxilla in the region of the maxillary antrum. The roentgen findings are those of large radiolucent expanding lesion, which is usually found in young patients ranging from 10 to 30 years of age. At first the lesions are usually entirely destructive and therefore radiolucent. The wall is clearly defined. Later some calcification is noted within the tumor. *Osteoid osteoma* may occasionally involve the mandible, where its typical roentgen appearance is usually diagnostic. *Hemangioma* of the jaw also presents an appearance typical of this lesion in other flat bones.

MALIGNANT TUMORS

Osteosarcoma and *chondrosarcoma* rarely occur in the jaw and their appearance there is similar to the appearance of these tumors elsewhere. As a rule, osteosarcoma of the mandible occurs 10 to 15 years later than does peripheral osteosarcoma, therefore it involves a somewhat older age group. As in other bones, there may be lytic or blastic tumors; a typical sunburst appearance may occur in the jaw. *Ewing's*

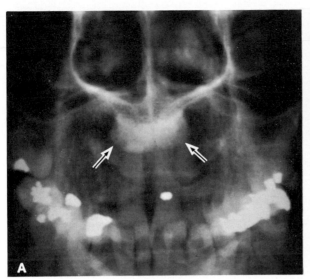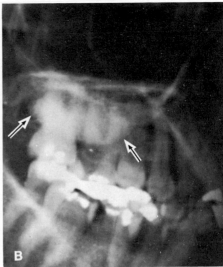

Fig. 35-14. Torus palatinus. **A.** Frontal projection showing the dense bone forming the torus extending downward from the palate **(arrows).** There is a poorly defined midline groove. **B. Arrows** outline the somewhat elongated bony mass in the hard palate in this lateral projection.

tumor is also found occasionally. The appearance of this tumor is similar to its appearance elsewhere (see Ch. 7). Solitary *plasma cell myeloma* (plasmacytoma) may occasionally arise in the jaw, producing a lytic expansile mass that is sometimes well marginated. *Multiple myeloma* develops eventually in most of these patients with solitary lesions. *Reticulum cell sarcoma* is rare in the jaw but occurs occasionally.

Carcinoma of the alveolar ridge or carcinoma arising in the maxillary antrum may involve the alveolus by direct extension. This results in destruction of bone in an irregular manner with no clearly defined wall and often with evidence of an associated soft-tissue mass (Fig. 35-15). In patients with carcinoma involving the alveolar ridge, there is often ulceration, and infection may involve the bone. Infection is characterized by sequestrum formation (Fig. 35-16). Fragments of devitalized bone separating or separated from the area of disease always are highly suggestive of osteomyelitis (see Ch. 6). Differentiation between infection and actual carcinomatous destruction of bone is sometimes difficult; biopsy is then required to make the diagnosis. The most common lesion of the jaw is a metastatic malignant tumor. Tumors of the lung, breast, and kidney are the most common primary source. In widespread multiple myeloma, lesions caused by this tumor may be visible. The manifestations are those of multiple areas of destruction without reaction in the osteolytic metas-

tases, which are far more common in the jaw than are blastic metastases.

INFECTIONS OF THE JAWS

Osteomyelitis may be of hematogenous origin but it is often secondary to dental infection and to carcinoma of the alveolus. Infection of bone may also follow jaw trauma and infection of the maxillary sinus. The roentgen findings of irregular bone destruction, sequestrum formation, periosteal reaction, and late sclerosis are similar to those of osteomyelitis elsewhere. Cellulitis adjacent to the mandible may cause periosteal new-bone formation without osteomyelitis. Chronic inflammations such as *tuberculosis* and *actinomycosis* may also involve the jaw, causing bone destruction. Soft-tissue involvement is common, especially in actinomycosis. Syphilis is rare but may cause a mixed lytic–sclerotic lesion of the jaw.

THE TEMPOROMANDIBULAR ARTICULATION

The temporomandibular articulation is examined with the patient's mouth open and closed, by the use of special projections and by means of tomography. Both joints are usually examined so that one can be

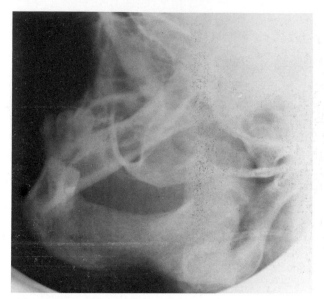

Fig. 35-15. Carcinoma eroding the mandible. Note the irregular destructive lesion on the inferior aspect of the body of the mandible just anterior to the angle. This was caused by direct extension of a squamous cell carcinoma in the submandibular region. There is no bone reaction and the outline is irregular.

compared with the other. More elaborate methods have been described as being very useful in dysfunction of the joint.[19] Arthrography has recently been reported as being helpful in demonstrating meniscal abnormalities of the temporomandibular joints in patients with joint dysfunction and minimal or no bony abnormality.[8] Occasionally we also use fluoroscopy and cinefluorography or video tape to study joint motion in certain patients with pain in the joints and no roentgenographic evidence of abnormality. Normally the articular surfaces are smooth and the mandibular condyle moves forward out of the glenoid fossa when the mouth is opened. The range of motion in the normal state is similar on the two sides and the appearances are similar but not necessarily identical (Fig. 35-17). There are variations in the formation of the glenoid fosssa ranging from a flat appearance to a deeply concave fossa. Pain upon motion of the jaw along with crepitation and limitation of motion are often secondary to dental disease and malocclusion which may not be evident on radiographic study. Effusion in the joint is manifested by widening of the joint space. Degenerative changes are similar to those noted in other joints, with some eburnation of joint surfaces and narrowing of the radiographic joint

space. Rheumatoid arthritis may involve these articulations, resulting in loss of joint space, irregularity, poor definition of joint surfaces, and destruction of subchondral bone. Ankylosing spondylitis is often accompanied by involvement of the temporomandibular joints with changes similar to those of rheumatoid arthritis including narrowing of the joint space, erosions of bone, decreased motion, secondary changes of demineralization, extensive sclerosis, and, at times, joint-space widening. These diseases may also lead to fibrous and, occasionally, to bony ankylosis. Fibrous ankylosis may also result from trauma and may be incomplete so that the range of motion is markedly diminished. Occasionally, bony ankylosis occurs, usually following septic arthritis. Roentgenograms show the continuity of bone between the condyle and glenoid fossa in this condition. *Pigmented villonodular synovitis* causes a smooth erosion of bone adjacent to the joint but is very rare. Clinically there is a soft-tissue mass in the vicinity of the joint, and this, in combination with smooth erosion, should suggest the lesion.[7]

THE SALIVARY GLANDS

Roentgen methods are used to study the salivary glands in patients suspected of having calculi, strictures, inflammatory disease, tumors, or sometimes, Sjogren's disease. The calculi are usually very dense and visualization is largely a matter of proper technique. Submaxillary glands and ducts are examined by placing an occlusal film in the mouth and using a submentovertex type of projection. Parotid calculi may be in the gland or duct. Intraoral, lateral extraoral, and anteroposterior or tangential, extraoral films are needed. Sialography can be used for localization if required.

Sialography. This examination consists of filling the salivary ducts of the parotid or submaxillary glands with an opaque medium; we use Pantopaque but Ethiodol may also be used. A preliminary film is taken to check for calcification. The duct is entered with a fine thin-walled Teflon tube with a tapered end. Often a dilator is not needed. The catheter is introduced for a distance of 1 to 3 cm. The catheter can be kept in place during the exposure. Some prefer using a blunt-tipped cannula that can also be taped in place. Local anesthesia (Xylocaine) may be used if necessary. When the parotid is to be examined, Stensen's duct can be catheterized for a short distance without much difficulty in most patients. Approxi-

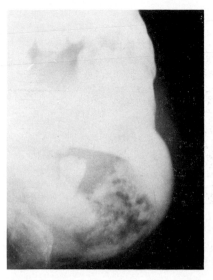
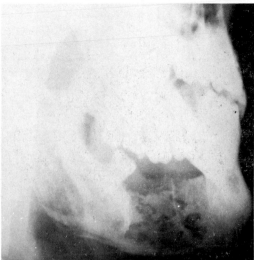

Fig. 35-16. Osteomyelitis of the mandible. Two projections showing irregular moth-eaten destruction of bone. There are a number of moderately dense sequestra forming a mosaic pattern in the area of disease.

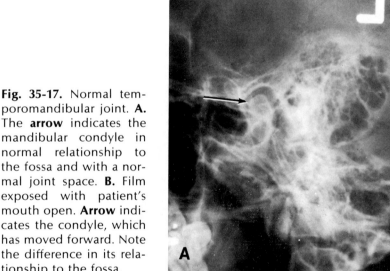
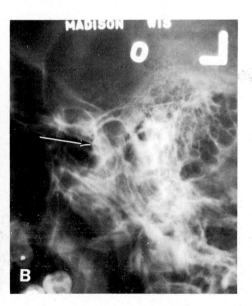

Fig. 35-17. Normal temporomandibular joint. **A.** The **arrow** indicates the mandibular condyle in normal relationship to the fossa and with a normal joint space. **B.** Film exposed with patient's mouth open. **Arrow** indicates the condyle, which has moved forward. Note the difference in its relationship to the fossa.

mately 1 to 2 cc of the desired radioopaque medium is injected under very low pressure or hydrostatic pressure and films of the parotid gland and duct area are obtained in lateral and frontal projections with the catheter left in place (Fig. 35-18). The examination is best completed under fluoroscopic control, then spot films can be exposed in suitable projections. We examine the submandibular gland much less frequently, and the injection of Wharton's duct is more difficult (Fig. 35-19). A fine dilator and a thin polyethylene catheter with guide wire are used; the catheter may be introduced for a distance of 2 to 5 cm and injection of 1 to 2 cc of an opaque medium is made under fluoroscopic control. Following this the films are checked. The patient is then given a few drops of lemon extract to stimulate salivary secretion and another set of films are obtained in 10 to 15 minutes to evaluate evacuation of the opaque medium. Subtraction techniques may be used when fine ductal detail is desired.[20] It is important to correlate the

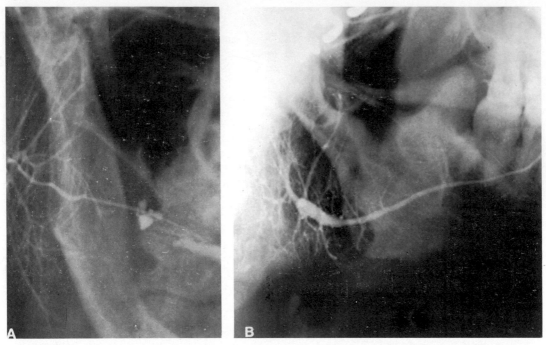

Fig. 35-18. Parotid sialogram—normal findings. **A.** Frontal projection showing the treelike branching of the ducts which are normal in caliber. **B.** Oblique projection showing findings similar to those in **A.**

Fig. 35-19. Submandibular sialogram. The duct is somewhat overdistended, and there is a considerable amount of opaque medium outlining the gland, indicating that more pressure was used than was necessary. Otherwise, the examination reveals no abnormality.

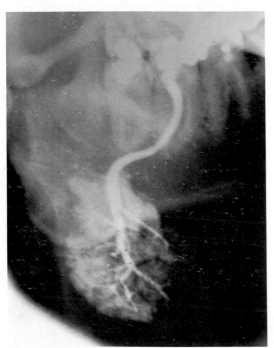

sialogram with the clinical findings. Ducts may be incompletely filled when obstructed by calculus; tumors in and adjacent to the parotid may displace the ducts; malignant tumor within the parotid gland characteristically causes irregular filling of the ducts. In Sjogren's syndrome, there may be edema, making it impossible to fill the acini; when the disease is more chronic, varying degrees of sialectasis (dilatation of salivary ducts) may be seen and, when present, provide a valuable aid in confirming the diagnosis.[4] Normally the glands empty in 30 minutes. Follow-up films can be obtained if desired, to study emptying of the gland. If the contrast substance remains in the gland more than 24 hours, abnormality is indicated.

THE NOSE AND NASOPHARYNX

Radiographic methods are useful in a number of conditions involving the nose and nasopharynx. In the infant with bilateral *choanal atresia*, respiratory distress is inevitable because the normal neonate is an obligate nasal breather. If this anomaly is suspected, the diagnosis can be confirmed by inserting a few drops of oily Dionosil into the patient's nasal cavities. A brow-up horizontal film will then show that the medium remains in the posterior nares, which are obstructed by the posterior atresia. Opaque intranasal masses, including ectopic intranasal teeth, foreign bodies, calcified polyps, and nasal "stones," can be detected on plain films. Soft-tissue masses such as enlarged adenoids, polyps, and tumors can also be outlined. Nasal packing in patients with epistaxis may cause retention of fluid in the paranasal sinuses, particularly the sphenoids, which can be detected on films exposed with the patient upright or on horizontal-beam films exposed with the patient recumbent.

Bone destruction involving the nasal septum and walls of the paranasal sinuses usually indicates malignant neoplasm or extensive inflammatory disease. Occasionally, benign nasal polyps may expand sufficiently to produce destruction of bone extending into the sphenoid or ethmoid areas. When this occurs, there is a strong likelihood of infection associated with the polyps, and, in some instances, there may be some sclerosis of bone as well as destruction, presumably a reaction to the infection. *Sarcoidosis* has also been reported as a cause of bone destruction involving the nasal septum and adjacent paranasal sinuses.[16] This destruction is associated with a soft-tissue mass and is a very unusual manifestation of sarcoidosis. *Midline lethal granuloma* is another non-neoplastic cause of bone destruction which characteristically arises in the nose and is associated with tissue necrosis leading to destruction of the nasal septum and, later, the adjacent sinuses.

Juvenile nasopharyngeal angiofibroma is a rare tumor observed in young boys. The plain-film findings include a large soft-tissue mass in the nasopharynx that often extends into the adjacent posterior nasal cavity. It may extend into the paranasal sinuses including the sphenoids, ethmoids, and the maxillary antra. Anterior bowing of the posterior wall of the maxillary sinus is a very charcteristic finding in this condition, and, when present in a young boy, is virtually diagnostic of angiofibroma. The bone destruction is a pressure-type erosion rather than one of invasive destruction, so the bony margins are usually sharp and dense. Tomograms are useful in defining the bone changes in addition to the soft-tissue mass. CT scanning is being used now in defining the soft tissue and bony components of these tumors. Biopsy is hazardous because of the tumor's marked vascularity. Angiography is usually carried out prior to surgery to outline the feeding vessels and thus facilitate the surgical approach. The arterial blood supply is now being embolized in some patients to decrease the blood loss at surgery.

There are several malignant lesions originating in the nasal cavity that also may cause destruction of the nasal septum and sometimes the walls of the adjacent sinuses. The hard palate also may be involved. Plain films usually demonstrate a soft-tissue nasopharyngeal mass associated with varying amounts of destruction of bone. Tomography and computerized tomography are very useful in the examination of these patients. Undifferentiated and squamous cell carcinoma are the most common of the tumors, but lymphosarcoma and cylindroma are found occasionally along with a rare extramedullary plasmacytoma. Roentgenographic examination is used to outline the soft-tissue and osseous extent of these tumors, most of which cause bone destruction. Occasionally, nasopharyngeal carcinoma will produce bone sclerosis. Meningiomas arising in the olfactory groove may extend downward to produce sclerosis in the nasal septum as well as in the base of the skull.

THE FACIAL BONES

The roentgen examination of the facial bones is used extensively for the diagnosis of fracture in patients who have had head and facial trauma. Inflammatory disease and tumor may also involve these structures. A number of different views are used, including those described for examination of the paranasal sinuses. The projections needed depend upon the problem (Fig. 35-20). Tomography is of definite value in the examination of the facial bones and is used extensively in the examination of patients with complicated fractures involving the orbital walls, the pterygoid processes, and the hard palate in addition to fractures of the petrous pyramids.

FRACTURES

Fractures of the bones of the face are commonly caused by direct trauma and may be severe and extensive. The roentgen signs of fracture of facial bones are comparable to those described for fractures elsewhere.

Nasal bone Fractures. A minimum of a lateral and an occlusal view are necessary in examination of the nose. Fractures of the nasal bones commonly occur in the anterior half; both bones are usually involved (Fig. 35-21). The fragments are depressed and displaced laterally in most instances. It is important not to mistake suture lines between the nasal bones and the frontal and maxillary bones for fractures. Diastasis of these sutures may occur, however. If all other

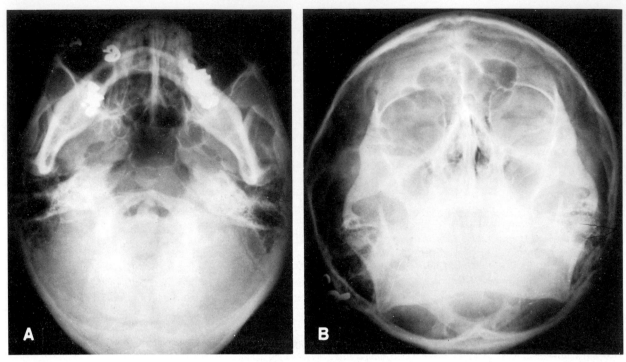

Fig. 35-20. The facial bones. **A.** Basal view of the skull and facial bones. **B.** Waters' view of the facial bones obtained especially to outline the zygomatic arches in this instance. This is a good projection to employ when zygomatic and facial bone fractures are suspected.

Fig. 35-21. Fracture of the nasal bone. The **arrow** indicates a fracture line. There is no significant displacement.

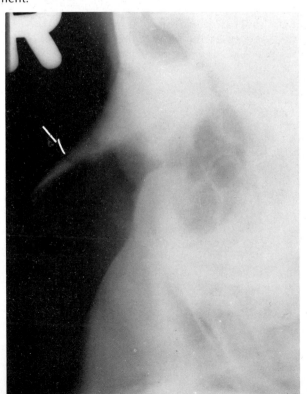

areas of the nasal bones, any radiolucent line that reaches the anterior cortex of the nasal bones must be considered to represent a fracture. It is important to check the anterior nasal spine of the maxilla since it may be fractured when the nose is injured. Unless the trauma is very local, it is also wise to obtain a Waters' view to check for adjacent facial bone injury which may be manifested by fluid or soft-tissue swelling in either antrum.

Maxillary Fractures. When there has been severe facial injury with suspected maxillary fracture, there are often injuries elsewhere which make roentgen examination difficult or may delay it for a time. We try to use a more or less standard set of exposures in these situations which includes a Water's view (stereo if possible), lateral, posteroanterior, and basal (submentovertical) stereo. A brow-up lateral view is useful if basal fracture is suspected to determine the presence of sphenoid sinus fluid. Then additional views are obtained if necessary after the initial films are checked. We depend upon polytomography to a large extent in the more complex injuries and usually start with anteroposterior films exposed at 5-mm intervals and obtain other sections as needed without moving the patient. There are numerous classifications of maxillary fractures; one of the oldest is the Le Fort (Table 35-1) which is still useful in describing these fractures (Fig. 35-22).

Obviously there are many variations, and unilateral fractures often occur. The alveolar processes may be involved without injury elsewhere. Dental fractures may occur. Clouding of maxillary sinuses is often present in fractures of the maxilla. As has been

indicated, we try to tailor the examination to the observed injury, using tomography very frequently.

Zygomatic Fractures. Injury in the zygomatic area may range from a local depressed fracture of the arch to a combination of injuries involving the frontozygomatic suture, the lateral wall and floor of the orbit, lateral wall of the maxillary sinus, and the region of the zygomatic-maxillary junction. Depression, comminution, and sutural separation are common (Fig. 35-23). The submentovertical view, in addition to a tangential, is useful in detecting depression of the zygomatic arch. Antral clouding is common in this group of injuries.

Orbital Fractures. Fractures of the medial or inferior orbital rim may be associated with fracture of the orbital floor, the so-called "blowout" fracture. The thin fragments of the orbital floor are displaced downward to encroach on the superior aspect of the maxillary sinus. Often there is an associated fracture of the lamina papyracca of the medial orbital wall in which case orbital emphysema may be observed. A Waters' view may show the bony fragments displaced downward or a similar displacement of the soft tissues of the floor of the orbit into the upper antrum. A "half" Waters' view, obtained at 20 degrees rather than at 37 degrees, is useful in this injury, since the central

Table 35-1. Classification of Maxillary Fractures (Le Fort)

LE FORT I. This is a transverse fracture through the maxillary sinus walls above the teeth; posteriorly it extends through the junction of the middle and lower third of the pterygoid processes of the sphenoid.

LE FORT II. This is a pyramidal fracture extending through the maxillary sinus in an oblique fashion to include the lower lateral sinus wall, the inferior orbital margin, the nasal bones in the region of the nasofrontal suture then downward and laterally in a similar fashion on the opposite side. Posteriorly the fracture terminates in the midportion of the pterygoid process (Fig. 35-22).

LE FORT III. This severe fracture extends from the region of the nasofrontal suture across the frontal processes of the maxillae, lacrimal bones, ethmoids, medial aspect of the inferior orbital fissure to the base of the pterygoid processes.

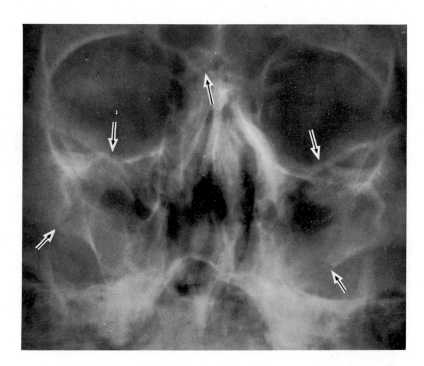

Fig. 35-22. Facial bone fractures (LeFort II). The **arrows** indicate the maxillary and orbital fracture sites. The fracture at the base of the nose is well defined on the right **(arrow)** but not on the left.

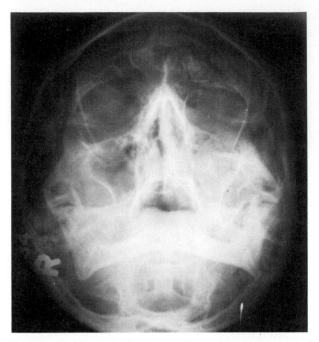

Fig. 35-23. Multiple fractures. Note the comminuted fracture of the left frontal bone extending into and including the roof of the left orbit. The left zygomatic arch is fractured and depressed. Compare it with the arch on the right side. The roof and lower lateral wall on the left maxillary antrum is also fractured, and there is clouding of the antrum as a result of hemorrhage and edema.

ray parallels the orbital floor and the small blowout fragments may be visualized (Fig. 35-24A). At times the fragments may be easily seen on a lateral view. If the antrum is opacified by disease or trauma, tomography is needed to outline the fragments and make the diagnosis. We obtain the initial tomograms at 5-mm intervals, check them, and add more levels if needed. There is usually no difficulty in making the diagnosis if proper films are available (Fig. 35-24B). There may be associated fractures elsewhere in the orbit or facial bones, so further roentgen examination may be needed. If orbital emphysema is present, fracture extending into the ethmoids or maxillary antrum is likely. Enophthalmos, which ultimately results, is not apparent in the immediate posttraumatic period because of edema and hemorrhage. Diplopia may be present to suggest the possibility of alteration in position of the globe in these patients.

Mandibular Fractures. The mandible is the facial bone most frequently fractured. Direct trauma is the cause in most instances. Since multiple fractures are common, when one fracture is visualized the remainder of the mandible should be examined closely. The most common fracture site is in the body of the mandible in the region of the cuspid tooth. When there is not much displacement the fracture line may not be visible in one plane, therefore two views should always be obtained at a 90 degree angle if possible (Fig. 35-25). The neck of the condylar process is particularly difficult to visualize in some patients. Con-

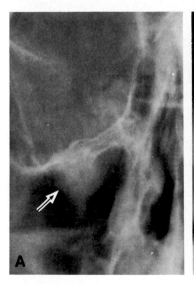
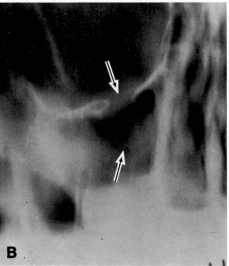

Fig. 35-24. Blow-out fractures of the orbit. **A.** Half Waters' view to show the pseudopolypoid mass extending downward into the right maxillary antrum from the floor of the orbit **(arrow). B.** Tomogram of another patient showing bone deficit in the orbital floor and a soft-tissue mass extending into the antrum **(arrows).**

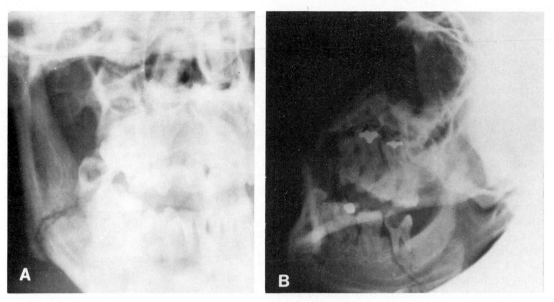

Fig. 35-25. Fracture of the body of the right mandible. Frontal **(A)** and lateral **(B)** projections clearly show the fracture line extending into the alveolus at the level of the second molar tooth.

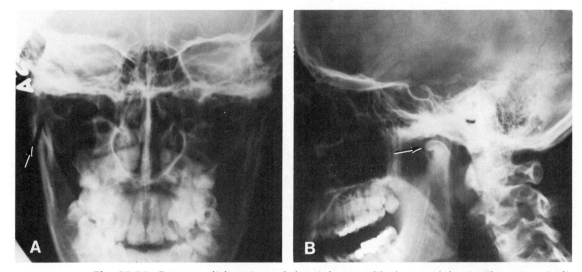

Fig. 35-26. Fracture dislocation of the right mandibular condyle. **A.** The **arrow** indicates the condylar fracture line. The tip of the condyle is medial to its normal position, but it is not well seen in this projection. **B.** The **arrow** indicates the mandibular condyle which is rotated and displaced anteriorly and inferiorly.

dylar fracture is particularly important in children under 3 years of age, since there may be a bone growth retardation leading to severe micrognathia and resultant facial deformity. The deformity is moderate when the injury occurs at age 3 to 6 years and minimal after 12 years. If a fracture in this area is suspected, special views used to visualize temporomandibular joints are sometimes of value in addition to the routine frontal and lateral projection. We use a combination of Panorex examination and sometimes Panoramix along with routine mandibular projections in patients with jaw injury. Occasionally, tomograms are used when the area cannot be clearly visualized in any other manner. There is often dislocation of the condyle, associated with fracture of the neck of the condylar process (Fig. 35-26). The combination of bilateral condylar neck fractures and a fracture near the symphysis may cause an apparent widening or flaring of the mandible.[3] The mandible appears to be too wide when compared with the maxilla. This is an important sign, since the anterior support of the tongue is lost. As a result, there may be airway obstruction due to posterior displacement of the tongue. In such an instance the fracture is an unstable one that often requires immediate intubation to prevent airway obstruction.

REFERENCES AND SELECTED READINGS

1. BECKER MH, KOPF AW, LANDE A: Basal cell nevus syndrome: its roentgenologic significance. Am J Roentgenol 99: 817, 1967
2. FREIMANIS AK: Fractures of the facial bones. Radiol Clin North Am 4: 341, 1966
3. GERLOCK AJ JR: The flared mandible sign of the flail mandible. Radiology 119: 299, 1976
4. GONZALEZ L, MACKENZIE AH, TARAR RA: Parotid sialography in Sjögren's syndrome. Radiology 97: 91, 1970
5. GORLIN RJ, PINDBORG JJ, CLAUSEN FP et al: The calcifying odontogenic cyst—a possible analog of the cutaneous calcifying epithelioma of Malherbe; an analysis of 15 cases. Oral Surg 15: 1235, 1962
6. HOUSTON IB, SHOTTS N: Rutherfurd's syndrome. A familial oculo-dental disorder. Acta Paediatr Scand 55: 233, 1966
7. LAPAYOWKER MS, MILLER WT, LEVY WM et al: Pigmented villonodular synovitis of the temporomandibular joint. Radiology 108: 313, 1973
8. LYNCH TP, CHASE DC: Arthrography in the evaluation of the temporomandibular joint. Radiology 126: 667, 1978
9. MERRILL V: Atlas of Roentgenographic Positions, Vol II. St. Louis, Mosby, 1967
10. PAVSEK EJ: Mandibulofacial dysostosis (Treacher Collins syndrome). Am J Roentgenol 79: 598, 1958
11. PINDBORG JJ: A calcifying epithelial odontogenic tumor. Cancer 11: 838, 1958
12. ROLAND MN, PEARL N: Traumatic injuries to the teeth of children. Ann Radiol (Paris) 18: 407, 1975
13. SHAFER WG: Cysts, neoplasms, and allied conditions of odontogenic origin. Semin Roentgenol 6: 403, 1971
14. STAFNE EC: Oral Roentgenographic Diagnosis, 3rd ed. Philadelphia, Saunders, 1969
15. STEINER RM, GOLDSTEIN BH, GOLD L: The medial mandibular bone concavity (Stafne's defect). Radiology 130: 344, 1979
16. TRACHTENBERG SB, WILKINSON EE, JACOBSON G: Sarcoidosis of the nose and paranasal sinuses. Radiology 113: 619, 1974
17. UNGER JD, UNGER GF: Fractures of the pterygoid processes accompanying severe facial bone injury. Radiology 98: 311, 1971
18. VIA WF JR: Radiology of the jaws: diseases involving the teeth. Semin Roentgenol 6: 370, 1971
19. YUNE HY, HALL JR, HUTTON CE et al: Roentgenologic diagnosis in chronic temporomandibular joint dysfunction syndrome. Am J Roentgenol 118: 401, 1973
20. YUNE HY, KLATTE EC: Current status of sialography. Am J Roentgenol 115: 420, 1972
21. ZIZMOR J, SMITH B, FASANO C et al: Roentgen diagnosis of blow-out fractures of the orbit. Am J Roentgenol 87: 1009, 1962

INDEX

U